Abrams' Angiography

Vascular and Interventional Radiology

Abrams' Angiography

Vascular and Interventional Radiology

FOURTH EDITION

Stanley Baum, MD

EDITOR

Eugene P. Pendergrass Professor of Radiology
and Chairman, Department of Radiology
University of Pennsylvania School of Medicine
Chairman, Department of Radiology
Hospital of the University of Pennsylvania
Philadelphia

VOLUME II

Little, Brown and Company

BOSTON   NEW YORK   TORONTO   LONDON

Library of Congress Cataloging-in-Publication Data

Abrams' angiography : vascular and interventional radiology. — 4th
  ed. / Stanley Baum, editor.
     p. cm.
   "With introductory comments by Herbert L. Abrams."
   Includes bibliographical references and index.
   ISBN 0-316-08408-5 (v. 1). — ISBN 0-316-08409-3 (v. 2). — ISBN
0-316-08467-0 (set)
   1. Angiography. 2. Interventional radiology. I. Abrams, Herbert L.
II. Baum, Stanley, 1929–   .
   [DNLM: 1. Angiography. WG 500 A157a 1997]
   RC691.6.A53A27 1997
   616.1'307572—dc20
   DNLM/DLC
   for Library of Congress   96-24525
                                     CIP

Vol. II ISBN 0-316-08409-3
Set ISBN 0-316-08467-0

Printed in the United States of America

EB-M

Editorial: Nancy E. Chorpenning, Deeth K. Ellis
Production Services: Julie Sullivan
Indexer: AlphaByte, Inc.
Production Supervisor: Michael A. Granger
Designer: Marty Tenney
Cover Designer: Louis C. Bruno, Jr.

To **Jeanne**

Contents

Volume I

I. General Considerations

Volume II

IV. The Abdomen and Pelvis

Section A: Lumbar Aortography

V. The Extremities and Lymphangiography

Section A: Angiography of the Extremities

Section B: Lymphangiography

Abrams' Angiography

Vascular and Interventional Radiology

Notice

The indications and dosages of all drugs in this book have been recommended in the medical literature and conform to the practices of the general medical community. The medications described do not necessarily have specific approval by the Food and Drug Administration for use in the diseases and dosages for which they are recommended. The package insert for each drug should be consulted for use and dosage as approved by the FDA. Because standards for usage change, it is advisable to keep abreast of revised recommendations, particularly those concerning new drugs.

IV

The Abdomen and Pelvis

41

Abdominal Aortography

MARTIN R. CRAIN
MARK W. MEWISSEN

*T*his chapter discusses the essential aspects of nonselective contrast abdominal aortography. The tools of angiography, including catheters, guidewires, contrast media, injectors, and filming methods, are dealt with in depth in other sections of this text, as are the complications of angiography, treatment of contrast reactions, and the preprocedural evaluation of candidates for angiography. This chapter focuses on the methods of catheterization of the abdominal aorta and the expected arterial anatomy of the abdomen and pelvis. It concludes with a description of alternative and noninvasive ways of imaging the abdominal arterial structures as the search for the ideal vascular imaging tool(s) continues.

Transfemoral Catheterization

The current practice of arteriography is an extension of the modification by Seldinger of earlier techniques.[1] Percutaneous catheterization of the aorta was first described by Peirce, who punctured the femoral artery with a large-bore needle through which he threaded a catheter into the aorta.[2] Seldinger subsequently refined the technique by describing passage of the catheter over the "leader" (wire) previously introduced through the puncture needle (Fig. 41-1). The "Seldinger technique" is the use of these three tools in that order; it does not specify the type of needle used or the number of walls punctured.

The common femoral artery is the most frequently used entry site for the percutaneous approach because of its accessibility, the ease of compression against the femoral head for hemostasis, and the low rate of significant complication when punctured. The skin entry site is chosen so that an oblique cephalad course (approximately 45-degree angle to the skin) results in arterial entry at a level between the inguinal ligament above and the bifurcation of the common femoral artery below (Fig. 41-2). When viewed with perpendicular fluoroscopy, the skin entry site is seen at the bottom

of the femoral head and the arteriotomy at or just inferior to the middle of the femoral head. It is better to rely on the fluoroscopic bony landmarks for puncture guidance[3] than to use the position of the inguinal crease, which can vary depending on age and weight. The inguinal crease does *not* demarcate the course of the inguinal ligament. Entry into this segment of the common femoral artery takes advantage of the surrounding protective femoral sheath and helps avoid the intra- and extraperitoneal bleeding associated with high punctures above the inguinal ligament[3] and the potential for creating an arteriovenous fistula between multiple crossing arterial and venous branches when puncture is made below the femoral bifurcation.

After sterile preparation and draping, local anesthesia is administered with the injection of 1 percent lidocaine down to and alongside the vessel wall in the same trajectory that the needle and catheter will follow. The patient will be more comfortable if the subcutaneous layers are infiltrated before the intracutaneous wheal is raised. All subsequent aspects of the procedure should be pain-free.

A small skin stab with a no. 11 scalpel blade, with or without spread of the subcutaneous tissues by a small hemostat, allows for easier catheter passage. The needle is directed along the course of the femoral artery at an angle to the skin. Arterial pulsations are usually transmitted through the needle and become the most reliable guide for needle direction as one gains experience. A single-wall puncture with a beveled hollow needle may be performed, or both walls can be punctured with a trocar-cannula needle followed by slow withdrawal of the cannula after trocar removal (see Fig. 41-1). The single-wall technique is favored when endovascular therapy is contemplated, such as thrombolytic therapy or angioplasty with concomitant anticoagulation. The needle may be lowered to lie more parallel to the skin for the gentle introduction of the guidewire after pulsatile blood return is obtained (see Fig 41-1C). If any resistance to wire advancement is encountered, several maneuvers may be tried to avoid

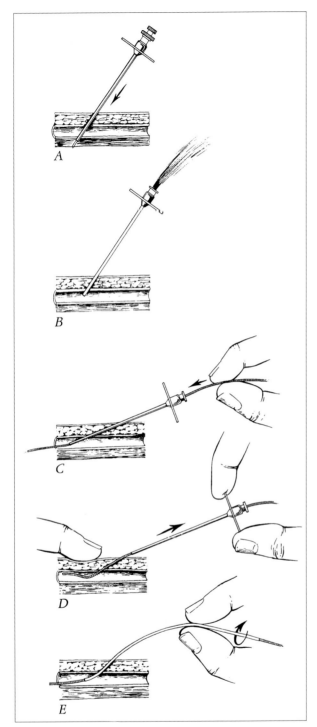

Figure 41-1. Technique for percutaneous catheterization.

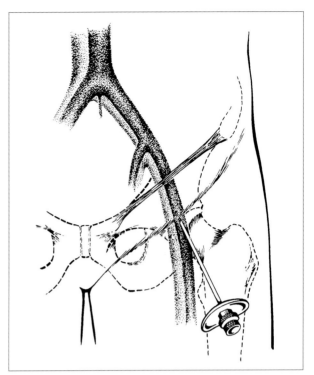

Figure 41-2. Relationship of the inguinal crease, inguinal ligament, and positioning of the percutaneous needle into the femoral artery.

The wire should be advanced carefully to avoid disruption of plaque. When the wire reaches the aorta, the needle is removed while hemostasis is maintained with the third, fourth, and fifth fingers and the thumb and index finger hold the guidewire. The catheter is then fed over the guidewire into the vessel with rotation (see Fig. 41-1E) and advanced to the aorta over the wire. Iliac artery tortuosity, plaques, and stenoses are not unusual and may preclude easy access to the abdominal aorta. In such instances, torquable curved-tip wires and catheters as well as "road-mapping" imaging capabilities greatly facilitate atraumatic access into the aorta. Should the catheter occlude flow while across a high-grade stenosis, heparin should be administered immediately to prevent thrombosis of the vessel while the study is being performed.

Direct puncture of prosthetic bypass grafts is safe[4] so long as the graft has had time to become fully incorporated into the subcutaneous tissues (generally several weeks). Scar tissue and tough graft material actually limit the spread of hematoma in the surrounding tissues, and inadequate hemostasis at the arteriotomy site in such patients usually results in direct external bleeding rather than occult hematomas.

Abdominal aortography should be performed with a multi-side-hole catheter to prevent forceful injection

subintimal passage and dissection. The hub of a beveled needle can be rotated to redirect the wire, or the hub can be angled in a medial or lateral direction if the vessel has been entered tangentially. Small injections of contrast medium may also help direct needle angulation in such cases.

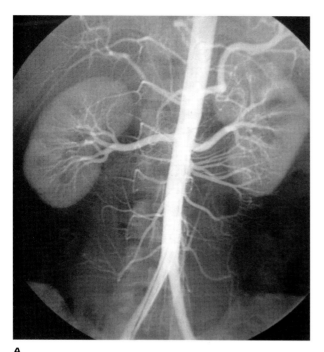

A

Figure 41-3. Aortograms obtained with catheter placed in the proximal abdominal aorta. (A) An anteroposterior view provides good visualization of the celiac branches, the proximal superior mesenteric artery branches, and the renal arteries. (B) The origins of the celiac and superior mesenteric arteries are best visualized with a lateral projection.

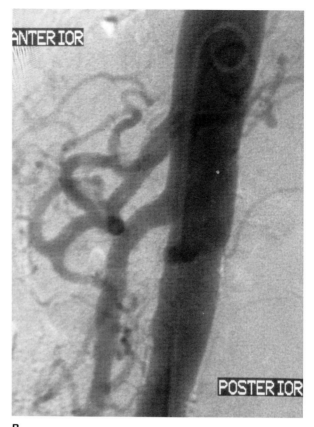

B

under atherosclerotic plaque and to avoid high-pressure injection of small branches. The most frequently used catheters are of the pigtail or tennis racket designs. The catheter should be positioned to include the most proximal aspect of the aorta and its branches to be studied. Typically, the thoracolumbar junction is chosen for visualization of the celiac and superior mesenteric arteries (Fig. 41-3A). The catheter is placed immediately below these vessels for optimal viewing of renal arterial anatomy (Fig. 41-4); location just above the aortic bifurcation will allow the best visualization of the pelvis.

Contrast injection rates should match the flow rates of the vessels injected. In most instances, 20 ml per second for a total volume of 40 ml will provide excellent opacification of the upper abdominal aorta and its branches. Adjustments can be made in cases of extensive atherosclerotic disease or decreased cardiac output, in which case the injection rate may be reduced accordingly. Similarly, somewhat larger volumes can be used to adequately fill large, slowly flowing abdominal aortic aneurysms.

Catheters should be periodically flushed with a heparinized solution to limit accumulation and subsequent embolization of aggregated platelet material. All

other angiographic equipment should be cleaned before being introduced into the arterial system.

Before catheter removal, all acquired angiographic data should be reviewed to ensure that no additional view is needed. The catheter is then removed and compression is applied directly over the skin puncture site

Figure 41-4. Aortogram obtained with pigtail catheter placement at the level of the renal arteries. Note the accessory renal artery to the lower pole of the right kidney.

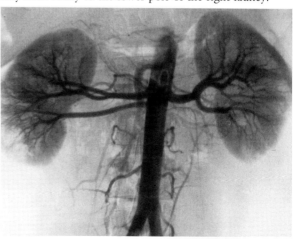

and the arterial entry site to achieve hemostasis. Pressure may be slowly eased in the latter portions of the compression period. Pressure is usually maintained for a minimum of 10 minutes for routine diagnostic procedures. The most reliable method for ensuring excellent hemostasis is the application of manual digital pressure, although several compression devices exist that are satisfactory *so long as proper observation by experienced personnel is maintained.*

Transaxillary Catheterization

The axillary approach may be necessary in patients with arteriosclerotic occlusive disease in the aortoiliofemoral system. Recent aortofemoral grafts may also preclude the transfemoral approach.

The left axillary approach is preferred over the right because the catheter does not cross the right brachiocephalic or left common carotid artery origins when catheterization from the left subclavian artery into the descending aorta is performed. The arm is abducted with the hand under the patient's head (Fig. 41-5). Careful lidocaine infiltration is advised to avoid the brachial plexus. The patient will immediately report an "electric shock" or pain down the arm if the brachial plexus is violated.

The actual puncture is made into the high or proximal brachial artery just beyond the axillary fold.[5] The

Figure 41-5. Position of patient for percutaneous axillary catheterization.

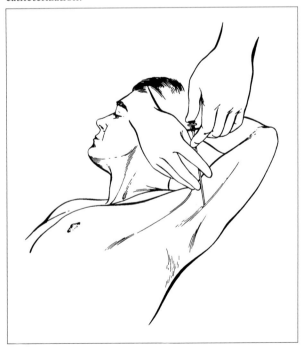

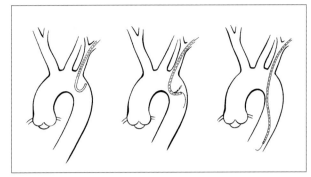

Figure 41-6. Axillary artery catheterization. The curved tip of the catheter is directed posterolaterally to the left for easier access to the descending aorta.

brachial artery can be mobile, and transmitted pulsations through the needle may not be as obvious as with the femoral artery.

In older patients with atherosclerotic disease and elongation of the transverse aortic arch, antegrade catheterization of the aorta can be difficult. Torquing the tip of a pigtail, sidewinder, or other angled catheter will direct the guidewire posterolaterally to the left and down the aorta (Fig. 41-6).

Hemostasis is extremely important in the transaxillary approach. Careful compression (not obliteration) at the puncture site is advised, especially because there is no firm or bony floor against which to compress the artery. Monitoring the radial artery pulse is helpful to assess the proper amount of compression. If delayed bleeding occurs within the axillary neurovascular sheath, early surgical axillary sheath decompression may be necessary to avoid permanent neurologic deficit.[6]

Translumbar Catheterization

Translumbar aortography was first described by dos Santos in 1929.[7,8] It remains a relatively safe procedure for contrast visualization of the aorta and its lower branches, although the need to resort to this approach is relatively uncommon with current catheter and wire technology applied to femoral and axillary sites. It is of paramount importance to exclude patients who are at risk of bleeding because of anticoagulation or abnormal coagulation factors. In addition, the inability to compress the puncture site makes this approach contraindicated when percutaneous intervention is contemplated. However, it is still indicated for patients who have diffuse atherosclerotic occlusive disease, which may prevent catheterization via other access sites.

With the patient lying prone, the 12th left thoracic rib is located by palpation or fluoroscopy. The skin is entered 2 cm below the inferior margin of this rib, 8 to 12 cm to the left of the midline spinous processes. Local anesthesia is administered, a small skin stab is made, and an 18-gauge sheathed needle 18 to 24 cm in length[9–11] is advanced so that it points at the ventral margin of the second to third lumbar vertebral body. When the anterolateral margin of the vertebral body is reached, the needle is withdrawn and redirected slightly more ventrally (Fig. 41-7). With angled fluoroscopy, it is possible to puncture the aorta without first engaging the vertebral body. When the aortic pulsations are felt, the aortic wall is penetrated with a short (1-cm), controlled stab of the needle. When pulsatile blood flow emerges, a guidewire is advanced cephalad or caudad through the needle into the aorta and the sheath is guided over the guidewire. Angiography is then performed with injection through the sheath, usually at a rate of 8 to 12 ml per second for a total of 25 to 30 ml of contrast.

Normal Arterial Anatomy of the Abdominal Aorta and Its Major Branches

Figures 41-8 and 41-9 are diagrammatic representations of the normal aorta and its abdominal and pelvic arterial branches. The schematic drawings are based, in part, on the original work of Muller and Figley.[12] In the remainder of the chapter, the numbers in parentheses that follow the artery names in the text and the numbers in other figures refer to those in Figures 41-8 and 41-9.

So-called typical patterns of the abdominal and pelvic arterial tree are seen in a slight majority of cases and are presented here. However, major and minor variations should be expected. As an aid in the identification of any branch, it is useful to search the radiograph in the general region of its expected distribution and then to work back from that point toward the origin. For further details of vascular anatomic structure, several excellent reference sources are available.[13–19]

Abdominal Aorta

The abdominal aorta begins as it emerges through the diaphragm and ends at its bifurcation into the common iliac arteries. It usually lies directly anterior and slightly to the left of the vertebral column midline (Fig. 41-10A).

The suprarenal internal luminal diameter is on aver-

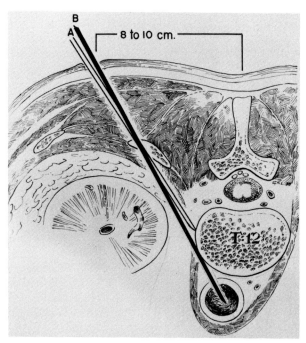

Figure 41-7. Transverse section of prone patient during left lumbar approach to abdominal aorta. The white needle (*A*) indicates the course the needle takes to meet the vertebral body. The black needle (*B*) shows repositioning of the needle to have it slide along the margin into the aorta. The usual level of entry is into the infrarenal aorta at L2-L3, although infrarenal aortic aneurysm or occlusion occasionally necessitates suprarenal entry at T12 as illustrated here.

age 25 mm and should not exceed 30 mm.[20,21] Immediately below the origins of the large visceral branches and the renal arteries, the aorta becomes significantly narrower. It decreases to approximately 15 mm at the bifurcation. Although the limits of normal are broad, any increase in the size of the distal lumen is abnormal.

Celiac Artery

The first major branch of the abdominal aorta is the celiac artery, which arises from the ventral surface of the aorta (see Figs. 41-3B and 41-10B) at the level of T12 or L1. Classically, the celiac trunk trifurcates into the splenic (5), common hepatic (13), and left gastric (11) arteries (see Fig. 41-8).

The splenic artery provides the dorsal pancreatic artery (6) proximally, then the pancreatica magna (7), and finally the left gastroepiploic (10) and several short gastric arteries (9) before entering the splenic hilum (8). These latter vessels are best shown with selective splenic arteriography. The splenic artery runs a tortuous course because it lies on the craniodorsal surface of the body and tail of the pancreas (see Fig. 40-10A

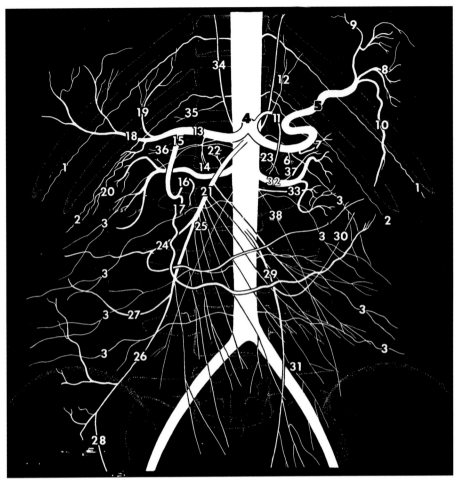

Figure 41-8. Radiographic anatomy of the abdominal aorta. Arteries: *1,* intercostals; *2,* subcostals; *3,* lumbar; *4,* celiac; *5,* splenic; *6,* dorsal pancreatic; *7,* pancreatic magna; *8,* terminal branches to spleen; *9,* short gastric; *10,* left gastroepiploic; *11,* left gastric; *12,* esophageal; *13,* common hepatic; *14,* right gastric; *15,* gastroduodenal; *16,* anterosuperior pancreaticoduodenal; *17,* right gastroepiploic; *18,* right hepatic; *19,* left hepatic; *20,* cystic; *21,* superior mesenteric; *22,* inferior pancreaticoduodenal; *23,* inferior pancreatic; *24,* middle colic; *25,* intestinal (jejunal and ileal); *26,* ileocolic; *27,* right colic; *28,* appendiceal; *29,* inferior mesenteric; *30,* left colic; *31,* sigmoid; *32,* renal; *33,* accessory renal; *34,* inferior phrenic; *35,* superior suprarenal; *36,* middle suprarenal; *37,* inferior suprarenal; *38,* internal spermatic or ovarian. Note that in this illustration, the ileocolic and right colic arteries represent a variation from currently accepted nomenclature as described in the text. (From Muller RF, Figley MM. The arteries of the abdomen, pelvis, and thigh. AJR 1957;77:296. Used with permission.)

and B). The splenic vein is just caudal to the artery (see Fig. 41-10B and C).

The common hepatic artery travels to the right and becomes the proper hepatic artery after giving rise to the small right gastric (14) and larger gastroduodenal (15) arteries. Before terminating as the right gastroepiploic artery (17), the gastroduodenal artery contributes anterior and posterior branches to the superior portion of the pancreaticoduodenal arcade (16). The right gastroepiploic artery courses along the greater curvature of the stomach to anastomose with the left gastroepiploic branch of the splenic artery. The proper hepatic artery terminates by dividing into the right (18) and left (19) hepatic arteries, with the cystic artery (20) usually arising from the right hepatic branch. The main hepatic artery lies anterior to the portal vein (see Fig. 41-10C). Occasionally, the left gastric artery contributes to the left hepatic circulation.

Superior Mesenteric Artery

The superior mesenteric artery (21) originates immediately below the celiac trunk at the L1 level (see Figs. 41-3B and 41-10C). The angiographic details of the

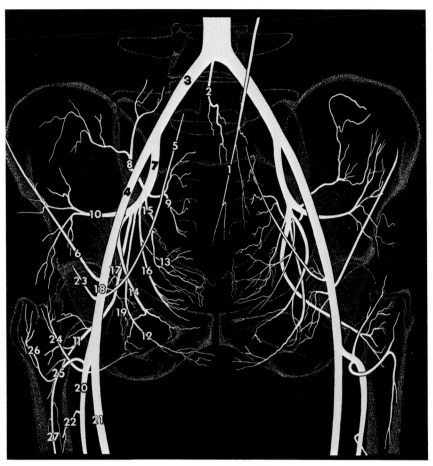

Figure 41-9. Radiographic anatomy of the arteries of the pelvis. Arteries: *1,* superior hemorrhoidal; *2,* middle sacral; *3,* common iliac; *4,* external iliac; *5,* inferior epigastric; *6,* deep circumflex; *7,* internal iliac; *8,* iliolumbar; *9,* lateral sacral; *10,* superior gluteal; *11,* inferior gluteal; *12,* internal pudendal; *13,* middle hemorrhoidal; *14,* obturator; *15,* uterine; *16,* vesical; *17,* superficial epigastric; *18,* common femoral; *19,* external pudendal; *20,* deep femoral (profunda femoris); *21,* superficial femoral; *22,* perforator; *23,* superficial circumflex iliac; *24,* medial femoral circumflex; *25,* lateral femoral circumflex; *26,* lateral femoral circumflex, ascending; *27,* lateral femoral circumflex, descending. (From Muller RF, Figley MM. The arteries of the abdomen, pelvis, and thigh. AJR 1957;77:296. Used with permission.)

superior mesenteric branches are best visualized with selective arteriography. From an aortogram, only pathology affecting the proximal portion of the vessel can be appreciated. For instance, it is not unusual to visualize the inferior pancreaticoduodenal (22) artery, the first branch of the superior mesenteric artery, particularly when it provides flow via the pancreaticoduodenal arcades to reconstitute the hepatic arterial circulation distal to a proximal celiac flow-limiting lesion. A "replaced" right hepatic artery, or the common hepatic or gastroduodenal arteries, may arise aberrantly early in the course of the superior mesenteric artery, which also can be demonstrated on nonselective aortography.

The superior mesenteric artery, which typically supplies the entire small bowel and the colon to the splenic flexure, is best demonstrated with selective arteriography. Proximal branches which often project to the right of the main trunk of the superior mesenteric artery are the inferior pancreaticoduodenal trunk (22) and the more variable middle colic artery (24) with its branches toward the right to the hepatic flexure and toward the left to the splenic flexure. Nearly the entire small bowel is then supplied by 12 to 20 parallel jejunal and ileal (intestinal) arteries (25) which nearly always project to the left of the main trunk. Some controversy has existed regarding the naming of peripheral superior mesenteric branches, and it should be noted that there is some discrepancy between the depiction in Figure 41-8 and the currently accepted nomenclature

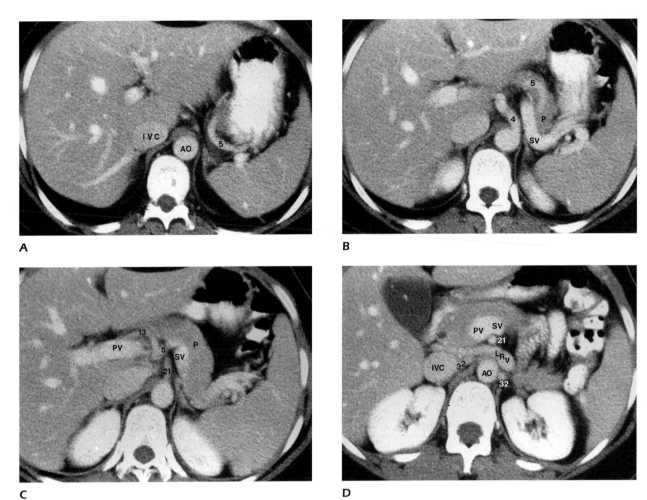

A

B

C

D

Figure 41-10. Axial CT images from the upper abdomen for three-dimensional correlation. Arterial numbering corresponds with Figure 41-8. Abdominal structures: *AO*, aorta; *IVC*, inferior vena cava; *P*, pancreas; *SV*, splenic vein; *PV*, portal vein; *LRV*, left renal vein. (A) The distal splenic artery (5) lies cephalad to the pancreatic tail. (B) Celiac (4) origin under the diaphragmatic crura. The splenic artery lies along the superior aspect of the pancreas, and the splenic vein is seen from the splenic hilum dorsal to the pancreas. (C) Ceceliac bifurcation inferior to the celiac origin, and superior mesenteric (21) origin dorsal to the pancreas. The hepatic artery (13) lies anterior to the portal vein. (D) View showing the left renal traversing the "nutcracker" between the aorta and the superior mesenteric artery; the splenoportal venous confluence anterior to the superior mesenteric artery; the right renal artery (32) origin from the anterolateral surface of the aorta and coursing posterior to the inferior vena cava; and the more vertical left renal artery (32) origin.

as put forward in the definitive work by VanDamme and Bonte.[17-19] The most constant distal branch from the main trunk is the ileocolic artery which projects to the right, arises at the transition from jejunal to ileal branches, terminates in cecal branches, and gives off small ileal branches, the appendiceal artery (28), and a superior branch feeding the entire ascending colon in the majority of subjects.[17-19] Infrequently seen is a separate right colic branch,[17-19] and this is the variant shown in Figure 41-8. Finally, the terminal branch arising straight off the superior mesenteric artery is a distal ileal artery.

Renal Arteries

The renal arteries (32) arise opposite each other from the lateral or anterolateral aspect of the aorta at the L1-L2 level about 2 cm below the superior mesenteric artery. The right renal artery courses posterior to the inferior vena cava (see Fig. 41-10D).

Multiple renal arteries occur in about 20 percent of cases, more often on the left.[22] Most frequently they arise from the aorta below the main artery (see Fig. 41-4), although their origin may be above the main renal artery or even aberrantly from the iliac arteries.

They usually enter the kidney parenchyma at its nearest point instead of accompanying the main artery into the hilum.

Inferior Mesenteric Artery

The inferior mesenteric artery (29), which originates from the left ventrolateral surface of the aorta anywhere between L1 and L4, is a smaller vessel not frequently seen with nonselective aortography. Its course is usually downward and almost parallel to the aorta on its left. It gives rise to the left colic artery (30), which bifurcates into ascending and descending divisions. It also contributes sigmoid branches (31) before terminating in the pelvis as the superior hemorrhoidal artery (1) (see Fig. 41-9).

Paired Lateral Branches

The inferior phrenic arteries (34) (see Fig. 41-8) usually arise high on the abdominal aorta just above or lateral to the celiac artery, and may spring from a common trunk, as separate paired branches, or even from the celiac artery.[23] They course sharply upward along the diaphragmatic crura.

The suprarenal or adrenal circulation is supplied from three separate sources. The superior suprarenal arteries (35) are small branches of the inferior phrenic arteries, and the middle suprarenal arteries (36) usually arise directly from the aorta. The largest adrenal vessels are the inferior suprarenal arteries (37), which originate from the renal arteries.[24,25]

The paired internal spermatic (testicular) or ovarian arteries (38) usually originate from the aorta just below the renal arteries. These delicate vessels are characterized by their lack of branches and their long, direct descent.

Segmental Branches

The segmental branches, which include the paired intercostal arteries (1), the subcostal arteries (2), and the four pairs of lumbar arteries (3), are the only major branches arising from the posterior surface of the aorta. Their origins are located immediately adjacent to each other. The costal branches run in the neurovascular groove along the inferior surface of the ribs. The lumbar arteries are recognized by their serpentine course (Fig. 41-11) and characteristic association with the lateral margins of the upper four lumbar vertebral segments. In Figure 41-11, the middle sacral artery (2), the last aortic branch, can be seen at the bifurcation; the fifth lumbar arteries may arise from this vessel.

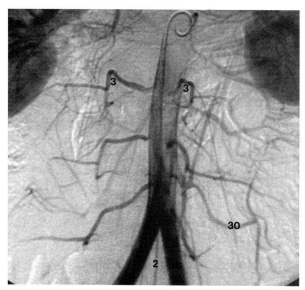

Figure 41-11. Aortogram of the lower abdominal aorta clearly showing the origins and course of the lumbar arteries (3, Fig. 41-8). Note also the middle sacral artery (2, Fig. 41-9) at the aortic bifurcation and the branch of the inferior mesenteric artery supplying the descending colon (30, Fig. 41-8).

Common Iliac Arteries

The abdominal aorta usually terminates at the L4 level, bifurcating into the right and the left common iliac arteries (3). The common iliac arteries usually give no major branches detectable by arteriography, although they may give rise to displaced renal arteries or to the iliolumbar artery, which normally arises from the internal iliac (hypogastric) artery. The common iliac arteries bifurcate into the external iliac (4) and the internal iliac (7) arteries (see Fig. 41-9) after a varying distance of 2 to 6 cm at the L5-S1 level.

External Iliac Artery

The external iliac artery curves smoothly down across the lateral sacrum and sacroiliac joint and near the iliopectineal line of the pelvic inlet. Its course is ventral as well as inferior and slightly lateral.

Just above the level of the inguinal ligament, the external iliac artery gives rise to the deep circumflex iliac artery (6), which ascends superiorly and laterally in a fairly straight line, and the inferior epigastric artery (5), which ascends superiorly and medially. At this point, the vessel continues as the common femoral artery (18).

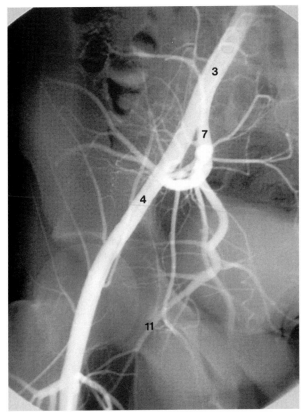

Figure 41-12. Left anterior oblique angiogram of the right iliac bifurcation into the internal (7, Fig. 41-9) and external (4) iliac arteries.

Internal Iliac Artery

The origin of the internal iliac (hypogastric) artery (7) is often obscured by the overlying external iliac artery in the anteroposterior projection. These vessels are best separated with a contralateral oblique view (Fig. 41-12).

The internal iliac artery usually divides into anterior and posterior divisions. The posterior trunk gives rise to one or two lateral sacral arteries (9), which in turn furnish the segmental branches to the sacral foramina. Next, the posterior division furnishes the iliolumbar branch (8) with its iliac and lumbar ramifications. The posterior trunk continues posteriorly through the sciatic notch as the superior gluteal artery (10) and inferior gluteal arteries (11) (see Fig. 41-12).

The anterior trunk of the internal iliac artery contributes the remaining pelvic arteries. The obturator artery (14) may be identified by tracing back from its terminal branches encircling the obturator foramen. The internal pudendal artery (12) usually crosses the obturator foramen inferior to the obturator artery and terminates as arteries to the penis and scrotum or the labia. The inferior gluteal artery (11) originates with

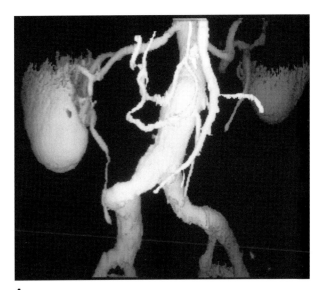

A

B

Figure 41-13. Three-dimensional reconstruction CT of lower abdominal and pelvic arterial anatomy. The technique employs rapid intravenous contrast bolus and helical CT scanner technology. (A) Shaded surface rendering technique with anteroposterior display shows an infrarenal abdominal aortic aneurysm, renal and superior mesenteric arteries, pancreaticoduodenal arcade vessels, and tortuous iliac arteries. Contrast-opacified lower renal poles and proximal ureters are also depicted. (B) Rotation of the data into the right posterior oblique projection lays out the tortuous iliac arteries. (Courtesy of W. Dennis Foley, M.D.)

either the superior gluteal of the posterior division or the internal pudendal artery of the anterior division. Its laterally descending posterior course parallels the axis of the femoral neck, and it is often projected over the bone or just medial to it (see Fig. 41-12).

The middle hemorrhoidal (13) and vesical (16) arteries are obscure and inconstant in position. The uterine artery (15) comes off high on the anterior trunk and may be identified by its coiled terminal azygos branches.

Conclusion

Angiography of the abdominal aorta should only be considered in patients in whom a therapeutic intervention, surgical or endovascular, is contemplated for the treatment of a variety of vascular processes, such as symptomatic atherosclerotic disease or aneurysmal degeneration. Although it is a safe imaging test in experienced hands, its invasiveness and cost prohibit its use for routine screening and follow-up examinations. For that reason, new imaging techniques have continued to evolve in an attempt to accurately and reliably predict variables that affect outcome of a major aortic intervention. Ongoing refinements in magnetic resonance angiography and three-dimensional computed tomography (CT) imaging techniques (Fig. 41-13) will undoubtedly play a major role in the preoperative evaluation of the abdominal aorta and will probably replace catheter aortography in many instances.

Acknowledgments

The current version of this chapter is based on the earlier work of our associate, Elliot O. Lipchik, M.D., and the late Stanley M. Rogoff, M.D. We have attempted to retain as much of their excellent original substance as possible while updating the material where appropriate. We thank Dr. Lipchik for giving us the opportunity to collaborate on this work.

References

1. Seldinger SI. Catheter replacement of the needle in percutaneous arteriography. Acta Radiol 1953;39:368.
2. Peirce EC II. Percutaneous femoral artery catheterization in man with special reference to aortography. Surg Gynecol Obstet 1951;93:56.
3. Rupp SB, Vogelzang RL, Nemcek AA Jr, Yungbluth MM. Relationship of the inguinal ligament to pelvic radiographic landmarks: anatomic correlation and its role in femoral arteriography. J Vasc Intervent Radiol 1993;4:409.
4. Eisenberg RL, Mani RL, McDonald EJ Jr. The complication rate of catheter angiography by direct puncture through aorto-femoral bypass grafts. AJR 1976;126:814.
5. Lipchik EO, Sugimoto H. Percutaneous brachial artery catheterization. Radiology 1986;160:842.
6. Dudrick S, Masland W, Mishkin M. Brachial plexus injury following axillary artery puncture. Radiology 1967;88:271.
7. dos Santos R, Lamas A, Pereira-Caldas J. Arteriografia da aorta e dos vasos abdominais. Med Contemp 1929;47:93.
8. dos Santos R, Lamas A, Pereira-Caldas J. L'arteriographie des membres de l'aorte et de ses branches abdominales. Soc Nat Chir Bull Mem 1929;55:587.
9. Amplatz K. Translumbar catheterization of the abdominal aorta. Radiology 1963;81:927.
10. Carlin RA, Amplatz K. Downstream aortography. AJR 1970;109:536.
11. Stocks LO, Halpern M, Turner AF. Complete translumbar aortography: the Teflon sleeve technique. AJR 1969;107:835.
12. Muller RF, Figley MM. The arteries of the abdomen, pelvis, and thigh. AJR 1957;77:296.
13. Kadir S. Atlas of normal and variant angiographic anatomy. Philadelphia: Saunders, 1991.
14. Michels NA. Blood supply and anatomy of the upper abdominal organs with a descriptive atlas. Philadelphia: Lippincott, 1955.
15. Nebesar RA, Kornblith PL, Pollard JJ, Michels NA. Celiac and superior mesenteric arteries: a correlation of angiograms and dissections. Boston: Little, Brown, 1969.
16. Reuter SR, Redman HC. Gastrointestinal angiography. Philadelphia: Saunders, 1972.
17. Nemcek AA Jr, Vogelzang RL. Introduction to angiography of the hollow viscera. In: Gore RM, Levine MS, Laufer I. Textbook of gastrointestinal radiology. Philadelphia: Saunders, 1994:140–150.
18. VanDamme JP, Bonte J. Vascular anatomy in abdominal surgery. New York: Thieme, 1990.
19. VanDamme JPJ, Van der Schuren G. Re-evaluation of the colic irrigation from the superior mesenteric artery. Acta Anat 1976;95:578–588.
20. Goldberg BB, Lehman JS. Aortosonography: ultrasound measurement of the abdominal and thoracic aorta. Arch Surg 1970;100:652.
21. Goldberg BB, Ostrum BJ, Isard HJ. Ultrasonic aortography. JAMA 1966;198:353.
22. Boijsen E. Angiographic studies of the anatomy of single and multiple renal arteries. Acta Radiol (Stockh) 1959;183(Suppl):1.
23. Merklin RJ, Michels NA. The variant renal and suprarenal blood supply with data on the inferior phrenic, ureteral and gonadal arteries. J Int Coll Surg 1958;29:41.
24. Edsman G. Angionephrography and suprarenal angiography. Acta Radiol (Stockh) 1957;155(Suppl):1.
25. Toni R, Mosca S, Favero L, Ricci S, Roversi R, Toni G, Vezzadini P. Clinical anatomy of the suprarenal arteries: a quantitative approach by aortography. Surg Radiol Anat 1988;10:297.

42

Complications of Angiography and Interventional Radiology

JONATHAN M. LEVY
SAMUEL J. HESSEL

The last decade has seen revolutionary changes in the practice of angiography. Digital imaging, nonionic contrast material, and large-field-of-view, C-arm-mounted image intensifiers have made the production of high-quality angiographic images much easier. Small-diameter (4 French and 5 French) catheters and new guidewire technology have facilitated superselective catheterization and decreased procedure times compared to previous techniques.

Along with these advances have come a host of new techniques that have combined to create a new species of radiologist—the interventionalist. The spectrum of interventional radiology now encompasses the entire field of medicine, from the treatment of intracranial tumors and vascular malformations to the biopsy and drainage of lesions anywhere in the body. As might be expected, with these techniques have come new complications. Before beginning a procedure, it is important for the angiointerventionalist to understand the nature and treatment of these potential complications. Such knowledge improves care at critical junctures and allows the physician to act quickly and decisively when a problem arises. It also ensures that adequate information is provided to the patient as part of the informed consent procedure.

Complications of Diagnostic Angiography

The American College of Radiology, with advice from the Society of Cardiovascular and Interventional Radiology, has developed a set of standards for diagnostic arteriography.[1] The standards include thresholds for angiographic complications for both institutions and individual physicians (Table 42-1). These thresholds are not meant to reflect ideals but are levels at which concern must be given to the quality of care provided.

Complications can generally be divided into three categories: systemic complications, complications related to the puncture site, and complications related to catheters and guidewires. Although there is necessarily some overlap, this schema provides a framework for reviewing the complications attributable to vascular procedures.

Systemic Complications

Idiosyncratic and Anaphylactoid Reactions to Contrast Media

Adverse reactions to the administration of contrast material can be mild, moderate, or severe (Table 42-2). Moderate contrast reactions may occur in as many as 5 to 12 percent of patients.[2] The authors' experience suggests that if all the mild reactions in Table 42-1 were documented they would occur in a large percentage of patients.

Serious contrast reactions are infrequent, occurring in 1 or 2 patients per 1000 examinations.[2] The latest reports suggest that the death rate from high- and low-osmolar contrast materials is equivalent, at approximately 0.9 per 100,000 examinations.[2] Angiography-related contrast-induced nephropathy has decreased in incidence since the advent of intraarterial digital subtraction angiography.[3]

The recognition and treatment of contrast reactions require continual observation of patients during angiography. Patients having angiographic examinations usually receive intravenous analgesics. All patients should be continuously monitored with ECG, blood pressure, and pulse oximetry. A fully equipped emergency cart is a requirement in all angiography-interventional suites. This allows quick access to needed medications and rapid treatment of patients with complications.

Most mild contrast reactions can be treated expectantly, with continued reassurance of the patient. Moderate reactions usually require treatment, and

Table 42-1. Complications of Diagnostic Arteriography Thresholds

Department Indicators	
Puncture site complications	
Hematoma (requiring transfusion, surgery, or delayed discharge)	<3.00%
Occlusion	<0.50%
Pseudoaneurysm	<0.50%
Arteriovenous fistula	<0.10%
Catheter-induced complications (other than puncture site)	
Distal emboli	<0.50%
Arterial dissection or subintimal passage	<2.00%
Subintimal injection of contrast media	<1.00%
Cerebral arteriography	
All neurologic complications	<4.00%
Permanent neurologic complications	<1.00%
Contrast reactions	
All idiosyncratic reactions	<3.00%
Major reactions	<0.50%
Contrast material–related death	<0.01%
Nonidiosyncratic reactions	<5.00%
(Cardiac decompensation, hypotension, severe nausea or vomiting, bradycardia, etc., resulting in unexpected admission, delayed discharge, or transfer to an intensive care unit.)	
Contrast-induced renal failure	<10.00%
(Elevation in baseline serum creatinine or blood urea nitrogen requiring care that delays discharge, requires unexpected admission or readmission, or that results in permanent impairment of renal function.)	
Individual Physician Indicators	
Unexpected readmission to the hospital, unexpected transfer to an intensive care unit, or delayed discharge due to a complication of an arteriographic procedure	<5.00%
Puncture site or injection site complications	<5.00%
All neurologic complications	<4.00%
Permanent neurologic complications	<1.50%
Contrast material–induced renal failure	<10.00%

From Spies JB, et al. Standard for diagnostic arteriography in adults. Standards of Practice Committee of the Society of Cardiovascular and Interventional Radiology. J Vasc Intervent Radiol 1993;4:385–395. Used with permission.)

severe reactions often mandate hospitalization. H_1-receptor blockers (such as Benadryl) and epinephrine (both in subcutaneous and intravenous dosages) should be instantaneously available. For detailed descriptions of the treatment of adverse reactions, the reader is referred to publications of the American College of Radiology.[2]

Renal Failure

Radiographic contrast material has long been known to cause renal failure in a small but significant number of patients. The most recent studies suggest that up to 12 percent of hospital-acquired renal insufficiency is caused by contrast media.[4] However, many different definitions of renal failure—tied to specific increases in serum creatinine levels—have been employed to identify affected patients. Thus the true incidence of this complication is not clearly defined and depends in substantial part on the definition of *azotemia* or *renal failure* used.[5] Contrast-induced renal failure manifests as acute tubular necrosis, with oliguria occurring within 24 hours after injection.[6] Renal function almost always returns to normal within 2 or 3 weeks.[7] Dialysis is required in less than 0.15 percent of cases.[6]

Many predisposing factors have been suggested as increasing the risk of contrast-related renal failure (Table 42-3), but there is no general agreement as to whether any one of these is a relative or absolute

Table 42-2. Reactions to Contrast Material

Mild	Moderate	Severe
Nausea, vomiting	Pulse change	Potentially life-threatening moderate signs
Cough	Hypotension	
Heat (warmth)	Hypertension	Unresponsiveness
Headache	Dyspnea-wheezing	Convulsions
Dizziness	Bronchospasm	Arrhythmias
Anxiety	Laryngospasm	Cardiac arrest
Altered taste		
Itching		
Pallor		
Flushing		
Chills		
Shaking		
Sweats		
Rash (hives)		
Nasal stuffiness		
Swelling of eyes or face		

Adapted from ACR Committee on Drugs and Contrast Media. Manual on iodinated contrast media. Reston, VA: American College of Radiology, 1991. Used with permission.

Table 42-3. Risk Factors for Contrast-Induced Renal Failure

Age	Hyperuricemia
Renal insufficiency	Exposure to other nephrotoxins
Diabetes mellitus	Repeated exposure to contrast media
Multiple myeloma	Large volume of contrast
Anemia	Intraarterial vs. intravenous
Proteinuria	Male sex
Abnormal liver function	Cardiovascular disease
Volume depletion	Hypertension
Dehydration	Renal transplantation

Adapted from Cronin RE. Southwestern internal medical conference: renal failure following radiologic procedures. Am J Med Sci 1989;298:342–356. Used with permission.

contraindication to contrast administration.[4-8] One study by D'Elia et al. showed that the only significant risk factor for patients having angiograms was preexisting azotemia.[9] However, another study, by Moore et al.,[10] showed that underlying renal insufficiency was not a risk factor for contrast-induced nephrotoxicity. It may be possible to lessen the deleterious effects of contrast material in patients with preexisting renal insufficiency by infusing dopamine (2.5–3.0 µg/kg/min) before or during the angiographic procedure.[11,12]

Diabetes mellitus seems to be a risk factor only in those patients with preexisting renal insufficiency.[9,13] Type II (adult-onset) diabetics are significantly less likely to develop renal failure than those with type I (insulin-dependent) disease.[14]

The overall risk of contrast-induced renal failure in patients with multiple myeloma is small. In the absence of proteinuria, patients with myeloma and normal renal function probably do not have an increased risk for renal failure.[5] The hydration status of all angiography patients should be assessed before examination, and studies on patients in a state of dehydration should be avoided.

Complications Related to the Use of Nonionic Versus Ionic Contrast Material

It is generally agreed that newer, low-osmolarity contrast media cause fewer reactions and have an important role in preventing postprocedure renal insufficiency.[15-17] Although a nonionic contrast medium such as iohexol (Omnipaque 350) causes significantly fewer contrast reactions than ionic media,[18] the ionic dimer ioxaglate (Hexabrix 320) may be less nephrotoxic than the nonionic media.[19] Multiple studies[18,20,21] suggest a reduced incidence of severe reactions when nonionic contrast materials are used. Both ionic and nonionic contrast media have anticoagulant properties, but nonionic contrast media are much less active in retard-

ing coagulation, in both catheters and syringes.[22-27] For this reason, when stasis is likely, such as during subselective arteriography, continuous flush systems and/or an ionic dimer (ioxaglate) should be used.

Infection

Infection, either systemic or at the puncture site, does not appear to be a significant complication of angiography. Hessel et al.[28] reported an incidence of endocarditis of 0.003 percent of patients after transfemoral angiography, and no significant puncture site infections in 118,591 examinations. Four patients had fever and chills, with no other sequelae. Postarteriography fever and chills are invariably limited in duration, and therefore are probably underreported.

Ameli et al. studied postoperative infections in patients having groin operations with and without prior arterial puncture.[29] They found no difference in the number of infections and concluded that angiography does not cause an increase in postoperative sepsis. As long as good sterile technique is observed, the incidence of infection related to angiographic procedures should be very low. Prophylactic antibiotics are not recommended before diagnostic angiography.[30]

Complications at the Puncture Site

Puncture site complications due to arterial catheterization include hemorrhage, thrombosis and/or vessel obstruction, fistula, pseudoaneurysm formation, spasm, and femoral neuralgia syndrome. Most of these are immediately apparent. However, recognition of pseudoaneurysm or fistula formation may be delayed. Most patients requiring surgery for puncture site complications have pain as the principal symptom.[31] Any lasting pain in this area should alert the angiographer to search for a cause.

Hematoma and Hemorrhage

It has been suggested in the cardiology literature that the number of femoral hematomas that require surgery is equal to the number that do not.[32] The authors believe that, on an all-inclusive basis, angiography entry-site hematomas are a relatively common occurrence. However, significant hematomas requiring surgery or transfusion are distinctly uncommon.

The incidence of hematomas requiring therapy has varied between 0.26 and 1.5 percent in previous series.[28,33] Puncture of the superficial femoral artery, or of the common femoral artery at an aberrant site, appears to contribute to the formation of a clinically significant hematoma.[31,34] This may be due to difficulty in compressing the femoral artery when the puncture is not made over the femoral head. Radiologists performing angiography should thoroughly familiarize themselves with anatomic landmarks. An understanding of the relationship of the inguinal ligament and femoral crease to the femoral artery should prevent aberrant punctures.

When operator experience and differences in training are taken into account, there is no relationship between needle tip shape or one- or two-walled puncture and subsequent hematoma formation.[35,36] Large hematomas have been shown to be significantly related to patient weight in some studies[37] but not in others.[31] There is no relationship to the size of the catheter employed.[37]

Puncture Site Thrombosis and Occlusion

Puncture site arterial occlusion is a relatively uncommon complication, reported in 0.14 percent of femoral punctures.[28] The incidence of occlusion in transaxillary cases was significantly higher in that paper. A study done by Siegelman et al. in 1968[38] showed a high incidence of pericatheter thrombi at the completion of femoral angiograms. The number of occlusions and/or emboli reported today is much lower than in the past, largely because of heparinization and meticulous attention to flushing of angiographic catheters.[33] Although systemic heparinization is used routinely during coronary angiography at many institutions,[39] it has been shown that the low doses of heparin used in angiographic solutions produce detectable systemic effects.[40] Full systemic heparinization is not used routinely in most angiographic suites. Since there is marked enhancement of blood clotting in glass syringes, plastic syringes should always be used for contrast and flush solutions.[24,25]

Arteriovenous Fistula

Puncture site arteriovenous fistula (AVF) is rarely reported in the literature and appears to represent only a tiny proportion of puncture site complications, with an incidence of 0.01 percent in one large study.[28] Most fistulas have occurred after cardiac catheterization or pulmonary angiography.[41] The great majority of fistulas connect the deep or superficial femoral artery with the venae comitantes[42] (Fig. 42-1). It is therefore important to localize arterial punctures to the common femoral artery, usually at the level of the head of the femur. It has also been suggested that simultaneous arterial and venous access, as often occurs during cardiac procedures, predisposes to AVF because of hematoma formation in the space between the punctured vessels.[43]

Symptoms of femoral AVF may appear months or years after the angiogram and may include palpable thrill, pulsating mass, or limb claudication due to

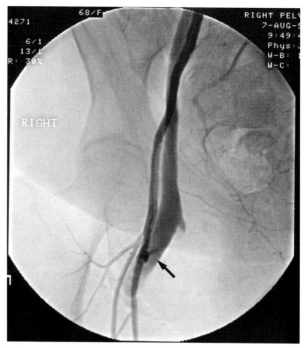

Figure 42-1. A 68-year-old woman had a coronary angiogram and developed right leg claudication shortly thereafter. Follow-up arteriogram shows a jet of an arteriovenous fistula (*arrow*) from the proximal superficial femoral artery to the femoral vein. Note the relationship of low puncture site to the femoral head.

"steal" from the femoral artery. Surgery has traditionally been required for correction. With the advent of newer invasive techniques, more peripheral fistulas are being described.[44] The authors have seen a peroneal artery-to-vein fistula following attempts at laser angioplasty (Fig. 42-2). It has been hypothesized that the midperoneal artery is particularly susceptible to this complication because of fixation of the vessel at the origin of a large nutrient artery supplying the fibula.[45]

Pseudoaneurysm

Pseudoaneurysms have historically been considered a rare sequela of arterial catheterization. Hessel et al. found an incidence of 0.01 percent.[28] However, a study of 38,822 femoral punctures by Roberts et al. in 1987 reported a 0.2 percent incidence after cardiac catheterization and a 0.1 percent incidence after radiologic procedures.[46] This relative incidence has been confirmed by others.[31,47] It is thought that the increased incidence in more recent studies is due to the use of large introducing sheaths and heparin, as well as to the wider use of angioplasty. There is an association between pseudoaneurysm formation and low puncture (distal to the common femoral artery).[48]

Small pseudoaneurysms may close spontaneously

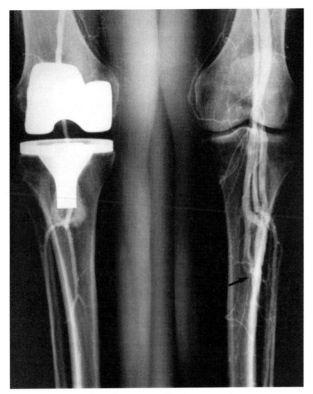

Figure 42-2. Arteriovenous fistula secondary to an attempted laser angioplasty. Note the position of the fistula (*arrow*) between the midperoneal artery and its vena comitante.

without intervention.[49] Larger and/or painful lesions require treatment. In a study by Graham et al., 12 of 50 false aneurysms ruptured 1 to 6 days after catheterization, with a mean of 2.8 days.[50] Patient age, peripheral vascular disease, and elevated liver enzymes were correlated with rupture.

The traditional treatment of pseudoaneurysm is surgical repair.[46] More recently, several reports have described treatment by ultrasound-guided manual compression.[47,51] This technique requires visualizing the aneurysm with color Doppler ultrasound and compressing it with the probe until flow in the aneurysm is halted. Visualization during treatment allows arterial patency to be maintained. Cycles of compression last 10 minutes (or 20 minutes in patients who have received anticoagulants) and are repeated until all flow into the pseudoaneurysm ceases.[47] This method can be employed to treat many femoral pseudoaneurysms nonsurgically. A brachial pseudoaneurysm has also been treated in this manner.[52] Chronic pseudoaneurysms and suprainguinal and infected lesions should be approached surgically.[53] Ultrasound is also important in evaluating pulsatile groin masses because it excludes

transmission through a hematoma and avoids surgical exploration of hematoma.[31]

Spasm

Arterial spasm may occur at the puncture site or at the catheter tip and usually is not a significant complication. However, particularly after brachial arteriography and in children, puncture site spasm can be limb-threatening.[54] Significant spasm may also occur in trifurcation vessels during angioplasty.

Spasm can be controlled by drugs in most cases. Sublingual or intravenous nifedipine[55] has been employed to decrease spasm during angioplasty. Intra-arterial nitroglycerine also produces relief of spasm, and the authors prefer this method because it is rapid and controllable. Severe spasm can be treated with intraarterial administration of such agents as Priscoline, reserpine, and prostaglandin E_1, which have more prolonged effects.[56,57] Papaverine should never be used intraarterially because the combination of this medication and nonionic contrast material can cause thrombosis in vivo.[58]

Femoral Neuralgia Syndrome

The femoral neuralgia syndrome is a late sequela of surgical repair of the femoral artery.[59] It is usually associated with pseudoaneurysm repair and has been reported only after coronary procedures. Patients complain of paroxysmal groin pain radiating down the thigh, associated with hyperesthesia. The neuralgia gradually improves over the course of 6 weeks to a year. Once other procedure-related complications are excluded, reassurance and support with analgesics are the indicated treatment. Femoral neuralgia syndrome is thought to result from stretching of the anterior cutaneous branches of the femoral nerve.[59] Although this syndrome has not been reported after noncardiac procedures, analogous pain occurs in some patients after angiography and also appears to be self-limited.

Complications Related to Catheters and Guidewires

Embolization

Arteriography-induced embolization includes embolization of clots formed in or on catheters. Trauma to the vessel wall can also dislodge cholesterol plaques or clot, which then flows distally. Potential embolic materials also include foreign bodies from equipment such as sponges, plastic emboli from catheters or guidewires, and air emboli due to poor technique.[60,61] Embolization probably occurs frequently during angiographic procedures, but the event usually causes no symptoms. However, when embolization occurs during cerebral arteriography, the consequences are more serious.

Hessel et al. reported a total neurologic complication rate of 0.23 percent due to transfemoral carotid arteriography.[28] This included motor weakness, transient ischemic attack and stroke, aphasia, blindness, and seizures. Most of the symptoms were transient. Another large study by Earnest et al. in 1984 reported a neurologic complication rate of 2.6 percent, with a 0.6 percent permanent complication rate.[62] Age, elevated serum creatinine level, and the use of more than one catheter were significantly correlated with an increase in complications.

The complication rate of cerebral arteriography using an axillary or brachial approach is higher than with femoral puncture, approaching 3.5 percent (0.7 percent permanent) in a recent review.[63] The American College of Radiology Standard suggests a maximum complication rate of less than 4 percent and a permanent complication rate of less than 1 percent (see Table 42-1).

Continuous attention should be paid to catheter flushing during arteriography, and catheter time should be kept to a minimum.[64] Continuous flush systems are used at many institutions, but care should be taken to forcefully flush catheters with multiple side holes, because continuous flush systems may only clear the proximal side holes.[61] Systemic heparinization should be considered in all patients at significant risk for embolic events. Hydrophilically coated guidewires have been shown to be significantly less thrombogenic than steel spring guides.[65] Heparin has been used to coat catheters, but it is not clear whether this has any significant effect on clot formation, and heparin-coated catheters are very expensive.[65,66]

Another, relatively rare manifestation of embolization after arteriography is the multiple cholesterol emboli syndrome (MCES). This may be an acute, catastrophic event or an insidious and chronic process.[5] Symptoms are listed in Table 42-4. The syndrome usually occurs in men who have marked atheromatous disease of the aorta. The true incidence of MCES is hard to determine, but at least one study has suggested that it is not uncommon.[67] The prognosis is usually poor, but some patients have survived after prolonged dialysis.[68]

Iatrogenic Dissection

Dissection of the arterial wall can occur spontaneously, or secondary to intimal damage caused by guidewires, catheters, or angioplasty balloons (Fig. 42-3). Clinically significant dissections have been reported in 1 to 7 percent of angioplasties.[69] In the authors' experi-

Table 42-4. Multiple Cholesterol Emboli Syndrome

Acute or catastrophic form
  Agitation, sweating
  Pain in legs or feet
  Abdominal and back pain
  Numbness or paralysis of extremities
  Skin discoloration (livedo reticularis and purple toes)
  Acute hypertension
  Acute renal failure
  Hypotension
  Death
Chronic or noncatastrophic form
  Malignant or episodic hypertension
  Postangiography or postoperative chronic renal failure
  Acute pancreatitis
  Myopathy
  Peritonitis, bowel ischemia (melena, hematochezia)
  Livedo reticularis
  Gangrene of extremity

From Cronin RE. Southwestern internal medicine conference: renal failure following radiologic procedures. Am J Med Sci 1989;298:342–356. Used with permission.

ence, this has been most common in the iliac artery. If there is occlusion or extravasation, early surgical treatment is mandatory, and in some cases occluded vessels can be opened with a Fogarty balloon.[70] If dissection is present without occlusion or bleeding, the angioplasty catheter can be reinflated in an attempt to "tack down" the intimal flap.[71] If this is not possible, an atherectomy catheter can be used to remove the flap, or an intravascular stent can be placed across the dissection.[72,73] We believe that stents should be used for iliac artery dissections, where the lumen size is large and vessel perforation cannot be tolerated. In the femoral arteries, atherectomy should be attempted.

Catheters and guidewires should always be visualized under fluoroscopy as they are advanced. This allows for the immediate detection of any obstruction to passage and prevents large subintimal tears. Another potential cause of dissection is placement of angulated catheters through arterial sheaths.[74] This abrades the arterial wall at the junction of sheath and vessel. Such dissections can be avoided by inserting catheters with guidewires in place.

Complications of Specific Procedures

Translumbar Aortography

Translumbar aortography has generally been replaced by femoral arteriography using the Seldinger technique. Direct aortic arteriography does not allow control of the puncture site and is of limited value if intervention is contemplated. However, it continues to be employed in some situations, particularly by vascular surgeons.

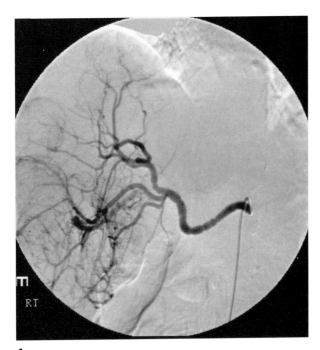

A

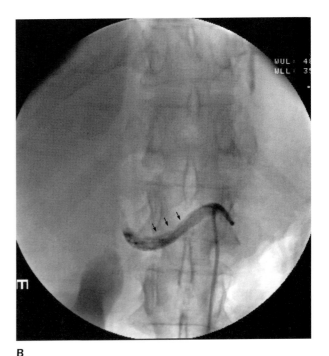

B

Figure 42-3. (A) Hepatic arteriogram before attempted embolization of hepatic metastasis. (B) During subselective manipulation of the guidewire, a long dissection of the he- patic artery was produced (*arrows*), which terminated the procedure. In most cases, dissections of the hepatic artery resolve spontaneously.

The largest study of the complications of this tech- nique, done in 1976, found seven major complications (0.05 percent) and two deaths (0.014 percent), an in- cidence equal to or slightly lower than that for femoral arteriography.[75] Major complications in the 14,550 cases studied included transpleural puncture in four patients, which produced significant hemothorax, three cases of severe retroperitoneal hemorrhage, and one patient who became paraplegic. "Minor" compli- cations included intravasation and extravasation of contrast material. Vascular surgeons performed all of the arteriograms surveyed.

A study of radiologists performing translumbar aor- tograms at many institutions[28] revealed a complication rate of 2.89 percent, significantly higher than the 1.73 percent complication rate of transfemoral angiography in the same sample. This difference may be due to the experience of the investigators or to other local factors. Its importance has been minimized because in the ma- jority of patients presently studied interventions must be performed for peripheral vascular disease, which mandates access via the femoral route.

Special care should be taken in choosing the level of puncture for translumbar aortography. Scrupulous attention must be paid to bleeding and clotting times. Because of the course of the needle puncture, compli- cations related to entrance into the splanchnic, renal, or lumbar arteries may occur. Nikolic et al. reported a case in which the translumbar needle transected the inferior mesenteric artery, necessitating surgical re- pair.[76] Delayed or persistent pain after translumbar puncture should alert the radiologist to the possibility of bleeding.

Transbrachial Arteriography

Complications related to brachial puncture are more frequent than with femoral arteriography. Grollman and Marcus[77] studied transbrachial selective arte- riograms in 72 patients and found a 7 percent inci- dence of major complications, including 3 patients who required surgery for brachial artery thrombosis. Another study found an 11 percent incidence in pa- tients who had direct catheter insertion, and it recom- mended placement of a 5 French arterial sheath through a high puncture (10 cm proximal to the ante- cubital crease) to reduce the number of complica- tions.[78] Most angiographers believe that brachial punc- ture should be reserved for those patients who have significant contraindications to femoral access.

If wire and catheter exchanges are contemplated, placement of a vascular sheath will reduce arterial trauma.[79] Administration of antispasmodic medica- tions, such as intraarterial nitroglycerin or sublingual nifedipine, should also be considered in patients at risk for thrombosis.

Transaxillary Arteriography

Arteriography by the transaxillary route, like brachial arteriography, has a significantly higher complication rate than femoral access.[28] In one recent series,[80] 13 percent of patients had brachial plexus injuries after the procedure. The axillary approach has been used when femoral access is not possible due to absent pulses, femoral artery aneurysm, severe aortoiliac disease, or previous failure.[81] The approach has also been used in patients who have had arterial grafts. However, a recent paper has shown that the complication rate for the axillary approach exceeds that for femoral arteriography through a graft,[82] although the complication rate is lower than for direct-stick brachial arteriography. Because of the higher complication rates, we believe the femoral route should be used whenever possible.

As at other sites, local complications are primarily related to thrombosis and hematoma, with the latter being more common and more serious. Hematoma in the axilla is more problematic than elsewhere because of the tight fascial compartments and proximity to the brachial plexus. The frequency of upper extremity nerve injuries after axillary puncture has been reported as 0.4 to 9.5 percent.[80,83] The neuropathy usually involves both the sensory and motor nerves of the hand, and spares the upper arm.[83]

Nerve injury due to axillary hematoma probably results from compression in what has been termed the *medial brachial fascial compartment*.[83] Since hematomas that occur distal to this tight compartment do not produce neurologic symptoms, low brachial artery entry may protect against complications. Patients should be instructed to report any symptoms of pain or weakness after axillary arteriograms. Those with sensory symptoms (paresthesias) can usually be treated expectantly, but any motor weakness should prompt surgical decompression of the axilla.[83]

Pulmonary Angiography

The complications related to pulmonary angiography have been recently reviewed as part of the Prospective Investigation of Pulmonary Embolism Diagnosis (PIOPED) study.[84] Of 1111 patients undergoing pulmonary studies, there were 5 deaths (0.5 percent), 4 other cases requiring cardiopulmonary resuscitation or intubation, 3 cases of renal failure requiring dialysis, and 2 significant puncture site hematomas. The frequency of complications was not related to the presence or absence of pulmonary emboli. Older patients were more likely to have decreases in renal function, but this is a characteristic of all procedures employing

Table 42-5. Nonmajor or Minor Complications of Pulmonary Angiography in 1111 Patients

Respiratory distress (prompt response to drugs)	4
Renal dysfunction (response to fluid and/or drugs)	10
Angina (monitored in CCU)	2
Hypotension (prompt response to drugs or fluid)	2
Pulmonary congestion (prompt response to drugs)	4
Urticaria, itching, or periorbital edema	16
Hematoma (not requiring transfusion)	9
Arrhythmia (spontaneous conversion or prompt response to drugs)	6
Subintimal contrast stain	4
Narcotic overdose (treated with naloxone)	1
Nausea and vomiting	1
Right bundle branch block	1
Total	60

From Stein PD, et al. Complications and validity of pulmonary angiography in acute pulmonary embolism. Circulation 1992;85: 462–468. Used with permission.

contrast material. "Minor" complications, some of which were life-threatening, are shown in Table 42-5.

Although pulmonary hypertension has been reported as a significant risk in pulmonary angiography,[85] there was no relationship between complications and pulmonary arterial pressure in the PIOPED trial.[84] The shift from main pulmonary artery injection to selective studies has made pulmonary hypertension less of a risk factor.

During passage of catheters through the right heart, extra systoles occur in almost every patient. Significant arrhythmias are much more infrequent. These include ventricular tachycardia, ventricular fibrillation, right bundle branch block, complete heart block, paroxysmal atrial tachycardia, and bradycardia.[85] Patients with irritable myocardia can be given 50 to 100 mg of lidocaine intravenously immediately before or during the procedure to decrease cardiac irritability. Simply asking the patient to cough repeatedly often alleviates arrhythmias without medication. Patients with preexisting left bundle branch block should probably have a venous pacemaker in the atrium before pulmonary artery catheterization.[86] Patients being treated for arrhythmias with amiodarone should be watched carefully. Acute respiratory failure and death have been reported after pulmonary angiography in patients taking this medication.[87]

In a nonteaching hospital study involving only 10 arteriograms per year, 3 perforations of the right atrium occurred, all without sequelae.[88] Perforation of the right ventricle or outflow tract occurred in 1 percent of patients in a 1980 study,[85] but in no patients in the PIOPED study reported in 1992.[84] We believe this decrease is due to the general acceptance of

Grollman-type pigtail catheters,[89] which do not recoil on contrast injection. A single case of pulmonary artery dissection after contrast injection has been reported in a patient with pulmonary hypertension, but this did not cause any significant morbidity.[90]

Complications of Interventional Radiology

The subspecialty of interventional radiology is one of the youngest in medicine. In the past several years, radiologists have assumed direct patient care responsibilities and developed new treatment modalities that save patients (and the medical care system) time, pain, and money. With any new endeavor comes the negative—complications heretofore not seen in the radiology department must be recognized and treated. Because many of the newer interventional procedures benefit small numbers of patients and because controlled, prospective studies are lacking in most instances, descriptions of complications are often anecdotal. Nevertheless, an understanding of the types and mechanisms of complications in interventional procedures has obvious value in avoidance and treatment.

The Head and Neck

Intracranial Embolization

Intracranial interventional procedures are fraught with potential hazards. The overall complication rate for embolization procedures in neuroradiology is 6.7 percent, and the mortality rate is 1.3 percent.[91] Procedures have been developed at a limited number of centers, which often have the only significant experience in a given technique. However, training programs are producing interventional neuroradiologists, and this suggests that these procedures may become more widespread in the near future.

Efforts have been directed at treating unclippable aneurysms, dural arteriovenous fistulas (AVFs), carotid-cavernous fistulas, and arteriovenous malformations (AVMs).[92] Meningiomas can be preoperatively infarcted to reduce blood loss during surgery.[93] Serious complications are to be expected in a significant number of patients. A team approach with neurosurgeons and neurologists, as well as detailed discussions of potential risks and benefits with the patient, is strongly recommended before undertaking these procedures. Arteriograms should be performed under local anesthesia with constant neurologic evaluation to prevent untoward effects.

Aneurysm, Fistula, and Malformation. Complica-

tions associated with attempts at aneurysm occlusion occur in up to 20 percent of patients, even in the largest centers.[94] Higashida et al., in a study of 215 patients with inoperable aneurysms,[95] had 21 deaths (9.8 percent) and 16 strokes (7.4 percent) attributable to balloon embolization. Complications relate to ischemia caused by balloon compression of the vessel, occlusion of the carotid artery, distal emboli, and hemorrhage due to aneurysm rupture.[96–98] Distal embolization may sometimes occur due to dislodgement of thrombus within the aneurysm; it may be best to wait 6 weeks after discovery of the aneurysm before treatment to allow clot organization or lysis to occur.[94,95]

Some patients experience the acute onset of vascular headache as the balloon is inflated, but this symptom usually lasts less than 10 minutes.[99] The use of calibrated leak detachable balloons[94] allows test inflations to judge neurosensory effects and may result in a lower complication rate than coil embolization.

Dural arteriovenous fistulas heal spontaneously in 10 to 60 percent of cases.[92,100] Depending on symptoms, the remainder require treatment. Because most dural AVFs are supplied by external carotid branches, complications are less ominous than in AVMs or aneurysms. Embolization of cavernous sinus AVFs can produce an inflammatory reaction in the orbit, which can be treated with steroids and anticoagulants.[101] Cranial nerve palsies can result from embolization of the occipital or ascending pharyngeal artery.[92]

Carotid-cavernous fistulas arise either spontaneously or after trauma. Complications are similar to those seen with dural AVFs but also include the risk of cerebrovascular embolization because the approach is through the internal carotid artery.

Cerebral arteriovenous malformations may be treated with surgery, radiation, or embolization alone. Because only 10 to 15 percent of AVMs are amenable to complete cure by embolization,[92] most patients have embolization followed by radiation or surgery.[102,103] Preoperative embolization effectively converts malformations into smaller lesions, which have lower complication rates at surgery.[104] Immediate or delayed hemorrhage occurs in 4 to 15 percent of patients, and neurologic deficits in 5 to 16 percent.[104,105] Hemorrhage may be related to catheter penetration of the subarachnoid space.[106] The mortality rate related to the procedure should be approximately 1 percent.[102]

Meningioma. Preoperative embolization of meningiomas has been performed in an effort to reduce operative bleeding, save involved dural sinuses, and/or allow for more precise delineation of surgical planes.[93] Embolization must be done with relatively small (50–150 μm) particles to produce significant tumor ischemia.[107] Patients premedicated with steroids have less postprocedure edema, and this may have a protective effect.[107] The use of small particles requires superselective catheterization to avoid scalp necrosis.[107] Liquid material should not be used because this can penetrate small collateral channels between internal and external circulations.[93] Facial palsy can follow middle meningeal artery occlusion.[108]

Extracranial Embolization

Embolization has been used for the treatment of facial arteriovenous fistulas and malformations, massive epistaxis, juvenile angiofibroma, and parathyroid adenoma. Reflux of embolic material must be carefully avoided because flow of emboli into the internal carotid vascular territory is disastrous. Preembolization arteriograms should be studied carefully to exclude vascular anastomoses between the external and internal carotid circulation. As in other embolization procedures, particular attention to slow and careful infusion of embolic material is required as the end vessels are obliterated and flow slows in the proximal vessel.[109,110]

In a series of 20 preoperative embolizations of juvenile nasopharyngeal angiofibromas, Deschler et al.[111] reported no complications related to embolization with polyvinyl alcohol particles. When the tumor extends into the skull base and either directly involves or receives significant arterial supply from the internal carotid artery, balloons may be used to temporarily occlude the internal carotid artery to test for collateral circulation.[111]

Thyroid Biopsy

The complication rate of thyroid biopsy is very low, with hematoma formation the most common untoward event.[112,113] Occasionally, vascular proliferation may occur in postbiopsy hematomas, resulting in development of cavernous hemangioma or hemangioendothelioma.[112,114] There has been a reported case of needle tract seeding of a papillary carcinoma.[115]

The Lung

Bronchial Artery Embolization

Embolization of the bronchial arteries is performed to treat recurrent hemoptysis, most often due to bronchiectasis. Other causes of bronchial hemorrhage are tuberculosis, pulmonary abscess, and central neoplasm.

Novak[91] reported an overall complication rate of 2.7 percent in 846 patients embolized for hemoptysis. Spinal cord infarction has been reported in two cases, and one of these was secondary to embolization of an intercostal artery.[116,117] The incidence of transverse my-

elitis as a sequela of bronchial artery embolization is decreasing, probably because of the use of nonionic contrast material and improvements in technique.[118] It is important to map the bronchial circulation before embolization and to establish that no spinal feeding vessels arise from the artery to be embolized. Particular care should be taken when studying the right intercostal arteries. Right fifth intercostal artery injections have produced a significant percentage of the small incidence of transverse myelitis following embolizations.[118,119] Left main stem bronchial stenosis[120] and bronchoesophageal fistula[121] have been reported after bronchial artery embolization. These may have been due to bronchial wall ischemia related to the procedure. Use of larger embolic particles may prevent these complications.

Pulmonary Arteriovenous Fistula Embolization

Pulmonary arteriovenous malformations (PAVMs) may be single or multiple. Most of the multiple fistulas are seen in patients with Rendu-Osler-Weber disease (hereditary hemorrhagic telangiectasia, or HHT).[122] Fistulas cause paradoxical emboli, right-to-left shunts, and occasional hemoptysis. Treatment consists of embolizing the PAVMs with detachable balloons, coils, or both.

Migration of embolic material into the systemic circulation is a major potential complication of PAVM embolization. In a review of 45 patients, Remy-Jardin et al.[123] reported 1 case of embolization of an occluding coil to the mitral valve, which necessitated immediate surgery. White et al.[124] described 2 balloon migrations in a study of 76 patients. The balloon lodged in the hepatic artery in one case and in the internal iliac artery in the second. No treatment was necessary. If coil or balloon migration occurs, prompt manual compression of the carotid arteries may help prevent embolization into the head.

Other complications of PAVM occlusion include air embolus, hemorrhage, and pleurisy.[123,124] Air embolism and hemorrhage can be avoided by careful technique, ensuring that blood can be aspirated from the catheter before contrast injection or embolization. Pleurisy is almost always self-limited and does not constitute a significant complication. Many patients with Rendu-Osler-Weber disease have complex, multiple organ involvement. Those with protean manifestations should be considered for transfer to institutions that have teams trained in the treatment of this malady.

Percutaneous Lung Biopsy

Common complications of transthoracic lung biopsy include pneumothorax and hemoptysis, both of which are usually not problematic.[125] Rare complications include air embolism and deposition of tumor cells in the needle tract.[126]

Asymptomatic pneumothorax is the most common complication of transthoracic lung biopsy, having been reported in 16.1 to 60 percent of patients undergoing the procedure.[125–133] Most pneumothoraces occur immediately after biopsy, and almost all are seen within 4 hours.[131] Accordingly, chest films should be taken at these intervals or when symptoms occur. Pneumothorax is much more common after biopsy in patients with chronic obstructive lung disease.[134,135] Small pneumothoraces usually require no treatment and can be observed expectantly. If there is no increase in the pneumothorax on the 4-hour postbiopsy film, the authors routinely send outpatients home with instructions to return immediately if pain or dyspnea occurs. These patients return for a follow-up film at 24 hours to check for resolution of the pneumothorax.

Symptomatic air leaks, including tension pneumothorax and large pneumothorax in patients with chronic lung disease,[125] have been reported in 0.4 to 11.5 percent of procedures.[126–132] Almost all significant leaks can be detected immediately after the procedure,[131] and routine postprocedure fluoroscopy of the pulmonary apex should be done on every patient. If symptomatic pneumothorax occurs, rapid placement of a small chest tube is a simple procedure (Fig. 42-4). Chest tubes can usually be removed in 24 to 48

hours.[132] If the small-caliber tube fails to eliminate the pneumothorax in a few days, a larger chest tube is probably required.[132]

A rare complication of pneumothorax is pulmonary torsion, in which the lung rotates in the hemithorax, compromising bronchial and pulmonary circulation. This entity usually requires prompt surgical treatment, although the two cases reported after lung biopsy did not produce sufficient compromise to necessitate operation.[136,137]

The incidence of pneumothorax can be decreased by careful attention to biopsy technique. The procedure should be planned to cross the shortest distance of lung.[125] Adjusting the needle path so it crosses fibrotic areas or pleural attachments rather than lung decreases the incidence of pneumothorax.[125,138] Patients who are kept with the biopsied side down for 1 hour after the procedure have a lower rate of pneumothorax.[128] There is no significant difference in incidence with large versus small needles, but there is a higher incidence with multiple passes.[125] Placement of a blood patch on needle withdrawal has not been shown to decrease the incidence of pneumothorax.[129,130] Recently, Engeler et al. reported the use of compressed collagen foam plugs to reduce the rate of postprocedure pneumothorax,[139] but this has not been confirmed at other institutions.

The incidence of significant hemoptysis due to lung

Figure 42-4. (A) Film taken immediately after percutaneous lung biopsy in a patient with onset of shortness of breath. Note the medial displacement of the pulmonary mass and the pneumothorax (*arrows*). The mediastinum is displaced to the right. (B) Film taken after a small-bore chest tube was placed. The mediastinum and descending aorta have shifted back into the midline.

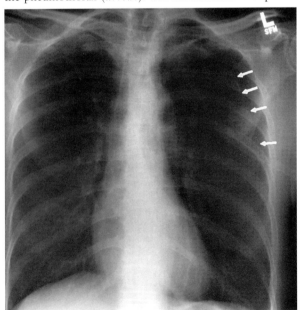

A

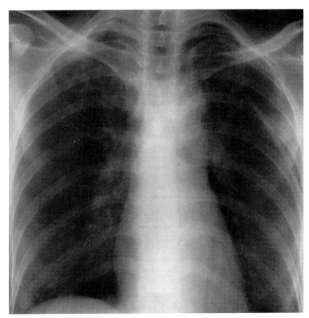

B

biopsy has decreased in recent years,[125] most likely because of refinement of the technique. Berquist et al. reported a twofold increase in hemoptysis in central as compared to peripheral lesions.[140] Haaga[125] recommends that uncooperative patients and those with pulmonary hypertension or on anticoagulant medications be excluded from lung biopsy. He insists that patients taking aspirin or other platelet inhibitors be required to stop the medication for 1 week before lung biopsy because of the risk of hemorrhage. Westcott[141] believes that significant hemoptysis almost never occurs and describes only a single case after biopsy with a 20-gauge or smaller needle. Our experience parallels that of Westcott.

If significant hemorrhage occurs, the patient should be immediately placed in the decubitus position with the biopsied side down.[125] Oxygen can be administered through a nasal cannula until control is established via a double-lumen endotracheal tube, if necessary.

Air embolism during lung biopsy is a rare event. Its occurrence has been related to the Valsalva maneuver, positive pressure ventilation, or coughing.[125,142] The time during which the biopsy needle is open to the air should be kept to a minimum to decrease the chances of air entering a pulmonary vein. The operator's finger can be used to cover the needle hub during removal and replacement of the obturator. If air embolism is suspected, the patient should immediately be placed in the Trendelenburg position with the left side down. This can (at least theoretically) trap air in the apex of the right ventricle and prevent it from embolizing further.[143] Nasal oxygen should be given. Hyperbaric oxygen therapy has been used in patients with air embolism in an attempt to reduce the size of the air bubbles and improve oxygenation.[142,144]

Seeding of the biopsy tract with malignant cells is a very rare complication.[145] Although malignant cells may be deposited in the needle tract in a high percentage of cases, actual metastasis to the tract is extremely uncommon.[146]

The Abdomen

Abdominal Biopsy

The overwhelming majority of abdominal masses that can be imaged are amenable to percutaneous biopsy. Diagnosis can be established in 70 to 95 percent of cases.[147] Major complications of biopsy include hemorrhage, pneumothorax, bile leak, infection, and seeding of the needle tract.[147,148] Fatal carcinoid crisis has been reported after biopsy of hepatic metastasis.[149] Transient fever, hematuria, and pain are minor complications, which usually resolve without treatment.

Major complications should occur in less than 2 percent of all cases,[147] and large studies of biopsies done under ultrasound guidance report a major complication rate of less than 0.2 percent.[150–152] These same studies had a mortality rate of 0.018 to 0.038 percent.

Seeding of the tract during liver biopsy may be underreported.[153] In an extensive review of the literature done by Smith,[152] 10 of the 23 instances of needle tract seeding occurred after biopsies of pancreatic malignancies.

The most common cause of death after percutaneous biopsy is hemorrhage. In a large study by Fornari et al.,[150] both deaths were due to hemorrhage after biopsy of hepatocellular carcinoma in cirrhotic livers. Because superficial hepatic lesions may bleed into the peritoneal cavity, biopsy of such lesions should be planned to cross as much uninvolved hepatic parenchyma as possible before entering the lesion.[152] If postprocedure bleeding is suspected, the patient should be scanned with computed tomography (CT), because CT is more accurate than ultrasound in evaluating for fresh blood.[148] As in other interventional procedures, persistence of pain after biopsy should prompt the search for a cause.

Although complications related to pancreatic biopsy are relatively rare,[152,154] they are more serious than in other organ biopsies because of the sequelae of pancreatitis. In a study of 184 patients undergoing pancreatic biopsy, Mueller et al.[155] reported severe pancreatitis in 5 cases (3 percent). Three of the 5 patients had biopsy-proven normal glands. One of the patients died. These authors believe that the incidence of pancreatitis after biopsy is increasing because refinements in technique have allowed the procedure to be applied to smaller lesions.

Abscess Drainage

Percutaneous abscess drainage was first used in postoperative patients. Now that it is often employed as a primary treatment, the number of surgical procedures performed has decreased. Abscesses in the peritoneal cavity and retroperitoneum, as well as within any of the abdominal organs, can be drained percutaneously. Multilocular abscesses may require placement of multiple drains.[147]

Studies that discuss abscess drainage procedures report major complications in less than 5 percent of cases.[147,156–159] These include systemic infection, perforation of an abdominal viscus with or without fistula formation, hemorrhage, and death. Minor complications, including pain, wound infection, pneumothorax, and catheter dislodgement, have an occurrence rate of 5 to 15 percent.[147,156–158] As in abdominal biopsy, complications are often more serious in procedures involving the pancreas. It is important to differentiate pancreatic phlegmon from abscess because premature attempts at pancreatic drainage have resulted in significant hemorrhage.[159]

Pyopneumothorax can occur after nephrostomy[160] or after other procedures in the upper abdomen. This is a potentially devastating event. In all cases the puncture site and tract must be carefully selected to avoid crossing the pleural space. It is extremely important for the interventionalist to understand that some patients will not have a safe access route to the abscess because of intervening viscus or vessels.[158] In this small percentage of patients, surgical abscess drainage should be done.

Percutaneous Nephrostomy and Nephrolithotomy

Percutaneous Nephrostomy. Complications of percutaneous nephrostomy include pain, bleeding, infection, urinoma, penetration of adjacent viscera, and failure to establish drainage.[161,162] Older studies documented major complications in 4 percent of cases and minor complications in 15 percent.[163] More recent reviews[147,164] describe each group of complications—bleeding, bacteremia, and urinoma—as occurring in 2 to 5 percent of cases. Today, almost all complications are not life-threatening.

Bleeding during or after nephrostomy is usually self-limited.[161,162] Cronan et al.[165] reported 8 clinically unsuspected hematomas (13 percent) in 62 consecutive nephrostomies, but none of these required surgical intervention or transfusion. The incidence of hematomas can be minimized by a posterolateral approach, which avoids traversing major vessels.[166] When bleeding is significant, a larger nephrostomy tube or balloon catheter can be used to tamponade the tract. This procedure will often stop the bleeding. Laceration of a major renal vessel is distinctly uncommon and can be treated by angiography with embolization.[167,168] If the bleeding site is not seen at angiography, the nephrostomy tube should be removed over a wire and the arteriogram repeated.[169]

Avoidance of infection, as in all interventional procedures, is best accomplished by careful attention to sterile technique. Antibiotic coating of catheters has not been of value.[170] However, the use of systemic antibiotics, both before and during the procedure, reduces the incidence of infection.[162] Because many nephrostomies are done to treat urosepsis, occasional spread of the existing inflammatory process is unavoidable.

Urinoma may follow procedures in which multiple punctures are made or when there is extravasation due to surgical trauma or obstruction. Urinomas may be drained percutaneously.[147] When there is a persistent leak, simultaneous placement of a nephrostomy tube and/or a ureteral stent often results in closure with complete resolution.[171]

Hopper and Yakes[172] studied the posterior intercostal approach for nephrostomy and determined that there was relatively little risk that the liver or spleen would be punctured. However, the pleural space would be crossed 29 percent of the time on the right and 14 percent on the left, even with the puncture done in the 11th intercostal space during expiration. Percentages rose for inspiration punctures and at the 10th intercostal space. A subcostal approach is safer and avoids potential complications.

Nephroduodenal fistulas have been reported as a rare complication of percutaneous nephrostomy.[173,174] Most cases probably result from transrenal puncture, with creation of a tract between the collecting system and the gastrointestinal tract. Sepsis may play a role in establishing the fistulous tract.[173] Nephrectomy was required in both the reported cases.[173,174] Erosion of a catheter from the perinephric space into the duodenum has also been reported.[175] This condition resolved after the catheter was repositioned.

Another potential complication of percutaneous nephrostomy is inability to remove the nephrostomy tube. The authors have removed encrusted tubes by cutting the hub and then placing an introducing sheath or peel-away catheter over the tube into the kidney. This reestablishes the tract and allows for manipulation and subsequent removal of the tube. Others[176] have placed a second nephrostomy adjacent to the problematic one and used this second tract to free the nephrostomy tube. Nosher et al.[170] reported a 17 percent incidence of inadvertent catheter withdrawal, which was more common in patients in critical care units. The use of retention loop catheters and sewing the catheter to the skin in patients who are comatose or uncooperative should decrease the incidence of complication.

In an effort to reduce the complication rate of nephrostomy, fine guidewire-catheter systems have been developed that allow one to enlarge tracts created by 21-gauge needles into standard catheter access routes.[177] Such systems use 0.018-inch platinum-tipped guidewires, which have fragile tips. These can be detached relatively easily from the wire mandrel.[178] Guidewires should not be pulled back through the needle or stiffening cannula if resistance is felt. Rather, the unit should be removed as a whole and another puncture performed.

Percutaneous Nephrolithotomy. As in nephrostomy, complication rates for nephrolithotomy have probably declined over time because of the learning curve involved in performing the procedure. Page and Walker[179] recently reported a complication rate of 3.6 percent for the entire procedure and a 0.9 percent complication rate for creation of the nephrostomy tract. This is lower than the rates reported in older series.[164] Significant bleeding is the only major complication of the procedure,[179] although failure of access may unnecessarily expose the patient to anesthesia and/or result in an open procedure. Autonomic hyperreflexia, with a sudden increase in blood pressure, has been reported in a paraplegic patient during nephrolithotomy.[180] This syndrome is controlled by administrating alpha- and beta-adrenergic blockers and terminating the procedure.

The Liver and Biliary Tree

Transcatheter Tumor Ablation

Hepatic artery embolization has been used as a primary method of tumor ablation and as an adjunct to chemotherapy. Since the hepatic artery is particularly susceptible to dissection (see Fig. 42-3), particular care should be taken in manipulating the catheter and guidewire in this vessel. As with other procedures, general complications as previously described apply to hepatic artery angiography.

The most common complication of hepatic embolization is postembolization syndrome.[181–183] It consists of pain and fever and is seen in almost every patient. The pain can begin immediately with the first infusion of embolic material or up to 3 days after the procedure. It lasts 7 to 10 days after the procedure. Intravenous analgesics are usually required for the first 24 to 48 hours. Nausea and vomiting occur in up to 50 percent of patients[181] and occasionally are associated with abdominal distention. All of these subside with treatment of symptoms.

Infarction of the gallbladder is another recognized complication of hepatic embolization. In most cases, this is an incidental finding at subsequent laparotomy, at which a scarred, contracted gallbladder is found.[184] However, acute cholecystitis necessitating surgery has been reported.[185,186] Changes in amylase levels, reflecting damage to the pancreas, have also been reported.[187] In treatment regimens using 5-fluorouracil (5-FU), gastrointestinal ulcers have been reported in up to 29 percent of patients.[188] To avoid these complications, embolic material should be infused as selectively as possible, and the procedure should be terminated before reflux of embolic material occurs. Biloma[189] and hemorrhage due to rupture of the liver[190] have also been reported after chemoembolization, but these are rare complications.

Intrahepatic gas is sometimes observed after embolization procedures, but this is usually due to necrosis and/or blood breakdown in the tumor and should not be mistaken for abscess formation.[191] Noninflammatory gas does not increase postprocedure pain, but infection greatly exacerbates symptoms. Administration of antibiotics reduces the risk of infection after embolization to approximately 2 percent.[192] Pulmonary oil embolization has been reported after Lipiodol infusion for treatment of hepatocellular carcinoma in 6 of 336 patients treated (1.8 percent).[193] One of these patients died of respiratory arrest. Oil embolization occurs to some extent in all patients receiving intrahepatic Lipiodol, and the potential benefits of the procedure should be weighed against the small probability of serious complication.

Embolization of hepatic carcinoid metastases can produce carcinoid crisis.[183] The crisis manifests as profound hypotension that is refractory to usual medications and difficult to reverse.[149] Immediate treatment should consist of volume expansion and intravenous administration of 50 µg of octreotide acetate (Sandostatin, Sandor Pharmaceuticals). Precipitation of the crisis can be avoided, or its effects lessened, by giving patients 50 to 400 µg of Sandostatin per day for 7 days before the procedure and 100 µg subcutaneously just before embolization.[194]

Percutaneous Ablation of Liver Tumors

Percutaneous CT- or ultrasound-guided ethanol injection has been used in the treatment of hepatocellular carcinoma, and more recently for ablation of liver metastases.[195] Because needles must traverse the peritoneal cavity, patients with ascites and/or significant clotting deficiencies should not have this procedure. Pain often occurs on injection of ethanol. Patients may have low-grade fevers for several days after the procedure, but this condition usually does not require treatment. In a study of 1413 ethanol injections performed on 190 patients by Shiina and Niwa,[195] there were three intraperitoneal hemorrhages, one significant pleural effusion, and one hemothorax. All of these resolved without treatment. Others have reported rare cases of jaundice and hepatic infarction after the procedure.[196,197] Tumor seeding of the needle track has also been reported.[198,199] Patient cooperation and accurate localization of the needle tip are the most important factors in reducing the number of complications from this procedure.

Percutaneous Transhepatic Cholangiography

Complications of percutaneous transhepatic cholangiography (PTC)—including sepsis, bile leak, and hemorrhage—occur in 5 to 15 percent of cases.[200,201] The complication rate has been markedly reduced in recent years because of the development of smaller, "skinny" needles.[147] Fluoroscopic determination of the position of the costophrenic sulcus should be made before puncture to avoid crossing of the pleural space. Observation of the needle path during insertion will avoid unintended deviation of the tip, thereby lowering the frequency of complications.[201] Patients with ascites and/or infection should be expected to have a higher complication rate.[200] Preprocedure antibiotics should be given to all patients, and care should be taken to avoid overdistention of the biliary tree with contrast material. Bleeding parameters should be checked before the procedure, and any abnormalities should be corrected if possible. However, the authors have found no increased incidence of hemorrhagic complications in "skinny needle" PTC in patients with borderline bleeding and clotting values.

The great majority of complications of PTC are minor and controllable. Some patients have transient pain during the procedure, probably from capsular irritation by the contrast material,[200] which can be alleviated with medication.

Biliary Drainage

Biliary drainage, with insertion of larger catheters across the liver, has a higher complication rate than cholangiography. Major complications (sepsis, hemorrhage, pneumothorax, and death) occur in 2 to 5 percent of cases.[147] Minor complications, including fever, pain, wound infection, catheter obstruction, or leakage, are seen in 20 to 40 percent of patients.[147]

Steps should be taken to avoid producing bacteremia in all patients undergoing percutaneous biliary drainage. Preprocedural administration of intravenous antibiotics and the addition of gentamycin to the contrast solution are helpful. When a dilated ductal system is entered, it is important to decompress the system before injecting significant amounts of contrast, because forceful injection promotes intravasation of infected bile and may cause septicemia. Suction drainage of the biliary tree should be instituted for 12 to 24 hours, even when an internal stent is placed, to reduce the chance of infection. In the authors' experience, septicemia is the most common cause of morbidity after biliary procedures.

The use of smaller-gauge needles for initial puncture of the liver has decreased the incidence of significant bleeding from biliary drainage procedures.[147] Balloon or large-bore catheters can be used to tamponade significant bleeding, and arteriography with embolization can stop hemorrhage not controllable by other methods.[169] Pneumothorax can be avoided by careful selection of the entry site and by suspension of respiration during punctures.

Biliary catheters have a high rate of obstruction compared to nephrostomies because of the viscous nature of bile. Patients (and/or their families) with potential long-term indwelling catheters should be taught to irrigate the catheters using sterile technique. We recommend maintenance of biliary catheters by forceful injection of 10 ml of sterile saline once every other day.

Removal of Common Duct Stones

Retained common duct stones can be removed through an existing T-tube tract or via transhepatic puncture. This procedure is usually done on an outpatient basis and has a morbidity rate of less than 5 percent.[147] Potential complications are the same as those of PTC and biliary drainage (Fig. 42-5).

Percutaneous Cholecystostomy

Percutaneous puncture and drainage of the gallbladder are most often performed in patients with acute cholecystitis who are not suitable for immediate surgery.[147] Early reports[182] suggested a complication rate of approximately 8 percent, with the most common problem being bradycardia and hypotension due to vagal stimulation. This complication can be treated with atropine and intravenous fluid.[202] Bile peritonitis and bleeding are uncommon complications. As in other interventional procedures, the complication rate has decreased with improvements in technique and equipment. CT or ultrasound should be used to define the "bare area" of the gallbladder where it is attached to the liver, and this portal should be used for transhepatic puncture. Puncture of the "bare area" avoids bile leakage and facilitates passage of guidewires and catheters.

Percutaneous Gastrostomy

The major complication rate of percutaneous gastrostomy should be less than 5 percent. In a study of 252 patients by Halkier et al.,[203] four patients (1.6 percent) required laparotomy for peritonitis, and one patient had a significant gastrointestinal hemorrhage. One of the patients with peritonitis died. Others[204] have treated peritoneal irritation with parenteral antibiotics, thus avoiding surgery.

Minor complications occur in less than 5 percent of cases and consist of peritoneal irritation without sepsis, leakage with spill into the peritoneum, small bowel perforation, stomal infection, and aspiration.[203] Occasionally, the guidewire and/or catheter may loop in the peritoneal cavity between the skin and stomach and cause loss of access. In these cases, a second puncture can usually be made and the procedure continued.[205] Use of the Cope retention suture[206] pulls the

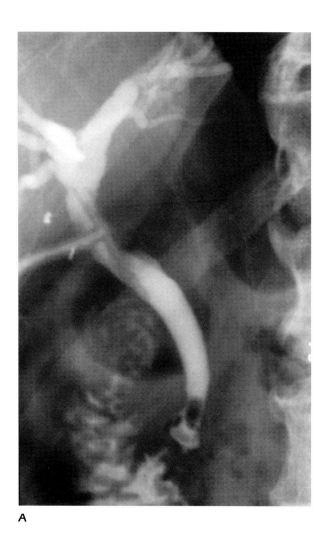

A

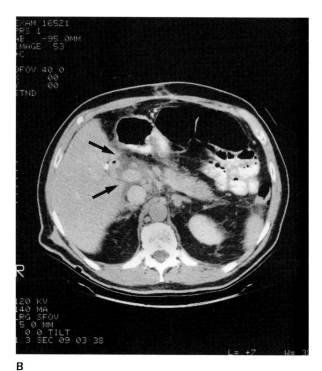

B

Figure 42-5. (A) Patient with retained stone in the common bile duct. (B) The patient developed midabdominal pain 2 days after percutaneous stone retrieval. CT scan shows inflammatory process enveloping the pancreatic head and portal region (*arrows*).

Figure 42-6. A 67-year-old man developed acute rest pain and decreased pulse shortly after a cardiac angioplasty. The symptoms were caused by an embolus (*arrow, left*) in the popliteal artery. After pulsed thrombolysis (*right*), the embolus has been dissolved.

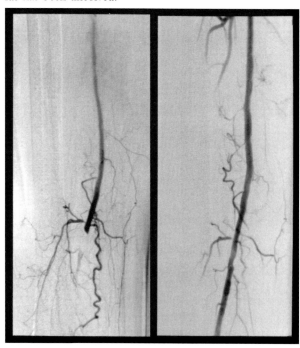

stomach to the anterior abdominal wall and avoids loss of the tract during dilatation and tube passage.

Complications of Peripheral Angiography and Interventions

Transluminal Angioplasty

Peripheral Angioplasty

General complications of peripheral angioplasty include perforation or disruption of the vessel, hemorrhage, thrombosis, distal embolization, dissection, and pseudoaneurysm formation.[207] The immediate complication rate in a series of angioplasties performed by Armstrong et al.[208] was 9 percent. In this series, complications were distal embolization (Fig. 42-6), bleeding, dissection, thrombotic occlusion, and vessel rupture. In a series of 667 iliac angioplasties, serious complications occurred in 3.9 percent of cases.[209]

These included death (0.3 percent), operation (1.0 percent), and delay in discharge (2.6 percent). Another study comparing inpatient and outpatient peripheral angioplasties showed that complication rates were not significantly different.[210] Major complications occurred in 8.3 percent of inpatients, 5.0 percent of outpatients, and 5.6 percent of those patients followed on a 1-day-care floor.

Pain during balloon inflation occurs in many patients. There is no correlation between the severity of pain and the tightness of the stenosis, but severe pain should suggest dissection or rupture of the vessel.[211,212] In the authors' experience, persistence of pain after balloon deflation, particularly in the iliac arteries, suggests dissection or vessel rupture and should prompt the search for a cause. If extravasation is seen, the balloon catheter should be reinflated across the lesion, and surgical backup should be called. Hopefully, development of covered arterial stents will allow for treatment of this complication in the angiography suite.

Balloon rupture during angioplasty could potentially cause disruption of the vessel, but in the authors' experience this has not occurred. Detachment of the angioplasty balloon from the catheter shaft is an unusual event and has become rare with improvements in catheter materials. Nevertheless, since this complication can still occur,[213] the integrity of balloon catheters should be checked after use. If intravascular cathe-

ter fragments are present, they can usually be removed using standard retrieval methods (Fig. 42-7).

Dissection and/or vessel occlusion during angioplasty produces a problem that must be addressed immediately. As mentioned in the diagnostic angiography section of this chapter, iliac dissection should first be approached by reinflating the angioplasty balloon in an attempt to "tack down" the dissection.[71] If this is not successful and the dissection causes a significant decrease in flow, placement of an intravascular stent may salvage the procedure.

Dissections of the superficial femoral artery (SFA) should be approached in the same manner. However, if the dissection cannot be "tacked down," atherectomy rather than stent placement should be attempted, because the incidence of intimal hyperplasia after SFA stenting is unacceptably high.[214] If a channel cannot be reestablished, popliteal puncture and retrograde placement of a catheter and wire should be considered, because this may salvage an unsuccessful antegrade procedure.[215]

Late complications of angioplasty include delayed bleeding and morbidity secondary to closure of the vessel. Thrombosis is significantly more common than restenosis after angioplasty of SFA occlusion.[216] Aneurysm and infected pseudoaneurysm have both been reported at the site of angioplasty,[217,218] but these are unusual complications. Death occurred within 30 days of femoropopliteal angioplasty in 0.8 percent of patients

Figure 42-7. (A) A 44-year-old woman had a central venous line placed for infusion of chemotherapeutic agents. A catheter fragment detached and embolized to the right lower lobe (*arrows*). (B) *Arrow* demonstrates Amplatz gooseneck snare engaging the catheter fragment, which was pulled out through a sheath in the femoral vein. (Courtesy of John F. Cardella, M.D.)

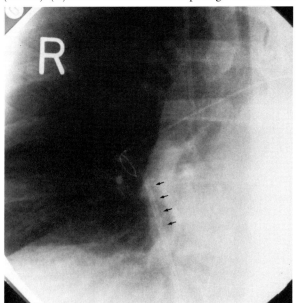

A

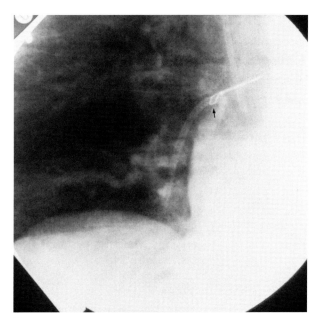

B

followed for late complications.[219] Nonfatal systemic morbidity occurred in 7.1 percent, and local morbidity in 1.6 percent, in this study. Advanced age and indication (limb salvage versus claudication) were predictive of increased mortality.

It is important to place the complication rate of angioplasty in perspective when considering the risk-benefit ratio of the procedure in relation to other forms of treatment. An interesting study by Bergan et al.[220] compared late complications of surgery and angioplasty in prospectively randomized patients with peripheral vascular disease. Mortality for surgical patients was 13.1 percent per year versus 8.4 percent for those having angioplasty, with significant differences in cardiac and renal disease. These data have been substantiated in the surgical literature.[221]

Renal Angioplasty

Complications of renal angioplasty include thrombosis, dissection, branch occlusion, and marked arterial spasm. Frank rupture of the artery has been reported[222,223] but is distinctly uncommon. Chronic corticosteroid therapy may predispose the renal artery to rupture during angioplasty.[222] All of these events may cause further deterioration in renal function, which is almost always compromised in patients with renal artery stenosis. Verapamil (200–1500 μg), given intraarterially before angioplasty, has been shown to decrease the complication rate.[224] The authors routinely use intraarterial nitroglycerin (100–200 μg) and heparin (1000–5000 units) to prevent spasm and thrombosis. Perforation of the right renal vein[225] and dissection of the abdominal aorta[226,227] have been reported after renal angioplasty. It is important to obtain a CT scan of the abdomen in any patient experiencing significant pain or falling blood pressure after renal angioplasty.

Acute occlusion of the renal artery during an attempt at angioplasty presents a more immediate problem than occlusions in the peripheral circulation, since the kidney is an end organ with a relatively poor collateral vascular supply. If a wire can be negotiated across the occluded segment, consideration should be given to the use of a reperfusion catheter,[228] which bypasses the obstruction and allows flow into the kidney until surgical backup can be obtained.

Finally, all patients with significant hypertension should be watched carefully after successful renal angioplasty so that hypotensive episodes can be recognized and treated appropriately.

Brachiocephalic Angioplasty

Angioplasty of the carotid arteries has not been routinely performed because of concerns about cerebral embolization. Recent review articles[229,230] suggest that permanent neurologic damage occurs in a very small number of patients, and that this low incidence may make the risks acceptable as compared to surgery. Complications that do not cause permanent deficits include transient ischemic symptoms, asymptomatic dissection, and arterial spasm.[229]

Vertebrobasilar artery angioplasty is becoming a more frequent procedure in patients with posterior fossa ischemic symptoms. Higashida et al.[231] reported a 7.1 percent incidence of permanent sequelae in a series of 41 patients. These consisted of stroke in 2 patients and a ruptured vessel in one. Transient complications (9.5 percent) were vessel spasm and cerebral ischemia, each of which occurred in 2 patients.

Percutaneous angioplasty has become the treatment of choice for symptomatic stenosis of the subclavian artery.[232] Recently, Mathias et al.[233] have shown that subclavian occlusion is also amenable to angioplasty and has a success rate of 83 percent. The risk of embolization is low, in the range of 3 percent.[234] If there is embolic debris, it flows into the arm, where consequences are less significant than from cerebral embolization. Patients with preexisting antegrade flow in the vertebral artery may be at significantly greater risk for cerebral embolization during subclavian or innominate angioplasty than those with steal physiology.[235] Some authors[236] have recommended temporary balloon occlusion of the vertebral artery during angioplasty to reduce the chance of cranial embolization.

Hyperperfusion syndrome is a rare complication following angioplasty of brachiocephalic arteries.[237] This syndrome is thought to be due to an increase in intracranial vascular perfusion pressure caused by angioplasty, analogous to the syndrome seen after repair of intracranial arteriovenous malformations.[238] In its milder form, patients develop unilateral headache after angioplasty. Cerebral edema and hemorrhage have been reported with this syndrome. Blood pressure should be carefully controlled in patients experiencing symptoms after angioplasty. Discontinuance of anticoagulants and/or antiplatelet agents should be strongly considered until symptoms abate.

Lasers, Atherectomy, and Stents

Vascular lasers, stents, and atherectomy devices have been developed in an effort to improve the success rate and long-term patency of coronary, renal, and peripheral artery interventions. Since the total number of reported cases using these modalities remains relatively small, no rigorous statements can be made about complication rates. However, the properties of the devices suggest that the complication rates will necessarily be higher than those of balloon angioplasty. Because these devices require large introducing sheaths relative to angioplasty balloon catheters, all of the puncture site complications detailed earlier in this chapter should be expected to occur. Further, because of the current state of development and factors related to the learning curve, an increased incidence of perforation, distal embolization, hemorrhage, and vessel occlusion would be expected to occur when such new systems are used.

Long-term (1-year) patency rates after laser angioplasty of the femoral artery are not significantly different from those of traditional therapy.[239] In a multicenter trial involving 129 patients,[240] complications of fluorescence-guided pulsed dye laser angioplasty included perforation (19 percent), hematoma (5 percent), thrombosis (4 percent), and distal embolization (4 percent). In a study of excimer laser angioplasty,[241] technical failure occurred in 11 of 26 patients (42 percent) and resulted in 5 femoropopliteal bypasses. Six perforations and 3 arteriovenous fistulas occurred in this series as well. "Hot tip" lasers also have been shown to have significant complication rates.[242,243] Perforation is only considered a significant complication when it aborts the procedure.[244]

Femoral hematomas appear to be more common in patients who are having laser angioplasty, and have been reported in 38 percent of 52 patients undergoing percutaneous procedures in a study in the surgical literature.[245] An intimal flap in the superficial femoral artery after laser angioplasty is associated with a decreased long-term patency rate.[246] Atherectomy or "tack down" procedures should be considered if a flap is seen. The authors believe, as we reported in 1989,[247] that lasers have very limited use in the peripheral vascular system.

Atherectomy devices have been used to treat asymmetric arterial stenoses and lesions resistant to conventional balloon angioplasty. Complication rates for the Simpson atherectomy catheter (Peripheral Systems Group), the most frequently used device, have varied from 3 to 21 percent, a higher level than that of conventional balloon angioplasty.[248] Groin complications should be expected more often when using this catheter, which requires placement of a large vascular sheath. Amputation of the guidewire tip of the newer, over-the-wire Simpson device has been reported.[249] We have also experienced this complication. A vascular snare retrieved the guidewire tip in our case. Pseudoaneurysm has also been reported after Simpson atherectomy.[250] Complication rates for the Kensey catheter (Theratek) have ranged from 15 to 35 percent, and for the Rotablator (Heart Technology), from 0 to 35

percent.[248] We believe that atherectomy is a viable alternative to angioplasty in a small number of carefully selected patients. This procedure should be approached with the knowledge that complication rates are relatively high.

Intravascular stents have been used to maintain patency in both the arterial and venous systems, as well as in the urinary and biliary tracts. Two stent systems have been used in significant numbers in the United States: the Wallstent (Schneider) and the Palmaz stent (Johnson & Johnson Interventional Systems). In the US Wallstent Trial,[251] the complication rate in 227 patients was 16 percent, with a 30-day mortality rate of 0.9 percent. A European study of 125 patients[252] had a complication rate of 4.9 percent for iliac stents and 35 percent for femoral stents. Complications in this study included ipsilateral and contralateral embolism, aortic dissection, and a large groin hematoma. Palmaz[253] reported 18 complications in his first 171 cases (10.5 percent). These included groin hematoma, distal embolization, extravasation, transient renal failure, subintimal dissection, and pseudoaneurysm. The Palmaz stent has been employed in the treatment of renal artery stenosis in a large multicenter study.[254] Access site complications in this population were higher than those of patients undergoing angioplasty. Strecker et al.[255] have reported a high incidence of acute complications and restenoses, compared to balloon angioplasty, in their series of 340 patients treated with the tantalum Strecker stent. This device has not been widely used in the United States.

Vascular stents are a useful adjunct to balloon angioplasty and should be used in the iliac artery in cases of total occlusion and after unsuccessful attempts at angioplasty. The routine use of stents results in an unacceptable risk-benefit ratio compared with that of older, proven, and less expensive techniques.

Thrombolytic Therapy

Complications of thrombolytic therapy include hemorrhage, distal embolization, pericatheter thrombosis, and allergic or idiosyncratic reactions to the thrombolytic agent.[256] Obviously, potential complications also include all those associated with arteriography in general, which are described in preceding sections of this chapter. A study in the surgical literature[257] of 138 thrombolytic procedures found complications in 60 cases (43 percent), 8 of which resulted in death. These authors found that physician errors resulted from mismanagement of bleeding complications, mistakes in patient selection, and failure to adhere to the thrombolysis protocol. Studies from the radiologic literature[258,259] have significantly lower complication rates.

It is important that any physician performing these procedures have experience in arteriography and its complications, as well as an understanding of the thrombolytic process.

The incidence of hemorrhage during arterial thrombolysis has decreased in recent years, primarily because of new protocols for the administration of urokinase and tissue-type plasminogen activator.[258–261] Significant hemorrhage requiring transfusion affects less than 15 percent of patients, and death has occurred in less than 1 percent of reported cases.[262] Although clinical considerations may prompt thrombolysis in any patient if circumstances warrant,[263] contraindications to the procedure (Table 42-6) should be weighed against potential benefits before therapy is instituted.

Monitoring of coagulation parameters during thrombolysis is controversial. Preprocedural measurement of thrombin time, fibrinogen, partial thromboplastin time, and prothrombin time has been advocated to exclude patients with preexisting coagulopathies.[256] Thrombin time[264] and fibrinogen levels[263] have been used to evaluate the state of systemic thrombolysis. In one study, three of five patients who bled had partial thromboplastin times (PTT) greater than 150 seconds and fibrinogen levels between 100 and 200 mg/dl.[265] It is prudent to monitor fibrinogen levels in patients undergoing thrombolysis to ensure that the fibrinogen level remains higher than 100 mg/dl. If the level falls below 200 mg/dl, PTT should be added. However, it is important to understand that elevated laboratory values do not accurately predict the occurrence or severity of hemorrhage.[262,266]

The vast majority of hemorrhagic complications during thrombolysis occur at the arterial puncture site.[246,262,263] These can almost always be controlled by direct compression, and the thrombolysis continued if clinically necessary. Obviously, bleeding at distant sites such as the gastrointestinal tract or brain mandates discontinuance of the infusion. This is usually all that is required. If bleeding continues, fresh-frozen plasma or cryoprecipitate can be given to restore circulating fibrinogen.[262]

Distal embolization of clot fragments is often asymptomatic in the lower extremities. However, particularly in patients with diminished outflow, embolization can worsen the ischemia. Continued infusion of thrombolytic agent will often dissolve tiny emboli and resolve the complication. If distal ischemia persists, surgical consultation should be obtained.[262]

Pericatheter thrombosis is more likely when catheters are maintained for long periods of time in vessels with slow flow.[262,267] In older series, incidence rates as high as 26 percent have been reported.[268]

Table 42-6. Contraindications to Fibrinolytic Therapy

Absolute
  Known active internal bleeding
  Recent (<2 months) cerebrovascular infarct or hemorrhage
  Intracerebral tumor, vascular malformation, or abscess
Relative
  Major
    Recent (<10 days) major surgery, obstetric delivery
    Recent serious gastrointestinal bleed
    Recent serious trauma
    Uncontrolled severe hypertension (≥200 systolic, ≥110 diastolic)
  Minor
    Bleeding diathesis
    Recent minor trauma
    Left heart thrombus
    External cardiac massage
    Bacterial endocarditis
    Severe hepatic or renal disease
    Pregnancy

From Risius B, Graor RA. Thrombolytic therapy. In: Taveras JM, Ferrucci JT. Radiology: diagnosis—imaging—intervention. Philadelphia: Lippincott, 1992;2(146):1–14. Used with permission.

Short-duration pulsed lysis methods should produce less pericatheter thrombosis. Most thrombolytic catheters are placed through vascular sheaths. In the authors' experience, very slow infusion of small quantities of heparinized saline (5000 units in 1000 ml of normal saline) into the sideport of the sheath has prevented this complication in the great majority of patients.

Septic arthritis of the knee has been reported after long-term arterial thrombolysis,[269] but this complication is unusual. Much more common are anaphylactoid reactions, including fever, chills, and bronchospasm, which have been reported in up to 42 percent of patients treated with streptokinase.[266] Because urokinase is a human-derived protein, no such reactions were expected with this agent.[270] However, rigors during urokinase infusion have been observed in a growing number of cases, and, in one series from New Zealand,[271] four out of six patients undergoing thrombolysis experienced the complication. Pretreatment with antihistamines and acetaminophen may decrease the severity of the rigors. Intravenous administration of Demerol during the reaction rapidly abates it.[272] Severe reactions may be treated with H_1 and H_2 blockers such as famotidine.[273] All such reactions should be reported to the Urokinase Reaction Registry,[272] which is gathering data to determine the incidence rate.

Vena Cava Filter Placement

Once the province of vascular surgeons, vena cava filter insertion has become a relatively routine radiologic

Table 42-7. Complications of Vena Cava Filter Insertion

	Stainless Steel Greenfield	Titanium Greenfield[a]	Amplatz	Bird's Nest[a]	Vena-Tech	Simon Nitinol
Total number of patients reported	469	72	30	568	210	245
Recurrent pulmonary embolus (%)	19/469 (4)	2/72 (3)	3/30 (10)	15/568 (3)	3/210 (1)	10/245 (4)
Caval patency (%)	446/469 (95)	19/22 (95)	17/22 (77)	551/568 (97)	195/210 (93)	9/12 (75)
Caval penetration (%)	NR[b]	0/22 (0)	3/26 (12)	NR[b]	0/28 (0)	4/12 (33)
Migration (%)	164/469 (35)	3/50 (6)	0/27 (0)	Original Model (9)	2/72 (3)	5/241 (3)
Recurrent DVT[c] (%)	NR[b]	1/6 (17)	4/21 (19)	NR[b]	8/25 (32)	1/9 (11)

[a]Currently available model.
[b]NR = not reported.
[c]DVT = deep venous thrombosis.
Stainless steel Greenfield filter data from Greenfield LJ, DeLucia A III. Endovascular therapy of venous thromboembolic disease. Surg Clin North Am 1992;72: 969–989. Data on other filters from Ferris EJ, McCowan TC, Carver DK, McFarland DR. Percutaneous inferior vena caval filters: follow-up of seven designs in 320 patients. Radiology 1993;188:851–856. Used with permission.

procedure. Complications associated with the procedure include hematoma, occlusion, or fistula at the venotomy site, filter fracture, misplacement or migration, and penetration of the caval wall.[274] A recent review of the literature[275] found that filter complications were relatively common but that life-threatening complications were distinctly rare. Only four deaths from filter insertion had been reported to 1992,[275] a death rate of 0.16 percent of cases published. Complication rates of the available filter designs have been studied by Greenfield and DeLucia,[276] and by Ferris et al. (Table 42-7).[277]

Insertion site thrombosis has been reported at rates varying between 11 and 41 percent with the older, stainless steel Greenfield filter.[274,278,279] The 24 French tract required for placement of this filter probably increased the incidence of vascular injury. Newer filters require significantly smaller-diameter tracts. Large-diameter venous catheters also predispose to air embolism, although this appears to be a rare complication.[274]

Late complications of filter placement are caval occlusion and embolization of the filter. Wall penetration and caval occlusion are more likely related to the type of filter employed than to any deficiency in technique. Pericardial tamponade has been reported after misplacement of a Greenfield filter in the right atrium[280] and after migration of a Bird's Nest filter.[281]

Although infrarenal filter placement is usually recommended, suprarenal placement is not contraindicated and may be the placement of choice in women who are of childbearing age.[282] In young patients and in suprarenal placements, use of the Greenfield filter should be strongly considered because of its historical long-term patency rate.[266] It is important to measure the width of the vena cava before filter insertion to prevent filter migration. For venae cavae larger than 28 mm, bilateral iliac vein filter placement[283] or the Bird's Nest filter[284] should be used. When the infrarenal cava is short, use of the Simon Nitinol filter[285] should be considered, because this filter has the shortest vertical length.

Asymmetry of filter struts has been reported in 5.4 percent of titanium Greenfield filter placements[286] but has been more common in our experience. However, strut asymmetry does not appear to affect the efficacy of the device.[274] Having the patient perform a Valsalva maneuver as the filter is placed maximally distends the cava and optimizes strut placement.

Misplaced filters have been retrieved percutaneously in many cases.[287-290] Filters with conical ends, such as the Greenfield and Vena-tech devices, can be manipulated by placing an Amplatz snare (Microvena Corporation) through the filter, snaring the cephalad end, and retracting the snare.[289] An embolized filter in the right heart has been followed for 7 years in an elderly patient.[291] Surgical retrieval should therefore be balanced against the patient's condition.

This chapter cannot be all-inclusive. New and innovative procedures are being continually developed, and each of these will have some level of complication. The more the interventionalist understands the nature of existing complications and how to limit their numbers, the more he or she will be prepared to best serve the patient.

References

1. Spies JB, et al. Standard for diagnostic arteriography in adults. Standards of Practice Committee of the Society of Cardiovascular and Interventional Radiology. J Vasc Intervent Radiol 1993;4:385–395.
2. ACR Committee on Drugs and Contrast Media. Manual on iodinated contrast media. Reston, VA: American College of Radiology, 1991.
3. Waugh JR, Sacharias N. Arteriographic complications in the DSA era. Radiology 1992;182:243–246.
4. Hou SH, Bushinsky DA, Wish JB, Cohen JJ, Harrington JT. Hospital-acquired renal insufficiency: a prospective study. Am J Med 1983;74:243–248.
5. Cronin RE. Southwestern internal medicine conference: renal failure following radiologic procedures. Am J Med Sci 1989; 298:342–356.
6. Westhoff-Bleck M, Bleck JS, Jost S. The adverse effects of angiographic radiocontrast media. Drug Saf 1991;6:28–36.
7. Gussenhoven MJE, Ravensbergen J, van Bockel JH, Feuth JDM, Aarts JCNM. Renal dysfunction after angiography; a risk factor analysis in patients with peripheral vascular disease. J Cardiovasc Surg 1991;32:81–86.
8. Billstron A, Hietala S.-O, Lithner F, Merikanto J, Wirell M, Wirell S. Nephrotoxicity of contrast media in patients with diabetes mellitus. Acta Radiol 1989;30:509–515.
9. D'Elia JA, et al. Nephrotoxicity from angiographic contrast material: a prospective study. Am J Med 1982;72:719–725.
10. Moore RD, et al. Frequency and determinants of adverse reactions induced by high-osmolality contrast media. Radiology 1989;170:727–732.
11. Hans B, Hans SS, Mittal VK, Khan TA, Patel N, Dahn MS. Renal functional response to dopamine during and after arteriography in patients with chronic renal insufficiency. Radiology 1990;176:651–654.
12. Hall KA, et al. Contrast-induced nephrotoxicity: the effects of vasodilator therapy. J Surg Res 1992;53:317–320.
13. Parfrey PS, et al. Contrast material–induced renal failure in patients with diabetes mellitus, renal insufficiency, or both. N Engl J Med 1989;320:143–149.
14. Shieh SD, Hirsch SR, Boshell BR, Pino JA, Alexander LJ, Witten DM, Friedman EA. Low risk of contrast media–induced acute renal failure in nonazotemic type 2 diabetes mellitus. Kidney 1982;21:739–743.
15. Lautin EM, et al. Radiocontrast–associated renal dysfunction: a comparison of lower-osmolality and conventional high-osmolality contrast media. AJR 1991;157:59–65.
16. Morris TW. X-ray contrast media: where are we now, and where are we going? Radiology 1993;188:11–16.
17. McClennan BL, Stolberg HO. Intravascular contrast media. Ionic versus nonionic: current status. Radiol Clin North Am 1991;29:437–454.
18. Vacek JL, Gersema L, Woods M, Bower C, Beauchamp GD. Frequencies of reactions to iohexol versus ioxaglate. Am J Cardiol 1990;66:1277–1278.
19. Campbell DR, Flemming BK, Mason WF, Jackson SA, Hirsch DJ, MacDonald KJ. A comparative study of the nephrotoxicity of iohexol, iopamidol and ioxaglate in peripheral angiography. J Can Assoc Radiol 1990;41:133–137.
20. Scherberich JE, Fischer A, Rautschka E, Kollath J, Riemann H. Nephrotoxicity of high and low osmolar contrast media: case control studies following digital subtraction angiography in potential risk patients. Fortschr Geb Rontgenstr Nuklearmed Erganzungsbd 1989;128:91–94.
21. Nikonoff T, Skau T, Berglund J, Nyberg P, et al. Effects of femoral arteriography and low osmolar contrast agents on renal function. Acta Radiol 1993;34:88–91.
22. Hwang MH, Piao ZE, Murdock DK, Messmore HL, Giardina JJ, Scanlon PJ. Risk of thromboembolism during diagnostic and interventional cardiac procedures with nonionic contrast media. Radiology 1990;174:453–457.
23. Dawson P. Contrast agents, red cells, coagulation, and the angiographer. Invest Radiol 1990;25:S117–S118.
24. Grabowski EF. A hematologist's view of contrast media, clotting in angiography syringes and thrombosis during coronary angiography. Am J Cardiol 1990;66:23F–25F.
25. Grabowski EF, Kaplan KL, Halpern EF. Anticoagulant effects of nonionic versus ionic contrast media in angiography syringes. Invest Radiol 1991;26:417–421.
26. Corot C, Cornillac A, Belleville J, Eloy R. European Clotting Group: scanning electron microscopic analysis of catheters during routine angiographic procedures. Invest Radiol 1991; 26:S96–S100.
27. Casalini E. Role of low-osmolality contrast media in thromboembolic complications: scanning electron microscopy study. Radiology 1992;183:741–744.
28. Hessel SJ, Adams DF, Abrams HL. Complications of angiography. Radiology 1981;138:273–281.
29. Ameli FM, Knackstedt J, Provan JL, St. Louis EL. The effect of femoral arteriography on the incidence of groin contamination and postoperative infections. Ann Vasc Surg 1990;4: 328–333.
30. Shawker TH, Kluge RM, Ayella RJ. Bacteremia associated with angiography. JAMA 1974;229:1090–1092.
31. Lilly MP, Reichman W, Sarazen AA Jr, Carney WI Jr. Anatomic and clinical factors associated with complications of transfemoral arteriography. Ann Vasc Surg 1990;4:264–269.
32. Dodek A, Boone JA, Hooper RO, Kavanagh-Gray D, Macdonald IL, Peretz DI. Complications of coronary arteriography. Can Med Assoc J 1983;128:934–936.
33. Lang EK. A survey of the complications of percutaneous retrograde arteriography. Radiology 1963;81:257–263.
34. Altin RS, Flicker S, Naidech HJ. Pseudoaneurysm and arteriovenous fistula after femoral artery catheterization: association with low femoral punctures. AJR 1989;152:629–631.
35. Frood LR, Smith DC, Pappas JM, Elvin PK, Westengard JC, Saukel GW. Use of angiographic needles with or without stylets: pathologic assessment of vessel walls after puncture.
36. Reuter SR, Redman HC. Gastrointestinal angiography. Philadelphia: Saunders, 1972:9.
37. Cragg AH, Nakagawa N, Smith TP, Berbaum KS. Hematoma formation after diagnostic angiography: effect of catheter size. J Vasc Intervent Radiol 1991;2:231–233.
38. Siegelman SS, Caplan LH, Annes GP. Complications of catheter angiography: study with oscillometry and "pullout" angiograms. Radiology 1968;91:251–253.
39. Walker WJ, Mundall SL, Broderick HG, Prasad D, Kim J, Ravi JM. Systemic heparinization for femoral percutaneous coronary arteriography. N Engl J Med 1973;288:826–828.
40. Glickstein MF, McLean GK, Sussman SK. Optimizing heparin utilization in angiographic flush solutions. Angiology 1990;41:825–828.
41. Almgren B, Karacagil S, Nybacka O. Arteriovenous fistula following transfemoral angiography. Aust N Z J Surg 1990;60: 549–550.
42. Marsan RE, McDonald V, Ramamurthy S. Iatrogenic femoral arteriovenous fistula. Cardiovasc Intervent Radiol 1990;13: 314–316.
43. Thadani U, Pratt AE. Profunda femoral arteriovenous fistula after percutaneous arterial and venous catheterization. Brit Heart J 1971;33:803–805.
44. Davidson JT. Peroneal arteriovenous fistula: a complication of Fogarty catheter thromboembolectomy. Am Surg 1989; 55:616–618.
45. Mavor GE, Walker MG, Dahl DP, Pegg CAS. Damage from the Fogarty balloon catheter. Br J Surg 1972;59:389–391.
46. Roberts SR, Main D, Pinkerton J. Surgical therapy of femoral artery pseudoaneurysm after angiography. Am J Surg 1987; 154:676–680.
47. Fellmeth BD, Roberts AC, Bookstein JJ, Freishlag JA, For-

sythe JR, Buckner NK, Hye RJ. Postangiographic femoral artery injuries: nonsurgical repair with US-guided compression. Radiology 1991;178:671–675.

48. Rapoport S, Sniderman KW, Morse SS, Proto MH, Ross GR. Pseudoaneurysm: a complication of faulty technique in femoral arterial puncture. Radiology 1985;154:529–530.

49. Kotval PS, Khoury A, Shah PM, Babu SC. Doppler sonographic demonstration of the progressive spontaneous thrombosis of pseudoaneurysms. J Ultrasound Med 1990;9:185–190.

50. Graham AN, Wilson CM, Hood JM, Barros D'Sa AA. Risk of rupture of postangiographic femoral false aneurysm. Br J Surg 1992;79:1022–1025.

51. Feld R, Patton GM, Carabasi RA, Alexander A, et al. Treatment of iatrogenic femoral artery injuries with ultrasound-guided compression. J Vasc Surg 1992;16:832–840.

52. Kehoe ME. US-guided compression repair of a pseudoaneurysm in the brachial artery. Radiology 1992;182:896.

53. Dorfman GS, Cronan JJ. Postcatheterization femoral artery injuries: is there a role for nonsurgical treatment? Radiology 1991;178:629–630.

54. Tonkin ILD. Special preparations and considerations for pediatric angiography and interventional procedures. In: Taveras JM, Ferrucci JT. Radiology: diagnosis—imaging—intervention. Philadelphia: Lippincott, 1992;2(149):1–15.

55. Olbert F, Karnel F. Techniques of percutaneous transluminal angioplasty. In: Dondelinger RF, Rossi P, Kurdziel JC, Wallace S, eds. Interventional radiology. New York: Thieme, 1990:550–563.

56. Levy JM, Joseph RB, Bodell LS, Nykamp PW, Hessel SJ. Prostaglandin E_1 in hand angiography. Am J Roentgenol 1983;141:1043–1046.

57. Levy JM, Ibrahim F, Nykamp PW, Weiland DE. Prostaglandin E_1 for treatment of ergot intoxication. Cardiovasc Intervent Radiol 1984;7:28–30.

58. Pallan TM, Wulkan IA, Abadir AR, Flores L, Chaudry MR, Gintautas J. Incompatibility of Isovue 370 and papaverine in peripheral arteriography. Radiology 1993;187:257–259.

59. Hallett JW Jr, Wolk SW, Cherry KJ Jr, Gloviczki P, Pairolero PC. The femoral neuralgia syndrome after arterial catheter trauma. J Vasc Surg 1990;11:702–706.

60. Kido DK, King PD, Manzione JV, Simon JH. The role of catheters and guidewires in the production of angiographic thromboembolic complications. Invest Radiol 1988;23:S359–S365.

61. Dawson P, Strickland NH. Thromboembolic phenomena in clinical angiography: role of materials and technique. J Vasc Intervent Radiol 1991;2:125–132.

62. Earnest F, Forbes G, Sandok BA, Piepgras DG, Faust RJ, Ilstrup DM, Arndt LJ. Complications of cerebral arteriography: prospective assessment of risk. AJR 1984;142:246–253.

63. Gagliardi JM, Batt M, Avril G, Declemy S, et al. Neurologic complications of axillary and brachial catheter arteriography in atherosclerotic patients: predictive factors. Ann Vasc Surg 1990;4:546–549.

64. Thromboembolism during angiography. Lancet 1992;339:1576–1578.

65. Leach KR, Kurisu Y, Carlson JE, Repa I, et al. Thrombogenicity of hydrophilically coated guide wires and catheters. Radiology 1990;175:675–677.

66. Raininko R, Soder H. Clot formation in angiographic catheters—an in vitro comparative study. Effects of heparin and protein coating of the catheter. Acta Radiol 1993;34:78–82.

67. Ramirez G, O'Neill WM, Lambert R, Bloomer A. Cholesterol embolization: a complication of angiography. Arch Intern Med 1978;138:1430–1432.

68. McGowan JA, Greenberg A. Cholesterol atheroembolic renal disease. Am J Nephrol 1986;6:135–139.

69. Gardiner GA, Meyerovitz MG, Stokes KR, Clouse ME, Harrington DT, Bettman MA. Complications of transluminal angioplasty. Radiology 1986;159:201–208.

70. Train JS, Dan SJ, Mitty HA, Dikman SH, Harrington EB, Miller CM, Jacobson JH. Occlusion during iliac angioplasty: a salvageable complication. Radiology 1988;168:131–135.

71. Murphy TP, Dorfman GS, Segall M, Carney WI Jr. Iatrogenic arterial dissection: treatment by percutaneous transluminal angioplasty. Cardiovasc Intervent Radiol 1991;14:302–306.

72. Maynar M, et al. Percutaneous atherectomy as an alternative treatment for postangioplasty obstructive intimal flaps. Radiology 1989;170:1029–1031.

73. Becker GJ, et al. Angioplasty-induced dissections in human iliac arteries: management with Palmaz balloon-expandable intraluminal stents. Radiology 1990;176:31–38.

74. Raphael MJ, Donaldson RM. A new complication of coronary arteriography. Cathet Cardiovasc Diagn 1990;21:55–57.

75. Szilagyi DE, Smith RF, Elliot JP Jr, Hagerman JH. Translumbar aortography: a study of safety and usefulness. Arch Surg 1977;112:339–342.

76. Nikolic G, Pervulov S, Stanojevic M, Pashu-Cerecina V, Draganic M, Cirkovic S, Kamenica S. An uncommon complication of translumbar aortography. AJR 1991;156:408.

77. Grollman JH Jr, Marcus R. Transbrachial arteriography: techniques and complications. Cardiovasc Intervent Radiol 1988;11:32–35.

78. Watkinson AF, Hartnell GG. Complications of direct brachial artery puncture for arteriography: a comparison of techniques. Clin Radiol 1991;44:189–191.

79. Andersen PE Jr. Brachialis Seldinger puncture with use of an introducer sheath. Br J Radiol 1985;58:777–778.

80. AbuRahma AF, et al. Complications of arteriography in a recent series of 707 cases: factors affecting outcome. Ann Vasc Surg 1993;7:122–129.

81. McIvor J, Rhymer JC. 245 transaxillary arteriograms in arteriopathic patients: success rate and complications. Clin Radiol 1992;45:390–394.

82. AbuRahma AF, Robinson PA, Boland JP. Safety of arteriography by direct puncture of a vascular prosthesis. Am J Surg 1992;164:233–236.

83. Smith DC, Mitchell DA, Peterson GW, Will AD, Mera SS, Smith LL. Medial brachial fascial compartment syndrome: anatomic basis of neuropathy after transaxillary arteriography. Radiology 1989;173:149–154.

84. Stein PD, et al. Complications and validity of pulmonary angiography in acute pulmonary embolism. Circulation 1992;85:462–468.

85. Mills SR, Jackson DC, Older RA, Heaston DK, Moore AV. The incidence, etiologies, and avoidance of complications of pulmonary angiography in a large series. Radiology 1980;136:295–299.

86. Miller SW, Waltman AC. The pulmonary circulation. In: Taveras JM, Ferrucci JT. Radiology: diagnosis—imaging—intervention. Philadelphia: Lippincott, 1993;1(70):1–5.

87. Malden ES, Tartar VM, Gutierrez FR. Acute fatality following pulmonary angiography in a patient on an amiodarone regimen—a case report. Angiology 1993;44:152–155.

88. Bernard SA, Jones BM, Stuckey JG. Pulmonary angiography in a non-teaching hospital over a 12-year period. Med J Aust 1993;158:213.

89. Stein MA, Winter J, Grollman JH Jr. The value of the pulmonary-artery-seeking catheter in percutaneous selective pulmonary arteriography. Radiology 1975;144:299–304.

90. van Beek EJ, Kuyer PM, Reekers JA. Dissection of pulmonary artery as a complication of pulmonary angiography. Rofo Fortschr Geb Rontgenstr Neuen Bildgeb Verfahr 1993;6:599–600.

91. Novak D. Complications of arterial embolization. In: Dondelinger RF, Rossi P, Kurdziel JC, Wallace S, eds. Interventional radiology. New York: Thieme, 1990:314–322.

92. Manelfe C, Lasjaunias P, Halbach VV, Mark AS. Embolization in the brain. In: Dondelinger RF, Rossi P, Kurdziel JC, Wallace S, eds. Interventional radiology. New York: Thieme, 1990:396–420.

93. Latchaw RE. Preoperative intracranial meningioma embolization: technical considerations affecting the risk-to-benefit ratio. AJNR 1993;14:583–586.

94. Higashida RT, Halbach VV, Barnwell SL, Dowd C, Dormandy B, Bell J, Hieshima GB. Treatment of intracranial aneurysms with preservation of the parent vessel: results of percutaneous balloon embolization in 84 patients. Am J Neuroradiol 1990;11:633–640.

95. Higashida RT, Halbach VV, Dowd CF, Barnwell SL, Heishima GB. Intracranial aneurysms: interventional neurovascular treatment with detachable balloons—results in 215 cases. Radiology 1991;178:663–670.

96. Knuckey NW, Haas R, Jenkins R, Epstein MH. Thrombosis of difficult intracranial aneurysms by the endovascular placement of platinum-Dacron microcoils. J Neurosurg 1992;77: 43–50.

97. Guglielmi G, et al. Endovascular treatment of posterior circulation aneurysms by electrothrombosis using electrically detachable coils. J Neurosurg 1992;77:515–524.

98. Hodes JE, et al. Endovascular occlusion of intracranial vessels for curative treatment of unclippable aneurysms: report of 16 cases. J Neurosurg 1991;75:694–701.

99. Martins IP, Baeta E, Paiva T, Campos J, Gomes L. Headaches during intracranial venovascular procedures: a possible model of vascular headache. Headache 1993;33:227–233.

100. Endo S, Koshu K, Suzuki J. Spontaneous regression of posterior fossa dural arteriovenous malformation. J Neurosurg 1979;51:715–717.

101. Lasjaunias P, Halimi P, Lopez-Ibor L, Sichez JP, Hurth M, De Tribolet N. Traitement endovasculaire des malformations vasculaires durales (MVD) pures "spontanées": revue de 23 cas explorés et traités entre mai 1980 et octobre 1983. Neurochirurgie 1983;30:207–223.

102. Vinuela F, et al. Combined endovascular embolization and surgery in the management of cerebral arteriovenous malformations: experience with 101 cases. J Neurosurg 1991;75: 856–864.

103. Pasqualin A, Scienza R, Cioffi F, Barone G. Treatment of cerebral arteriovenous malformations with a combination of preoperative embolization and surgery. Neurosurgery 1991; 29:358–368.

104. Jafar JJ, Davis AJ, Berenstein A, Choi IS, Kupersmith MJ. The effect of embolization with N-butyl cyanoacrylate prior to surgical resection of cerebral arteriovenous malformations. J Neurosurg 1993;78:60–69.

105. Fournier D, TerBrugge KG, Willinsky R, Lasjaunias P, Montanera W. Endovascular treatment of intracerebral arteriovenous malformations: experience in 49 cases. J Neurosurg 1991;75:228–233.

106. Purdy PD, Batjer HH, Samson D. Management of hemorrhagic complications from preoperative embolization of arteriovenous malformations. J Neurosurg 1991;74:205–211.

107. Wakhloo AK, Juengling FD, Velthoven VV, Schumacher M, Henning J, Schwechheimer K. Extended preoperative polyvinyl alcohol microembolization of intracranial meningiomas: assessment of two embolization techniques. AJNR 1993;14: 571–582.

108. Bentson J, Rand R, Calcaterra T, Lasjaunias P. Unexpected complications following therapeutic embolization. Neuroradiology 1978;16:420–423.

109. Platzbecker H, Kohler K. Embolization in the head and neck region. Acta Radiol 1991;377(Suppl):25–26.

110. Lasjaunias P. Nasopharyngeal angiofibromas: hazards of embolization. Radiology 1980;136:119–123.

111. Deschler DG, Kaplan MJ, Boles R. Treatment of large juvenile nasopharyngeal angiofibroma. Otolaryngol Head Neck Surg 1992;106:278–284.

112. Tsang K, Duggan MA. Vascular proliferation of the thyroid: a complication of fine-needle aspiration. Arch Pathol Lab Med 1992;116:1040–1042.

113. Atkinson BF. Fine needle aspiration of the thyroid. Monogr Pathol 1993;35:166–199.

114. Axiotis CA, Merino MJ, Ain K, Norton JA. Papillary endothelial hyperplasia in the thyroid following fine-needle aspiration. Arch Pathol Lab Med 1991;115:240–242.

115. Hales MS, Hsu FS. Needle tract implantation of papillary carcinoma of the thyroid following aspiration biopsy. Acta Cytol 1990;34:801–804.

116. Remy J, Marache P, Lemaitre L, Lafitte JJ, Tonnel AB, Voisin C. Accidents de l'embolisation dans le traitement des hemoptysies. Nouv Presse Med 1978;7:4306.

117. Vujic I, Pyle R, Parker E, Mithoefer J. Control of massive hemoptysis by embolization of intercostal arteries. Radiology 1980;137:617–620.

118. Roberts AC. Bronchial artery embolization therapy. J Thorac Imaging 1990;5:60–72.

119. Kardijiev V, Symeonov A, Chankow I. Etiology, pathogenesis, and prevention of spinal cord lesions in selective angiography of the bronchial and intercostal arteries. Radiology 1974; 112:81–83.

120. Girard P, Baldeyrou P, Lemoine G, Grunewald D. Left mainstem bronchial stenosis complicating bronchial artery embolization. Chest 1990;97:1246–1248.

121. Munk PL, Morris DC, Nelems B. Left main bronchial-esophageal fistula: a complication of bronchial artery embolization. Cardiovasc Intervent Radiol 1990;13:95–97.

122. White RI. Pulmonary arteriovenous malformations: how do we diagnose them and why is it important to do so? Radiology 1992;182:633–635.

123. Remy-Jardin M, Wattinne L, Remy J. Transcatheter occlusion of pulmonary arterial circulation and collateral supply: failures, incidents and complications. Radiology 1991;180:699–705.

124. White RI, et al. Pulmonary arteriovenous malformations: techniques and long-term outcome of embolotherapy. Radiology 1988;169:663–669.

125. Haaga JR. Percutaneous lung biopsy. In: Mueller PR, ed. Syllabus. A categorical course in diagnostic radiology: interventional radiology. Oak Brook, IL: Radiological Society of North America, 1991:23–34.

126. Westcott JL. Percutaneous transthoracic needle biopsy. Radiology 1988;169:593–601.

127. Lalli AF, McCormack LJ, Zeich M, Reich NE, Belovich D. Aspiration biopsies of chest lesions. Radiology 1978;127:35–40.

128. Moore EH, Shepard JA, McLoud TC, Templeton PA, Kosiuk JP. Positional precautions in needle aspiration lung biopsy. Radiology 1990;175:733–735.

129. Bourgouin PM, Shepard JO, McLoud TC, Spizarny DL, Dedrick CG. Transthoracic needle aspiration biopsy: evaluation of the blood patch technique. Radiology 1988;166:93–95.

130. Herman SJ, Weisbrod GL. Usefulness of the blood patch technique after transthoracic needle aspiration biopsy. Radiology 1990;176:395–397.

131. Perlmutt LM, Braun SD, Newman GE, Oke EJ, Dunnick NR. Timing of chest film follow-up after transthoracic needle aspiration. AJR 1986;146:1049–1050.

132. Perlmutt LM, Braun SD, Newman GE, Cohan RH, Saeed M, Sussman SK, Dunnick NR. Transthoracic needle aspiration: use of a small chest tube to treat pneumothorax. AJR 1987; 148:849–851.

133. Klein JS. Thoracic intervention. Curr Opin Radiol 1992;4: 94–103.

134. Fish GD, Stanley JH, Miller KS, Schabel SI, Sutherland SE. Postbiopsy pneumothorax: estimating the risk by chest radiography and pulmonary function tests. AJR 1988;150:71–74.

135. Miller KS, Fish GB, Stanley JH, Schabel SI. Prediction of pneumothorax rate in percutaneous needle aspiration of the lung. Chest 1988;93:742–745.

136. Graham RJ, Heyd RL, Raval VA, Barrett TF. Lung torsion after percutaneous needle biopsy of lung. AJR 1992;159:35–37.

137. Callol L, et al. Total pulmonary torsion without vascular compromise—a case report. Angiology 1992;43:529–538.

138. Haramati LB, Austin JHM. Complications after CT-guided needle biopsy through aerated versus nonaerated lung. Radiology 1991;181:778.

139. Engeler CE, Hunter DW, Castaneda-Zuniga W, Tashjian JH, Yedlicka JW, Amplatz K. Pneumothorax after lung biopsy: prevention with transpleural placement of compressed collagen foam plugs. Radiology 1992;184:787–789.

140. Berquist TH, Bailey PB, Cortese DA, Miller WE. Transthoracic needle biopsy: accuracy and complications in relation to location and type of lesion. Mayo Clin Proc 1980;55:475–481.

141. Westcott JL. Lung biopsy. In: Dondelinger RF, Rossi P, Kurdziel JC, Wallace S, eds. Interventional radiology. New York: Thieme, 1990:9–17.

142. Tolly TL, Feldmeier JE, Czarnecki D. Air embolism complicating percutaneous lung biopsy. AJR 1988;150:555–556.

143. Marco AP, Furman WR. Anesthetic problems: venous air embolism, airway difficulties, and massive transfusion. Surg Clin North Am 1993;73:213–228.

144. Murphy BP, Harford FJ, Cramer FS. Cerebral air embolism resulting from invasive medical procedures: treatment with hyperbaric oxygen. Ann Surg 1985;201:242–245.

145. Sanders C. Transthoracic needle aspiration. Clin Chest Med 1992;13:11–16.

146. Seyfer AE, Walsh DS, Graeber GM, Nuno IN, Eliasson AH. Chest wall implantation of lung cancer after thin-needle aspiration biopsy. Ann Thorac Surg 1989;48:284–286.

147. Mueller PR, vanSonnenberg E. Interventional radiology in the chest and abdomen. N Engl J Med 1990;322:1364–1374.

148. Charboneau JW. US-guided biopsy. In: Mueller PR, ed. Syllabus. A categorical course in diagnostic radiology: interventional radiology. Oak Brook, IL: Radiological Society of North America, 1991:9–16.

149. Bissonnette RT, Gibney RG, Berry BR, Buckley AR. Fatal carcinoid crisis after percutaneous fine-needle biopsy of hepatic metastasis: case report and literature review. Radiology 1990;174:751–752.

150. Fornari F, Civardi G, Cavanna L, et al. Complications of ultrasonically guided fine-needle abdominal biopsy: results of a multicenter Italian study and review of the literature. Scand J Gastroenterol 1989;24:949–955.

151. Nolsoe C, Nielsen L, Torp-Pedersen S, Holm HH. Major complications and deaths due to interventional ultrasonography: a review of 8000 cases. JCU 1990;18:179–184.

152. Smith EH. Complications of percutaneous abdominal fine-needle biopsy. Radiology 1991;178:253–258.

153. John TG, Garden OJ. Needle track seeding of primary and secondary liver carcinoma after percutaneous liver biopsy. HPB Surg 1993;6:199–204.

154. Smith EH. Is percutaneous biopsy a hazard? An update. Presented at the annual meeting of the Radiological Society of North America, Chicago, IL, 1987.

155. Mueller PR, et al. Severe acute pancreatitis after percutaneous biopsy of the pancreas. AJR 1988;151:493–494.

156. Gerzof SG, Johnson WC, Robbins AH, Nasbeth DC. Expanded criteria for percutaneous abscess drainage. Arch Surg 1985;120:227–232.

157. Gerzof SG, Robbins AH, Johnson WC, Birkett DH, Nasbeth DC. Percutaneous catheter drainage of abdominal abscesses: a five-year experience. N Engl J Med 1981;305:653–657.

158. vanSonnenberg E, Ferrucci JT Jr, Mueller PR, Wittenberg J, Simeone JF. Percutaneous drainage of abscesses and fluid collections: technique, results, and applications. Radiology 1982; 142:1–10.

159. Lang EK, Springer RM, Glorioso LW III, Cammarata CA. Abdominal abscess drainage under radiologic guidance: causes of failure. Radiology 1986;159:329–336.

160. Lang EK. Renal, perirenal, and pararenal abscesses: percutaneous drainage. Radiology 1990;174:109–113.

161. Banner MP. Interventional radiology in the kidney. In: Mueller PR, ed. Syllabus. A categorical course in diagnostic radiology: interventional radiology. Oak Brook, IL: Radiological Society of North America, 1991:35–47.

162. Cochran ST, Barbaric ZL, Lee JJ, Kashfian P. Percutaneous nephrostomy tube placement: an outpatient procedure? Radiology 1991;179:843–847.

163. Stables DP, Ginsberg NJ, Johnson ML. Percutaneous nephrostomy: a series and review of the literature. AJR 1978;130: 75–82.

164. Lang EK. Percutaneous nephrostolithotomy and lithotripsy: a multi-institutional survey of complications. Radiology 1987; 162:25–30.

165. Cronan JJ, Dorfman GS, Amis ES, Denny DF Jr. Retro-peritoneal hemorrhage after percutaneous nephrostomy. AJR 1985;144:801–803.

166. Hruby W. Percutaneous nephrostomy. In: Dondelinger RF, Rossi P, Kurdziel JC, Wallace S, eds. Interventional radiology. New York: Thieme, 1990:234–235.

167. Koonings PP, Teitelbaum GP, Finck EJ, Schlaerth JB. Renal artery laceration secondary to percutaneous nephrostomy catheter placement. Gynecol Oncol 1991;40:164–166.

168. Peene P, Wilms G, Baert AL. Embolization of iatrogenic renal hemorrhage following percutaneous nephrostomy. Urol Radiol 1990;12:84–87.

169. Routh WD, Tatum CM, Lawdahl RB, Rösch J, Keller FS. Tube tamponade: potential pitfall in angiography of arterial hemorrhage associated with percutaneous drainage catheters. Radiology 1990;174:945–949.

170. Nosher JL, Ericksen AS, Trooskin SZ, Needell GS, Harvey RA, Greco RS. Antibiotic bonded nephrostomy catheters for percutaneous nephrostomies. Cardiovasc Intervent Radiol 1990;3:102–106.

171. Matalon TA, Thompson MJ, Patel SK, Ramos MV, Jensik SC, Merkel FK. Percutaneous treatment of urine leaks in renal transplantation patients. Radiology 1990;174:1049–1051.

172. Hopper KD, Yakes WF. The posterior intercostal approach for percutaneous renal procedures: risk of puncturing the lung, spleen, and liver as determined by CT. AJR 1990;154: 115–117.

173. Morris DB, Siegelbaum MH, Pollack HM, Kendall AR, Gerber WL. Renoduodenal fistula in a patient with chronic nephrostomy drainage: a case report. J Urol 1991;146:835–837.

174. Culkin DJ, Wheeler JS Jr, Canning JR. Nephroduodenal fistula: a complication of percutaneous nephrolithotomy. J Urol 1985;134:528–530.

175. Sacks D, Banner MP, Meranze SG, Burke DR, Robinson M, McLean GK. Renal and related retroperitoneal abscesses: percutaneous drainage. Radiology 1988;167:447–451.

176. Koolpe HA, Lord B. Eccentric nephroscopy for the incarcerated nephrostomy. Urol Radiol 1990;12:96–98.

177. Cope C. Conversion from small (0.018-in.) to large (0.039-in.) guidewires in percutaneous drainage procedures. AJR 1982;138:170–171.

178. Quinn SF, Morse S. Complications from 0.018-in. floppy platinum-tip guidewires. AJR 1990;154:1103–1104.

179. Page JE, Walker WJ. Complications attributable to the formation of the track in patients undergoing percutaneous nephrolithotomy. Clin Radiol 1992;45:20–22.

180. Chang CP, Chen MT, Chang LS. Autonomic hyperreflexia in spinal cord injury patient during percutaneous nephrolithotomy for renal stone: a case report. J Urol 1991;146: 1601–1602.

181. Tylén U. Angiographic management of malignant tumors in the thorax, abdomen and bones. In: Dondelinger RF, Rossi P, Kurdziel JC, Wallace S, eds. Interventional radiology. New York: Thieme, 1990:443–461.

182. Therasse E, et al. Transcatheter chemoembolization of progressive carcinoid liver metastasis. Radiology 1993;189:541–547.

183. Marlink RG, Lokich JJ, Robins JR, Clouse ME. Hepatic arterial embolization for metastatic hormone-secreting tumors. Cancer 1990;65:2227–2232.

184. Kuroda C, et al. Gallbladder infarction following hepatic transcatheter arterial embolization. Radiology 1983;149:85–89.

185. Simons RK, Sinanan MN, Coldwell DM. Gangrenous cholecystitis as a complication of hepatic artery embolization: case report. Surgery 1992;112:106–110.

186. Nakamura H, Kondoh H. Emphysematous cholecystitis: a complication of hepatic artery embolization. Cardiovasc Intervent Radiol 1986;9:152–153.

187. Khan KN, Nakata K, Shima M, Kusumoto Y, et al. Pancreatic tissue damage by transcatheter arterial embolization for hepatoma. Dig Dis Sci 1993;38:65–70.

188. Pentecost MJ. Regional therapies for unresectable hepatic malignancies. Presented at the 1993 Meeting of the Western Angiographic and Interventional Society, Portland, Oregon, September 29–October 3, 1993.

189. Inoue Y, Nakamura H, Takashima S, Yamazaki K, et al. Biloma following transcatheter oily chemoembolization. Radiat Med 1991;9:57–60.

190. Bilbao JI, Ruza M, Longo JM, Lecumberri FJ. Intraperitoneal hemorrhage due to rupture of hepatocellular carcinoma after transcatheter arterial embolization with Lipiodol: a case report. Eur J Radiol 1992;15:68–70.

191. Marks WM, Filly RA. Computed tomographic demonstration of intraarterial air following hepatic artery ligation. Radiology 1979;132:665–666.

192. Pentecost MJ. Unresectable hepatic malignancy: regional infusion and embolization. In: Cope C, ed. Current techniques in interventional radiology. Philadelphia: Current Medicine, 1994:6.1–6.9.

193. Chung JW, Park JH, Im JG, Han JK, Han MC. Pulmonary oil embolism after transcatheter oily chemoembolization of hepatocellular carcinoma. Radiology 1993;187:689–693.

194. Stokes KR, Stuart K, Clouse ME. Hepatic arterial chemoembolization for metastatic endocrine tumors. J Vasc Intervent Radiol 1993;4:341–345.

195. Shiina S, Niwa Y. Percutaneous ethanol injection therapy in the treatment of liver neoplasms. In: Cope, C, ed. Current techniques in interventional radiology. Philadelphia: Current Medicine, 1994:3.1–3.14.

196. Sheu JC, Sung JL, Huang GH, et al. Intratumor injection of absolute ethanol under ultrasound guidance for the treatment of small hepatocellular carcinoma. Hepatogastroenterology 1987;34:255–261.

197. Fujimoto T. The experimental and clinical studies of percutaneous ethanol injection therapy (PEIT) under ultrasonography for small hepatocellular carcinoma. Acta Hepatol Jpn 1988;28:52–59.

198. Goletti O, De Negri F, Pucciarelli M, Sidoti F, Bertolucci A, Chiarugi M, Seccia M. Subcutaneous seeding after percutaneous ethanol injection of liver metastasis. Radiology 1992;183:785–786.

199. Cedrone A, Rapaccini GL, Pompili M, Grattagliano A, Aliotta A, Trombino C. Neoplastic seeding complicating percutaneous ethanol injection for treatment of hepatocellular carcinoma. Radiology 1992;183:787–788.

200. Mueller PR, vanSonnenberg E, Simeone JF. Fine-needle transhepatic cholangiography: indications and usefulness. Ann Intern Med 1982;97:567–572.

201. Mueller PR, Harbin WP, Ferrucci JT Jr, Wittenberg J, vanSonnenberg E. Fine-needle transhepatic cholangiography: reflections after 450 cases. AJR 1981;136:85–90.

202. vanSonnenberg E, Wing VW, Pollard JW, Casola G. Life-threatening vagal reactions associated with percutaneous cholecystostomy. Radiology 1984;151:377–380.

203. Halkier BK, Ho C, Yee ACN. Percutaneous feeding gastrostomy with the Seldinger technique: review of 252 patients. Radiology 1989;171:359–362.

204. Ho CS, Gray RR, Goldfinger M, Rosen IE, McPherson R. Percutaneous gastrostomy for enteral feeding. Radiology 1985;156:349–351.

205. Wills JS, Oglesby JT. Percutaneous gastrostomy: further experience. Radiology 1985;154:71–74.

206. Suggested instructions for placement of the Cope gastrointestinal suture anchor. Bloomington, IN: Cook, 1988.

207. Belli AM, Cumberland DC, Knox AM, Procter AE, Welsh CL. The complication rate of percutaneous peripheral balloon angioplasty. Clin Radiol 1990;41:380–383.

208. Armstrong MW, Torrie EP, Galland RB. Consequences of immediate failure of percutaneous transluminal angioplasty. Ann R Coll Surg Engl 1992;74:265–268.

209. Johnston KW. Iliac arteries: reanalysis of results of balloon angioplasty. Radiology 1993;186:207–212.

210. Struk DW, Rankin RN, Eliasziw M, Vellet AD. Safety of outpatient peripheral angioplasty. Radiology 1993;189:193–196.

211. Korogi Y, Takahashi M, Bussaka H, Hatanaka Y. Percutaneous transluminal angioplasty: pain during balloon inflation. Br J Radiol 1992;65:140–142.

212. Chong WK, Cross FW, Raphael MJ. Iliac artery rupture during percutaneous angioplasty. Clin Radiol 1991;43:142–143.

213. Selby JB Jr, Oliva VL, Tegtmeyer CJ. Circumferential rupture of an angioplasty balloon with detachment from the shaft: case report. Cardiovasc Intervent Radiol 1992;15:113–116.

214. Hagen B. Long term outcome of femoral stenting with Strecker stents. Presented at the 1993 meeting of the Western Angiographic and Interventional Society, Portland, OR, September 29–October 3, 1993.

215. McCullough KM. Retrograde transpopliteal salvage of the failed antegrade transfemoral angioplasty. Australas Radiol 1993;37:329–331.

216. Jørgensen B, Meisner S, Holstein P, Tønnesen KH. Early rethrombosis in femoropopliteal occlusions treated with percutaneous transluminal angioplasty. Eur J Vasc Surg 1990;4:149–152.

217. Cooper JC, Woods DA, Spencer P, Procter AE. The development of an infected false aneurysm following iliac angioplasty. Br J Radiol 1991;64:759–760.

218. Vive J, Bolia A. Aneurysm formation at the site of percutaneous transluminal angioplasty: a report of two cases and a review of the literature. Clin Radiol 1992;45:125–127.

219. Hunink MG, et al. Risks and benefits of femoropopliteal percutaneous balloon angioplasty. J Vasc Surg 1993;17:183–194.

220. Bergan JJ, Wilson SE, Wolf G, Deupree RH. Unexpected, late cardiovascular effects of surgery for peripheral artery disease. Arch Surg 1992;127:1119–1124.

221. Boba A. On survival rates in surgical treatment for ischaemic leg. Br J Surg 1979;66:293.

222. Ashenburg RJ, Blair RJ, Rivera FJ, Weigele JB. Renal arterial rupture complicating transluminal angioplasty: successful conservative management. Radiology 1990;176:583–584.

223. Olin JW, Wholey MH. Rupture of the renal artery nine days after percutaneous angioplasty. JAMA 1987;257:518–520.

224. Rossi G, Feltrin GP, Miotto D, Semplicini A, Casolino P, Mozzato MR, Pessina AC. Percutaneous transluminal renal angioplasty: influence of complications on long-term blood pressure results. J Hypertens 1985;3(Suppl):S461–S463.

225. Sharma S, Arya S, Mehta SN, Talwar KK, Rajani M. Renal vein injury during percutaneous transluminal renal angioplasty in nonspecific aortoarteritis. Cardiovasc Intervent Radiol 1993;16:114–116.

226. Gendler R, Mitty HA. Case report: evolution of a type B aortic dissection following renal artery angioplasty. Mt Sinai J Med 1993;60:330–332.

227. Dorsey DM, Rose SC. Extensive aortic and renal artery dissection following percutaneous transluminal angioplasty. J Vasc Intervent Radiol 1993;4:493–495.

228. Kim D, Porter DH, Siegel JB, Shapiro ME, Strom TB, Glotzer DJ. Use of a reperfusion catheter after angioplasty dissection for salvage of ischemic renal allograft: case report. Cardiovasc Intervent Radiol 1991;14:179–182.

229. Brown MM. Balloon angioplasty for cerebrovascular disease. Neurol Res 1992;14(Suppl):159–163.

230. Kachel R, Basche S, Heerklotz I, Grossmann K, Endler S. Percutaneous transluminal angioplasty (PTA) of supra-aortic ar-

teries especially the internal carotid artery. Neuroradiology 1991;33:191–194.

231. Higashida RT, Tsai FY, Halbach VV, Dowd CF, Smith T, Graser K, Hieshima GB. Transluminal angioplasty for atherosclerotic disease of the vertebral and basilar arteries. J Neurosurg 1993;78:192–198.

232. Millaire A, Trinca M, Marache P, de Groote P, Jabinet J-L, Ducloux G. Subclavian angioplasty: immediate and late results in 50 patients. Cathet Cardiovasc Diagn 1993;29:8–17.

233. Mathias KD, Luth I, Haarmann P. Percutaneous transluminal angioplasty of proximal subclavian artery occlusions. Cardiovasc Intervent Radiol 1993;16:214–218.

234. Mathias K. Percutaneous transluminal angioplasty of the supra-aortic arteries. In: Dondelinger RF, Rossi P, Kurdziel JC, Wallace S, eds. Interventional radiology. New York: Thieme, 1990:564–583.

235. Sharma S, Kaul U, Rajani M. Identifying high-risk patients for percutaneous transluminal angioplasty of subclavian and innominate arteries. Acta Radiol 1991;32:381–385.

236. Koike T, Minakawa T, Abe H, Takeuchi S, Sasaki O, Nishimaki K, Tanaka R. PTA of supra-aortic arteries with temporary balloon occlusion to avoid distal embolism. Neurol Med Chir (Tokyo) 1992;32:140–147.

237. Mandalam KR, Rao VR, Neelakandhan KS, Kumar S, Unnikrishnan M, Mukhopadhyay S. Hyperperfusion syndrome following balloon angioplasty and bypass surgery of aortic arch vessels: a report of 3 cases. Cardiovasc Intervent Radiol 1992; 15:108–112.

238. Spetzler RF, Wilson CB, Weinstein P, Mehdorn M, Townsend J, Telles D. Normal perfusion pressure breakthrough theory. Clin Neurosurg 1978;25:651–672.

239. Belli AM, Cumberland DC, Procter AE, Welsh CL. Followup of conventional angioplasty versus laser thermal angioplasty for total femoropopliteal artery occlusions: results of a randomized trial. J Vasc Intervent Radiol 1991;2:485–488.

240. Douek PC, Leon MB, Geschwind H, Cook PS, Selzer P, Miller DL, Bonner RF. Occlusive peripheral vascular disease: a multicenter trial of fluorescence-guided, pulsed dye laser-assisted balloon angioplasty. Radiology 1991;180:127–133.

241. McCarthy WJ, Vogelzang RL, Nemcek AA Jr, Joseph A, Pearce WH, Flinn WR, Yao JST. Excimer laser-assisted femoral angioplasty: early results. J Vasc Surg 1991;13:607–614.

242. Aburahma AF, Kennard W. Yag laser-assisted thermal balloon angioplasty: our early experience at Charleston Area Medical Center. W V Med J 1990;86:242–245.

243. Owen ER, Moussa SA, Lewis JD, Wilkins RA. Peripheral laser assisted angioplasty: results, complications and follow-up. J R Coll Surg Edinb 1990;35:75–79.

244. Reekers JA, Sprangers RL, van de Kley AJ. Angioplasty after laser perforation. Cardiovasc Intervent Radiol 1991;14:113–114.

245. Criado FJ, Queral LA, Patten P, Rudolphi D. Laser angioplasty in the lower extremities: an early surgical experience. J Vasc Surg 1990;11:532–535.

246. Rankin RN, Vellet AD, Munk PL. Excimer-laser-assisted angioplasty in chronic femoropopliteal occlusion: the significance of an intimal flap in predicting reocclusion. Can Assoc Radiol J 1993;44:257–261.

247. Levy JM, Hessel SJ, Horsley WW, Cook GC, Dickey JE. Value of laser-assisted angioplasty in the community hospital. Radiology 1989;170:1017–1018.

248. McLean GK. Percutaneous peripheral atherectomy. J Vasc Intervent Radiol 1993;4:465–480.

249. Naik K, Chalmers N, Gillespie IN. Amputation of the fine guidewire tip during atherectomy using the Simpson over-the-wire peripheral atherectomy catheter. Cardiovasc Intervent Radiol 1993;16:193–194.

250. Matsumoto AH, Selby JB Jr, Ladika JE Jr, Tegtmeyer CJ. Pseudoaneurysm formation following directional atherectomy. J Vasc Intervent Radiol 1993;4:283–286.

251. Martin EC, Katzen B. US Wallstent trial in the peripheral vascular system. Presented at the 1993 meeting of the Western

Angiographic and Interventional Society, Portland, OR, September 29–October 3, 1993.

252. Günther RW. Wallstents for the treatment of iliac and femoral stenoses and occlusions—mid-term results. Presented at the 1993 meeting of the Western Angiographic and Interventional Society, Portland, OR, September 29–October 3, 1993.

253. Palmaz JC, et al. Placement of balloon-expandable intraluminal stents in iliac arteries: first 171 procedures. Radiology 1990;174:969–975.

254. Rees CR. Renal stents, results of multicenter trial. Presented at the 1993 meeting of the Western Angiographic and Interventional Society, Portland, OR, September 29–October 3, 1993.

255. Strecker EP, Hagen B, Liermann D, Kuhn FP, Roth FJ. Iliac, subclavian and mesenteric artery stenting with flexible tantalum stents. Presented at the 1993 meeting of the Western Angiographic and Interventional Society, Portland, OR, September 29–October 3, 1993.

256. Katzen BT, van Breda A. Local arterial thrombolysis. In: Dondelinger RF, Rossi P, Kurdziel JC, Wallace S, eds. Interventional radiology. New York: Thieme, 1990:633–644.

257. Hirshberg A, Schneiderman J, Garniek A, Walden R, Morag B, Thomson SR, Adar R. Errors and pitfalls in intraarterial thrombolytic therapy. J Vasc Surg 1989;10:612–616.

258. McNamara TO, Bomberger RA, Merchant RF. Intraarterial urokinase as the initial therapy for acutely ischemic lower limbs. Circulation 1991;83(Suppl):I120–I121.

259. Roberts AC, Valji K, Bookstein JJ, Hye RJ. Pulse-spray pharmacomechanical thrombolysis for treatment of thrombosed dialysis access grafts. Am J Surg 1993;166:221–225.

260. Bookstein JJ, Valji K. "How I do it": pulse-spray pharmacomechanical thrombolysis. Cardiovasc Intervent Radiol 1992; 15:228–233.

261. Decrinis M, Pilger E, Stark G, Lafer M, Obernosterer A, Lammer J. A simplified procedure for intra-arterial thrombolysis with tissue-type plasminogen activator in peripheral arterial occlusive disease: primary and long-term results. Eur Heart J 1993;14:297–305.

262. Risius B, Graor RA. Thrombolytic therapy. In: Taveras JM, Ferrucci JT. Radiology: diagnosis—imaging—intervention. Philadelphia: Lippincott, 1992;2(146):1–14.

263. Holden RW, Becker GJ. Principles of fibrinolytic therapy. In: Taveras JM, Ferrucci JT. Radiology: diagnosis—imaging—intervention. Philadelphia: Lippincott, 1992;2(145):1–20.

264. Bell WR, Meek AG. Guidelines for the use of thrombolytic agents. N Engl J Med 1979;301:1266–1270.

265. Sheiman RG, Phillips DA. Combined effects of urokinase and heparin on PTT values during thrombolytic therapy. Angiology 1993;44:114–122.

266. Graor RA, Risius B, Young JR, Geisinger MA, Zelch MG, Smith JAM, Ruschhaupt WF. Low dose streptokinase for selective thrombolysis: systemic effects and complications. Radiology 1984;152:35–39.

267. Becker BJ, et al. Low dose fibrinolytic therapy. Radiology 1983;148:663–670.

268. Eskridge JM, Becker GJ, Rabe FE, Richmond BD, Holden RW, Yune JY, Klatte EC. Catheter-related thrombosis and fibrinolytic therapy. Radiology 1983;149:429–432.

269. Patel AG, Wilson NV, Kakkar VV. Septic arthritis of the knee: complication of intra-arterial thrombolytic therapy. Eur J Vasc Surg 1993;7:580–581.

270. Mathey DG, Schofer J, Sheehan FH, Becher H, Tilsner V, Dodge HT. Intravenous urokinase in acute myocardial infarction. Am J Cardiol 1985;55:878–882.

271. Matsis P, Mann S. Rigors and bronchospasm with urokinase after streptokinase. Lancet 1992;340:1552.

272. van Breda A, Rholl KS, Parker BC. Urokinase Reaction Registry. Urokinase Registry/Alexandria Hospital, Department of Radiology, 4320 Seminary Road, Alexandria, VA 22304.

273. Vidovich RR, Heiselman DE, Hudock D. Treatment of uro-

kinase-related anaphylactoid reaction with intravenous famotidine. Ann Pharmacother 1992;26:782–783.

274. Cho KJ, Proctor MC, Greenfield LJ. Efficacy and problems associated with vena cava filters. In: Cope C, ed. Current techniques in interventional radiology. Philadelphia: Current Medicine, 1994:8.1–8.17.

275. Becker DM, Philbrick JT, Selby JB. Inferior vena cava filters: indications, safety, effectiveness. Arch Intern Med 1992;152:1985–1994.

276. Greenfield LJ, DeLucia A III. Endovascular therapy of venous thromboembolic disease. Surg Clin North Am 1992;72:969–989.

277. Ferris EJ, McCowan TC, Carver DK, McFarland DR. Percutaneous inferior vena caval filters: follow-up of seven designs in 320 patients. Radiology 1993;188:851–856.

278. Rose BS, Simon DC, Hess ML, Van Aman, ME. Percutaneous placement of the Kimray-Greenfield vena cava filter. Radiology 1987;165:373–376.

279. Pais SO, Mirvis SE, De Orchis DF. Percutaneous insertion of the Kimray Greenfield filter: technical considerations and problems. Radiology 1987;165:377–381.

280. Lahey SJ, Meyer LP, Karchmer AW, Cronin J, Czorniak M, Maggs PR, Nesto RW. Misplaced cava filter and subsequent pericardial tamponade. Ann Thorac Surg 1991;51:299–301.

281. Rogoff PA, Hilgenber AD, Miller SL, Stephan SM. Cephalic migration of the bird's nest inferior vena cava filter: report of two cases. Radiology 1992;184:819–822.

282. Greenfield LJ, Cho JK, Proctor MC, Sobel M, Shah S, Wingo J. Late results of suprarenal Greenfield vena cava filter placement. Arch Surg 1992;127:969–973.

283. Ramchandani P, Zeit RM, Koolpe HA. Bilateral iliac vein filtration: an effective alternative to caval filtration in patients with megacava. Arch Surg 1991;126:390–393.

284. Reed R, Teitelbaum G, Taylor F, Pentecost MJ, Roehm JOF. Use of the bird's nest filter in oversized inferior venae cavae. J Vasc Intervent Radiol 1991;2:447–450.

285. Simon M, et al. Simon nitinol inferior vena cava filter: initial clinical experience. Radiology 1989;172:99–103.

286. Greenfield L, et al. Results of a multicenter study of the modified hook titanium Greenfield filter. J Vasc Surg 1991;14:253–257.

287. Braun MA, Collins MB, Sarrafizadeh M, Koslow AR. Percutaneous retrieval of tandem right atrial Greenfield filters. AJR 1991;157:199.

288. Sadighi P, Frost E. Retrieval of Greenfield filter from the right atrium. Ann Vasc Surg 1992;6:173–175.

289. Siegel EL, Robertson EF. Percutaneous retrieval of a free-floating titanium Greenfield filter with an Amplatz goose neck snare. J Vasc Intervent Radiol 1993;4:565–568.

290. Malden ES, et al. Transvenous retrieval of misplaced stainless steel Greenfield filters. J Vasc Intervent Radiol 1992;3:703–708.

291. Rodriguez LF, Saltiel FS. Long-term follow-up of ectopic intracardiac Greenfield filter. Chest 1993;104:611–612.

43

The Abnormal Abdominal Aorta: Arteriosclerosis and Other Diseases

MICHAEL J. HALLISEY
STEVEN G. MERANZE

Arteriosclerosis is a progressive disorder that develops over many years. The earliest lesions of arteriosclerosis can be found in children by the age of 3,[1] but the prevalence of this disease increases dramatically in older age groups, affecting 5 percent of patients in their fifties and 20 percent of patients in their seventies.[2] Three types of lesions are seen in arteriosclerotic disease[1,3]:

1. *Fatty streaks* are smooth, flat, or slightly elevated lesions caused by lipid-containing macrophages and smooth muscle cells ("foam cells").
2. *Fibrous plaques* are elevated lesions caused by fibrous connective tissue covering the foam cells that protrude and narrow the arterial lumen.
3. *Complicated plaques* are fibrous plaques that have calcified and undergone hemorrhage, ulceration, and/or thrombosis.

The cells of the blood vessel wall, namely, the smooth muscle cells and endothelial cells, play an active role in the pathogenesis of these plaques of arteriosclerosis. These cells interact with plasma lipoproteins and circulating platelets and macrophages. Specific growth factors and mediators can activate and accelerate proliferation of the lipid-containing smooth muscle cells in the intima of the aorta. Although arteriosclerotic plaques can cause narrowing in small vessels because of their space-occupying features, these plaques usually cause more significant morbidity in the aorta because of thinning of the media. The thinning of the aortic media can lead to weakening of the aortic wall, aneurysm formation, accumulation of mural thrombus, and subsequent ulceration, rupture, or atheroembolism.[3]

Patients with symptomatic arteriosclerotic disease of the aortoiliac junction usually present in their fifties. Moreover, in 30 percent of all patients with symptomatic peripheral vascular disease, the lesions are located in the aorta.[4,5] Certain risk factors predispose to plaque formation and/or accelerated arteriosclerosis. Lipoprotein metabolism and transport play a major role in lipid deposition and plaque development.[6–8] Elevations in very-low-density lipoproteins (VLDLs) and low-density lipoproteins (LDLs) appear to increase atherogenic potential, whereas elevations in high-density lipoproteins (HDLs) may actually protect against arteriosclerosis.[9–15] Hypertension increases the risk and severity of arteriosclerotic occlusive disease.[16–19] This predisposition in hypertensive patients may be due to alterations in normal hemodynamics; hypertension may result in turbulence, alteration in laminar blood flow, and changes in arterial wall pressure.[19] Cigarette smoking also predisposes to plaque formation and an acceleration of arteriosclerosis.[19–25] Another primary risk factor for arteriosclerosis is diabetes mellitus, although this change appears to be more significant in smaller, more peripheral vessels than in the abdominal aorta.[26]

The abdominal aorta, frequently the aortoiliac junction, is one of the most common sites of arteriosclerosis. The symptoms of aortoiliac arteriosclerotic disease can be elucidated from the patient's history and objectively measured by noninvasive physiologic testing.[27] Most symptomatic patients demonstrate diffuse arteriosclerotic aortic disease that extends into the iliac arteries and frequently into the femoral and popliteal arteries. A small subgroup of patients—frequently women smokers in their forties or fifties with diffusely small aortas—demonstrate focal aortic stenoses without significant arteriosclerotic plaque in their distal runoff.[28–30]

Aortoiliac occlusive disease may demonstrate symptoms that are characteristic to their location. Although calf claudication may be present in these patients, complaints of thigh and buttock ischemia may also be evident. Male patients may present with impotence. Aortic aneurysm formation may result in a pulsatile abdominal mass; aortic thrombus may predispose to distal emboli and a blue toe syndrome.

Treatment of symptomatic arteriosclerosis of the aorta is based on the severity, etiology, and location of the lesions. Darling et al. have classified arteriosclerotic occlusive lesions of the aorta as types I to III.[31] Type I disease is segmental arteriosclerotic stenoses limited to the abdominal aorta and common iliac arteries. These patients with focal aortoiliac disease are frequently women smokers under 50 years of age[28,29]; they have a low prevalence of diabetes and a high prevalence of hypercholesterolemia.[32] An early menopause is seen in 50 percent of these patients.[33] Type II disease is aortic, iliac, and femoral disease extending to the level of the groin. However, the majority of symptomatic patients present with type III, or multisegment arteriosclerotic stenoses involving the femoropopliteal and tibial arteries in addition to aortoiliac disease. These patients are frequently elderly males with an increased prevalence of diabetes mellitus and hypertension.[31]

Current treatment options for symptomatic arteriosclerosis of the aorta include percutaneous transluminal angioplasty and surgical bypass procedures. Extraanatomic procedures include axillofemoral bypass.[5] The axillofemoral bypass is performed during the excision of mycotic aortic aneurysms or infected aortic grafts, to repair an aortoenteric fistula, or for patients with high-risk medical problems who may not be adequate candidates for larger intraabdominal surgical procedures. Anatomic bypass procedures include aortoiliac endarterectomy and aortofemoral bypass. Aortic endarterectomy is performed for focal arteriosclerotic stenoses in the absence of aneurysmal disease. The procedure is now performed less frequently because many of these lesions may be amenable to percutaneous transluminal angioplasty.[29] Moreover, aortic endarterectomy achieves the best results in patients who do not have other significant atherosclerotic stenoses in the peripheral vessels; these patients may be ideal candidates for percutaneous transluminal angioplasty.[5,29,34] Aortofemoral bypass is now the most frequently performed surgical procedure for inflow revascularization. This procedure is best performed with an end-to-end graft in the presence of significant multilevel segmental arteriosclerotic disease involving the aorta and/or iliac arteries.[5,35] The cumulative 5-year survival rate following surgical revascularization is approximately 70 percent; concomitant arteriosclerosis of the cerebral and coronary vessels results in a significant mortality in these patients with aortoiliac disease.[4,36-38]

Although magnetic resonance imaging (MRI)[39] and spiral computed tomography (CT)[40] have been used in the evaluation of the abdominal aorta, angiography remains the most effective diagnostic method for evaluating arteriosclerotic stenoses or occlusions. Angiography provides important information regarding distal runoff vessels, collateral vessels, associated occlusions, or stenoses of major visceral arteries; furthermore, percutaneous transluminal angioplasty can be performed at the same time as the diagnostic arteriogram. Hemodynamically significant stenoses due to arteriosclerotic vessel narrowing can be estimated by angiography when the stenosis is severe or mild.[41] In moderately severe stenoses (50–75 percent narrowing) the angiographic appearance may not accurately reflect the hemodynamic significance,[42,43] but simultaneous pressure measurements without or with intraarterial vasodilators can identify unsuspected significance to arteriosclerotic stenoses.

Angiographic Signs of Arteriosclerosis

Angiography of the abdominal aorta can demonstrate findings that reflect the morphologic changes of arteriosclerosis. The arteriogram should include views that clearly define the severity, location, and extent of the arteriosclerotic disease. Intraarterial vasodilators and pressure measurements should be used to determine the hemodynamic significance of focal arteriosclerotic lesions. The examiner should have a working knowledge of the characteristic signs of arteriosclerotic disease. These include (1) diffuse long segment narrowing, (2) irregular vascular contour, (3) calcification of vessels, (4) eccentric changes in contrast density, (5) diffusely dilated or tortuous vessels, (6) focal saccular or aneurysmal dilatations, and (7) occluded segments. The actual arteriosclerotic plaque is frequently more severe than is demonstrated by the arteriogram; therefore, the most subtle findings of arteriosclerotic plaque on the arteriogram should receive further hemodynamic evaluation with vasodilators or additional views.

Diffuse Segmental Vascular Narrowing

Smooth, long segment narrowing of the abdominal aorta can be deceptive, hiding the underlying circumferentially arteriosclerotic plaque protruding into the arterial lumen. A focal aortic stenosis can demonstrate smooth margins due to plaque surrounding the lumen of the aorta (Fig. 43-1). The arteriogram will also demonstrate focal areas of constriction, dilatation, or irregular vessel margins, which represent arteriosclerotic plaques interrupting the smooth segmental nar-

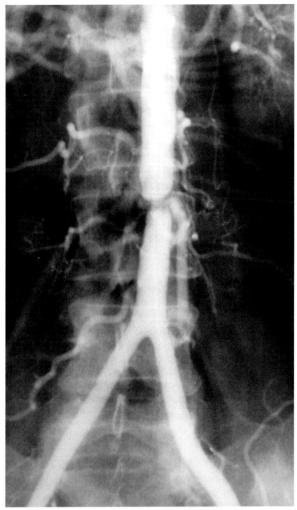

Figure 43-1. Circumferential narrowing of the abdominal aorta secondary to a focal arteriosclerotic plaque resulted in significant hip, thigh, and calf claudication in this 40-year-old patient. Note that the location of the lesion is near the origin of the inferior mesenteric artery, an important landmark in arteriosclerotic disease of the aorta.

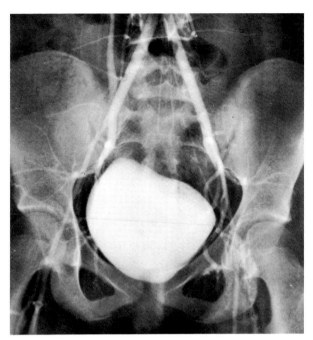

Figure 43-2. Although arteriosclerosis is more common, diffuse narrowing of the arteries may also be secondary to congenital hypoplasia. The common femoral arteries are diffusely narrowed on both sides in this 13-year-old girl. Hypertension had been present at least since early childhood, with increasing claudication.

rowing of the aorta. When the plaques become large enough, they can cause turbulence, stasis, and occlusion of the vessel.

Segmental luminal narrowing of a vessel, including the abdominal aorta, may be seen in the presence of a dissecting aneurysm, mural thrombus within an aneurysm, aortitis,[44-46] fibromuscular dysplasia, congenital hypoplasia (Fig. 43-2), midaortic syndrome (Fig. 43-3),[47] retroperitoneal fibrosis (Fig. 43-4),[48] coarctation, or hypercalcemia,[49-51] or it may be secondary to radiation therapy. Severe arteriosclerotic plaque disease can lead to diffuse vessel narrowing, which can

then lead to thrombosis (Fig. 43-5) of the aorta; usually collateral vessels provide blood flow around the stenoses to the pelvis or lower extremities (Fig. 43-6). The abdominal aorta can demonstrate luminal narrowing in Takayasu disease and other nonspecific arteritis. Angiographic examination of the aortic arch for associated major vessel involvement should be undertaken[44-46,52]; although the differentiation from midaortic syndrome may be difficult, Takayasu arteritis demonstrates a propensity for "flame-shaped" narrowing of the great vessels.

Irregular Vascular Contours

The native arterial luminal diameter should taper in a smooth and gradual manner as arteries branch into more peripheral and smaller vessels. Any change in this smooth tapering suggests arteriosclerosis (see Fig. 43-6). This also includes abrupt narrowing or dilatation as the aorta branches into the common iliac arteries. In addition, mass effect on the aorta due to an extravascular retroperitoneal mass can cause an abrupt change in the diameter of the contrast column.

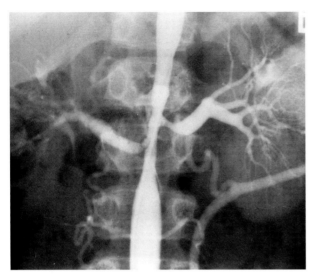

Figure 43-3. Midaortic syndrome is a rare disorder manifest as diffuse severe narrowing of the abdominal aorta. The narrowing frequently extends into the mesenteric and renal vessels.

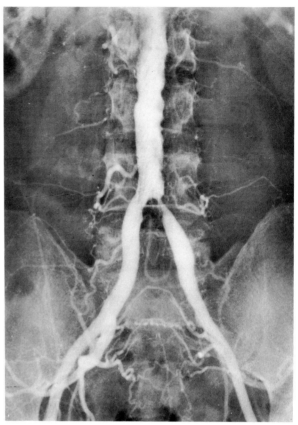

Figure 43-4. Retroperitoneal fibrosis can cause focal, smooth narrowing of the proximal common iliac artery. In this case the fibrotic process extended up the retroperitoneal space on the left, also involving the left ureter. Also note the classic arteriosclerotic irregularities and notches of the abdominal aorta. (From Neistadt A, Jones T, Rob C. Vascular system involvement by idiopathic retroperitoneal fibrosis. Surgery 1966;59:950. Used with permission.)

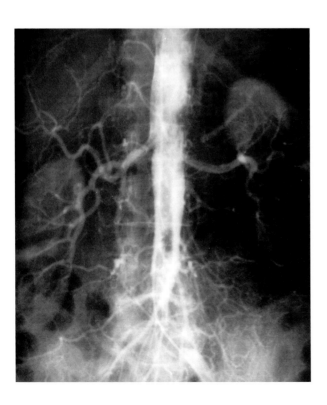

Figure 43-5. Diffuse vessel narrowing and occlusion can be due to arteriosclerosis with vessel thrombosis. Although this thrombus was secondary to a paradoxical embolus, the mass effect led to slowing and stasis of normal flow. A large filling defect is seen in the central lumen of the aorta with occlusion at the level of the aortic bifurcation due to acute thrombus accumulation.

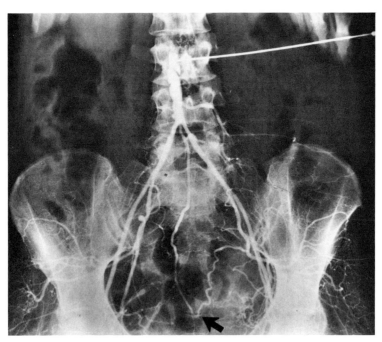

Figure 43-6. Diffuse arteriosclerosis. The common iliac and common femoral vessels are slender and smooth, but the ragged aortic column and the narrowed common iliac origins are signs of diffuse arteriosclerosis. Also note the abrupt and irregular change in the contour of the midportion of the abdominal aorta; these changes in aortic diameter are not smooth or gradual and suggest arteriosclerosis. The prominence of the middle sacral artery and its inosculation (*arrow*) with the left lateral sacral artery is a clue to collateralization around a significant stenosis of the left common iliac origin. There is a diffuse decrease in the contrast density in the left iliac artery due to decreased flow across the stenosis.

Vessel Wall Calcification or Filling Defects in the Contrast Column

Degenerative changes within the aortic plaques, including intraplaque hemorrhage or calcification, are typical findings in arteriosclerosis (Figs. 43-6 and 43-7). Although the plaque hemorrhage cannot be visualized radiographically, the calcification may be recognized on the preliminary films for the arteriogram. Calcification of the wall of the aorta is not diagnostic of vessel thrombosis but suggests arteriosclerosis; moreover, severe arteriosclerosis can occur in large vessels without obvious calcification.[53] Adherent thrombus along the wall of the aorta can also lead to nicks or filling defects in the contrast column. The thrombi may project into the lumen, but the examiner may not realize that these filling defects are not of arteriosclerotic origin (Figs. 43-8 and 43-9).[54] Arteriosclerotic plaque size may have greater significance in peripheral vessels than in the aorta, and calcification of smaller vessels may be a more significant sign of obstruction than calcification within the aorta.[29] Patients with chronic renal failure are prone to metastatic calcification of small vessels due to secondary hyperparathyroidism.

Figure 43-7. A scout film from an arteriogram (with the angiographic catheter in the aorta) demonstrates diffuse severe arteriosclerotic calcification of the abdominal aorta. Note the heavily calcified splenic artery in the left upper quadrant above the opacified left renal pelvis, as well as the heavily calcified iliac arteries.

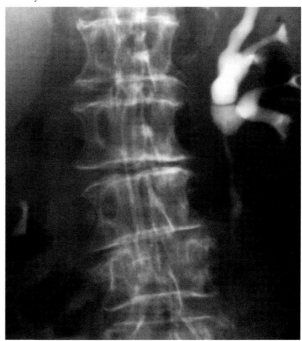

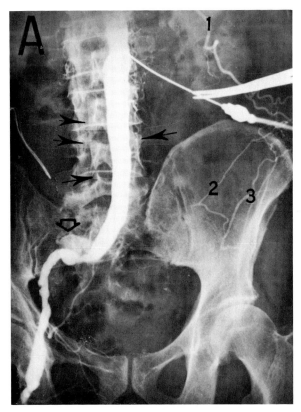

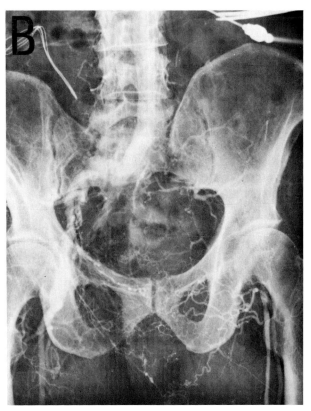

Figure 43-8. (A) A thrombus within a calcified abdominal aneurysm (*solid arrows*) narrows the remaining lumen of the aorta. There is thrombosis and occlusion of the lower lumbar, the left iliac, and the common femoral arteries. Note the faintly opacified internal iliac artery aneurysm (*open arrow*). Collateral circulation has developed in response to the occlu-

sion on the left; the numbers refer to the subcostal arteries (*1*) and the circumflex iliac branches (*2, 3*). (B) A film several seconds later reveals opacification of the left superficial and deep femoral arteries from the collateral vessels seen in (A) and probably from the pudendal and inferior hemorrhoidal vessels.

Eccentric Changes in Contrast Column Density

Although arteriosclerotic plaque is often in an eccentric location within the abdominal aorta, the plaque can occur anywhere around the concentric wall of this vessel. Because the aorta is a three-dimensional structure, routine oblique or biplane views should be obtained to evaluate the anterior or posterior aorta for plaque accumulation (Figs. 43-6, 43-9, 43-10, and 43-11).[55,56] Severe arteriosclerotic plaques may accumulate on the anterior or posterior wall of the aorta and remain undetected on frontal arteriograms because the lateral diameter of the aorta appears normal. However, a subtle eccentric variation in the contrast column of the aortogram may suggest the presence of

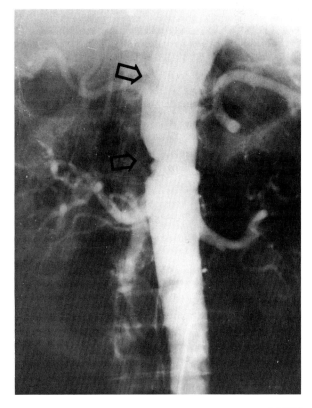

Figure 43-9. An abdominal aortogram demonstrates contour deformities and mural filling defects (*arrow*) of adherent mural thrombi. Subtle eccentric variations in the contrast column suggest arteriosclerotic plaque in the anterior or posterior wall of the infrarenal aorta. (From Lindsey SM, Maddison FF, Towne JB. Heparin-induced thromboembolism: angiographic features. Radiology 1979;131:771–774. Used with permission.)

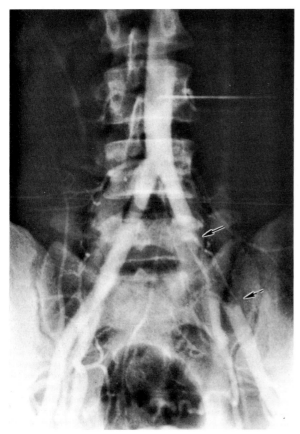

Figure 43-10. Thrombus in the left common iliac artery extending for a short distance into the external iliac artery (*arrows*). This was an acute occurrence in a patient with long-standing rheumatic heart disease. The aorta and other vessels have normal, smooth, parallel walls. Decreased density in the midportion of the right common iliac artery suggests anteroposterior narrowing or thrombus.

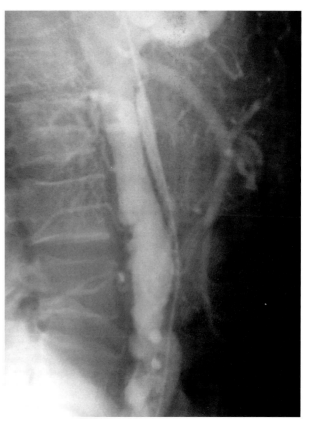

Figure 43-11. Since arteriosclerotic plaque is frequently located on the posterior wall of the aorta, angiography of the abdominal aorta should be performed with several views for more accurate delineation of the arteriosclerosis. This lateral view demonstrates the irregular notching due to arteriosclerosis on the posterior wall of the aorta.

arteriosclerotic plaque or mural thrombi on the anterior or posterior wall of the vessel.[57] There are limitations to frontal aortograms, and inconspicuous but hemodynamically significant arteriosclerotic plaques on the anterior or posterior wall of the aorta can be overlooked. Eccentric intimal dissections secondary to the trauma of a lap seat belt injury or a dissecting aortic aneurysm may be overlooked if only the frontal aortogram is obtained.[58,59]

Diffusely Dilated or Tortuous Vessels

Arteriosclerosis can be manifest as diffuse dilatation and tortuosity of the vessels (Fig. 43-12). The wall of the aorta and the iliac vessels are altered histologically by the arteriosclerotic plaque, and the internal elastic membrane may be fragmented. When there is diffuse dilatation, the vessels are usually not narrowed by the arteriosclerotic plaque but appear lengthened and very

tortuous; this diffuse tortuosity and lengthening may be seen in very young patients.[60,61] Arteriosclerosis of the aorta may result in small, short saccular dilatations or discrete aneurysms (Fig. 43-13). These dilatations should be distinguished from protruding collections of contrast within ulcerated portions of the arteriosclerotic plaque.

Aneurysms

Aneurysmal dilatation of the abdominal aorta is a manifestation of arteriosclerosis. Aneurysms of the aorta are discussed in Chapter 44.

Occlusions

Acute thrombosis of the aortoiliac junction is usually the result of progressive accumulation of arteriosclerotic plaque and narrowing of the aorta.[57,62,63] The arteriosclerotic plaque alone does not necessarily occlude the vessel; thrombus frequently accumulates in a very

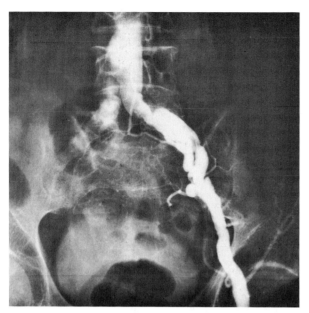

Figure 43-12. Irregular aneurysmal dilatation and marked tortuosity, particularly in the iliac arteries, is a manifestation of arteriosclerotic disease.

narrow channel as a result of turbulence and slowing of flow. The diameter of a blood vessel can be reduced by up to 70 percent of normal without reducing adequate blood flow through the vessel[64]; in the larger aorta an 82 percent luminal narrowing due to arteriosclerotic plaque results in only a 50 percent reduction in blood flow.[29,57,65] The patient may tolerate long-standing claudication and may not show signs of severe ischemia until complete occlusion develops.[57,66]

Collaterals will develop in the presence of a slowly progressive arteriosclerotic narrowing of the abdominal aorta. As the narrowing of the vessel reaches a critical stenosis or occlusion, the collateral reserve may prevent manifestation of significant changes in the patient's symptoms. In contrast, acute occlusion of a vessel due to an embolus may result in acute ischemia of the lower extremity. Aortoiliac stenoses or thromboses can be manifest as claudication of the hips, buttocks, and thighs; the patient may also have chronic low back or abdominal pain, impotence, and calf pain (Figs. 43-14 through 43-16).

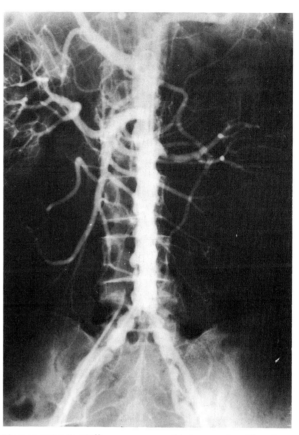

Figure 43-13. Diffuse, severe, multiple saccular dilatations and plaques of the abdominal aorta and iliofemoral arteries. This arteriosclerotic disease process also involved the lower thoracic aorta but spared the superficial femoral and popliteal arteries. Note the severe narrowing of the first portion of the left renal artery. (Courtesy of Frank E. Maddison, M.D.)

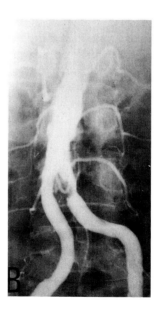

Figure 43-14. Tortuosity of the aorta and iliac arteries is a finding in patients with arteriosclerosis. The aorta shows the ragged outlines of arteriosclerosis, and the iliac arteries show the moderate tortuosity of arteriosclerosis. There is a localized narrowing in the common iliac artery on the left with compensatory hypertrophy of the ipsilateral lumbar artery.

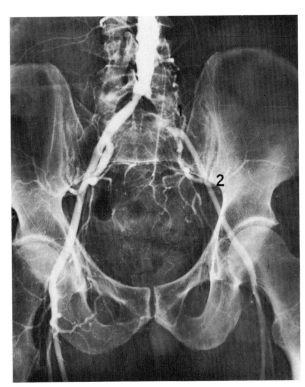

Figure 43-15. Chronic localized iliac thrombosis in a 60-year-old man with claudication of the left hip and gluteal regions. Note the decreased density of the entire left iliofemoral system, indicating a slower or decreased flow of blood. The important collateral vessels arise from the left lumbar, iliolumbar (*1*), and superior gluteal (*2*) arteries.

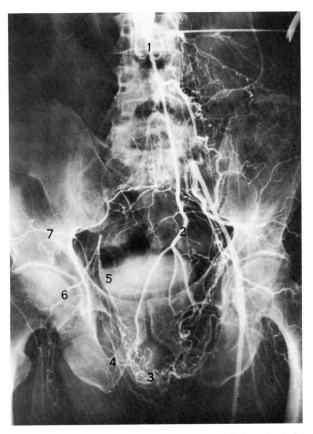

Figure 43-16. Chronic aortoiliac occlusion below the inferior mesenteric artery. The principal affluent collateral vessel is the inferior mesenteric artery (*1*) with its superior hemorrhoidal branch (*2*). Through rich rectal and perirectal anastomoses, the inferior hemorrhoidal (*3*), internal pudendal (*4*), middle hemorrhoidal (*5*), inferior gluteal (*6*), and superior gluteal (*7*) branches of the internal iliac artery are refilled bilaterally.

Arteriosclerotic plaque originating in an aortic aneurysm can embolize distally and can result in angiographically demonstrable occlusions.[67] However, in cholesterol embolism syndrome the small vessels that are occluded by microemboli usually will not visualize on the arteriogram. Cholesterol crystals may embolize to the kidneys, gastrointestinal tract, pancreas, or foot vessels and may be the result of catheter manipulation in the aorta during arteriography.[68–70]

Arteriography of the aorta should at least include views of the iliac and femoral vessels. If the patient demonstrates diffuse aortoiliac disease, an aortofemoral bypass may be indicated. The bypass graft is most often performed as an end-to-end graft from the infrarenal aorta to the common femoral arteries. The femoral arteries should be evaluated for focal areas of plaque accumulation. Moreover, a focal iliac stenosis may be identified and treated with percutaneous transluminal angioplasty before repair of an abdominal aortic aneurysm. Percutaneous transluminal angioplasty may be used as the treatment of select cases of focal aortic stenoses in the absence of significant iliac and femoral arteriosclerotic disease.[29]

Chronic Aortoiliac Thrombosis

Leriche syndrome is a term used to describe a clinical spectrum of abnormalities related to partial obstruction (Figs. 43-16 and 43-17) or complete obstruction of the aorta.[53,62,71–75] In the original description by Leriche, these symptoms included (1) lower extremity weakness without claudication; (2) global atrophy of the lower extremities without trophic changes of the nails or skin; (3) delayed wound healing; (4) absence of the aortic, iliac, femoral, and foot pulses; (5) persistent foot and leg pallor, unrelieved by dependency; and (6) vasculogenic impotence, manifest as the inability to maintain an erection. Leriche also described this syndrome as more common in young, adult males.[71,72] Patients whose symptoms fit the complete spectrum are not common; furthermore, patients with chronic aortoiliac thrombosis may demonstrate some, but not

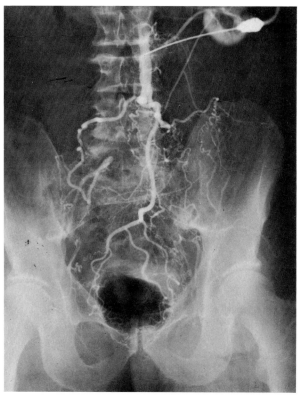

Figure 43-17. The presence, location, and patency of the inferior mesenteric artery in the presence of aortic occlusion is very important for collateral circulation. A translumbar aortogram demonstrates obstruction of the abdominal aorta just distal to the inferior mesenteric artery. Note the aberrant left renal artery to the lower pole. The lower lumbar arteries and inferior mesenteric artery serve as large affluent collateral vessels. Both femoral arteries were seen to be reconstituted on a later film. The patient underwent a successful aortofemoral bypass.

all, of these symptoms depending on the quality of collateral circulation to the pelvis and lower extremities.[76]

Complete Aortic Occlusion

Complete occlusion of the aorta requires a rich collateral circulation to supply the pelvis and lower extremities. The renal arteries frequently remain patent when the aorta occludes; however, in chronic aortic occlusion the renal and mesenteric arteries frequently demonstrate significant arteriosclerotic changes.[76] Although rare, total occlusion of the aorta above the level of the renal arteries[77] requires that the mesenteric vessels and lower aorta be supplied by collateral vessels traversing the wall of the thorax and abdomen (Figs. 43-18 and 43-19).

Midaortic syndrome (see Fig. 43-3),[47] coarctation

of the aorta,[49,78] and syphilis can cause occlusion at or near the renal arteries. Thrombosis of an abdominal aortic aneurysm (Fig. 43-20) and severe arteriosclerotic disease of the iliac vessels or aorta may also result in occlusion of the aorta below the renal arteries. The inferior mesenteric artery is an important landmark in the presence of complete occlusion of the abdominal aorta (see Fig. 43-17).[79] In approximately 50 percent of patients, the aortic occlusion extends into the common iliac arteries but begins below the inferior mesenteric artery, which remains patent and may enlarge to provide collateral supply below the occlusion. Occlusion of the abdominal aorta above the inferior mesenteric artery may result in significant collateralization from epigastric and intercostal arteries that opacify upon injection of the ascending thoracic aorta. The superior mesenteric artery, via the middle colic to left colic anastomosis, fills the inferior mesenteric artery, which can then provide collateral blood flow below the occlusion. Although it is difficult to determine whether an occluding thrombus formed at the site of a narrowed vessel is a result of an embolus,[80] more often than not chronic aortic occlusion is due to chronic arteriosclerotic diseases at the aortoiliac junction that leads to thrombosis extending retrograde into the terminal aorta.[62,73,81,82] Depending on the location of the occlusion, the progression of disease, and the demand for lower extremity blood flow, collateral vessels will hypertrophy to provide arterial supply around the occlusion.

Collateral Pathways

Although the arteriogram of the abdominal aorta should include the origin of the stenosis or occlusion, careful attention should be given to the size, number, and location of collateral vessels because they may provide important information relating to the severity of arteriosclerotic stenoses. For example, hypertrophy of the mesenteric or lumbar arteries may be in response to an occlusive arteriosclerotic plaque in the distal aorta or iliac vessels. Further investigation may reveal subtle defects or arteriosclerotic irregularities in the contrast column of the aorta; these suggest significant aortic or iliac stenosis, particularly in the presence of prominent collateral branch arteries. The arteriogram should include the major branch arteries that provide collateral supply (Fig. 43-21). The study should also be timed to demonstrate significant filling of collateral vessels and the location of distal reconstitution of major arterial branches.

An understanding of the potential collateral circulation in occlusion of the aorta is helpful.[83,84] A collateral

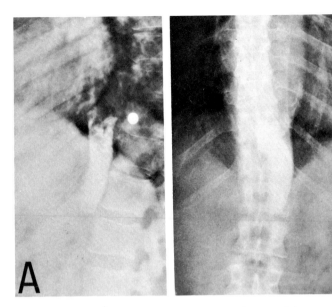

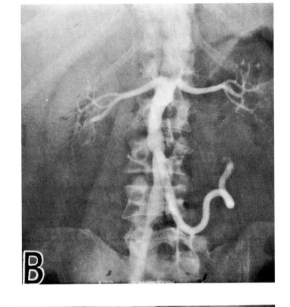

Figure 43-18. Calcified thrombosis with occlusion of the abdominal aorta localized to a segment above the origins of the renal arteries. (A) Anteroposterior and lateral roentgenograms show smoothly marginated, dense calcification within the lumen of the aorta from the 11th thoracic vertebra to the 1st lumbar vertebra. (B) A retrograde aortogram (there were good femoral artery pulsations) shows abrupt, convex obstruction to the contrast material corresponding exactly to the inferior limit of the calcified thrombus. (C) A hypertrophied branch of the inferior mesenteric artery courses to the left and joins with and fills the proximal portion of the middle colic branch of the superior mesenteric artery. Later films showed opacification of the main trunk of the superior mesenteric artery and its intestinal branches. (From Lipchik EO, et al. Obstruction of the abdominal aorta above the level of the renal arteries. Radiology 1964;82:443. Used with permission.)

branch originating from the patent main vessel above the stenosis or occlusion is called an *affluent* vessel. A collateral branch that receives incoming blood from the affluent artery and reconstitutes distal blood flow around a stenosis is called an *effluent* artery. *Inosculation* occurs when there is direct communication between affluent and effluent arteries. In some cases there may be a network of intermediate vessels communicating between the main affluent and effluent collateral arteries. In contrast, a *retiform anastomosis* is a fine network of small intervening collateral vessels that connect the affluent and effluent arteries.

The continuous and rapid flow of blood from an affluent vessel into an effluent vessel in an inosculation provides more direct and continuous flow of blood around a block or stenosis than a retiform anastomosis (see Fig. 43-6). In the presence of inosculation, the contrast column will define prominent affluent or ef-

Figure 43-20. Aortic occlusion due to thrombosis of a large aneurysm. A left axillary artery approach was used to place a catheter in the upper abdominal aorta. (A) Both renal arteries and the superior mesenteric artery are patent. (B) The superior mesenteric artery supplies the distal inferior mesenteric artery via branches of the middle colic artery (*arrow*). ▶ There was later faint opacification of distal femoral vessels. This 68-year-old man had a typical Leriche syndrome, and his most troublesome complaints were pain and fatigue of both legs and feet.

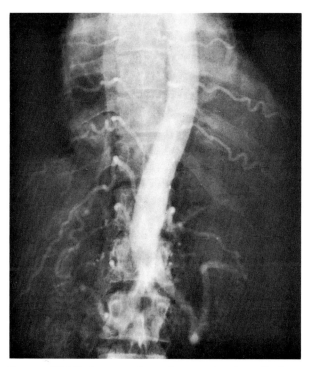

Figure 43-19. Intercostal arteries coursing laterally from the aorta are an important source of collateral blood flow in response to arteriosclerotic occlusive disease. Aortogram shows dilated, tortuous intercostal arteries that serve as important collateral vessels in overcoming obstruction of the abdominal aorta in a 57-year-old woman.

fluent vessels without a significant change in opacification. However, as the collateral blood flows into a retiform anastomosis, there is an inevitable decrease in pressure, flow, and opacification. The retiform anastomosis may not be identifiable on the arteriogram, but its presence can be suspected by the locations of the respective affluent and effluent vessels. In aortoiliac arteriosclerosis, prominent collateralization can be seen between the lumbar and iliolumbar arteries (Figs. 43-22 and 43-23; see also Figs. 43-15 and 43-20). Other significant examples of inosculation are seen between obturator and medial femoral circumflex arteries (Figs. 43-24 and 43-25; see also Fig. 43-22), between the iliolumbar and deep circumflex iliac arteries (Fig. 43-26), and between the superior gluteal artery and the ascending branch of the lateral femoral circumflex artery (Figs. 43-21, 43-26, and 43-27). Collateral pathways may provide a clue to the significance and location of aortoiliac arteriosclerotic disease.

Collateral Circulation in Aortoiliac Occlusion

Collateral arteries can provide blood flow around aortoiliac arteriosclerotic disease through a complex network of visceral or parietal arteries involving the thorax, abdomen, pelvis, or lower extremities. Figure

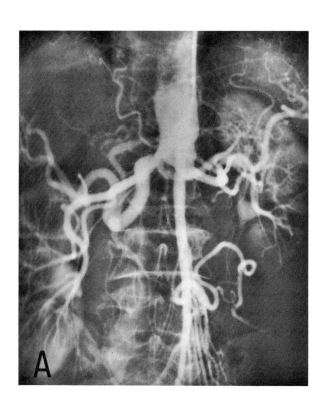

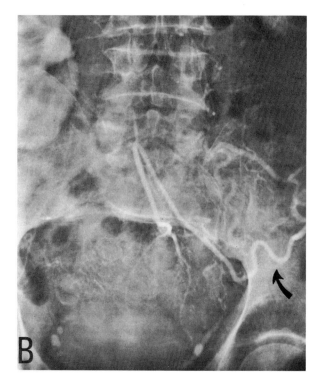

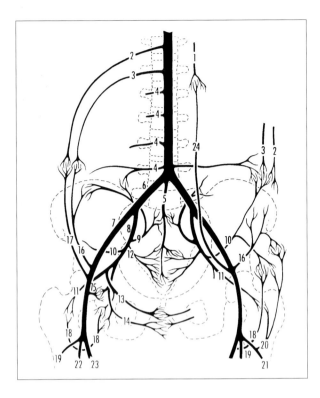

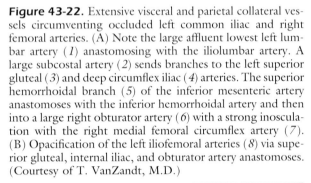

Figure 43-21. Schematic diagram of the major potential parietal pathways of collateral circulation demonstrated in aortoiliofemoral occlusive disease. Arteries: superior epigastric, *1;* intercostal, *2;* subcostal, *3;* lumbar, *4;* middle sacral, *5;* common iliac, *6;* external iliac, *7;* internal iliac, *8;* iliolumbar, *9;* superior gluteal, *10;* inferior gluteal, *11;* lateral sacral, *12;* obturator, *13;* internal pudendal, *14;* external pudendal, *15;* deep iliac circumflex, *16;* superficial iliac circumflex, *17;* medial femoral circumflex, *18;* lateral femoral circumflex, *19;* lateral ascending branch, *20;* lateral descending branch, *21;* profunda femoris, *22;* superficial femoral, *23;* inferior epigastric, *24.* (From Muller RF, Figley MM. The arteries of the abdomen, pelvis and thigh. AJR 1957;77:296. Used with permission.)

Figure 43-22. Extensive visceral and parietal collateral vessels circumventing occluded left common iliac and right femoral arteries. (A) Note the large affluent lowest left lumbar artery (*1*) anastomosing with the iliolumbar artery. A large subcostal artery (*2*) sends branches to the left superior gluteal (*3*) and deep circumflex iliac (*4*) arteries. The superior hemorrhoidal branch (*5*) of the inferior mesenteric artery anastomoses with the inferior hemorrhoidal artery and then into a large right obturator artery (*6*) with a strong inosculation with the right medial femoral circumflex artery (*7*). (B) Opacification of the left iliofemoral arteries (*8*) via superior gluteal, internal iliac, and obturator artery anastomoses. (Courtesy of T. VanZandt, M.D.)

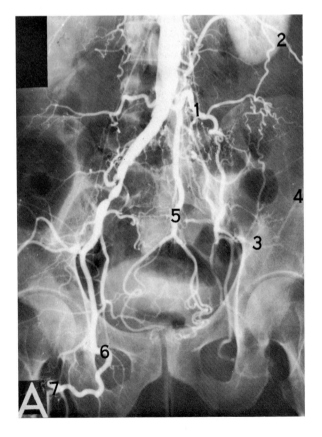

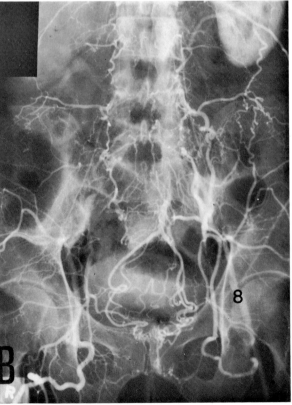

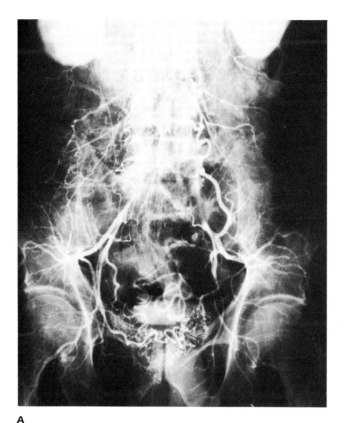

A

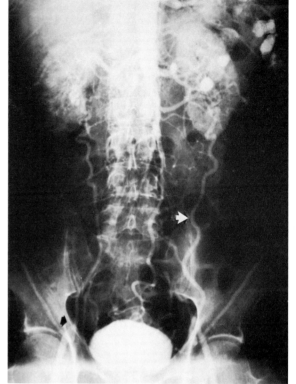

B

Figure 43-23. The epigastric arteries are an important source of collateral circulation in aortoiliac occlusion. (A) An upper abdominal aortogram demonstrates complete occlusion of the lower aorta and both common iliac arteries and extensive collateral vessels to the internal iliac systems. The femoral arteries were not opacified at any time after this injection. (B) The second injection of contrast material into the ascending aorta shows good opacification of dilated epigastric arteries (*upper arrow*) reconstituting the femoral arteries (*lower arrow*). (Courtesy of Frank Maddison, M.D.)

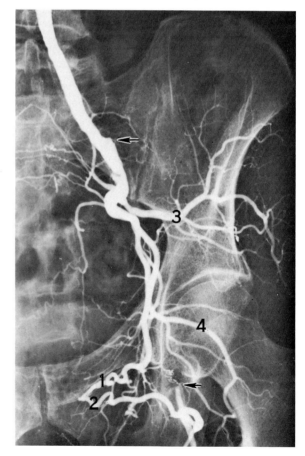

Figure 43-24. Left common and external iliac and superficial femoral artery obstruction (*between arrows*) with refilling of the deep femoral artery (*lower arrow*) via internal iliac affluent vessels. Note the large direct connection (inosculation) between the obturator (*1*) and medial femoral circumflex (*2*) arteries. The superior gluteal artery (*3*) is dilated, but its eventual anastomosis is not yet visible in this phase of the arteriogram. (It usually anastomoses via its ascending branch with the lateral femoral circumflex artery.) The inferior gluteal artery (*4*) is also quite dilated and helps supply the deep femoral artery. These parietal collateral vessels are unusually dilated because the inferior mesenteric and iliolumbar arteries were blocked.

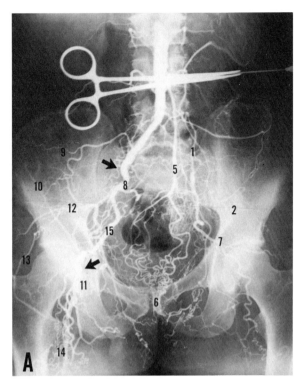

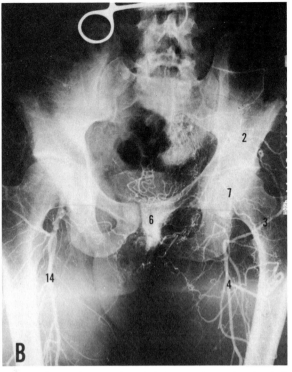

Figure 43-25. Chronic aortoiliofemoral obstruction. Note the importance of serial radiographs in defining extensive visceral and parietal collaterals. (A) On the patient's left there is a complete block of the iliofemoral system above the inguinal region. There are three main affluent channels to the left side: the left lumbar branches anastomose both with the left iliolumbar artery's lumbar branch (*1*) and with the left superior gluteal (*2*) and inferior gluteal (*7*, A) arteries, which in turn feed the lateral femoral circumflex artery (*3*, B) and thereby help to refill the left femoral artery (*4*, B). The superior hemorrhoidal arteries (*5*) inosculate around the rectum (*6*) with the middle and inferior hemorrhoidal arteries, which act as intermediates across the effluent branches of the left deep femoral artery (*4*, B). The sacral arteries also help to transmit blood to the deep femoral artery via anastomoses with the lumbar artery and again into the left inferior gluteal branch (*7*, B). On the right side there is an occlusion of the external iliac artery (*upper arrow*). However, inosculating collaterals between the iliac branch (*9*) of the iliolumbar and the deep circumflex iliac arteries (*10*) refill the right common femoral artery (*11*). (B) The later arterial phase shows that the superior gluteal artery (*13*, A; *3*, B) also fill the deep femoral arteries (*14*). The hypogastric artery (*15*) communicates directly with the common femoral artery (*lower arrow*, A). In subsequent films, both distal superficial femoral and popliteal arteries were fully patent.

43-21 is a schematic diagram of the major parietal pathways of collateral circulation.

Visceral-Systemic Collateral Network

Depending on the location of the aortic stenosis or occlusion, the inferior or superior mesenteric arteries can deliver blood flow to collateral vessels below the area of narrowing or occlusion (see Figs. 43-17, 43-18, and 43-20).

The inferior mesenteric artery can provide affluent collateral flow around a distal aortic occlusion through the superior hemorrhoidal branch to rich communications in the middle and inferior hemorrhoidal arteries supplying the perirectal region. These middle and inferior hemorrhoidal arteries can then anastomose with all branches of the internal iliac arteries except the iliolumbar.[83,84] Retrograde flow in the internal iliac artery preserves antegrade flow into the external iliac artery as long as there is no significant arteriosclerotic disease present. If there is an occlusion of the external iliac artery, collateral vessels can also reconstitute the common femoral artery in the groin. This rectal and hemorrhoidal collateral network appears to be more prominent in aortic occlusion than in common iliac occlusions.

Arteriosclerosis of the aorta is frequently located at or near the origin of the inferior mesenteric artery.[29,82] In the presence of a distal aortic occlusion, a critical stenosis of the inferior mesenteric artery may prevent reconstitution or slow collateral blood flow into the external iliac artery. Selective catheterization of the visceral arteries may be necessary to demonstrate distal

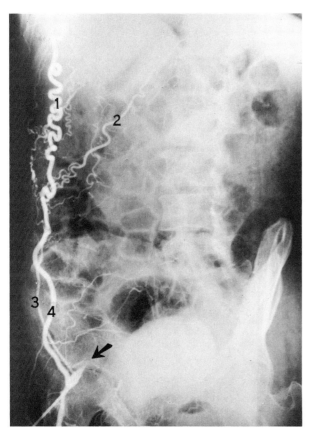

Figure 43-26. Obstruction of the right common iliac artery in a 52-year-old man who had a distal aorto–bilateral common iliac graft. The common femoral artery is occluded down to the needle site (*arrow*) in the right common femoral artery. Collateral anastomoses between the intercostal (*1*), subcostal (*2*), deep iliac circumflex (*3*), and superficial iliac circumflex (*4*) arteries are demonstrated. (From Friedenberg MJ, Perez CA. Collateral circulation in aorto-ilio-femoral occlusive disease: as demonstrated by a unilateral percutaneous common femoral artery needle injection. AJR 1965; 94:145. Used with permission.)

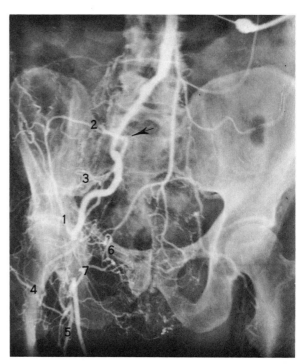

Figure 43-27. Internal iliac artery obstruction on the right. There are also obstructions involving a segment of the right common femoral artery and the iliofemoral system on the left. A large deep circumflex iliac artery (*1*) arises from the external iliac artery and refills the iliac branch of the iliolumbar artery (*2*) back to its common origin (*arrow*) with the superior gluteal and inferior gluteal (*3*) arteries (poorly opacified). The common femoral artery obstruction is reconstituted by an anastomosis between the refilled gluteal vessels and the lateral femoral circumflex branches (*4*) back into the deep femoral artery (*5*). The inosculation from the obturator artery (*6*) to the medial femoral circumflex artery (*7*) is evident.

runoff in the presence of visceral to systemic collaterals.[79]

If the occlusion is above the inferior mesenteric artery, the left branch of the middle colic artery originating from the superior mesenteric artery can deliver blood flow into the intermediate left colic branch of the inferior mesenteric artery (see Fig. 43-20).[81,83-85] When there is a direct communication (see Fig. 43-6) between the left branch of the middle colic artery into the left colic artery, this is called the *meandering mesenteric artery* or *central anastomotic artery*.[85] The inferior mesenteric artery then supplies the lower extremity through collaterals originating in the hemorrhoidal network.

Systemic-Systemic (Parietal) Collateral Network

Many parietal vessels can act as important affluent channels of collateral blood flow around an aortic occlusion (Figs. 43-28; see also Figs. 43-19, 43-23, and 43-24). Although the parietal collateral network is less common than the visceral network, the angiographic catheter must be placed in the thoracic aorta to visualize the affluent intercostal arteries, which can anastomose with the effluent deep iliac circumflex and lumbar vessels. These vessels, in turn, can both reconstitute the common femoral artery (see Fig. 43-28). However, the lumbar arteries may anastomose to the iliolumbar artery; from the iliolumbar artery, blood flows retrograde into the superior gluteal to the internal iliac and then antegrade in the external iliac artery.[81,86-87]

The Winslow pathway is a collateral channel origi-

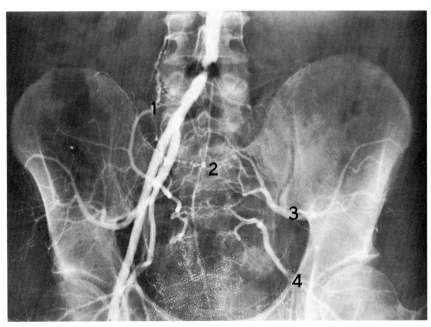

Figure 43-28. Left aortoiliofemoral occlusion in a 50-year-old man complaining of claudication of the left lower extremity. A translumbar aortogram shows transpelvic lateral sacral collateral vessels (*2*) from the right side opacifying the superior (*3*) and the inferior (*4*) gluteal arteries of the left internal iliac artery. The large right-sided gluteal arteries are also an expression of the severity of the stenosis of the origin of the right common iliac artery. Note the anastomoses of the iliolumbar artery (*1*) with the fourth lumbar artery on the right.

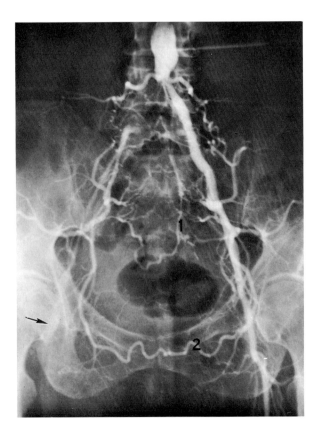

nating from the affluent intercostal and internal mammary arteries; this pathway provides blood flow into the epigastric arteries (see Fig. 43-23), which flows retrograde into the external iliac arteries.[88,89] Recent data suggest a sex-linked male preponderance for the development of thoracic collaterals in the presence of severe aortoiliac disease.[90] This may be due to the rich collateral network from the internal iliac vessels available in women; moreover, women who have undergone a hysterectomy are more likely to have thoracic collaterals in aortoiliac occlusion. A filling defect in the contrast column of the external iliac artery may be seen on a pelvic arteriogram when there is retrograde flow in the inferior epigastric artery.[81] If this filling defect (due to inflow of nonopacified blood into the femoral artery on an abdominal aortogram) is identified or if there is no visualization of pelvic collaterals, the angiographic catheter should be placed into the aortic arch;

Figure 43-29. Translumbar aortogram with placement of the needle into a small lower abdominal aortic aneurysm shows occlusion of the common iliac artery on the right. The internal iliac artery on the right is filled mainly via collateral vessels from the left lateral sacral (*1*) and left internal pudendal (*2*) arteries. There is faint opacification of the right common femoral artery (*arrow*). Additional serial films showed patent femoral and popliteal arteries.

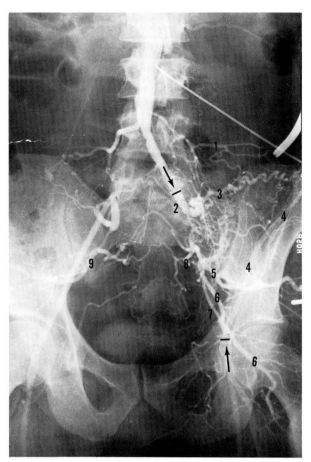

Figure 43-30. Left external iliac artery (*2*) obstruction (*between arrows*) as well as occlusion of the proximal main trunk of the internal iliac artery. The right common iliac artery is also occluded. The left fourth lumbar artery (*1*) is anastomosing with other retroperitoneal vessels in the sacral region and with the deep circumflex iliac artery (*4*). The coiled iliac portion (*3*) of the iliolumbar artery helps supply the superior gluteal artery (*5*), which in turn supplies the inferior gluteal (*6*), internal pudendal (*7*), and lateral sacral (*8*) arteries. The lateral sacral artery enables the sacral network to nourish the opposite superior gluteal artery via the lateral sacral artery (*9*) below the right common iliac occlusion.

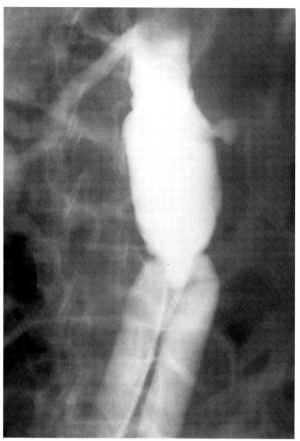

Figure 43-31. Dimplelike defect in the abdominal aorta caused by an aortoenteric fistula. This patient had undergone previous iliac surgery and had an abdominal aortic aneurysm.

an arteriogram of the ascending aorta or subclavian vessels is indicated to evaluate for an aortic occlusion with reconstitution of the external iliac artery via Winslow pathway.

Lumbar Arteries

The lumbar arteries may be the most common and important affluent collateral vessels in aortoiliac arteriosclerotic disease. The lumbar arteries will originate from the aorta above the level of the obstruction and course laterally; they commonly communicate with the iliolumbar and superior gluteal branches of the in-

ternal iliac artery (Fig. 43-29; see also Figs. 43-22 and 43-27), causing retrograde flow into the internal iliac artery, which then reconstitutes the external iliac artery (Fig. 43-30). A second parietal network of arteries originates in the lumbar arteries and courses through the abdominal wall anteriorly and the spine posteriorly; these collaterals supply the superior and inferior epigastric arteries, which then reconstitute the profunda femoral artery.[91] Careful attention to the location and origin of prominent collateral vessels will provide information about the circuitous routes through which blood will flow around a stenosis or occlusion. Significant variability can exist from patient to patient in the collateral network; parietal and visceral arterial networks can communicate at variable locations along their course to reconstitute a vessel below the arteriosclerotic occlusion. However, the presence of collateral vessels provides important information about the severity and significance of an aortic obstruction. A large collateral artery may suggest a more severe arteriosclerotic plaque than is evident by the changes in the contrast column alone.

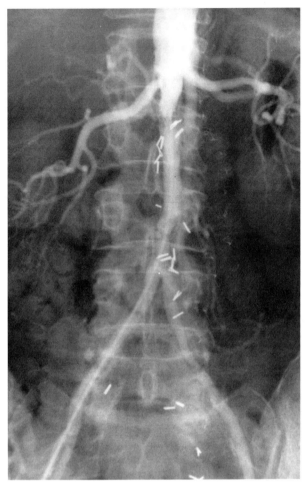

Figure 43-32. Diffuse irregular narrowing of the infrarenal abdominal aorta. This patient had undergone thromboend-arterectomy over 10 years previously for a focal abdominal aortic arteriosclerotic plaque. A clue to the cause of the diffuse narrowing is the multiple metallic clips used during the surgical procedure.

Postoperative Aortic Arteriography

Aortofemoral bypass is the most frequently performed surgical procedure for inflow revascularization. The graft is best performed as an end-to-end graft beginning in the infrarenal aorta above the level of the inferior mesenteric artery. In patients who have undergone an aortofemoral bypass, the arteriogram should include views of the proximal anastomosis.

Aortoenteric fistula is a complication of aortic surgery in patients who have had complicated or emergent surgical bypasses for abdominal aortic aneurysm or multiple procedures for severe arteriosclerotic disease. The most common site of the fistula is from the proximal aortic graft into the duodenum.[92] These patients may present with intestinal bleeding, and an aor-

togram (Fig. 43-31) may demonstrate a dimplelike defect in the wall of the aorta. Direct flow of contrast from the aorta into the intestine is only rarely seen.

With the advent of successful percutaneous transluminal angioplasty of the abdominal aorta, thromboendarterectomy of the aorta for arteriosclerosis is less commonly performed. However, some patients may exhibit defects in the abdominal aorta many years following thromboendarterectomy (Fig. 43-32). These defects may be irregularity, nicks, abrupt contour changes, and diffuse narrowing as seen in primary arteriosclerosis of the aorta.

References

1. Consigney PM. Pathogenesis of atherosclerosis. In: 1993 International Symposium on Vascular Diagnosis and Intervention. Miami Beach, FL, January 25–28, 1993:33–36.
2. Criqui MH, Fronek A, Barrett-Connor E, et al. The prevalence of peripheral arterial disease in a defined population. Circulation 1985;71:510–515.
3. Schoen FJ. Atherogenesis, endovascular therapy and restenosis. In: 1992 First International Symposium on Cardiovascular and Interventional Radiology. Boston, October 13–16, 1992:2–14.
4. McDaniel MD, Cronenwett JL. Basic data related to the natural history of intermittent claudication. Ann Vasc Surg 1989; 3:273–277.
5. Perler BA. Aortoiliac disease: surgical options and results. In: 1993 International Symposium on Vascular Diagnosis and Intervention. Miami Beach, FL, January 25–28, 1993:95–100.
6. The Pooling Project Research Group. Relationship of blood pressure, serum cholesterol, smoking habit, relative weight and ECG abnormalities to incidence of major coronary events. J Chron Dis 1978;31(4):201–306.
7. Keys A. Coronary heart disease in seven countries. Circulation 1970;41(4 Suppl):I40–211.
8. Grundy SM, Bilheimer D, Blackburn H, et al. Rationale of the diet-heart statement of the American Heart Association. Circulation 1982;65(4):839A–854A.
9. Gofman J, Jones H, Strisower B. Blood lipids in human atherosclerosis. Circulation 1951;S:119–134.
10. Gofman J, Glazier F, Tamplin A. Lipoproteins, coronary heart disease and atherosclerosis. Physiol Res 1954;34:589–607.
11. Borrie P. Type III hyperlipoproteinemia. Br Med J 1969; 2(658):665–667.
12. Hessel LW, Vermeer BJ, Polan MK, et al. Primary hyperlipoproteinemia in xanthomatosis. Clin Chim Acta 1976;69(3):405–416.
13. Ross AC, Zilversmit DB. Chylomicron remnant cholesteryl esters as the major constituent of very low density lipoproteins in plasma of cholesterol-fed rabbits. J Lipid Res 1977;18(2):169–181.
14. Krause RM. Regulation of high density lipoprotein levels. Med Clin North Am 1982;66(2):403–430.
15. Pomrehn P, Duncan B, Weissfeld L, et al. The association of dyslipoproteinemia with symptoms and signs of peripheral arterial disease: The Lipids Research Clinics Program Prevalence Study. Circulation 1986;73(Suppl I):100–107.
16. Dawber TR, ed. The Framingham Study: the epidemiology of atherosclerotic disease. Cambridge: Harvard Univ Press, 1980: 1–257.
17. Strong JP. Atherosclerotic lesions. Arch Path Lab Med 1992; 116:1268–1275.

18. Sternby NH. Atherosclerosis in a defined population: an autopsy survey in Malmo, Sweden. Acta Pathol Microbiol Scand 1968;194:5.
19. Glagor S. Hemodynamic risk factors: mechanical stress, mural architecture, medial nutrition and vulnerability of arteries to atherosclerosis. In: Wissler, Geer JC, eds. The pathogenesis of atherosclerosis. Baltimore: Williams & Wilkins, 1972:164–199.
20. Wilens SL, Plair CM. Cigarette smoking and arteriosclerosis. Science 1962;138:975–977.
21. Sackett DL, Gibson RW, Brass ID, et al. Relation between aortic atherosclerosis and the use of cigarettes and alcohol. N Engl J Med 1968;279(26):1413–1420.
22. Strong JP, Richards ML, McGill HC Jr, et al. On the association of cigarette smoking with coronary and aortic atherosclerosis. J Atheroscler Res 1969;10(3):303–317.
23. Strong JP, Richards ML. Cigarette smoking and atherosclerosis in autopsied men. Atherosclerosis 1976;23:451–476.
24. Tracey RE, Toca VT, Strong JP, et al. Relationship of raised atherosclerotic lesions to fatty streaks in cigarette smokers. Atherosclerosis 1981;38:347–357.
25. Kannel WB, McGee DL. Update on some epidemiologic features of intermittent claudication: the Framingham study. J Am Geriatr Soc 1985;33:13–18.
26. Branch FN, Abbott RD, Kannel WB. Diabetes, intermittent claudication and risk of cardiovascular events. Diabetes 1989;38:504–509.
27. Fronek A, Johansen KH, Dilley RB, et al. Noninvasive physiologic tests in the diagnosis and characterization of peripheral arterial occlusive disease. Am J Surg 1973;126:205–214.
28. Tegtmeyer CJ, Kellum CD, Kron IL, et al. Percutaneous transluminal angioplasty in the region of the aortic bifurcation. Radiology 1985;157:661–665.
29. Hallisey MJ, Meranze SG, Parker BC, et al. Percutaneous transluminal angioplasty of the abdominal aorta. J Vasc Intervent Radiol 1994;5:679–687.
30. Palmaz JC. Predictive value of angiographic disease: statistical analysis of 455 cases. In: Fifth Annual International Symposium on Vascular Diagnosis and Intervention. Miami Beach, FL, January 25–28, 1993:67–68
31. Darling RC, Brewster DC, Hallett JW Jr, et al. Aorto-iliac reconstruction. Surg Clin North Am 1979;59(4):565–579.
32. Freidman SA, Novack S, Thomson GE. Arterial calcification and gangrene in uremia. N Engl J Med 1969;280:1392–1394.
33. Freidman SA, Holling HE, Roberts B. Etiologic factors in aortoiliac and femoropopliteal vascular disease: Leriche syndrome. N Engl J Med 1964;27:1382–1385.
34. Darling RC. Peripheral arterial surgery. N Engl J Med 1969;280:141–146.
35. Brewster DC, Perler BA, Robison JG, et al. Aortofemoral graft for multilevel occlusive disease: predictors of success and need for distal bypass. Arch Surg 1982;117:1593–1600.
36. Donaldson MC. Atherosclerosis: a vascular surgeon's view of appropriate therapeutic triage. In: First International Symposium on Cardiovascular and Interventional Radiology. Boston, October 13–16, 1992:24–32.
37. Hertzer NR, Beven EG, Young JR, et al. Coronary artery disease in peripheral vascular patients. A classification of 1000 coronary angiograms and results of surgical management. Ann Surg 1984;199(2):223–233.
38. Manson JE, Tosteson H, Ridker PM, et al. The primary prevention of myocardial infarction. N Engl J Med 1992;326:1406–1416.
39. Arlart IP, Guhl L, Edelman RR. Magnetic resonance angiography of the abdominal aorta. CVIR 1992;15:43–50.
40. Bautz W, Strotzer M, Lenz M, et al. Preoperative evaluation of the vessels of the upper abdomen with spiral CT: comparison with conventional CT and arterial DSA. Radiology 1991;181(P):261.
41. Lipchik EO, Rob CG, Schwartzberg S, et al. Obstruction of the abdominal aorta above the level of the renal arteries. Radiology 1964;82:443–446.
42. Castaneda-Zuniga W, Knight L, Formanek A, et al. Hemodynamic assessment of obstructive aortoiliac disease. AJR 1976;127:559–561.
43. Udoff EJ, Barth KH, Harrington DP, et al. Hemodynamic significance of iliac artery stenosis: pressure measurements during angiography. Radiology 1979;132:289–293.
44. Gotsman MS, Beck W, Schrire V. Selective angiography in arteritis of the aorta and its major branches. Radiology 1967;88:232–248.
45. Liu YQ, Du JH. Aorto-arteritis: further angiographic study of 231 cases. Chin Med J 1982;95:15–20.
46. Liu YQ. Radiology of aortoarteritis. Radiol Clin North Am 1985;23(4):671–688.
47. Lewis VD III, Meranze SG, McLean GK, et al. The midaortic syndrome: diagnosis and treatment. Radiology 1988;167:111–113.
48. Haynes IG, Simon J, West RJ, et al. Idiopathic retroperitoneal fibrosis with occlusion of the abdominal aorta treated by transluminal angioplasty. Br J Surg 1982;69:432–433.
49. Kittrege RD, Anderson JW. Coarctation of the lower thoracic and abdominal aorta. Radiology 1962;79:799–803.
50. Martin JF, Yount EH. Coarctation of the abdominal aorta: report of a case illustrating the value of aortography as a diagnostic aid. AJR 1956;76:782–786.
51. Pyolrala K, Heinonen O, Koskelo P. Coarctation of the abdominal aorta: review of 27 cases. Am J Cardiol 1960;6:650–652.
52. Sano K, Aiba T, Saito I. Angiography in pulseless disease. Radiology 1970;94:69–74.
53. deWolfe JA, LeFevre, Humphries AW, et al. Intermittent claudication of the hip and the syndrome of chronic aortoiliac thrombosis. Circulation 1954;9:1–16.
54. Lindsey SM, Maddison FE, Towne JB. Heparin-induced thromboembolism: angiographic features. Radiology 1979;131(3):771–774.
55. Sethi GK, Scott SM, Takaro T. The value of multiple-plane angiography in the assessment of aortoiliac disease. South Med J 1977;70(1):43–46.
56. Thomas ML, Andress MR. Value of oblique projections in translumbar aortography. AJR 1972;116(1):187–193.
57. Wylie EJ, McGuinness JS. The recognition and treatment of arteriosclerotic stenosis of major arteries. Surg Gynecol Obstet 1953;97:425–433.
58. Campbell DK, Austin RF. Seat-belt injury: injury of the abdominal aorta. Radiology 1969;92:123–124.
59. Moshyedi AC, Baxter J. Seat-belt injury of the abdominal aorta. AJR 1993;160:661–662.
60. Beuren AJ, Hort W, Kalbfleisch H, et al. Dysplasia of the systemic and pulmonary arterial system with tortuosity and lengthening of the arteries. Circulation 1969;39(1):109–115.
61. Ertugrul A. Diffuse tortuosity and lengthening of the arteries. Circulation 1967;36(3):669–672.
62. Beckwith R, Huffman ER, Eiseman B, et al. Chronic aortoiliac thrombosis: a review of 65 cases. N Engl J Med 1958;258:721–726.
63. Lowenberg EL. Changing concepts of the pathology and management of acute arterial occlusion of the lower extremities. South Med J 1958;51:35–42.
64. Kunkel P, Stead EA Jr. Blood flow and vasomotor reactions in the foot in health, in arteriosclerosis, and in thromboangiitis obliterans. J Clin Invest 1938;17:715–723.
65. Eiseman G, Waggener HU. Role and interpretation of arteriograms in atherosclerosis and atherosclerotic aneurysms. Arch Surg 1957;74:934–943.
66. Mann FC, Herrick JF, Essex HE, et al. The effect on the blood flow of decreasing the lumen of a blood vessel. Surgery 1938;4:249–252.
67. Flory CM. Arterial occlusions produced by emboli eroded aortic atheromatous plaques. Am J Pathol 1945;21:549–565.
68. Kassirer JP. Atheroembolic renal disease. N Engl J Med 1969;280:812–818.
69. Colt HG, Begg RJ, Saporito JJ. Cholesterol emboli after cardiac catheterization. Medicine 1988;67(6):389–400.

70. Kennedy A, Cumberland D, Gaines P. The pathology of cholesterol embolism arising as a complication of intra-aortic catheterization. Histopathology 1989;15:515–521.
71. Leriche R, Kunlin J, Boely C. Lesions arteritiques des iliaques et de l'aorte d'apres 90 aortographies. Lyon Chir 1950;45:5–26.
72. Leriche R. Des obliterations arterielles hautes (obliteration de la terminaison de l'aorte) commes causes des insuffisances circulatoires des membres inferieurs. Bull Mem Soc Chir Paris 1923;49:1404–1407.
73. Gottlob R. Uber Thrombosen der Aorta and der Iliacalarterien. Arch Klin Chir 1952;272:408–428.
74. Wylie EJ, Goldman L. The role of aortography in the determination of operability in arteriosclerosis of the lower extremities. Ann Surg 1958;148:325–342.
75. Boender AC, Perlberger RR. An attempt to classify the collateral systems in total occlusions at different levels of the lumbar aorta and pelvic arteries: causes and consequences. Radiol Clin 1977;46:348–363.
76. Julian O. Chronic occlusion of aorta and iliac arteries. Surg Clin North Am 1960;40:139–151.
77. Sequeira JC, Beckman CT, Levin DC. Suprarenal aortic occlusion. AJR 1979;132:773–776.
78. Martin JF, Yount EH. Coarctation of the abdominal aorta: report of a case illustrating the value of aortography as a diagnostic aid. AJR 1956;76:782–786.
79. Bron KM. Thrombotic occlusion of the abdominal aorta. AJR 1966;96(4):887–895.
80. Schenk EA. Pathology of occlusive disease of the lower extremities. Cardiovasc Clin 1973;5:287–310.
81. Muller RF, Figley MM. The arteries of the abdomen, pelvis and thigh. AJR 1957;77:296–311.
82. Leriche R. De la resection du carrefour aortoiliaque avec double sympathectomie lombaire pour thrombose arteritique de l'aorte: le syndrome de l'obliteration termino-aortique par arterite. Presse Med 1940;48:601–604.
83. Edwards EA, LeMay M. Occlusion patterns and collaterals in arteriosclerosis of the lower aorta and iliac arteries. Surgery 1955;38:950–963.
84. Krupski WC, Sumchai A, Effeney DJ, et al. The importance of abdominal wall collateral blood vessels. Arch Surg 1984;119:854–857.
85. Moskowitz M, Zimmerman H, Felson B. The meandering mesenteric artery of the colon. AJR 1964;92:1088–1099.
86. Elliott RV, Peck ME. Thrombotic occlusion of aorta as demonstrated by translumbar aortograms. JAMA 1952;148:426–431.
87. Friedenberg MJ, Perez CA. Collateral circulation in aorto-iliofemoral occlusive disease: as demonstrated by a unilateral percutaneous femoral artery needle injection. AJR 1965;94:145–158.
88. Gottlob R. Uber die "Ascendierende Arteriographie," Zugleich ein Beitrag zur Auswertung Aortographischer Bilder. Arch Klin Chir 1954;277:483–489.
89. Chait A. The internal mammary artery: an overlooked collateral pathway to the leg. Radiology 1976;121:621–624.
90. Conrad C, Corfidsen MT, Fries J. Sex-linked pattern of collaterals in iliac artery occlusive disease. Acta Radiol Diagn 1986;27(2):195–198.
91. Rian RL, Eyler WR. Aortic, iliac and visceral arterial lesions. Radiol Clin North Am 1967;5:409–432.
92. Peck JJ, Eidemiller LR. Aortoenteric fistulas. Arch Surg 1992;127:1191–1194.

44

Aneurysms of the Abdominal Aorta

DANA R. BURKE

Aneurysms of the abdominal aorta are relatively common, producing significant morbidity and mortality throughout the world. Despite great advances in the diagnosis and treatment of aneurysms, they cause an estimated 15,000 deaths per year in the United States and are the 10th leading cause of death in men over 55 years of age.[1,2] The incidence and mortality from abdominal aortic aneurysms have increased over the last 30 years.[3] Despite extensive experience and research, considerable controversy remains over the causes of abdominal aortic aneurysms, their natural history, and the most appropriate strategies for diagnosing and treating this lethal disease.

Etiology

Abdominal aortic aneurysms are defined as focal dilatations of the aorta to 1.5 times the diameter of the aorta at the renal arteries. Alternatively, a diameter of greater than 3.5 cm is used (Fig. 44-1). With the exception of those aneurysms caused by infection, trauma, or rare connective tissue diseases, abdominal aortic aneurysms have long been felt to be caused by atherosclerosis.[4] Atherosclerotic plaques are present within aneurysmal segments of the aorta to variable degrees, aneurysmal and stenotic vascular disease share certain risk factors.[5] Aneurysms are 5 to 10 times more common in men than in women, and up to 60 percent of patients with aneurysms have a history of hypertension or evidence of hypertension at autopsy. High serum cholesterol is also a risk factor, and smokers may have as much as an eightfold increase in risk compared to nonsmokers.[4–8] These similarities in risk factors and the high prevalence of coronary artery disease in patients with aneurysms convinced early investigators that abdominal aortic aneurysms are primarily a manifestation of atherosclerotic disease, and this theory is widely supported.[7]

Challenges to the traditional theory have come from epidemiologic, biochemical, and genetic research. The epidemiologic evidence is that, whereas the incidence of coronary artery disease and stroke have decreased since the mid-1960s, the incidence of abdominal aortic aneurysms has increased during this same time period.[1,3] Others have noted that patients with aneurysms tend to have generalized arteriomegaly, are significantly older, and have had a lower incidence of peripheral vascular symptoms compared with patients with stenotic aortic disease. They are also less likely to have late graft failure after repair than are patients with occlusive atherosclerotic disease.[9,10] Other research has shown that the walls of aneurysms contain less collagen and elastin and an increase in elastase compared with normal or atherosclerotic aortas.[11,12] Familial cases of abdominal aortic aneurysm are not uncommon, suggesting that there may be a genetic component as well.[13] Immediate relatives of patients with aneurysms have a much higher risk of developing aneurysms, particularly if they are children of an affected mother.[14] Some investigators feel that the genetic component of aneurysmal disease could be as high as 70 percent.[15] However, atherosclerosis is so prevalent that it clearly will tend to coexist with other disease processes even without having a direct causal relationship. The etiology of abdominal aortic aneurysms is probably multifactorial, involving an interplay of genetic, biochemical, and environmental risk factors.

Incidence

The incidence of abdominal aortic aneurysms in patients aged 60 years is 2 to 4 percent and increases with age. As mentioned, men have a 5- to 10-fold higher incidence than women.[1,3,5,6] The incidence of aneurysms is increasing, in part because more small aneu-

1073

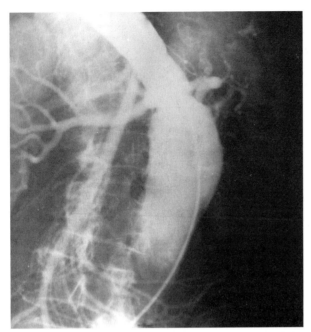

Figure 44-1. Typical infrarenal fusiform aneurysm of abdominal aorta. The aneurysm lumen demonstrated on this angiogram measures 1.5 times the diameter of the aorta at the level of the renal arteries. (Courtesy of James Spies, M.D.)

rysms are being detected. However, larger and symptomatic aneurysms have also increased by a factor of 2 to 3 over the last 30 years, indicating a true increase in incidence.[3,16] With the increased incidence has come a documented increase in mortality from aneurysms.[16]

Pathology

About 90 percent of abdominal aortic aneurysms arise below the level of the main renal arteries. They are usually fusiform in configuration, but saccular aneurysms are not uncommon (Fig. 44-2). Forty to 70 percent of aneurysms extend to involve one or more of the common iliac arteries. Hypogastric, femoral, and popliteal aneurysms are associated with abdominal aortic aneurysms, with each having an approximately 5 percent incidence in this population. Aneurysms usually contain mural thrombus due to nonlaminar flow within the diseased segment.[2,8,17,18] The aneurysm wall consistently demonstrates thinning of the media, and fragmentation and loss of elastic tissue are characteristic. The intimal involvement with atherosclerotic plaque varies from 25 to 70 percent.[1,2,4,10] Those patients with arteriomegaly, an extreme form of aneurysmal tendency, demonstrate the most loss of elastin and the least involvement with atherosclerotic plaque.[10,19]

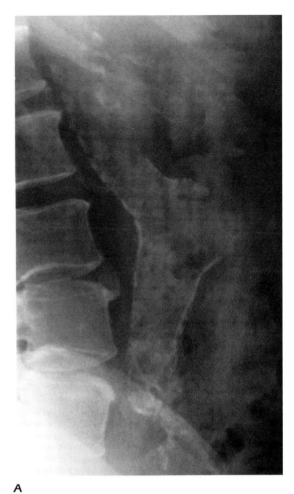

A

Figure 44-2. Nonpalpable saccular aneurysm discovered incidentally during carotid angiography. (A) Lateral scout view clearly defines the aneurysm because of heavy calcification. (B) Lateral aortogram demonstrates the patency of the superior mesenteric and inferior mesenteric (*arrow*) arteries, that the aneurysm begins well below the renal arteries, and that there is no intraluminal thrombus. (C through F) CT images at the level of the renal arteries (C), at the level of the aneurysm (D), just caudal to the origin of the inferior mesenteric artery (E), and in the common iliac arteries (F). These CT images clearly demonstrate the cephalocaudal extent of the aneurysm. Note the thin, although calcified, wall of the aneurysm and the crisp interface with adjacent retroperitoneal fat. Images (C) and (F) suggest calcified renal and iliac stenoses, but the angiogram demonstrated that these vessels were widely patent.

Inflammatory aneurysms are a variant of the abdominal aortic aneurysm in which there is marked thickening of the aneurysmal wall with striking fibrosis in the adjacent retroperitoneum. This produces adherence of adjacent structures to the anterior wall of the aneurysm, thereby complicating the surgical treatment. The incidence of inflammatory aneurysm reported in the literature ranges from 4½ to 23 percent.[17,20,21] The etiology of the fibrosis is unknown.

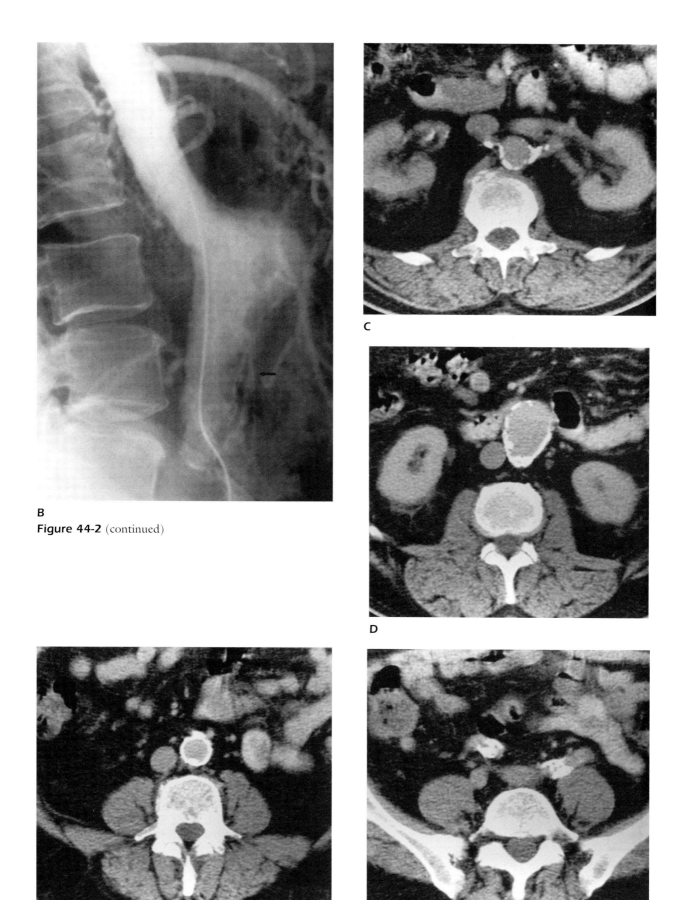

B

Figure 44-2 (continued)

C

D

E

F

Inflammation from chronically leaking blood and an autoimmune reaction to components of plaque have been proposed, but convincing evidence is lacking for either theory. The risk factors for inflammatory aneurysm do not seem to differ from those for standard aortic aneurysm. In one 30-year review of 127 patients, 7.6 percent of the patients had a family history of aneurysm, 92 percent were smokers, 50 percent had hypertension, and the male-female ratio was 30:1.[20]

Extension of the inflammatory aneurysmal process into the iliac arteries occurs in one-third to one-half of patients. The duodenum, inferior vena cava, left renal vein, and left ureter are usually involved within the inflammatory process. The overall size of these aneurysms, including the marked wall thickening, tends to be large—6 to 8 cm at the time of operation. The wall thickening is due almost entirely to adventitial thickening in the anterior and lateral walls of the aorta (Fig. 44-3). The media is thin and shows the typical fragmentation and loss of elastic tissue. There is usually

Figure 44-3. Inflammatory abdominal aortic aneurysm. (A and B) Transverse and longitudinal sonograms demonstrate the intensely echogenic aortic wall surrounded by a hypoechoic mantle of inflammatory tissue. (C) CT scan before contrast administration shows soft tissue thickening of the wall peripheral to the intimal calcification anteriorly and laterally but not posteriorly. Contrast this with the aneurysm wall in Figure 44-2. (D) Following contrast administration, there is intense enhancement of the thickened aortic wall, indicating active inflammation. Note the four layers of this process: enhancing lumen, rim of nonenhancing thrombus, calcified aortic wall, uniformly enhancing inflammatory mass. (From Cullenward MJ, et al. Inflammatory aortic aneurysm [periaortic fibrosis]: radiologic imaging. Radiology 1986;159:75–82. Used with permission.)

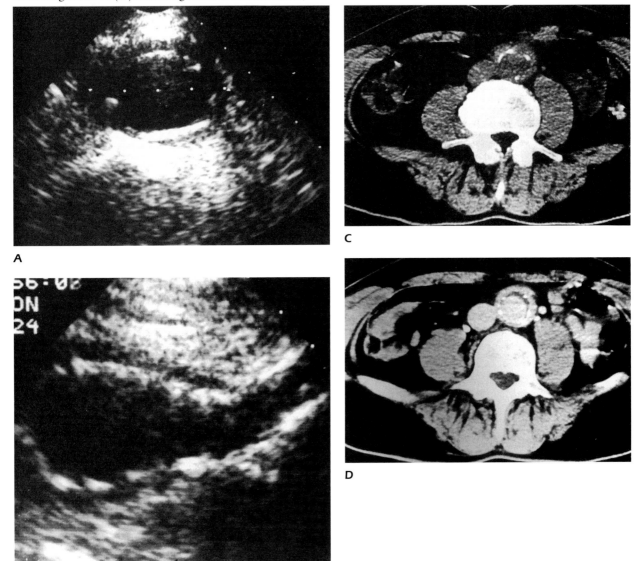

A

B

C

D

considerable involvement of the intimal surface with atherosclerotic plaque. Overall wall thickness is two to four times normal. Within the thickened adventitia and media there is an intense inflammatory infiltrate of lymphocytes and plasma cells with evidence of endarteritis of the vasa vasorum. This inflammatory picture is nonspecific and resembles the inflammatory process seen in Takayasu and giant-cell arteritides.[20] Whereas the anterior and lateral walls are thickened, there is often striking thinning of the posterior wall, and complete erosion of the posterior wall is noted in 5 to 10 percent of patients, along with exposure of the anterior spinal ligament.[20,21]

Mycotic aneurysms represent 1 to 2 percent of aneurysms of the abdominal aorta. The underlying etiology is focal destruction of the aortic wall by an infectious process. Historically, these aneurysms were most commonly caused from septic emboli from bacterial endocarditis.[22] Contiguous spread from adjacent infectious processes such as osteomyelitis and direct implantation of bacteria inadvertently during surgery or from penetrating trauma are the other recognized mechanisms of pathogenesis. *Salmonella* and *Staphylococcus aureus* are the most common etiologic agents. The primary risk factor for mycotic aneurysm is intravenous drug use. Other risk factors include altered flow dynamics such as valvular disease, coarctation, and atherosclerosis, and conditions that depress immunocompetence, such as alcoholism, diabetes mellitus, autoimmune disease, and chemotherapy or steroid treatment.[23] However, a direct invasion of normal endothelium can oc-

cur, particularly with *Salmonella*.[24,25] Up to half the patients have negative blood cultures, and a primary infectious source is often not found.[22,23]

Mycotic aneurysms tend to be lobulated and saccular, arising from the upper abdominal aorta near the margins of the renal and superior mesenteric arteries or near the aortic bifurcation (Fig. 44-4). Virulent organisms produce rapid destruction of the aortic wall with the formation of a pseudoaneurysm and early rupture. More indolent organisms tend to cause a true aneurysm because all layers of the aortic wall are damaged less rapidly. At histology the intima is destroyed and there is infiltration of the media and intima with a severe acute inflammatory process. Destruction of muscle and elastic tissue leads to the rapid dilatation.[22-25]

Syphilitic aneurysms were once the most common type of aneurysm but have become rare with the worldwide success at preventing and treating syphilis.[4,26,27] Syphilitic aneurysms usually involve the proximal abdominal aorta and tend to be saccular[26,28,29] (Fig. 44-5).

Other rare causes of abdominal aortic aneurysms include trauma and aortitis.[30]

Clinical Presentation

Aneurysms of the abdominal aorta are usually asymptomatic until they acutely expand or rupture. The percentage of asymptomatic aneurysms has increased over

Figure 44-4. Mycotic aneurysm in elderly patient presenting with back pain, chills and fever, and pulsatile abdominal mass. (A) Abdominal CT scan demonstrates opacification of the aneurysm (*An*) at the level of the renal arteries separate from a calcified nondilated aorta (*ao*). There is also an infarction of the left kidney (*arrowhead*). The paraaortic low-attenuation mass surrounding the aorta and the aneurysm does not enhance. This represented hematoma and inflammatory tissue from contained rupture of the aneurysm.

(B) Aortogram demonstrates two saccular aneurysms arising eccentrically from the aorta and impeding flow in the left renal artery, accounting for the findings of infarction on the CT. The larger aneurysm arises laterally, and the smaller aneurysm (*arrows*) arises anteriorly. The proximal location and saccular appearance are typical of mycotic aneurysms. (From Gonda RL Jr, Gutierrez OH, Axoda MVU. Mycotic aneurysms of the aorta: radiologic features. Radiology 1988;168: 343. Used with permission.)

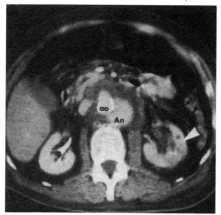

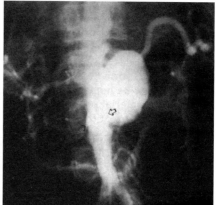

A

B

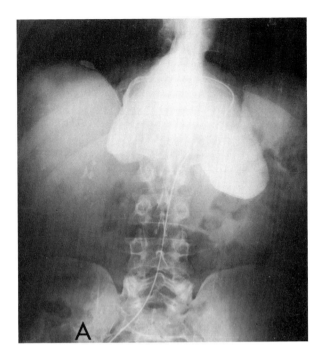

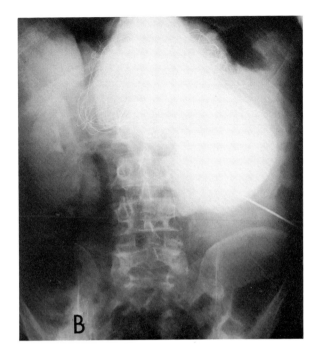

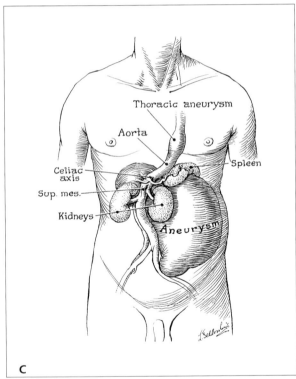

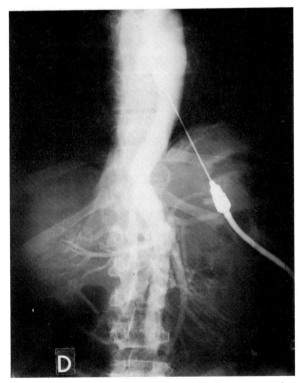

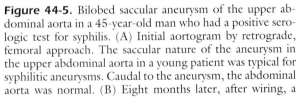

Figure 44-5. Bilobed saccular aneurysm of the upper abdominal aorta in a 45-year-old man who had a positive serologic test for syphilis. (A) Initial aortogram by retrograde, femoral approach. The saccular nature of the aneurysm in the upper abdominal aorta in a young patient was typical for syphilitic aneurysms. Caudal to the aneurysm, the abdominal aorta was normal. (B) Eight months later, after wiring, a translumbar aortogram demonstrates that the aneurysm has increased in all diameters. Note that the translumbar needle has directly punctured the aneurysm. (C) Sketch of operative findings. A separate fusiform aneurysm of the descending thoracic aorta was also found. (D) Aortogram 1 month after surgery for thoracic and abdominal components.

time as improvements in imaging have allowed the discovery of smaller aneurysms and the percentage of syphilitic aneurysms has decreased. Aneurysms are often discovered in the radiologic evaluation of abdominal pain and back pain, which are so common in the elderly population. Before the development of cross-sectional imaging, only 25 to 30 percent of aneurysms were reported to be asymptomatic, but this is because many aneurysms remained undetected until they became large enough to be easily palpable and/or symptomatic.[17,26,29] Small asymptomatic aneurysms may be palpable in nonobese patients on physical examination, but up to two-thirds of aneurysms greater than 4 cm in diameter are undetected by physical examination.[31–33] Twenty to 40 percent of patients with aneurysms have peripheral vascular ischemic symptoms that bring them to medical attention; the aneurysm is then discovered during vascular evaluation.[34–36]

Symptoms are more likely to occur in larger aneurysms, commonly manifesting as a dull ache in the periumbilical region or lower back.[5,8] Acute, intermittent exacerbations of this pain may represent small leaks from aneurysms over time. As the aneurysm size increases, it can impinge upon adjacent structures, with radiation of pain to the thigh or groin sometimes reported. Gastrointestinal symptoms are frequently recorded in patients with large aneurysms, including anorexia, nausea, vomiting, and symptoms of diverticulitis or irritable bowel. The other common set of symptoms mimics pathology in the genitourinary tract, where the pain simulates renal colic, perinephric abscess, prostatitis, testicular torsion, or epididymitis.[26,27,29,37,38]

Ruptured Aneurysms

Ruptured aortic aneurysms are virtually always symptomatic, with a classic presentation being severe abdominal pain, an enlarging pulsatile mass, and shock. However, this triad of symptoms is present in 50 percent or less of patients. The presenting symptoms can be confusing and will differ depending on the site of rupture. Most ruptures occur into the retroperitoneum from the posterior lateral aspect of the aneurysm (Fig. 44-6). Retroperitoneal rupture can

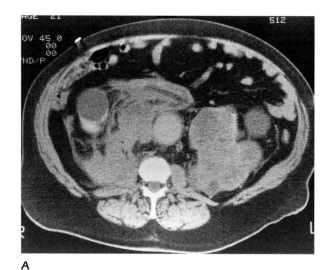

A

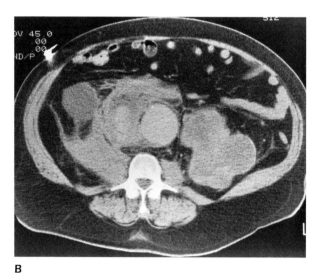

B

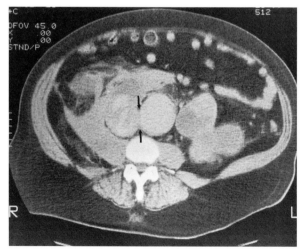

C

Figure 44-6. Ruptured aneurysm. (A) CT scan showing a large retroperitoneal soft tissue mass displacing the right kidney anteriorly. The aorta at this level measures 4 cm. There is a large, multiloculated, left lower pole renal cyst. (B) Six-centimeter aneurysm. The high attenuation within the periaortic soft tissue indicates acute hemorrhage. (C) Point of rupture in posterior lateral wall of a 6-cm aneurysm (*arrows*). Again, there is evidence of recent hemorrhage.

mimic acute pancreatitis, aortic dissection, renal colic, or acute disk herniation. Intraperitoneal rupture can mimic perforated peptic ulcer, volvulus, pancreatitis, mesenteric thrombosis, and bowel perforation with peritonitis.[38-40] Rupture directly into the intestinal lumen occurs most commonly in the duodenum but is fortunately an uncommon complication. Rapid exsanguination often ensues, but, if the leak is slower, the presentation can mimic peptic ulcer or diverticular bleeding because melena is uniformly present.[38,41] A rare, but dramatic, presentation follows rupture directly into the inferior vena cava. These patients usually have swelling of the lower extremities with engorged veins and high output cardiac failure. On physical examination there is a loud continuous murmur over the abdomen[41,42] (Fig. 44-7).

Inflammatory Aneurysms

The clinical presentation of inflammatory abdominal aortic aneurysm differs from the usual presentation in that a strikingly increased percentage of patients are symptomatic without having leaking or rupture. Most series report that two-thirds of the patients have chronic abdominal pain, and some feel that weight loss

Figure 44-7. Abdominal aortogram reveals a saccular infrarenal abdominal aortic aneurysm with an arteriovenous fistula extending from the distal aorta and right common iliac artery to the right common iliac vein and inferior vena cava. The trilobed venous pseudoaneurysm is seen to compress the inferior vena cava, partially obstructing flow. (From Raabe R, et al. Aorta/peripheral arteries: radiographic and clinical findings in unusual abdominal aortic aneurysms. Cardiovasc Intervent Radiol 1986;9:176–181. Used with permission.)

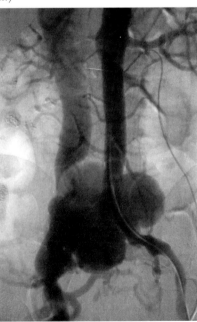

is a significant component of this disease. Genitourinary symptoms can follow from incorporation of the ureter in the periaortic inflammatory process.[19-21] Up to 20 percent of patients will have hydronephrosis.[21] In some series an elevated erythrocyte sedimentation rate was also suggestive of inflammatory aneurysm in patients with known aneurysms. Clinical evidence of associated arterial occlusive disease was present in 44 percent of patients in one large series.[20]

Mycotic Aneurysms

Mycotic aneurysms usually present with nonspecific symptoms such as fever, chills, weakness, and malaise. Larger aneurysms are more likely to be symptomatic, causing back pain or urologic complaints. Blood cultures may be negative in almost one-half of cases. The typical location in the suprarenal aorta should strongly suggest the diagnosis. Because of the nonspecific symptoms and the tendency to early rupture, a high index of suspicion is essential for diagnosis and surgical treatment before rupture[22-24] (Fig. 44-8).

Syphilitic Aneurysms

The age at presentation for syphilitic aneurysms tends to be younger than for the usual abdominal aortic an-

Figure 44-8. Mycotic saccular aneurysm of the right common iliac artery due to a *Salmonella* infection. This 60-year-old man had an acute history of night sweats, shaking, chills, and low back pain radiating to the groin and extending to the right lower abdominal quadrant. The initial diagnosis was perforating appendicitis. The right fourth lumbar artery (*arrow*) is dilated, an angiographic indication of poor flow of blood through the right iliac system due to compression from the aneurysm. The aneurysm was successfully repaired with a Dacron graft.

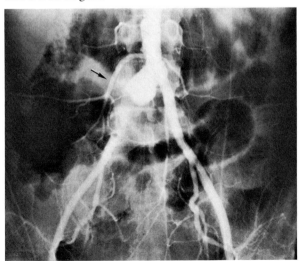

eurysm. These aneurysms are also more likely to produce symptoms unrelated to leaking or rupture. The increase in symptomatology is related to their location in the upper abdomen, where they impress on adjacent organs and erode the spine (see Fig. 44-5).[26-29]

Natural History

Considerable controversy exists as to the natural history of aneurysms of the abdominal aorta. Rates of expansion and risks of rupture differ widely in published series. Autopsy-based series tend to have higher estimated risks of rupture for given aneurysm size.[27,28,39] Darling reported an incidence of 18 percent for aneurysms 5 cm or less in diameter, 20 percent for those between 5 and 7 cm in diameter, 60 percent for those between 7 and 10 cm, and 95 percent for those over 10 cm.[39] Several clinical studies have followed patients with untreated abdominal aortic aneurysms. In Estes' series, 63 percent of the patients died from rupture of the aneurysm.[26] However, a recent retrospective clinical study estimated a 1 percent 6-year cumulative incidence of rupture for aneurysms less than 4.0 cm, a 2 percent incidence for those 4.0 to 4.9 cm, and a 20 percent incidence for those 5.0 cm or greater.[43] Referral center series tend to publish higher rates of growth and risks of rupture than do community-based studies, particularly for aneurysms less than 5 cm in diameter.[44,45] Annual rates of growth of 2 to 8 mm are reported, with the high values for larger aneurysms, whose walls are under greater tension because of their increasing diameter, according to the law of Laplace.[46] There is considerable individual variation among patients in the rate of growth and the risk of rupture, further confounding the issue (Figs. 44-9 and 44-10). Most physicians agree that aneurysms greater or equal to 5 cm in diameter should be electively repaired.

Radiographic Evaluation

Detection and Serial Evaluation

Standard projection radiographs done for back pain or abdominal pain (Fig. 44-11) or as part of an intravenous pyelogram (Fig. 44-12) or barium study can detect calcification of the wall of an aneurysm in approximately 50 percent of cases.[32,47] Before cross-sectional imaging was developed, the size of aneurysms over time was monitored with plain radiographs, primarily on the basis of the mass effect produced on adjacent

organs or displacement of the aortic wall calcification.[47,48]

Ultrasound is the imaging study that detects the majority of unsuspected aneurysms during the course of evaluating patients for other abdominal problems. Aneurysms detected or suspected on plain films are confirmed and evaluated with an ultrasound examination. The examination should be done with the highest-megahertz transducer that provides adequate penetration, usually 5.0 or 3.5 MHz. Care must be taken to provide axial and sagittal images that are perpendicular and parallel to the long axis of the aneurysm, respectively. Because of elongation and buckling of the aneurysm, the long axis of the aneurysm is often not parallel to the long axis of the patient's body, and oblique scanning can produce inaccurate measurements. With good technique, however, ultrasound depicts the length and diameter of aneurysms with great accuracy and is the preferred method for monitoring the size of aneurysms until a decision to operate is made (Fig. 44-13).[6,33,49] With color flow and Doppler techniques, experienced ultrasonographers can frequently determine the relationship of the aneurysm to the renal arteries and iliac arteries (Fig. 44-14), but this level of expertise is not widely available.

Once an aneurysm has been detected, its size should be monitored with repeat ultrasound examinations at 6-month intervals. If the aneurysm appears to be expanding rapidly (more than 3 mm between examinations), the follow-up study interval should be reduced to 3 months.

If suboptimal imaging with ultrasound is obtained, usually because of obesity or excessive bowel gas, computerized tomography (CT) scanning without contrast is indicated.

Preoperative Evaluation

Once ultrasound has demonstrated a rapid increase in aneurysm diameter or enlargement to 5 cm, the patient is a candidate for elective aneurysm repair.

CT scanning with intravenous contrast is requested by most surgeons before operation. The abdomen and pelvis should be scanned at 1-cm intervals as rapidly as possible during mechanical injection of iodinated contrast at a rate of 2 to 4 ml per second for a total volume of 100 of 150 ml. CT scanning not only confirms the maximum diameter of the aneurysm but also reliably defines the craniocaudal extent of the aneurysm and determines whether it involves the iliac arteries (Fig. 44-15). The intravenous contrast enhancement makes it easier to detect renal arteries and their relationship to the aneurysm (see Fig. 44-24) and

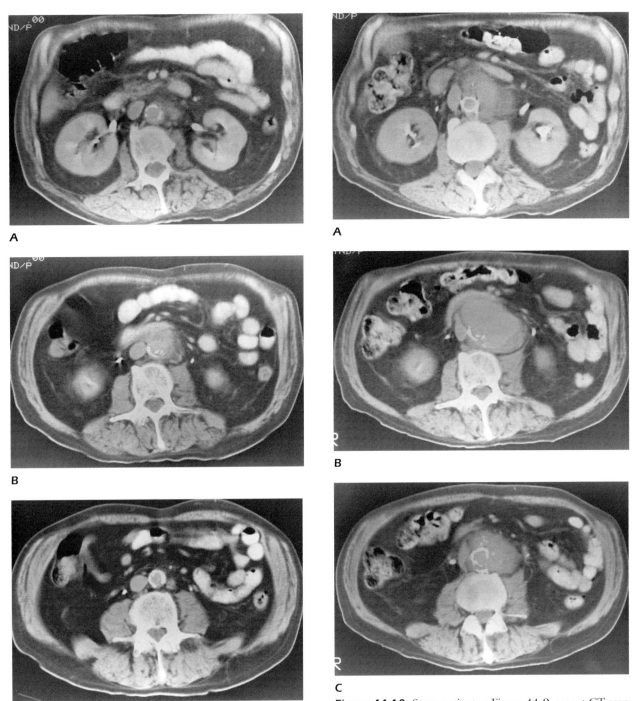

Figure 44-9. This 70-year-old man had an abdominal CT scan as part of an evaluation for abdominal pain. (A) Calcified normal-caliber aorta in upper abdomen. (B) Three-centimeter aneurysm. The lack of crisp interface between the aneurysm and retroperitoneal fat did not cause alarm at this time because of the small size of the aneurysm. This in retrospect probably represented a small leak from the aneurysm. (C) Normal-caliber aorta distal to the aneurysm with crisp interface with adjacent retroperitoneal fat.

Figure 44-10. Same patient as Figure 44-9; repeat CT scan following acute exacerbation of abdominal pain 12 days later. (A to C) Images from the same levels as in Figure 44-9 clearly show a large amount of abnormal soft tissue in the retroperitoneum with disruption of the ring of calcium within the wall of the aorta due to rupture of this 3-cm aneurysm.

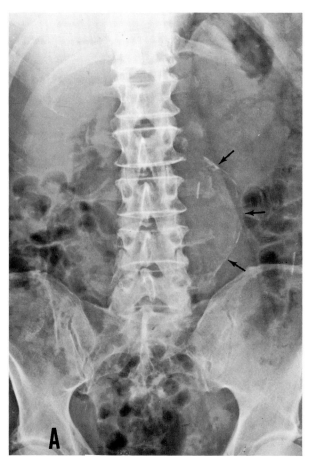

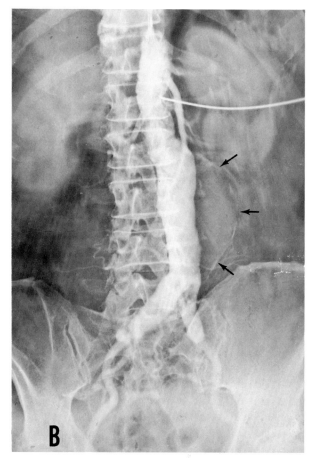

Figure 44-11. (A) Film done to evaluate abdominal pain shows the typical curvilinear calcification in a large lower abdominal aortic aneurysm (*arrows*). (B) Translumbar aortogram demonstrates the lumen of the aneurysm, which also

extends into the common iliac arteries. The portion of the aneurysm between the opacified lumen and the calcified wall is occupied by thrombus. This patient also had a popliteal artery aneurysm.

demonstrates the enhancing fibrosis of inflammatory aneurysms well[17,49] (see Fig. 44-3). CT also gives an overview of the abdomen and retroperitoneum and can demonstrate the relationship of the ureters and renal veins to the aneurysm. Standard CT scanning is relatively poor at demonstrating the number of renal arteries when they are multiple, or at assessing for stenotic disease in the visceral or iliac branches (see Fig. 44-2C and F and Fig. 44-15A).[49-52]

Angiography is a minimally invasive but very safe method to evaluate the abdominal aorta, its branches, and peripheral vasculature.[35,53,54] The procedure is usually performed from a femoral artery or occasionally a brachial artery approach using a small (4 or 5 French) multiple side hole catheter. In current practice translumbar aortography is seldom performed because of limited catheter positioning for optimizing the study, increased patient discomfort, and increased risks compared with peripheral-access, small-catheter angiography.

Figure 44-12. A 59-year-old man complained of dull, aching pains in the left back and buttock, radiating to the thigh. Film from an intravenous pyelogram demonstrates marked displacement without obstruction of the left ureter (*black arrow*) by an aneurysm 5 cm in diameter (*white arrows*).

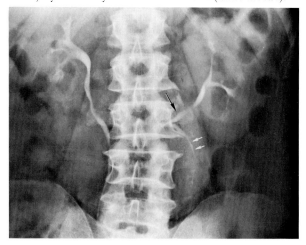

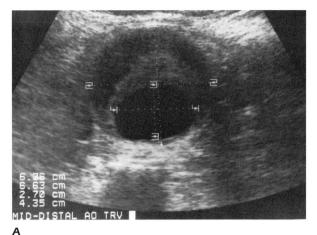

A

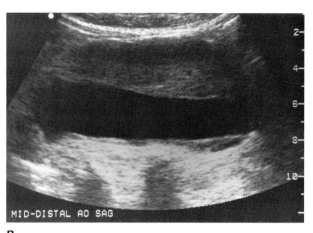

B

Figure 44-13. Ultrasound of abdominal aorta using 3.5-MHz transducer. (A) Axial image allows precise measurement of the aneurysm diameter in the transverse and anteroposterior dimensions. Echogenic thrombus is easily distinguished anterior to the remaining patent lumen. (B)

True longitudinal image through the aneurysm showing a large amount of thrombus anterior to the remaining lumen. The aneurysm was greater than 6 cm. (Courtesy of Barbara J. Dinsmore, M.D.)

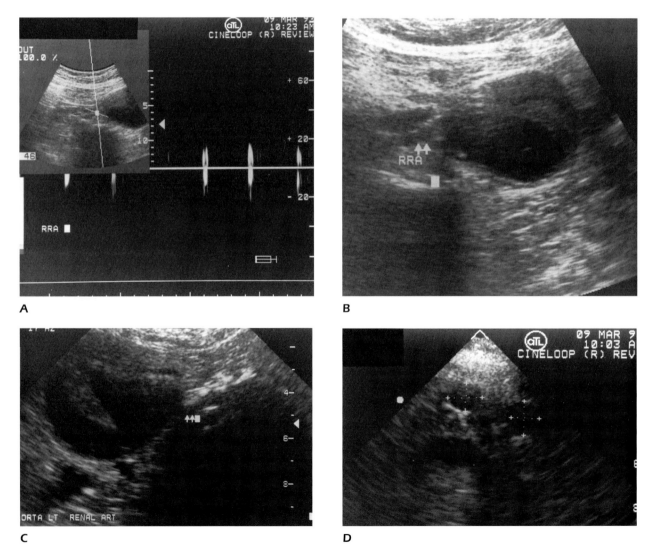

A

B

C

D

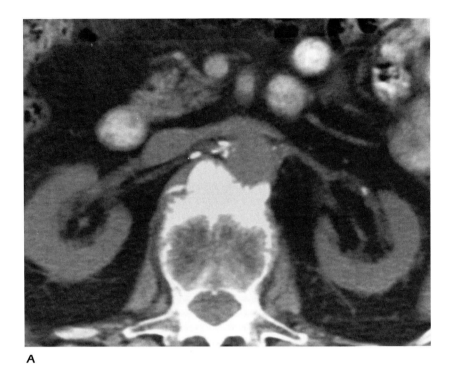

A

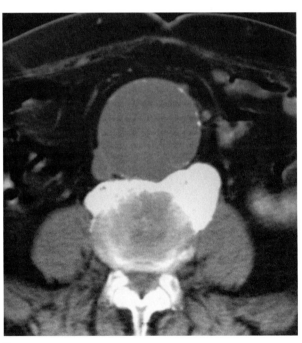

B

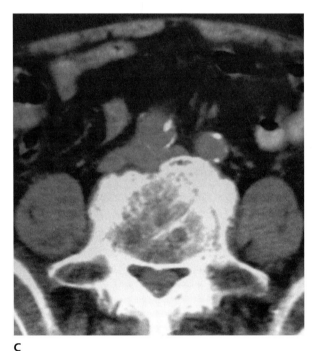

C

Figure 44-15. Preoperative evaluation of abdominal aortic aneurysm using CT. (A) The origins of both renal arteries are clearly seen arising from a normal-caliber aorta, indicating an infrarenal location of the aneurysm. No right renal artery stenosis was present on the angiogram. (B) Thin-walled 6-cm aneurysm with no evidence of inflammatory wall thickening or retroperitoneal leak. (C) The right common iliac artery is also involved with the aneurysm, indicating the need for a bifurcation graft.

◄ **Figure 44-14.** Ultrasound demonstration of relationship of branch vessels to aneurysm. (A) Doppler probe being used to identify right renal artery by its arterial flow pattern. (B) Closeup showing right renal artery (*RRA*) arising from the aneurysmal portion of the aorta. (C) The left renal artery (*white arrows*) also arises from the aneurysm. Doppler also demonstrated patency of this vessel. (D) The aneurysm involves the common iliac arteries with thrombus in the anterior aspect of the right iliac artery. (Courtesy of Barbara J. Dinsmore, M.D.)

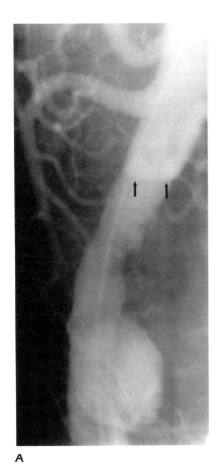

A

Angiography is routinely done as an outpatient study, with 4 to 6 hours of postprocedure bedrest before discharge.[55]

Films of the aorta are acquired in the frontal and lateral views during injection of 40 ml of contrast at 15 to 20 ml per second in the upper abdominal aorta. The lateral view is needed to assess the origins of the celiac and superior mesenteric arteries as well as the patency of the inferior mesenteric artery, or to identify the collaterals that reconstitute the inferior mesenteric artery's circulation if the origin is occluded (Fig. 44-16). Filling of the inferior mesenteric artery may require injection directly into the distal aorta because contrast layering can lead to nonopacification of a patent inferior mesenteric artery and a false sense that it is occluded (Fig. 44-17). Frontal or preferably oblique

Figure 44-16. Biplane abdominal aortogram from right femoral approach. (A) Lateral aortogram demonstrates widely patent celiac axis and superior mesenteric arteries in the upper abdominal aorta. The renal arteries arise well above the aneurysm (*arrows*). (B) Anteroposterior aortogram shows that the renal arteries are widely patent, that the inferior mesenteric artery is patent (*arrow*), and that the aneurysm ends above the aortic bifurcation. (C) Persistent opacification of aneurysm lumen. Patency of the left third and fourth lumbar arteries (*arrows*) indicates that the left posterior lateral wall is not involved with the aneurysm. (Courtesy of James Spies, M.D.)

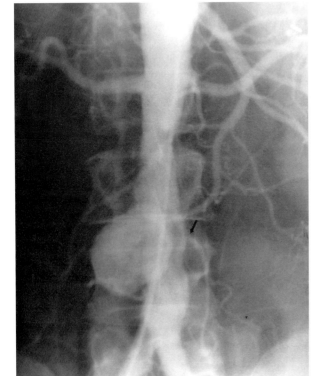

B

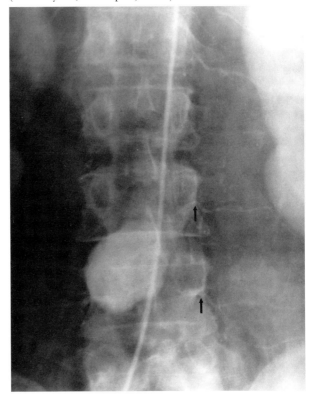

C

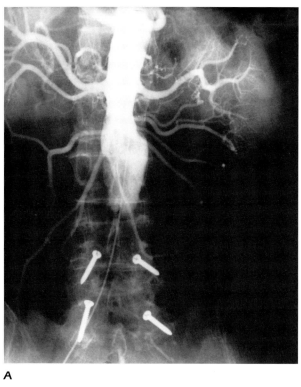

A

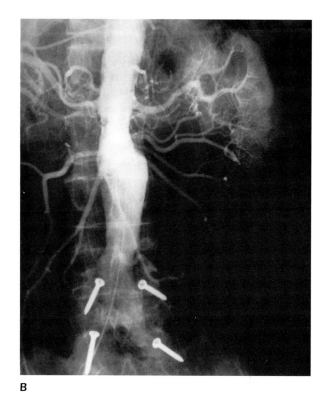

B

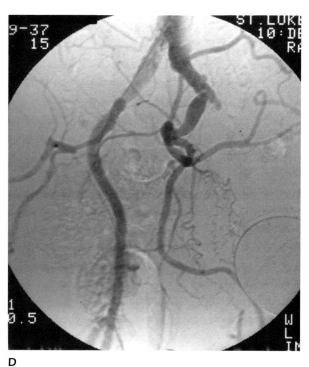

C

D

Figure 44-17. Low aortic injection to define visceral artery anatomy. (A) Early phase of aortogram demonstrates single arteries to each kidney but no arterial supply to the lower pole of the left kidney. (B) Midarterial phase opacifies the aneurysm lumen and the large left fourth lumbar artery but not the inferior mesenteric artery or collateral supply to its distribution via the arch of Riolan or marginal artery of Drummond. Arterial supply to the left lower pole of the kidney is not identified. (C) Digital right anterior oblique angiogram after withdrawing the catheter into the aneurysm.

The inferior mesenteric artery is now well demonstrated (*arrow*) because contrast is now in contact with the anterior wall of the aorta, where the inferior mesenteric artery arises. The stenotic left lower pole renal artery arises just cephalad to the inferior mesenteric artery (*arrowhead*). It was reimplanted at surgery. (D) Steep right anterior oblique pelvic angiogram shows complete occlusion of the left external iliac artery, indicating the need to extend the graft to a left femoral artery.

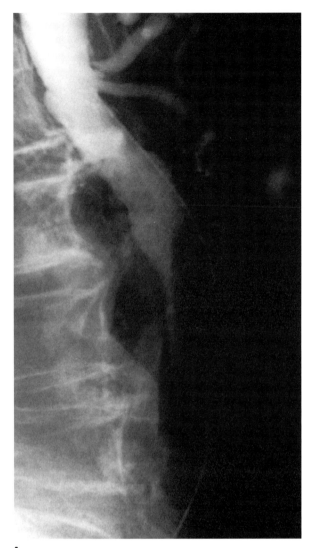

A

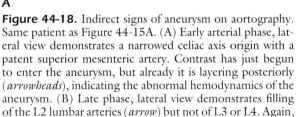

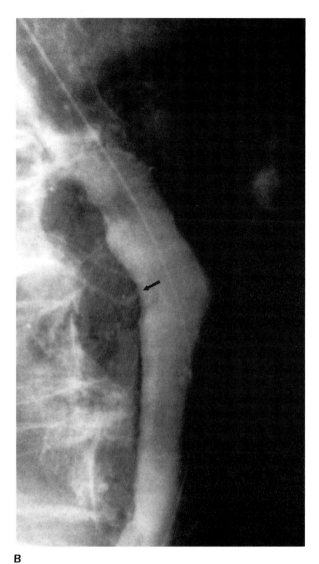

B

Figure 44-18. Indirect signs of aneurysm on aortography. Same patient as Figure 44-15A. (A) Early arterial phase, lateral view demonstrates a narrowed celiac axis origin with a patent superior mesenteric artery. Contrast has just begun to enter the aneurysm, but already it is layering posteriorly (*arrowheads*), indicating the abnormal hemodynamics of the aneurysm. (B) Late phase, lateral view demonstrates filling of the L2 lumbar arteries (*arrow*) but not of L3 or L4. Again,

the contrast layers posteriorly to the catheter. (C) Late phase, anteroposterior view shows angulation of the lumen, straight smooth interface between the contrast and thrombus, and absence of filling of the lower lumbar arteries. Even without the information provided on the CT scan, the presence of an aneurysm is obvious from the angiographic findings.

views of the pelvis to include the common femoral arteries are performed while injecting 15 to 25 ml of contrast at 5 to 10 ml per second. In patients with peripheral ischemic symptoms, runoff angiography is included, tailored to the individual patient. The study is filmed with conventional technique, or preferably with digital subtraction technique. Sixteen-inch, high-resolution image intensifiers with 1024 matrix digital systems produce images that approach the resolution

of conventional film angiograms yet require much less contrast and allow significantly shortened examination times.

Aortography directly demonstrates the patent lumen of the aneurysm. The lumen may range in size from "normal" diameter to full aneurysm diameter, depending on the amount of intraluminal thrombus. When the remaining lumen approximates normal aortic diameter, the presence of an aneurysm is usually

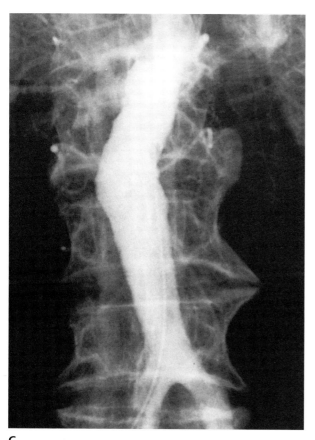

C

Figure 44-18 (continued)

indicated by one or more indirect signs. As contrast enters the aneurysm, there is marked slowing of its progression due to abnormal flow dynamics within the aneurysm, and the contrast quickly layers posteriorly. Characteristic signs are abrupt angulation of the lumen; a straight, smooth interface between the contrast and thrombus; absence of lumbar arteries; mass effect upon the adjacent organs; and calcification within the wall (Fig. 44-18).[35,50,56]

The routine use of angiography before surgery was debated even before the emergence of excellent cross-sectional imaging.[34,35,47] The proponents of routine preoperative angiography feel that it provides information that is essential or useful in planning surgery in up to 60 percent of patients. Angiography is particularly useful in demonstrating the number and location of aberrant renal arteries and in detecting stenotic disease of renal and mesenteric vessels; it also identifies collateral visceral circulation (Fig. 44-19; see also Fig. 44-17) and stenotic or aneurysmal disease of the pelvic and peripheral arteries (Figs. 44-20 and 44-21).[18,34,36] Others believe that the information regarding the number of renal arteries and the status of the visceral circulation can be determined by inspection and palpation at the time of operation and reserve preoperative angiography for those patients with lower extremity claudication, suspected renovascular hypertension,

Figure 44-19. Right lower pole accessory renal artery. (A) Anteroposterior abdominal aortogram from left femoral puncture shows early branching of the main right renal artery but nonopacification of the lower pole of the right kidney. The fusiform infrarenal aneurysm is well demonstrated. (B) Closeup of later arterial phase demonstrates a stenotic right lower pole renal artery arising below the aneurysm just above the aortic bifurcation (*arrowheads*). Because of the stenosis there is very slow flow within this vessel. It was treated with endarterectomy and reimplantation during repair of the aneurysm with a tube graft. Because the vessel courses posteriorly to the aneurysm, it would have been sacrificed if it had not been identified preoperatively on the angiogram.

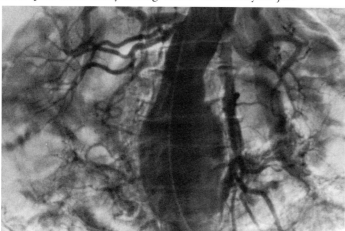

A

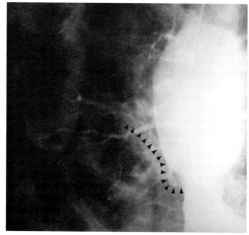

B

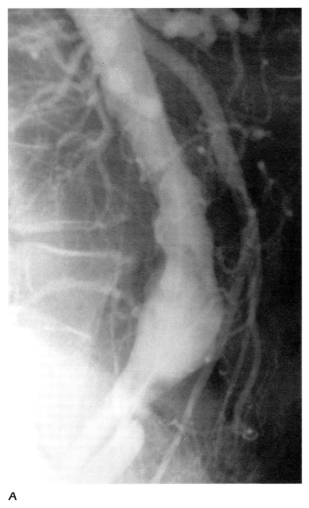

A

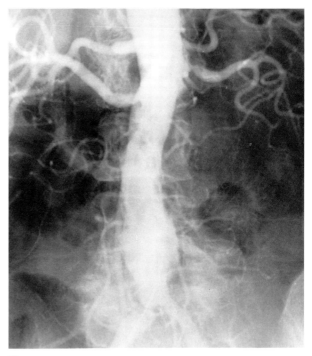

B

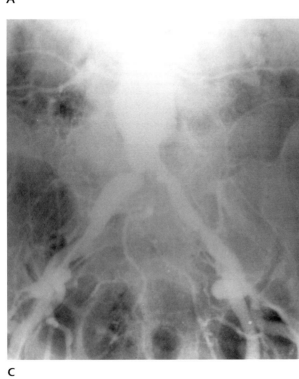

C

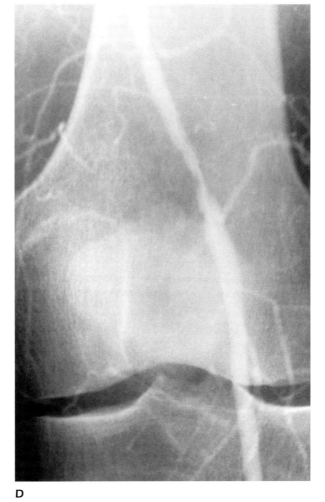

D

visceral angina, aneurysms involving the juxtarenal or suprarenal aorta, suspected aneurysms of the femoral or popliteal vessels, and horseshoe kidney.[50,56]

Magnetic resonance imaging (MRI) provides excellent depictions of aneurysms of the abdominal aorta as well as of large visceral branches using conventional spin-echo techniques. It can demonstrate the findings in multiple planes in addition to the axial (Fig. 44-22).[49,50,52,57] It requires no intravenous contrast. However, it is limited in detecting multiple renal arteries and shares the limitation of standard CT in detecting visceral and iliac stenotic disease. Because MRI is significantly more expensive than CT and currently provides limited additional information, it is not widely used for preoperative assessment.[49,57,58] However, patients with severe allergy to iodinated contrast agents or poor renal function can be safely and effectively evaluated with MRI rather than contrast-enhanced CT.

Early reports on magnetic resonance angiography suggest that it could replace angiography in certain situations.[59] As these techniques are refined, MRI may play an increasing role in the evaluation of abdominal aortic aneurysms.

Spiral volumetric computed tomography (spiral CT) is a recently developed technique that provides continuous scanning during 360-degree gantry rotation while the patient is simultaneously moving through the gantry. Intravenous contrast is injected while the area of interest is scanned over 30 seconds. This method produces information that can provide three-dimensional images as well as images in any plane desired.[60] The technique is particularly well suited for evaluating abdominal aortic aneurysms because of its high resolution, lack of motion and flow artifacts, accurate depiction of all iliac, renal, and mesenteric branches, and short procedure time of 20 minutes (Fig. 44-23). Stenoses of aortic branches are particularly well demonstrated, giving spiral CT a distinct advantage over CT, ultrasound, and MRI.[60,61] However, it is not practical for evaluating the peripheral vasculature because its coverage is limited to 40 cm or less. Improved x-ray tube capacity and detector sensitivities

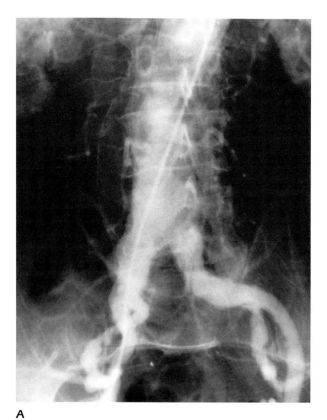

A

Figure 44-21. Abdominal aortic aneurysm with multiple associated aneurysms. (A) Late arterial phase of abdominal aortogram shows distal abdominal aortic aneurysm extending into the common iliac arteries bilaterally.

are expected to improve resolution and anatomic coverage in the future.

The choice of preoperative imaging modality depends on the preference of the surgeon, the presence of newer technologies such as spiral CT and MRI, and the availability of the expertise to apply newer technologies and interpret the information they provide. If noninvasive imaging technology continues to improve and the expertise in its use becomes more widespread, the need for catheter angiography in the presurgical

---

◀ **Figure 44-20.** A 75-year-old man with high blood pressure, severe right lower extremity claudication, and abdominal aortic aneurysm demonstrated on ultrasound. Lateral (A) and anteroposterior (B) views of the aortogram demonstrate a 4-cm distal abdominal aortic aneurysm. There is a high-grade left renal artery stenosis producing poststenotic dilatation, indicating its hemodynamic significance. Renal vein renin sampling confirmed renovascular hypertension. (C) A pelvic angiogram demonstrates the aneurysm but also shows right common iliac origin stenosis with poststenotic or separate aneurysmal dilatation of the right common iliac artery. (D) Lower extremity angiogram also shows high-grade right popliteal artery stenosis, which in conjunction with the iliac lesion and poor inflow due to the aneurysm accounted for the patient's severe right lower extremity claudication. The patient was successfully treated with aortoiliac graft. After surgery the left renal artery stenosis and right popliteal artery stenosis were successfully treated with angioplasty.

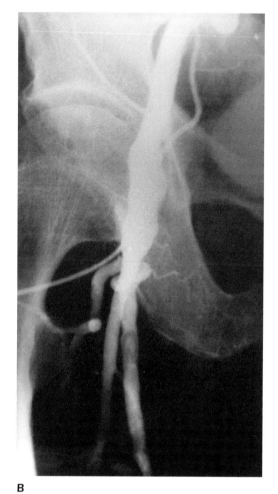

B

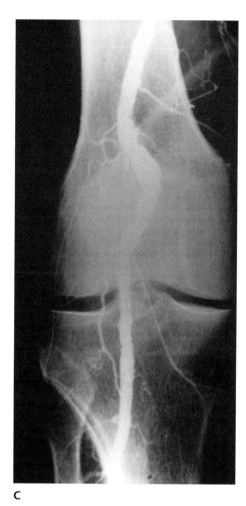

C

Figure 44-21 (continued). (B) Right lower extremity angiogram demonstrates right common femoral artery aneurysm. The left common femoral artery was also abnormally dilated. (C) The popliteal artery demonstrates the characteristic angulation and luminal dilatation of a popliteal artery aneurysm. (Courtesy of James Spies, M.D.)

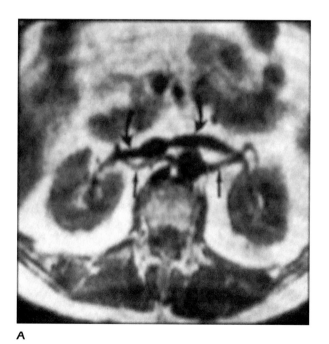

A

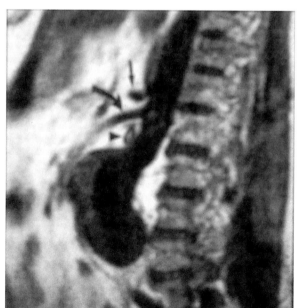

B

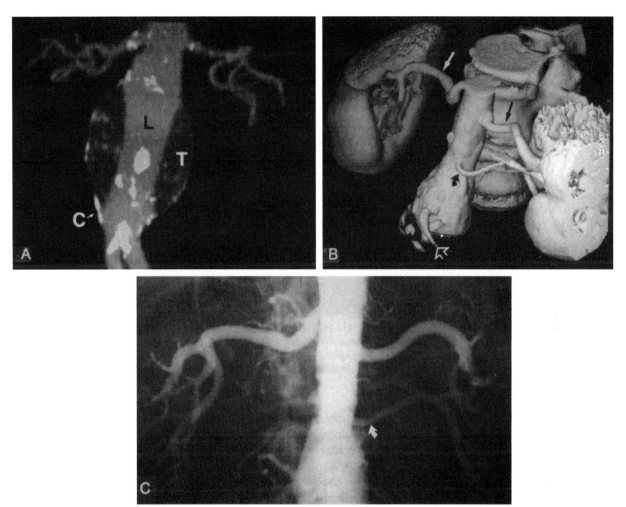

Figure 44-23. Three-dimensional spiral computed tomographic angiogram. (A) Maximum intensity projection of abdominal aortic aneurysm demonstrates contrast-filled lumen (*L*), mural thrombi (*T*), and mural calcifications (*C*). (B) Left anterior oblique shaded-surface display of another patient with an abdominal aortic aneurysm. Although the main renal arteries (*straight arrows*) arise above the neck of the aneurysm, the small left accessory renal artery (*curved arrow*) and patent inferior mesenteric artery (*open arrow*) arise from the anterior aspect of the aneurysm. (C) Conventional aortogram of same patient as in (B). (From Rubin GD, Walker PJ, Drake MD, et al. Three-dimensional spiral computed tomographic angiography: an alternative imaging modality for the abdominal aorta and its branches. J Vasc Surg 1993;18:656. Used with permission.)

evaluation of aortic aneurysms should be greatly reduced in the future.

Recently a new procedure, endoluminal grafting, has been used to treat aortic aneurysms. This method requires the precise placement of a graft anchored with metal stents inside the aorta from a femoral artery approach using fluoroscopic guidance. Since the operating physician does not have the opportunity to directly visualize or palpate the aorta and its branches, this technique requires more thorough preprocedure and postprocedure imaging than does standard surgical repair. Currently, patients are routinely evaluated before and after the procedure with CT—usually spiral CT—and angiography (personal communication,

◄ **Figure 44-22.** Magnetic resonance imaging of aortic aneurysm. (A) Axial T1-weighted image, 600/32 (TR/TE), at level of renal hilus shows renal arteries (*straight arrows*) and renal veins (*curved arrows*). The aorta is normal in size (compare with Fig. 44-15). (B) Sagittal image, 600/32, shows the aortic aneurysm. The superior mesenteric artery (*curved arrow*), celiac axis (*straight arrow*), and left renal vein (*arrowhead*) are also seen. (From LaRoy LL, Cormier PJ, Matalon TAS, et al. Imaging of abdominal aortic aneurysms. AJR 1989;152:785–792. Used with permission.)

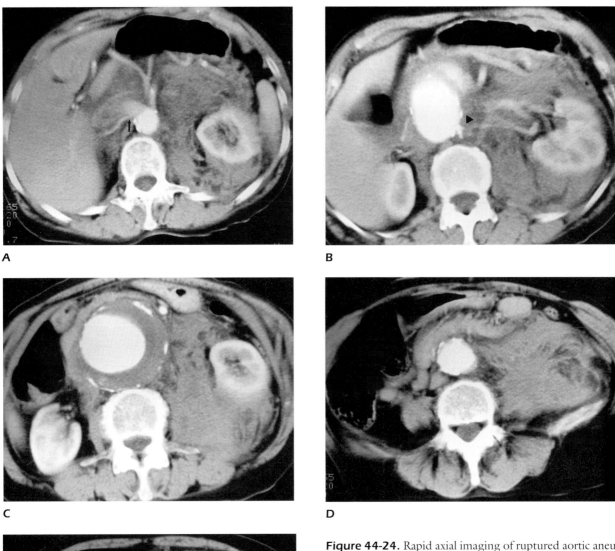

Figure 44-24. Rapid axial imaging of ruptured aortic aneurysm with spiral CT. (A) Upper abdominal image demonstrates a large amount of abnormal retroperitoneal density from the ruptured aneurysm. The superior mesenteric artery and right renal artery (*arrow*) arise above the aneurysm. (B) The left renal artery (*arrowhead*) arises from the upper portion of the aneurysm. Contrast enhancement facilitates this identification. The left kidney is displaced laterally and anteriorly by the large retroperitoneal hematoma. (C) The maximum diameter of the aneurysm is 8 cm. There is a large amount of mural thrombus. (D) The aorta returns to nearly normal caliber before the aortic bifurcation. (E) The iliac arteries are not aneurysmal. This patient was scanned with the spiral CT technique from the diaphragm to the sacroiliac joints in 22 seconds. On the basis of this study, the surgeon knew that he could perform a tube graft rather than the more time-consuming bifurcation graft, but that he needed to re-implant the left renal artery. The operation was successful.

Dr. Michael Drake). As this technique evolves, the role of preprocedural and follow-up imaging will be clearly defined.

Evaluation of Suspected Leaking or Ruptured Aneurysm

Radiologic imaging should not be performed on hemodynamically unstable patients, particularly if they have known aneurysms. These patients should be transported to the operating room as rapidly as possible because even several minutes' delay can be critical. However, many patients with leaking or contained rupture will remain hemodynamically stable for hours or even days, allowing time for rapid evaluation with ultrasound or, preferably, CT.[29,39,41] Many patients with known aneurysms who develop acute abdominal or back pain have other etiologies of the pain that may not be best treated with emergency laparotomy, such as pancreatitis, mesenteric ischemia, or renal colic. In the past a CT scan of the abdomen and pelvis took 45 to 60 minutes, introducing an unacceptable delay in the evaluation of a potentially rapidly lethal disease. With current generation of CT scanners, particularly those using slip ring technology (spiral CT), the entire abdomen can be scanned in less than 1 minute, with the round trip to the CT scanner consuming 10 minutes or less (Fig. 44-24). If rapid CT imaging is available, hemodynamically stable patients can be safely scanned emergently to confirm the diagnosis before the operation.

The CT diagnosis of ruptured aneurysm depends on the identification of an aneurysm associated with high-attenuation paraaortic fluid collections, usually displacing the kidneys anteriorly (see Figs. 44-6 and 44-24). Intravenous contrast is not needed to make the diagnosis of rupture but can help differentiate rupture from other causes of paraaortic fluid such as abscess. Contrast enhancement can provide additional information relevant to surgery concerning the relationship of the aneurysm to branch vessels and variant vascular anatomy, particularly of the inferior vena cava and left renal vein. CT can also diagnose other paraaortic pathology causing back pain, such as adenopathy or retroperitoneal fibrosis.[62,63] In one series of 65 patients suspected of ruptured aneurysm, 18 patients had the CT findings of rupture and were taken promptly to surgery, with a mortality of only 25 percent. The remainder of the patients had no aneurysms, had aneurysms repaired electively with no mortality, were not surgical candidates, or were found to have other diagnoses on CT scanning.[63]

Angiography is usually not recommended in cases of suspected rupture of aortic aneurysms because CT, in general, provides more information in a shorter time. However, the angiographic findings of rupture are well documented from before the era of excellent cross-sectional imaging. These include contrast accumulation outside the calcified wall of the aneurysm or projecting away from an otherwise smooth-walled lumen with pooling of this extravasated contrast after washout of the intraluminal contrast[40] (Fig. 44-25). An unusual type of rupture is one into the inferior vena cava or left renal vein, usually a retroaortic renal vein.[64] The resulting aortovenous fistula presents classically with abdominal pain and pulsatile mass associated with lower extremity edema and high-output heart failure.[41] The angiogram demonstrates the aneurysm and the exact point of connection of the arteriovenous fistula (see Fig. 44-7). These angiogram findings are characteristic and are needed for planning operative repair.

Evaluation of Postoperative Complications

Postoperative infection of aortic prosthetic grafts occurs in 1 to 2 percent of patients overall but is three times as common if the aneurysm has ruptured preoperatively.[65] The most common organism is *Staphylococcus epidermidis.* The signs and symptoms of infected grafts are nonspecific and include fever, abdominal pain, malaise, pulsatile mass, and draining sinus. The patient may present within days of surgery or months or even years later.[65,66]

Anastomotic pseudoaneurysms occur from failure of the suture line caused by suture breakdown or excess tension on the anastomosis. They may also occur secondary to infection of the graft.[65,67]

Aortoenteric fistula occurs following suture line breakage from graft infection and then erosion into bowel. The duodenum is the most commonly involved portion of the gastrointestinal tract.[65,66]

CT scanning is the best method for evaluating the complications of aortic graft surgery. Perigraft hematoma and gas are normal findings in the immediate postoperative period. Complete resolution of hematomas usually occurs within 3 months, and all ectopic gas should be reabsorbed by 3 to 4 weeks.[66] The CT findings of graft infection are perigraft fluid, soft tissue density, or ectopic gas beyond this time period or increasing in amount over time (Fig. 44-26).[65,66] Aortoenteric fistulas do not have specific findings, but in these cases ectopic gas and focal bowel wall thickening suggest the diagnosis (Fig. 44-27). However, graft infection can be present without any abnormalities

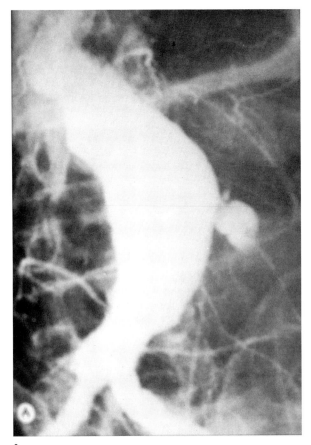

A

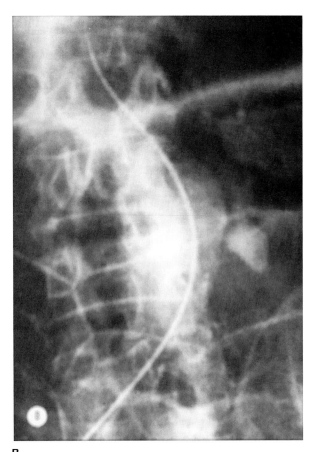

B

Figure 44-25. Ruptured 10-cm aortic aneurysm. (A) Aortogram showing infrarenal fusiform abdominal aortic aneurysm. The opacified lumen measured 4.5 cm. Note the irregular area of extravasation extending laterally to the remainder of the lumen. (B) Late phase showing retention of contrast in the area of extravasation. At surgery a 10-cm aneurysm was found that had ruptured into the retroperitoneum on the left. (From Chisolm AJ, Sprayregen S. Angiographic manifestations of ruptured abdominal aortic aneurysms. Am J Roentgenol 1976;127:769. Used with permission.)

noted on radiologic imaging.[65,66] Pseudoaneurysms can be detected with ultrasound, CT, or MRI.[67] Angiography is usually performed after diagnosis to help plan the operative repair (Fig. 44-28).

Screening for Abdominal Aortic Aneurysm

Screening of patients with radiologic imaging to detect unsuspected abdominal aortic aneurysms is a controversial issue. The extremely high morbidity and mortality from ruptured aneurysm (75–90 percent) compared with the very minimal morbidity and mortality from elective repair (5 percent) suggests that detection before rupture is critical.[32] In addition, it is a growing public health problem because the mortality from aneurysms of the abdominal aorta is increasing.[3,33] The problem is compounded by the fact that as many as 50 percent of aneurysms 5 cm or greater in diameter are undetected by physical examination, and most aneurysms are asymptomatic up to the time of rupture.[31,33] For these reasons, ultrasound screening of high-risk groups, such as hypertensive white males who smoke, has been recommended.[6,32] However, despite the relatively low cost of ultrasound, this would be an extremely expensive undertaking because of the low prevalence of the disease in the at-risk population.[31,47] The cost-effectiveness of such a program would depend on the value society places on saving a life and on carefully selecting the population to be screened on the basis of age, sex, family history, and risk factors.[6,31–33, 68]

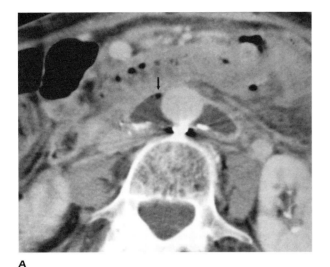

A

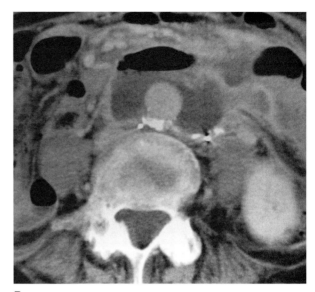

B

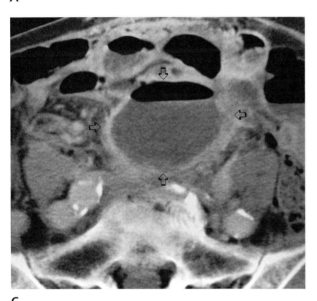

C

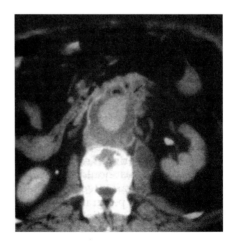

D

Figure 44-26. This patient had fever and an elevated white count 1 month after aneurysm repair. (A) Image through proximal graft demonstrates opacification of the graft, indicating patency. There is fluid around the graft, along with a tiny amount of gas (*arrow*). As isolated findings these are not definitive for graft infection at this interval after surgery.

(B) However, lower images demonstrate a large amount of periaortic fluid with a large air-fluid level (*arrowheads*). (C) Caudal to the aortic bifurcation there is an abscess with an air-fluid level (*open arrows*). These findings are conclusive evidence of graft infection. (D) The patient was treated with graft resection and extraanatomic bypass (*large arrow*).

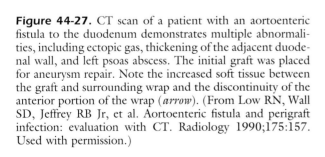

Figure 44-27. CT scan of a patient with an aortoenteric fistula to the duodenum demonstrates multiple abnormalities, including ectopic gas, thickening of the adjacent duodenal wall, and left psoas abscess. The initial graft was placed for aneurysm repair. Note the increased soft tissue between the graft and surrounding wrap and the discontinuity of the anterior portion of the wrap (*arrow*). (From Low RN, Wall SD, Jeffrey RB Jr, et al. Aortoenteric fistula and perigraft infection: evaluation with CT. Radiology 1990;175:157. Used with permission.)

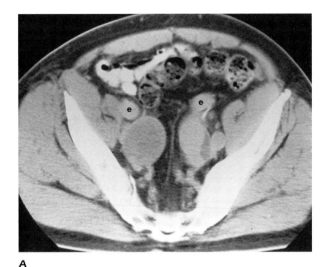

A

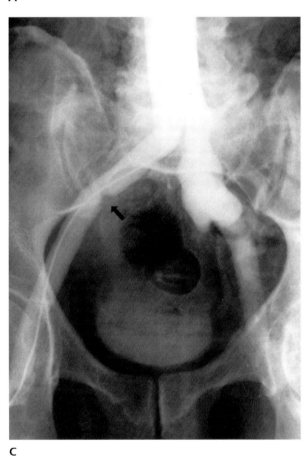

C

B

Figure 44-28. Anastomotic pseudoaneurysms following aortofemoral graft. (A) Axial CT image with contrast at level of lower sacroiliac joint. Two iliac aneurysms are identified posterior to the external iliac arteries (*e*). The right aneurysm is completely thrombosed, as indicated by the lack of opacification. The left is only partially thrombosed. (B) Image 2 cm caudal to (A). Both aneurysms are thrombosed. They are medial to the internal iliac arteries (*i*). These were incidental findings on CT done to evaluate abdominal pain. (C) Preoperative angiogram shows only irregularity at the anastomosis of the right limb because of complete thrombosis of this pseudoaneurysm (*arrow*). On the left the only partially thrombosed pseudoaneurysm is clearly demonstrated and corresponds well with the CT images.

References

1. Reilly JM, Tilson MD. Incidence and etiology of abdominal aortic aneurysms. Surg Clin North Am 1989;69:705–711.
2. Reuler JB, Kumar KL. Abdominal aortic aneurysm. J Gen Intern Med 1991;6:360–366.
3. Melton LJ III, Bickerstaff LK, Hollier LH, et al. Changing incidence of abdominal aortic aneurysms: a population-based study. Am J Epidemiol 1984;120:379–386.
4. Blakemore AH, Voorhees AB Jr. Aneurysm of the aorta: a review of 365 cases. Angiology 1954;5:209–231.
5. Swinton NW Jr, Jewell ER, Tsapatsaris NP. Abdominal aortic aneurysms. Cardiol Clin 1991;9:483–488.
6. Thurmond AS, Semler HJ. Abdominal aortic aneurysm: incidence in a population at risk. J Cardiovasc Surg 1986;27:457–460.
7. Reed D, Reed C, Stemmermann G, et al. Are aortic aneurysms caused by atherosclerosis? Circulation 1992;85:205–211.
8. Ruberti U, Scorza R, Biasi GM, et al. Nineteen year experience on the treatment of aneurysms of the abdominal aorta: a survey of 832 consecutive cases. J Cardiovasc Surg 1985;26:547–553.
9. Tilson M, Stansel H. Differences in results for aneurysm vs occlusive disease after bifurcation grafts. Arch Surg 1980;115:1173–1175.
10. Tilson M, Dang C. Generalized arteriomegaly: a possible predisposition to the formation of abdominal aortic aneurysms. Arch Surg 1981;116:1030–1032.
11. Sumner D, Hokanson D, Strandness D. Stress-strain characteristics and collagen-elastin content of abdominal aortic aneurysms. Surg Gynecol Obstet 1970;130:459–466.

12. Cannon D, Read R. Blood elastolytic activity in patients with aortic aneurysms. Ann Thorac Surg 1982;34:10–15.
13. Johansen K, Koepsell T. Familial tendency for abdominal aortic aneurysms. JAMA 1986;256:1934–1936.
14. Cole C, Barber G, Bouchard A, et al. Abdominal aortic aneurysm: the consequences of a positive family history. Can J Surg 1989;32:117–120.
15. Powell J, Greenhalgh R. Multifactorial inheritance of abdominal aortic aneurysms. Eur J Vasc Surg 1987;1:29–31.
16. Lilienfeld DE, Gunderson PD, Sprafka JM, et al. Epidemiology of aortic aneurysms: I. Mortality trends in the United States, 1951 to 1981. Arteriosclerosis 1987;7:637–643.
17. Cullenward MJ, Scanlan KA, Pozniak MA, et al. Inflammatory aortic aneurysm (periaortic fibrosis): radiologic imaging. Radiology 1986;159:75–82.
18. Bunt TJ, Cropper L. Routine angiography for abdominal aortic aneurysm: the case for informed operative selection. J Cardiovasc Surg 1986;27:725–727.
19. Thomas ML. Arteriomegaly. Br J Surg 1971;58:690–697.
20. Pennell RC, Hollier LH, Lie JT, et al. Inflammatory abdominal aortic aneurysms: a thirty-year review. J Vasc Surg 1985;2:859–869.
21. Boontje AH, van den Dungen JJAM, Blanksma C. Inflammatory abdominal aortic aneurysms. J Cardiovasc Surg 1990;31:611–616.
22. Weintraub RA, Abrams HL. Mycotic aneurysms. AJR 1968;102:354–362.
23. Gonda RL Jr, Gutierrez OH, Axoda MVU. Mycotic aneurysms of the aorta: radiologic features. Radiology 1988;168:343.
24. Kario K, Mizuno Y, Kanatsu K, et al. Infected abdominal aortic aneurysm due to salmonella: CT evaluation. Clin Imaging 1991;15:261–264.
25. Flamand F, Harris KA, DeRose G, et al. Arteritis due to salmonella with aneurysm formation: two cases. Can J Surg 1992;35:248–252.
26. Estes JE Jr. Abdominal aortic aneurysm: a study of one hundred and two cases. Circulation 1950;11:258–264.
27. Brindley P, Stembridge VA. Aneurysms of the aorta: a clinicopathologic study of 369 necropsy cases. Am J Pathol 1956;32:67–82.
28. Gliedman ML, Ayers WB, Bestal BL. Aneurysms of the abdominal aorta and its branches: a study of untreated patients. Ann Surg 1957;146:207–215.
29. Boyes-Barratt BG. Symptomatology and prognosis of abdominal aortic aneurysm. Lancet 1957;2:716–720.
30. Hills EA. Behcet's syndrome with aortic aneurysms. Br Med J 1967;4:152–154.
31. Bergqvist D, Bengtsson H. Should screening for abdominal aortic aneurysms be advocated? Acta Chir Scand 1990;555(Suppl):89–97.
32. Allen PIM. Screening for abdominal aortic aneurysm. Biomed Pharmacother 1988;42:451–454.
33. Norman PE, Castleden WM, Lawrence-Brown MMD. Screening for abdominal aortic aneurysms. NZJ Surg 1992;62:333–337.
34. Kwaan JHM, Connolly JE, Vander Molen R, et al. The value of arteriography before abdominal aneurysmectomy. Am J Surg 1977;134:108–114.
35. Rösch J, Keller FS, Porter JM, et al. Value of angiography in the management of abdominal aortic aneurysm. Cardiovasc Radiol 1978;1:83–94.
36. Brewster DC, Retana A, Waltman AC, et al. Angiography in the management of aneurysms of the abdominal aorta: its value and safety. N Engl J Med 1975;292:822–825.
37. Moore WS, Preger L, Hall AD. Abdominal aortic aneurysms. Calif Med 1968;108:345–349.
38. Blum L. Ruptured aneurysm of abdominal aorta. NY State J Med 1968;39:2061–2066.
39. Darling RC. Ruptured arteriosclerotic abdominal aortic aneurysms: a pathologic and clinical study. Am J Surg 1970;119:397–401.
40. Chisolm AJ, Sprayregen S. Angiographic manifestations of ruptured abdominal aortic aneurysms. Am J Roentgenol 1976;127:769.
41. Bower TC, Cherry KJ Jr, Pairolero PC. Unusual manifestations of abdominal aortic aneurysms. Surg Clin North Am 1989;69:745–753.
42. Beall BC Jr, Cooley DA, Morris GC Jr, et al. Perforation of arteriosclerotic aneurysms into inferior vera cava. Arch Surg 1963;86:137–146.
43. Guirguis EM, Barber GG. The natural history of abdominal aortic aneurysms. Am J Surg 1991;162:481–483.
44. Katz DA, Littenberg B, Cronenwett JL. Management of small abdominal aortic aneurysms: early surgery vs watchful waiting. JAMA 1992;268:2678–2686.
45. Nevitt MP, Ballard DJ, Hallett JW Jr. Prognosis of abdominal aortic aneurysms: a population-based study. N Engl J Med 1989;321:1009–1013.
46. Limet R, Sakalihassan N, Albert A. Determination of the expansion rate and incidence of rupture of abdominal aortic aneurysms. *J Vasc Surg* 1991;14:540–548.
47. Hodges PC. Radiology: roentgenographic manifestations of abdominal aortic aneurysm. Postgrad Med 1964:A-77–A-82.
48. Janower ML. Ruptured arteriosclerotic aneurysms of the abdominal aorta: roentgenographic findings on plain films. N Engl J Med 1962;265:12–15.
49. LaRoy LL, Cormier PJ, Matalon TAS, et al. Imaging of abdominal aortic aneurysms. AJR 1989;152:785–792.
50. Bandyk DF. Preoperative imaging of aortic aneurysms: conventional and digital subtraction angiography, computed tomography scanning, and magnetic resonance imaging. Surg Clin North Am 1989;69:721–735.
51. Papanicolaou N, Wittenberg J, Ferrucci JT Jr, et al. Preoperative evaluation of abdominal aortic aneurysms by computed tomography. AJR 1986;146:711–715.
52. Pavone P, Di Cesare E, Di Renzi P, et al. Abdominal aortic aneurysm evaluation: comparison of US, CT, MRI, and angiography. Magn Reson Imaging 1990;8:199–204.
53. Hessel SJ, Adams DF, Abrams HL. Complications of angiography. Radiology 1981;138:273–281.
54. Cragg AH, Nakagawa N, Smith TP, et al. Hematoma formation after diagnostic angiography: effect of catheter size. J Vasc Intervent Radiol 1991;2:231–233.
55. Katzen BT, Van Breda A, Rholl KS, et al. Outpatient femoral arteriography: results in 1000 patients. J Intervent Radiol 1987;2:141–143.
56. Gordon DH, Martin EC, Schneider M, et al. The complementary role of sonography and arteriography in the evaluation of the atheromatous abdominal aorta. Cardiovasc Radiol 1978;1:165–171.
57. Flak B, Li DKB, Ho BYB, et al. Magnetic resonance imaging of aneurysms of the abdominal aorta. AJR 1985;144:991–996.
58. Kandarpa K, Piwnica-Worms D, Chopra PS, et al. Prospective double-blinded comparison of MR imaging and aortography in the preoperative evaluation of abdominal aortic aneurysms. J Vasc Intervent Radiol 1992;3:83–89.
59. Kim D, Edelman RR, Kent KC, et al. Abdominal aorta and renal artery stenosis: evaluation with MR angiography. Radiology 1992;174:727–731.
60. Rubin GD, Walker PJ, Drake MD, et al. Three-dimensional spiral computed tomographic angiography: an alternative imaging modality for the abdominal aorta and its branches. J Vasc Surg 1993;18:656.
61. Galanski M, Prokop M, Chavan A, et al. Renal arterial stenoses: spiral CT angiography. Radiology 1993;189:185–192.
62. Rosen A, Korobkin M, Silverman PM, et al. CT diagnosis of ruptured abdominal aortic aneurysm. AJR 1984;143:265–268.
63. Kvilekval KHV, Best IM, Mason RA, et al. The value of computed tomography in the management of symptomatic abdominal aortic aneurysm. J Vasc Surg 1990;12:28–33.
64. Raabe R, Lawrence PF, Luers PR, et al. Aorta/peripheral arteries: radiographic and clinical findings in unusual abdominal aortic aneurysms. Cardiovasc Intervent Radiol 1986;9:176–181.

65. Hermreck AS. Prevention and management of surgical complications during repair of abdominal aortic aneurysms. Surg Clin North Am 1989;69:869–895.

66. Low RN, Wall SD, Jeffrey RB Jr, et al. Aortoenteric fistula and perigraft infection: evaluation with CT. Radiology 1990;175: 157.

67. Guinet C, Buy J, Ghossain MA, et al. Aortic anastomotic pseudoaneurysms: US, CT, MR, and angiography. J Comput Assist Tomogr 1992;16:182–188.

68. Quill DS, Colgan MP, Sumner DS. Ultrasonic screening for the detection of abdominal aortic aneurysms. Surg Clin North Am 1989;69:713–719.

45

Renal Angiography: Techniques and Hazards; Anatomic and Physiologic Considerations

ERIK BOIJSEN

Four decades have passed since Seldinger[1] published his method of percutaneous catheterization of the femoral arteries. The advantages and risks of this technique have been analyzed in detail, and the literature on this subject is extensive. The basic technique has not changed over the years, but the complications of percutaneous renal angiography have been markedly reduced. The technical improvements responsible for this change include developments in needle, guidewire, and catheter design; in radiographic equipment for catheterization and documentation; and in new contrast media. This change is welcome, because the renal angiographic procedure is not, and can never be, completely free from risks for the patient. It is therefore rational to reduce the number of renal angiographic examinations and replace them with noninvasive imaging methods, which are less traumatic, give more information about the renal parenchyma and renal function, and are cost-effective. Nevertheless, despite technical advances in ultrasound with duplex and color Doppler imaging,[2,3] in magnetic resonance imaging (MRI),[4,5] and recently also in computed tomographic (CT) angiography,[6] these techniques cannot completely replace conventional renal angiography. For a short period intravenous digital subtraction angiography (DSA) was considered an acceptable alternative, but it was soon realized that intraarterial contrast deposition was a requirement for adequate information on the renal vasculature[7,8] and intraarterial DSA is now considered to belong to the group of conventional angiographic techniques.

Many of the complications of renal angiography can be avoided with proper technique, since most complications occur because of lack of experience and improper handling of the material.[9,10] Because renal angiography will continue to be used, perhaps mainly for therapeutic reasons, there is reason to analyze and discuss proper technique and how complications can be avoided.

Preparation

The patient should be well informed about why and how the procedure is performed and what discomfort he or she may experience. There is no reason to frighten the patient by talking about all the complications that can occur, but the patient should know that there are certain but very small risks with the method and that these must be accepted for proper treatment.

It should be clear that the radiologist has full responsibility for the examination. The radiologist should refuse to perform angiography if there is any indication that the patient will not tolerate the procedure or feels that the reason for the examination is not adequate. The case history and the previous clinical and radiologic examinations should be carefully reviewed before a decision is made to perform angiography.

The bowel should be cleansed in a routine way. During the day of the examination, the patient should be allowed light meals and a free intake of fluids to prevent dehydration. The patient's groin should be shaved before he or she is sent to the angiography suite.

Since it is important that the patient is relaxed during the examination, a sedative should be given if the patient is tense. To this should be added 0.5 mg of atropine to prevent any vasovagal reflex that can occur in predisposed patients. Before the procedure is started, the blood pressure should be recorded and the pulsations of the artery distal to the puncture site should be checked.

Puncture Site

In renal angiography, the femoral artery is the most common entrance site for the catheter. However, because modern guidewires and catheters have smaller dimensions than they did a decade ago, both translumbar and transbrachial approaches are gaining popularity, especially for introducing 4 to 5 French (1.27- to 1.59-mm) catheters.[11–16] The transbrachial approach appears especially promising because the general tendency is to perform these procedures on an outpatient basis.[14] The translumbar approach is rarely used for renal angiography, and the transaxillary approach is outdated because of the high complication rate.[9]

After local anesthesia is given, the common femoral or brachial artery is punctured with a needle varying in size between 18 gauge (1.28 mm) and 21 gauge (0.82 mm), depending on the guidewire and catheter and the artery into which they will be introduced. The common femoral artery should be punctured below the inguinal ligament, which is situated just above the inguinal crease, except in obese patients, in whom the ligament may be high above the crease.[10,17] At this level, the common femoral artery passes anterior to the medial part of the femoral head, where it can be efficiently compressed after catheter extraction. The brachial artery is punctured 2 to 3 cm above the antecubital crease on an extended and supinated arm.[14] The left brachial artery is usually punctured because it is easier to pass the catheter to the descending aorta from the left side.

Guidewires, Catheters, and Catheterization Technique

Guidewires vary in size and construction. Most guidewires have a J-shaped flexible tip to negotiate tortuosity and to avoid subintimal passage or perforation.[18] The common size used for the femoral artery has been 0.89 mm, but the smaller guidewires, 0.45 or 0.81 mm,[13,14] are often used for lumbar renal aortography, from either the femoral artery or the brachial artery. Improvements in guidewires include increased rigidity for better torque control and for facilitating catheter introduction[13]; a movable core for increased flexibility[19]; platinum coating for increased visibility[20]; and Teflon coating with a central canal for interventional radiography.[21]

The guidewire should never be allowed to pass into the artery against resistance. When the guidewire tip is in the iliac or central brachial-subclavian arteries or in the aorta, the needle is retracted, slight pressure is applied over the entrance, and the previously selected

catheter is passed over the guidewire. All guidewires are thrombogenic. Heparin coating has been shown to render them temporarily resistant to thrombus deposition.[22–26] Further developments are the hydrophilically coated guidewires, which are slippery and reduce thrombus formation.[27,28]

The *catheter* used for renal angiography depends on the indication for the examination. Two main types of catheters are used, one for aortic injection and one for selective renal angiography. Originally, the catheter introduced for aortic injection was of polyethylene with an end hole. The tip was positioned at the level of origin of the renal arteries. The drawback of this type of catheter was that a large part of the bolus of contrast medium reached the splanchnic arteries, with consequent reduction of information regarding the renal vasculature. To reduce the jet effect, side holes were introduced and the tapered tip was occluded[29] (see Fig. 49-11).

Other variations of the catheter design for semi-selective aortography (*Etagen-Aortographie*) were developed. A loop catheter[30,31] (a catheter with no end hole but two side holes, introduced via a Teflon sheath[32]) and a catheter with a long, tapered tip[33] (later called a *pigtail catheter*[34]) were developed. Another type of catheter had two side holes close to the top hole; the top of the catheter was placed in one renal artery and the two side holes were positioned in the aorta close to the opposite renal artery.[35,36] However, with the high injection rate required for renal aortography (20 ml per second), there is an obvious risk of subintimal deposition of contrast medium in the catheterized renal artery. Since renal artery dissection was also observed with this technique, the use of this catheter was abandoned.[36] The radiopaque catheter most commonly used for renal angiography has a 6 or 7 French outer diameter, which means it can deliver contrast medium at a rate of about 20 ml per second when it is placed in the lumbar aorta. As mentioned previously, there is a tendency to reduce the size of the catheters to 4 or 5 French because technical developments have made them tolerate high injection pressure. Smaller catheters are also easy to find on the monitor because of the higher resolution in the imaging system. These "high-flow" catheters can accept flows up to 30 ml per second and are well suited for total or nonselective renal angiography.[12,13,37–39] Because the thrombogenicity and vessel trauma mainly depend on catheter size, there is reason to believe that the complication rate can be almost completely eliminated at the puncture site with the use of these smaller catheters.[13]

It is generally agreed that in renal angiography an aortic injection of contrast medium should precede selective angiography and the selective method should be performed only if the expected information is not obtained by the survey angiogram. Selective angiography is rarely needed if the quality of the aortic study is good. A good aortic study can be obtained in most cases if *semiselective renal angiography* is performed. The catheter used for this purpose is a thin-walled radiopaque catheter (outer diameter/inner diameter, 2.2/1.45 mm) with a 3-cm tapered part (outer diameter/inner diameter, 1.4/1.0 mm). The catheter has six side holes just proximal to the tapered part (Figs. 45-1 and 45-2A,B). The tip of the catheter is positioned in one of the main renal arteries. When contrast medium is delivered at a rate of 20 ml per second, approximately the same amount passes through the top hole as through each side hole. When the usual total amount of 30 ml per second is injected, about 5 ml passes through the top hole over a period of 1.5 seconds, and 25 ml is deposited in the aorta, close to the opposite main renal artery (Fig. 45-3D; see also Figs. 45-2A and B, 45-9, 45-10, 45-11, and 49-2). Thus both selective angiography and nonselective renal angiography are achieved at the same time. If necessary, the tip of the catheter then can be positioned in the contralateral renal artery to gain more detailed information about that kidney. The tapered tip of the catheter should be formed so that it follows as closely as possible the course of the renal artery. Therefore, a slight bend on the most distal part is appropriate (see Figs. 45-1 and 45-2). The rather slow rate of injection into the catheterized renal artery guarantees an atraumatic injection of contrast medium. We have found this technique advantageous in, for example, renal hypertension, particularly when marked stenosis is present, because the thin catheter tip can pass such a stenosis without interfering with the blood flow.

The pigtail catheter has been used for nonselective renal angiography with great advantage compared with many other varieties. However, the tip of this catheter has been reported to enter an intercostal artery during contrast medium injection, with consequent spinal cord damage.[40] The reason for this problem seems to be that the tapered part, which is curved, straightens as a result of the jet effect. The straightening does not occur with a semiselective catheter because the main bend is in the more rigid part of the catheter.

Hawkins[37,39] and Cope[13] have shown that adequate high flow is obtained with 4 and 5 French catheters, and the catheters will remain in the same position during the entire injection period if appropriate application of side holes is made. The catheters will not whip or recoil, and subintimal injection of contrast medium can be avoided.

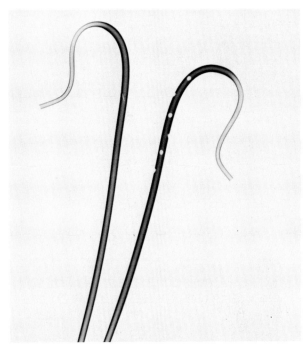

Figure 45-1. Catheter design for selective and semiselective renal angiography.

Selective renal angiography requires an exchange of catheters. The same type of catheter may be used as for semiselective angiography, but without side holes (see Figs. 45-1, 45-2C and D, and 45-3E). The catheter has a tapered distal part with an outer diameter of 1.4 mm. Consequently, the distal part of the catheter does not have a very sharp and rigid tip, as do other selective catheters. Both 3 and 4 French catheters can also be used for selective renal angiography with or without the use of the telescope technique with 6 French catheters; these larger catheters are mainly used in interventional angiography, where balloon catheters are also useful.[13,20,21,41-45]

Complications due to Guidewires and Catheters

Subintimal Dissection

Although rarely reported, subintimal dissection of the renal artery has serious consequences for the patient[36,46-52] (Fig. 45-4; see also Fig. 45-3). It may cause instant, severe hypertension, which must be treated with arterial repair or nephrectomy. If the occlusion is not complete, watchful waiting and anticoagulant therapy and repeated scintigraphic checks may be the best treatment.[36,53] It is said that the lesion occurs more often in patients with atherosclerosis or fibromuscular dysplasia with hypertension, but it may occur in any

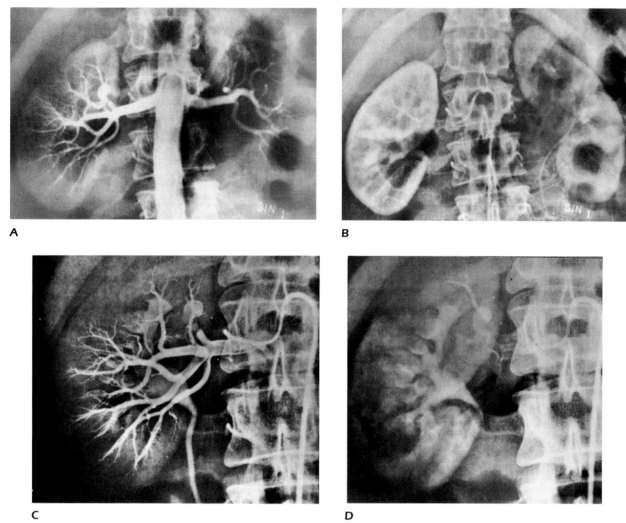

A

B

C

D

Figure 45-2. Renovascular hypertension due to short stenosis in cranial branch of ventral artery with a jet aneurysm. (A and B) Semiselective right renal angiography, arterial and capillary phases. Note the delayed circulation in the branch supplying the anterior part of the upper pole. The catheter is shaped according to the course of the renal artery. (C and D) Selective angiography with a tapered catheter without side holes. Two micrograms of angiotensin was given before the contrast medium injection. Note the marked delay in the perfusion of the ischemic segment. A 1-mm-long stenosis and a jet aneurysm are well demonstrated.

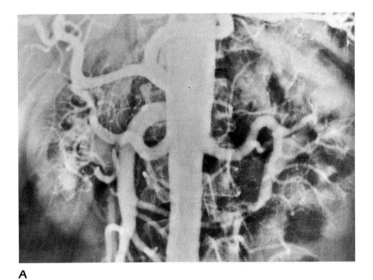

A

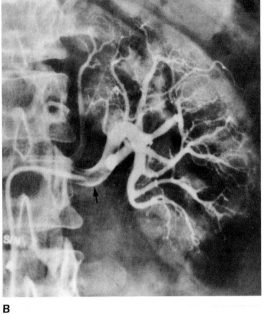

B

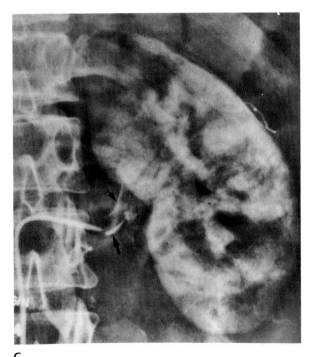

C

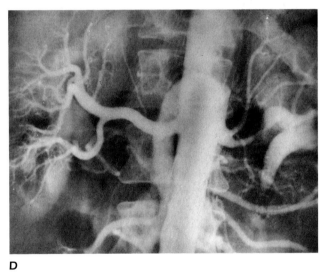

D

Figure 45-3. A 37-year-old man examined because of hematuria. (A) Nonselective renal angiography and (B and C) selective left renal angiography, arterial and nephrographic phases. No abnormality is observed. The sleevelike subintimal deposit of contrast medium (*arrows*) at the tip of the catheter was not recorded. The patient returned 2 years later with severe hypertension. (D) Semiselective right renal angiography and (E) selective left renal angiography reveal marked narrowing of the left main stem extending into the dorsal artery.

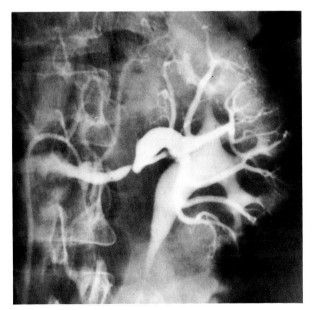

E

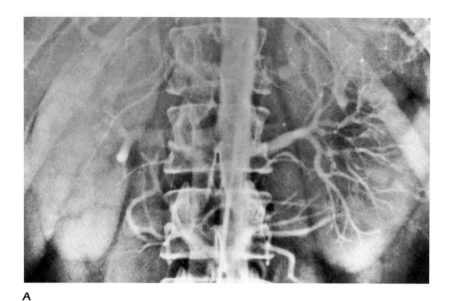

A

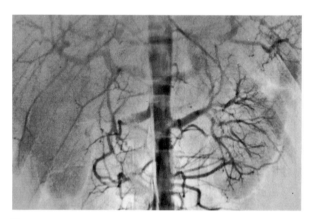

B

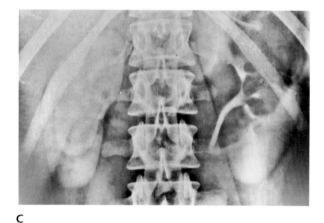

C

Figure 45-4. Hematuria and massive proteinuria were the main indications for renal angiography in this 20-year-old woman. At selective test injection into the right renal artery, a subintimal deposit of contrast medium occurred. The catheter was removed, and a nonselective aortogram was performed a few minutes later. (A) A nonselective renal angiogram and (B) a subtraction film of the same show that the contrast medium in the almost normal appearing renal artery on the right is in fact subintimally located and that there is complete occlusion of flow through the right kidney. (C) A urogram made 10 minutes later shows that the nephrographic effect is still present on the right as a consequence of the subintimal dissection.

age group. Subintimal dissection occurs much more often than reported, a fact that becomes obvious in a well-controlled prospective study.[53,54] Many of the cases are not reported because they are not recognized at the time of examination (Fig. 45-5; see also Fig. 45-3), particularly when there is only a thin, sleevelike contrast deposit subintimally.

To avoid subintimal dissection, it is advantageous to use a catheter with a 2- to 3-cm-long tapered part. The catheter used for selective angiography must have no side holes; if side holes are present, a small artery may constrict around the tip even when there is free flow. Injection of contrast medium into an ischemic kidney will cause renal damage.[55–57]

During injection, not only may the contrast medium pass subintimally from the tip of the catheter, but the renal artery may be perforated by the jet effect of the contrast medium.[58] The tip of the catheter may also recoil into a small adrenal or capsular artery originating from the first part of the renal artery, with consequent extravasation (Fig. 45-6). In addition, the guidewire may pass subintimally or even perforate an artery during its passage to the aorta. A smooth passage of a flexible J guidewire usually prevents compli-

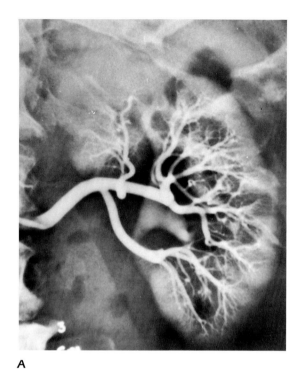

A

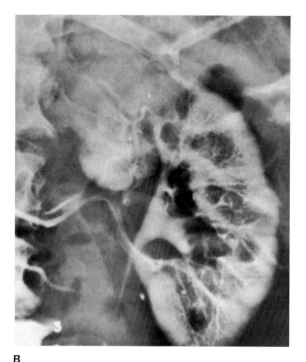

B

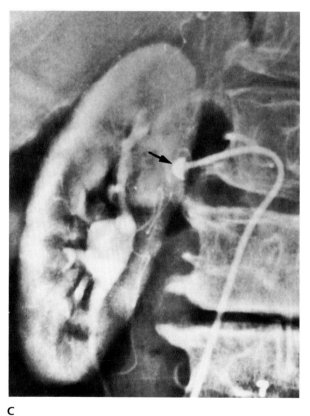

C

Figure 45-5. Subintimal injection of contrast medium into the left and right renal arteries. (A and B) An arterial and a late arterial left renal angiogram reveals a sleevelike deposit of contrast medium at the tip of the catheter not recognized at the time of examination. (C) A nephrographic phase of selective right renal angiography in the right posterior oblique position shows a small deposit of contrast medium at the tip of the catheter (*arrow*). The complications had no deleterious consequences.

cations. The smaller guidewires reduce this risk further.

Thromboembolic Consequences

Like guidewires, catheters are thrombogenic. Scanning electron microscopy and other methods have shown that fibrin deposition on the catheter is a rule. The original catheters, with a rugged surface, were very thrombogenic, whereas the smoother, nonopaque catheters were less thrombogenic.[22,26,58–61] Catheters activate the coagulation system, causing increased platelet adhesiveness and a consumption of fibrinogen. The length and diameter of the catheter (i.e., the amount of catheter surface exposed to blood) is related to the amount of fibrin deposited.[62,63] Consequently, the frequency of complications due to thromboembolism is related to the type of catheter used, an observation that explains the wide range in the incidence of thromboembolic complications reported in the literature.

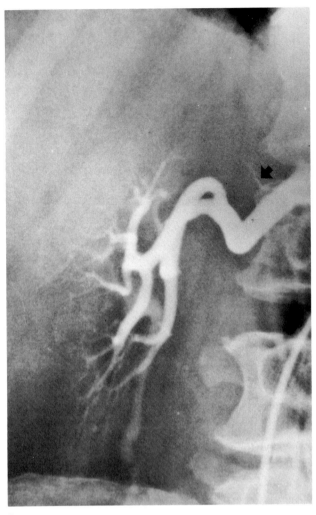

A

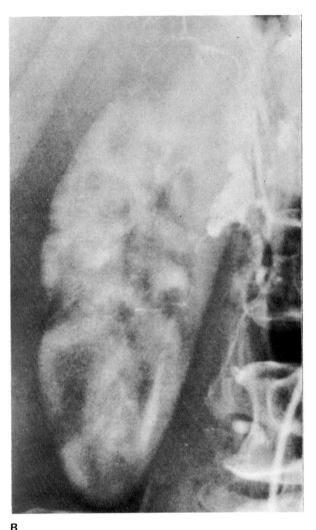

B

Figure 45-6. Rupture of a capsular artery. (A and B) Selective right renal angiography in the right posterior oblique position, arterial and capillary phases. During the contrast medium injection, the tip of the catheter recoiled into a small capsular artery (*arrow*, A), with resultant extravasation. The patient had severe pain, followed by marked hypotension, which was difficult to treat.

Commercially made catheters now have a smoother surface than those previously used. An in vitro test comparing catheters made of nylon, polyamine polymer, polyethylene, and polyurethane for thrombogenicity showed minimal differences among the catheters. The effect of heparinization of the catheters was obvious but of short duration.[64] Catheters coated with hydrophilic plastics had no reduced thrombogenicity compared with nylon, whereas heparinization had a striking effect when tested in dogs.[28]

Complications caused by catheters are mainly of two types. The most frequently recorded complication occurs when the catheter is withdrawn and the deposits on it are sloughed off. This phenomenon occurs in practically every instance but seldom gives rise to ischemic symptoms. Occlusion at the puncture site or more distally in the leg resulting in loss of pulse or symptoms occurs in 0.1 to 1.2 percent of cases.[9,65–70] Pullout arteriography and oscillometry result in higher rates of this complication.[71–73]

The second most common type of thromboembolic complication occurs when a clot within the catheter is released and causes embolism (Fig. 45-7).[74–76] This event occurs particularly when the guidewire has to be reintroduced for catheter exchange. With modern interventional embolization techniques, renal embolism is not considered as serious a complication as it was previously. Furthermore, both immediate hepa-

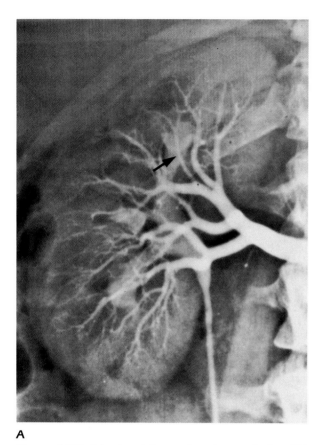

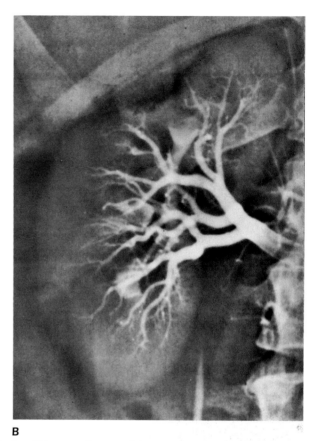

A **B**

Figure 45-7. Selective right renal angiogram before (A) and after (B) an occlusion of the interlobar artery (*arrow*) that supplies mainly the third anterior lobe. An embolus was released from the catheter during a prolonged investigation.

rinization and transcatheter embolectomy have proved successful in treating this complication.[77,78] Thromboembolism can be prevented by heparinizing the patient.[5,79-81] The recommended dose is 45 units of heparin per kilogram of body weight to a maximum of about 3000 units given through the catheter at the start of the procedure.[80,81] At the completion of the examination, protamine sulfate can be given.[82,83] Other workers have recommended the infusion of low-molecular-weight dextran as an effective method of preventing coagulation.[84] Heparin coating of the catheters is still another method,[85] but it has the drawback of prolonging the necessary compression time after catheter removal.[86]

Clot formation can be reduced dramatically with the technique mentioned in text preceding. In modern renal angiography, however, there is rarely any complication of this kind in the adult patient, and therefore no need for the more expensive heparin-coated catheters.[53] On the other hand, systemic heparinization is a precaution that should be routinely employed in every catheterization procedure.

Other Complications due to Guidewires and Catheters

Fatal complications are extremely rare but do occur, even with modern techniques and contrast media.[9,53,65,67,73] *Thromboembolic occlusion* requiring surgery in debilitated patients is one potentially fatal complication; another is *retroperitoneal hemorrhage* due to catheter or guidewire perforation of the iliac arteries or lumbar aorta. No doubt, preexisting severe disease is the main factor in fatal outcomes.[68]

Complications at the puncture site can be serious. One such complication is the *subintimal passage* of the guidewire or catheter, or perforation of the artery, a lesion that may cause thrombosis, false aneurysm, or arteriovenous fistula.[9,10,53,65,66,69] *Guidewire breakage* is another complication, though rare.[66,67,69,87]

Hematoma formation occurs frequently, and a large hematoma may require surgery.[9,53,65-67,69] Hematomas may be particularly problematic in patients with hypertension; they may occur later, when the patient has been sent back to the hospital bed. In a prospective series, serious delayed bleeding occurred in 0.5 percent of the patients examined by various types of abdominal angiography.[53] With the assistance of ultrasonography, early complications may be controlled through graded compression of the femoral artery,[88] and in selected cases an arteriovenous fistula may be treated nonsurgically.[89]

Thrombosis of the femoral vein as a consequence of abdominal angiography is rarely reported.[69,90] It is surprising that this complication does not occur more often, considering the fact that the patients in question are old and bedridden, have poor perfusion of the legs, and have a hematoma that compresses the vein. In a prospective search for this complication in a highly selected group of 20 patients, Widestadt et al. found only one patient with a thrombosis secondary to a large hematoma.[90] However, pulmonary embolism has been observed as perfusion scintigram defects in about one-third of all patients undergoing transfemoral arteriography with 6.5 to 8 French catheters.[91]

Subintimal injection of contrast medium into the renal artery, mentioned previously, may also occur in the abdominal aorta or the iliac arteries. It was once regarded as a frequent complication,[69,92-94] but has become much less frequent with the technique recommended in text preceding.

Embolization due to clot formation has also been mentioned previously. In advanced atherosclerosis, plaque may be dislodged and embolized to various vascular beds.[95-98] Cholesterol embolization causes a characteristic syndrome that may occur spontaneously or follow aortic surgery. Despite the large number of angiographic procedures performed, cholesterol embolization appears to be a rare complication.[99] The classical features are lower limb livedo reticularis and ischemia due to arteriolar or small artery branch occlusion with preserved pulses. Deterioration of renal function is the most common result secondary to renal embolization and infarction.[99-101] The syndrome usually occurs after a complicated angiographic procedure but may also be observed in a simple angiography of short duration.[101] Renal failure after an angiographic procedure is not an uncommon complication; it is usually attributed to the contrast medium but may also be secondary to cholesterol embolization. This complication occurs more often than reported because the emboli are too small to be observed or to cause symptoms.

Foreign materials, such as surgical glove powder and cotton fiber, were previously reported in the kidneys after selective renal angiography.[69,102-104] This complication usually occurred because foreign material fell into the open bowls that had been used in flushing the catheters; the complication was eliminated after closed reservoir-tubing systems were introduced. Glass particles and other material have been found to contaminate contrast media,[105,106] and particulate contamination of all kinds of fluid administration sets and cannulas has been observed.[107] The thrombogenicity of catheters and guidewires has been mentioned above; in addition, the rough surfaces of the equipment contribute to the release of particles.[25] At experimental selective renal angiography, the particles have caused renal infarction.[108]

Contrast Medium

Techniques

The delivery rates and the amounts of contrast medium are generally adjusted to the renal blood flow rate, the size of the patient, and the size of the lumbar aorta. The method of contrast administration used is also important. Intravenous digital subtraction angiography (DSA) is still used in many centers as a screening technique, but, with less traumatic arterial catheterization, intraarterial DSA will eventually be the method of choice, replacing full-size, film-screen radiography as well as 100-mm photofluorography. At intraarterial DSA the iodine concentration is reduced by almost 50 percent as compared with the other techniques.[109,110] In nonselective renal DSA, 30 to 40 ml of nonionic or ionic contrast medium containing 150 mg iodine per milliliter is injected at a rate of 20 ml per second. In selective renal DSA, 8 to 10 ml of a contrast agent (100 mg iodine/ml) is injected at a rate of 5 ml per second, and in nondigital documentation a low-osmolar agent (200 mg iodine/ml) is used. In renal disease with reduced blood flow, the amount of contrast medium and the injection rate should be reduced. Thus, in severe renal disease, 3 to 4 ml injected at a rate of 2 to 3 ml per second may be sufficient. On the other hand, 30 to 40 ml may be delivered at a rate of 15 ml per second in a kidney that has a richly vascularized carcinoma, when the main purpose is to determine whether the renal vein has been invaded by tumor. However, this determination is now made with noninvasive imaging.

In selected patients, *vasoconstrictors* may be used to obtain additional information[111-114] (see Fig. 45-2). The most reliable information is obtained with a dose of 0.5 to 2.0 μg of angiotensin injected 10 to 15 seconds before the contrast medium injection.

Toxicity

Intravenous as well as intraarterial injection of contrast agents may cause acute renal failure or dysfunction.

Unless specifically looked for, the dysfunction will not be recognized because there is only a slight or moderate increase of plasma creatinine, peaking about 24 to 36 hours after the contrast medium injection and returning to preangiographic levels within 5 to 7 days. True renal failure after angiography is rare but has been observed in 0.5 to 12 percent of cases.[115-117] The role of cholesterol embolization in renal failure after angiography is not known (see text preceding). In reports on the general complications of angiography, none or very few cases of renal failure have been mentioned.[9,65,69,118] The reason for this discrepancy is that a slight or moderate azotemia and short-term oliguria may pass undetected. Acute renal failure is almost always reversible. The oliguria usually lasts for no longer than 72 hours.[119] However, it may be fatal for a patient at risk. An increasing number of cases of acute renal failure after angiography were reported during the 1970s when the amount of contrast agent given to each patient was increasing and the total number of renal angiographic examinations reached a peak.[115-117,120-124]

Certain factors increase the risk of renal failure after the delivery of contrast medium.[116] Advanced age, a past or current reduction in renal function, dehydration, hyperuricemia, diabetes (particularly insulin-dependent), cardiovascular disease when combined with digoxin medication, and large doses of contrast media are important risk factors that should be considered before renal angiography is done.[115,117,125-128] The renal parenchyma may also be destroyed if the contrast agent is injected into an ischemic kidney (as in renal artery stenosis, angioplasty, transplanted donor kidney).[55,57,129-131]

Toxicity is related to the concentration, osmolality, and volume of the contrast medium and to the contact time and the number of injections.[132-134] The least concentrated contrast medium adequate to the diagnostic task should be used. Therefore, intraarterial DSA should be preferred because the iodine concentration can be diminished, thus reducing both general toxicity and osmolality. Large doses of contrast media accidentally injected into the renal artery have not caused significant damage to the kidney[135-137]; however, clinical and experimental evidence indicates that there is a short period of decreased renal function and signs of reversible renal damage. Transient enzyme excretion suggests that there is tubular damage,[138-141] and signs of cell injury and regeneration have been observed.[142]

Injection of contrast medium into the renal artery causes a number of changes in renal function that have been observed particularly well in experimental studies but also in humans. High-osmolar contrast media cause a decreased glomerular filtration rate and creatinine clearance, increased permeability of the glomeruli with increasing amounts of albumin in the urine, and renal tubular dysfunction.[126,128,143-148] In humans, an "osmotic nephrosis" has been observed in biopsies performed within a week of arteriography[149]; in infants, tubular changes and even medullary necrosis have been observed.[150] The nephrotoxic changes also occur with the low-osmolar media (nonionics and ionic dimers), but they are less intense and occur less frequently.

With the development of nonionic contrast media, a number of experimental and clinical prospective studies have been undertaken to find the difference, if any, in nephrotoxicity among the various contrast agents. These studies have focused mainly on the creatinine level in plasma, with varying results. From none to up to 40 percent of patients have shown signs of renal dysfunction after angiography, with the highest levels consistently occurring after the administration of high-osmolar ionic contrast media.[127,128,140,148,151-159] The great variations in the incidence of acute renal dysfunction found in the literature depend on a number of factors. One is the time after angiography that the creatinine level in plasma is determined. A second factor is that the definition of acute renal dysfunction based on the creatinine increase varies, and only a few investigators have used sophisticated methods such as creatinine clearance and serial radionuclide renograms to estimate the change in renal function.[126,128,148] A third factor is the fact that intraarterial injection does not always mean that the contrast medium reaches the kidneys undiluted. A fourth factor is the different concentrations of contrast media used. A fifth and perhaps the most important factor is that the prevalence of insulin-dependent diabetics and patients with azotemia varies in different series. These two groups almost always show some reduction in renal function after angiography, but the changes are not observed to the same extent with the low-osmotic when compared with the high-osmotic agents.[128,156-158]

The exact mechanism of the nephrotoxic effects of the contrast medium is not definitely known. Most of the effects can be related to the response of the vascular bed. Probably the increased stiffness of the red blood cells is an important factor, in addition to hyperosmolality and viscosity.[160] Abnormal rigidity of red blood cells is also caused by nonionic contrast media, although not to the same extent as with high-osmolar media. Another factor of importance is the interaction of nonionic contrast media with blood. Aggregates and clots are formed by these agents.[161,162] However, it has been convincingly shown that these red blood cell formations are easily dispersed and without clinical significance.[163]

Hypertonicity certainly plays an important role, since the nephrotoxic effect is higher when contrast medium is injected on the arterial side than on the venous side. It should be noted that nonionic contrast media are hyperosmolar in relation to blood, but to a lesser extent than the high-osmolar ionic media. This fact could explain the lower nephrotoxic effect of the nonionic media when they are injected on the arterial side. When contrast media are injected intravenously, there is no hypertonic effect when they reach the renal artery and yet there is a deterioration of renal function in azotemic patients.[164,165] Because of the lower general toxicity of nonionic media, the nephrotoxic effects are also lower when the media are injected intravenously.[165]

The renal vascular bed does not respond to contrast medium injection in the same way that other vascular beds do. There is no unanimous description of the changes in renal blood flow, but in all cases described there is a decreased flow.[166-171] In most reports, the increased resistance is observed at 10 to 15 seconds after injection and lasts for 1 to 15 minutes. During the first few seconds the kidney volume is reduced, and a prolonged period of renal distention follows.[172]

The pathophysiology of acute renal failure is complex. It can be explained by reversible damage of the vascular endothelium, which causes protein to leak from the glomeruli and into the tubular ducts. Plugging of the ducts, in combination with the osmotic effects of the contrast medium in the ducts and extracellular fluid, explains the increased renal size. The intrarenal pressure rises because the high resistance of the renal capsule causes an increased resistance to flow. The increased contact time of the contrast medium with the tubular cells and a certain anoxia can explain the tubular damage. Thus the decreased flow does not necessarily mean that vasoconstriction is present, but there is evidence that the renin-angiotensin system is activated during selective renal angiography.[169,173]

Vasoconstriction may be observed at renal angiography either as a localized, short, concentric ring at the tip of the catheter or as a long segment of fusiform narrowing. A third type of vasoconstriction involves multiple small cortical perfusion defects (Fig. 45-8).[174-176] Because the most common cause is a malpositioning of the catheter in the renal artery, these defects disappear when a vasodilating drug is given or when the catheter's position is corrected.

Spasm of the cortical arteries is also observed if the renal artery is clamped or if intraarterial vasoconstric-

Figure 45-8. Cortical arterial spasm due to malpositioning of the catheter in the renal artery. (A and B) Selective left renal angiography, early and late arterial phases. Observe that the tip of the catheter causes bulging of the arterial wall (*arrow,* A), with secondary spasm of the cortical arteries and irregular perfusion, which was not demonstrated at nonselective renal angiography.

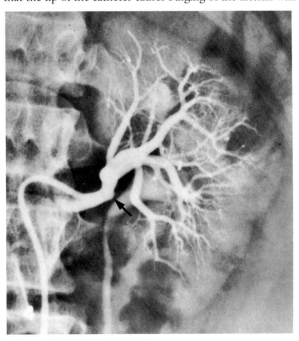

A

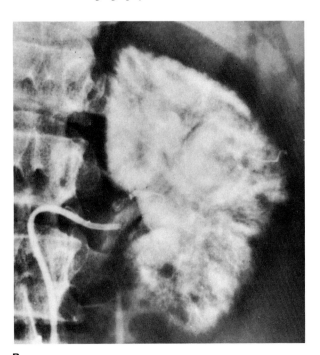

B

tors are given before the contrast medium injection.[177,178] Similar perfusion defects are observed when angiography is performed during hypotension or shock due to hemorrhage.[179] It should be recognized that the use of vasoconstrictors in combination with contrast media increases the risk of renal damage.[180,181]

Radiographic Technique

Radiographic technique varies with the actual situation and the indications for renal angiography. It should always begin with proper positioning of the catheter to obtain as much information as possible about the lumbar aorta and the renal arteries. As mentioned, the most precise information is obtained with a semiselective technique. After a test injection of 10 ml of contrast medium (to check the position of the catheter), the patient is positioned over a film changer. Ordinary radiographic techniques are used (1) to prevent unnecessary scattered irradiation (by compression of the abdomen and careful collimation) and (2) to arrive at the best possible geometry (the patient should be positioned as close as possible to the film changer). The generator should be capable of giving exposures below 0.10 second at 70 to 75 kV.

The modern angiographic laboratory is equipped with a C or U arm and a carbon fiber tabletop for abdominal and peripheral angiographic or interventional procedures.[182] A 35-cm image intensifier tube, which can be electronically switched to lower fields, is positioned opposite the x-ray tube. The intensifier can swiftly be replaced by a Puck changer for full-size documentation, but today most renal angiograms are documented via the image intensifier. Either a 100-mm camera is used for direct photography of the output screen or the image is converted into digital form via the television camera. Serial 100-mm photofluorography gives as good a resolution as full-size film, the dose is lower, and the smooth operation with the small format is attractive.[183] Furthermore, the patient does not need to move for different views because the C or U arm can be moved for any selected projection. However, the digital technique is usually the first choice because with the improved resolution obtained with the 1024^2 matrix this imaging technique has many advantages.

When possible, a selective angiogram should be performed with 3× magnification (Figs. 45-9 and 45-10). To lower the radiation dose to the skin, the number of exposures can be decreased to cover only the later arterial and early nephrographic phases.[184–187]

Nonselective or Semiselective Renal Angiography

During the arterial phase, two frames per second give enough information in most cases. Because the injection time is about 1.5 seconds, usually six frames over 3 seconds cover the arterial phase. To cover the nephrographic and venous phases, one frame every other second (i.e., six frames over 12 seconds) is sufficient. Particularly in hypertension, it is important to visualize the origin of the renal arteries from the aorta. Because the arteries often arise from the anterolateral aspect of the aorta, oblique films may be necessary. If the semiselective technique is used, the catheter tip is positioned in the left renal artery in the right posterior oblique projection and in the right renal artery in the left posterior oblique projection.

Selective Renal Angiography

Selective renal angiography is performed only when the expected information has not been obtained or when a selective study can be expected to give more information. Thus selective angiography is done when vasoactive drugs are used or when large doses of contrast medium are required for venous demonstration. The injection time for a normal selective renal angiogram is 1 to 2 seconds. Usually, four frames over 2 seconds cover the arterial phase, and four frames over 8 seconds cover the nephrographic and venous phases. If vasoconstrictors are injected before the contrast medium, a slower injection rate and longer intervals between the exposures are recommended. Also, when large doses of contrast medium are injected for tumor analysis, one exposure every other second suffices for arterial and venous information.

Anatomic Considerations

Renal angiography gives essential information about the morphology of the renal vasculature, the renal cortex, and any abnormal states in the kidney and its vicinity. It also gives information about renal hemodynamics and vascular physiology. With the development of noninvasive radiologic methods, the indications for renal angiography have diminished markedly. Renal angiography is still necessary, however, to determine an adequate approach in vascular disease states of various forms as well as before surgery or interventional radiologic procedures. It is therefore just as important today as it was a few years ago to have detailed knowledge about the renal angiogram in order not to misinterpret the many normal variations as renal pathology.

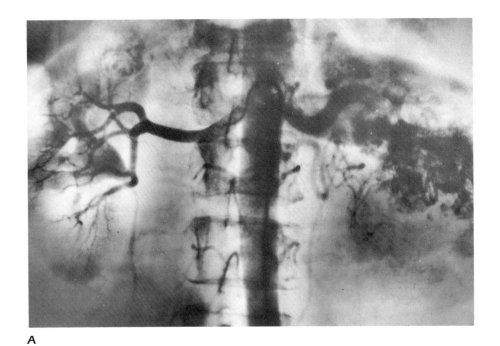

A

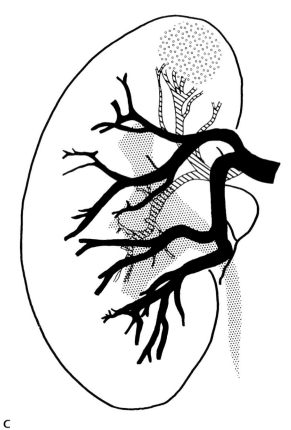

B

C

Figure 45-9. (A) Semiselective and (B) 2× magnification selective right renal angiography in a patient with renal carcinoma on the left and a small metastasis in the right upper renal pole. (C) A typical distribution of the ramifications of the dorsal artery (*hatching*). The dorsal artery supplies the entire superior pole, including the metastasis and the posterior intermediate part. A small middle capsular artery is observed.

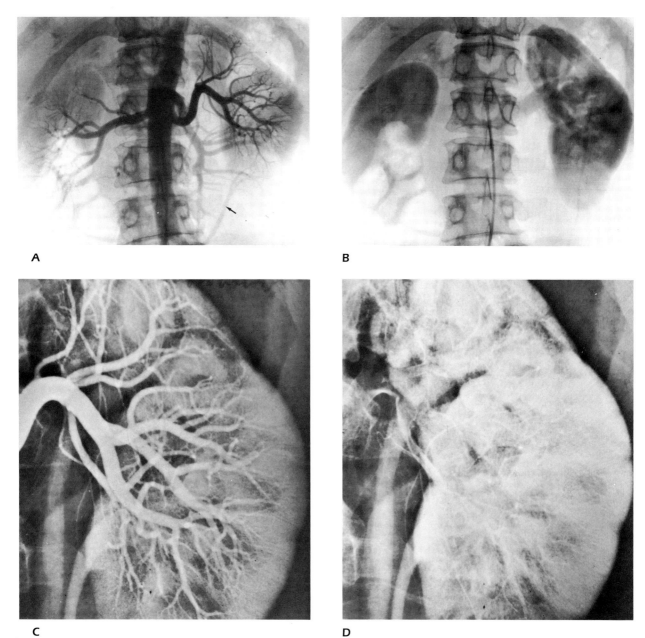

Figure 45-10. Double renal pelvis with hydronephrosis and parenchymal reduction of the left upper pole. (A and B) Semiselective renal angiography in the arterial and venous phases. Note the reduced width of the segmental branches to the upper pole, the lower polar artery from the common iliac artery on the left (*arrow,* A), and the early origin of a superior segmental polar artery on the right. (C and D) 3× magnification, 0.1-mm focal spot. Arterial and cortical glomerular nephrographic phases. The summation effect of the interlobular arteries and the glomerular tufts is well observed in the normal intermediate and lower parts. Slight cortical indentations are noted on the lateral surface, and there is marked reduction of the cortex in the upper pole. Pelvic and capsular arteries are seen.

The renal angiogram is composed of the arterial, nephrographic, and venous phases. When contrast medium is injected into the lumbar aorta or into the renal artery, serial filming is performed to cover these phases.

Arterial Phase

An aortic injection should precede selective renal angiography to determine the many variations in origin, number, and size of the renal arteries. An injection of contrast medium well above the renal arteries also gives information about the difference in flow to the kidneys, which, with modern technique, quickly gives reliable information about the renal blood flow.[188–194] An aortic injection at the level of the renal arteries or as a semiselective study (see Fig. 45-9) as a rule gives the information required for therapeutic considerations. If, however, there is a need for more precise information, selective angiography, with magnification if available, should follow. To perform only selective injection would be more comfortable for the patient, but the many variations in the renal blood supply would cause unpredictable problems and would give false information about the renal vessels and parenchyma.[195]

Origin

The renal artery or, if multiple arteries are present, the main renal artery arises from the lumbar aorta at the level of L1 and L2. The right renal artery usually arises somewhat higher than the left renal artery, and both usually take their origin from the anterolateral part of the aorta.[196,197] An origin of the renal artery at the level of T11 is rare.[198]

Course

Because of its rather constant origin, the renal artery has a varying course, depending on the site of the kidney. Thus, in ptosis, the renal artery has a steep caudolateral course to the renal hilus. In cranial ectopia, the renal artery takes a steep cranial course.[199] Multiple arteries are common; they are discussed in Chapter 49.

Caliber

The caliber of the single renal artery varies within rather wide limits. In the adult patient, the diameter varies between about 5 and 10 mm, as measured on the renal angiogram, with values for the female in the lower part of the range.[174,200] The diameter or cross-sectional area of the renal artery reflects the function of the renal parenchyma and thus the renal blood flow.[201–204] Vasoactive substances changing renal blood flow also change the caliber of the renal artery. With an increased blood flow there is dilatation,[205,206] and with decreased blood flow there is a reduced width.[207,208] The main renal artery has mainly elastic tissue in its wall and may therefore increase in width with increased blood pressure and peripheral resistance.[209] This increase may be observed in malignant hypertension, or the artery may be of normal width despite reduced parenchyma (Fig. 45-11).

As a consequence of aging and arteriosclerosis, various changes occur in the main stem. The width is usually reduced owing to senile involution of the parenchyma, but increased width and tortuosity are often encountered. Increased tortuosity may be regarded as a progression of the changes present in the cortical vessels and arcuate arteries in old age, when the normal tapering disappears. Tortuosity starts in the interlobar arteries.[210,211] Tortuosity of the extrahilar parts of the renal artery and its branches is in fact more common than is usually observed in renal angiography[212] because the posterolateral course of the renal artery from the aorta to the renal hilus cannot be fully appreciated in the anteroposterior projection. The normal movements of the kidney from the supine to the erect position require, of course, a certain adaptability of the renal pedicle.

Branches of the Renal Artery and the Segmental Supply

The renal artery branches into two, three, or more arteries before it enters the renal hilus. In the normal renal angiogram, the pattern of arborization is smooth and regular (Fig. 45-12). The vessels taper toward the periphery. The branches pass anteriorly and posteriorly to the renal pelvis in the renal sinus. Branches are also observed to the upper pole, the suprarenal gland, and the renal capsule without crossing the renal pelvis. A separate branch to the lower pole is even more common, but this artery crosses the renal pelvis usually on the anterior side. Within the renal sinus, the vessels, whether anterior or posterior, rebranch and give rise to a variable number of interlobar arteries that spread out around the minor calices. Each interlobar artery gives off arcuate arteries, which, in the distal part, run parallel to the renal surface. The arcuate arteries give off the interlobular arteries, which course peripherally in the cortex (Fig. 45-13). They give rise to numerous afferent arterioles to the glomeruli. Selective renal angiography can give information about the renal arterial tree up to this point; the efferent arteriolae and the vasa recta cannot be distinguished.

Many attempts have been made to define a segmental supply of the primary branches of the renal artery by both anatomic dissections and angiography.[196,212,216–220] There are various opinions regarding this segmental

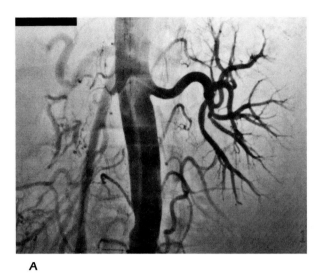

A

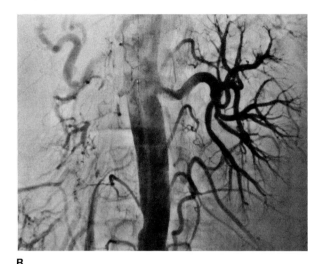

B

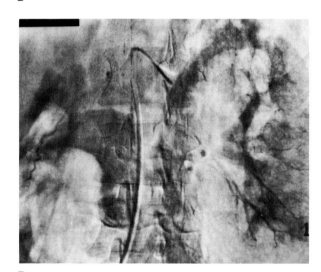

C

D

Figure 45-11. Semiselective left renal angiography in a patient with severe malignant hypertension and occlusion of the right renal artery. After the end of the injection of 30 ml of contrast medium, the subtraction films presented were exposed in the following order: (A) 0.1 second, (B) 0.6 second, (C) 3 seconds, and (D) 6.2 seconds. The left renal artery is of normal width despite a marked reduction in renal functioning and an increased resistance to flow. The interlobar and arcuate arteries are still observed 6.2 seconds after the end of the injection. The nephrographic phase is poor, and there is no demarcation of the cortex.

distribution. To understand the ramification and distribution of the renal artery branches, a few facts must be understood. One is that the renal artery branches are end-arteries; that is, they have their definite field of supply. Another is that the large variations that exist depend entirely on the macroarchitecture of the kidney. Seven anterior and seven posterior pyramids with the surrounding cortex form seven pairs of lobes.[221] Because the kidney during its fetal stage has to accommodate to surrounding structures, the pyramids undergo fusions and deviations that give the final shape to the kidney. It is therefore the distal branches in the sinus of the kidney, the *interlobar arteries* that run close to the septa of Bertin, that represent the true seg-

mental lobar supply and from which six to eight arcuate arteries arise and enter the kidney tissue at the interphase between the cortex and the medulla (see Fig. 45-13).[214] Each lobe is supplied by at least two interlobar arteries that can be traced backward to the renal hilus, where they join to form segmental vessels, which thus supply more than one lobe.

In an attempt to systematize the segmental supply of the renal artery, the author has suggested that there are four main segments made up of two polar and two intermediate segments (Fig. 45-14).[216] Because each interlobar artery supplies two adjacent lobes, the segmental distribution is not limited to the exact border of the lobes. Nevertheless, it is of practical value to

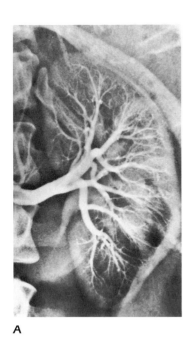

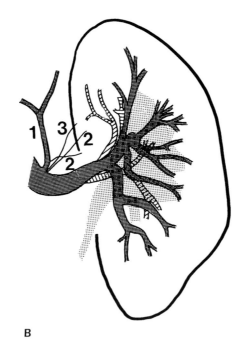

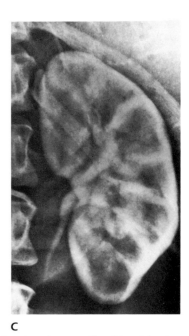

A   B   C

Figure 45-12. Normal selective left renal angiography. (A and B) Arterial phase. (C) Late cortical nephrogram and early venous phase. A common trunk for the inferior phrenic (*1*), superior capsular (*2*), and adrenal arteries (*3*) arises early from the renal artery. The dorsal artery (*hatching,* B) arises as the first renal branch and supplies the posterior lobes in the upper and intermediate parts of the kidney. The cortex is thin, and the columns of Bertin are prominent.

have this segmental orientation to understand the variations of the normal anatomy. The intermediate segments are made up of three anterior and three posterior lobes, and the upper and lower polar segments are made up of two pairs of lobes each. The main value of this suggestion is that it can be used to identify a dorsal artery supplying the intermediate posterior seg-

ment and a ventral artery going to the corresponding anterior segment. The interlobar arteries are thus subsegmental arteries. Because of the position of the kidney in the body, the ventral artery in the anteroposterior projection always supplies the lateral border, and the dorsal artery always supplies the medial border of the intermediate part of the kidney (see Figs. 45-9 and

Figure 45-13. Diagrammatic presentation of the blood supply of the renal parenchyma. *1,* Interlobar arteries; *2,* arcuate arteries; *3,* interlobular arteries; *4,* afferent arteries; *5,* peritubular plexus; *6,7,* arteriolae rectae; *8,* perforating arteries; *9,* spiral arteries. (Adapted from Davidson,[213] Hodson,[214] and Meiisel and Apitzsch.[215] Used with permission.)

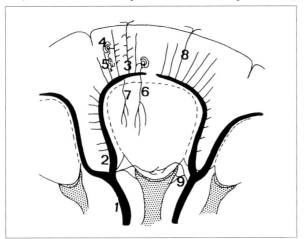

Figure 45-14. The four renal segments as they are projected on the renal surface according to Boijsen. (From Boijsen E. Angiographic studies of the anatomy of single and multiple renal arteries. Acta Radiol (Stockh) 1959;Suppl 183. Used with permission.)

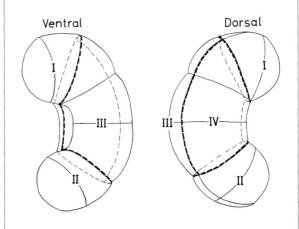

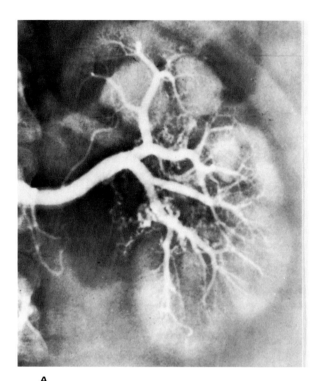

A

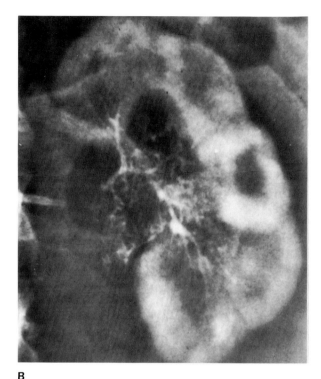

B

Figure 45-15. Dorsal renal artery ligated at pyelolithotomy. (A) At selective renal angiography, only ventral artery branches are filled in addition to numerous wide pelvic arteries that serve as collateral vessels to the dorsal artery. In the renal sinus, the ventral branches do not cross each other. (B) In the nephrographic phase, the distribution of the dorsal artery branches is well observed. Note the lobulation, mainly the result of the reduced volume of the dorsal parenchyma.

45-12). From there on, the vessels can be traced back to their origin from the renal artery, where certain characteristics appear. One characteristic is that the branches of the ventral artery do not, as a rule, cross each other; nor do the branches of the dorsal artery in the renal sinus. Another characteristic is that the dorsal artery is usually smaller in caliber and appears as a branch of the renal artery, whereas the ventral artery appears more as a direct continuation of the renal artery. Furthermore, the dorsal artery appears as the first branch of the renal artery in some 50 percent of kidneys. These are simple observations, but they are easily overlooked in, for example, a kidney whose dorsal artery has been ligated (Fig. 45-15).[222,223] Because of the ligation, the dorsal lobes are reduced in size, and the ventral lobes are hyperplastic. The kidney may still be of normal size.

The variations of the supply of the upper and lower poles are many (Figs. 45-16 and 45-17). There may be only two branches, one dorsal artery supplying the posterior lobes and one ventral artery supplying the anterior lobes; but this phenomenon occurs only in some 15 percent of kidneys. Most often, the ventral artery supplies the entire lower pole as well as the anterior intermediate part, a phenomenon that occurs in some 60 percent of kidneys. The dorsal artery supplies the entire upper pole and the posterior intermediate segment in about 20 percent of kidneys, but it rarely supplies the anterior part of the lower pole.

Course in the Renal Sinus

The dorsal and ventral arteries are very close when they enter the upper part of the renal hilus. They often appear to squeeze the ramus of the renal pelvis to the upper pole (Fig. 45-18). At this point, a vascular impression is often observed in the renal pelvis.[216,224–228] A combination of dilatation and papillary destruction of the upper pole and a vascular impression of the upper ramus has been falsely regarded as an obstruction to flow that causes pain.[226,229] Surgery has been performed on the crossing artery because of this combination. Vascular impressions causing obstruction to flow from the upper pole probably can occur only when a large aneurysm is present or when a mass displaces the artery.[230] Aneurysms usually cause deformation of the upper part of the renal pelvis, which may cause differential diagnostic problems.[231]

The dorsal artery usually follows the posterior border of the renal hilus in a caudal direction (Fig. 45-19).[216,232] This point is of importance in renal surgery

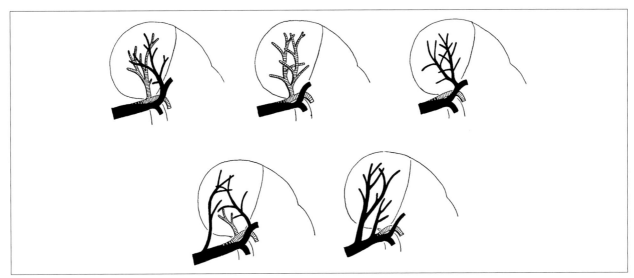

Figure 45-16. Left upper renal pole showing common variations of arterial supply. (From Boijsen E. Angiographic studies of the anatomy of single and multiple renal arteries. Acta Radiol (Stockh) 1959;Suppl 183. Used with permission.)

Figure 45-17. Left lower pole showing common variations in origin, course, and field of supply of the lower polar artery. (From Boijsen E. Angiographic studies of the anatomy of single and multiple renal arteries. Acta Radiol (Stockh) 1959;Suppl 183. Used with permission.)

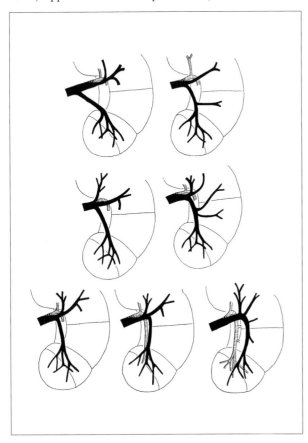

because access to the renal pelvis is often from the posterior aspect of the kidney, and so the artery may be severed (see Fig. 45-15).[222,223,233] In hydronephrosis or in space-occupying lesions of the renal sinus, the displacement can rarely be appreciated in an anteroposterior view, whereas in a true lateral view of the kidney vascular displacement is obvious (Fig. 45-20).

Arcuate and Cortical Arteries

In most angiograms, the arcuate arteries are the last branches of the renal artery that can be observed. In high-quality angiograms (particularly magnification angiograms), however, the summation effect of the interlobular arteries as well as the glomerular tufts is observed (see Figs. 45-9 and 45-10). The distance between the arcuate arteries running parallel to the renal surface and their closest distance to this surface give information about the amount of renal cortex present. (The interlobular arteries and the glomeruli are considered in the discussion of the nephrographic phase.)

Capsular and Pelvic Arteries

In the arterial phase, adrenal capsular and renal pelvic arteries are also observed (Fig. 45-21). The renal capsular artery system is composed of three basic pathways: superior, medial, and inferior capsular arteries. They rarely all take their origin from the single renal artery. They are easy to define because the rate of flow through these arteries is slower than that through the renal parenchymal arteries and because contrast material is more persistent in them during the nephrographic phase.

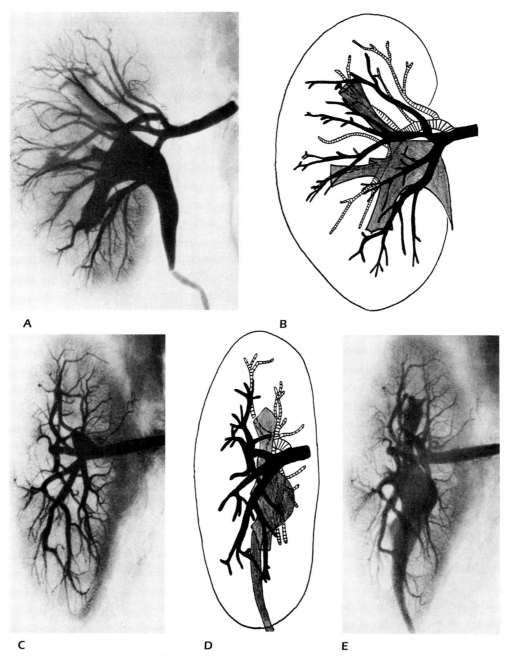

Figure 45-18. Autopsy specimen, right kidney. (A and B) True "frontal" projection. (C to E) True "lateral" projection. Observe how close the ventral and dorsal arteries are to each other and to the renal pelvis in the renal sinus. The upper ramus is squeezed between the two vessels.

The superior capsular artery (see Fig. 45-12), which is observed in about one-third of all selective renal arteriograms, usually arises together with the inferior adrenal artery from the first part of the single renal artery and follows a characteristic tortuous path over the superior pole of the kidney. It may arise together with all the adrenal arteries and the inferior phrenic artery as a common trunk from the first part of the renal artery, from the angle between the aorta and the renal artery, from a supplementary upper polar artery, or directly from the aorta.

The middle capsular arteries arise from the renal artery or its main branches, usually in the renal hilus. To reach the anterior and posterior aspects of the kidney, the middle capsular arteries pass medially before they spread in the perirenal fat (Fig. 45-22; see also Fig. 45-9).

The inferior capsular artery is rarely observed at

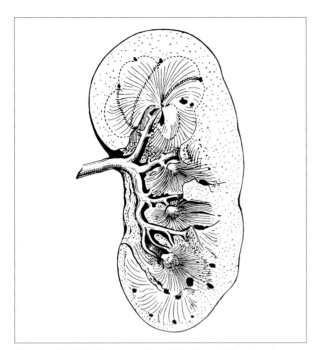

Figure 45-19. Course and ramification of the dorsal artery in the sinus according to Hou-Jensen. (From Hou-Jensen H. Die Verästelung der Arteria renalis in der Niere des Menschen. Z Anat Entwicklungsgesch 1930;91:1. Used with permission.)

selective renal angiography because it usually takes its origin from the gonadal artery or from an inferior polar artery arising from the aorta.

Perforating capsular arteries also exist. They arise from arcuate and interlobular arteries (see Fig. 45-22).[216,234] They may be important collateral pathways in occlusive disease. These arteries are most often observed in advanced nephropathy.

The pelvic arteries arise as tiny twigs from the branches of the renal artery in the renal sinus and form a network on the renal pelvis and calices.[235] They are too small to be seen at angiography, mainly because the accumulation of contrast medium in the nephrographic phase "hides" these very small vessels. In occlusive disease, they may enlarge markedly and then have a characteristic tortuous appearance (see Fig. 45-15). The ureteric or pelviureteric artery is usually observed as a very small artery running medially and caudally from one of the main branches of the renal artery (see Fig. 45-22).

The importance of the perirenal and pelvic arterial supply of the kidney has been well demonstrated in anatomical dissection studies and in various disease entities.[234,236–241]

Nephrographic Phase

Four different stages of the nephrographic phase can be distinguished: the cortical arteriogram, the glomerulogram, the cortical nephrogram, and the general nephrogram.

The accumulation of contrast medium in the renal cortex appears simultaneously with the filling of the interlobular arteries. The *cortical arteriogram* (i.e., the point at which the contrast medium is observed in the interlobular arteries) lasts for less than 0.5 second because the vessels are quickly obscured by the increasing density of the cortex. The normal disappearance time of contrast medium from the renal arterial tree is approximately 1.0 second (0.5–2.0 seconds) after the end of the injection in selective renal angiography. Often the interlobular arteries cannot be seen in high-quality renal angiograms because the timing of the exposures is not correctly related to the short period they are visible. The interlobular arteries arise at right angles from the arcuate arteries at approximately 3-mm intervals.[242] They run parallel and straight toward the renal surface. What is really seen in the cortical arteriogram is probably a composite of groups of interlobular arteries because of overlapping.[186,207]

With 3× magnification and with a fine focus of less than 0.2 mm, the interlobular arteries and glomeruli more than 100 μm in diameter can be observed (see Figs. 45-9 and 45-10). What is seen are not single glomeruli but a composite of glomerular tufts.[186] Thus with the magnification technique, in the early nephrographic phase a peppery appearance that depends on the filling of the glomeruli with contrast medium can be seen.[243]

The *glomerulogram* lasts for about 1 to 2 seconds. The glomerulus acts as an aneurysm and stores the contrast medium temporarily because the diameters of the afferent and efferent arteriolae are one-third to one-fifth of the diameter of the glomerulus.[242] Because of overlapping, they seem to vary in size, being largest (2–3 mm) in the renal hilus and subcortically. By counting the glomeruli in certain areas, it seems possible to obtain highly accurate information about glomerular function. The glomerulogram represents only that part of the glomerular population that is most promptly perfused and that probably represents the fast component of the ^{133}Xe clearance curve.[242]

After 1 to 2 seconds, the background density increases to such an extent that the glomeruli can no longer be seen. The *cortical nephrogram* becomes more homogeneous because the tubular filtrate, the cortical capillaries, and the peritubular spaces also become opacified. In normal kidneys, during the cortical

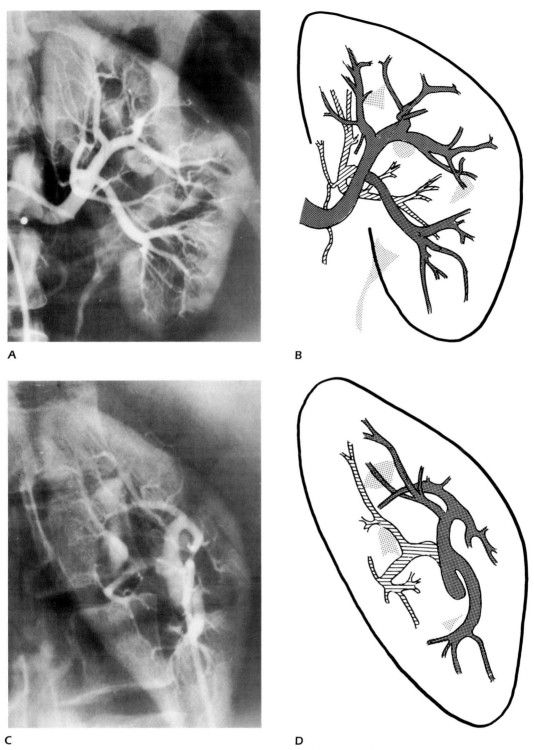

Figure 45-20. Abscess of the renal sinus that compresses the renal pelvis. (A and B) In the anteroposterior projection, displacement of the sinus branches can hardly be discerned. (C and D) In a true lateral view of the kidney, the segmental and interlobar branches are at a great distance from each other, and they are arch-shaped because of the expansive lesion in the sinus.

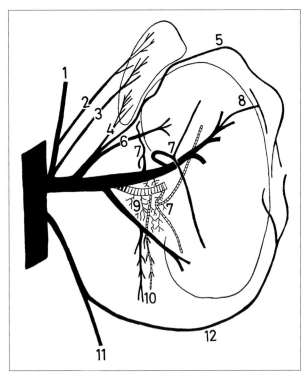

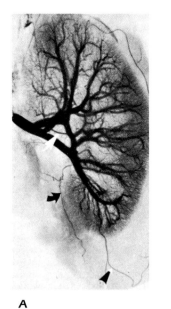

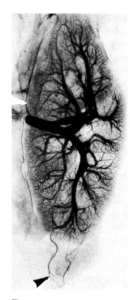

A   **B**

Figure 45-22. Autopsy specimen. A view corresponding to in vivo (A) frontal and (B) true lateral views of the kidney. The middle capsular arteries (*white arrowheads*) arise from the dorsal artery and supply the fatty capsule posterior to the kidney. A wide perforating artery (*black arrowheads*) arises from an arcuate artery in the lower pole. The ureteric artery (*arrow*) branches from the lower polar artery. (From Boijsen E. Angiographic studies of the anatomy of single and multiple renal arteries. Acta Radiol (Stockh) 1959;Suppl 183. Used with permission.)

Figure 45-21. Diagram showing adrenal capsular and pelvic arteries that are frequently observed in the renal angiogram. *1,* Inferior phrenic artery; *2–4,* arteries to the adrenal gland; *5,* superior capsular artery; *6,* sublobular branch to the upper pole arising from the superior capsular–inferior adrenal artery; *7,* middle capsular arteries; *8,* perforating artery; *9–10,* pelvic and ureteric arteries; *11–12,* spermatic and inferior capsular arteries. (From Boijsen E. Angiographic studies of the anatomy of single and multiple renal arteries. Acta Radiol (Stockh) 1959;Suppl 183. Used with permission.)

nephrogram the cortex is well distinguished from the medulla and the renal surface is also well defined. The renal surface appears smooth, but shallow indentations between each lobe may be identified. Somewhat deeper fissures are often noted between the intermediate part and the superior and inferior poles. Fetal lobulation, represented by deep fissures between the lobes, is rarely observed.[220,244] If marked lobulation is present, it is more often due to abnormal situations, such as central scarring or hyperplasia (see Fig. 45-15). This type of cortical fissure should be distinguished from the irregularities caused by cortical destruction.

The cortical width and the total cortical volume can be estimated and can be used to obtain accurate information about the amount of functioning parenchyma.[245,246] The columns of Bertin are usually well outlined, giving good information about the position of the various lobes (see Fig. 45-12).[216] The cortex is somewhat thicker in the poles (where it is about 10

mm) than in the intermediate parts (where it is 7–8 mm).[245]

The density of the cortical nephrogram depends on the amount and the rate of injection of contrast medium given and the functional capacity of the kidney. The high density of the cortical nephrogram lasts about 4 seconds. It is followed by a *general nephrogram,* during which the density of the cortex steadily decreases over a period of 10 to 15 seconds. The border between the cortex and medulla then gradually disappears. During this period, the contrast medium is washed out of the cortical vessels and extracellular spaces, and it appears in the lumina of the pyramids and their vascular compartments. The slow disappearance rate has been said to be due partly to the relatively large amount of contrast medium in the tubular cells that is washed out to the peritubular capillaries and partly to the stagnation of the filtered contrast medium in the lumina of the nephrons.[247] It is more probable that the contrast medium is retrieved from the extracellular space. After about 20 seconds, a steady state of the nephrographic phase is observed for about 2 minutes, which is due to recirculation and to the slow transport through the lumina of the nephrons.

Venous Phase

Even if small intrarenal veins can sometimes be observed at magnification angiography,[242] they usually cannot be distinguished in an angiogram performed with routine technique. The reason is that the high extraction of contrast medium from the blood results in a rather poor concentration of the medium in the veins. Furthermore, the dense cortical nephrogram prevents demonstration of the veins. Therefore the larger collecting veins in the renal sinus are also poorly demonstrated (see Figs. 45-10 and 45-12).

The normal appearance time of the renal veins is approximately 3.50 seconds (1.75–5.00 seconds) after the onset of injection in the renal artery, with the peak density at 8 seconds (6–10 seconds). Contrast medium is retained in the veins for about 20 seconds.[207] The retardation of the contrast medium in the renal vein is in accordance with the slow disappearance of contrast medium from the cortex.

The normal anatomy of the intrarenal and extrarenal parts of the renal vein usually cannot be defined with accuracy. With high doses of contrast medium, the extrarenal part may be reasonably well defined, but this technique can be accepted only in situations in which nephrectomy is planned. In selected cases, renal phlebography is a far better method for defining the anatomy.

Physiologic Considerations

Injection of contrast medium into the renal artery is an unphysiologic technique that is bound to cause changes in the renal blood flow.[166,169,248] The high viscosity and osmolality, the changes in the blood corpuscles, and the sudden increase in pressure at the injection are all factors of importance to remember when evaluating renal morphology and function by angiography. Nevertheless, an aortic or selective injection of contrast medium gives information about renal function that cannot be obtained by other methods. Several of these parameters were mentioned before; they are briefly recapitulated:

1. The *size* of the renal artery and its branches is a crude but nevertheless good indication of renal function. It should be remembered, however, that in acute or subacute renal failure, the renal artery is of normal width. Also, in hypertension or atherosclerosis the renal artery may be of normal size despite the reduction in cortical flow.
2. The intrarenal arterial pattern shows so many variations that reliable information can be obtained only when local changes are present. General age-related changes are particularly difficult to evaluate.
3. A reflux of contrast medium to the aorta during selective injection at the rate of 8 to 10 ml per second usually indicates an increased resistance to flow. Use of a spillover flowmeter combined with cinefluorography can give semiquantitative information.[249]
4. The transit time of contrast medium through the renal arterial tree is another parameter that can be used to give certain information about the blood flow. In particular, local changes in blood flow may be appreciated, but these cannot be quantified.
5. The degree of accumulation of contrast medium in the cortical nephrogram and the cortical width are crude but nevertheless practical and often-used criteria for quickly evaluating renal function. The cortical volume can be estimated.[245,246]
6. The number of glomeruli in a defined area can be counted to give quantitative information about renal functioning.[242]
7. The appearance time of contrast in the renal vein and the width of the vein give less important information about renal function.

Counting the number of glomeruli, using the spillover technique, and estimating the cortical volume can give some quantitative information about renal blood flow and functioning parenchyma, but on the whole, with this method, the renal arteriogram gives limited information. Because the arterial tree of the kidney responds in a rather limited manner to a variety of diseases, the renal arteriogram is not informative enough about early changes in the renal parenchyma. Age-related changes also have to be included in the evaluation, which makes a diagnosis of parenchymal disease even more difficult. One cannot predict, therefore, the state of the arteriolar bed on the basis of angiographic data alone.[227,250] During selective catheterization of the renal artery, quantitative information can be obtained by the dye dilution technique[251,252] or with the radioactive gas washout technique.[253] Methods based on the linear velocity of the flow have been developed using either cinedensitometry or videodensitometry.[188,254] Another method is the videodensitometric measurement of iodine in the cortex.[254,255] More recently, simpler techniques have been developed; one is the determination of the relative blood flow with a videodilution technique in which the renal blood flow is measured as a fraction of the cardiac output.[190]

Although angiography has been used in research for estimating renal blood flow, it has had little practical clinical impact. Digital angiography offers a variety of methods for this purpose[191-194] but is not used often in practice, mainly because the flow can be estimated by noninvasive methods and without contrast media.

Conventional ultrasound does not offer information about renal blood flow, but, with the addition of the Doppler technique, spectral analysis of flow direction and velocity can be obtained. The addition of color Doppler supports the graphic tracing. However, the spatial resolution is not adequate for detailed analysis of the main renal arteries except in a limited number of cases, and supplementary arteries are usually overlooked.[256] On the other hand, flow velocity and vascular resistance can be estimated in peripheral branches down to the level of the arcuate arteries to discriminate significant primary and secondary vascular disease.[2,257] However, abdominal gas and adipositas often limit the value of ultrasound studies.

With the recent improvements in magnetic resonance imaging (MRI) of the renal vessels and estimation of renal blood flow, reliable information seems to be possible. A good correlation has been found between blood flow measurements made with phase-contrast cine MRI and clearance with p-aminohippurate.[258]

Like renal angiography, the noninvasive imaging methods give information of renal function by estimating renal blood flow. More important is the information obtained about the renal parenchyma, without the addition of contrast media. Both ultrasonography and MRI show a distinction between the renal cortex and medulla, which is also observed on CT after intravenous injection of contrast medium. With the intravenous bolus of contrast agent, time-density curves can be recorded in the renal parenchyma during CT,[259-261] and an image of the active cortical volume can be obtained. Similarly, experimental and clinical experience show that time-signal intensity curves and dynamic imaging can be obtained during MRI.[262-268]

References

1. Seldinger SI. Catheter replacement of the needle in percutaneous arteriography: a new technique. Acta Radiol 1953;39:368–376.
2. Scoutt LM, Zawin ML, Taylor KJW. Doppler US: Part II. Clinical applications. Radiology 1990;174:309–319.
3. Foley DW, ed. Color Doppler flow imaging. Boston: Andover, 1991.
4. Lewin SL, Laub B, Hausmann R. Three-dimensional time-of-flight MR angiography: applications in the abdomen and thorax. Radiology 1991;179:261–264.
5. Kent KC, Edelman RR, Kim D, et al. Magnetic resonance imaging: a reliable test for the evaluation of proximal atherosclerotic renal arterial stenosis. J Vasc Surg 1991;13:311–318.
6. Rubin GD, Dake MD, Napel SA, et al. Three-dimensional spiral CT angiography of the abdomen: initial clinical experience. Radiology 1993;186:147–152.
7. Crummy AB, Stieghorst MF, Turski PA, et al. Digital subtraction angiography: current status and use of intraarterial injection. Radiology 1982;145:303–307.
8. Dawson P. Digital subtraction angiography—a critical analysis. Clin Radiol 1988;39:474–477.
9. Hessel SJ, Adams DF, Abrams HL. Complications of angiography. Radiology 1981;138:273–281.
10. Rapoport S, Sniderman KW, Morse SS, et al. Pseudoaneurysm: a complication of faulty technique in femoral arterial puncture. Radiology 1985;154:529–530.
11. Grollman JH Jr, Marcus R. Antegrade translumbar aortography. Radiology 1984;153:249–250.
12. van Schaik JPJ, Hawkins IF. Translumbar catheter redirection using a tip-deflector technique. Radiology 1985;155:829–830.
13. Cope C. Minipuncture angiography. Radiol Clin North Am 1986;24:359–367.
14. Gritter KJ, Laidlaw WW, Peterson NT. Complications of outpatient transbrachial intraarterial digital subtraction angiography: work in progress. Radiology 1987;162:125–127.
15. Patel YD. Technical development: a modified pigtail catheter for transbrachial aortography. Clin Radiol 1990;41:128–129.
16. Baudouin CJ, Belli AM, Peck RJ, Cumberland DC. The complications of high brachial artery puncture. Clin Radiol 1990;42:277–280.
17. Grier D, Hartnell G. Percutaneous femoral artery puncture: practice and anatomy. Br J Radiol 1990;63:602–604.
18. Judkins MP, Kidd HJ, Frische LH, Dotter CT. Lumen-following safety J-guide for catheterization of tortuous vessels. Radiology 1967;88:1127–1130.
19. Smith TP, Derauf BJ, Darcy MD, et al. Movable core guide wire: evaluation of improved model. Radiology 1986;159:552–553.
20. Meyerovitz MF, Levin DC, Boxt LM. Superselective catheterization of small-caliber arteries with a new high-visible steerable guide wire. Am J Radiol 1985;144:785–786.
21. Sos TA, Cohn DJ, Srur M, et al. A new open-ended guide wire/catheter. Radiology 1985;154:817–818.
22. Formanek G, Frech RS, Amplatz K. Arterial thrombus formation during clinical percutaneous catheterization. Circulation 1970;41:833–839.
23. McCarty RJ, Glasser SP. Thrombogenicity of guide wires. Am J Cardiol 1973;32:943–946.
24. Ovitt TW, Durst S, Moore R, Amplatz K. Guide wire thrombogenicity and its reduction. Radiology 1974;111:43–46.
25. Anderson JH, Gianturco C, Wallace S, et al. Anticoagulation techniques for angiography: an experimental study. Radiology 1974;111:573–576.
26. Roberts GM, Roberts EE, Davies RL, Lawrie BW. Thrombogenicity of arterial catheters and guide wires. Br J Radiol 1977;50:415–418.
27. Takayasu K, Muramatsu Y, Moriyama N, et al. Plastic-coated guide wire for hepatic arteriography. Radiology 1988;166:545–546.
28. Leach KR, Kurisu Y, Carlson JE, et al. Thrombogenicity of hydrophilically coated guide wires and catheters. Radiology 1990;175:675–677.
29. Olin T. Studies in angiographic technique. Thesis, University of Lund, Malmö, 1963.
30. Mannila TO, Wiljasalo M. Semiselective renal arteriography. Invest Radiol 1967;2:176–178.
31. Owitt TW, Amplatz K. Semiselective renal angiography. AJR 1973;119:767–769.
32. Hettler M. Angiographische Probleme und Möglichkeiten: II. Der perkutane Arterienkatetermismus mit an der Spitze verschlossenem Katheter als Grundlage der Etagen-Aortographie. ROEFO 1960;92:198–206.
33. Boijsen E, Judkins MP. A hook-tail "closed-end" catheter for percutaneous selective cardioangiography. Radiology 1966;87:872–877.
34. Judkins MP. Percutaneous transfemoral selective coronary angiography. Radiol Clin North Am 1968;6:467–492.

35. Erikson U. On the technique of selective renal arteriography. Aust Radiol 1973;17:316–317.
36. Talner LB, McLaughlin AP, Bookstein JJ. Renal artery dissection: a complication of catheter angiography. Radiology 1975;117:291–295.
37. Hawkins IF, Haseman MK, Gelfand PN. Single mini-catheter for abdominal aortography and selective injection. Radiology 1979;132:755–757.
38. Rees CR, Merchun G, Becker GJ, et al. In vitro study of high-pressure catheters and various contrast agents. Radiology 1988;166:53–56.
39. Hansen EC, Hawkins MC, Hawkins IF Jr, et al. New high-flow "cloud" catheter for safer delivery of contrast material. Radiology 1989;173:461–464.
40. Brodey PA, Doppman JL, Bisaccia LJ. An unusual complication of aortography with the pig-tail catheter. Radiology 1974;110:711.
41. ApSimon HT, Hartley DE: Embolization of small vessels with a double-lumen microballoon catheter: Part I. Design and construction. Radiology 1984;151:55–57.
42. ApSimon HT, Hartley DE, Maddren L, Harper C. Embolization of small vessels with a double-lumen microballoon catheter: Part II. Laboratory, animal and histological studies. Work in progress. Radiology 1984;151:59–64.
43. Rosen RJ. A new catheter for selective and superselective angiography. Cardiovasc Intervent Radiol 1986;9:49–51.
44. Hosoki T, Hashimoto T, Masuike M, et al. Slippery coaxial catheter system. Radiology 1989;171:858–859.
45. Okazaki M, Higashihara H, Koganemaru F, et al. Emergent embolization for control of massive hemorrhage from a splanchnic artery with a new coaxial catheter system. Acta Radiol 1992;33:57–62.
46. Hare WSC, Kincaid-Smith P. Dissecting aneurysm of the renal artery. Radiology 1970;97:255–263.
47. Gill WB, Cole AT, Wong RJ. Renovascular hypertension developing as a complication of selective renal arteriography. J Urol 1972;107:922–924.
48. Reiss MD, Bookstein JJ, Bleifer KH. Radiologic aspects of renovascular hypertension: IV. Arteriographic complications. JAMA 1972;221:374–378.
49. Bergentz SE, Faarup P, Hegedüs V, et al. Diagnosis of hypertension due to occlusion of a supplemental renal artery; its localization, treatment by removal from the body, microsurgical repair and reimplantation: a case report. Ann Surg 1973; 178:643–647.
50. Engberg A, Erikson U, Killander A, et al. An unusual complication of selective renal angiography: a case presentation. Aust Radiol 1974;18:304–307.
51. Gewertz BL, Stanley JC, Fry WJ. Renal artery dissections. Arch Surg 1977;112:409–414.
52. Delin A, Fernström I, Swedenborg J. Intimal dissection of the renal artery following selective angiography: report of two cases and review of the literature. Vasa 1979;8:78–82.
53. Sigstedt B, Lunderquist A. Complications of angiographic examinations. AJR 1978;130:455–460.
54. Jonsson K, Lunderquist A, Pettersson H, Sigstedt B. Subintimal injection of contrast medium as a complication of selective abdominal angiography. Acta Radiol 1977;18:55–64.
55. Smiddy FG, Anderson GK. Tolerance of the kidneys to the contrast medium Urografin. Br J Urol 1960;32:156–159.
56. Farry PJ, Beale LR, Macbeth WAAG. Intrarenal extravasation complicating selective vessel angiography. N Z Med J 1970; 72:17–18.
57. Obrez I, Abrams HL. Temporary occlusion of the renal artery: effects and significance. Radiology 1972;104:545–556.
58. Olbert F, Denck H, Wicke L. Komplikationen bei Katheterangiographien: Ursachen und deren Behandlung. Wien Med Wochenschr 1973;123:293–298.
59. Jacobsson B, Bergentz SE, Ljungqvist U. Platelet adhesion and thrombus formation on vascular catheters in dogs. Acta Radiol 1969;8:221–227.
60. Nachnani GH, Lessin LS, Motomyia T, Jensen WN. Scanning electron microscopy of thrombogenesis on vascular catheter surfaces. N Engl J Med 1972;286:139–140.
61. Schlossman D. Thrombogenicity of vascular catheters. Thesis, University of Gothenburg, Sweden, 1972.
62. Jacobsson B, Schlossman D. Thromboembolism of leg following percutaneous catheterization of femoral artery for angiography: predisposing factors. Acta Radiol 1969;8:109–118.
63. Yellin AE, Shore EH. Surgical management of arterial occlusion following percutaneous femoral angiography. Surgery 1973;73:772–777.
64. Raininko R, Söder H. Clot formation in angiographic catheters—an in vitro comparative study: effects of heparin and protein coating of the catheter. Acta Radiol 1993;34:78–82.
65. Lang EK. A survey of the complications of percutaneous retrograde arteriography: Seldinger technique. Radiology 1963; 81:257–263.
66. Halpern M. Percutaneous transfemoral arteriography: an analysis of the complications in 1,000 consecutive cases. Am J Roentgenol 1964;92:918–934.
67. Saur HT. Komplikationen bei der indirekten (perkutanen Katheter-) Methode der Aortographie: Folgerungen in Bezug auf ihre Anwendung. Roentgen-blaetter 1966;19:305–308.
68. Baum S, Stein GN, Kuroda KK. Complications of "No arteriography." Radiology 1966;86:835–838.
69. Folin J. Complications of percutaneous femoral catheterization for renal angiography. Radiologe 1968;8:190–196.
70. Moore CH, Wolma FJ, Brown RW, Derrick JR. Complications of cardiovascular radiology: a review of 1204 cases. Am J Surg 1970;120:591–593.
71. Siegelman SS, Caplan LH, Annes GP. Complications of catheter angiography: study with oscillometry and "pull out" angiograms. Radiology 1968;91:251–253.
72. Jacobsson B, Paulin S, Schlossman D. Thromboembolism of leg following percutaneous catheterization of the femoral artery for angiography. Acta Radiol 1969;8:97–108.
73. Cramer R, Morre R, Amplatz K. Reduction of the surgical complication rate by the use of a hypothrombogenic catheter coating. Radiology 1973;109:585–588.
74. Edling NPG, Ovenfors CO. Risks in selective renal catheterization and arteriography: an experimental study in dogs. Acta Radiol 1964;2:241–249.
75. Hartmann HR, Newcomb AW, Barnes A, Lowman RM. Renal infarction following selective renal angiography. Radiology 1966;86:52–56.
76. Morrow J, Amplatz K. Embolic occlusion of the renal artery during aortography. Radiology 1966;86:57–59.
77. McConnel RW, Fore WW, Taylor A. Embolic occlusion of the renal artery following arteriography: successful management. Radiology 1973;107:273–274.
78. Buxton DR Jr, Mueller CF. Removal of iatrogenic clot by transcatheter embolectomy. Radiology 1974;111:39–41.
79. Porstmann W, Geisser W. Die retrograde Katerisierung des linken Ventrikels in der A. femoralis und der A. carotis communis dextra: Zwei sich ergänzende Methoden, ihre Indikationen und Ergebnisse. ROEFO 1959;91:14–24.
80. Wallace S, Medellin H, DeJongh D, Gianturco C. Systemic heparinization for angiography. Am J Roentgenol 1972;116:204–209.
81. Antonovic R, Rösch J, Dotter CT. The value of systemic arterial heparinization in transfemoral angiography: a prospective study. Am J Roentgenol 1976;127:223–225.
82. Dotter CT, Keller FS, Rösch J, Buschman RW. The value of protamine following heparin-covered angiography: double-blind placebo-controlled study. Radiology 1980;135:229–230.
83. Porstmann W, Wierny L, Warnke H, et al. Catheter closure of patent ductus arteriosus: 62 cases treated without thoracotomy. Radiol Clin North Am 1971;9:203–218.
84. Langsjoen PH, Best EB. Studies in the prevention of complications of angiography. Am J Roentgenol 1969;106:425–433.

85. Cramer A, Frech RS, Amplatz K. A preliminary human study with a simple non-thrombogenic catheter. Radiology 1971; 100:421–422.

86. Eldh P, Jacobsson B. Heparinized vascular catheters: a clinical trial. Radiology 1974;111:289–292.

87. Cope C. Intravascular breakage of Seldinger spring guide wires. JAMA 1962;180:1061–1063.

88. Fellmeth BD, Roberts AC, Bookstein JJ, et al. Postangiographic femoral artery injuries: nonsurgical repair with US-guided compression. Radiology 1991;178:671–675.

89. Dorfman GS, Cronan JJ. Postcatheterization femoral artery injuries: is there a role for nonsurgical treatment? Radiology 1991;178:629–630.

90. Widestadt BM, Bergentz SE, Boijsen E. Catheter angiography and venous thrombosis. Acta Radiol 1976;17:773–776.

91. Yasuno M, Onodera T, Kawata R, et al. Pulmonary embolism as a complication of transfemoral arteriography: incidence, symptoms and prevention. Jpn Circ J 1984;48:439–444.

92. Davidsen HG, Gudbjerg CE, Thomsen G. Complications of selective angiocardiography and percutaneous transarterial aortography. Acta Chir Scand (Suppl) 1961;283:161–181.

93. Gudbjerg CE, Christensen J. Dissection of the aortic wall in retrograde lumbar aortography. Acta Radiol 1961;55:364–368.

94. Gilbert GJ, Melnick GS. Pathophysiology of subintimal hematoma formation during retrograde arteriography. Radiology 1965;85:306–318.

95. Harrington JT, Sommers SC, Kassirer JP. Atheromatous emboli with progressive renal failure: renal arteriography as the probable inciting factor. Ann Intern Med 1968;68:152–166.

96. Lonni YGW, Matsumoto KK, Lecky JW. Postaortographic cholesterol (atheromatous) embolization. Radiology 1969; 93:63–65.

97. Sieniewicz DJ, Moore S, Moir FO, McDade DF. Atheromatous emboli to the kidneys. Radiology 1969;92:1231–1240.

98. Schwartz S, Waters L. Cholesterol embolization. Radiology 1973;106:37–41.

99. Gaines PA, Cumberland DC, Kennedy A, et al. Cholesterol embolization: a lethal complication of vascular catheterization. Lancet 1988;I:168–170.

100. Rosansky SJ, Deschamps EG. Multiple cholesterol emboli syndrome. Am J Med Sci 1984;288:45–48.

101. Henderson MJ, Manhire AR. Case report: cholesterol embolization following angiography. Clin Radiol 1990;42:281–282.

102. Adams DF, Olin TB, Kosek J. Cotton fiber embolization during angiography: a clinical and experimental study. Radiology 1965;84:678–681.

103. Yunis EJ, Landes RR. Hazards of glove powder in renal angiography. JAMA 1965;193:304–305.

104. Kay JM, Wilkins RA. Cotton fibre embolism during angiography. Clin Radiol 1969;20:410–413.

105. Brekkan A, Lexow PE, Woxholt G. Glass fragments and other particles contaminating contrast media. Acta Radiol 1975;16:600–608.

106. Winding O. Intrinsic particles in angiographic contrast media. Radiology 1980;134:317–320.

107. Williams A, Barnett MJ. Particulate contamination in intravenous fluids, administration sets and cannulae. Pharmacol J 1973;211:190–204.

108. Winding O, Grønvall J, Faarup P, Hegedüs V. Sequelae of intrinsic foreign-body contamination during selective renal angiography in rabbits. Radiology 1980;134:321–326.

109. Dalla Palma L, Stacul F, Pozzi-Mucelli R. Criteria for choice and use of contrast media in intraarterial DSA. Eur J Radiol 1985;5:62–67.

110. Naisby GP, Owen JP, Alexander TW, et al. Transfemoral digital subtraction angiography: are diluted high osmolar contrast media acceptable? Acta Radiol 1991;32:137–140.

111. Abrams HL. The response of neoplastic renal vessels to epinephrine in man. Radiology 1964;82:217–224.

112. Ekelund L, Göthlin J, Lunderquist A. Diagnostic improvement with angiotensin in renal angiography. Radiology 1972; 105:33–37.

113. Ekelund L. Pharmako-Angiographie der Niere. Radiologe 1973;13:279–282.

114. Bookstein JJ, Ernst CB. Vasodilatory and vasoconstrictive pharmacoangiographic manipulation of renal collateral flow. Radiology 1973;108:55–59.

115. Older RA, Miller JP, Jackson DC, et al. Angiographically induced renal failure and its radiographic detection. Am J Roentgenol 1976;126:1039–1045.

116. Byrd L, Sherman RL. Radiocontrast-induced acute renal failure: a clinical and pathophysiologic review. Medicine 1979; 58:270–279.

117. Swartz RD, Rubin JE, Leeming BW, Silva P. Renal failure following major angiography. Am J Med 1978;65:31.

118. Robertson PW, Dyson ML, Sutton PD. Renal angiography: a review of 1750 cases. Clin Radiol 1979;20:401–409.

119. Alexander RD, Berkes SL, Abuelo JG. Contrast media induced oliguric renal failure. Arch Intern Med 1978;138:381.

120. Borra S, Hawkins D, Duguid W, Kaye M. Acute renal failure and nephrotic syndrome after angiocardiography with meglumine diatrizoate. N Engl J Med 1971;284:592.

121. Kovnat PJ, Lin KY, Popky G. Azotemia and nephrogenic diabetes insipidus after arteriography. Radiology 1973;108:541–542.

122. Port FK, Wagoner RD, Fulton RE. Acute renal failure after angiography. Am J Roentgenol 1974;121:544–550.

123. Weinrauch JA, Healy RW, Leland OS, et al. Coronary angiography and acute renal failure in diabetic azotemic nephropathy. Ann Intern Med 1977;86:56.

124. Krumlovsky FA, Simon N, Santhanam S, et al. Acute renal failure—association with administration of radiographic contrast material. JAMA 1978;239:128.

125. Lang EK, Foreman J, Schlegel JU, et al. The incidence of contrast medium induced acute tubular necrosis following arteriography. Radiology 1981;138:203–206.

126. Gates GR, Green GS. Transient reduction in renal function following arteriography: a radionuclide study. J Urol 1983; 129:1296–1307.

127. Lautin EM, Freeman NJ, Schoenfeld AH, et al. Radiocontrast-associated renal dysfunction: incidence and risk factors. Am J Radiol 1991;157:49–58.

128. Katholi RE, Taylor GJ, Woods WT, et al. Nephrotoxicity of nonionic low-osmolality versus ionic high-osmolality contrast media: a prospective double-blind randomized comparison in human beings. Radiology 1993;186:183–187.

129. Weibull H, Törnqvist C, Bergqvist D, et al. Reversible renal insufficiency after percutaneous transluminal angioplasty (PTA) of renal artery stenosis. Acta Chir Scand 1984;150: 295.

130. Weibull H, Cederholm C, Almén T, et al. Does cerebral angiography of cadaveric kidney donors interfere with graft function? Acta Radiol 1987;28:451–455.

131. Cederholm C, Almén T, Bergqvist D, et al. Acute renal failure in rats: interaction between contrast media and temporary renal arterial occlusion. Acta Radiol 1989;30:321–326.

132. Idbohrn H, Berg N. On the tolerance of the rabbit's kidney to contrast media in renal angiography: a roentgenologic and histologic investigation. Acta Radiol 1954;42:121–140.

133. Mudge GH. Some questions on nephrotoxicity. Invest Radiol 1970;5:407–423.

134. Almén T. Relations between chemical structure, animal toxicity and clinical adverse effects of contrast media. In: Enge I, Edgren J, eds. Patient safety and adverse events in contrast medium examinations. Amsterdam: Science Publishers BV, 1989.

135. Laubscher WML, Raper FP. A report of a case of the injection of a massive dose of Urografin into the renal artery. Br J Urol 1960;32:160–164.

136. Sidd JJ, Decter A. Unilateral renal damage due to massive contrast dye injection with recovery. J Urol 1967;97:30–32.

137. Pepper HW, Korobkin MT, Palubinskas AJ. Massive injection

of contrast medium into a renal artery segment: a case report. Radiology 1974;112:273–274.

138. Talner LB, Rushmer HN, Coel MN. The effect of renal artery injection of contrast material on urinary enzyme excretion. Invest Radiol 1972;7:311–322.

139. Goldstein EJ, Feinfeld DA, Fleischner GM, Elkin M: Enzymatic evidence of renal tubular damage following renal angiography. Radiology 1976;121:617–619.

140. Albrechtsson U, Hultberg B, Larusdottir H, et al. Nephrotoxicity of nonionic contrast media in aorto-femoral angiography. Acta Radiol 1985;26:615–618.

141. Skovgaard N, Holm J, Hemmingsen L, et al. Urinary protein excretion following intravenously administered ionic and nonionic contrast media in man. Acta Radiol 1989;30:517–520.

142. Evensen A, Skalpe IA. Cell injury and cell regeneration in selective renal arteriography in rabbits: a preliminary report. Invest Radiol 1971;6:299–303.

143. Kaude J, Nordenfelt I. Influence of nephroangiography on ^{131}I-hippuran nephrography. Acta Radiol 1973;14:69–81.

144. Sorby WA, Hoy RJ. Renal arteriography and renal function. Aust Radiol 1968;12:25.

145. Danford RO, Talner LB, Davidson AJ. Effect of graded osmolalities of saline solution and contrast media on renal extraction of PAH in the dog. Invest Radiol 1969;4:301.

146. Holtås S, Almén T, Tejler L. Proteinuria following nephroangiography: III. Role of osmolality and concentration of contrast medium in renal arteries in dogs. Acta Radiol 1978;19:401–407.

147. Törnqvist C, Almén T, Golman K, et al. Renal function following nephroangiography with metrizamide and iohexol: effects on renal blood flow, glomerular permeability and filtration rate and diuresis in dogs. Acta Radiol 1985;26:483–489.

148. Mason RA, Arbeit LA, Girow F. Renal dysfunction after arteriography. JAMA 1985;253:1001–1004.

149. Moreau JF, Droz D, Sabto J, et al. Osmotic nephrosis induced by water-soluble tri-iodinated contrast media in man: a retrospective study of 47 cases. Radiology 1975;115:329–336.

150. Gruskin AB, Detliker OH, Wolfish NM, et al. Effects of angiography on renal function and histology in infants and piglets. J Pediatr 1970;76:41–48.

151. Kumar S, Hull JD, Lathi S, et al. Low incidence of renal failure after angiography. Arch Intern Med 1981;141:1268–1270.

152. Martin-Paredero V, Dixon SM, Baker JD, et al. Risk of renal failure after major angiography. Arch Surg 1983;118:1417–1420.

153. Cruz C, Hricak H, Samhouri F, et al. Contrast media for angiography: effect on renal function. Radiology 1986;158:109–112.

154. Miller DL, Chang R, Wells WT, et al. Intravascular contrast media: effect of dose on renal function. Radiology 1988;167:607–611.

155. Moore RD, Steinberg EP, Powe NR, et al. Frequency and determinants of adverse reactions induced by high-osmolality contrast media. Radiology 1989;170:727–732.

156. Billström Å, Hietala SO, Lithner F, et al. Nephrotoxicity of contrast media in patients with diabetes mellitus. Acta Radiol 1989;30:509–515.

157. Gomes AS, Lois JF, Baker JD, et al. Acute renal dysfunction in high-risk patients after angiography: comparison of ionic and non-ionic contrast media. Radiology 1989;170:65–68.

158. Lautin EM, Freeman NJ, Schoenfeld A, et al. Radiocontrast-associated renal dysfunction: a comparison of lower-osmolality and conventional high-osmolality contrast media. Am J Roentgenol 1991;157:59–65.

159. Niconoff T, Skau T, Berglund J, et al. Effects of femoral arteriography and low osmolar contrast agents on renal function. Acta Radiol 1993;34:88–91.

160. Aspelin P. Effect of ionic and non-ionic contrast media on red blood cell morphology and rheology. Thesis, University of Lund, Malmö, 1976.

161. Raininko R, Ylinen SL. Effect of ionic and non-ionic contrast media on aggregation of red blood cells in vitro: a preliminary report. Acta Radiol 1987;28:87–92.

162. Robertson HJF. Blood clot formation in angiographic syringes containing nonionic contrast media. Radiology 1987;163:621–622.

163. Dawson P. Contrast agents, red cells, coagulation and the angiographer. Invest Radiol 1990;25(Suppl):S117–S118.

164. Smith HJ, Levorstad K, Berg J, et al. High dose urography in patients with renal failure: a double blind investigation of iohexol and metrizoate. Acta Radiol 1985;26:213–220.

165. Harris KG, Smith TP, Cragg AH, et al. Nephrotoxicity from contrast material in renal insufficiency: ionic versus nonionic agents. Radiology 1991;179:849–852.

166. Aperia A, Broberger O, Ekengren K. Renal hemodynamics during selective renal angiography. Invest Radiol 1968;3:389–396.

167. Talner LB, Davidson AJ. Renal hemodynamic effects of contrast media. Invest Radiol 1968;3:310.

168. Sherwood T, Lavender JP. Does renal blood flow rise or fall in response to diatrizoate? Invest Radiol 1969;4:327–328.

169. Caldicott WJ, Hollenberg NK, Abrams HL. Characteristics of response of renal vascular bed to contrast media: evidence of vasoconstriction induced by renin-angiotensin system. Invest Radiol 1970;5:539–547.

170. Katzberg RW, Morris TW, Burgener FA, et al. Renal renin and hemodynamic responses to selective renal artery catheterization and angiography. Invest Radiol 1977;12:381–388.

171. Morris TW, Katzberg RW, Fischer HW. A comparison of the hemodynamic responses to metrizamide and meglumine/sodium diatrizoate in canine renal angiography. Invest Radiol 1978;13:74–78.

172. Dorph S. Changes in renal size following intraarterial administration of water-soluble contrast medium. Invest Radiol 1974;9:487–492.

173. Young DB, Rostorfer HH. Renin release responses to acute alterations in renal arterial osmolality. Am J Physiol 1973;225:1003.

174. Edsman G. Angionephrography and suprarenal angiography. Acta Radiol (Stockh) 1957;Suppl 155.

175. Albrechtsson U, Tylén U. Spasm of cortical arteries as a complication to selective nephroangiography. Acta Radiol 1978;19:785–791.

176. Spriggs DW, Brantley RE. Recognition of renal artery spasm during renal angiography. Radiology 1978;127:363–366.

177. Elkin M, Meng CH. Angiographic study of the effect of vasopressors—epinephrine and levarterenol—on renal vascularity. Am J Roentgenol 1965;93:904–915.

178. Elkin M, Meng CH. The effects of angiotensin on renal vascularity in dogs. Am J Roentgenol 1965;98:927–934.

179. Kupic EA, Abrams HL. Renal vascular alterations induced by hemorrhagic hypotension: preliminary observations. Invest Radiol 1968;3:345.

180. Redman HC, Olin TB, Saldeen T, Reuter SR. Nephrotoxicity of some vasoactive drugs following selective intra-arterial injection. Invest Radiol 1966;1:458–464.

181. Knapp R, Hollenberg NK, Busch GJ, Abrams HL. Prolonged unilateral acute renal failure induced by intra-arterial norepinephrine infusion in the dog. Invest Radiol 1972;7:164–173.

182. Levin DC, Dunham L. New equipment considerations for angiographic laboratories. Am J Roentgenol 1982;139:775–780.

183. Aakhus T, Lantto L, Kolmannskog F, et al. Comparison of image intensifier photofluorography and full-size radiography in abdominal angiography. Acta Radiol 1981;22:39–47.

184. Sakuma S, Ikeda H, Ayakawa Y, et al. Angiography with direct fourfold magnification. Invest Radiol 1969;4:310–316.

185. Stein HL. Direct serial magnification. Renal arteriography: a clinical study. J Urol 1973;109:967–970.

186. Bookstein JJ, Davidson AJ, Hill GS, et al. The small renal vessels. In: Hilal SK, ed. Small vessel angiography. St. Louis: Mosby, 1973.

187. Boijsen E, Maly P. Vergrösserungstechnik in der abdominellen Angiographie. Radiologe 1978;18:167–171.

188. Silverman NR. Television fluorodensitometry: technical consideration and some clinical application. Invest Radiol 1970; 5:35–40.

189. Lantz B. Relative flow measured by roentgen videodensitometry in hydrodynamic model. Acta Radiol 1975;16:503–519.

190. Link DP, Lantz BMT, Foerster JM, et al. New videodensitometric method for measuring renal artery blood flow at routine angiography: validation in the canine model. Invest Radiol 1979;14:465–470.

191. Kruger RA, Anderson RE, Koehler PR, et al. A method for the noninvasive evaluation of cardiovascular dynamics using a digital radiographic device. Radiology 1981;139:301–305.

192. Heintzen PH, Brennecke R, Bürsch JH, et al. Quantitative analysis of structure and function of the cardiovascular system by roentgen-video-computer techniques. Mayo Clin Proc 1982;57(Suppl):78–91.

193. Kruger RA, Bateman W, Yu Liu P, Nelson JA. Blood flow determination using recursive processing: a digital radiographic method. Radiology 1983;149:293–298.

194. Swanson DK, Myerowitz PD, Hegge JO, Watson KM. Arterial blood-flow waveform measurement in intact animals: new digital radiographic technique. Radiology 1986;161:323–328.

195. Köhler R. Incomplete angiogram in selective renal angiography. Acta Radiol 1963;1:1011–1031.

196. Engelbrecht HE, Keen EN, Fine H, et al. The radiological anatomy of the parenchymal distribution of the renal artery. S Afr Med J 1969;43:826–834.

197. Aubert J, Koumare K. Variations of origin of the renal artery. Eur Urol 1975;1:182–188.

198. Doppman J. An ectopic renal artery. Br J Radiol 1967;40: 312.

199. Lundius B. Intrathoracic kidney. AJR 1975;125:675–681.

200. Wójtowicz J. Relationship of the surface parameters of the kidney to the size of the renal artery. Invest Radiol 1967;2: 231–242.

201. Idbohrn H. Renal angiography in experimental hydronephrosis. Acta Radiol (Stockh) 1956;Suppl 136.

202. Widén T. Renal angiography during and after unilateral ureteric occlusion. Acta Radiol (Stockh) 1958;Suppl 162.

203. Kittredge RD, Hemley SD, Kanick V, Finby N. The atrophic renal artery. AJR 1964;92:309.

204. Ludin H, Elde M, Fehr H, Thoelen H. Correlation of renal size, renal artery calibre, and effective renal plasma flow in man. Acta Radiol 1967;6:296–302.

205. Freed TA, Hager H, Vinik M. Effects of intra-arterial acetylcholine on renal arteriography in normal humans. AJR 1968; 104:312–318.

206. Ozer H, Hollenberg NK. Renal angiographic and hemodynamic responses to vasodilators: a comparison of five agents in the dog. Invest Radiol 1974;9:473–478.

207. Abrams HL. The kidney: quantitative derivates of renal radiologic studies: an overview. Invest Radiol 1972;7:240–279.

208. Newhouse JH, Hollenberg NK. Vascular characteristics of unilateral acute renal failure in the dog: assessment with vasodilators and antagonists to angiotensin and norepinephrine. Invest Radiol 1974;9:241–251.

209. Kupic EA, Gibbons PD, Leavitt T. Angiographic studies of the canine kidney following intravenous injection of methedrine: a preliminary report. Invest Radiol 1974;9:404–407.

210. Ljungqvist A. The intrarenal arterial pattern in the normal and diseased human kidney. Acta Med Scand 1963;174:1–38.

211. Davidson AJ, Talner LB, Downs WM III. A study of the angiographic appearance of the kidney in an aging normotensive population. Radiology 1969;92:975–983.

212. Hegedüs V. Arterial anatomy of the kidney: A three-dimensional angiographic investigation. Acta Radiol 1972;12:604–618.

213. Davidson AJ. Radiological diagnosis of renal parenchymal disease. Philadelphia: Saunders, 1977.

214. Hodson CJ. The logic of the blood supply to the kidney. In: Margulis AR, Gooding CA, eds. Diagnostic radiology. San Francisco: University of California Press, 1978.

215. Meiisel P, Apitzsch DE. Atlas der Nierenangiographie. Berlin: Springer-Verlag, 1978.

216. Boijsen E. Angiographic studies of the anatomy of single and multiple renal arteries. Acta Radiol (Stockh) 1959;Suppl 183.

217. Graves FT. The anatomy of the intrarenal arteries and its application to segmental resection of the kidney. Br J Surg 1954; 42:132.

218. Graves FT. The anatomy of the intrarenal arteries in health and disease. Br J Surg 1956;43:605.

219. Poisel S, Spängler HP. Die Verästelungstypen der Arteria renalis in Hinblick auf die arterielle Blutversorgung des Parenchyms der Niere: Ein Beitrag zum Problem der sogennanten Nierensegmente. Acta Anat 1970;76:516–529.

220. Sykes D. The correlation between renal vascularization and lobulation of the kidney. Br J Urol 1964;36:549–555.

221. Löfgren F. Das topographische System der malpigischen Pyramiden der Menschenniere. Thesis, University of Lund, Malmö, 1949.

222. Hellström J. Uber die Varianten der Nierengefässe. Z Urol Chir 1928;29:253.

223. Andersson I. Renal artery lesions after pyelolithotomy: a potential cause of renovascular hypertension. Acta Radiol 1976; 17:685–695.

224. Baum S, Gillenswater JY. Renal artery impression on the renal pelvis. J Urol 1966;95:139–145.

225. Rusiewicz E, Reilly BJ. The significance of isolated upper pole calyceal dilatation. J Can Assoc Radiol 1968;19:179–182.

226. Fraley EE. Dismembered infundibulopyelostomy: improved technique for correcting vascular obstruction of the superior infundibulum. J Urol 1969;101:144–148.

227. Gill WM Jr, Pudvan WR. Arteriographic diagnosis of renal parenchymal disease. Radiology 1970;96:81–84.

228. Gold JM, Bucy JG. Fraley's syndrome with bilateral infundibular obstruction. J Urol 1974;112:299–301.

229. Fraley EE. Vascular obstruction of superior infundibulum causing nephralgia: a new syndrome. N Engl J Med 1966; 275:1403–1409.

230. Boijsen E, Link DP. Arteriography before needle puncture of renal hilar lesions. J Urol 1977;118:237–239.

231. Ekelund L, Boijsen E, Lindstedt E. Pseudotumor of the renal pelvis caused by renal artery aneurysm. Acta Radiol 1979;20: 753–761.

232. Hou-Jensen H. Die Verästelung der Arteria renalis in der Niere des Menschen. Z Anat Entwicklungsgesch 1930;91:1.

233. Andersson I, Boijsen E, Hellsten S, Linell F. Lesions of the dorsal renal artery in surgery for renal pelvic calculus. Eur Urol 1979;5:343–346.

234. Eliska O. The perforating arteries and their role in the collateral circulation of the kidneys. Acta Anat 1968;70:184–201.

235. Douville E, Hollinshead WH. The blood supply of the normal renal pelvis. J Urol 1955;73:906–912.

236. Merklin RJ, Michels NA. The variant renal and suprarenal blood supply with data on the inferior phrenic, ureteral, and gonadal arteries. J Int Coll Surg 1958;29:41–76.

237. Boijsen E, Folin J. Angiography in the diagnosis of renal carcinoma. Radiologe 1961;1:173–191.

238. Boijsen E, Folin J. Angiography in carcinoma of the renal pelvis. Acta Radiol 1961;56:81–93.

239. Abrams HL, Cornell SH. Patterns of collateral flow in renal ischemia. Radiology 1965;84:1001–1012.

240. Meyers MA, Freidenberg RM, King MC, Meng CH. The significance of the renal capsular arteries. Br J Radiol 1967;40: 949–956.

241. Yune HY, Klatte EC. Collateral circulation to an ischemic kidney. Radiology 1976;119:539–546.

242. Cope C, Raja RM, Isard HJ. Correlation of glomerulography

and renal function in hypertension. Radiology 1974;110:15–19.

243. Takaro T. Clinical renal glomerulography. Radiology 1968; 90:1203–1204.

244. Cooperman LH, Lowman RM. Fetal lobulation of the kidneys. AJR 1964;92:273–280.

245. Hegedüs V, Faarup P. Cortical volume of the normal human kidney: correlated angiographic and morphologic investigations. Acta Radiol 1972;12:481–496.

246. Hegedüs V, Ravnskov U. Cortical volume in apparently normal kidneys. Scand J Urol 1972;6:159–165.

247. Bolin H. Contrast medium in kidney during angiography: a densitometric method for estimation of renal function. Acta Radiol (Stockh) 1966;Suppl 257.

248. Tadavarthy SM, Castaneda W, Amplatz K. Redistribution of renal blood flow caused by contrast media. Radiology 1977; 122:343–348.

249. Olin T, Redman HC. Spillover flow-meter: a preliminary approach. Acta Radiol 1966;4:217–222.

250. Davidson AJ, Talner LB. Lack of specificity of renal angiography in the diagnosis of renal parenchymal disease: a point of view. Invest Radiol 1973;8:90–95.

251. Lingårdh G, Muth T, Olin T. Renal blood flow in dogs studied by means of a dye-dilution technique. Scand J Urol Nephrol 1969;3:281–290.

252. Göthlin J, Olin T. Dye dilution technique with nephroangiography for the determination of renal blood flow and related parameters. Acta Radiol 1973;14:113–117.

253. Barger AC, Herd JA. Physiology in medicine: the renal circulation. N Engl J Med 1971;284:482–490.

254. Deininger HK, Heuck F, Vanselow K. The determination of the circulation in normal human kidneys by means of angiocinedensitometry. Ann Radiol 1978;21:365–367.

255. Erikson U, Lörelius LE, Ruhn G. Determination of the renal blood flow by videodensitometry. Ann Radiol 1978;21:363–364.

256. Berland LL, Koslin DB, Routh WD, Keller FS. Renal artery stenosis: prospective evaluation of diagnosis with color duplex US compared with angiography. Work in progress. Radiology 1990;174:421–423.

257. Stavros AT, Parker SH, Yakes WF, et al. Segmental stenosis of the renal artery: pattern recognition of tardus and parvus abnormalities with duplex sonography. Radiology 1992;184: 487–492.

258. Sommer G, Noorbehesht B, Pelc N, et al. Normal renal blood flow measurement using phase-contrast cine magnetic resonance imaging. Invest Radiol 1992;27:465–470.

259. Treugut H, Nyman U, Hildell J. Sequenz-CT: frühe Dichteveränderungen der gesunden Niere nach Kontrastmittelapplikation. Radiologe 1980;20:558–562.

260. Ishikawa I, Onouchi Z, Saito Y, et al. Renal cortex visualization and analysis of dynamic CT curves of the kidney. J Comput Assist Tomogr 1981;5:695–701.

261. Jaschke WR, Gould RG, Cogan MG, et al. Cine-CT measurement of cortical renal blood flow. J Comput Assist Tomogr 1987;11:779–784.

262. Pettigrew RI, Avruch L, Dannels W, et al. Fast-field-echo MR imaging with Gd-DTPA: physiologic evaluation of the kidney and liver. Radiology 1986;160:561–563.

263. Kikinis R, von Schulthess GK, Jäger P, et al. Normal and hydronephrotic kidney: evaluation of renal function with contrast-enhanced MR imaging. Radiology 1987;165:837–842.

264. Carvlin MJ, Arger PH, Kundel HL, et al. Acute tubular necrosis: use of Gadolinium-DTPA and fast MR imaging to evaluate renal function in the rabbit. J Comput Assist Tomogr 1987;11:488–495.

265. Carvlin MJ, Arger PH, Kundel HL, et al. Use of Gd-DTPA and fast gradient-echo and spin-echo MR imaging to demonstrate renal function in the rabbit. Radiology 1989;170:705–711.

266. Choyke PL, Frank JA, Girton ME, et al. Dynamic Gd-DTPA-enhanced MR imaging of the kidney: experimental results. Radiology 1989;170:713–720.

267. Munechika H, Sullivan DC, Hedlund LW, et al. Evaluation of acute renal failure with magnetic resonance imaging using gradient-echo and Gd-DTPA. Invest Radiol 1991;26:22–27.

268. Hamed MM, Hamm B, Ibrahim ME, et al. Dynamic MR imaging of the abdomen with gadopentetate dimeglumine: normal enhancement patterns of the liver, spleen, stomach and pancreas. AJR 1992;158:303–307.

46

Renal Tumor Versus Renal Cyst

HERBERT L. ABRAMS
CLEMENT J. GRASSI

The ability to diagnose carcinoma of the kidney accurately is of particular importance because renal mass lesions are frequently encountered, requiring nephrectomy if malignant and renal tissue conservation if benign. Although histologic certainty is achieved only after a piece of tissue has been examined, imaging approaches to the kidney are so well developed that a high accuracy of diagnosis is now possible in most cases. Because several methods of radiologic investigation are available, the contribution of each method must be carefully defined. Intravenous urography, ultrasonography, computed tomography, radionuclide renography, angiography, renal venography, and magnetic resonance imaging are all available methods of studying the kidney, and each makes its particular contribution. Before critical management decisions can be made, one must consider the strengths and weaknesses of each modality and the degree of certainty that is required.

This chapter discusses the application of angiography to the evaluation of the nature of renal mass lesions and also indicates the relative contributions of other imaging methods.

Tumors

Tumors of the kidney account for about 1 percent of cancer deaths,[1] and renal cell carcinoma accounts for 3 percent of all adult cancers.[2] A number of features sometimes render diagnosis complex and therapy challenging. Renal cell carcinoma may be characterized by such nonurologic symptoms and signs as polycythemia, fever, weight loss, hypertension, and hypercalcemia suggesting hyperparathyroidism. It is one of the few tumors in which regression of the metastases has been reported after removal of the primary carcinoma.[3,4]

Renal tumors are variously characterized as primary or secondary; benign or malignant; epithelial or nonepithelial; parenchymal, pelvic, or capsular; and ma-

ture or immature. Although each of these classifications is useful, the relatively simple classification of Table 46-1 places the most important tumors in focus. Wilms tumor, renal cell carcinoma, and transitional cell carcinoma are the tumors of greatest importance clinically. Renal cell carcinoma constitutes approximately 80 to 83 percent; transitional cell, 7 to 10 percent; Wilms tumor, 5 to 6 percent; and miscellaneous tumors, 3 to 4 percent of clinically recognizable renal neoplasms.[5,6] In autopsy material benign renal tumors of both epithelial and mesenchymal origin are found far more commonly than malignant tumors.[7]

Wilms Tumor

Wilms tumor (nephroblastoma, adenomyosarcoma) is derived from embryonal renal tissue and is a mixture of connective, epithelial, and muscular elements. It is by far the most common renal tumor of infants and children; two-thirds of the cases of Wilms tumor are observed before the age of 3, and three-fourths before the age of 5. This explains the unusual double-peak incidence of malignant renal tumors in the first and the sixth decades of life. The tumor occurs twice as often in males as in females.

Pathology

These bulky tumors are the largest tumors of children, and they are characterized by rapid growth, early metastasis, and direct extension to neighboring organs. Metastases are found most commonly in the lung, but they also occur in the liver, bone, lymph nodes, and central nervous system (Table 46-2).[8,9] Both kidneys are involved in 2 to 8 percent of cases, either with double primary tumor or metastasis. By the time of clinical recognition, at least 20 percent of patients have metastases.

The tumors are usually solid in consistency, opaquely white on cut section, and lobular (Fig. 46-1). The larger tumors may have areas of necrosis, hem-

Table 46-1. Classification of Renal Tumors

	Primary Tumors		Metastatic Tumors
Benign	**Malignant**		
Epithelial	Epithelial		Epithelial
Adenoma	Renal cell carcinoma (parenchymal)		Especially from lung and breast carcinoma,
Nonepithelial	Transitional or squamous cell carcinoma		but also from other primary carcinomas
Fibroma	(pelvic)		Nonepithelial
Leiomyoma	Nonepithelial		Lymphoma
Neurogenic tumor	Wilms tumor		Melanoma
Angioma	Sarcoma of different cell types		Sarcoma
Hamartoma			

orrhage, and cyst formation. Histologically, the dominant cells are primitive spindle cells and round cells (resembling a sarcoma containing epithelial tubules), smooth and striated muscle cells, connective tissue, and sometimes cartilage and osseous tissue. Although the spindle-shaped cells resemble fibroblasts on light microscopy, their ultrastructure is such that some of them appear to be undifferentiated epithelial cells, such as those seen in the developing metanephros.[10]

Symptoms and Signs

The most common manifestation of Wilms tumor that brings the patient to the physician's attention is abdominal swelling or distention, frequently observed by the parent or by the pediatrician on routine physical examination (Table 46-3). About one-half of cases are discovered in this way, but 90 percent of patients have a palpable mass on physical examination.[11] Pain is a less common presenting symptom in children; it is very likely secondary to the mechanical effect of the tumor mass, stretching of the renal capsule, or bleeding into the tumor. Fever and hematuria may also signal the presence of the tumor. Hypertension has been commonly noted, perhaps on the basis of local ischemia caused by the renal mass.

On physical examination, the mass is commonly felt, enabling a presumptive diagnosis. Ascites and

swelling of the limbs may be observed if the tumor is large enough to compress or invade the inferior vena cava. The child may seem ill and look emaciated by the time the tumor is suspected.

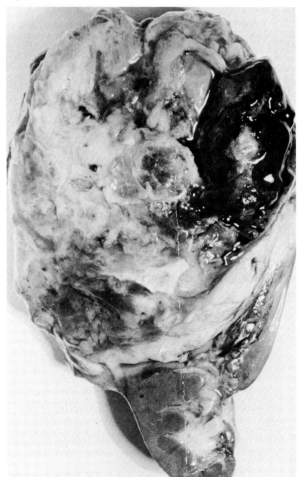

Figure 46-1. Gross pathologic appearance of Wilms tumor. Most tumors are lobular and opaquely white on cut section. They may have areas of necrosis, hemorrhage, and cyst formation. Note that the tumor has virtually replaced the kidney in this case.

Table 46-2. Extrarenal Metastases in 59 Patients with Wilms Tumor

Site of Metastases	Number of Patients	Percentage of Patients
Lung	28	47
Liver	8	14
Bone	7	12
Spinal cord	1	2
Retroperitoneum	1	2

Data from Clark et al.[8] and Westra et al.[9]

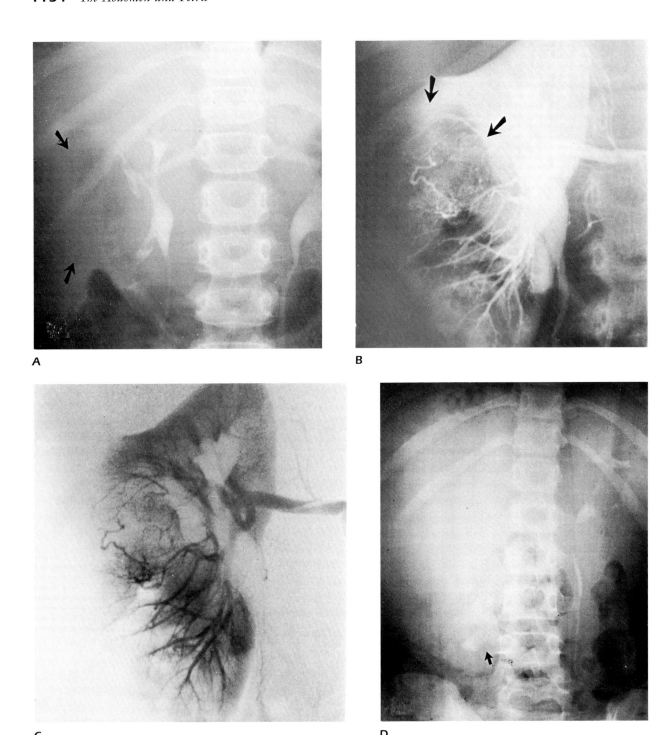

C   **D**

Figure 46-2. Wilms tumor. (A to C) Hypovascular localized mass. (A) Urogram. Note the displacement and distortion of the middle and lower pole calices and clear evidence of a mass (*arrows*). (B and C) Angiogram. Although the tumor (*arrows*) is not highly vascular, irregular, coiled, randomly distributed tumor vessels are visible; they are particularly well shown on the subtraction film (C). (D to F) Hypervascular Wilms tumor invading the inferior vena cava. (D) Urogram.

The collecting system is displaced caudally (*arrow*), and a large mass fills the right upper quadrant. (E) Arteriogram. A highly vascular renal tumor involves much of the total volume of the kidney. The renal artery is displaced to the left. (F) Inferior vena cavogram. A large tumor embolus fills the suprarenal segment of the inferior vena cava (*arrows*). (Courtesy of Kenneth Fellows, M.D.)

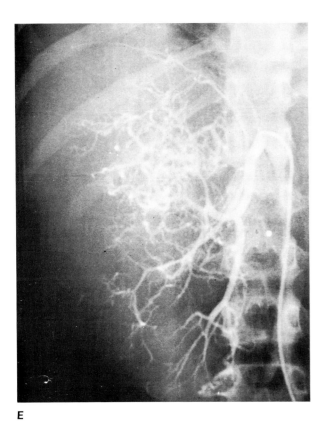

E

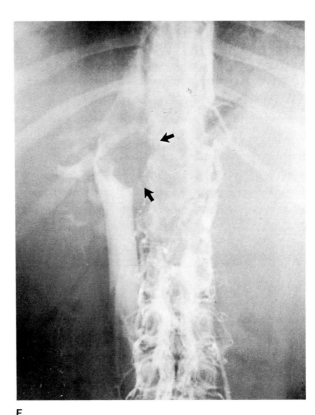

F

Figure 46-2 (continued).

Diagnostic Evaluation

Intravenous Urography. Urography is the initial and most important confirmatory diagnostic procedure in suspected Wilms tumor (Fig. 46-2; Table 46-4).[8,9,12] The examination demonstrates, in varying degrees in different patients, enlargement of the kidney by a mass; displacement, narrowing, flattening, elongation, bizarre distortion, or obliteration of the infundibula and calices; impingement on and compression of the renal pelvis; displacement and compression of the ureter, and at times a nonfunctioning kidney. Displacement of the adjacent viscera may be observed, depending on the size of the mass.

Ultrasound. Ultrasound studies should be performed to determine whether the mass is solid or cystic. Infantile polycystic disease, multicystic kidney, and hydronephrosis of the kidney or of the upper pole of a double kidney may simulate Wilms tumor, but all

Table 46-3. Incidence of Symptoms and Signs in Wilms Tumor

Symptom or Sign	Percentage of Patients Showing Symptom or Sign
Palpable mass	90
Hypertension	60
Abdominal pain	20
Anorexia, nausea, vomiting	16
Fever	10
Gross hematuria	6

Adapted from Snyder WH Jr, Hastings TA, Pollack WF. Retroperitoneal tumors. In: Mustard WR, et al, eds. Pediatric surgery. 2nd ed. Chicago: Year Book, 1969;2:1020.

Table 46-4. Urographic Signs in Wilms Tumor

Sign	Total Number of Patients	Number Showing Sign	Percentage Showing Sign
Renal mass	50	48	96
Calcification	81	9	11
Nonfunctioning kidney	72	13	18
Distortion of carices or infundibula	12	4	33
Stretching of carices or infundibula	12	3	25
Compression of pelvis	12	2	—
Displacement and compression of pelvis and/or ureter	12	2	—
Hydronephrosis	12	2	—

Adapted from Clark,[8] Westra et al.,[9] and Lalli et al.[12]

three masses are relatively anechoic or demonstrate complex sonographic patterns.

Computed Tomography and Magnetic Resonance Imaging. Computed tomography (CT) and magnetic resonance imaging (MRI) have been used widely for children with abdominal mass lesions. Each method provides important information on the size, location, texture, and extent of a mass and presents graphic information about its relationship with other viscera. Their use has sharply diminished the need for angiography in many cases.

Renal Arteriography. Arteriography in Wilms tumor may demonstrate a mass that is moderate-sized (see Fig. 46-2A to C) to huge (see Fig. 46-2D to F) and that involves a variable volume of the kidney and sometimes displaces it strikingly. The tumor may appear to be well encapsulated (see Fig. 46-2C and D) or diffusely infiltrating (see Fig. 46-2E). Because Wilms tumor may involve both kidneys, arteriography is frequently done bilaterally. The important arteriographic findings are as follows (Table 46-5; see Fig. 46-2):

1. Stretching of vessels.
2. Narrowing of vessels.
3. Displacement of vessels.
4. Amputation of vessels.
5. Encasement of vessels.
6. Presence of tumor vessels. Wilms tumor varies from a relatively avascular or hypovascular tumor (see Fig. 46-2B and C) to a moderately hypervascular mass (see Fig. 46-2E).
7. At times, metastases to the liver, retroperitoneal nodes, or other adjacent organs.

Arteriography is useful not only to confirm the diagnosis but also to assess the extent of tumor, liver metastases, bilaterality, response to therapy, and recurrence. Angiography usually distinguishes Wilms tumor from hydronephrosis and multicystic kidneys (small, displaced, or widely spread vessels; no tumor vessels).[8] Although most cases of Wilms tumor can readily be separated from neuroblastoma, in some instances it is difficult, if not impossible, to make the distinction, as noted in text following.

Chest films should always be obtained before angiography to determine the presence or absence of pulmonary metastases.

Inferior Vena Cavography and Renal Venography. Because these bulky tumors frequently invade the renal veins and the inferior vena cava when they are large (see Fig. 46-2F), venography is rewarding in delineating the extent of involvement and the surgical requirements. Percutaneous transfemoral cavography can be done initially and then followed by selective renal ve-

Table 46-5. Angiographic Signs in Wilms Tumor

Sign	Total Number of Patients	Number Showing Sign
Tumor vessels	12	7
Avascular area	12	4
Stretching of intrarenal vessels	12	1
Hypovascular area	12	1

Adapted from Clark RE, Moss AA, DeLorimer AA, et al. Arteriography of Wilms' tumor. AJR 1971;113:476.

nography if needed. The vein may be compressed, displaced, or invaded. With invasion, the wall has a ragged or irregular appearance.

Differential Diagnosis

Hydronephrosis produces renal enlargement, but a site of obstruction can usually be delineated on urography and the dilated collecting system of hydronephrosis is generally diagnostic. Arteriography may show the characteristic features: displaced, narrow vessels without encasement, amputation, or tumor vascularity.

Infantile polycystic disease may simulate Wilms tumor. It is usually bilateral, and it involves most of both kidneys. Urography is helpful but not necessarily diagnostic. Ultrasonography may be useful.

Whereas Wilms tumor involves the intrarenal structures and alters the appearance of the renal pelvis and calices, *neuroblastoma* usually displaces the kidney because it is extrarenal in origin. Neuroblastoma may sometimes infiltrate the kidney, however, and Wilms tumor may at times appear as a localized mass. The distinction, therefore, is not always clear. Calcification is somewhat more common in neuroblastoma than in Wilms tumor.

Other renal tumors, renal abscesses, and intraabdominal masses in infancy that arise from the liver, pancreas, retroperitoneum, and ovary must also be considered in the differential diagnosis.

Treatment

Surgical removal is the primary treatment of choice. Irradiation is useful in the postoperative period and is important in inoperable tumors, tumors that have metastasized, and bilateral tumors. Chemotherapy, particularly with actinomycin D, has demonstrated the importance of adjunctive therapy in these tumors and is recognized as part of the management.

Prognosis

The overall survival for children with disease confined to the kidney, perinephric tissue, and abdominal lymph nodes is 78 percent at 2 to 4 years. Even with widespread metastatic disease, a 50 percent survival rate can be achieved.[13]

Renal Cell Carcinoma

In 1883 Grawitz described renal cell carcinoma in the mistaken belief that it arose from the adrenal gland. The terms *hypernephroma* and *Grawitz tumor* were applied to the tumor, and they have been difficult to dislodge. The concept that this tumor arises from renal tubular epithelial cells has received support from electron microscopic studies that demonstrate many striking similarities between the cells of renal cell carcinoma and normal epithelial cells of the proximal convoluted tubules.[10] This concept is generally accepted, and the term *renal cell carcinoma* (or *renal adenocarcinoma*) seems most appropriate. This tumor constitutes 85 percent of renal malignancies,[5,7,14] has a peak incidence in the sixth decade,[14] and is more common in males. Its presence as a second primary carcinoma in elderly patients with carcinoma of other organs has been described.[1]

Pathology

Although the size varies greatly, often the tumor is bulky and larger than the remaining normal kidney (Fig. 46-3). The surface is usually white or yellow, knobby or irregular, and covered by dilated veins. The tumor often appears to be well demarcated from adjacent renal tissue, although it may have spread beyond its capsule. On cut section, the highly vascular nature of the tumor is evident, and areas of necrosis and hemorrhage are visible. Renal vein invasion, which is common, is a poor prognostic sign.

Microscopically, the tumor usually consists of clear cells or mixtures of clear and granular cells (Fig. 46-4) arranged variously, in sheets or tubules or in papillary fashion. Calcification is present in 5 to 10 percent of cases. In general, the more anaplastic and the larger the tumor, the poorer is the prognosis.

Metastases are found in all sites, but they are most common in the lung, bone, lymph nodes, liver, adrenal glands, and contralateral kidney, in descending order of frequency.[15] At times, metastasis to the bone is the initial manifestation of the tumor.[7]

Staging is important and is clearly related to the prognosis. A simple approach to staging is that of Flocks and Kadesky[16]:

Figure 46-3. Gross pathologic appearance of renal cell carcinoma. The tumor is located in the midportion of the kidney. More medially, it has a somewhat meaty appearance, and laterally it is white and opaque (*arrows*), with an area of necrosis. Note the relatively well defined separation from the adjacent normal renal tissue despite the fact that the tumor has spread well beyond its apparent capsule. Multiple blood vessels are visible in the cut section.

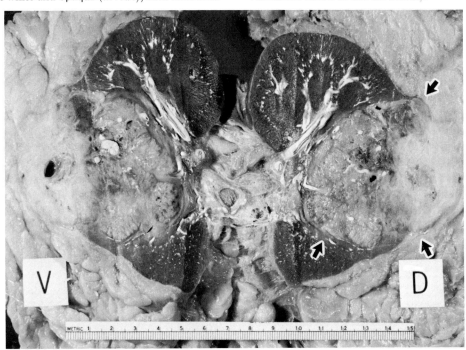

Table 46-6. Symptoms and Signs of Renal Cell Carcinoma in the Peter Bent Brigham Series

	Total Number of Patients	Number Showing Symptom or Sign	Percentage Showing Symptom or Sign
Hematuria	80	36	45
Hematuria as first symptom	80	25	31
Painless hematuria	80	15	19
Pain	81	31	38
Pain as first symptom	81	11	14
Palpable mass	84	39	46
Palpable mass as first symptom	84	11	13
Polycythemia	84	3	4
Hypertension	57	19	33

Adapted from Crocker DW. Renal tumors. In: Sommers SC, ed. Kidney pathology decennial. New York: Appleton-Century-Crofts, 1975:609.

Stage I: Limited to renal capsule
Stage II: Invasion of the renal pedicle or perirenal fat
Stage III: Regional lymph node involvement
Stage IV: Distant metastases demonstrable

Symptoms and Signs

Hematuria, pain, and a mass (or "swelling") are the three common symptoms of renal cell carcinoma (Table 46-6). In one series (Peter Bent Brigham Hospital, PBBH), *hematuria,* the most common symptom, was found in about one-half of the patients.[7,17] It was usu-ally gross, intermittent, and associated with blood vessel invasion or involvement of the renal pelvis or both.

Pain was noted slightly less often. It was commonly dull and continuous, but it was acute and severe when associated with hematuria. Pain was observed in over 40 percent of patients with renal capsular extension.

A *palpable mass* was detected in slightly less than 50 percent of patients. In this group, the patient noted the mass as the presenting symptom 25 percent of the time. No tumors under 3 cm were felt; 35 percent of the tumors that were 3 to 10 cm and 70 percent of the tumors that were over 10 cm were palpable.

Nonspecific symptoms (weakness, fatigue, fever, weight loss, and anorexia) were common and frequently anteceded the development of hematuria, pain, or mass. Polycythemia was found in 3.6 percent of PBBH patients, compared to 2 to 3 percent in the literature.[18] Because polycythemia may appear clinically as polycythemia vera, all such patients should probably be screened with intravenous urography or renal ultrasound. The polycythemia is thought to be associated with the production of a factor stimulating erythropoiesis.[19]

Hypertension was observed in one-third of the patients in the PBBH series, but its relationship to the tumor was uncertain. Hypercalcemia is known to occur in patients with documented skeletal metastases but also (rarely) in the absence of bone involvement. In such patients, the tumor may secrete its own parathormone.[7]

Besides *polycythemia* and *hypercalcemia,* other paraneoplastic syndromes include *pyrexia,* thought to be due to ectopic hormone secretion and observed in as

Figure 46-4. Renal cell carcinoma: microscopic pathology. (A) Low power. The large tumor embolus in the blood vessel (*arrows*) demonstrates the classic appearance of a renal cell carcinoma. The black material in the large vessels adjacent to the tumor embolus is postmortem injectate. (B) High power. Typical clear cells are visible throughout the section.

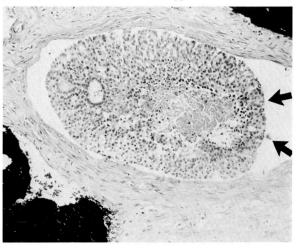

A

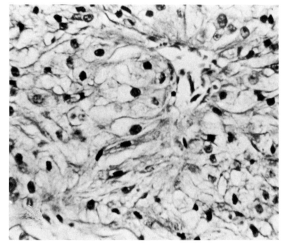

B

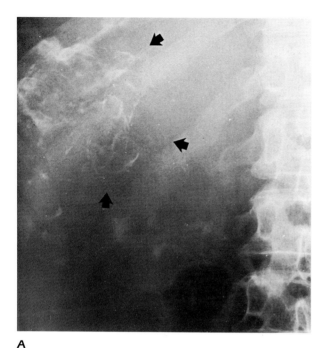

A

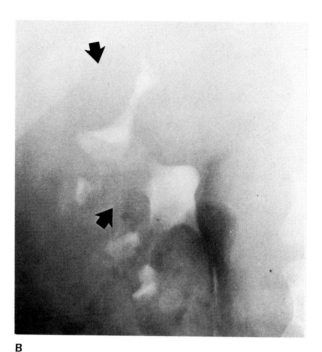

B

Figure 46-5. Renal cell carcinoma: plain films and urograms. (A) Calcification: plain film of the right kidney. There is an amorphous calcification that is more or less curvilinear but is irregularly placed in a large mass in the right kidney (*arrows*); it represents a renal cell carcinoma. (B) Infiltrating carcinoma, upper pole. This urogram demonstrates a mass in the right upper pole as well as compression and distortion of the calices and infundibula (*arrows*). (Compare with polycystic disease, Fig. 46-18A.)

many as 20 percent of patients,[17,20] and *hepatic dysfunction*, which has occurred in as many as 15 percent of patients in whom liver metastases were not demonstrated.[17,21]

Left-sided varicocele, when present, is caused by left renal and testicular vein obstruction by the tumor.

Finally, *metastatic lesions* can give rise to manifestations (e.g., bone pain or central nervous system signs) that depend on the location of the secondary deposits. In 17 percent of the PBBH patients, metastases were the source of the initial symptoms.

Renal cell carcinoma may also be asymptomatic. In the PBBH series, 19 patients (more than 20 percent) had no symptoms referable to their tumors. The tumors were found at autopsy in 6 patients, at surgery in 3, on routine physical examination in 6, at intravenous urography in 3, and on laboratory analysis prompted by an elevated sedimentation rate in 1.[7] In other series of patients examined during life, the rates of discovery in asymptomatic patients ranged from 5 to 31 percent, with most rates in the range of 8 to 15 percent.[22-24] In autopsy series, asymptomatic renal cell carcinoma has been noted in as many as 66 percent of cases.[25]

Diagnostic Evaluation

The sequence of the diagnostic procedures depends on the presenting symptoms. If significant hematuria is the first symptom, cystoscopy may be important in determining whether the source is above the bladder and, if so, from which ureter. In general, however, intravenous urography is the first imaging procedure employed.

Intravenous Urography. The preliminary film may show increased renal size, localized renal mass, an irregularly nodular surface, or calcification (Fig. 46-5A), which occurs in 5 to 10 percent of tumors examined pathologically[7] and radiologically[26-30] (Table 46-7). Eccentric tumors may produce displacement and rotation of the kidney.

Table 46-7. Plain Film in Renal Tumor

	Total Number of Patients	Number Showing Sign	Percentage Showing Sign
Irregular renal outline	209	153	73
Obstruction of psoas shadow	35	14	40
Renal displacement	25	8	32
Renal enlargement or mass	176	35	20
Calcification	411	40	10

Adapted from Ettinger and Elkin,[26] Kikkawa and Lasser,[27] Graham,[28] Folin,[29] and Woodruff et al.[30]

Table 46-8. Urographic Signs in Renal Tumors

Sign	Total Number of Patients	Number Showing Sign	Percentage Showing Sign
Obliteration of pelvic or caliceal lumen	67	37	55
Extrinsic compression of calices or pelvis	209	93	44
Intraluminal filling defect	189	68	36
Diminished functioning	1,202	396	33
Caliectasis or pyelectasis	167	22	13
Hydronephrosis	251	28	11
Displacement of ureter	176	19	11
Nonvisualization of kidney	269	29	11
Elongation of pelvis and calices	167	17	10

Adapted from Ettinger and Elkin,[26] Kikkawa and Lasser,[27] Graham,[28] Folin,[29] and Woodruff et al.[30]

With opacification of the collecting system, the mass is better delineated by its effect on the calices. The following changes may be seen: displacement, narrowing, distortion, stretching, invasion, obliteration, and amputation of the calices and infundibula (Fig. 46-5B). Blunted calices may also be evident when the infundibulum is compressed or invaded by the renal mass (Table 46-8).

The renal pelvis may be displaced, flattened, distorted, elevated, depressed, or obliterated. It may contain filling defects that must be distinguished from renal pelvic neoplasms, clots, and stones. At times, the bizarre and distorted appearance of the collecting system simulates polycystic kidney; however, this is invariably bilateral. If the tumor is localized and produces displacement and compression of the calices, it may be difficult to distinguish from a cyst on conventional urography. Nephrotomography may then be used, although renal ultrasound is the method of choice to confirm the presence of a cyst.

Overall, intravenous urography is a very useful imaging modality. Its sensitivity for small lesions, however, is low.[31,32] One cannot rely on a negative excretory urogram to exclude a renal tumor in a patient with unexplained hematuria or other clinical signs strongly suggestive of a renal neoplasm.

Isotope Imaging. Nuclear medicine's role in neoplastic disease of the kidney is a secondary one. One important area is the differentiation between mass and hypertrophied renal column or unusual shape.[33] Although oncocytoma has been reported to concentrate hippuran,[34] no malignant tumor has demonstrated uptake. When the presence of a mass is uncertain and pseudotumor is suspected, isotope imaging may play an important role with imaging by glucoheptonate or DMSA scan.[33] Because such pseudotumors as dromedary humps, fetal lobulation, lobular compensatory hypertrophy, and prominent columns of Bertin have functioning parenchyma, they do not produce a defect (a cold spot) with such radionuclides, unlike tumors and cysts (Fig. 46-6). Thus isotope imaging in this situation may confirm the innocuous nature of the urographic finding.

Ultrasonography. The main role of sonography is to further characterize renal lesions detected with other studies, especially to distinguish cystic from solid renal lesions. It is useful in evaluating the renal mass that is homogeneous and has a density greater than water, and ultrasound can be used to distinguish a solid renal mass from a hemorrhagic cyst.[35]

Ultrasonography is more sensitive than excretory urography, especially for masses less than 3 cm in diameter.[32] Its limitations include operator dependency and the fact that the quality of the images may vary widely according to the body habitus of the patient.

Computed Tomography. CT is useful for evaluating indeterminate masses and for distinguishing solid renal masses from cystic renal masses. Since the attenuation coefficient of tumor is significantly higher than that of fluid (cyst), the distinction can be made both on the basis of the image attained and on the quantitative assessment of x-ray absorption (Fig. 46-7). The method is used for indeterminate renal masses found with ultrasonography, and CT is more sensitive than ultrasound for masses less than 2 cm in size.[32] When urographic or sonographic results are positive, CT has considerable value in demonstrating the precise extent and volume of the tumor, the lymph node involvement, and the involvement of adjacent tissues.[36,37] Retroperitoneal and inferior vena caval involvement are delineated accurately, especially after contrast enhancement (see Fig. 46-7B and C). CT also has a role in confirming apparently negative urographic findings when clinical suspicion of a lesion is high.[32]

Magnetic Resonance Imaging. MRI has provided additional specific capabilities and should be considered complementary to CT for renal imaging. In the evaluation of cysts, for example, MRI is helpful in characterizing the lesion if the fluid within the cystic mass has the signal characteristics of simple fluid; if signal intensity is similar to normal urine, then cysts can be identified as benign.[38,39] MRI has been found to be approximately equivalent to CT for detecting and characterizing renal masses in a comparative study of 38 patients and 114 lesions.[40] However, it is limited by motion-induced artifacts and the failure to confidently define calcifications. Its advantages over CT include

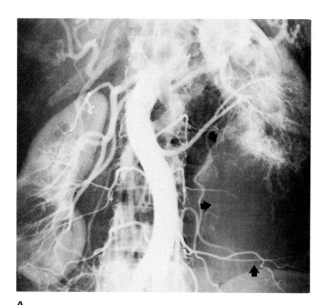

A

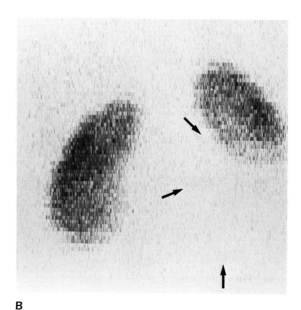

B

Figure 46-6. Renal carcinoma: arteriogram and renal iso-tope scan. (A) Renal arteriogram. A huge mass is present in the lower pole of the left kidney (*arrows*). Later films demonstrated multiple tumor vessels in the mass. (B) Isotope scan.

The lower pole in the region of the tumor mass shows no perfusion and no function (*arrows*). This picture is consistent with that of a known renal mass replacing renal tissue, but it is by no means pathognomonic of carcinoma.

higher contrast resolution, which may allow for the detection of smaller lesions and better characterization of cystic versus solid lesions; better determination of the hemorrhage into a cyst; and enhancement of tumor thrombus (vascular invasion) and adenopathy (Fig. 46-8).[40,41] Gadolinium-enhanced imaging renders an even higher lesion detection rate and, when combined with the fat-saturation technique, is more sensitive for detecting small lesions (less than 2 cm) than is unenhanced MRI.[42]

Table 46-9. Arteriographic Findings in Renal Cell Carcinoma

Finding	Total Number of Patients	Number Showing Finding	Percentage Showing Finding
Tumor vessels	312	278	92
Displacement of renal artery or its branches	105	96	91
Early venous filling	58	51	88
Enlarged renal artery	158	90	57
Enlarged capsular vessels	236	114	48
Nonvisualization of renal vein	347	158	46
Tumor stain	165	51	31
Venous collateral vessels	198	68	34
Distinct tumor edge	230	46	20

Adapted from Boijsen and Folin,[45] Cornell and Dolan,[46] Folin,[47] and Watson et al.[44]

Angiography. The majority of renal cell carcinomas are hypervascular and are readily diagnosed by angiography in 94 to 97 percent of cases (Fig. 46-9, Tables 46-9 and 46-10).[43,44] Characteristically, the angiogram will delineate the disordered tumor vascular bed and the limits of the renal mass lesion.[45–47] The tumor size varies from a few centimeters to a huge mass displacing the kidney and adjacent viscera. Bilateral arteriography should be performed because renal cell carcinoma may metastasize to the contralateral side or may occur as bilateral primary lesions.

The most characteristic finding on angiography is the presence of "tumor" vessels, which are irregular, tortuous, randomly distributed, variable in size, and

Table 46-10. Vascularity of Renal Cell Carcinoma as Judged by Angiography

Degree of Vascularity	Number of Cases
Avascular	6
Minimal vascularity	16
Moderate vascularity	16
Marked vascularity	62
Total	100

Adapted from Watson RC, Fleming RJ, Evans JA. Arteriography in the diagnosis of renal carcinoma. Radiology 1968;91:888.

Text continues on page 1146

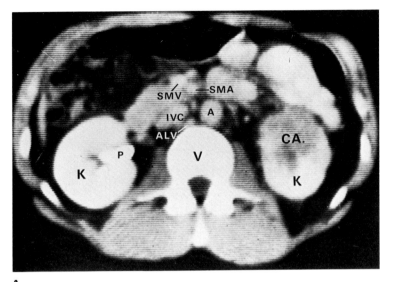

A

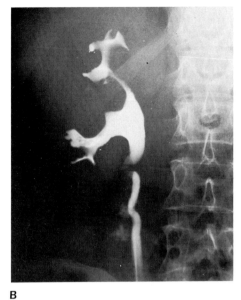

B

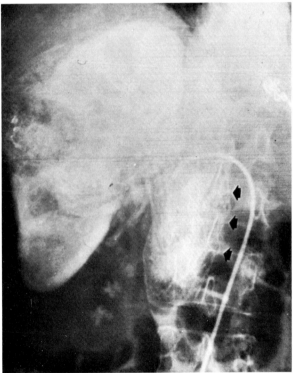

C

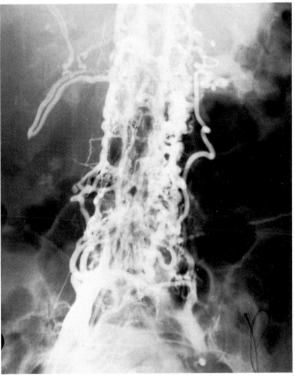

D

Figure 46-7. Renal carcinoma. (A) CT scan obtained in the supine position through the midportion of the kidneys. The right kidney is homogeneously opacified, and contrast material fills the renal pelvis. On the left side, however, only the lower pole shows normal opacification, while the upper pole and the midportions of the kidney demonstrate diminished concentration and an irregular mottled appearance (*CA*). This appearance is characteristic of renal neoplasm. *K*, kidney; *P*, pelvis of kidney; *A*, aorta; *ALV*, ascending lumbar vein; *IVC*, inferior vena cava; *SMV*, superior mesenteric vein; *SMA*, superior mesenteric artery; *V*, vertebral body. (B to I) Renal cell carcinoma with extension into the renal vein and the inferior vena cava. (B) Retrograde urogram. There

is gross distortion of the infundibula, pelvis, and collecting system of the midportion and upper pole of the kidney. Complete amputation of the midpole infundibulum is visible. (C) Selective renal arteriogram, venous phase. The hypervascular renal cell carcinoma demonstrated in the earlier phase has invaded the renal vein and the inferior vena cava (*arrows*). Multiple striated, contrast-filled tumor vessels are visible extending into a large tumor thrombus below the level of the renal hilus. (D) Femoral venogram. There is complete obstruction of the inferior vena cava, which is invaded by renal cell carcinoma. The vertebral venous plexuses and the ascending lumbar veins are opacified as the major avenues of blood return from the lower extremities.

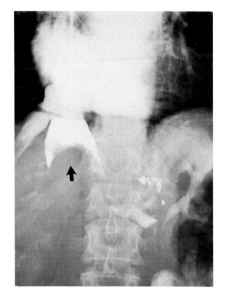

E

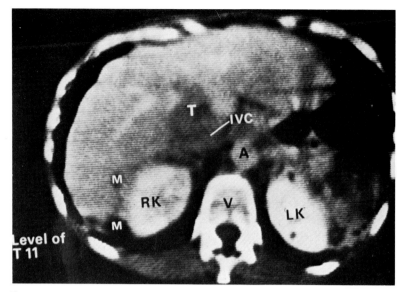

F

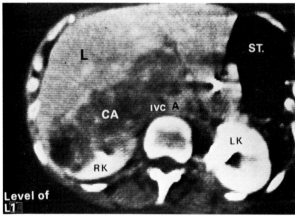

G

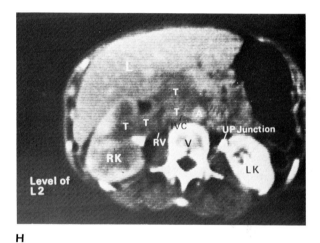

H

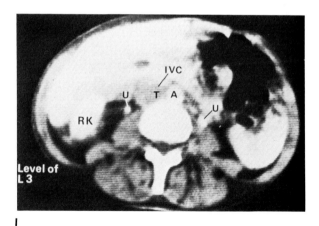

I

Figure 46-7 (continued). (E) Inferior vena cavogram. Opacification of the cephalic portion of the inferior vena cava has been accomplished through trans-right-atrial catheterization. In this way, the upward extent of the tumor is shown (*arrow*). This information may be of great importance to the surgeon because it tells precisely where resection of the cava is essential during nephrectomy and tumor removal. (F) CT scan at the level of T11. The right kidney (*RK*) is opacified, but its ventral portion is invaded by a tumor (*T*) that extends into the inferior vena cava (*IVC*). Note the two metastases (*M*) in the adjacent liver. *A*, aorta; *LK*, left kidney; *V*, vertebral body. (G) CT scan at the level of L1. Extensive replacement of a large portion of the right kidney by the renal cell carcinoma (*CA*) is apparent. It extends into the retroperitoneum, with tumor thrombus in the inferior vena cava. *L*, liver; *ST*, stomach. (H) CT scan at the level of L2. Less involvement of the right kidney is visible, but the tumor mass extends well into the retroperitoneum (*T*) and involves the renal vein (*RV*). (*I*) CT scan at the level of L3. Although both ureters (*U*) are visible, the tumor thrombus (*T*) in the inferior vena cava is still clearly demarcated at the level of the lower pole of the right kidney.

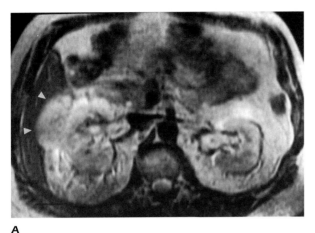

A

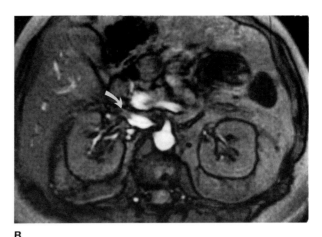

B

Figure 46-8. Renal cell carcinoma: MRI. Selected images from (A) spin-echo TR 2000/TE 80, and (B) axial gradient-echo 30-degree, TR 33/TE 12 of the kidneys. (A) A large (8 × 10 cm) mass arises from the inferior pole of the right kidney (*arrowheads*). (B) Low signal abnormality in the right renal vein (*arrow*) represents either tumor or bland thrombus; it extends to its junction with the inferior vena cava.

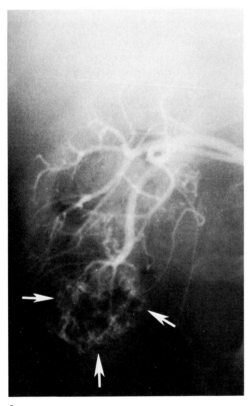

A

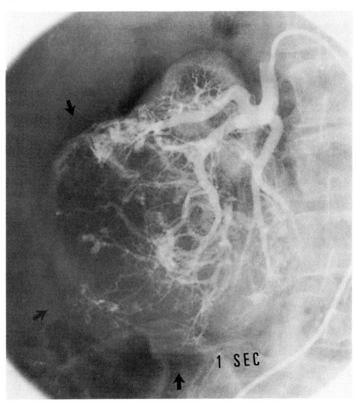

B

Figure 46-9. Renal carcinoma: angiographic appearance. (A) Localized carcinoma. A 4-cm renal carcinoma is delineated in the lower pole of the right kidney (*arrows*). In contrast to the normal arborizations of the upper and middle poles, the tumor vessels are coiled and randomly distributed, with small lakes of contrast density. (B to D) Arteriovenous shunting in a carcinoma. (B) A large renal cell carcinoma (*arrows*) replaces much of the lower and middle segments of the right kidney. Contrast the normal cortical and interlobular vessels in the upper pole of the right kidney with the unusual vessels in the lower pole, which are not only tortuous, coiled, beaded, and irregular in caliber but are also distributed randomly throughout the mass. Some segments of the mass are far more vascular than others. (C) At 2.5 seconds, the tumor is becoming densely stained, although contrast material remains within the arterial bed. Simultaneously, filling of the left renal vein and the inferior vena cava (*arrow*) is demonstrated by arteriovenous shunting. (D) At 7 seconds, large veins over the surface of the kidney are visible (*arrows*), reflecting the marked increase in blood flow to the kidney rather than renal vein obstruction. Contrast this situation with that shown in (F). (E and F) Renal carcinoma with renal vein obstruction. The kidney's almost complete replacement by a renal carcinoma diffusely spread throughout the parenchyma is reflected in the extensive network of tumor vessels and neovascularity in all segments of the kidney. The venous phase (F) shows no evidence of a discrete renal vein. Instead, there is a huge network of collateral channels (*arrows*), indicating renal vein obstruction by the tumor. This suspicion was confirmed at nephrectomy.

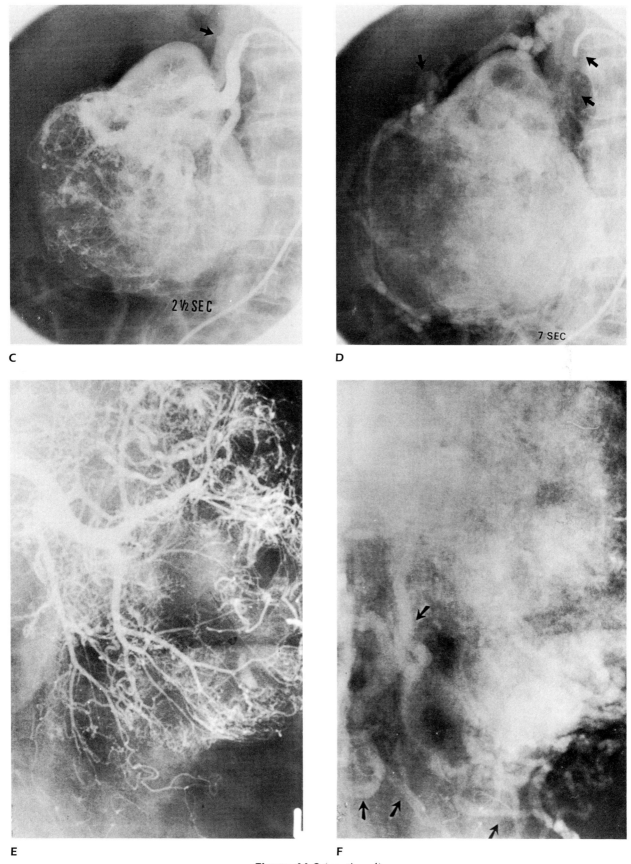

C

D

E

F

Figure 46-9 (continued).

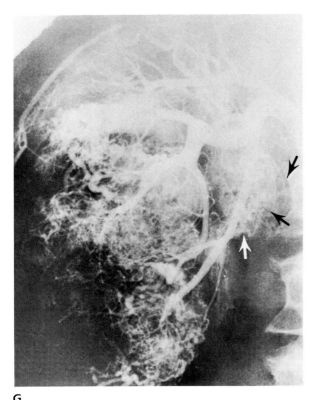

G

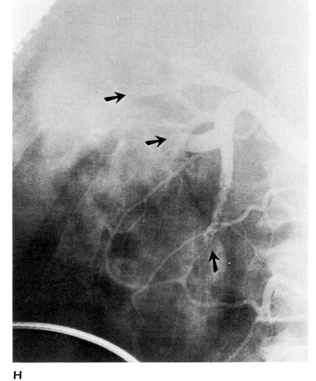

H

Figure 46-9 (continued). (G and H) Large hypervascular carcinoma. The selective renal arteriogram (G) demonstrates remarkable hypervascularity in the renal cell carcinoma, with medial filling of a tumor mass adjacent to the pelvis of the kidney (*arrows*). Because this patient required nephrectomy and because it was desirable to diminish blood loss, Gelfoam was instilled through the selective catheter as multiple emboli (*arrows*, H). Thus the hypervascular mass was rendered ischemic, and the surgeon could work in a relatively bloodless field.

unpredictable in branching. Although some tumors are hypovascular, the most common findings are as follows:

1. Increased vascularity (see Fig. 46-9A, B, E, G).
2. "Random" distribution of vessels, in contrast to the uniform distribution of normal renal vessels (see Fig. 46-9E).
3. Tortuous vessels, with absence of normal tapering (see Fig. 46-9B and C).
4. Dilated vessels, with pooling of contrast material in "lakes" (see Fig. 46-9B and G).
5. Arteriovenous communications (see Fig. 46-9B and C; see also Fig. 46-13B).
6. Encasement of arteries. The margins are irregular and appear fixed and unchanging during different phases of the heart cycle. This finding is more characteristic of transitional cell than of renal cell carcinoma.
7. Staining of the tumor mass during the capillary phase (see Fig. 46-9D and F).
8. Pooling of contrast in venous lakes.

9. Neoplastic response to epinephrine (Figs. 46-10 through 46-12). If 6 to 10 µg of epinephrine is injected arterially before contrast injection, the normal renal vessels contract, whereas the tumor vascular bed exhibits a lessened vasoconstrictor response. Thus the tumor bed opacifies, whereas normal kidney tissue does not. This selectivity provides better demarcation of the tumor mass, confirms the diagnosis when it is in doubt, and at times establishes a positive diagnosis when conventional arteriography is inconclusive (see Figs. 46-10 and 46-11).[48] The relative lack of response by the tumor vascular bed is probably associated with the primitive muscular and elastic tissue in the walls of some tumor vessels.[49,50]
10. Renal vein invasion and/or obstruction by tumor (Fig. 46-13; see also Fig. 46-9E and F).

Once the diagnosis of carcinoma has been made, a large volume (25 ml) of contrast agent may be injected selectively to obtain better visualization of the veins. Tumor vessels within the vein may be delineated and

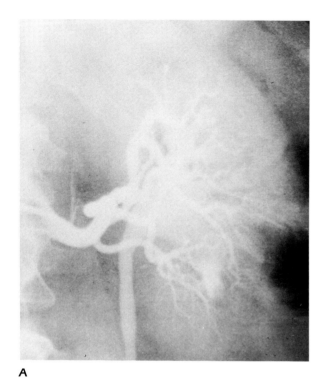

A

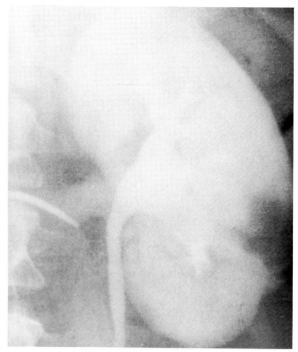

B

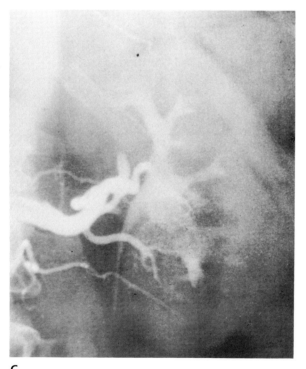

C

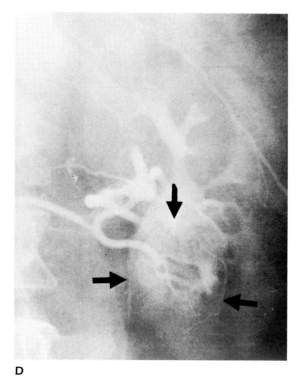

D

Figure 46-10. Renal cell carcinoma: the use of epinephrine arteriography. (A) Selective renal arteriogram without epinephrine in a patient with hematuria. Arterial phase. No evidence of a neoplasm is visible. (B) Nephrogram. The nephrogram appears normal. (C) Epinephrine arteriogram, 2 seconds. Diminished flow is evident through all parts of the renal vascular bed, with only a few branches visible extending to the parenchyma, just caudal to the renal pelvis. (D) Epinephrine arteriogram, 4.5 seconds. A discrete renal cell carcinoma impinging on the caudal margin of the pelvis is demonstrated (*arrows*). (Courtesy of Ronald Castellino, M.D.)

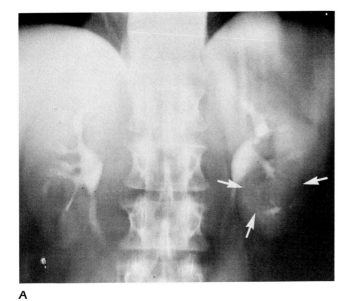

A

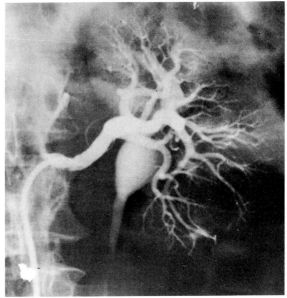

B

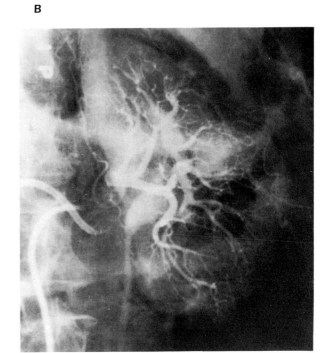

D

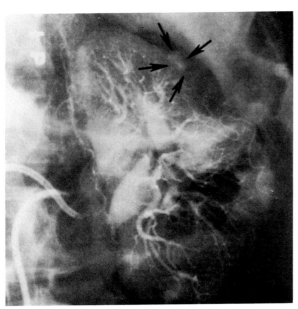

C

E

Figure 46-11. Renal carcinoma: epinephrine arteriogram. The patient entered the hospital for evaluation of hematuria. (A) Urogram. A mass is visible (*arrows*) in the lower pole of the kidney; its appearance is suggestive of a cyst. (B) Selective renal arteriogram. The vessels to the lower pole are displaced around a smooth, round mass. No tumor vessels or encasement is visible. (C) Nephrographic phase. A lucent area in the lower pole suggests a cyst. In addition, a localized invagination just above the midportion of the lateral border of the kidney resembles a prior infarct with scarring. (D) Epinephrine arteriogram, 1 second. There is no filling of the vessels to the cortex of the kidney. (E) Epinephrine arteriogram, 2.5 seconds. The interlobar renal arteries remain opacified, but now a small local area of increased density (*arrows*) extends beyond the margin of the kidney adjacent to the upper pole. Surgical exploration revealed that this lesion was a renal cell carcinoma. A benign simple cyst was present in the lower pole of the kidney. (Courtesy of Ernest Ferris, M.D.)

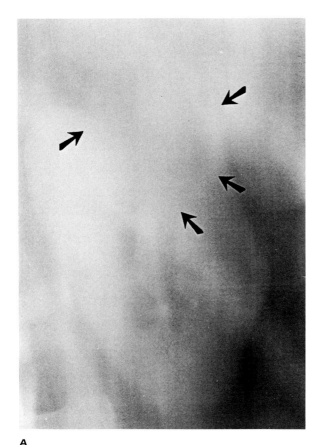

A

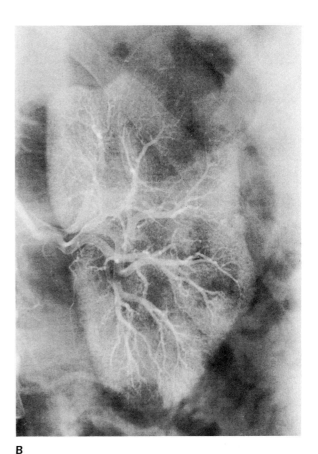

B

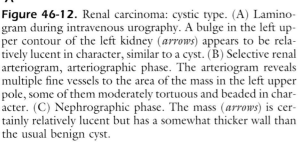

C

Figure 46-12. Renal carcinoma: cystic type. (A) Laminogram during intravenous urography. A bulge in the left upper contour of the left kidney (*arrows*) appears to be relatively lucent in character, similar to a cyst. (B) Selective renal
arteriogram, arteriographic phase. The arteriogram reveals
multiple fine vessels to the area of the mass in the left upper
pole, some of them moderately tortuous and beaded in character. (C) Nephrographic phase. The mass (*arrows*) is certainly relatively lucent but has a somewhat thicker wall than
the usual benign cyst.

so establish the presence of invasion. Failure to opacify
the renal vein is not conclusive evidence of tumor invasion; demonstration of a large venous collateral network is strongly suggestive.[51]

Avascular renal cell tumors, although less common,
may resemble benign cysts. Often tumor vessels will
be apparent.

Renal tumors may invade renal arteries and produce
massive hemorrhage, suggesting a huge renal tumor
(Figs. 46-14 and 46-15). At times, the tumor itself
may be quite small (see Fig. 46-15), and the mass effect may be predominantly that of the hematoma.

In addition to having diagnostic usefulness, renal
arteriography furnishes the surgeon with important
preoperative anatomic knowledge of the renal vascular
bed. Its accuracy is high, approximately 95 percent.[52]

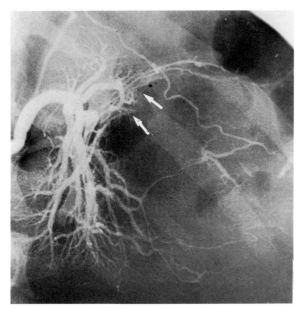

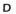

D

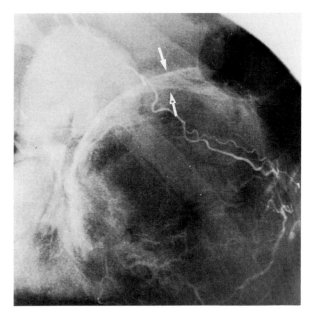

E

Figure 46-12 (continued). Exploratory surgery revealed a renal cell carcinoma. (D to F) Large cystic carcinoma. (D) Arterial phase shows obvious draping and stretching of vessels over a large mass in the lateral aspect of the left kidney (*arrows*). Multiple vessels are clumped together in the upper and lower margins of the mass, and a large capsular vessel runs over its surface and communicates with other capsular branches. (E) Nephrographic phase. At 7 seconds it is apparent (*arrows*) that the cyst wall is significantly thicker than that of a benign cyst and that there is contrast material in the vessels supplying tissue in the medial and caudal aspects of the cyst mass. (F) Postepinephrine film. After administration of epinephrine, there is virtually no flow to the normal renal vessels. The vessels to the cystic mass (*arrows*) are relatively well filled with contrast agent, suggesting that they are neoplastic. Note the staining of the medial caudal margin of the tumor. Surgery revealed an extensive cystic renal carcinoma.

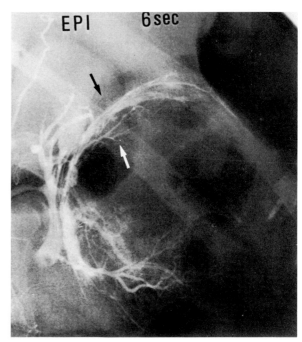

F

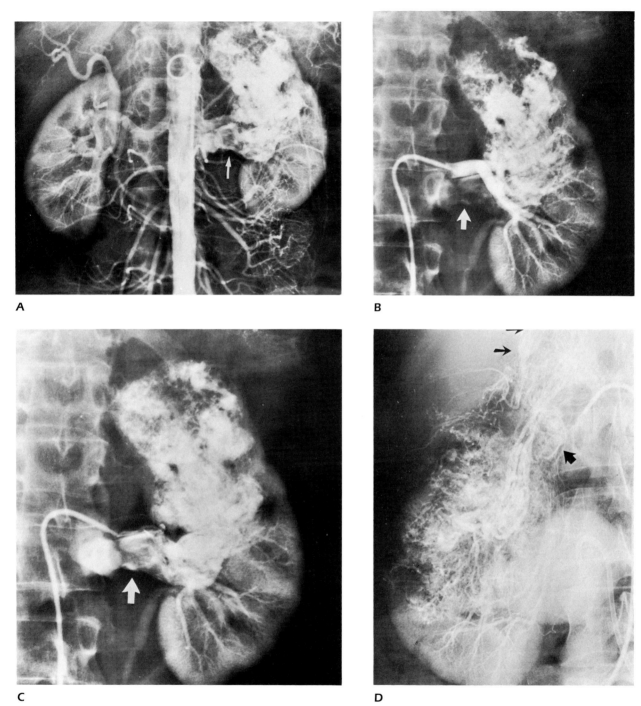

A

B

C

D

Figure 46-13. Renal cell carcinoma with renal vein invasion. (A) Aortogram. Dense staining of the neoplasm involving the upper two-thirds of the left kidney is apparent. In addition, the tumor has invaded the left renal vein (*arrow*). (B) Selective renal arteriogram, 1 second. While the artery is still opacified, arteriovenous shunting has occurred with renal vein opacification (*arrow*). (C) Selective renal arteriogram, 2 seconds. A large tumor thrombus is visible in the left renal vein (*arrow*). (D) Selective renal arteriogram in a patient with renal cell carcinoma, 2.5 seconds. Note the typical renal cell carcinoma extension into the vena cava as denoted by the malignant vessels extending far outside the kidney (*arrows*) and directly into the region of the inferior vena cava.

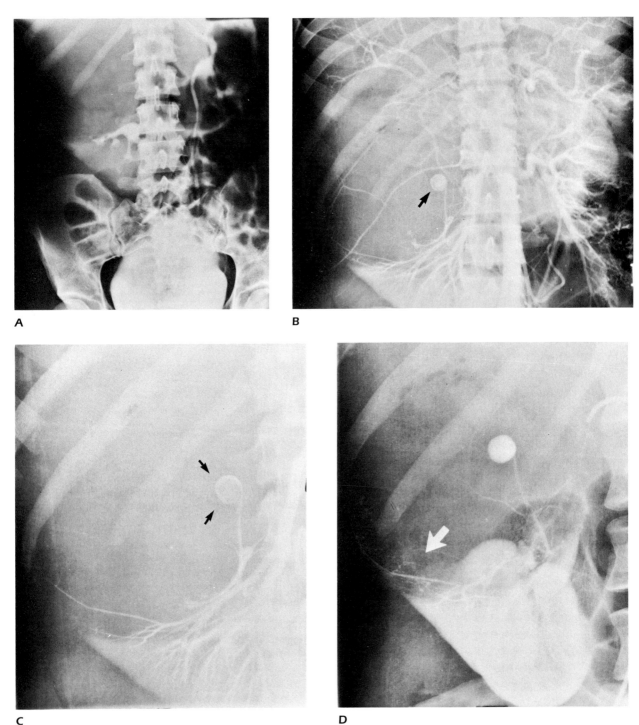

A

B

C

D

Figure 46-14. Renal cell carcinoma, with intrarenal hemorrhage. This patient entered the hospital with gross hematuria. (A) Urogram. The right kidney is markedly displaced and depressed by what appears to be a huge mass in its upper midportions. This area lacks the nephrographic effect. (B) Aortogram. The apparent mass lesion is generally avascular, except for a discrete collection of contrast material fed by a small branch vessel of the lower pole renal arteries (*arrow*). (C) Selective renal arteriogram. The collection of contrast represents a pseudoaneurysm (*arrows*), presumably in the middle of a large hemorrhagic mass. (D) Selective renal arteriogram, 3.5 seconds. The pseudoaneurysm is now densely opacified. In addition, abnormal vessels are seen (*arrow*) at the edge of the large mass, displacing and distorting the right kidney. A nephrectomy demonstrated a renal cell carcinoma with a massive intrarenal hematoma in the center of a necrotic area of tumor. (Courtesy of R. R. Freeman, M.D.)

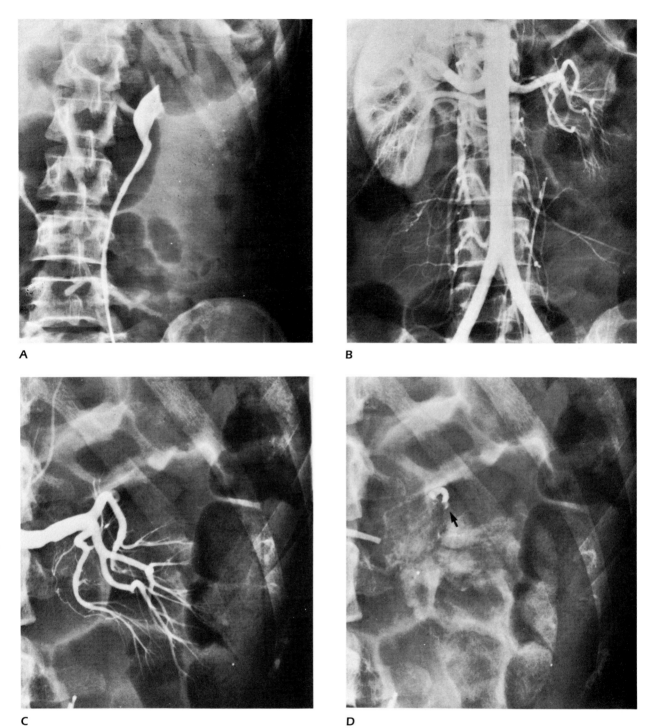

Figure 46-15. Renal cell carcinoma with hemorrhage. This 35-year-old woman had a 24-hour history of severe left flank pain. An intravenous urogram revealed a nonfunctioning left kidney. (A) Retrograde left urogram. Extrinsic compression of the renal pelvis, with kinking of the ureteropelvic junction. No contrast material fills the caliceal system. (B) Aortogram. There is profound slowing of the flow through the left kidney as compared to the right. (C) Selective renal arteriogram. The small vessels failed to fill, and the renal cortex is not opacified. No arterial filling to the upper pole of the kidney is apparent. (D) Nephrogram. At 8 seconds, the nephrogram is faint. Persistent contrast filling of a single arterial branch is visible (*arrow*).

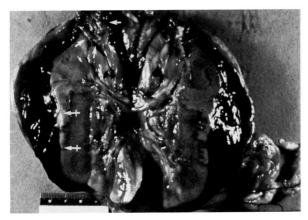

E

Figure 46-15 (continued). (E) Pathologic specimen. There was a 3-cm, highly vascular, infarcted upper pole renal cell carcinoma (*white arrows*) that had produced massive subcapsular hemorrhage. A large, tense, subcapsular hematoma (*barred arrows*) was present. Thus, although there was clearly a mass lesion, the findings were those of increased intrarenal resistance due to a large collection of blood within the renal capsule.

Even the demonstration of renal vein occlusion does not preclude surgery, although it is important to confirm the finding preoperatively.

Because angiography of the contralateral kidney is mandatory, the presence or absence of undetected abnormalities can also be determined. Metastases are often hypervascular, resembling the pattern of the primary tumor.

Inferior Vena Cavography and Renal Venography. Because of the common tendency of renal cell carcinoma to invade the renal vein and the inferior vena cava and because CT, MRI, and arteriography are not always conclusive with regard to renal vein involvement, cavography and renal venography may afford important information to the surgeon about the extent of the tumor (see Chapter 52).[53] The theoretical objection that renal venography may encourage the spread of tumor has not been borne out in the authors' experience.

Other Radiologic Procedures. A chest examination for pulmonary metastases and a bone scan for osseous metastases are essential for the evaluation of patients with renal cell carcinoma. Bone scans are more accurate than radiographic skeletal surveys, and they improve clinical staging.[54]

Differential Diagnosis

The differential diagnosis of renal cell carcinoma includes all mass lesions of the kidney. In lymphomatous infiltration, a "palisadelike" appearance may be observed, with small abnormal arteries and a tumor blush; in Hodgkin disease, the appearance may resemble that of an infiltrative neoplasm, with abnormal vessels indistinguishable from those in hypovascular renal cell carcinoma.[55] Vascular tumors need to be differentiated from hamartomas (which is not always possible) and from other benign vascular tumors, such as those of neurogenic origin. The hypovascular and cystic tumors may resemble benign solitary cysts.

Inflammatory lesions, such as renal abscess (Fig. 46-16) and xanthogranulomatous pyelonephritis (Fig. 46-17), may mimic renal cell tumors. With abscesses or inflammatory masses, one finds an increase in the size and number of capsular vessels, an abnormal intrarenal circulation manifested by slow and diminished blood flow, stretching of the interlobar branches, loss of the cortical-medullary border, and loss of the kidney outline (see Fig. 46-16). Typical tumor vessels of renal cell carcinoma are not observed, and no arteriovenous shunts are present. The distinction from cystic or hypovascular tumors may be difficult.[56]

The urographic appearance of polycystic kidney may be similar to that of infiltrating carcinoma, but its angiographic appearance is different (Figs. 46-18 and 46-19).

Treatment

Radical nephrectomy is the conventional treatment; partial nephrectomy with "benchtop" surgery is used in selected cases for renal tissue conservation. Irradiation plays a role in the management of the inoperable patient, the patient in whom surgery is known to have removed the tumors incompletely, and the patient who requires palliation of osseous or pulmonary metastases. Transcatheter selective renal embolization has also been employed. Both nonhormonal and hormonal antitumor chemotherapies have been tried in carcinoma of the kidney with metastatic disease, but there is no evidence that objective tumor regression has occurred.[17]

Renal Pelvic Tumors

Tumors of the renal pelvis, occurring mostly in the sixth and seventh decades of life, account for 7 to 8 percent of all malignant renal tumors. Although there are different histologic types, the transitional cell carcinoma predominates, accounting for over 80 percent of pelvic tumors.

Pathology

Transitional cell carcinoma is almost invariably papillary (Fig. 46-20). It is invasive and frequently reaches the lymphatics and invades the renal vein. It metasta-

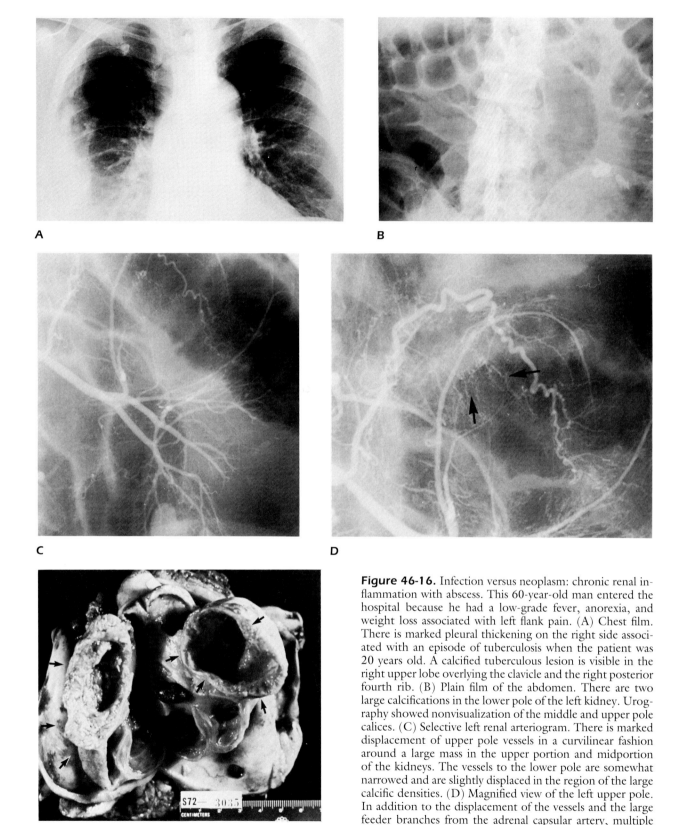

Figure 46-16. Infection versus neoplasm: chronic renal inflammation with abscess. This 60-year-old man entered the hospital because he had a low-grade fever, anorexia, and weight loss associated with left flank pain. (A) Chest film. There is marked pleural thickening on the right side associated with an episode of tuberculosis when the patient was 20 years old. A calcified tuberculous lesion is visible in the right upper lobe overlying the clavicle and the right posterior fourth rib. (B) Plain film of the abdomen. There are two large calcifications in the lower pole of the left kidney. Urography showed nonvisualization of the middle and upper pole calices. (C) Selective left renal arteriogram. There is marked displacement of upper pole vessels in a curvilinear fashion around a large mass in the upper portion and midportion of the kidneys. The vessels to the lower pole are somewhat narrowed and are slightly displaced in the region of the large calcific densities. (D) Magnified view of the left upper pole. In addition to the displacement of the vessels and the large feeder branches from the adrenal capsular artery, multiple thin, irregularly ramifying branches are visible within the mass lesion (*arrows*).

Figure legend continues on next page.

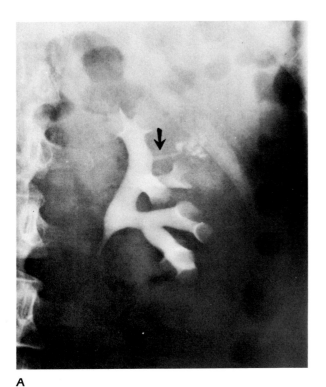

A

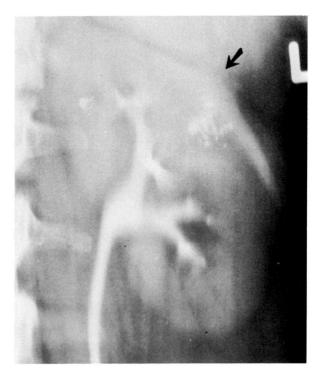

B

Figure 46-17. Localized xanthogranulomatous pyelonephritis. (A) Intravenous urogram. Calcification was present on the plain film, and the infundibulum extending to the area of amorphous calcification was stretched and narrowed (*arrow*). (B) Tomogram during urography. A small mass was apparent (*arrow*) extending from the region of the calcification. (C) Selective renal arteriogram. Somewhat irregular vessels (*arrows*) are visible in the area of the mass, extending through the renal margin. Although these vessels are slightly irregular, they do not have the appearance of classic neoplastic vessels, but carcinoma could not be excluded. Pathologic examination of tissue obtained by a wedge resection of the area demonstrated a localized area of xanthogranulomatous pyelonephritis in association with calculi.

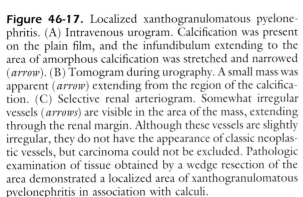

Figure 46-16 (continued). A few irregularly coiled branches are also opacified. No lakes, no premature venous opacification, and no evidence of typical so-called malignant vessels can be seen. Nevertheless, an avascular renal cell carcinoma must be considered seriously, as must a large transitional cell carcinoma. Furthermore, in view of the known history of tuberculosis, the possibility of tuberculous pyonephrosis must be entertained (a diagnosis that is untenable without calcification in the involved area; in addition, the characteristic amputation of vessels associated with tuberculosis is not visible). Finally, the possibility that the picture is that of a chronic abscess in an individual with chronic pyelonephritis and calculus formation in the lower pole clearly requires serious consideration. Because of the continuing fever and the nonvisualization of the left kidney on urography, nephrectomy was performed. (E) Pathologic specimen. Pathologic examination revealed a large, thick-walled abscess in the left upper pole with inflammatory changes throughout much of the kidney (*arrows*).

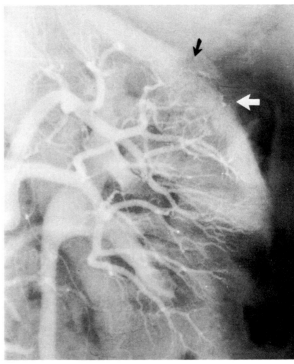

C

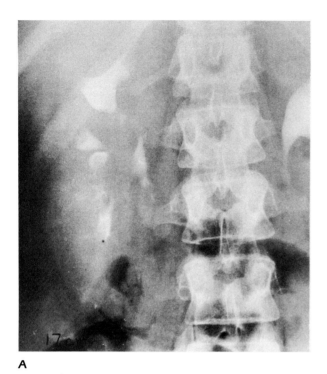

A

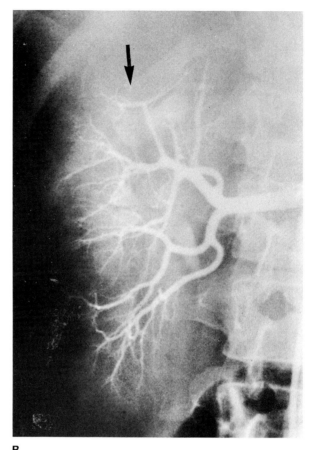

B

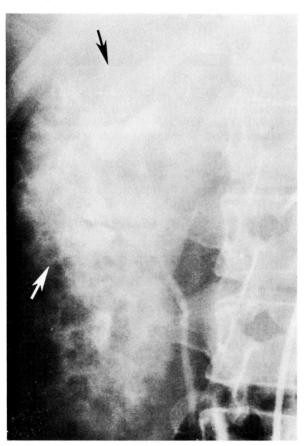

C

Figure 46-18. Polycystic kidney. (A) Urogram shows dilatation and separation of the calices and rather marked deformity of the infundibula and the pelvis of the kidney. The appearance is not dissimilar to that of infiltrating carcinoma (compare with Fig. 46-8F and G). (B) Selective renal arteriogram. In multiple areas of the kidney, the renal arteries appear displaced and stretched around local small masses. In the upper pole, a larger mass (*arrow*) is apparent. (C) Nephrographic phase. The larger cyst in the upper pole (*black arrow*) is well defined. Multiple lucent areas visible throughout the kidney stretch from the upper pole to the lower pole and present a mottled appearance (*white arrow*). This is the classic appearance of polycystic kidney.

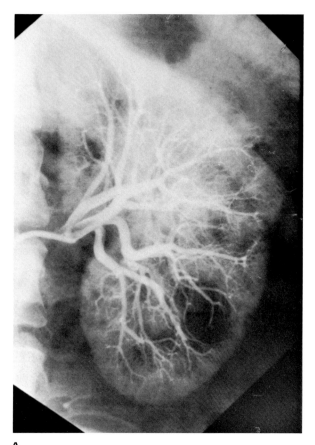

A

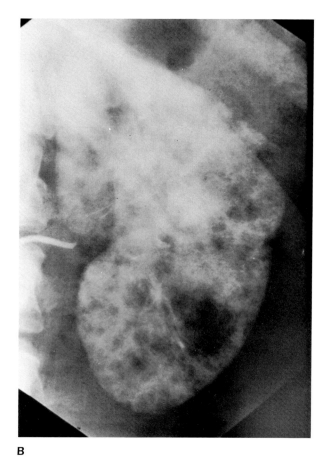

B

Figure 46-19. Polycystic kidney. The urogram was normal, except for the increased size of the kidney. (A) Selective renal arteriogram, 1.5 seconds. There is a slight displacement of multiple branches of the renal arteries throughout the kid- neys. (B) At 3.5 seconds, multiple lucent areas are visible, representing cysts of varying size and a polycystic kidney. Cysts may be so small that they do not necessarily cause ma- jor abnormalities of the collecting system in some patients.

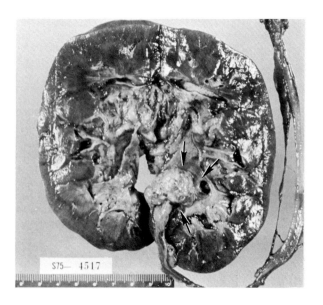

sizes to the retroperitoneum, lungs, liver, and bones. Squamous cell carcinoma (which comprises about 15 percent of renal pelvic tumors) is commonly papillary, but it may be solid and flat. It is frequently associated with calculus and infection. Mucin-producing adeno- carcinoma is a more rare tumor of the renal pelvis.

Symptoms and Signs

Hematuria, by far the most common symptom,[57] is found in more than 80 percent of patients with transi- tional cell carcinoma. It was the first symptom in 13 of 14 patients at the Brigham Hospital.[7] Pain was pres- ent in less than one-third of the patients, and none of

Figure 46-20. Transitional cell carcinoma: gross appear- ance. Transitional cell carcinoma is almost invariably papil- lary. It is invasive, frequently reaching the lymphatics and invading the renal vein. It is visible in the bisected kidney as a verrucous mass in the renal pelvis (*arrows*). The patient's presenting symptom was hematuria.

A

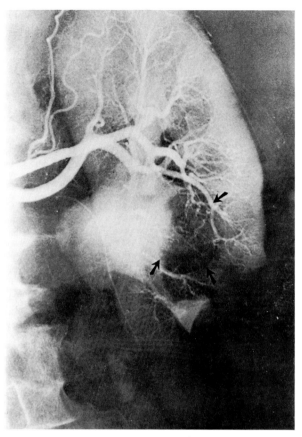

B

Figure 46-21. Renal pelvic carcinoma. (A) Urogram. An irregular mass apparently originates in the renal pelvis and presents an irregular margin laterally (*arrows*). It extends into the infundibulum to the lower pole with consequent slight dilatation of the calix to the lower pole. The appearance is strongly suggestive of a transitional cell carcinoma of the renal pelvis. (B) Selective renal arteriogram. This patient had two vessels to the kidney. Only the upper vessel is opaci- fied; the supplementary artery supplying the lower pole is unfilled. Note that there are a number of small irregular vessels representing tumor vessels adjacent to the area of irregularity in the renal pelvis (*arrows*). The presence of these abnormal vessels demonstrates clearly that the tumor mass extends laterally into the parenchyma despite the fact that it has arisen in the renal pelvis.

the patients had a palpable mass. Squamous cell carcinoma and adenocarcinoma cause bleeding in the late stages and are sometimes discovered only because of the association with stone, infection, or hydronephrosis.

Diagnostic Evaluation

Intravenous Urography. The classic urographic finding is a filling defect in the renal pelvis (Fig. 46-21 and Table 46-11). The defect varies in size and in the extent of deformity of the renal pelvis. Infundibular obstruction, mass, hydronephrosis, and nonvisualization of the collecting system are also observed (Fig. 46-22).

Ultrasonography and Computed Tomography. If the tumor has extended into the kidney, ultrasonography may be useful in demonstrating the presence of

an echoic mass, leading to the presumptive diagnosis of carcinoma. Computed tomography not only depicts the degree of involvement of the kidney but also may

Table 46-11. Intravenous Urography in Renal Pelvic Carcinoma

Finding	Number of Patients
Filling defect	15
Infundibular obstruction	3
Mass	4
Hydronephrosis	5
Nonvisualization	8
Total	35

Adapted from Cummings KB, Correa RJ Jr, Gibbons RP, et al. Renal pelvic tumors. J Urol 1975;113:158.

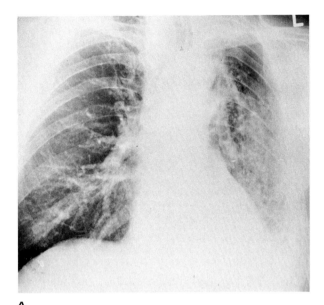

A

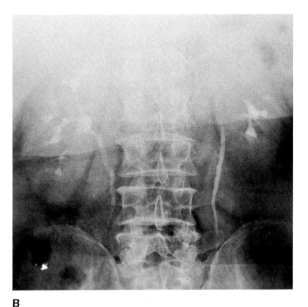

B

Figure 46-22. Transitional cell carcinoma of the kidney: differential diagnosis from tuberculosis. (A) Chest film. There is decreased volume of the left hemithorax associated with pulmonary fibrous lesions and pleural thickening as the residue of a tuberculous infection. (B) Urogram. The lower pole calices on the left are normal, but there is nonvisualization of the upper pole calices. The infundibulum to the middle calix is obliterated.

show the deformity of the renal pelvis of the mass lesion involving and surrounding the renal pelvis and, at times, the upper ureter.

Cystoscopy, Retrograde Pyelography, and Cytologic Examination of the Urine. If heavy bleeding is the initial symptom, cystoscopy may be helpful in determining whether the source is in the bladder or above it. If no bladder source is defined, it may identify which ureter drains the blood. Because transitional cell carcinoma frequently seeds in the ureter, retrograde pyelography may be helpful if the ureter is not visualized. During cystoscopy and ureteral catheterization, urine samples should be collected for cytologic examination, which is helpful when positive.

Angiography. Selective renal arteriography may be helpful in establishing the diagnosis, clarifying the extent of the disease, and depicting the vascular anatomy preoperatively. Relatively few of these tumors are localized to the renal pelvis or collecting system. Frequently they infiltrate the kidney and at times produce the picture of an infiltrative disorder, without hypervascularity. Most of these tumors are hypovascular, but in many of them some tumor vessels may be defined (see Fig. 46-21B), particularly if magnification and epinephrine arteriography are performed. Vascular encasement and a tumor blush are relatively common (see Fig. 46-22 and Table 46-12),[58] and arteriovenous shunting is not observed. The degree of main vascular involvement may be very extensive, and at times amputation of branch renal arteries is an important finding. In half of the cases, the pelviureteric artery is enlarged.[58]

Renal Venography. Renal venography may be used in demonstrating venous encasement by renal pelvic carcinoma when the diagnosis is in doubt (Fig. 46-23). It also establishes the presence or absence of major renal vein invasion.

Differential Diagnosis

A filling defect in the renal pelvis may be a tumor, a blood clot, or a calculus. When the tumor extends into the parenchyma, it may resemble renal cell carcinoma, benign renal tumors, renal tuberculosis, and other

Table 46-12. Angiographic Findings in 22 Cases of Renal Pelvic Carcinoma

Finding	Number of Patients with Finding	Percentage of Patients with Finding
Prominent pelvico-ureteral artery	12	55
Neovascularity	18	82
Blush	18	82
Vessel encasement	16	73
Arteriovenous shunting	0	—

Adapted from Rabinowitz J, Kinkhabwala M, Himmelfarb E, et al. Renal pelvic carcinoma: an angiographic re-evaluation. Radiology 1972;102:551.

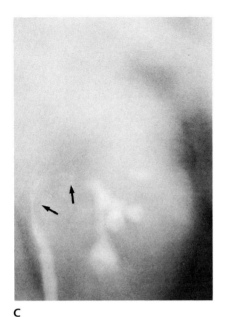

C

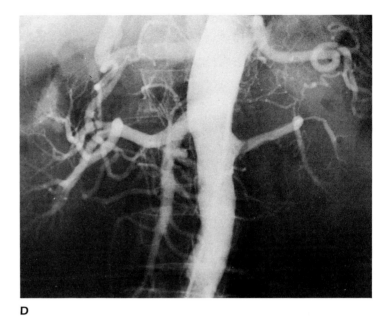

D

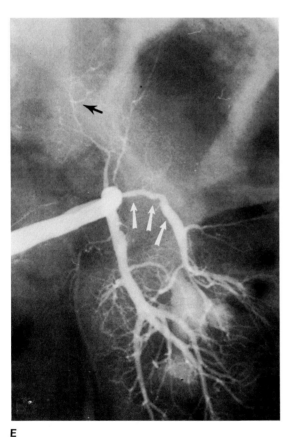

E

Figure 46-22 (continued). (C) Laminogram. Marked narrowing of the pelvis of the kidney and of the upper ureter is seen (*arrows*). A single calix is seen in the midportion of the kidney, with no visualization of the infundibulum. (D) Abdominal aortogram. The right kidney appears normal. The left kidney demonstrates narrowed vessels, as to an atrophic kidney. (E) Selective renal arteriogram. Encasement of the central branches of the renal artery, particularly involving the branch to the midportion of the kidney (*white arrows*), is visible. Multiple small branches extend to the upper pole of the left kidney (*black arrow*). With the history of tuberculosis, the amputation of vessels, and the impingement on infundibula, the possibility of chronic tuberculous pyonephrosis in the upper portion of the kidney was considered. Epinephrine arteriography showed tumor vessels. Nephrectomy then was performed; the pathologic diagnosis was transitional cell carcinoma.

Treatment

Nephrectomy and ureterectomy are the treatment of choice.

Other Tumors

Adenoma

The adenomas are the most common benign renal tumors; many are found incidentally on examination of renal tissue at autopsy or in surgical specimens.[59] They are composed of small, uniform epithelial cells and have a papillary growth pattern. Preoperative distinction between large adenomas and renal cell carcinoma can be difficult because some adenomas have malignant features.[13]

chronic inflammatory processes. Infundibular narrowing may be produced by transitional cell carcinoma, by inflammation, or even by vascular imprints. Arteriography can establish the relationship of the vascular bed to the involved infundibulum (Fig. 46-24).

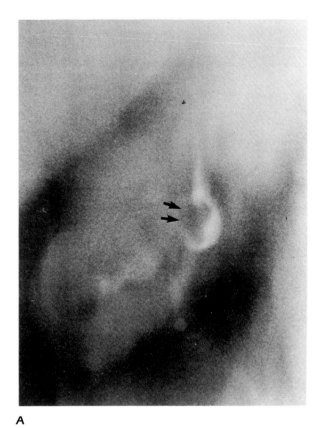

A

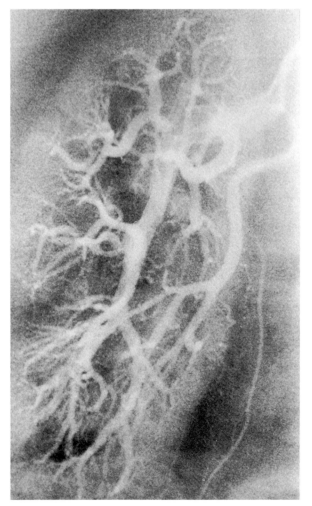

B

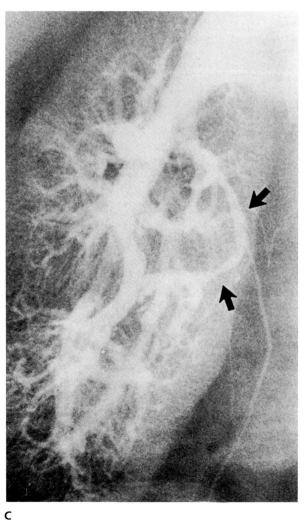

C

Figure 46-23. Renal venography in a renal pelvic carcinoma. The patient entered the hospital because of hematuria. (A) Intravenous urogram: laminographic section. A lobulated filling defect is visible in the pelvis of the kidney (*arrows*). (B) Selective renal arteriogram. No definite abnormalities are visible, although there is a suggestion of a slight irregularity at the lateral edge of the dorsal renal arterial branch extending to the lower pole. (C) Selective renal venogram. Gross irregularity and encasement of the renal venous branch adjacent to the pelvis of the kidney is apparent (*arrows*). These findings confirm the malignant nature of the filling defect visible in the pelvis, which might otherwise have been a clot or stone on the basis of the radiographic appearance alone. (Courtesy of Stanley Baum, M.D.)

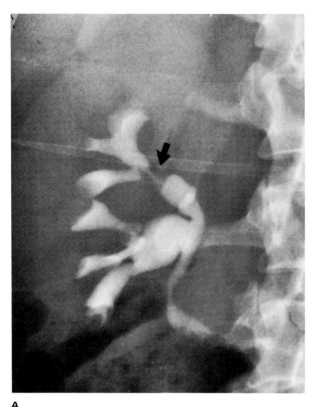

A

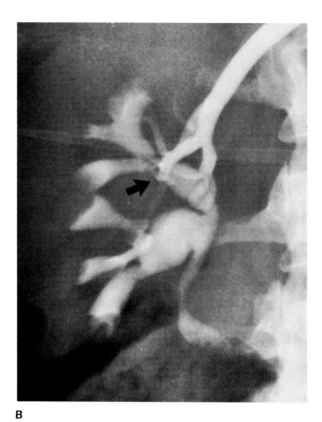

B

Figure 46-24. Infundibular narrowing by a renal artery branch. (A) Intravenous urogram. There is gross narrowing of the infundibulum to the upper pole (*arrow*) (and the absence of any other evidence of infection) in a patient with hematuria. The possibility of neoplasm must be considered, although inflammatory stenosis, such as that caused by tu-berculosis, and vascular compression are also diagnostic possibilities. (B) The narrowing of the infundibulum (*arrow*) represents a vascular impression caused by the ventral branch of the renal artery. It could readily be eliminated with ureteral compression and altered positioning of the patient.

Adenomas rarely cause symptoms during life, but they may grow to considerable size and be discovered as a mass on a urographic examination. A report of five cases indicated the presence of caliceal distortion in three, renal displacement in three, and calcification in one. Two of the tumors were lucent, and three were dense. Angiography in renal adenoma shows increased vascularity in some cases, but with vessels less bizarre than in carcinoma; decreased vascularity may occur with a faint blush or the appearance of a cyst; and a third type of adenoma has a relatively normal appearance.[60] Because these tumors are benign, conservative therapy is warranted if the diagnosis can be established with sufficient tissue by percutaneous ultrasonically guided biopsy.

Hamartoma

Renal hamartoma (angiomyolipoma) is of greatest importance because it is difficult to differentiate from hypervascular clear cell carcinoma. The tumors associated with tuberous sclerosis present little diagnostic problem: 60 to 80 percent of patients with such tu-mors have multiple lesions in their kidneys in association with adenoma sebaceum and the classic features of the syndrome. Solitary tumors almost invariably come to surgery. Most occur in females. Pathologically, the tumor is composed of smooth muscle, fat, and angiomatous tissue.

The symptoms are often vague, and the tumor is commonly found on a urogram as part of a general examination. Flank pain may be noted in some patients, and occasionally there may be hematuria. In a small percentage of cases, the presence of fat in a renal mass suggests the diagnosis on the plain film. Calcification may be found. With filling of the collecting system during intravenous urography, a renal mass is defined that displaces and distorts the calices but rarely amputates the calices and infundibula. When the hamartoma is associated with tuberous sclerosis or there are multiple hamartomas, the appearance is similar to that of adult polycystic disease. Nephrotomography may reveal low-density areas produced by fat (Fig. 46-25), and CT of the tumor is most helpful in defining the invariable lipomatous component.[61,62]

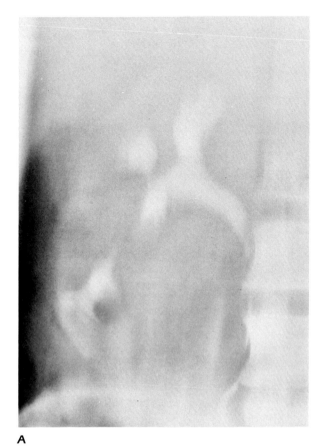

A

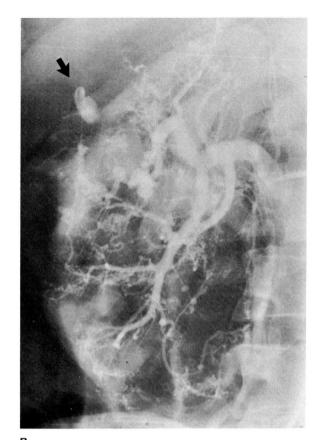

B

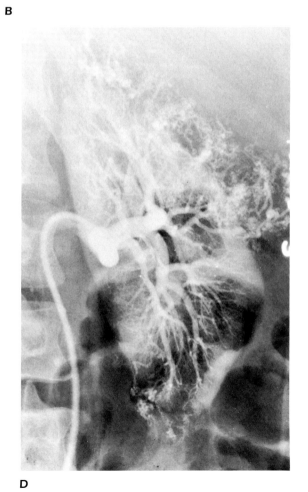

C

D

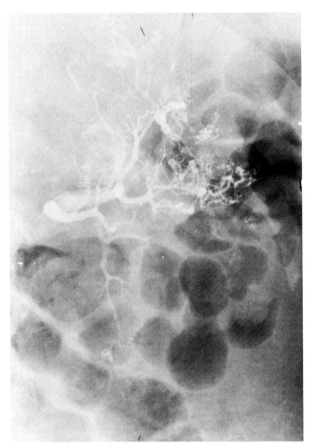

Figure 46-25. Renal hamartomas in a patient with tuberous sclerosis. (A) Tomogram of the right kidney during urography. The collecting system is grossly distorted, with the appearance of multiple masses. A number of lucent areas, particularly in the lateral aspect of the kidney, suggest the presence of fat. (B) Selective right renal arteriogram. A bizarre vascular pattern is apparent, characterized especially by multiple saccular aneurysms (*arrow*) throughout the tumor masses. (C) Selective left renal arteriogram. Large vascular masses are present in both the upper and lower poles of the kidney, with the characteristically distorted vascular bed associated with hamartoma. The multiple aneurysms demonstrated in this view are considered characteristic of the vascular pattern in hamartoma. (D) Selective left renal arteriogram, left posterior oblique position. The abnormal vessels are visible extending well outside the projected normal renal contour. (E) Selective epinephrine arteriogram. Only the abnormal vessels fill, while the normal renal arteries demonstrate failure of opacification in their midportion and distal portion. Because these vessels are relatively primitive and have relatively less muscle tissue than normal vessels, they fail to respond the way normal vessels do to epinephrine. When multiple tumors of this type are seen in the presence of tuberous sclerosis, the diagnosis of hamartoma is readily made. An isolated hamartoma, on the other hand, may resemble renal cell carcinoma, and the high fat content shown on CT in particular may be useful.

The characteristic angiographic appearance is that of hypervascularity, a large feeder artery, tortuous vessels that may be circumferentially arranged in the arterial phase, and multiple aneurysms with a "sunburst" or "whorled" appearance in the nephrographic and venous phases (see Fig. 46-25). Arteriovenous shunting is not observed, but filling of lakes is commonly observed. Although the findings have been said to be characteristic,[63] hamartoma cannot be definitively distinguished from carcinoma on the basis of angiography.

Other Benign Tumors

Fibromas, leiomyomas, and neurogenic tumors, such as neurofibroma or schwannoma of the kidney (Fig. 46-26), sometimes reach considerable size and may be highly vascular, suggesting a malignant tumor.

Metastases

Ten percent of all patients who die of carcinoma have renal metastases.[15] The primary sites include the breast, lung, and other organs (Table 46-13). The metastases urographically appear as mass lesions and angiographically resemble the angioarchitecture of the primary tumor. Although metastatic renal tumors are at least twice as common as primary tumors at autopsy, they come to clinical attention far less often. This is explained by the fact that metastasis to the kidney is part of a disseminated neoplastic process in which the involvement of other viscera frequently is the critical issue for the patient.[64]

Renal Pseudotumors

A number of conditions mimic tumors of the kidney and require recognition if elaborate diagnostic proce-

Table 46-13. Primary Site of Carcinomas Metastasizing to Kidney in 781 Consecutive Autopsied Cases

Primary Site	Number of Cases	Number of Cases with Renal Metastases	Percentage of Cases with Renal Metastases
Kidney	34	8	24
Lung	160	36	23
Breast	167	21	13
Stomach	119	12	11
Pancreas	32	3	9
Colon	118	9	8
Ovary	64	3	5
Rectum	87	3	3
Total	781	95	12

Adapted from Abrams HL, Spiro R, Goldstein N. Metastases in carcinoma: analysis of 1,000 autopsied cases. Cancer 1950;3:74.

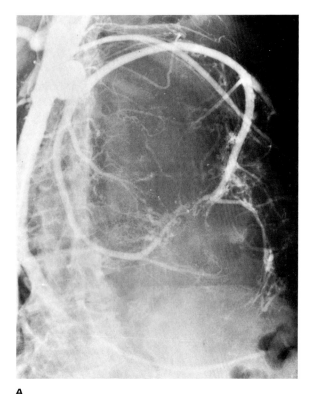

A

B

Figure 46-26. Neurogenic tumor of the kidney. The patient presented with increasing distention of his left lower abdomen and the sensation of a mass. Microscopic hematuria was present. The urogram demonstrated nonfunction of the left kidney, with a large mass apparently associated with the left kidney. (A) Aortogram, 1.5 seconds shows gross displacement of the major renal arteries and the beginning fill-ing of some abnormal vessels. (B) Aortogram, 3 seconds. A huge number of tortuous, randomly distributed vessels are opacified, a finding that is strongly suggestive of a malignant neoplasm. A nephrectomy was performed. The tumor demonstrated the classic histology of a schwannoma, a neurogenic tumor. Highly vascular neurogenic tumors are difficult to distinguish from classic renal cell carcinomas.

dures and surgery are to be avoided. Among these is prominent columns of Bertin, or focal cortical hyperplasia, which represents a projection of normal renal cortical tissue into the renal sinus (Figs. 46-27 and 46-28). The majority occur between the middle and upper pole calices and are marginated medially because of surrounding renal sinus fat. Caliceal stretching and deformity may be present, but arteriography demonstrates no tumor vessels, and there is a homogeneous, well-circumscribed nephrographic blush.[65] On glucoheptonate or DMSA renal scanning, pseudotumors reveal functioning renal parenchyma without defect.[33]

Congenital lobulation is a common anatomic variant most often observed in the middle segment of the lateral margin of the kidney. It may mimic a renal mass and/or suggest cortical atrophy secondary to focal pyelonephritis or renal infarction.

Renal fibrolipomatosis is associated with excessive fat in the renal sinus producing pelvocaliceal deformities suggestive of tumor or cyst.

Focal or diffuse renal hypertrophy may follow infection, trauma, infarction, or obstruction and may suggest a mass on urography because of distortion of the calices or altered renal contour (Fig. 46-29). These variants demonstrate no tumor vessels on angiography and frequently have associated signs of the predisposing conditions, such as chronic pyelonephritis.

The "dromedary hump" of the left kidney is now generally recognized as a normal variation, possibly caused by the adjacent spleen.

Other lesions that may simulate tumors, such as parapelvic cysts (Fig. 46-30), hydronephrosis of the upper pole of a duplicated collecting system,[66] intrarenal abscesses, intrarenal hematomas, and xanthogranulomatous pyelonephritis, require careful and critical evaluation before a neoplasm can be excluded.

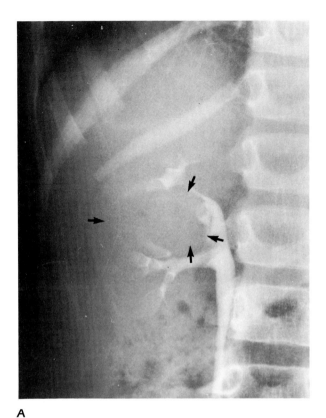

A

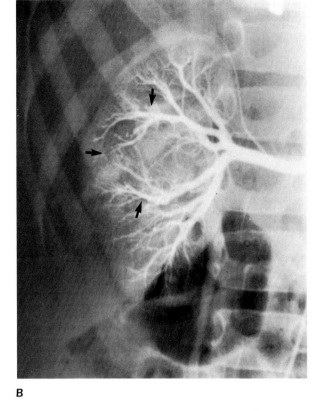

B

Figure 46-27. Renal pseudotumor. (A) Urogram. An apparent mass is visible on the right (*arrows*), separating the infundibulum to the midportion of the kidney from the infundibulum to the upper pole. (B) Selective renal arteriogram. There is separation of interlobar branches in the region of the "mass" shown on urography (*arrows*). No tumor vessels are visualized. (C) Nephrographic phase. A dense area in the midportion of the kidney (*arrows*) represents a large column of Bertin, an infolding of renal cortical tissue that has no pathologic significance. (Courtesy of H. Taybi, M.D.)

C

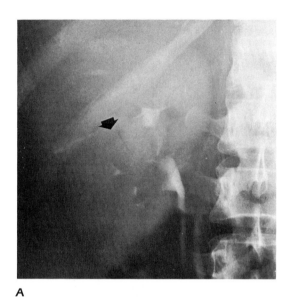

A

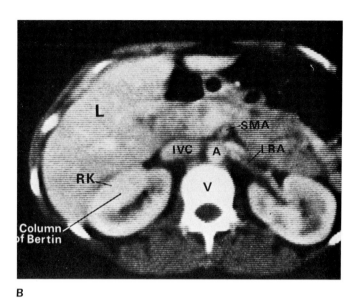

B

Figure 46-28. Renal pseudotumor. (A) Urogram demonstrates the separation of the upper pole and midpole calices by an apparent mass (*arrow*). (B) Computed tomogram. The "mass" lesion in the midportion of the right kidney is clearly defined as representing a column of Bertin, which is a normal variant.

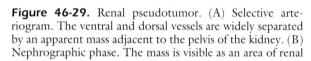

Figure 46-29. Renal pseudotumor. (A) Selective arteriogram. The ventral and dorsal vessels are widely separated by an apparent mass adjacent to the pelvis of the kidney. (B) Nephrographic phase. The mass is visible as an area of renal tissue (*arrows*), which represents compensatory hypertrophy in the presence of gross pyelonephritis involving the lower pole in particular but also the midportion of the kidney.

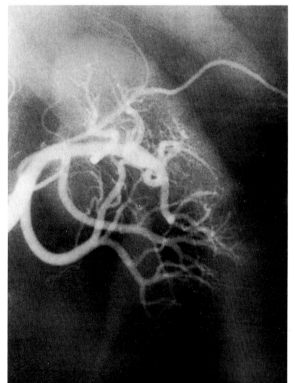

A

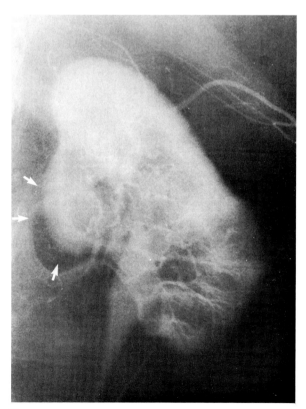

B

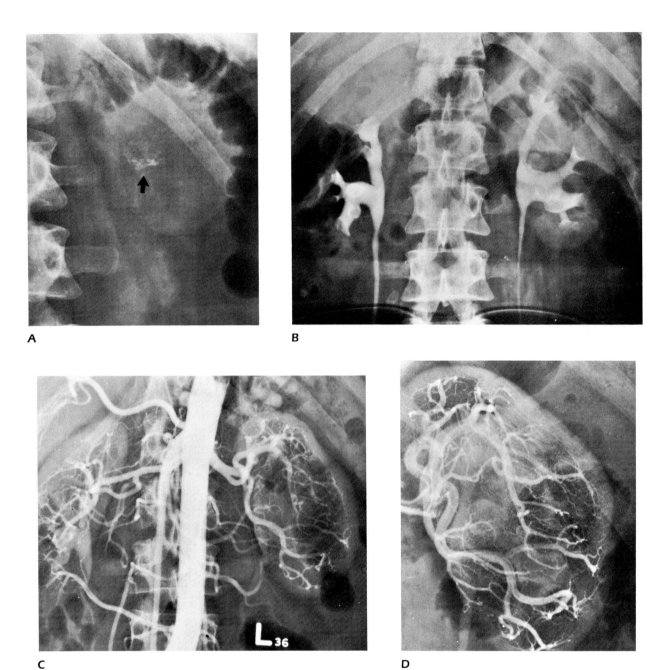

A

B

C

D

Figure 46-30. Renal pseudotumor. This 42-year-old man entered the hospital because of hematuria and hypertension. (A) Plain film shows amorphous calcification in the left kidney (*arrow*). (B) Urogram shows good concentration but evidence of a mass lesion on the left separating the upper and middle pole calices and compressing them. (C) Aortogram. The right kidney is normal, but the left kidney demonstrates splaying of vessels around a mass.

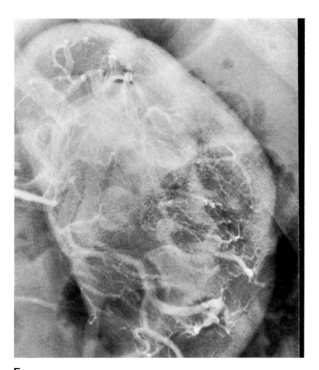

E

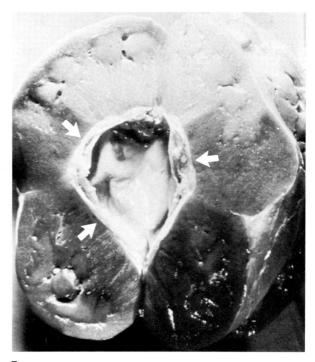

F

Figure 46-30 (continued). (D and E) Selective renal arteriograms with magnification. Multiple fine vessels are visible, none characteristic of renal cell carcinoma but presenting an unusual distribution for the renal circulation. (F) Specimen. On the assumption that the mass represented a renal tumor, a nephrectomy was performed. A 4-cm subcapsular posterolateral cyst showing fibrosis and focal calcification and ossification was found (*arrows*). It produced compression of the superior portion of the pelvis and calices.

Renal Cysts

The subject of renal cystic disease is complex and beset with varying terms and classifications. Solitary renal cysts are of central importance in their resemblance, as renal masses, to renal neoplasms and therefore require detailed discussion. Congenital renal cystic disease may present as a renal mass lesion in infancy. Polycystic kidney is reviewed in the early pages of this chapter, in the discussion of the differential diagnosis of renal cell carcinoma.

Incidence

Renal cysts are common in autopsies of adults over the age of 50[67] but are observed in no more than 1 to 2 percent of patients at urography.[68] They are seen at all ages but most commonly in the sixth and seventh decades.

Pathology

The cysts are smooth, thin-walled masses that contain a clear serous fluid of low specific gravity (Fig. 46-31).

They vary markedly in size and volume and may contain up to a liter of fluid. Cysts are covered by the renal capsule, and they usually lie more or less laterally. As they enlarge, they compress adjacent renal parenchyma. The cyst wall is no more than 1 to 2 mm in thickness and is lined with cuboidal epithelium. There has been much dispute as to the incidence of carcinoma arising from the cyst wall. Most observers consider the figure of 1 percent reliable,[69] but estimates as high as 7 percent have been reported.[70]

Symptoms and Signs

Small or modest-sized cysts rarely cause symptoms and are usually detected as incidental findings on the intravenous urogram. Large cysts may be associated with bulging of the flank and flank discomfort. Local pain may be produced by stretching of the renal capsule. Occasionally polycythemia[71] or hypertension[72] appear to be associated with simple renal cysts. One patient with a renal cyst had hypertension of 6 years' duration with a high ipsilateral renal vein renin value. Aspiration of the cyst was associated with a prompt remission in hypertension with a diastolic pressure of 80 mm throughout 9 months of follow-up.[73]

Diagnostic Evaluation

Intravenous Urography

The plain film demonstrates a smooth mass protruding from the renal border. So-called eggshell calcification—a thin, smooth, curvilinear calcific density—is typical of simple renal cyst and is observed in 2 to 3 percent of cysts; unfortunately, it may also be observed (rarely) in carcinoma.[74]

The early nephrographic film of 10 to 30 seconds is useful in depicting an avascular mass within the kidney. With contrast in the collecting system, varying degrees of deformity are demonstrated (Fig. 46-32). If the cyst is small, lateral, and partially extrarenal, the urographic appearance may be normal. More often, with moderate-sized-to-large cysts the calices are displaced, compressed, or "splayed." The infundibula may be narrowed or stretched. With large cysts, the caliceal system may be clumped or grouped in a relatively small portion of the kidney. The pelvis may be compressed, flattened, or distorted. The axis of the kidney can be shifted in any direction.

In general, no matter how great the impression on the collecting system, the calices remain delicate and sharp (unless infundibular obstruction occurs) and show no sign of irregularity or invasion. Similarly, the margins of the infundibula are smooth, even when narrowed, and are not irregular. Except for the nephrographic phase, which may strongly suggest the cystic character of the lesion, the urographic features cannot definitively distinguish cyst from solid tumor.

Nephrotomography

Nephrotomography has been widely applied to the evaluation of renal masses.[68,75] In approximately 85 percent of cases it establishes the diagnosis of renal cyst.[76]

Like ultrasonography, nephrotomography is a screening procedure, and to some extent it duplicates the diagnostic data derived from sonography. Nephrotomography provides useful supportive information but is rarely definitive, except in small, peripheral cysts in which the appearance is unequivocal.

Ultrasonography

Real-time ultrasound is a major noninvasive advance in the evaluation of renal masses and complements the urogram in the diagnostic workup. The classic cyst is entirely lacking in internal echoes at both high and low sensitivity levels, and the posterior cyst wall is smooth and well defined. "Through transmission" of echoes deep to the cyst is characteristic. The accuracy of ultrasonography in simple cysts is 90 to 95 percent.[68]

In some cystic lesions, such as abscesses, necrotic

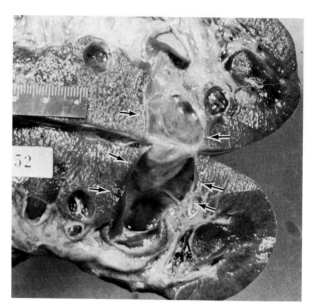

Figure 46-31. Gross pathology of a renal cyst. The kidney has been hemisected. The cyst (*arrows*) extends to the lateral edge of the kidney. It is smooth and thin walled and contains a clear, serous fluid of low specific gravity. In general, cysts vary markedly in size and volume and may contain up to a liter of fluid. Cysts are covered by the renal capsule and usually lie more or less laterally. As they enlarge, they compress adjacent renal parenchyma. The cyst wall is no more than 1 to 2 mm in thickness and is lined with cuboidal epithelium. There has been much dispute as to the incidence of carcinoma arising from the cyst wall. Most observers consider the figure of 1 percent reliable,[14] but estimates as high as 7 percent have been reported.[47]

or hemorrhagic tumors, multiple cysts, and hydronephrosis, a complex sonographic pattern is observed with both cystic and solid (echoic) elements. Finally, the sonogram may indicate a solid mass, typical of tumor. If a solid or complex pattern is observed, contrast-enhanced CT or MRI should follow.

Computed Tomography

Because a cyst contains fluid, it attenuates the x-ray beam less than solid tissue does. This difference allows a reliable distinction of cyst from tumor to be made by CT scanning (Fig. 46-33).

Angiography

The angiographic criteria of simple renal cyst are well established. A sharply defined radiolucent mass with a thin, smooth wall (1 mm in thickness) and an acute angle at the junction of cyst wall and renal cortex forming a "beak" is characteristic of a cyst (Fig. 46-34). Angiography has a high degree of accuracy, but it very occasionally may be misleading in the presence of avascular or cystic tumors. If any of the classic diagnostic

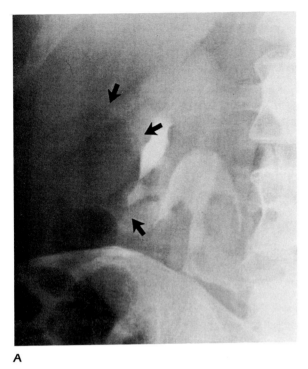

A

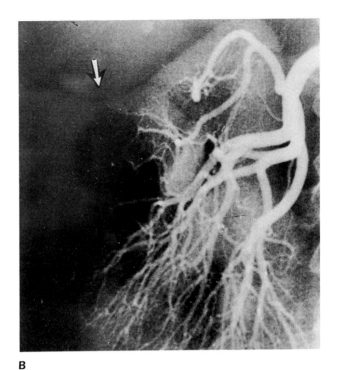

B

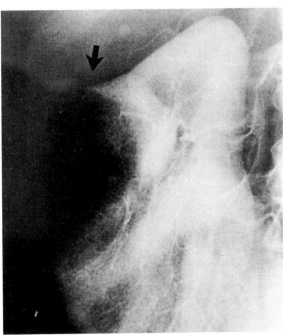

C

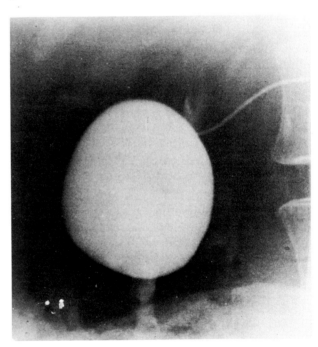

D

Figure 46-32. Renal cyst. (A) Urogram. A smooth, lucent mass at the lateral border of the right kidney (*arrows*) compresses and displaces the upper pole and midpole calices. (B) Selective renal arteriogram. The vessels to the lucent area are sharply displaced, and a so-called beak (*arrow*) characteristic of a renal cyst is seen. (C) Nephrographic phase. The beak (*arrow*) is well visualized, as are the striking lucency and absence of neoplastic vessels. Nevertheless, the entire wall of the cyst could not be visualized, and so a cyst puncture was undertaken. (D) Renal cyst puncture. The smoothly outlined ovoid collection of contrast agent represents a benign cyst. Fluid for cell and fat analyses was obtained, but no malignant cells were found. It is essential in cyst puncture that the area of the contrast-filled cyst fully account for any filling defect on the urogram.

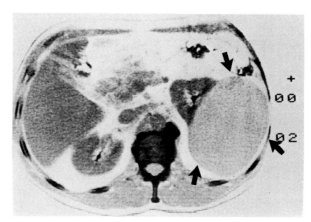

Figure 46-33. Renal cyst: computed tomogram. A large mass is visible in the left kidney (*arrows*), displacing normal parenchyma medially. The right kidney, inferior vena cava, and aorta are clearly delineated. The mass in the left kidney has less density than does normal renal tissue and represents a renal cyst with a low mean value in Hounsfield units. In general, the density of a renal cyst is close to the density of water (zero), and the density of a renal tumor lies between that of a cyst and that of the normally opacified renal parenchyma after the intravenous injection of 50 to 100 ml of contrast agent. The normal parenchyma generally measures 80 to 100 Hounsfield units after opacification. (Courtesy of Stuart Segal, M.D.)

criteria are lacking, epinephrine arteriography should be undertaken to enhance the demonstration of tumor vessels.

Differential Diagnosis

Like renal cell carcinoma, renal cyst must be distinguished from all other renal masses. In particular, avascular or cystic renal cell carcinoma is the most important single diagnosis to establish because the treatment is radically different. Hydronephrosis of the upper pole of a kidney with a double collecting system at times may be confused with findings of a cyst (Fig. 46-35). Renal fibrolipomatosis may present a urographic image resembling that of either cyst or tumor.

Treatment

"Cysts should be explored surgically."[14] This older view has changed because most urologists are now reassured when the classic radiographic, sonographic, and CT criteria for simple cyst are definitely present. When the diagnostic criteria for simple cyst are present, conservative management is desirable. When the diagnosis is in doubt, exploration is mandatory.

Diagnostic Decision Tree in Renal Mass Lesions

For the patient with a renal mass lesion undergoing imaging evaluation, the stakes are reasonably high: the untreated tumor, mistakenly diagnosed as cyst, may spread locally, metastasize, and move the patient into the incurable group. The benign cyst that is mistakenly taken to surgery exposes the patient to significant morbidity and mortality. A mortality of 1.5 to 2.4 percent and a major morbidity of 30 percent have been reported.[77] It must be acknowledged that there is the possibility of leaving a renal carcinoma untreated, that is, failing to detect a carcinoma in the cyst. According to Sherwood and Trott, the likelihood is less than 1 in 1000.[78] Thus the importance of a systematic and efficient approach to diagnosis must be emphasized.

Most urologists have adopted their approach to renal masses. "With modern radiologic techniques . . . an asymptomatic renal mass can be diagnosed accurately. The non-operative approach is precise, has almost no morbidity and costs half as much as operative evaluation."[79]

The widening application of CT and MRI to the diagnosis of renal mass lesions has decreased the need for arteriography in most cases. CT is also very useful in accurate staging of the tumor. Furthermore, for patients over the age of 60, CT depicts multiple cysts rapidly and can confirm the diagnosis of cyst when the appearance is typical.

The problem of renal mass lesions is particularly acute in the aged. All too often the mass is discovered on the urogram performed for the patient with prostatic disease. In the older age group, the risk of renal exploration is higher. Scrupulous attention to the nonsurgical diagnostic management of such patients can forestall unnecessary surgery.

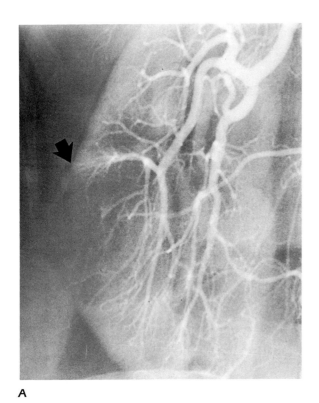

A

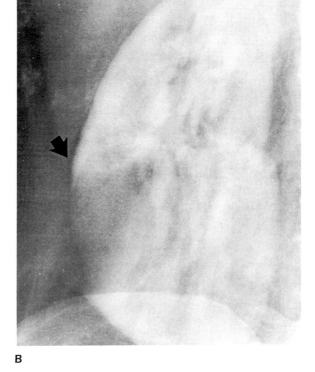

B

Figure 46-34. Renal cyst. (A) Arteriogram. Note the displacement of vessels and the avascular area (*arrow*). (B) Nephrogram. A "beak" (*arrow*) characteristic of a benign cyst is visible. (C) Cyst puncture. The cyst is opaque and accounts fully for the apparent mass seen on arteriography.

C

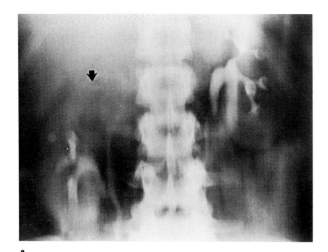

A

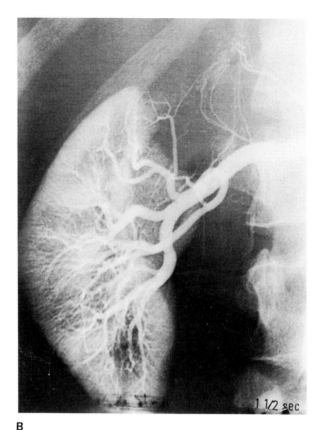

B

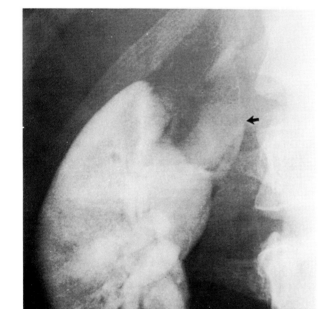

C

Figure 46-35. Hydronephrosis of the upper pole of a double collecting system. (A) Urogram. An apparent cyst (*arrow*) is visible in the upper pole in the kidney. Note that no calices extend above the midportion of the kidney and that there are fewer calices on the right side than on the left. (B) Selective renal arteriogram, arterial phase. A few small vessels extend from the main renal artery and its branches to surround the apparent upper pole cyst. (C) Nephrographic phase. A thin but definite curvilinear density (*arrow*) surrounding the apparent cystic area medially represents compressed parenchyma. Surgical exploration revealed a hydronephrotic upper pole of a double collecting system on the right.

References

1. Hadju SI, Berg JW, Foote FW. Clinically unrecognized, silent renal-cell carcinoma in elderly cancer patients. J Am Geriatr Soc 1970;18:443.
2. Cronin RE. Renal cell carcinoma. Am J Med Sci 1991;302: 249–259.
3. Everson TC. Spontaneous regression of cancer. Ann NY Acad Sci 1964;114:721.
4. Freed SL, Halperin JP, Gordon M. Idiopathic regression of metastases from renal cell carcinoma. J Urol 1977;118:538.
5. Lucke B, Schiumberger JS. Tumors of the kidney, renal pelvis, and ureter. In: Atlas of tumour pathology, Armed Forces Institute of Pathology, 1957. Sect. 8, Fasc. 33.
6. Robbins SL. Textbook of pathology with clinical application. 2nd ed. Philadelphia: Saunders, 1962.
7. Crocker DW. Renal tumors. In: Sommers, SC, ed. Kidney pathology decennial. New York: Appleton-Century-Crofts, 1975: 609.
8. Clark RE, Moss AA, DeLorimer AA, et al. Arteriography of Wilms' tumor. AJR 1971;113:476.
9. Westra P, Keiffer SA, Mosser DG. Wilms' tumor: a summary of 25 years of experience before actinomycin-D. AJR 1967; 100:214.
10. Tannenbaum M. Ultrastructural pathology of human renal cell tumors. In: Sommers SC, ed. Kidney pathology decennial. New York: Appleton-Century-Crofts, 1975:647.
11. Snyder WH Jr, Hastings TA, Pollack WF. Retroperitoneal tumors. In: Mustard WR, Ravitch MM, Snyder WH Jr, Welch KS, Benson CD, eds. Pediatric surgery. 2nd ed. Chicago: Year Book, 1969;2:1020.
12. Lalli AF, Ahstrom L, Ericsson NO, et al. Nephroblastoma (Wilms' tumor): urographic diagnosis and prognosis. Radiology 1966;87:495.
13. Clark P, Anderson K. Tumors of the kidney and ureter. In: Blandy J, ed. Urology. London: Blackwell, 1976:391.
14. Damming CL, Harvard BM. Tumors of the urogenital tract. In: Campbell MF, Harrison JH, eds. Urology. Philadelphia: Saunders, 1970:885.
15. Abrams HL, Spiro R, Goldstein N. Metastases in carcinoma: analysis of 1,000 autopsied cases. Cancer 1950;3:74.
16. Flocks RH, Kadesky MC. Malignant neoplasms of the kidney: an analysis of 353 patients followed five years or more. J Urol 1958;79:196.
17. Lokich JJ, Harrison JH. Renal cell carcinoma: natural history and chemotherapeutic experience. J Urol 1975;114:371.
18. Smith H, Riches E. Haemoglobin values in renal carcinoma. Lancet 1963;1:1017.
19. Thorling EB, Ersbak J. Erythrocytosis and hypernephroma. Scand J Hematol 1964;1:38.
20. Chisholm GB, Ray RR. The systemic effects of malignant renal tumors. Br J Urol 1971;43:687.
21. Utz DC, Warren MM, Gregg JA, et al. Reversible hepatic dysfunction associated with hypernephroma. Mayo Clin Proc 1970;45:161.
22. Newman HR, Schulman ML. Renal cortical tumors: a 40-year statistical study. Urol Surv 1969;19:2.
23. Siegleman SS, Sprayregen S, Bosniak MA. Serendipity in the diagnosis of renal carcinoma. J Can Assoc Radiol 1972;23:251.
24. Skinner DG, Colvin RB, Vermillion CD. Diagnosis and management of renal cell carcinoma: a clinical and pathologic study of 309 cases. Cancer 1971;28:1165.
25. Bottiger LE, Hallberg D, von Schreeb T. Renal carcinoma as an accidental finding. Acta Chir Scand 1964;127:158.
26. Ettinger A, Elkin M. Value of plain film in renal mass lesions (tumors and cysts). Radiology 1954;62:372.
27. Kikkawa K, Lasser EC. "Ring-like" or "rim-like" calcification in renal cell carcinoma. AJR 1969;107:737.
28. Graham AP. Malignancy of the kidney: survey of 195 cases. J Urol 1947;58:10.
29. Folin J. Conventional roentgenography and urography in the diagnosis of renal tumors. Radiologe 1961;1:166.
30. Woodruff JH Jr, Chalek CC, Ottoman RE, et al. The roentgen diagnosis of renal neoplasms. J Urol 1956;75:615.
31. Dunnick NR. Renal lesions: great strides in imaging. Radiology 1992;182:305–306.
32. Warshauer DM, et al. Detection of renal masses: sensitivities and specificities of excretory urography/linear tomography, US, and CT. Radiology 1988;169:363–365.
33. Blaufox MD. Procedures of choice in renal nuclear medicine. J Nucl Med 1991;32:1301–1309.
34. Lee VW, Foster AJ, et al. Functional oncocytoma of the kidney: evaluation by dual-tracer scintigraphy. J Nucl Med 1987;28: 1911–1914.
35. Foster WL, Roberts L Jr, Halvorsen RA, Dunnick NR. Sonography of small renal masses with indeterminate density characteristics on computed tomography. Urol Radiol 1988;10:59–67.
36. Levine E, Lee KR, Weigel J. Preoperative determination of abdominal extent of renal cell carcinoma by computed tomography. Radiology 1979;132:395.
37. Williamson B Jr, Hattery RR, Stephens DH, et al. Computed tomography of the kidneys. Semin Roentgenol 1978;13: 249.
38. Marotti M, Hricak H, Fritzsche P, Crooks LE, Hedgcock MW, Tanagho EA. Complex and simple renal cysts: comparative evaluation with MR imaging. Radiology 1987;162:679–684.
39. Hartman DS, Aronson S, Frazer H. Current status of imaging indeterminate renal masses. Radiol Clin North Am 1991;29: 475–496.
40. Semelka RC, Shoenut JP, Krocker MA, MacMahon R, Greenberg HM. Renal lesions: controlled comparison between CT and 1.5 T MR imaging with nonenhanced and gadolinium-enhanced fat suppressed spin-echo and breath-hold FLASH techniques. Radiology 1992;182:425–430.
41. Choyke PL, Pollack HM. The role of MRI in diseases of the kidney. Radiol Clin North Am 1988;26:617–631.
42. Semelka RC, Hricak H, Stevens SK, Finegold R, Tomei E, Carroll PR. Combined gadolinium-enhanced and fat saturation MR imaging of renal masses. Radiology 1991;178:803–809.
43. Meaney TF. Errors in angiographic diagnosis of renal masses. Radiology 1969;93:361.
44. Watson RC, Fleming RJ, Evans JA. Arteriography in the diagnosis of renal carcinoma. Radiology 1968;91:888.
45. Boijsen E, Folin J. Angiography in the diagnosis of renal carcinoma. Radiology 1961;1:173.
46. Cornell SH, Dolan KD. Angiographic findings in renal carcinoma: analysis of 25 cases. J Urol 1967;98:71.
47. Folin J. Angiography in renal tumors: its value in diagnosis and differential diagnosis as a complement to conventional methods. Acta Radiol (Stockh) 1967;Suppl 267.
48. Bosniak MA, Ambos MA, Madayag MA, et al. Epinephrine-enhanced renal angiography in renal mass lesions: is it worth performing? AJR 1977;129:647.
49. Abrams HL. The response of neoplastic renal vessels to epinephrine in man. Radiology 1964;82:217.
50. Abrams HL, Obrez I, Hollenberg NK, et al. Pharmacoangiography of the renal vascular bed. Curr Probl Radiol 1971;1:1.
51. Whitley NO, Kinkhabwala M, Whitley JE. The collateral vein sign: a fallible sign in the staging of renal cancer. AJR 1974; 120:660.
52. Lang EK. The accuracy of roentgenographic techniques in the diagnosis of renal mass lesions. Radiology 1971;98:119.
53. Smith JC, Rösch J, Athanasoulis CA, et al. Renal venography in the evaluation of poorly vascularized neoplasms of the kidney. AJR 1975;123:552.
54. Cole AT, Mandell J, Fried FA, et al. The place of bone scan in the diagnosis of renal cell carcinoma. J Urol 1975;114:364.
55. Williams LH, Anastopoulos HP, Presant CA. Selective renal arteriography in Hodgkin's disease of the kidney. Radiology 1969;93:1059.
56. Koehler PR. The roentgen diagnosis of renal inflammatory

masses—special emphasis on angiographic changes. Radiology 1974;112:257.

57. Cummings KB, Correa RJ Jr, Gibbons RP, et al. Renal pelvic tumors. J Urol 1975;113:158.
58. Rabinowitz J, Kinkhabwala M, Himmelfarb E, et al. Renal pelvic carcinoma: an angiographic re-evaluation. Radiology 1972; 102:551.
59. Xipel JM. The incidence of benign renal nodules (in clinicopathologic study). J Urol 1971;106:503.
60. Holt RG, Neiman HL, Korsower JM, Newhouse J. Angiographic features of benign renal adenoma. Urology 1975;6: 764.
61. Hanse GC, Hoffman RB, Sample WF, et al. Computed tomography diagnosis of renal angiomyolipoma. Radiology 1978; 128:789.
62. Shawker TH, Horvath KL, Dunnick NR. Renal angiomyolipoma: diagnosis by combined ultrasound and computerized tomography. J Urol 1979;121:675.
63. McCallum RW. The pre-operative diagnosis of renal hamartoma. Clin Radiol 1975;26:257.
64. Ben-Menachem Y, Marcos J, Wallace S, et al. Angiography of renal metastases. Br J Radiol 1974;47:869.
65. Popky GL, Bogash M, Pollack H, et al. Focal cortical hyperplasia. J Urol 1969;102:657.
66. Olsson O. Renal malformation. In: Abrams HL, ed. Angiography. 2nd ed. Boston: Little, Brown, 1971:823.
67. Heptinstall RH. Pathology of the kidney. 2nd ed. Boston: Little, Brown, 1974.
68. Becker JA, Schneider M. Simple cyst of the kidney. Semin Roentgenol 1975;10:103.
69. Emmett JL, Levine SR, Woolner B. Co-existence of renal cyst and tumor: incidence in 1007 cases. Br J Radiol 1963;35:403.
70. Gibson TE. Interrelationship of renal cysts and tumors: report of three cases. J Urol 1954;71:241.
71. Cohen NN. Polycythemia associated with bilateral unilocular renal cysts. Arch Intern Med 1960;105:301.
72. Babja JC, Cohen MS, Sode J. Solitary intrarenal cyst causing hypertension. N Engl J Med 1974;291:343.
73. Rockson SG, Stone RA, Gunnells JC Jr. Solitary renal cyst with segmental ischemia and hypertension. J Urol 1974;112:550.
74. Daniel WW Jr, Hartman GW, Witten DM, et al. Calcified renal masses: a review of ten years' experience at the Mayo Clinic. Radiology 1972;103:503.
75. Pollack HM, Goldberg BB, Bogash M. Changing concepts in the diagnosis and management of renal cysts. J Urol 1974;111: 326.
76. Greene LF, Fraser RA, Hartman GW. Bolus nephrotomography in diagnosis of lesions of kidney. Urology 1976;7:221.
77. Kropp KA, Grayhack JT, Wendell RM, et al. Morbidity and mortality of renal exploration for cyst. Surg Gynecol Obstet 1967;125:803.
78. Sherwood TR, Trott PA. Needling renal cysts and tumors: cytology and radiology. Br Med J 1975;3:755.
79. Clayman RV, Williams RD, Fraley EE. Current concepts in cancer: the pursuit of the renal mass. N Engl J Med 1979;300:72.

47

Angiography of Renal Infection

MORTON A. BOSNIAK
MARJORIE A. AMBOS
RICHARD S. LEFLEUR

The past 15 to 20 years have seen extraordinary advances in diagnostic imaging as well as in percutaneous interventional techniques in the kidney. The addition of ultrasonography (US), computed tomography (CT), and needle aspiration techniques (aided by CT and US localization) has made possible an extremely high level of diagnostic accuracy in the evaluation of renal inflammatory diseases. Although a great amount of experience and knowledge has been gathered with angiography, this modality is no longer needed for diagnosis in renal inflammatory disease. Nevertheless, in the interest of completeness, this chapter describes and summarizes the angiographic findings in inflammatory disease of the kidney.

Many radiologic findings are associated with renal inflammatory disease. The process may be acute, subacute, or chronic, and either diffusely present throughout the kidney or localized. The disease may extend into the perirenal space or may be confined to the collecting system structures. The angiographic findings, which reflect this wide range of disease, depend on the stage of the inflammatory process, the etiologic agent, and the distribution of the disease in and around the kidney.

The following outline is used to organize the discussion of renal infection in this chapter:

1. Acute diffuse inflammation, including acute pyelonephritis (acute bacterial nephritis and acute suppurative pyelonephritis with microabscesses)
2. Renal abscess, including acute localized abscess (carbuncle), subacute to chronic localized abscess, and perinephric abscess (either primary or due to extension from renal abscess)
3. Chronic inflammation, diffuse and localized
   a. Xanthogranulomatous pyelonephritis, tumefactive and nontumefactive
   b. Tuberculosis
   c. Chronic atrophic pyelonephritis

4. Miscellaneous inflammatory conditions
   a. Infected cysts or caliceal diverticula
   b. Infected hydronephrosis, pyonephrosis (see Chapter 48)
   c. Fungous disease

Acute Pyelonephritis (Acute Bacterial Nephritis, Acute Suppurative Pyelonephritis)

Acute pyelonephritis is a renal parenchymal inflammation resulting from the spread of pathogenic organisms to the kidney, either by ascent up the ureter from the lower urinary tract or via the bloodstream. It has a wide range of radiologic and pathologic findings, depending on the severity of involvement.[1,2] With acute infection, there is an inflammatory response in the renal parenchyma with secondary edema resulting in kidney enlargement.[1,3] Gross examination of a kidney with acute pyelonephritis may reveal multiple microabscesses throughout the cortex. These range in size from approximately 1 to 5 mm and are most clearly seen on the subcapsular renal surface.[1,2] Microscopically, there are interstitial edema, hyperemia, and infiltrates of neutrophilic leukocytes between the tubules.[2] In a more severe form of pyelonephritis, previously termed *bacterial nephritis* or *acute suppurative pyelonephritis,* the inflammatory process is more extensive, with increased leukocyte infiltration and focal areas of tissue necrosis. Some pathologists refer to this latter condition as *phlegmon of the kidney.*[2] When acute pyelonephritis is focal in one portion of the kidney, the term *lobar nephronia* has been used.[4] In this entity, one specific segment or lobe of the kidney is infected, generally by *Escherichia coli.* No true abscess exists because there is no liquefaction or necrosis. It is felt that lobar nephronia is probably secondary to reflux.[4]

There has been considerable confusion as to the terminology used in cases of renal inflammation. It has been recently proposed that the term *acute focal pyelonephritis* be used instead of *lobar nephronia* and *severe pyelonephritis* be used to denote the more severe inflammation process that has been termed *bacterial nephritis*. For the remainder of this chapter, we will use this simplified terminology.

Histologic examination in cases of seemingly unilateral acute pyelonephritis has often revealed inflammatory changes in the contralateral kidney, suggesting that the infection is often bilateral but is subclinical on one side.[3]

Acute pyelonephritis is most commonly seen in females between the ages of 15 and 40.[5] Fever, chills, and flank pain are frequently present. Although the laboratory findings are variable, leukocytosis is often present, and analysis of the urine may show both white and red blood cells. The urine culture is frequently positive, and *E. coli* is often the offending organism, especially in patients with reflux.[5–7] A more severe form of pyelonephritis is frequently seen in diabetic females. In these patients, gram-negative organisms (most frequently *E. coli*) are cultured from both the urine and the blood.[2,7] It has been postulated that a more severe inflammatory process develops in diabetics because of an altered or diminished host response to infection.

In a patient with acute pyelonephritis, one of three courses occurs: (1) the inflammation may resolve completely, leaving a grossly normal kidney; (2) the inflammation may worsen into a more severe case of infection, possibly with microabscesses; or (3) the inflammation may go on to frank abscess formation.[2] The eventual outcome depends on a combination of therapy, host response, and organism involved.

Approximately 25 percent of patients having intravenous urography during an episode of acute pyelonephritis show one or more abnormal findings.[2,3,7] Urographic changes include focal or generalized renal enlargement, delayed filling of the collecting system, a decreased nephrogram, and a diminished density of contrast in the collecting system.[1,2,8] With appropriate antibiotic therapy, all these changes are reversible.[4] In the more severe cases there is often marked diminution in renal excretion of contrast material, with a faint nephrogram and a lack of caliceal visualization.[8–10]

It should be noted that most cases of pyelonephritis can be readily diagnosed by clinical and laboratory findings with treatment instituted without the use of imaging studies. However, when standard antibiotic treatment has not been successful or if the patient's presentation is unusually severe or atypical, imaging studies for diagnosis are often needed.

Sonographic findings in acute pyelonephritis are variable and depend to a large degree on the severity of the infection. Milder cases of pyelonephritis may show no significant changes on ultrasound studies, whereas more severe cases show enlargement of the kidney with loss of definition of the renal sinus (central echo complex). Areas of variable echotexture of the parenchyma can be seen with predominantly hypoechoic areas corresponding to parenchymal edema. US can detect associated hydronephrosis, focal abscess, or perirenal fluid collections, which are some of the important complications of acute pyelonephritis.[11–13]

CT is the most important and sensitive imaging technique in the diagnosis of pyelonephritis.[14–16] The study must be performed with intravenous contrast because abnormality of the nephrogram is the key finding that indicates renal parenchymal infection. A swollen kidney with a decreased nephrogram is seen in acute diffuse pyelonephritis. A number of the more common nephrographic patterns of diminished attenuation in the nephrogram may be seen, such as a striated nephrogram, poorly defined rounded areas of diminished attenuation, and wide bands of decreased nephrogram extending from the calices to the renal surface. These represent areas of edema, inflammatory debris, and vascular spasm caused by the inflammatory process. Focal areas of diminished attenuation with liquefaction and perirenal fluid collections indicating renal abscess or perirenal abscess are also readily visualized. One can also assess a functional aspect of the kidney by observing the amount and speed of contrast excretion by the infected kidney.

Renal scintigraphy (^{99m}Tc-DMSA) has also been used in diagnosing pyelonephritis. The technique is more sensitive than US or intravenous urography in detecting renal parenchymal infection but is not as specific as CT. Its main use has been to distinguish upper from lower urinary tract infection in children.[17]

Arteriography is rarely used in the diagnosis of acute pyelonephritis. However, a large experience with arteriography in this disease has been accumulated and is presented here to familiarize the reader with the vascular patterns in renal inflammatory disease.

Arteriography may show a spectrum of changes in acute pyelonephritis, depending on the severity of the infection and whether it is generalized or segmental. There are often stretching and attenuation of the intrarenal arteries secondary to parenchymal edema, as well as loss of the corticomedullary junction[18] (Fig. 47-1). In the subgroup of acute focal pyelonephritis, there is actual stretching of vessels around the infected lobe of tissue (Fig. 47-2).[4] In the nephrogram phase of the angiogram in acute pyelonephritis, two patterns may

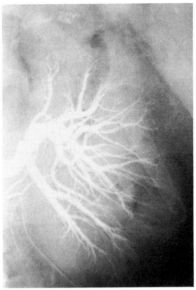
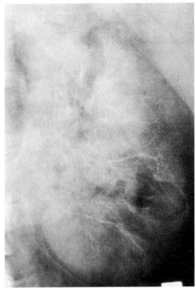
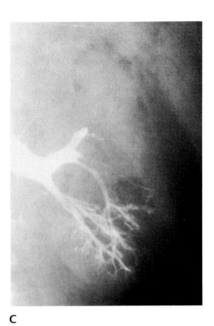

A **B** **C**

Figure 47-1. Case 1. Acute diffuse inflammation with microabscesses in a 61-year-old man with fever and left flank pain. No visualization of the left kidney was noted on urography. (A) Selective left renal arteriogram, arterial phase. The vessels are stretched in the swollen kidney but no focal abnormalities are seen. (B) Selective left renal arteriogram, late arterial, early nephrographic phase. A diffusely mottled and decreased nephrogram is seen, with loss of the corticomedullary junction and the suggestion of slow flow through the arterial system. (C) Left renal venogram (epinephrine-enhanced). Complete obstruction of the upper and middle pole veins can be seen, with attenuation and some stretching of the lower pole veins. It is evident that the findings on the venogram are more extensive than those on the arteriogram. Because of the left kidney's continued poor functioning, nephrectomy was performed. Pathologic examination of the removed kidney revealed a diffuse inflammatory process with several small focal abscesses, particularly in the upper portion of the kidney. (From Pingoud EG, Pais SO, Glickman M. Epinephrine renal venography in acute bacterial infection of the kidney. AJR 1979;133:665–669. Used with permission.)

be present. Multiple small lucencies, representing microabscesses, may be scattered throughout the parenchyma, giving the nephrogram a mottled appearance (Fig. 47-3). In other cases, there may be a series of alternately lucent and dense stripes in the cortex (striated nephrogram) (Fig. 47-4).[2,3,19] In the milder forms of acute pyelonephritis, normal angiograms may be seen.[3]

In the severe form of acute pyelonephritis, arteriographic changes are consistently present and are more severe.[9] The kidney is swollen, leading to marked stretching, splaying, and attenuation of the intrarenal arteries. The interlobar arteries and their branches are decreased in both number and caliber[2,9] (see Fig. 47-1), and slower flow is observed in the affected areas. In severe infection, the arteries are stretched around small inflammatory masses.[5] As in simple acute pyelonephritis, there is loss of the corticomedullary border, and the nephrogram may show mottled lucencies or cortical striations. In the more severe forms of the disease, the cortical striations are more consistently seen.[9,10] It has been suggested that these striations are

due to redistribution of blood flow away from the cortex as a result of obliteration of interlobular arteries by perivascular inflammatory cells,[5,9] whereas the loss of the corticomedullary border seen in acute pyelonephritis is due to cortical vasoconstriction.[3,20]

Follow-up urograms on patients with severe pyelonephritis who have been successfully treated with antibiotics may reveal global wasting with caliceal clubbing but without focal scarring.[9] In one study, follow-up angiograms on patients with treated severe pyelonephritis showed attenuation of the arterial tree.[21]

Several groups have suggested that renal venography is more valuable than arteriography in the diagnosis of acute pyelonephritis.[4,18,22,23] Because the walls of veins are more sensitive to surrounding disease than are arterial walls, it is felt that they may reflect earlier changes in the kidney.[4] Epinephrine-enhanced venography in acute pyelonephritis may reveal smooth narrowing or total occlusion of intrarenal veins. As on the arterial side, the parenchymal edema leads to stretching and attenuation.[23] These venous changes are not

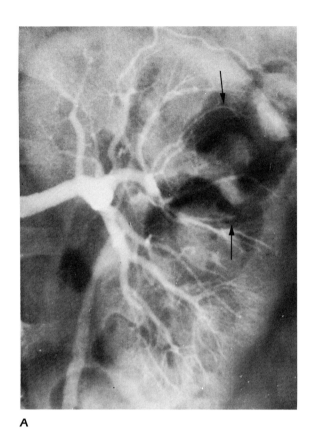

A

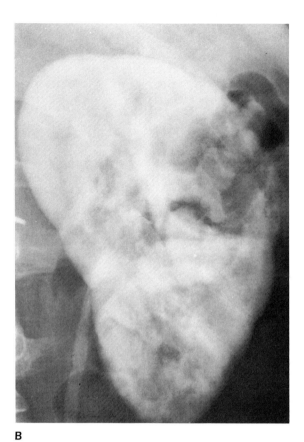

B

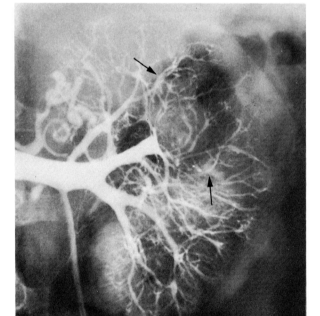

C

Figure 47-2. Case 2. Acute focal inflammation in a 43-year-old man with left renal colic and spiking temperatures. (A) Selective left renal arteriogram, arterial phase. A hypovascular mass is seen in the upper portion of the kidney with stretching of the interlobar branches around the mass (*arrows*), but there is no abnormal vascularity. (B) Selective left renal arteriogram, nephrographic phase. A diminished nephrogram with indistinct margins in the area of the mass is noted (it is somewhat obscured by overlying bowel gas). (C) Left renal venogram (epinephrine-enhanced). Narrowed, irregular veins in area of the localized inflammatory mass are well seen (*arrows*). Note that the veins are much more affected than the arteries. The patient was treated with antibiotics, and his symptoms disappeared in about a week. Follow-up studies revealed no abnormality in the kidney, except for a small upper pole scar. (From Pingoud EG, Pais SO, Glickman M. Epinephrine renal venography in acute bacterial infection of the kidney. AJR 1979;133:665–669. Used with permission.)

diagnostic of infection but, with an appropriate history and laboratory findings, are suggestive of infection.[18] Figures 47-1 and 47-2 demonstrate that the extent of the inflammatory disease is more clearly seen on venography than on arteriography. These observations, which have no application in the present evaluation of renal infection, are included for historical purposes and indicate the difficulty that was encountered in accu-

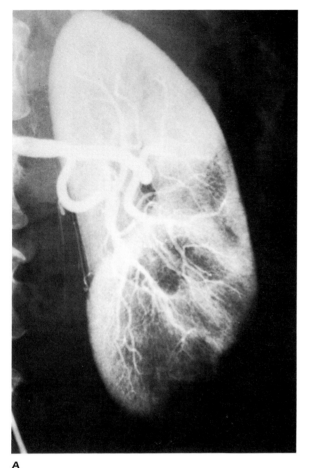

A

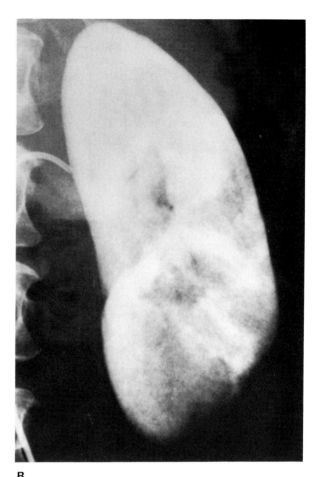

B

Figure 47-3. Case 3. Acute inflammation of the kidney in a 42-year-old woman with fever and flank pain. An intravenous urogram revealed swelling and fullness of the lower pole of the left kidney, as well as poor visualization of the lower pole calix. (A) Selective left renal arteriogram, arterial phase. Decreased vascularity in the lower pole of the kidney is noted, with areas of poor perfusion and slower flow of contrast medium. No distinct displacement of vessels is shown, however. (B) Selective left renal arteriogram, nephrographic phase. Multiple areas of decreased or absent nephrogram in the lower pole are seen, with loss of delineation of the corticomedullary junction and multiple defects in the contour of the kidney. At surgical exploration for possible drainage of abscess in the lower pole of the left kidney, a swollen, edematous kidney was noted. A left nephrectomy was performed because a neoplasm was suspected. Study of pathologic specimen revealed acute and chronic inflammation with edema and microabscesses but no gross collection of pus.

rately diagnosing renal inflammatory disease before the introduction of US and CT.

Renal Abscess

Bacterial invasion of the renal parenchyma may, in certain cases, progress to abscess formation. When this occurs, the earliest stage of the infection is edema with multiple microabscesses. These abscesses may then coalesce into a suppurative mass that progresses to frank liquefaction or necrosis.[1,5] At this point, a true abscess (renal carbuncle) is present, and it may follow one of three courses: (1) it may remain confined to the renal parenchyma; (2) it may break through into the perinephric space; or (3) it may extend into the renal collecting system.[1] The radiologic findings depend on the time at which the abscess is studied, that is, on whether the abscess is acute or chronic and whether it is confined to the parenchyma or has extended.

In the past, *Staphylococcus aureus* has been the most common organism found in renal abscesses. It generally involves the kidney via the hematogenous route.[6,24,25] Ascending infections may also cause abscess formation, and in these cases gram-negative organisms are commonly found.[6,26] Ascending infections most commonly affect kidneys that were previously damaged by calculi or other causes of hydronephro-

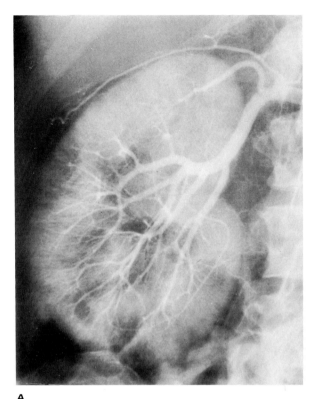

A

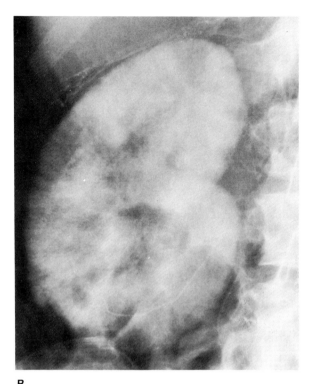

B

Figure 47-4. Case 4. Acute diffuse pyelonephritis in a 54-year-old man with right flank pain, fever, and leukocytosis. On urography a swollen right kidney was seen with faint visualization of the collecting system. (A) Selective right renal arteriogram, arterial phase. Stretching of the intrarenal branches and capsular artery is demonstrated. No focal ab-normality is noted. (B) Selective right renal arteriogram, nephrographic phase. A diffusely swollen kidney is seen, with loss of delineation of the cortical-medullary junction. Note the striated nephrogram pattern throughout (best seen along outer margin of kidney).

sis.[27] The spectrum of organisms causing renal abscesses has changed in recent years because of the earlier treatment of infections with antibiotics and the increase in the abuse of intravenous drugs associated with drug addiction.[7] Gram-negative bacteria, especially *E. coli, Pseudomonas,* and *Proteus,* are increasingly found to be the cause of renal abscesses.[7]

When the pathway of infection is the bloodstream, the bacteria lodge in the small intrarenal arteries and multiply there, forming microabscesses that may eventually coalesce to form a mass filled with pus.[1,26,28] The abscess, when new, lacks a well-defined wall and is less a true mass than an area of inflamed parenchyma.[28] At this early stage there may be an extension of the infection into the perirenal space or the renal collecting system.[29] When the abscess remains confined to the renal parenchyma, a wall forms around it. This wall is the result of fibroblastic proliferation and vascularization around the periphery of the inflammatory mass. In time, the wall thickens into a pseudocapsule with vascular connective tissue.[5] The chronic renal abscess is actually a necrotic mass surrounded by a broad zone of granulation tissue.[28]

Clinical Findings

Two different clinical pictures may be seen in renal abscesses, depending on whether the process is acute or chronic. If it is acute, the patient complains of fever, chills, and flank pain. If the abscess is secondary to a staphylococcal skin or respiratory infection or to dental work, it usually becomes evident 1 to 8 weeks following the primary episode.[27,30] Laboratory findings may include leukocytosis and an elevated erythrocyte sedimentation rate. Unless the abscess breaks through into the collecting system, urine culture and urinalysis are often unremarkable.[2,25] Chronic abscesses are more difficult diagnostic problems because they often develop insidiously, with minimal clinical and laboratory findings.[31] Localizing symptoms are rare, the history of a preceding infection is often overlooked, and the urine culture is usually negative.[31] Prior to the availability of modern imaging techniques, a correct preoperative diagnosis of renal abscess was made in only about 20 percent of cases based on clinical parameters.[24,32] With the introduction of angiography, the ability to correctly diagnose renal abscess preoperatively increased significantly. The subsequent development and use of US and CT and the more frequent and accurate use of needle aspiration has made the diagnosis of renal abscess even less of a problem. When the condition is correctly diagnosed, antibiotic therapy may be curative, although larger abscesses usually require drainage.[27]

Radiologic Findings

Radiologic findings in renal abscesses vary with the stage and extent of the process. The plain abdominal film often shows loss of the renal and psoas outlines on the affected side.[28,29] If the renal outline is seen, it may reveal generalized or focal enlargement.[33] Intravenous urography often demonstrates a diminished excretion of contrast material with decreased opacification of all or parts of the collecting system.[2,24] In a series of 22 patients with renal abscess, the urogram showed enlargement of the kidney in 7 and a distinct mass effect in 12.[29] With chronicity, mass lesions are more commonly found. Because of the necrosis within the abscess, an area of lucency may be seen on the urogram.[2] With extension into the perirenal space, the renal outline becomes hazy or blurred in the involved area.[1] Ultrasonography of an acute abscess may show a sonolucent area, with few or no internal echoes; as time passes, the abscesses become more echogenic. Perinephric involvement may also be demonstrated by US.[33,34] CT can also be helpful in the diagnosis of renal abscess. Perinephric extension is clearly seen and the diagnosis of perinephric abscess can be readily made. Most abscesses of the kidney can be diagnosed on CT studies without difficulty, particularly when combined with the clinical history. A localized mass with a central area of decreased attenuation is observed. The wall is thickened and hyperemic.[14,33] A small amount of air may be present on occasion, which would be diagnostic. The thickness of the wall is determined by the chronicity of the abscess. Occasionally chronic renal abscesses can be confused with a necrotic neoplasm by CT, particularly when the clinical history is not indicative of infection.[35] However, the great majority of renal abscesses can be readily diagnosed and confirmed by needle aspiration.

Angiographic findings in renal abscesses do, of course, vary with the stage and extent of the process. Occasionally, a mass may not be appreciated angiographically, even when one is suggested on urography.[26,28] An early, acute abscess suggests generalized edema rather than displaying a mass effect. Vessels are not displaced by the abscess but rather go through the involved area with some attenuation and stretching.[24,28,36] (The findings are similar to those described for acute, localized pyelonephritis.) There is slower flow through the vessels in the abscess and, as in other renal infections, loss of the corticomedullary junction.[2,28,36]

If the therapy is inadequate, the inflammatory process will progress, localize, and liquefy, leading to an acute, localized abscess—a carbuncle. At this stage, the abscess appears radiographically as a renal mass (Figs. 47-5 and 47-6). Angiographically, one sees stretching of vessels about the mass and often a zone of increased density surrounding the abscess, representing compression of the surrounding renal parenchyma. There is often loss of the sharp renal margin adjacent to the area of the infection.[26] The nephrogram may show a hazy blush in the area of the abscess, depending on the duration of the inflammatory process. When the process is chronic, there is an increase in the neovascularity and hyperemia, both in and around the abscess. The degree of neovascularity is variable. Some abscesses remain hypovascular, whereas others show considerable hyperemia.[28] When neovascularity is present, it is of a fine or reticular type. Although this pattern is not pathognomonic for infection, the vessels do tend to be more delicate and homogeneous than those seen in renal cell carcinoma.[31,37] Reports of positive epinephrine studies and early venous filling in abscesses further emphasize the difficulty of ruling out tumor.[28,38–40] Normal intrarenal arteries stretch around the abscess, as they do with any mass. Because of central necrosis, the abscess is lucent during the nephrogram, but there is a blush around the border that becomes more prominent as the abscess becomes more chronic. This blush is due to hyperemia in the granulation tissue in the wall around the abscess (Figs. 47-7 and 47-8).[24,29]

Extension into the Collecting System

If the acute abscess does not become walled off, it is free to break into either the collecting system or the perinephric space (Fig. 47-9). Extension into the collecting system usually occurs in chronic diseased kidneys with long-standing obstruction due to calculi. Angiography in these cases shows the changes of hydronephrosis—that is, stretching and attenuation of the arteries around the dilated calices. Because of the inflammatory process, however, neovascularity is often

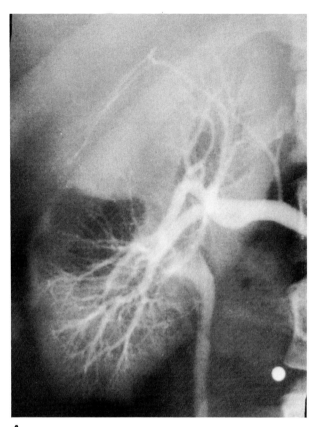

A

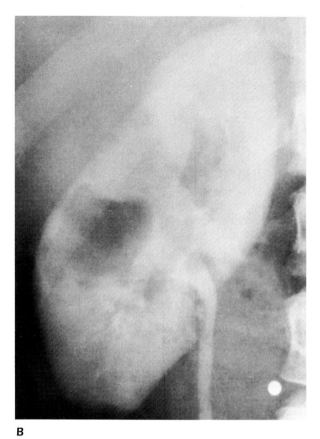

B

Figure 47-5. Case 5. Acute renal abscess in a 22-year-old heroin addict with fever, leukocytosis, and right flank pain. An intravenous pyelogram disclosed a mass in the lateral aspect of the midportion of the right kidney. (A) Selective right renal arteriogram, arterial phase. Poor visualization and flow in the vessels in the midportion of the right kidney in its lateral aspect are noted, with some elongation and straightening of the vessels on the outer margin of this hypovascular area. The capsular artery supplying the perinephric tissues adjacent to the hypovascular mass is hypertrophied. (B) Selective right renal arteriogram, nephrographic phase. There is loss of the nephrogram in the midportion of the kidney. Flattening of the lateral margin of the kidney in the involved area is noted, along with slight contrast staining in the perinephric space, which indicates subcapsular and perinephric extension of the abscess. At surgery, the abscess was drained.

present around the dilated calices, which have hazy borders (see Fig. 47-19).[41]

Perinephric Extension

More common than involvement of the collecting system is extension into the perinephric space with subsequent perinephritis. In fact, the perinephric process may often overshadow the parenchyma abscess (Figs. 47-10 through 47-12). With perirenal disease, the capsular vessels enlarge and are displaced away from the kidney. There is a distinct increase in both the size and number of capsular branches. A blush, often apparent in the perinephric space,[1,29] is due to reactive hyperemia about the inflammatory process and possible leakage of small amounts of contrast medium into the inflamed tissues through diseased capillaries. Although a perirenal abscess is generally secondary to a renal parenchymal abscess, it may arise either de novo or from other retroperitoneal infection. The perirenal process may be diffuse or localized. When localized, it generally occurs on the dorsolateral aspect of the kidney.[1]

Differentiation from Renal Carcinoma

Because chronic renal abscesses may have an insidious course, differential diagnosis may be a problem. The

Text continues on page 1192

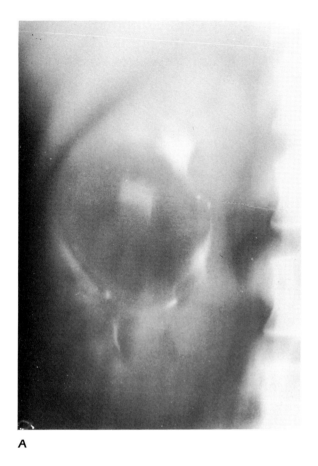

A

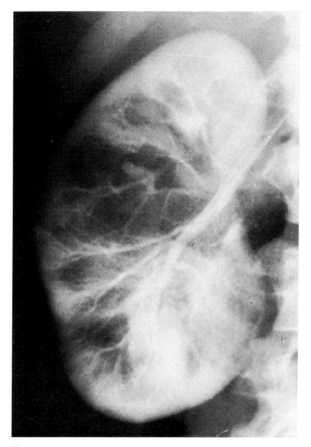

B

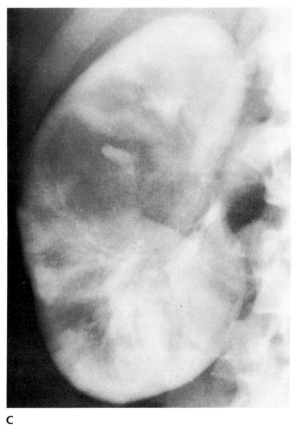

C

Figure 47-6. Case 6. Acute abscess of the kidney in a 24-year-old woman with juvenile diabetes who had acute right flank pain and a high fever. (A) Urogram with tomography of the right kidney. A large, fairly well demonstrated lucent mass is seen in the midportion of the kidney. (B) Selective right renal arteriogram, arterial phase. The mass is shown to be hypovascular, and stretching of major vessels around the mass is seen. Two smaller avascular areas are demonstrated at the lower pole of the kidney laterally. (C) Selective right renal arteriogram, nephrographic phase. Loss of the nephrogram is evident in the large mass in the center of the kidney and in smaller areas in its lower portion. At surgery, a large abscess filled with purulent material was evacuated. A culture revealed *Escherichia coli.*

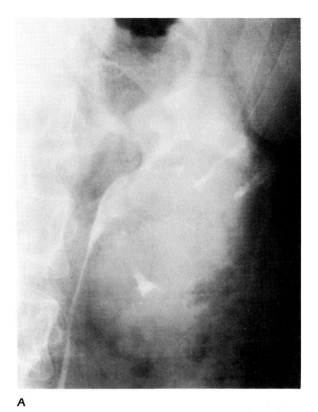

A

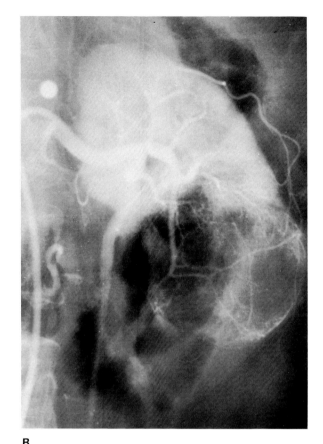

B

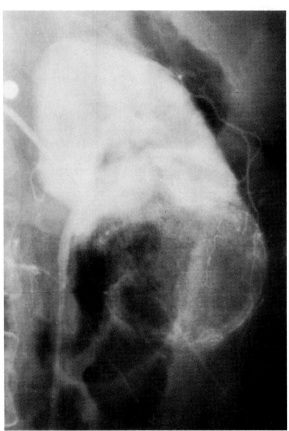

C

Figure 47-7. Case 7. Renal abscess in a 64-year-old woman with left flank pain and fever. (A) Urogram. A large mass is shown involving the middle and lower poles of the left kidney. (B) Selective left renal arteriogram, arterial phase. A hypovascular mass in the left kidney is well defined. Stretching of the vessels over and around the mass is evident, with hyperemia and neovascularity at the margin of the abscess. The lower margin of the kidney is not opacified because of the presence of an accessory renal artery. (C) Selective left renal arteriogram, nephrographic phase. A hypovascular mass in the lower pole of the left kidney is well defined. Some hyperemia along the margin of the abscess is seen, as well as slow flow and stasis of contrast material in the vessels along the abscess margin. A left nephrectomy was performed for acute and chronic abscess of the left kidney.

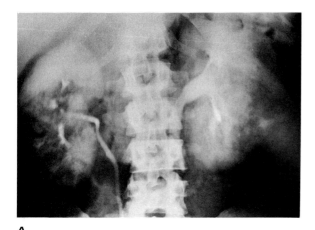

A

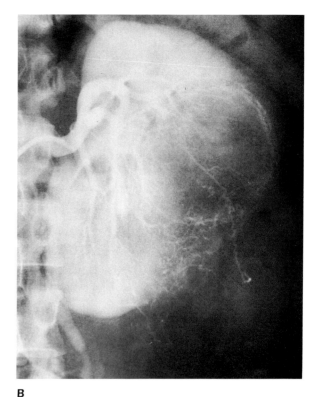

B

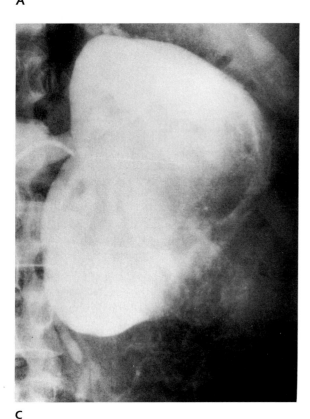

C

Figure 47-8. Case 8. Acute and chronic renal abscess angiographically indistinguishable from renal neoplasm. The patient, a 46-year-old man, had left flank pain but was without clear clinical symptoms or signs of infection. (A) Urogram. A large mass in the lateral aspect of the left kidney can be seen. (B) Selective left renal arteriogram, arterial phase. A large lucent mass occupies the lateral aspect of the left kidney. Vessels are stretched around the relatively hypovascular mass, with some hyperemia along the margins. Also seen are neovascularity with tortuous vessels inferior to the mass and some perforating capsular arteries extending into the perinephric space. (C) Selective left renal arteriogram, nephrographic phase. Extensive involvement of the kidney and extension into the perinephric space are seen. Some hyperemia and contrast blush are also seen. The mass has rotated the kidney and pushed the lower pole medially and anteriorly over the spine. The patient underwent a left radical nephrectomy after a preoperative diagnosis of renal cell carcinoma. The pathology examination revealed abscess of the left kidney with acute and chronic inflammatory changes.

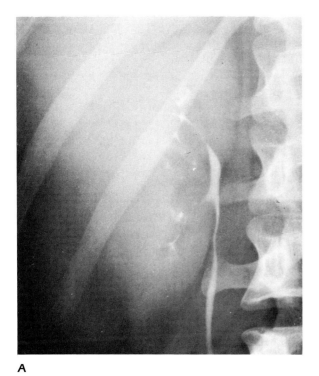

A

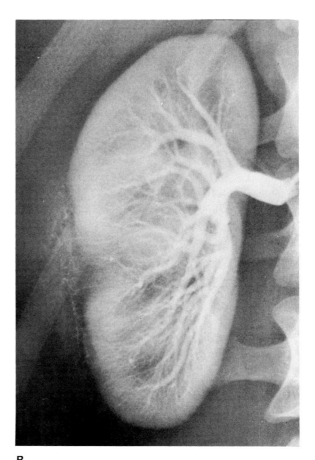

B

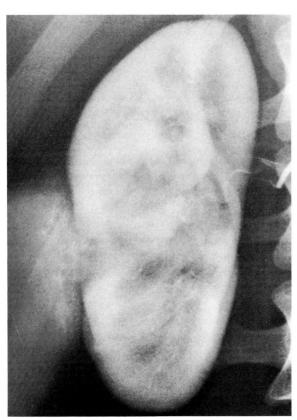

C

Figure 47-9. Case 9. Acute renal abscess with extension into the subcapsular and perirenal space. A 27-year-old man with flank pain and fever. (A) Urogram. A mass effect is noted along the lateral aspect of the right kidney. The lateral margin of kidney is poorly defined. (B) Selective right renal arteriogram, arterial phase. Flattening of the lateral aspect of the right kidney is seen. A defect in the cortex at this level is evident. Some delicate neovascularity is seen in the subcapsular and perirenal space in this area, with some tracking superiorly and inferiorly along the renal margin. (C) Selective right renal arteriogram, nephrographic phase. Flattening of the lateral aspect of the kidney is observed. A large blush of contrast medium is seen along the renal margin, indicating spread of the inflammation outside the cortex. Hyperemia and contrast blush are well demonstrated. An acute abscess was drained at surgery.

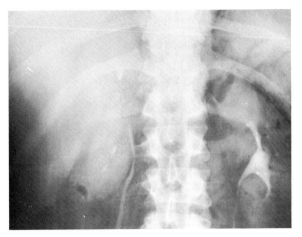

A

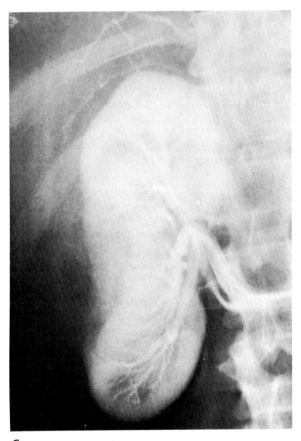

C

B

Figure 47-10. Case 10. Perinephric abscess. A 49-year-old man with flank pain and fever. (A) Urogram. A mass is seen flattening the lateral aspect of the right kidney and displacing the kidney medially. (B) Aortogram. Hypertrophy of a capsular artery (*upper arrow*), a branch of the inferior phrenic artery (*arrowhead*) (which in this case originates from the right renal artery), can be seen. The capsular artery inferior to the kidney is also visualized (*lower arrow*). Hyperemia and neovascularity lateral to the kidney are present. (C) Selective right renal arteriogram. Flattening of the lateral aspect of the kidney is apparent. No defect is present in the nephrogram, except for extrinsic pressure from the perinephric mass. Very little supply to the abscess from the renal vessels is visualized. (Some "flash filling" of the capsular vessels above the kidney can be seen because the catheter is deep within the renal artery, past the origin of the capsular vessels.) At surgery, a large perinephric abscess was drained.

Figure 47-12. Case 12. Chronic abscess. A 56-year-old woman who had a fever and a palpable right-sided abdominal mass. Urography revealed nonvisualization of the right kidney. (A) Selective right renal arteriogram, arterial phase. Distortion and stretching of the intrarenal vessels are seen. Stretching, palisading, and hypertrophy of the medial capsular vessels over the area of the renal pelvis are evident, as is filling of the vessels in the perirenal space inferiorly. (B) Selective right renal arteriogram, nephrographic phase. An irregular spotty nephrogram is present. The renal margin is indistinct, particularly medially, and there is a contrast medium blush in the perirenal areas that indicates extension of the inflammatory process outside the kidney. A chronic abscess involving the right kidney and chronic inflammation in the perinephric space were found at surgery. Some foam cells were seen histologically, suggesting a diagnosis of xanthogranulomatous pyelonephritis. (From Caplan LH, Siegelman SS, Bosniak MA. Angiography in inflammatory space-occupying lesions of the kidney. Radiology 1967;88:14–23. Used with permission.)

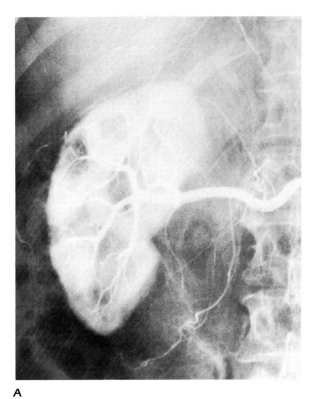

A

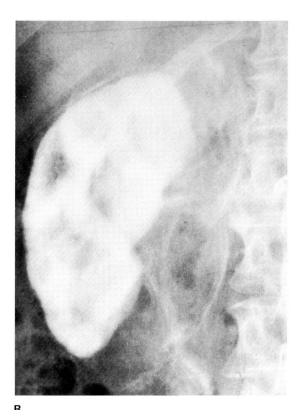

B

Figure 47-11. Case 11. Perinephric abscess. A 67-year-old diabetic with flank pain and fever. An intravenous urogram revealed nonvisualization of the right kidney. (A) Selective right renal arteriogram, arterial phase. The kidney is displaced laterally. The intrarenal vessels are intact, but there is increased filling of capsular vessels, which are stretched and separated from the kidney by the perirenal inflammatory mass. (B) Selective right renal arteriogram, nephrographic phase. The renal margin is hazy, particularly in the medial aspect of the kidney. Considerable blushing of the perirenal tissues is evident. At surgery, a large perinephric abscess was drained.

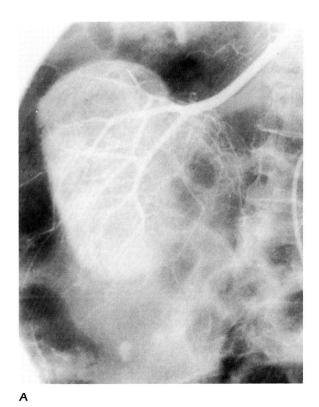

A

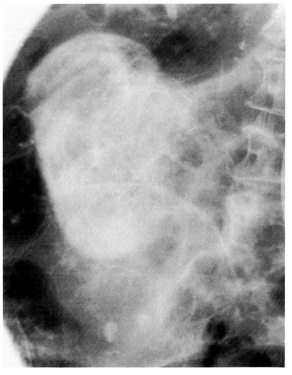

B

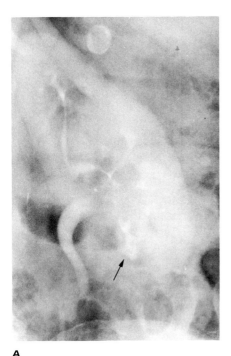
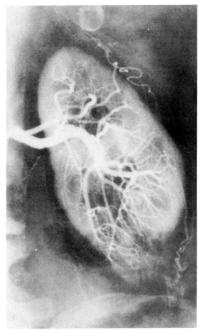
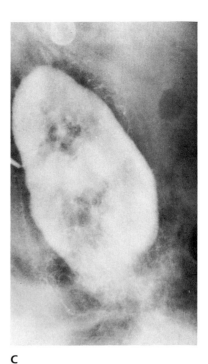

A   **B**   **C**

Figure 47-13. Case 13. Perirenal inflammation with abscess. A 61-year-old woman with left flank pain and fever. (A) Intravenous urogram. A calculus is present in the lower pole calix (*arrow*), and loss of the inferior renal margin is evident. A calcification in the splenic artery can be seen. (B) Selective left renal arteriogram, arterial phase. The intrarenal vessels are normal but slightly hypertrophied. A capsular artery feeding the perirenal tissues at the lower pole of the kidney is seen. Note the loss of margination of the kidney at the lower pole. (C) Selective left renal arteriogram, nephrographic phase. Hyperemia and blush at the inferior margin of the kidney are present, indicating an inflammatory reaction. No mass is evident, however, indicating an inflammation without abscess. Because no distinct mass was demonstrated, the patient was treated with antibiotics; after 1 week, her symptoms resolved.

major entity to be ruled out is a cystic or necrotic renal cell carcinoma, which may so closely resemble an abscess angiographically that definite differentiation may not be possible. Chronic inflammatory vascularity and tumor vascularity, although different pathologically, can usually not be differentiated angiographically.[31] In both conditions, increased vascularity, hyperemia, and contrast staining can be seen (Fig. 47-13; see also Fig. 47-8). Because the "wild-looking" (aneurysmally dilated and corkscrew-shaped) vessels seen in neoplasms are not seen in inflammatory masses, inflammation can usually be excluded if these vessels are present. However, in necrotic neoplasms without such bizarre vessels, differentiation becomes difficult. The use of epinephrine angiography was found not to be helpful because inflammatory neovascularity, like neoplastic vessels, does not respond to epinephrine as normal vessels do. (There probably is a quantitative difference in the response of inflammatory and neoplastic vascularity to epinephrine, but the difference is not great enough to be used angiographically.)[31,32,39]

In the past it was suggested that renal venography might be able to differentiate neoplastic from inflammatory disease by providing information about the venous involvement. Renal cell carcinoma tends to invade and extend into renal veins, whereas transitional cell carcinoma, squamous cell carcinoma, and other invasive neoplasms tend to constrict, encase, and amputate veins in the kidney.[42,43] In inflammatory disease, however, similar findings have been seen, including attenuation and occlusion of veins by extrinsic compression or by intraluminal thrombus formation.[4,22,23] Therefore, renal venography cannot be used to clearly differentiate severe inflammatory disease from neoplastic disease. On the other hand, if gross intraluminal occlusion of the main renal vein occurs, it is statistically likely that the disease is neoplastic.

Often a diagnosis of chronic abscess rather than carcinoma can be made only if the clinical features point to infection as the cause. *The possibility of abscess must be entertained if the diagnosis is to be made.* In such cases, if a diagnosis of abscess is suspected, needle aspiration is indicated. If pus is obtained, the abscess is identified and can be drained percutaneously.[44] If bloody debris is obtained, a neoplasm is likely and nephrectomy is in order.

Xanthogranulomatous Pyelonephritis

Xanthogranulomatous pyelonephritis is a rare form of renal inflammation that is usually seen in patients with obstruction secondary to long-standing calculi.[45-47] Why some patients with chronic obstruction develop not just simple hydronephrosis or even pyonephrosis but xanthogranulomatous pyelonephritis is not known. Clinically, these patients have flank pain and often a palpable mass. Because the process is generally severe and destroys the bulk of the kidney, nephrectomy is the usual therapy.[48]

Xanthogranulomatous pyelonephritis may involve the kidney in two ways, either diffusely, replacing the entire kidney, or as a focal (tumefactive) disease. The diffuse form, which is by far the most common, develops behind an obstructing renal pelvic calculus.[48,49] In one study, more than 70 percent of those with diffuse disease had calculi.[47] With focal disease, a localized portion of the kidney is involved and a history of calculi is not as common. Whether diffuse or focal, the pathologic process is the same. The renal parenchyma is replaced by xanthogranulomatous masses that have the gross appearance of yellow nodules scattered throughout the kidney. In addition to these masses, which are the hallmark of the process, small abscesses and areas of dense fibrous tissue may be seen. When diffuse involvement is present, all the calices are filled with purulent fluid and calculi.[45,46] Microscopically, lipid-laden macrophages or foam cells are present. Occasionally, plasma cells, lymphocytes, and multinucleated giant cells are all seen.[46,47] The glomeruli and tubules become atrophic.[45] *Bacillus proteus* is the most frequent pathogen found, but *E. coli* and *S. aureus* have also been cultured in this disease.[46]

The radiographic patterns of xanthogranulomatous pyelonephritis reflect the pathologic changes and are different in the diffuse and focal forms. In the diffuse disease, plain films of the abdomen often show enlargement of the renal outline and calculi.[45,46,48] The most common finding on intravenous urography is nonvisualization of the diseased kidney. Retrograde pyelography may demonstrate hydronephrosis or amputation of a portion of the collecting system,[45] or it may show extravasation of contrast material into the parenchyma due to the friable urothelium (Fig. 47-14). In focal xanthogranulomatous pyelonephritis, the kidney is visualized on urography and a mass is seen. The mass may distort the collecting system or renal outline and may be indistinguishable radiologically from a renal neoplasm or a chronic renal abscess.[46,48]

On US, a large kidney is seen with distortion of the central echo complex. Renal pelvic or caliceal calculi are usually identified, and calices containing pus or xanthomatous tissue produce low-level echoes simulating thickening renal parenchyma.[50,51] On CT one sees a large kidney containing calculi and low-attenuation areas throughout the parenchyma, indicating pus or xanthomatous tissue (characterized by foam cells, or fat-filled macrophages). The attenuation varies between -5 and 25 Hounsfield units, depending on the amount of xanthomatous tissue present. There is considerable perirenal tissue thickening, including Gerota fascia, and enlarged lymph nodes can often be seen in the retroperitoneum near the hilum of the kidney. The CT appearance is characteristic, and the diagnosis should be readily made.[50,52]

The angiographic findings vary with the stage and type of involvement. In the diffuse form of the disease, the findings are similar in many ways to those of simple hydronephrosis (Fig. 47-15; see also Fig. 47-14), with stretching and attenuation of intrarenal vessels.[45,48,53] However, unlike simple hydronephrosis, neovascularity due to the inflammatory process is present. During the later arterial phase, vessels are seen to be stretched around dilated calices and inflammatory masses.[54] The nephrogram may be either homogeneous or mottled. If it is mottled, the scattered lucencies again represent the calices and granulomas.[45,46,48] There may be areas of increased density in parts of the kidney representing residual normal parenchyma[54] or hyperemia due to the inflammatory reaction. The corticomedullary junction is not seen, and there may be prominent capsular and ureteric vessels.[48,53,54] These last changes are nonspecific and are seen with most chronic renal infections. Differential diagnosis of the angiogram in diffuse xanthogranulomatous pyelonephritis includes infected hydronephrosis or pyonephrosis[48]; however, the neovascularity is more prominent in xanthogranulomatous pyelonephritis. (US is helpful in differentiating the fluid-filled hydronephrosis from the more solid xanthogranulomatous pyelonephritis.)

A more difficult diagnostic problem occurs in the focal or tumefactive form of xanthogranulomatous pyelonephritis. Here, angiography is often unable definitely to rule out a hypovascular renal cell carcinoma.[47] The xanthogranulomatous mass, which closely resembles a chronic abscess, is generally avascular centrally but often has neovascularity and blush on the periphery. Wild vascularity is not present.[46,49] The problem is made more difficult because patients with the focal form of xanthogranulomatous pyelonephritis are often

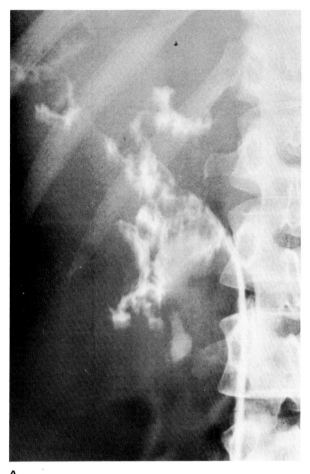

A

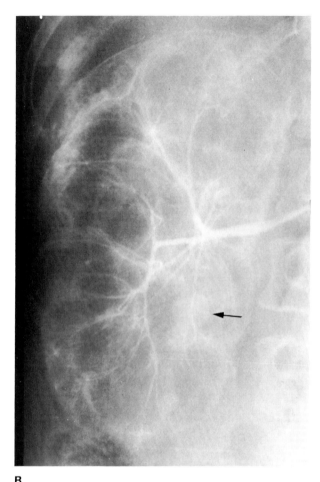

B

Figure 47-14. Case 14. Xanthogranulomatous pyelonephritis. A 44-year-old woman with right flank pain. An intravenous urogram revealed a nonfunctioning right kidney with staghorn calculi. (A) Right retrograde pyelogram. Extravasation of contrast material from the collecting system and into the kidney is noted. Large calculi in the right renal pelvis are somewhat obscured by the contrast material. (B) Right renal arteriogram, arterial phase. Stretching of the intrarenal vessels over the hypovascular masses is seen. The pattern resembles hydronephrosis, except that more vascularity and hyperemia are present. The *arrow* points to calculi. A right nephrectomy revealed a xanthogranulomatous pyelonephritic kidney.

the ones without chronic calculus disease and infection. Nephrectomy is indicated in extensive xanthogranulomatous pyelonephritis as well as in renal cell carcinoma, so that differentiation may not be critical, although a more radical approach should be taken with neoplasm. Localized disease can be treated by partial nephrectomy, but establishing this diagnosis preoperatively is difficult.

It should be noted that the diagnosis of xanthogranulomatous pyelonephritis is a pathologic diagnosis that often does not have relevance radiologically. Many cases of long-standing chronic inflammatory disease of the kidney show foam cells histologically and some yellow nodules of tissue on gross inspection, signs

that permit a pathologic diagnosis of xanthogranulomatous pyelonephritis to be made. The lesions shown in Figures 47-7, 47-8, 47-12, and 47-19 contained foam cells as well as small areas of yellow xanthogranulomatous tissue, but they were considered chronic abscesses with some associated changes of xanthogranulomatous pyelonephritis. Varying gradations of disease exist, and a distinction should be made between (1) the more extensive tumefactive xanthogranulomatous pyelonephritis, in which the focal areas of interstitial inflammation become confluent, forming a parenchymal mass, and (2) the more common minimal changes of xanthogranulomatous pyelonephritis seen in many cases of chronic inflammatory disease of the kidney.

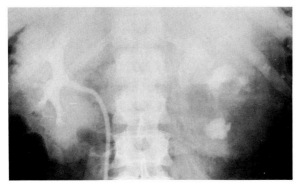

A

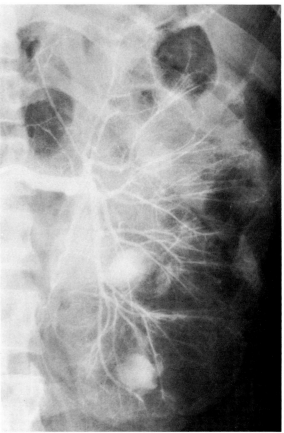

B

Figure 47-15. Case 15. Xanthogranulomatous pyelonephritis. A 48-year-old man with left flank pain and a palpable abdominal mass. (A) Intravenous urogram. Two large calculi are seen in a large, nonfunctioning left kidney. (B) Selective left renal arteriogram, arterial phase. Stretching of atrophic renal artery branches in an enlarged kidney is present. (C) Selective left renal arteriogram, nephrographic phase. Multiple hypovascular areas surrounded by hyperemic areas are seen. The pattern is similar to that in hydronephrosis, except for increased vascularity. A left nephrectomy revealed xanthogranulomatous pyelonephritis.

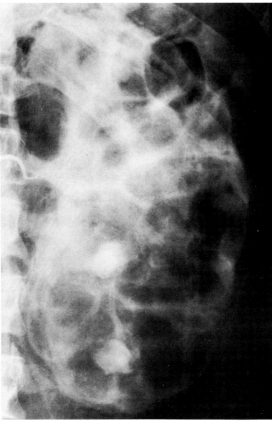

C

Tuberculosis

Tuberculosis usually involves the kidneys via the hematogenous route. The tuberculosis bacilli seed the kidneys, lodging in the glomerular and peritubular capillary beds. Often clinical symptoms do not occur, and healing takes place without residual effects. In some patients, however, there is erosion of the tuberculosis bacilli out of the vascular bed and into the tubules.

From the tubules there may be extension into, and eventual erosion of, the renal papillae. Cavities of varying sizes occur with or without connection to the collecting system. Granulomas also may form and grow large enough that they appear as renal masses on urography—but this is an unusual finding. A definite diagnosis of renal tuberculosis requires microscopic demonstration of acid-fast bacilli or culture of bacilli on appropriate media.[5]

The urographic findings in renal tuberculosis reflect the extent of the disease. In early renal involvement, the intravenous urogram is negative. The earliest urographic sign of renal tuberculosis is minimal irregularity of the minor calices due to papillary erosions. This irregularity may progress to extensive papillary necrosis with cavities of varying sizes filling on both intravenous urography and retrograde studies; however, not all cavities connect with the collecting system. Granulomatous masses or tuberculomas appear as solid masses distorting the collecting system or the renal outline. Calcification and fibrosis are the hallmarks of healing in tuberculosis and, as such, are often seen in the kidney. The fibrosis may lead to strictures of the infundibula or the renal pelvis and, if severe enough, will cause hydronephrosis as well as nonvisualization during urography.[5] An amputated calix with distal hydronephrosis secondary to fibrotic stricture of the infundibulum is one of the more characteristic findings.[55]

The US and CT findings depend on the type and extent of involvement. Localized hydronephrosis may be seen. Calcification is common in tuberculosis of the kidney, and its presence along with strictures and necrosis is highly suggestive of tuberculous involvement. Focal masses in the kidney are also noted, representing granulomatous masses or tuberculomas. By themselves, these lesions can be difficult to diagnose as being due to tuberculosis, but when combined with the other findings of calcification, stricture, and cavitary necrosis, the etiology becomes much clearer.[56,57] Occasionally, fine-needle aspiration biopsy is helpful in diagnosis.[58]

Angiography in renal tuberculosis demonstrates a variety of findings, all of which are relatively nonspecific. The basic pathologic process that causes changes in the intrarenal arteries is a periarteritis and an endarteritis. This inflammation leads to irregularity and poor filling of the renal arteries on angiography. Changes are first seen in the smaller vessels (i.e., the arcuate and interlobular arteries), but, with progression, the interlobar vessels are also affected.[59,60] There may be a decrease in the number of vessels that fill during angiography and obliteration of portions of the arterial tree[61,62] (Figs. 47-16 and 47-17). If a tuberculoma is present, there is stretching of vessels around the mass, but no neovascularity within it. The nephrographic phase of the angiogram in renal tuberculosis is usually heterogeneous or patchy, with areas of diminished density due to obliteration of portions of the vascular tree. Tuberculous cavities may appear as discrete lucencies in the nephrogram.[62] Although there is usually a general decrease in the renal vascularity, there may be hypertrophy of the peripelvic and capsular vessels secondary to the chronic inflammatory process.[60]

Figure 47-16. Case 16. Tuberculous right kidney. A 48-year-old man with hematuria. (A) Right retrograde pyelogram. Stricture of the lower pole infundibulum and nonfilling of the upper portion of the collecting system are demonstrated. (B) Selective right renal arteriogram, arterial phase. A decrease in the number of vessels in the upper pole of the kidney is seen. Amputation of some vessels (*arrows*) is evident, as is the loss of secondary branches. There is no evidence of a mass effect. (C) Selective right renal arteriogram, nephrographic phase. A greatly diminished nephrogram in the upper pole is noted. The tubercle bacillus was cultured from the urine.

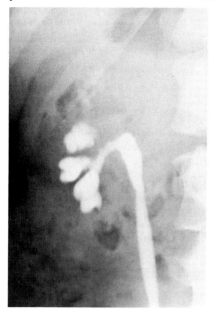

A

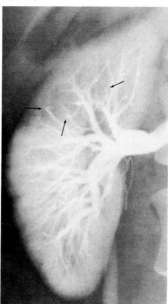

B

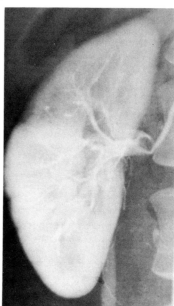

C

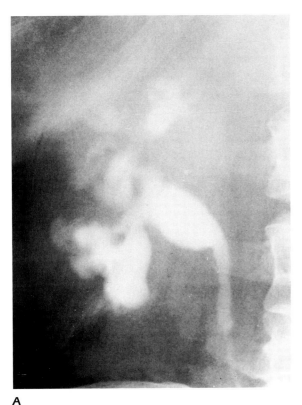

A

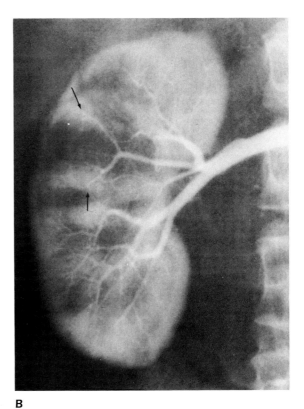

B

Figure 47-17. Case 17. Tuberculous right kidney. A 59-year-old man with hematuria. (A) Right retrograde pyelogram. Papillary necrosis of all the visualized papillary areas is evident, as are irregularity and distortion of the caliceal structures. (B) Right renal arteriogram. A decrease in the number of secondary and tertiary branches is evident, along with amputated vessels (*arrows*). Areas of diminished nephrogram are present. A right nephrectomy was performed. Extensive tuberculous destruction was noted in the excised specimen.

When a part of the kidney or the entire kidney becomes hydronephrotic due to collecting system strictures, the arterial pattern is one of stretched and attenuated vessels. This is again nonspecific and can be seen in any hydronephrotic kidney, regardless of the cause.[60]

The angiographic changes in renal tuberculosis that have been discussed are not consistently seen in all involved kidneys. In a series of 43 patients with renal tuberculosis, the most common angiographic findings were diminished vascularity in the involved portion of the kidney and pruning of the arterial tree. These findings were present in 74 percent; 65 percent showed parenchymal scarring, and 47 percent showed irregularity of the walls of the smaller arteries.[63] Again, it should be stressed that these angiographic findings are nonspecific and that the intravenous urogram is more diagnostic. Angiography is therefore generally not needed in the diagnostic workup of a patient with renal tuberculosis, but it may be useful in assessing the blood supply of the kidney if partial nephrectomy is contemplated in the treatment approach.

Chronic Atrophic Pyelonephritis

Although acute pyelonephritis generally affects the entire kidney, chronic atrophic pyelonephritis is a focal disease, involving a part or parts of one or both kidneys and sparing other portions. Although the cause and pathogenesis of this disease have not been established, most studies suggest that a combination of infection and reflux in early infancy leads to focal areas of renal infection and subsequent atrophy. Therefore, this condition is also called *reflux nephoropathy*. Although the infectious process is centered in the medullary portion of the kidney, the whole thickness of renal tissue is affected in scar formation.[5] Intravenous urography, US, and CT can demonstrate localized changes secondary to the scarring. Urography shows focal depressions in the renal outline, with distortion and clubbing of the underlying calices. These changes represent fibrosis and retraction of tissue.[64]

Angiography in chronic pyelonephritis shows arterial changes secondary to parenchymal loss and fibrosis (Fig. 47-18). There is a decrease in the size of the main

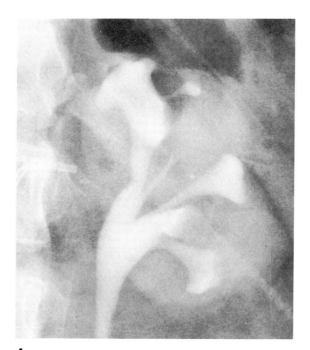

A

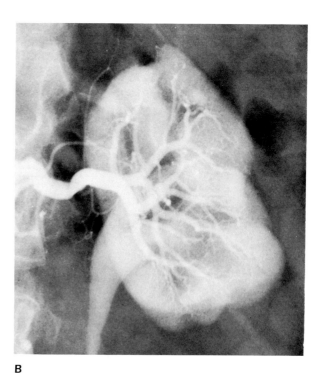

B

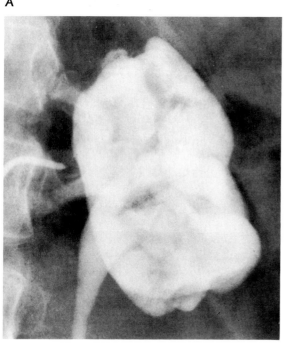

C

Figure 47-18. Case 18. Chronic pyelonephritis. A 42-year-old woman with a urinary tract infection. (A) Urogram. Scarring of the renal parenchyma can be seen associated with blunted calices. Some normal calices are seen, and in these areas the parenchyma is normal. (B) Selective left renal arteriogram, arterial phase. Distortion of the renal vasculature in the scarred areas is evident, with abrupt tapering of the vessels and loss of peripheral branches. (C) Selective left renal arteriogram, nephrographic phase. Scarring of the parenchyma is well demonstrated. Areas of hypertrophied normal tissue give a lumpy contour to the renal margin.

renal artery commensurate with the decrease in functioning renal mass.[62] The intrarenal arteries, which are also diminished in caliber, are crowded together because of the loss of parenchyma, thus becoming tortuous or corkscrewed.[20,62,64] These changes are nonspecific and can be seen in any entity that leads to renal fibrosis and scarring, such as nephrosclerosis or radiation nephritis.[20] Some areas of the chronic pyelonephritic kidney may show diminished vascularity due to fibrotic occlusion of vessels. The nephrogram demonstrates cortical scarring and areas of increased density due to the crowding together of vessels.[62] Early venous filling, which was seen in 9 of 11 patients in one series, may be secondary to the shunting of blood through the larger medullary veins.[65]

The renal scarring often leads to hypertrophy of uninvolved areas, which may then be confused with renal masses, so-called pseudotumors. Angiography can clearly show that the hypertrophied areas are normal renal parenchyma and not neoplastic. However, this information can be obtained by CT or nuclear medicine scanning in a less invasive fashion.

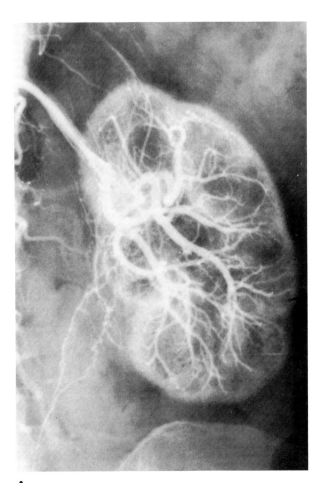

A

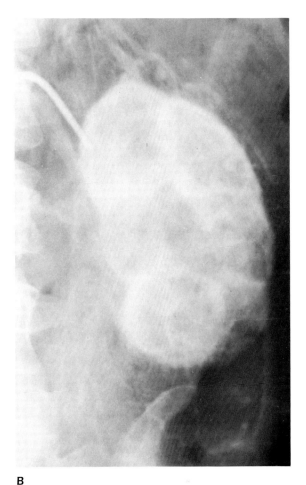

B

Figure 47-19. Case 19. Pyonephrosis (infected hydronephrosis). A 61-year-old woman with a high fever and left flank pain. No visualization of the right kidney was noted on intravenous pyelography. (A) Selective left renal arteriogram, arterial phase. Changes suggestive of mild hydronephrosis are seen, with some stretching of the interlobar branches over dilated caliceal structures. However, the usual atrophy of the peripheral vessels is not seen. In fact, there is a suggestion of increased vascularity. Prominent, enlarged, and tortuous pelvic arteries are seen supplying the pelvis and the upper ureter. (B) Selective left renal arteriogram, nephrographic phase. Hyperemia and staining in the perinephric spaces are present, along with filling of the capsular vessels. The changes of hydronephrosis, with irregular staining in the kidney, are seen. Contrast staining or blush in the wall of the pelvis is also seen. A left nephrectomy was performed for a diffusely infected and pyonephrotic kidney.

Miscellaneous Conditions

The remaining inflammatory conditions of the kidney include infected renal cyst, infected caliceal diverticulum, fungous disease, and infected hydronephrosis (pyonephrosis).

Infected renal cyst and *infected caliceal diverticulum* are comparatively rare phenomena. When a cyst becomes infected, the patient may have fever, chills, and flank pain. Sometimes leukocytosis or pyuria or both are present. The CT appearance is usually identical to that of an uninfected cyst, but the wall of the infected cyst may be seen to be hazier than expected. The US findings vary from an echo-free mass to a mass containing occasional low-level echoes or layered debris.[66]

Angiography demonstrates an avascular mass with a thin hypervascular rim. Inflammatory neovascularity is frequently seen around the rim, and the junction of cyst and normal parenchyma may be hazy. If the cyst is peripheral, there may be hypertrophy of a capsular artery.[67] If the lesion progresses and becomes extensive, however, the radiologic and pathologic findings are similar to those of an acute renal abscess.

Infected hydronephrosis, or *pyonephrosis,* which is depicted in Figure 47-19, is covered in the section on hydronephrosis.

Fungous disease is a comparatively rare infection in the kidney. The offending organisms are most commonly *Candida* and *Aspergillus*.[68,69] The patients affected are usually undergoing chemotherapy for malignancy, receiving steroid treatment while debilitated, or diabetic. The fungous disease usually involves the collecting system, with changes in the kidney usually secondary to obstruction. Occasionally, extensive involvement of the renal parenchyma occurs. Very little has been reported, however, about any angiographic findings, which would most closely resemble those existing in xanthogranulomatous pyelonephritis, infected hydronephrosis, or pyonephrosis.

Role of Angiography in Renal Inflammatory Disease

The role of angiography in the workup of the patient with inflammatory disease has undergone considerable change and is only occasionally used in radiologic diagnosis. This role has been taken over by US, CT, and needle aspiration. However, the angiographic patterns that were observed in renal inflammatory disease and are depicted in the chapter enable us to better understand the radiologic and pathologic findings seen in renal inflammatory disease.

Acknowledgments

We would like to thank Charles Smith, M.D., Babylon, New York, for Case 3; Marvin Hinke, M.D., Marshfield, Wisconsin, for Case 8; Richard Gordon, M.D., and Peter Sforza, M.D., New York, for Case 16; and Manuel Madayag, M.D., who performed many of the angiograms shown in this chapter.

References

1. Evans JA, Meyers MA, Bosniak MA. Acute renal and perirenal infections. Semin Roentgenol 1971;6:274–291.
2. Wicks JD, Thornbury JR. Acute renal infections in adults. Radiol Clin North Am 1979;17:245–260.
3. Silver TM, Kass EJ, Thornbury JR, et al. The radiological spectrum of acute pyelonephritis in adults and adolescents. Radiology 1976;118:65–71.
4. Rosenfield AT, Glickman MG, Taylor KJ, et al. Acute focal bacterial nephritis (acute lobar nephronia). Radiology 1979;132:553–561.
5. Davidson AJ, Hartman DS. Radiology of the kidney and urinary tract. 2nd ed. Philadelphia: Saunders, 1994:272.
6. Heptinstall RH. Pyelonephritis: pathologic features. In: Heptinstall RH, ed. Pathology of the kidney. 4th ed. Boston: Little, Brown, 1992:1489–1562.
7. Roberts JA. Pyelonephritis, cortical abscess and perinephric abscess. Urol Clin North Am 1986;13:637–645.
8. Kass EJ, Silver TM, Konnak JW, et al. The urographic findings in acute pyelonephritis: non-obstructive hydronephrosis. J Urol 1976;116:544–546.
9. Davidson AJ, Talner LB. Urographic and angiographic abnormalities in adult onset acute bacterial nephritis. Radiology 1973;106:249–256.
10. Davidson AJ, Talner LB. Late sequelae of adult onset acute bacterial nephritis. Radiology 1978;127:367–371.
11. Hoddick W, Jeffrey RB, Goldberg HI, et al. CT and sonography of severe renal and perirenal infections. AJR 1983;140:517–520.
12. Lee JKT, McClennan BL, Melson GL, et al. Acute focal bacterial nephritis: emphasis on gray scale sonography and computed tomography. AJR 1980;135:87–92.
13. Kass EJ, Fink-Bennett D, Cacciarelli AA, et al. The sensitivity of renal scintigraphy and sonography in detecting nonobstructive acute pyelonephritis. J Urol 1992;148:606–608.
14. Soulen MC, Fishman EK, Goldman SM, et al. Bacterial renal infection: role of CT. Radiology 1989;171:703–707.
15. Gold RP, McClennan BL, Rottenberg RR. CT appearance of acute inflammatory disease of the renal interstitium. AJR 1983;141:343–349.
16. Rauschkolb EN, Sandler CM, Patel S, et al. Computed tomography of renal inflammatory disease. J Comput Assist Tomogr 1982;6:502–506.
17. Bjorguinsson E, Majd M, Eggli KD. Diagnosis of acute pyelonephritis in children. Comparison of sonography and ^{99m}Tc-DMSA scintigraphy. AJR 1991;157:539–543.
18. Barth KH, Lightman NI, Ridolfi RL, et al. Acute pyelonephritis simulating poorly vascularized renal neoplasm: non-specificity of angiographic criteria. J Urol 1976;116:650–652.
19. Berliner L, Bosniak MA. The striated nephrogram in acute pyelonephritis. Urol Radiol 1982;4:41–44.
20. Hill GS, Clark RL. A comparative angiographic, microangiographic and histologic study of experimental pyelonephritis. Invest Radiol 1972;7:33–41.
21. Lillenfeld RM, Lande A. Acute adult onset bacterial nephritis: long-term urographic and angiographic follow-up. J Urol 1975;114:14–20.
22. Goldman ML, Gorelkin L, Rude JC, et al. Epinephrine renal venography in severe inflammatory disease of the kidney. Radiology 1978;127:93–101.
23. Pingoud EG, Pais SO, Glickman M. Epinephrine renal venography in acute bacterial infection of the kidney. AJR 1979;133:665–669.
24. Caplan LH, Siegelman SS, Bosniak MA. Angiography in inflammatory space-occupying lesions of the kidney. Radiology 1967;88:14–23.
25. Gadrinab NM, Lome LG, Presman D. Renal abscesses: role of renal arteriography. Urology 1973;2:39–42.
26. Klein DL, Filpi RG. Acute renal carbuncle. J Urol 1977;118:912–915.
27. Fair WR, Higgins MH. Renal abscess. J Urol 1970;104:179–183.
28. Rabinowitz JG, Kinkhabwala MN, Robinson T, et al. Acute renal carbuncle: the roentgenographic clarification of a medical enigma. AJR 1972;116:740–748.
29. Koehler PR. The roentgen diagnosis of renal inflammatory masses—special emphasis on angiographic changes. Radiology 1974;112:257–266.
30. Moore CA, Gangai MP. Renal cortical abscess. J Urol 1967;98:303–306.
31. Levin DC, Gordon D, Kinkhabwala M, et al. Reticular neovascularity in malignant and inflammatory renal masses. Radiology 1976;120:61–68.
32. Shenoy SS, Culver GJ, Arani DT. Renal carbuncle: stimulation of tumor response to epinephrine. Urology 1977;10:601–603.
33. Merenrich WM, Popky GL. Radiology of renal infection. Med Clin North Am 1991;75:425–469.
34. Goldman SM, Minkin SD, Naraval DC, et al. Renal carbuncle: the use of ultrasound in its diagnosis and treatment. J Urol 1977;118:525–528.

35. Bosniak MA. The current radiological approach to renal cysts. Radiology 1986;158:1–10.
36. Craven JD, Hardy B, Stanley P, et al. Acute renal carbuncle: the importance of preoperative angiography. J Urol 1974;111:727–731.
37. Salmon RB, Koehler PR. Angiography in renal and perirenal inflammatory masses. Radiology 1967;88:9–13.
38. Caro G, Meisell R, Held B. Epinephrine-enhanced arteriography in renal and perirenal abscess. Radiology 1969;92:1262–1264.
39. Kahn PC, Wise HM Jr. Simulation of renal tumor response to epinephrine by inflammatory disease. Radiology 1967;89:1062–1064.
40. Combs JA, Crummy AB, Cossman FP. Angiography in renal and pararenal inflammatory lesions: the significance of early venous filling. Radiology 1971;98:401–403.
41. Koehler PR, Nelson JA. Arteriographic findings in inflammatory mass lesions of the kidney. Radiol Clin North Am 1976;14:281–293.
42. Kahn PC. Selective venography in renal parenchymal disease. Radiology 1969;92:345–349.
43. Smith JC, Rösch J, Athanasoulis CA, et al. Renal venography in the evaluation of poorly vascularized neoplasms of the kidney. AJR 1975;123:552–556.
44. Sacks D, Banner MP, Meranze SG. Renal and related retroperitoneal abscesses: percutaneous drainage. Radiology 1988;167:447–451.
45. Gingell JC, Roylance J, Davies ER, et al. Xanthogranulomatous pyelonephritis. Br J Radiol 1973;46:99–109.
46. Strasberg Z, Jacobson S, Srolovitz H, et al. Xanthogranulomatous pyelonephritis: radiologic considerations. J Can Assoc Radiol 1970;21:173–177.
47. Malek RS, Elder JS. Xanthogranulomatous pyelonephritis: a critical analysis of twenty-six cases and of the literature. J Urol 1978;119:589–593.
48. Beachley MC, Ranniger K, Roth FJ. Xanthogranulomatous pyelonephritis. AJR 1974;121:500–507.
49. Vinik M, Freed TA, Smellie WAB, et al. Xanthogranulomatous pyelonephritis: angiographic considerations. Radiology 1969;92:537–540.
50. Subramanyam BR, Megibow AJ, Raghavendra BN, et al. Diffuse xanthogranulomatous pyelonephritis: analysis by computed tomography and sonography. Urol Radiol 1982;4:5–9.
51. Hartman DS, Davis CJ Jr, Goldman SM, et al. Xanthogranulomatous pyelonephritis: sonographic pathologic correlation of 16 cases. J Ultrasound Med 1984;3:481–488.
52. Goldman SM, Hartman DS, Fishman EK, et al. CT of xanthogranulomatous pyelonephritis. AJR 1984;142:963–967.
53. Rossi P, Myers DH, Furey R, et al. Angiography in bilateral xanthogranulomatous pyelonephritis. Radiology 1968;90:320–321.
54. Becker JA. Xanthogranulomatous pyelonephritis: a case report with angiographic findings. Acta Radiol 1966;4:139–144.
55. Kollins SA, Hartman GW, Carr DT, et al. Roentgenologic findings in urinary tract tuberculosis: a 10 year investigation. Am J Roentgenol 1974;121:487–500.
56. Perkumar A, Lattimer J, Newhouse JH, et al. CT and sonography of advanced urinary tract tuberculosis. AJR 1987;148:65–68.
57. Goldman SM, Fishman EK, Hartman DS, et al. Computed tomography of renal tuberculosis and its pathologic correlates. J Comput Assist Tomogr 1985;9:771–776.
58. Baniel J, Manning A, Leitman G. Fine needle cytodiagnosis of renal tuberculosis. J Urol 1991;146:689–691.
59. Frimann-Dahl J. Selective angiography in renal tuberculosis. Acta Radiol 1958;49:31–41.
60. Giusta PE, Watson RC, Shulman H. Arteriographic findings in various stages of renal tuberculosis. Radiology 1971;100:597–602.
61. Becker JA, Weiss RM, Lattimer JK. Renal tuberculosis: the role of nephrotomography and angiography. J Urol 1968;100:415–419.
62. Foster RS, Shuford WH, Weens HS. Selective renal arteriography in medical diseases of the kidney. AJR 1965;95:291–308.
63. Bjorn-Hansen R, Aakhus R. Angiography in renal tuberculosis. Acta Radiol 1971;11:167–176.
64. Friedenberg MJ, Eisen S, Kissane J. Renal angiography in pyelonephritis, glomerulonephritis and arteriolar nephrosclerosis. AJR 1965;95:349–363.
65. Becker JA, Kanter IE, Perl S. Rapid intrarenal circulation. AJR 1970;109:167–171.
66. Schneider M, Becker JA, Staiano S, et al. Sonographic-radiologic correlation of renal and perirenal infections. AJR 1976;127:1007–1014.
67. Cho KJ, Maklad N, Curran J, et al. Angiographic and ultrasonic findings in infected simple cysts of the kidney. AJR 1976;127:1015–1019.
68. Gerle RD. Roentgenographic features of primary renal candidiases: fungus ball of the renal pelvis and ureter. AJR 1973;119:731–738.
69. Michigan S. Genitourinary fungal infections. J Urol 1976;116:390–397.

48

Angiography of Hydronephrosis

MORTON A. BOSNIAK
RICHARD S. LEFLEUR
MARJORIE A. AMBOS

Although dilatation of the renal collecting system is usually the result of mechanical obstruction of the system somewhere along its course, nonobstructive causes, such as inflammation, atony, and neurogenic processes, may less frequently lead to the same changes.[1] With obstruction, the changes that are seen depend on the acuteness and duration of the pathologic process.[2] Animal experiments have shown that ligation of a ureter leads first to an increase in the pressure within the renal pelvis. Normal pelvic pressure is near zero; with total acute obstruction this pressure rises to 50 to 125 mmHg. Glomerular filtration decreases but does not stop completely in the acute phase, so that if intravenous contrast material is administered it is still excreted, but its passage through the collecting tubules is slowed. Because water is resorbed and the contrast material becomes more concentrated, a dense nephrogram results.[3,4]

Patients with acute obstruction have radiographic changes that reflect this state. Urography classically demonstrates a swollen, enlarged kidney with delayed function, diminished excretion of contrast material, and a dense nephrogram.[4,5] Significant dilatation of the pelvis and calices and parenchymal atrophy only occur with time. The large kidney with saclike calices, a huge pelvis, and markedly diminished parenchyma is the result of long-term partial obstruction or multiple episodes of obstruction.[2,5] The primary effect of the increased renal pelvic pressure of chronic obstruction is parenchymal atrophy. Two factors lead to this loss of tissue: (1) the relative ischemia of the kidney due to the increased pressure on the intrarenal arteries and (2) the direct effect of constant abnormal pressure on the renal parenchyma. Although this renal atrophy is global, it is first seen radiographically in the papilla. As the papilla atrophies, the corresponding calices enlarge, going from the classic Y configuration to a rounded shape and finally becoming clubbed. The end stage is a kidney with the merest shell of parenchyma, its major mass being saclike calices and a huge pelvis.[1]

Most cases of chronic hydronephrosis are secondary to obstruction of the ureteropelvic junction due to a congenital abnormality. Pathologic studies of these kidneys have shown a deficient muscle layer or abnormal direction of muscle bundles at the ureteropelvic junction that, in turn, is felt to lead to submucosal fibrosis and secondary muscular hypertrophy. These changes may occasionally be associated with an aberrant vessel or accessory vessels in the area. Other common causes of chronic hydronephrosis are calculi, urothelial carcinoma, and retroperitoneal processes.[6]

Findings on intravenous urography reflect the chronicity and severity of the obstructive process. In acute conditions, function is compromised but no significant dilatation or atrophy occurs. With time there is progressively decreased excretion of contrast material and delay in filling of the collecting system, so that films may have to be obtained up to 24 hours following administration of contrast material.[3] Eventually there is nonvisualization of the kidney and collecting system.[1] At that point, other techniques, such as retrograde pyelography, antegrade pyelography, ultrasonography, computed tomography (CT), nuclear medicine renal function studies, and angiography, may be necessary to evaluate the kidney further and to help decide on therapy.

In acute obstruction, leakage of urine from a renal calix into the renal sinus and into the retroperitoneum (or into the renal lymphatics) may occur, continuing until the obstruction is relieved. This phenomenon has been documented on urography in many cases, but how often this actually occurs is not known. In one series it was seen urographically in 22 to 33 percent of cases when higher doses of contrast material were used.[7]

This extravasation may act as a protective mechanism to decrease intrapelvic pressure. The ability of the kidney to protect itself by leaking urine into its renal sinus or lymphatics might help explain the varied end results in cases of renal obstruction. In some patients with long-standing ureteral obstruction, large hydronephrotic sacs develop, whereas in others small hydronephrotic sacs or atrophic small kidneys result. There are also various degrees of recovery of renal function when a long-standing ureteral obstruction is relieved.

Imaging of Hydronephrosis

The extent and etiology of hydronephrosis are studied and diagnosed by intravenous urography, retrograde pyelography, sonography, CT, nuclear medicine studies, and angiography. A discussion of the role of each of these techniques is beyond the scope of this presentation. Although angiography has only a minimal role in the imaging of the hydronephrotic kidney, its vascular appearance has been well established and is presented here to familiarize the reader with the angiographic findings and patterns in hydronephrosis.

Angiographic Findings

The angiographic findings in hydronephrosis depend on the severity and duration of the process. When selective renal angiography is performed on an acutely obstructed kidney, the findings are minimal, and often the angiogram is completely normal. However, the main renal artery branches can be stretched as the result of renal swelling and enlargement.[8] There may also be delayed filling of the secondary and tertiary branches of the intrarenal arteries due to increased intrarenal pressure from the obstruction. These findings are best seen on a midstream aortic injection because it is by comparison to the normal arteries in the contralateral kidney that subtle differences in filling may be noted (Fig. 48-1).

The angiographic changes in chronic hydronephrosis are more constant and more severe than in the acute phase, reflecting the greater dilatation of the collecting system and the parenchymal atrophy (Figs. 48-2 through 48-6). The first vessels affected are the small distal arteries. These are tapered and show decreased branching. As the process worsens, changes proceed proximally.[9] The intrarenal arteries are splayed, stretched, and narrowed as they pass around the dilated calices.[10,11] There is a decrease in the size and number of branches. Because of increased intrarenal pressure, circulation time through the vessels is slowed.[12] If the renal pelvis becomes extremely dilated, as in a tight ureteropelvic junction obstruction, the dorsal and ventral branches of the main renal artery are spread over it, and the main renal artery itself is pushed upward over the large pelvis (see Figs. 48-2 through 48-6).[10,13]

The nephrogram reflects the amount of functioning renal tissue; its integrity is important in determining whether a kidney is salvageable. In acute hydronephrosis, a good nephrogram is seen, but with time and atrophy it becomes progressively diminished, until eventually a nephrogram is no longer visualized. This decrease in functioning renal tissue is also reflected in the size of the main renal artery. As function diminishes, the renal artery and its branches atrophy.[14,15] In end-stage hydronephrosis, there is a small main renal artery, splayed and diminished intrarenal branches, and no functioning renal tissue.

The changes just mentioned are those of classic hydronephrosis; when they occur throughout the kidney, the angiographic diagnosis is obvious. However, hydronephrosis may be localized to one calix or segment of the kidney, appearing as a mass, and the condition may be more difficult to diagnose. In this localized form, the vessels are splayed and attenuated around the obstructed area. Although the appearance on urography is of a mass, the avascular nature, combined with contrast filling of the mass on delayed urogram films, will generally allow the correct diagnosis to be made (Figs. 48-7 through 48-10).[16] (Of course, sonography and CT would also clearly indicate that the "mass" is in reality localized hydronephrosis.)

Angiography in Infected Hydronephrosis and Pyonephrosis

When the collecting system of a hydronephrotic kidney becomes infected, other radiographic findings are superimposed on those of dilatation and atrophy. Whatever the level of function of the kidney, infection generally worsens it. Visualization of an infected or a pyonephrotic kidney is poor or nonexistent on intravenous urography. With the use of high-dose infusion techniques, better visualization was reported and some nephrogram or rim of density around the dilated calices was seen in about half the patients in one study.[17] If a retrograde pyelogram is done in pyonephrosis, in which pus fills the collecting system, a shaggy, bizarre pattern is seen as the contrast material mixes with the exudate.[1] Sonography and CT can be helpful in diagnosing infection in the hydronephrotic kidney by appreciating inflammatory debris in the infected urine and inflammatory reactive changes in the renal parenchyma and perirenal space.[18–20]

Text continues on page 1212

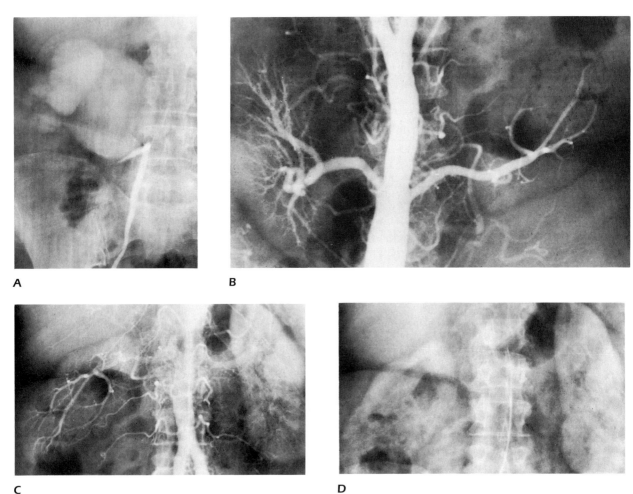

A

B

C

D

Figure 48-1. Case 1. Hydronephrosis with salvageable kidney in a 42-year-old woman with right-sided pain. (A) Retrograde pyelogram. A tight ureteropelvic junction obstruction with greatly dilated pelvis and calices is seen. (B) Aortogram, early arterial phase. The renal arteries are equal in size. The flow of contrast medium through the right kidney is slow as compared to its flow through the left. (C) Aortogram, later arterial phase. Delayed filling of the intrarenal vessels on the right can be seen. These vessels are stretched and somewhat attenuated. The nephrogram is already shown in the left kidney. (D) Aortogram, nephrogram phase. The nephrograms in both kidneys are similar. Surgical repair of the ureteropelvic junction obstruction on the right was performed, with return to normal function in the right kidney.

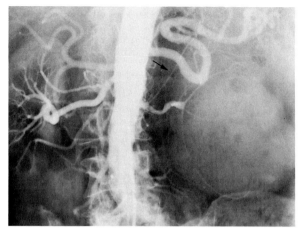

A

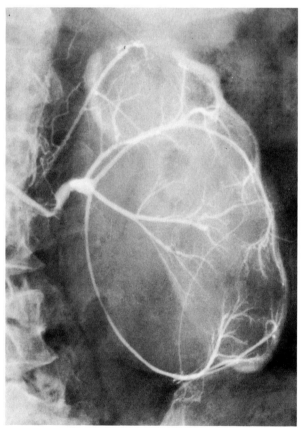

B

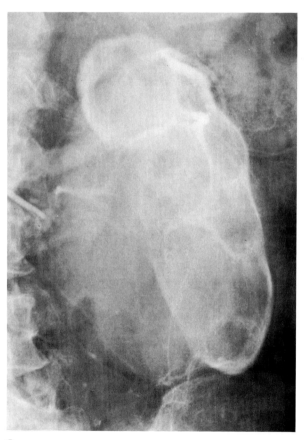

C

Figure 48-2. Case 2. Chronic hydronephrosis in a 59-year-old woman with a palpable left-flank mass. (A) Aortogram. An atrophic left renal artery is seen. Poor filling of vessels in the left kidney is noted, with sparse vascularity and stretching of filled vessels over a dilated pelvis. A superior polar artery is seen (*arrow*) supplying the upper pole of the left kidney. (B) Selective left renal arteriogram, arterial phase. Atrophic vascularity to the "shell" of the left kidney is well demon-strated. Diminished branches and stretching of vessels over a dilated collecting system are noted. Major branches of the renal artery are seen stretched over a dilated pelvis. (C) Selective left renal arteriogram, nephrogram phase. A minimal nephrogram in the remaining parenchyma is seen. Dilated calices are outlined by the opacified parenchyma. A left nephrectomy was performed.

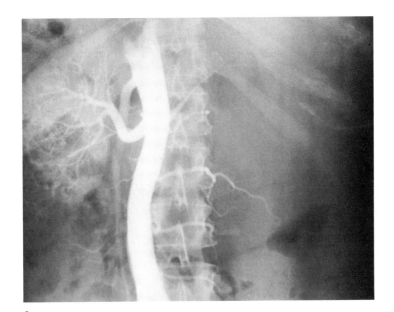

A

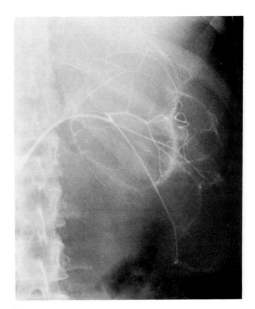

B

Figure 48-3. Case 3. Chronic hydronephrosis in a 45-year-old man with a palpable abdominal mass on the left. (A) Aortogram. Atrophy of the left renal artery is apparent, with minimal filling of the distal branches to the left kidney. A mass in the left flank is displacing the aorta to the right.

(B) Selective left renal arteriogram. Marked stretching of an atrophic left renal artery and branches is apparent. This appearance is characteristic of chronic hydronephrosis. At surgery, a large hydronephrotic sac was removed.

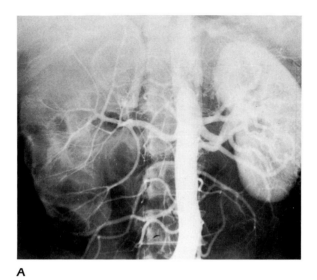

A

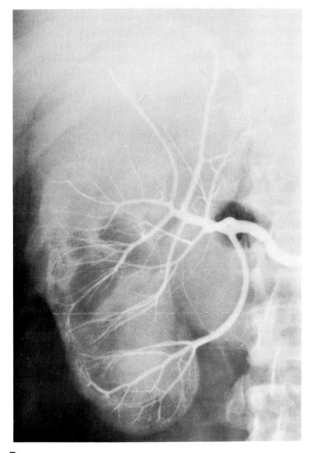

B

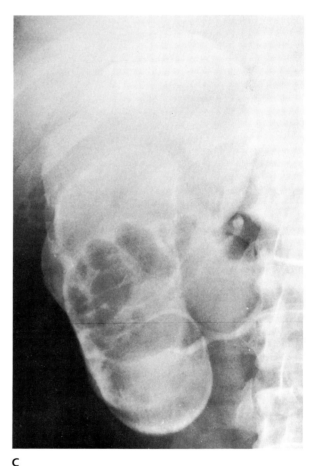

C

Figure 48-4. Case 4. Chronic hydronephrosis in a 31-year-old man with right flank pain. (A) Aortogram. An enlarged right renal contour and stretched atrophic vessels coursing over a hydronephrotic kidney are seen. (B) Selective right renal arteriogram, arterial phase. Characteristic stretched, splayed, and atrophied branches of the right renal artery are noted coursing over dilated caliceal structures. (C) Selective right renal arteriogram, nephrogram phase. A thin rim of parenchyma is opacified. A right nephrectomy was performed. The parenchyma of the pathologic specimen was 1 to 2 mm thick.

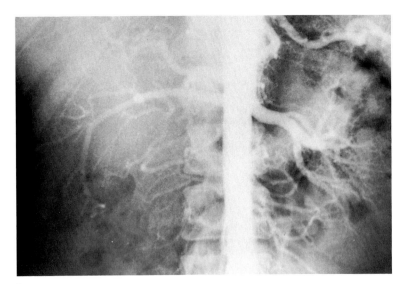

A

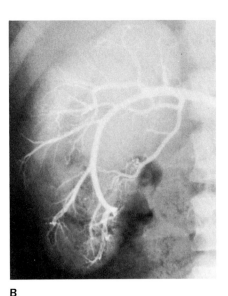

B

Figure 48-5. Case 5. Chronic hydronephrosis in a 22-year-old man with right flank pain. (A) Aortogram. Stretching of the right renal artery and its branches over a hydronephrotic right kidney is seen. (B) Selective right renal arteriogram. Stretching and atrophy of branches of the right renal artery can be seen, with some minimal parenchyma noted along the outer margin of the kidney. A right nephrectomy was performed. The parenchyma of the pathologic specimen was 0.1 to 1.0 cm thick.

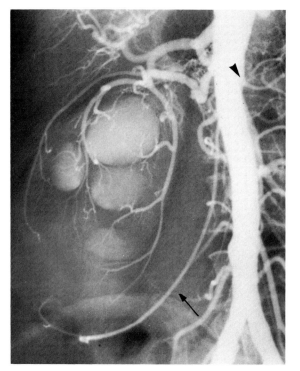

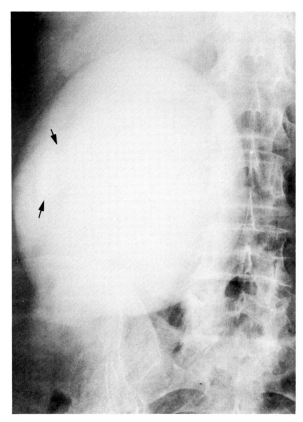

A

 B

Figure 48-6. Case 6. Chronic hydronephrosis in a 66-year-old patient with right-sided pain and a palpable mass in the right side of the abdomen. (A) Delayed film (2 hours) of intravenous urogram. There is a greatly dilated right renal pelvis indicating a ureteropelvic junction obstruction. Some filling of the dilated calices (*arrows*) can be seen through the opacified pelvis. (B) Aortogram, arterial phase. A kinked right renal artery is shown supplying a hydronephrotic right kidney. Atrophy and stretching of the peripheral branches are seen. The accessory renal artery courses inferiorly (*arrow*) and stretches around the dilated pelvis. An accessory renal artery is not obstructing the pelvis but is being pushed by the pelvis. Also note an atrophic left renal artery (*arrowhead*). An atrophic kidney was present on the left. (C) Aortogram, nephrogram phase. A thinned parenchyma but some nephrogram is apparent, along with dilated calices. At surgery, a plastic repair of the renal pelvis was performed, with great improvement in the right renal function.

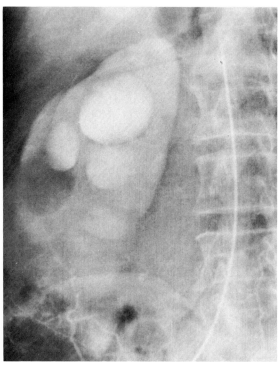

C

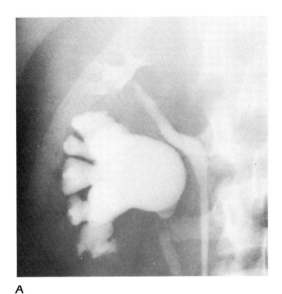

A

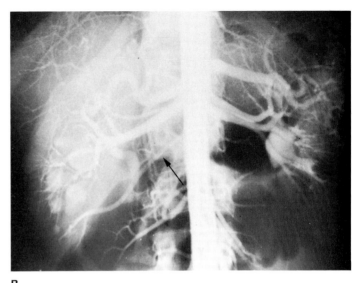

B

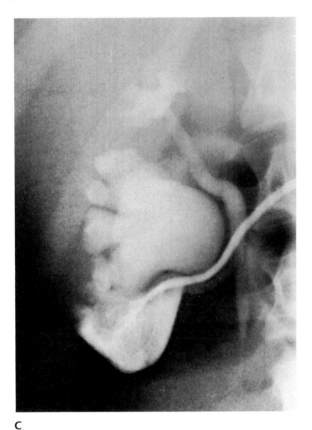

C

Figure 48-7. Case 7. Localized hydronephrosis caused by an accessory renal artery. A 19-year-old man with right flank pain. (A) Urogram, delayed film. A hydronephrotic lower collecting system is now opacified. A ureteropelvic junction obstruction is present. (B) Aortogram. Two renal arteries of about equal size to the left kidney are seen. A normal-sized right renal artery with a superior polar branch is filled. A smaller accessory renal artery is also seen (*arrow*) supplying the lower pole of the right kidney. (C) Selective study of the accessory right renal artery. The accessory artery to the lower pole crosses the pelvis of the lower pole collecting system, obstructing it. At surgery, a plastic repair of the obstruction was performed. The pelvis was placed anterior to the obstructing vessel.

Figure 48-9. Case 9. Localized hydronephrosis in a dupli- ▶ cated collecting system. A 50-year-old woman with left flank pain. The patient had had a hysterectomy 4 years previously. (A) Excretory urogram and antegrade pyelogram of a lower pole collecting system on the left. Hydronephrosis and hydroureter are seen in the lower pole collecting system of a duplicated system on the left. The right kidney and the upper pole left kidney are visualized secondary to the urogram. The hydronephrotic system on the left was not visualized on the urogram, and it was opacified by a percutaneous antegrade injection. The obstruction of the distal ureter on the left (by a surgical tie) is clearly seen. (B) Aortogram, arterial phase. The main renal artery to the left kidney is barely seen (*higher arrow*) on this film. A second atrophic renal artery (*lower arrow*) to the lower pole is noted. The atrophic branches are stretched. (C) Aortogram, nephrogram phase. The nephrogram of the normal upper pole is present intact. No nephrogram is seen in the lower portion of the kidney, except for a minimal rim at the lower pole (*arrow*) of the kidney. Note the overlying calcified mesenteric nodes. At surgery, the hydronephrotic lower pole was removed.

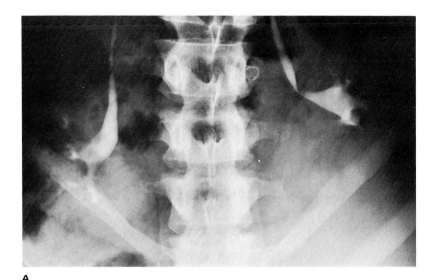

A

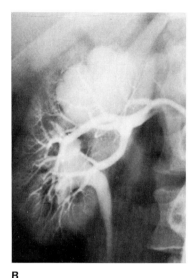

B

Figure 48-8. Case 8. Localized hydronephrosis in a duplicated collecting system. A 28-year-old woman with right-sided abdominal pain and infection. (A) Urogram. There is no visualization of the calices in the upper pole of the right kidney. (B) Selective right renal arteriogram. Localized hydronephrosis with dilated calices in the upper pole collecting system is seen. Atrophy of the branches to the upper pole is noted. Branches of the renal artery cross the upper pole collecting system and contribute to its obstruction. At surgery, a partial nephrectomy of the upper pole of the kidney was performed after it was determined that the plastic salvage would be technically difficult.

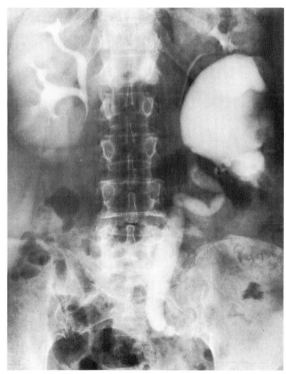

A

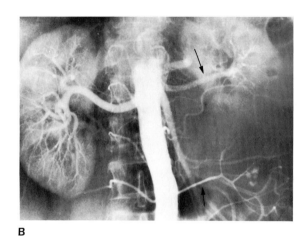

B

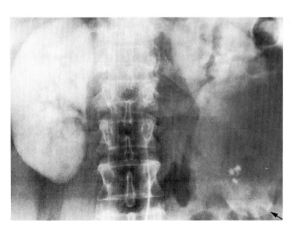

C

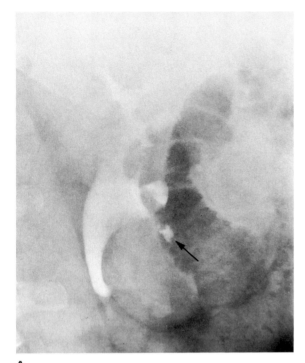

A

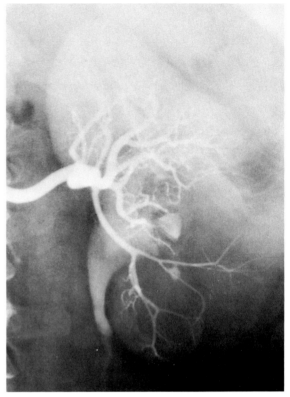

B

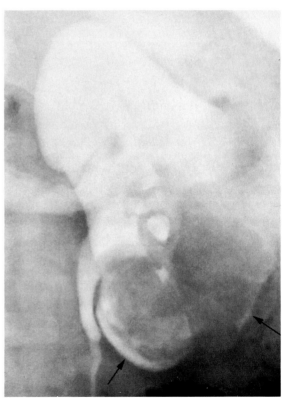

C

Figure 48-10. Case 10. Localized hydronephrosis due to a calculus. A 45-year-old man with left flank pain. (A) Urogram. A bulbous enlargement of the lower pole of the kidney is seen, with poor visualization of collecting system structures. The *arrow* points to a calculus seen on the preliminary film. (B) Selective left renal arteriogram, arterial phase. Atrophy and stretching of the branches to the lower pole of the kidney are seen. The upper pole vessels are normal. (C) Selective left renal arteriogram, nephrogram phase. A normal nephrogram is noted in the upper pole. Only the rim of the parenchyma is seen (*arrows*) surrounding the hydronephrotic lower lobe. A heminephrectomy of the lower pole of the left kidney was performed.

Angiography in pyonephrosis shows the previously described changes of hydronephrosis: atrophy of vessels, stretching and splaying of arteries around dilated calices, and a decrease in the number of terminal and parenchymal branches.[21] Added to this in many cases are inflammatory vascular changes. Small, fine, tortuous neovascularity may be present around the infected collecting system structures. The borders of the calices are ill defined and hazy. Zones of abnormal vessels in the capillary phase lead to areas of abnormal "blush" on the nephrogram (Fig. 48-11).[21–23] As in other chronic renal infections, there may be hypertrophy and increased tortuosity of periureteric and capsular arteries as they give rise to some of these inflammatory vessels.[21]

In summary, the angiographic picture reflects the pathologic picture and may range from a pattern like that of simple hydronephrosis to one of xanthogranu-

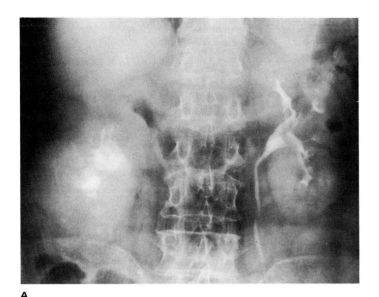

A

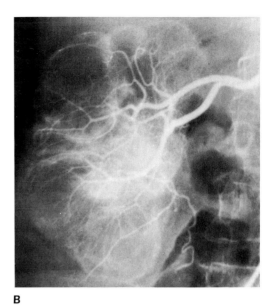

B

Figure 48-11. Case 11. Pyonephrosis. A 53-year-old woman with a high fever and right-sided discomfort. (A) Urogram. Calculi were seen on the preliminary film in the right kidney. No visualization of the contrast material is seen on the right. (B) Selective right renal arteriogram. The changes indicative of hydronephrosis are seen, with atrophy of the branches and stretching of the vessels over the hydronephrotic sacs. However, there is increased filling of the smaller branches, with hyperemia, and staining, which is indicative of an associated inflammation. A nephrectomy revealed a hydronephrotic sac filled with pus (pyonephrosis) and calculi.

lomatous pyelonephritis (see Chapter 47), with extensive inflammatory vascularity.

Use of Angiography to Determine the Cause of Hydronephrosis

A kidney that is not visualized on intravenous urography is generally assessed by the use of retrograde pyelography, ultrasonography, computed tomography, or, occasionally, antegrade pyelography. Ultrasonography has been found to be reliable in diagnosing chronic hydronephrosis, showing an echo-free mass with little surrounding parenchyma in the most severe cases or, in earlier stages, cystlike areas radiating out from the renal pelvis.[24,25]

Computed tomography can sensitively diagnose the existence of hydronephrosis and has proved accurate in determining the etiology of the obstruction, particularly when this is uncertain by retrograde pyelography or in cases when pyelography is not indicated.[26,27] Angiography's role in this regard has almost entirely been supplanted, although it is capable of diagnosing the cause of hydronephrosis in many cases, as depicted in Figure 48-12, where angiography demonstrates the hydronephrotic kidney and also tumor vascularity in the renal pelvis with extension into the ureter. In renal pelvic tumors, the artery to the renal pelvis and upper ureter may enlarge and give rise to this neovascularity. If the urothelial tumor invades the renal parenchyma, the previously normal intrarenal vessels in the involved area will be encased and often occluded.[28,29]

Angiography can also determine whether an aberrant or accessory vessel, either artery or vein, is the cause of the obstruction.[2,10,13] Numerous angiographic studies of patients with hydronephrosis have shown that they have a higher-than-average incidence of accessory renal vessels (see Figs. 48-6 and 48-7). The incidence of multiple renal arteries to a kidney is about 20 percent in the normal population. In patients with hydronephrosis due to structural congenital causes, the incidence is 40 percent.[13] Evidently, there is an embryologic association between the occurrence of ureteropelvic junction narrowing and the persistence of multiple renal vessels. Although at first it was presumed that the accessory vessel was usually the cause of the obstruction, surgical correlation has shown that it is uncommon for the accessory vessel to be responsible.[6,30,31] In one series of 39 patients with accessory renal arteries and hydronephrosis, an accessory vessel was found to be the cause of the obstruction in 14 patients. In another 3 patients in this series, the artery plus perivascular adhesions caused the narrowing, but

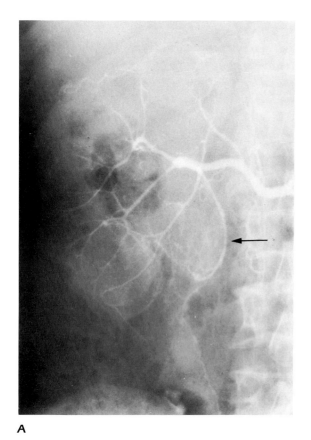

A

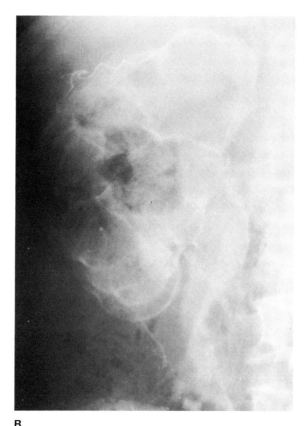

B

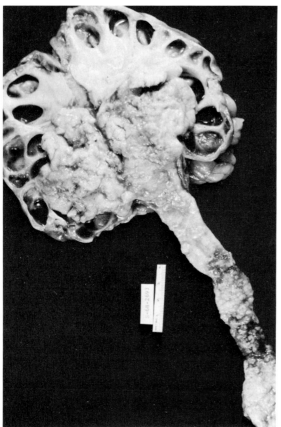

C

Figure 48-12. Case 12. Hydronephrosis secondary to renal pelvic carcinoma. A 65-year-old man with hematuria. A urogram revealed nonvisualization of the right kidney, and a right retrograde pyelogram could not be performed. (A) Selective right renal arteriogram, arterial phase. The typical changes of hydronephrosis, with atrophy and stretching of the intrarenal vessels over the dilated calices, are seen. A hypertrophied pelvic artery (*arrow*) gives off some tumorlike vessels in the renal pelvis and extends inferiorly to supply the ureter. (B) Selective right renal arteriogram, nephrogram phase. The hydronephrotic "shell" of the right kidney is seen. Also noted is a slight blush of tumor tissue in the renal pelvis and the upper ureter. (C) A pathologic specimen reveals hydronephrosis with extensive tumor in the renal pelvis and the ureter. (From Evans JA, Bosniak MA. The kidney. [Atlas of tumor radiology series.] Chicago: Year Book, 1971. Used with permission.)

in the other 22 patients the accessory vessel was in no way related to the hydronephrosis. In all cases in which the artery was a causal factor, it ran ventral to the renal pelvis and originated within 40 mm of the origin of the main renal artery. A polar branch with an early take-off from the main renal artery may also cause obstruction, and aberrant veins are also capable of producing enough pressure on the collecting system to lead to obstruction.[31]

Frequently, an accessory renal artery is present at an

obstructed ureteropelvic junction but the vessel itself is not the cause of the obstruction (see Fig. 48-6). The vessel may merely contribute to the obstruction of an already enlarging renal pelvis or may merely limit its extent of dilatation. When it must be decided preoperatively whether an artery is associated with a point of obstruction, comparisons of the angiogram and the intravenous urogram should enable one to make the determination. This can be more clearly demonstrated by performing arteriography after initially filling the renal pelvis with contrast media. The point of obstruction and the crossing vessel can then be well correlated (see Fig. 48-7).[10]

Angiography in Treatment Planning

In situations of ureteropelvic junction obstruction, angiography has played a role in determining whether the chronically obstructed kidney is salvageable. More recently, this evaluation has been made by determining parenchymal thickness as imaged by CT or by radionuclide studies. If a plastic repair to relieve the obstruction will not result in a functioning kidney, a simple nephrectomy can be performed. Multiple animal experiments have shown that the size of the main renal artery is a guide to potential recovery of function.[9,11,13,32,33] When the ureter is totally occluded, there is a progressive decrease in both the size of the main renal artery and the intensity of the nephrogram. Although these studies vary as to the exact length of time necessary for irreversible changes to occur, they generally agree that 30 to 40 days is the critical time. By this point, the artery has diminished in size to less than 50 percent of its original diameter. Once this critical value is reached, irreversible damage is done. No comparable data are available for humans; however, in cases of chronic hydronephrosis, diminution in the caliber of the renal artery has been a constant finding. When the main renal artery of the affected kidney has a caliber less than 50 percent of that of the contralateral vessel, there is little hope of restoring function to the hydronephrotic kidney.[11,13,33] However, if the decrease in the diameter of the main renal artery in the obstructed kidney has not reached 50 percent, release of the obstruction may result in a return of function of varying degrees (see Fig. 48-1). However, this is not necessarily true in every case. We have seen a number of examples of unsalvageable kidneys with main renal arteries greater than 50 percent of the original diameter in which at surgery no significant amount of renal tissue was present and in which nephrectomy was performed (see Figs. 48-4 and 48-5). Again, the above data are of interest in a historical sense. These angiographic criteria are not used in clinical decisions, which are determined more by clinical factors (patient's age, condition of opposite kidney, etc.), CT evaluation of parenchymal thickness, and the quality of the nephrogram and radionuclide studies of renal function.[34,35]

The amount of functioning parenchyma left in the hydronephrotic kidney is well evaluated by renal angiography because the intensity of the nephrogram is in effect the amount of functioning renal tissue.[8,10] The same experiments that demonstrated increasing atrophy of the renal artery with increasing time of occlusion also showed a decrease in the intensity of the nephrogram with time.[11,33] The density of the nephrogram gives a better understanding of the amount of functioning parenchyma in the kidney than does the visualization of the collecting system structures by urography. However, nuclear medicine techniques, including the use of ^{99m}Tc-DMSA and visualization of the quality of the nephrogram on CT, are now being increasingly used to determine the amount of residual functional renal tissue in these cases.

Finally, the angiogram is an important road map for the surgeon, particularly if he or she contemplates plastic repair and salvage of the hydronephrotic kidney. Complete knowledge of the vascular anatomy is essential for the best surgical results.

References

1. Emmett JL, Witten DM. Clinical urography. 3rd ed. Philadelphia: Saunders, 1971;1:369, 2:800.
2. Frimann-Dahl J. Angiography in hydronephrosis. In: Kincaid OW, ed. Renal angiography. Chicago: Year Book, 1966:209.
3. Bigongiari LR, Davis RM, Novak WG, Wick JD, Kass E, Thornbury JR. Visualization of the medullary rays on excretory urography in experimental ureteric obstruction. AJR 1977;129:89.
4. Elkin M, Boyarsky S, Martinez J, Kaplan N. Physiology of ureteral obstruction as determined by roentgenologic studies. AJR 1964;92:291.
5. Ney C, Friedenberg RM. Radiographic atlas of the genitourinary system. Philadelphia: Lippincott, 1966:114, 172.
6. Chahlaoui J, Herba MJ. Ureteropelvic junction obstruction in the adult. J Can Assoc Radiol 1977;28:40.
7. Bernardino ME, McClennan B. High dose urography: incidence and relationship to spontaneous peripelvic extravasation. AJR 1976;127:373.
8. Leary DJ, Templeton AW, Thompson IM, Sibala JL. Preoperative aortography in hydronephrosis. J Urol 1972;107:542.
9. Petasnick JP, Patel SK. Angiographic evaluation of the nonvisualizing kidney. AJR 1973;119:757.
10. Siegelman SS, Bosniak MA. Renal arteriography in hydronephrosis: its value in diagnosis and management. Radiology 1965;85:609.
11. Idbohrn H. Renal angiography in experimental hydronephrosis. Acta Radiol Suppl (Stockh) 1956;136.
12. Herdman JP, Jaco NT. The renal circulation in experimental hydronephrosis. Br J Urol 1950;22:52.

13. Olsson O. In: Abrams HL, ed. Angiography: 2nd ed. Boston: Little, Brown, 1971;2:785, 815.
14. Idbohrn H. Renal angiography in cases of delayed excretion in intravenous urography. Acta Radiol 1954;42:333.
15. Kauffmann G, Seib UC. Angiographische Differential diagnose der Hydronephrose. Radiologe 1975;15:457.
16. Bosniak MA, Scheff S, Kaufmann S. Localized hydronephrosis masquerading as renal neoplasm. J Urol 1968;99:241.
17. Watt I, Roylance J. Pyonephrosis. Clin Radiol 1975;27:513.
18. Fultz PJ, Hampton WR, Totterman SMS. Computed tomography of pyonephrosis. Abdom Imaging 1993;18:82–87.
19. Subramanyam BR, Raghavendra BN, Bosniak MA, et al. Sonography of pyonephrosis: a prospective study. AJR 1983;140:991–993.
20. Jeffrey RB, Laing FC, Wing VW, et al. Sensitivity of sonography in pyonephrosis: a re-evaluation. AJR 1985;144:71–73.
21. Koehler PR. The roentgen diagnosis of renal inflammatory masses—special emphasis on angiographic changes. Radiology 1974;112:257.
22. Wicks JD, Thornbury JR. Acute renal infections in adults. Radiol Clin North Am 1979;17:245.
23. Becker JA, Fleming R, Kanter I, Melicow M. Misleading appearances in renal angiography. Radiology 1967;88:691.
24. Marangola JP, Bryan PJ, Azimi F. Ultrasonic evaluation of the unilateral nonvisualized kidney. AJR 1976;126:853.
25. Sanders RC, Bearman S. B-scan ultrasound in the diagnosis of hydronephrosis. Radiology 1973;108:375.
26. Bosniak MA, Megibow AJ, Ambos MA, et al. Computed tomography of ureteral obstruction. AJR 1982;138:1107–1113.
27. Schwartz JM, Bosniak MA, Hulnick DH, et al. The use of computed tomography in the diagnosis of carcinoma of the renal pelvis causing ureteropelvic junction obstruction. Urol Radiol 1988;9:204–209.
28. Mitty HA, Baron MG, Feller M. Infiltrating carcinoma of the renal pelvis: angiographic features. Radiology 1969;92:994.
29. Rabinowitz JG, Kinkhabwala M, Himmelfarb F, Robinson T, Becker JA, Bosniak M, Madayag MM. Renal pelvic carcinoma: an angiographic re-evaluation. Radiology 1972;102:551.
30. Jewett HJ. Accessory renal vessels: their influence in certain cases of hydronephrosis. Surg Gynecol Obstet 1936;68:666.
31. Olsson O. Roentgen diagnosis of the urogenital system. Berlin: Springer-Verlag, 1973. Part 1:114, 319.
32. Hinman F, Morison DM. Experimental hydronephrosis: arterial changes in the progressive hydronephrosis of rabbits with complete ureteral obstruction. Surg Gynecol Obstet 1926;42:209.
33. Widen T. Renal angiography during and after unilateral ureteric occlusion: a long-term experimental study in dogs. Acta Radiol (Stockh) 1958;Suppl 162.
34. Kawamura J, Shinichi H, Yosida O, Fujita T, Yashushi I, Torizuka A. Validity of ^{99m}Tc dimercaptosuccinic acid renal uptake for an assessment of individual kidney function. J Urol 1978;119:305.
35. Blaufox MD, Fine E, Lee H-B, et al. The role of nuclear medicine in clinical urology and nephrology. J Nucl Med 1984;25:619.

49

Anomalies and Malformations

ERIK BOIJSEN

Multiple Renal Arteries

Multiple renal arteries are often present, particularly in malrotated and dystopic kidneys. In kidneys situated at a normal level, multiple arteries occur in anatomic dissection series in about 30 percent of cases.[1] In the angiographic literature, multiple renal arteries are reported to be observed in 20 to 27 percent of cases,[2-5] but lower figures are on record. The figures are lower at angiography than in dissection studies mainly because very small sublobar branches that pass from the aorta directly to the upper pole[6] often arise together with the superior capsular artery and adrenal arteries; at aortography these branches are too small to be noted or are misinterpreted as capsular arteries. These branches pass directly to the parenchyma without passing the renal hilus (Fig. 49-1).

The branches that pass directly to the parenchyma are usually called *pole* or *aberrant arteries,* whereas those passing through the hilus are called *hilar arteries.* Pole arteries can arise directly from the aorta or from hilar branches (see Figs. 45-3 and 45-10). The superior pole artery is most often encountered in dissection studies. In a thorough analysis, aortic superior pole arteries were found in 7 percent of cases and lower pole arteries were found in 5.5 percent. Polar branches from hilar arteries were found to the upper and lower pole in 12 percent and 1.4 percent, respectively.[1] In an angiographic series, extrahilar inferior pole arteries were found in 9 percent to arise from the aorta or the iliac arteries.[5]

In kidneys with multiple arteries, usually one main stem arises from the aorta at a normal level. Usually the main stem supplies anterior parts of the kidney and, most often also, at least the dorsal intermediate part. The most common extra artery from the aorta, here called the *supplementary artery,* passes through the hilus to the lower pole. In a clinical angiographic series, 72.5 percent of all supplementary arteries pass to the lower renal pole.[3] In most cases, this artery behaves as a lower pole artery arising from the renal ar-

tery, and it originates usually close to the main stem (Fig. 49-2). This vessel is of particular clinical importance because it usually passes on the anterior side of the ureteropelvic junction and may cause obstruction to the urinary flow. When it arises more distally from the aorta, the vessel has a horizontal course to the hilus and so does not cause mechanical obstruction. However, the concomitant vein may then cause the same type of obstruction (Fig. 49-3).

When the lower pole artery arises more distally from the aorta or the iliac arteries, it has a steep craniolateral course and may prevent the kidney from rotating to its final position (Fig. 49-4). The kidney is usually longer than normal but is situated at the normal place with the hilus directed anteriorly.

The supplementary arteries arising from the aorta are segmental or subsegmental arteries.[3,6] The most important one is thus the lower pole artery. The next most common supplementary artery is the one to the upper pole, but that artery usually supplies only a minor part, and, as mentioned previously, it is not fully represented in clinical angiography. In a clinical series, the supplementary dorsal artery was present as often as a superior pole artery (14 percent). A supplementary artery to the anterior intermediate segment was present in about 6 percent (see Fig. 49-1). The frequency of the supplementary arteries was above 100 percent in this series, because more than two arteries were present in 8 of the 152 kidneys with multiple arteries (see Figs. 49-1 and 49-4).

Anatomists are well aware that supplementary arteries may arise not only from the lumbar aorta and iliac arteries but also from a variety of abdominal vessels and may supply kidneys at a normal level. Among others, the superior and inferior mesenteric, celiac, middle colic, lumbar, and middle sacral arteries are described.[1,7,8] In the angiographic literature, few observations of this kind have been reported. A common trunk arising from the abdominal aorta at about normal level and supplying both kidneys has been observed,[9] as has a common trunk for both lower poles.[10]

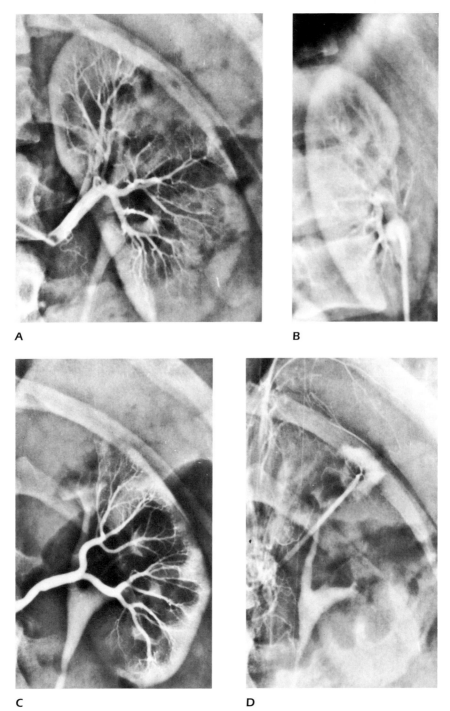

A

B

C

D

Figure 49-1. Normal kidney supplied by three branches arising from the aorta. (A and B) The arterial phase of a selective injection into the dorsal artery, which is the main renal artery; anteroposterior and lateral views. The entire posterior part and the anterior part of the superior lobe are supplied by the dorsal artery, except for a small area of the superior pole. (C and D) A selective injection (C) of the supplementary ventral artery and (D) of an artery with branches to the inferior phrenic artery, the adrenal gland, the renal capsule, and a small section of the upper pole.

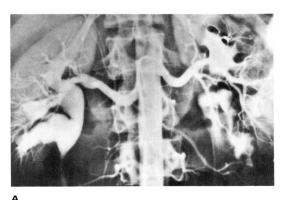

A

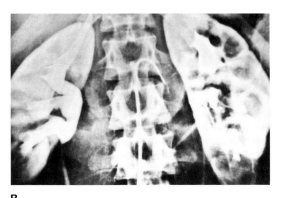

B

Figure 49-2. Hydronephrosis of the left kidney caused by a supplementary lower pole artery. (A and B) Semiselective left renal angiography, arterial and nephrographic phases. A lower pole artery arises from the aorta 3 cm below the main stem and is displaced in an arch, with convexity directed medially and distally.

Figure 49-3. Hydronephrosis of left kidney caused by a vein crossing the ureteropelvic junction. (A and B) Arterial and venous phases of semiselective renal angiography. The supplementary lower pole artery arises from the aorta 3.5 cm distal to the main stem. It passes almost horizontal to the lower part of the renal hilus. A concomitant lower pole vein (*arrow*) that is displaced in an arch, with convexity directed medially and distally, causes the obstruction.

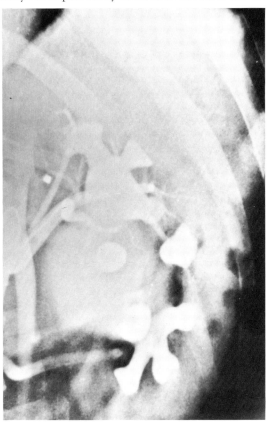

A

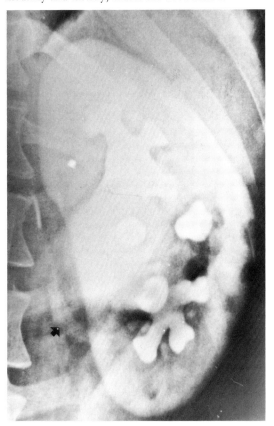

B

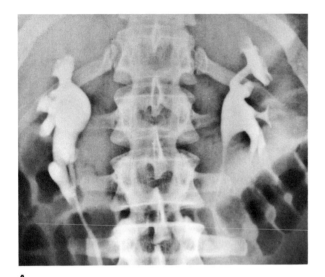

A

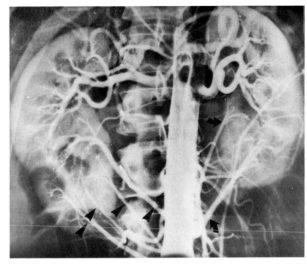

B

Figure 49-4. Incomplete rotation of the right kidney due to supplementary arteries. (A) Urogram. (B and C) Arterial and nephrographic phases. Both kidneys are at normal sites and are supplied by main stems that arise from the aorta at a normal level. The right kidney is long and is malrotated, with an atypical, broad lower pole that is supplied by four supplementary arteries (*arrowheads*) that arise from the lower aorta and the right iliac artery. The left lower pole is supplied by two supplementary arteries (*arrows*) that arise from the distal aorta, but the kidney is not malrotated.

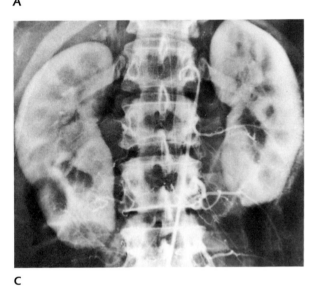

C

Figure 49-5. Diagram of the *rete arteriosum urogenitale*, formed by segmental arteries that supply the mesonephros and the later metanephros in early embryonal life. (From Felix W. Die Entwicklung der Harn- und Geschlechts-organe. In: Keibel K, Mall FP, eds. Handbuch der Entwicklungsgeschichte des Menschen. Leipzig: Hirzel, 1911;2:732. Used with permission.)

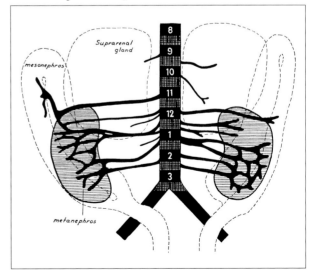

A supplementary artery arising from the contralateral renal artery[11-13] and a lower pole artery from the inferior mesenteric artery has also been reported.[14]

The wide variations in the origin and course of multiple renal arteries can be explained by the development of the mesonephric arteries (Fig. 49-5).[15] These arteries develop on each side of the aorta and are distributed from the sixth cervical to the third lumbar segments, where they form a network, the *rete arteriosum urogenitale*. In addition to the mesonephros, these arteries supply the adrenal, the metanephros (i.e., the final kidney), and the gonads. Eventually, some of the roots and part of the network degenerate, and the area that they previously supplied is taken over by a neighboring root. Finally, only one mesonephric artery at the level of L1 takes over the entire supply of the kidney. The mesonephric arteries may reach down to the L3 segment and persist, which may explain the presence of supplementary arteries down to this level. Renal arteries distal to L3 represent vessels that arose during the ascent of the metanephros but for some reason were not obliterated. The appearance of vascular anomalies is thus the result of unusual paths in the primitive vascular plexuses and the persistence of vessels normally obliterated.[16]

Renal Ectopy

The angiographic findings in malrotated and ectopic kidney have been presented in textbooks to a certain extent, but a comprehensive analysis is lacking. Besides the few case reports analyzing the cause of abdominal pain in ectopic kidney, only a few reports exist on the angiographic characteristics of these malformations.[3,17–20] The reason is, first, that ectopic kidney is rare (fused kidney occurs in some 0.2 percent and ectopic kidney in 0.1 percent of all autopsies), and, second, angiography is performed only before a planned operation on such a kidney.

It is generally assumed that caudal ectopic kidneys have multiple arteries, but that is not necessarily the case. Thus, in *horseshoe kidney,* one single artery to each kidney, including the bridge, has been observed.[6,21] Most often, however, multiple arteries are present in horseshoe kidney. The supplementary arteries arise below the main arteries from the lower aorta or iliac arteries, either as a single trunk to each side or as a main trunk to both sides of the bridge and the lower parts of the kidneys. Supplementary arteries arising above the main stem also occur (Fig. 49-6). In horseshoe kidney, the distribution of the intrarenal arteries can still be traced.[6] The bridging part usually contains renal parenchyma, but an "avascular" connective tissue connection may be present. The bridge probably causes the anterior location of the renal hilus in the same manner that the supplementary lower pole artery does in malrotated kidneys at normal level.[3]

The most common type of *fused kidney* is the horseshoe kidney, but a large variety exists, including crossed ectopia (Fig. 49-7), fused presacral kidney, and pelvic kidney (Figs. 49-8 and 49-9). The vascular supply of these malformations is unpredictable. The main renal supply originates below L3, which means that the vessels do not belong to the segmental mesonephric system, and the intrarenal distribution can no longer be systematized. Multiple arteries originating from the lower aorta or pelvic arteries are usually present to supply each kidney, but not always (Figs. 49-9 and 49-10).

In *lumbar ectopia,* one artery may arise from the lower part of the aorta passing behind the kidney and one may arise at the same level passing anterior to the kidney and enter anterior to it and enter the laterally situated hilus, which may explain the renal colic present (see Fig. 49-10). In other situations, an artery passing from the iliac artery to the lower pole of the malrotated kidney may be stretched in a certain position and cause nephralgia.[22]

Figure 49-6. (A and B) Horseshoe kidney supplied by two main renal arteries that also supply the parenchymatous bridge. A small supplementary artery (*arrow*) arises from the aorta just above the main renal artery.

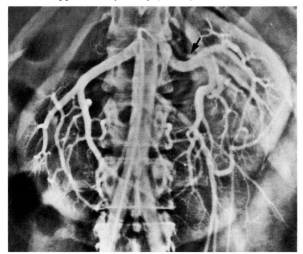

A

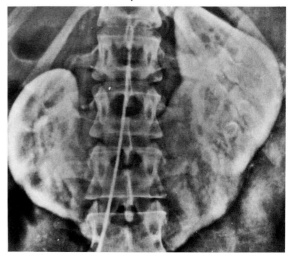

B

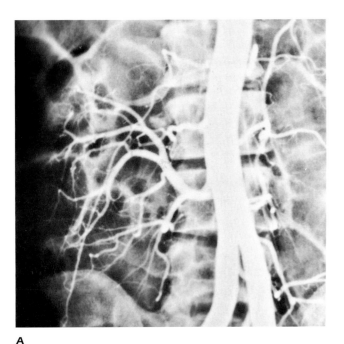

A

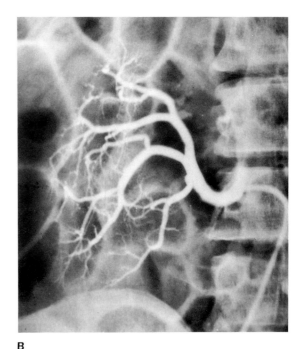

B

Figure 49-7. Lumbar ectopic, fused kidney on the right in a 38-year-old man with nephropathy and uremia. (A) At lumbar aortography, two arteries arising at the level of L4 supply the kidney, which measures 15 × 8 cm. No renal ar-teries are present on the left. (B) At selective angiography of the main artery, increased resistance of flow and poor cortical perfusion are observed.

Malformation of the Renal Parenchyma

Absence of any fetal or metanephrogenic tissue (*agenesia*) or the presence of only fetal nephrogenic structures (*aplasia*) may be an indication for angiography when other methods fail to explain the absence observed at urography or scintigraphy.[17–19,23,24] If a small renal artery is observed at lumbar aortography, it usually represents an adrenal artery, but it may also represent the very small blood supply of the *hypoplastic kidney* (Fig. 49-11). The acquired small kidney will also have a small renal artery. A distinction between this and the hypoplastic kidney could be that in acquired disease the origin of the renal artery retains its width.[25] The contralateral kidney is hyperplastic, and frequently multiple arteries are present,[17] or abnormalities are present in the renal pelvis (see Fig. 49-11). Anuria in a newborn may be an indication for angiography to show the bilateral absence of renal arteries.[17]

In *total renal dysplasia* of childhood, there is disturbed differentiation of nephrogenic tissue with persistence of structures inappropriate to the gestational age of the patient. It is the most common abdominal mass in the newborn infant and the most common cystic disorder of the kidney in children. At angiography, small renal vessels and poor perfusion have been observed.[26]

Dysplasia may be localized to one small part or to several parts of the kidney. At angiography, no cortical vessels are observed and the renal pelvis reaches the renal capsule (Fig. 49-12).

Renal hypoplasia and *dysplasia* are controversial definitions from a pathoanatomic point of view.[27–29] The Ask-Upmark kidney is one such entity.[30,31] For the radiologist, there appears to be no definite way to decide whether the lesion is a congenital malformation or a lesion that occurred in early childhood or during intrauterine life. However, when the lesion is combined with other abnormalities regarded as malformations, it appears more justified to describe a localized

Figure 49-8. Sacral ectopic, fused kidney that measures 15 × 7 × 12 cm. (A and B) Lumbar aortography, anteroposterior view. Three arteries supply the conglomerated kidney, which does not seem to have a hilus. The arteries arise from the distal aorta at the level of the bifurcation (*1, 2, 3*). The normally coursing short ureters are observed in the nephrographic phase (*arrows*, B). (C and D) Lateral view. The kidney makes an impression on the fundus of the bladder. ▶

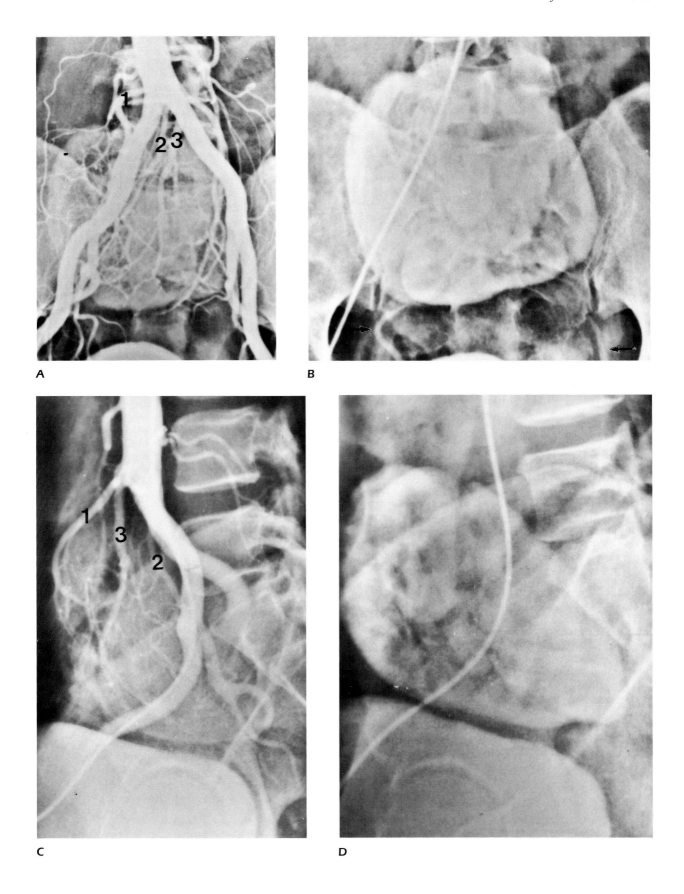

A

B

C

D

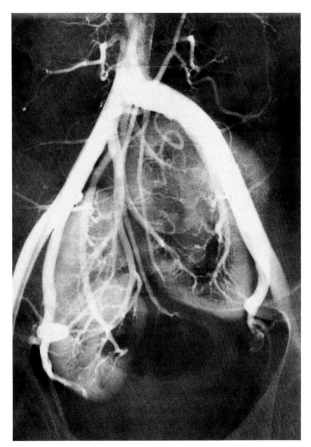

Figure 49-9. Partly fused pelvic kidney. Lower lumbar aortography, subtraction film. The right kidney is supplied by only one artery arising from the common iliac, and the left kidney is supplied by two arteries. The superior hemorrhoidal artery passes in a groove between the two kidneys.

absence of a lobe drained by a calix as a dysplasia (see Fig. 49-12) and a very small kidney as a hypoplasia (see Fig. 49-11).

Many classifications of *cystic disease* of the kidneys exist, and the literature is controversial and confusing.[32-35] It is not the purpose of this presentation to go into a deep analysis of these entities. Suffice it here to say that with the combination of angiography and urography a distinction can be made among medullary cystic disease, the common type of adult hereditary polycystic disease, adult polycystic disease, type Potter 3, and the cystlike dilatation of the tubules in medullary sponge kidney.

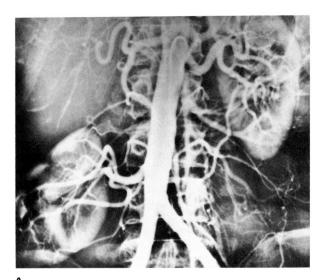

A

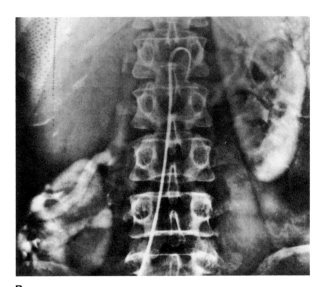

B

Figure 49-10. Palpable tumor and pain on right side was the main indication for urography in this 51-year-old woman. At urography, a right lumbar ectopic kidney with the hilus directed laterally was observed. (A and B) Lumbar aortography, arterial and venous phases. The left kidney is supplied by one artery at a normal level. The right ectopic kidney is supplied by only one artery, which arises at the level of the disk between L3 and L4. Probably one branch passes anterior and one branch passes posterior to the kidney before entering the laterally oriented hilus. Probably also, the two draining veins follow the same course.

Figure 49-12. Congenital focal dysplasia with local absence of cortical structures and with the calices reaching the renal surface. (A) Urography, tomographic cut, shows local absence of parenchyma in the superior pole and the intermediate part. (B) Selective renal angiogram, 2× magnification, subtraction film, shows localized absence of cortical vessels and glomeruli at the site of previously mentioned abnormalities but also in the lower pole. Marked localized hyperplasia between the absent cortical sections is evident. ▶

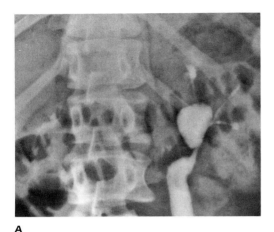

A

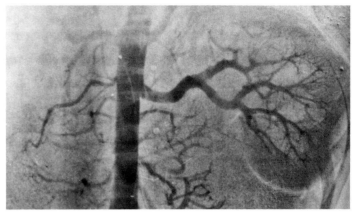

B

Figure 49-11. Hypoplastic right kidney and anomalous left renal collecting system in a hyperplastic kidney. (A) Urography. The 3 × 2 cm kidney on the right concentrates the contrast medium quite well. Three small infundibula with poorly developed calices drain into a wide confluent part of the renal pelvis on the left. (B and C) Lumbar aortography, subtraction film, arterial and capillary phases. One artery to each kidney arising at a normal level is demonstrated. The small right renal artery arises together with the inferior phrenic and adrenal arteries.

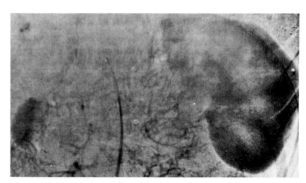

C

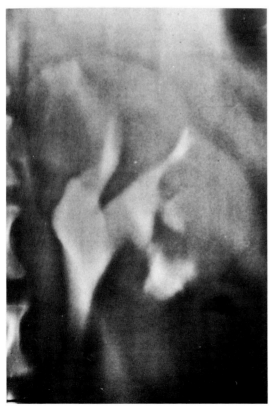

A

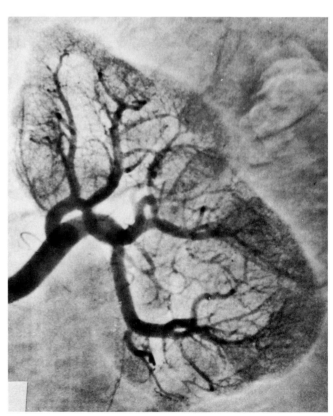

B

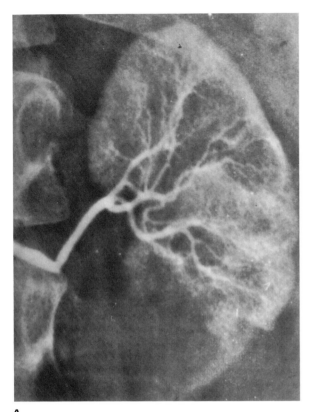

A

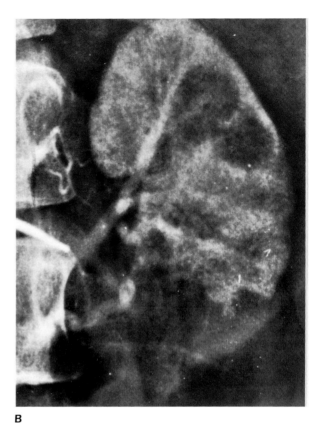

B

Figure 49-13. Medullary cystic disease, histologically verified in a 35-year-old uremic woman treated with hemodialysis for 4 years. (A and B) Selective left renal angiography of the main trunk, arterial and venous phases. The 7 × 3 cm kidney contains numerous small filling defects due to cystic dilatation of tubuli at the corticomedullary level, giving a honeycomb pattern. The cortical surface is not interrupted. Similar findings are observed on the right side.

In *medullary cystic disease,* or juvenile nephronophthisis, the kidneys are small. The renal arteries are thin, and in the nephrographic phase a marked cortical thinning is observed (Fig. 49-13). Filling defects of 1 to 2 mm in diameter are scattered through the kidney but spare the outermost cortical layer.[36] The lack of cortical interruption is thus the characteristic finding that is not observed in any other type of lesion.

The *common type of adult hereditary polycystic disease* differs completely from medullary cystic kidney disease (Fig. 49-14). The renal artery supplying a large kidney is reduced in caliber, and the cortical surface is interrupted by cysts of various size, which gives the nephrographic phase an extremely irregular appearance, the extent of which varies with the stage of the disease.[33,37,38]

In *adult polycystic disease, type Potter 3,* the cysts are not as numerous as in the common adult type, but the characteristic contrast-filled medullary cyst observed at urography is pathognomonic for this entity.[33,39] Focal dysplasia often is present.

In *medullary sponge kidney,* or benign tubular ectasia, the renal angiogram is normal.[39,40] Secondary pyelonephritis often occurs in this malformation of the papilla; when it does, angiography is, of course, abnormal.

In *hereditary nephritis* (Alport syndrome), there are diffuse fibrosis and tubular atrophy, mainly in the corticomedullary junction. Angiographically, the lesion is not distinguishable from other types of nephropathy (Fig. 49-15).[41]

Pseudotumor is a blanket term for different types of normal variations of the renal pelvis or parenchyma, ranging from fetal lobulation to impressions made by adjacent organs, such as the spleen or the liver.[42–45] The cause may also be an unusually large column of Bertin, which causes splaying of the renal calices, the infundibula, and the associated interlobar arteries.[42–44,46–48] At angiography, a well-circumscribed dense accumulation is observed and, often, a central lucency (Fig. 49-16). Other causes of pseudotumor may be (1) traction applied to the lower pole by a supplementary lower

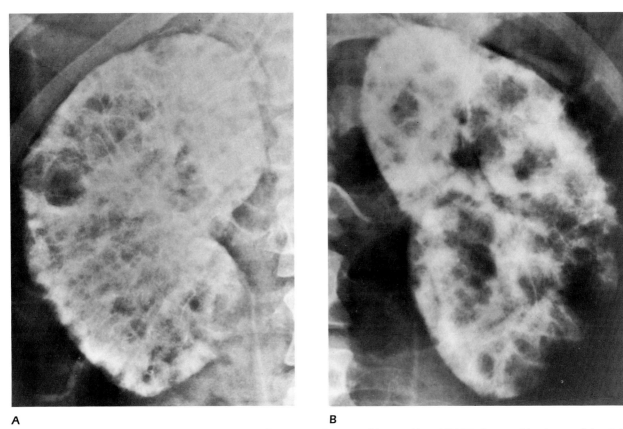

A   **B**

Figure 49-14. Early stage of hereditary polycystic disease in a 31-year-old man. (A and B) Nephrographic phases of the right and left kidneys. There are a large number of cysts of varying size with typical cortical distribution in the moderately enlarged kidney.

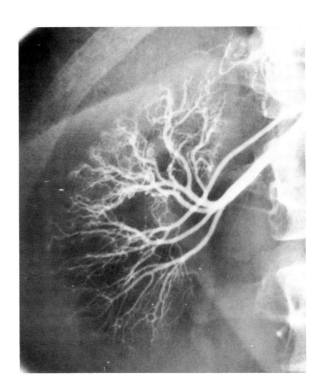

Figure 49-15. Hereditary nephritis (Alport syndrome). Selective angiography of the right kidney, arterial phase. The intrarenal arteries are crowded and reduced in caliber. The cortex is reduced, and marked resistance to flow is present. Similar findings are observed in the opposite kidney.

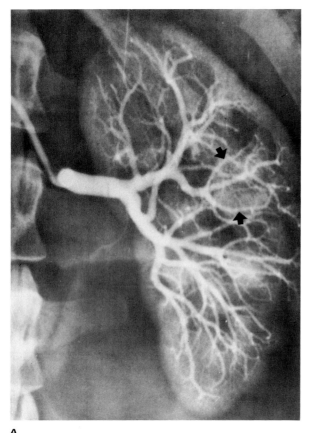

A

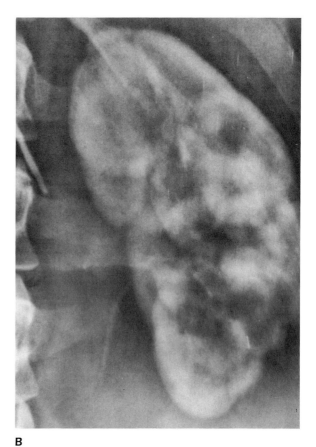

B

Figure 49-16. Arteritis in a 32-year-old woman with lupus. (A and B) At selective left renal angiography, arterial and nephrographic phases, the cortical surface is irregular because of small infarctions. In the intermediate part, the in- terlobar arteries (*arrows,* A) are slightly splayed by a pseu- dotumor, with central lucency. It is formed by a somewhat large column of Bertin.

pole artery in malrotated kidneys at the normal site[49] and (2) focal hyperplasia in a kidney with local destruc- tion of parenchyma (see Fig. 49-12).

Malformation of the Renal Pelvis

Primary congenital anomalies of the renal pelvis, such as megacalices or renal pelvic duplication, do not in- fluence the normal renal angiogram unless secondary disease affects the parenchyma (see Fig. 45-10).[50–52]

References

1. Merklin RJ, Michels NA. The variant renal and suprarenal blood supply with data on the inferior phrenic, ureteral and gonadal arteries. J Int Coll Surg 1958;29:41–75.
2. Edsman G. Angionephrography and suprarenal angiography. Acta Radiol (Stockh) 1957;Suppl 155.
3. Boijsen E. Angiographic studies of the anatomy of single and multiple renal arteries. Acta Radiol (Stockh) 1959;Suppl 183.
4. Fontaine R, Kieny R, Jurascheck F, Perez-Day C. Etude angio- graphique des artères rénales accessoires (polaires supérieures et inférieures indépendantes des artères rénales normales) et leur signification pathologique. Lyon Chir 1965;61:685–702.
5. Guntz M. Radio-anatomie de l'artère rénale: deductions chi- rurgicales. C Rendus Assoc Anat 1967;138:623–631.
6. Graves FT. Arterial anatomy of congenitally abnormal kidney. Br J Surg 1969;56:533–541.
7. Gillespie C, Miller LJ, Baskin M. Anomalous renal vessels and their surgical significance. Anat Rec 1916;11:77–86.
8. Poisel S, Spängler HP. Über aberrante und akzessorische Nie- renarterien bei Nieren in typischer Lage. Anat Anz 1969;124: 244–259.
9. Kónya A. An unusual congenital abnormality of the renal ar- tery: left renal artery arising from the right renal artery. Br J Radiol 1985;58:891–893.
10. Levine NO. An unusual renal artery anomaly: common origins of arteries to lower poles. Br J Radiol 1970;43:66–67.
11. Jeffery RF. Unusual origins of renal arteries. Radiology 1972; 102:309–310.
12. Libschitz H, Ben-Menachem Y, Kuroda K. Unusual renal vas- cular supply. Br J Radiol 1972;45:536–538.
13. Cederlund CG, Dimitrov N, Jonsson K, Carlsson S. Arterial supply of the left kidney from the right renal artery: a case re- port. ROEFO 1982;136:480–481.

14. Tisnado J, Amendola MA, Beachley MC. Renal artery originating from the inferior mesenteric artery. Br J Radiol 1979;52: 752–754.
15. Felix W. Die Entwicklung der Harn- und Geschlechts-organe. In: Keibel K, Mall FP, eds. Handbuch der Entwicklungsgeschichte des Menschen. Leipzig: Hirzel, 1911;2:732.
16. Arey LB. Developmental anatomy. 6th ed. Philadelphia: Saunders, 1954.
17. Olsson O, Wholey M. Vascular abnormalities in gross anomalies of kidneys. Acta Radiol 1964;2:420–432.
18. Bachmann D, Schäfer P. Nierenmissbildungen: angiographische Befunde. ROEFO 1967;107:50–59.
19. Thiemann KJ, Wieners H. Probleme der angiographischen Diagnostik von Agenesien, Aplasien, Fusionsanomalien und Ektopien der Niere. Radiologe 1970;10:108–118.
20. Dretler SP, Olsson C, Pfister RC. The anatomic, radiologic, and clinical characteristics of the pelvic kidney. J Urol 1971; 105:623–627.
21. Boatman DL, Cornell SH, Kölln CP. The arterial supply of horseshoe kidneys. AJR 1971;113:447–451.
22. Schwartz DT, Robbins S. Nephralgia due to an aberrant renal capsular vessel: case report. J Urol 1973;109:761–762.
23. Love L, Des Rosier RJ. Angiography of renal agenesis and dysgenesis. AJR 1966;98:137–142.
24. Hynes DM, Watkin EM. Renal agenesis—roentgenologic problem. AJR 1970;110:772–777.
25. Templeton AW, Thompson JM. Aortographic differentiation of congenital and acquired small kidneys. Arch Surg 1968;97: 114–117.
26. Newman L, Simms K, Kissane J, McAlister WH. Unilateral total renal dysplasia in children. AJR 1972;116:778–784.
27. Ericsson NO, Ivemark BJ. Renal dysplasia and pyelonephritis in infants and children: I. Arch Pathol 1958;66:255–263.
28. Ericsson NO, Ivemark BJ. Renal dysplasia and pyelonephritis in infants and children. II. Primitive ductules and abnormal glomeruli. Arch Pathol 1958;66:264–269.
29. Ljungqvist A, Lagergren C. The Ask-Upmark kidney. Acta Pathol Microbiol Scand 1962;56:277–283.
30. Ask-Upmark E. Über juvenile maligne Nephrosklerose und ihr Verhältnis zu Störungen in der Nierenentwicklung. Acta Pathol Microbiol Scand 1929;6:383–445.
31. Adler O, Rosenberger A. Radiologic aspects of Ask-Upmark kidney. ROEFO 1977;126:227–230.
32. Osathanondh V, Potter EL. Pathogenesis of polycystic kidneys: historical survey. Arch Pathol 1964;77:459–465.
33. Ivemark BJ, Lagergren C, Lindvall N. Roentgenologic diagnosis of polycystic kidney and medullary sponge kidney. Acta Radiol 1970;10:225–235.
34. Hatfield PM, Pfister RC. Adult polycystic disease of the kidneys (Potter type 3). JAMA 1972;222:1527–1531.
35. Cho KJ, Thornbury JR, Bernstein J, et al. Localized cystic disease of the kidney: angiographic-pathologic correlation. AJR 1979;132:891–896.
36. Mena E, Bookstein JJ, McDonald FD, Gikas PW. Angiographic findings in renal medullary cystic disease. Radiology 1974;110: 277–281.
37. Meaney TF, Corvalan JG. Angiographic diagnosis of polycystic renal disease. Cleve Clin J Med 1968;35:79–84.
38. Ettinger A, Kahn PC, Wise HM Jr. The importance of selective renal angiography in the diagnosis of polycystic disease. J Urol 1969;102:156–161.
39. Ebel KD, Olbring H. Zur Röntgendiagnostik der polyzystischen Nierendegeneration im Kindesalter. ROEFO 1969; 110:28–38.
40. Ekström T, Engfeldt B, Lagergren C, Lindvall N. Medullary sponge kidney. Stockholm: Almqvist & Wiksell, 1959.
41. Demetropoulos KC, Hoskins P, Rapp R. Angiographic study of hereditary nephritis (Alport's syndrome). Radiology 1973; 108:539–540.
42. Cooperman LR, Lowman RM. Fetal lobulation of the kidney. AJR 1964;92:273–280.
43. King MC, Friedenberg RM, Tena LB. Normal renal parenchyma simulating tumor. Radiology 1968;91:217–222.
44. Felson B, Moskowitz M. Renal pseudotumors: the regenerated nodule and other lumps, bumps and dromedary humps. AJR 1969;107:320–329.
45. Feldman AE, Pollack HM, Perri AJ Jr, et al. Renal pseudotumors: an anatomic-radiologic classification. J Urol 1978;120: 133–139.
46. Charghi H, Dessureault P, Drouin G, et al. Malposition of a renal lobe (lobar dysmorphism): a condition simulating renal tumor. J Urol 1971;105:326.
47. Gooding CA. Childhood renal pseudotumor: a case report. Radiology 1971;98:79–80.
48. Dacie JE. The "central lucency" sign of lobar dysmorphism (pseudotumor of the kidney). Br J Radiol 1976;49:39–42.
49. Kyaw MM, Newman H. Renal pseudotumors due to ectopic accessory renal arteries: the angiographic diagnosis. AJR 1971; 113:443–446.
50. Gittes RF, Talner LB. Congenital megacalices versus obstructive hydronephrosis. J Urol 1972;108:833–836.
51. Kittredge RD, Levin DC. Unusual aspect of renal angiography in ureteric duplication. AJR 1973;119:805–811.
52. Talner LB, Gittes RF. Megacalyces: further observations and differentiation from obstructive renal disease. AJR 1974;131: 473–486.

50

Angiography and Embolization in Renal Trauma

RICHARD G. FISHER
YORAM BEN-MENACHEM

Renal injuries are not uncommon in patients with abdominal trauma. The most frequent presenting clinical sign is hematuria, but the amount of bleeding is usually a poor indicator of the degree of renal injury.[1] In pedicle injuries, hematuria may be absent in over one-third of cases.[2] Imaging is essential for further evaluation in order to stage the degree of injury and plan appropriate therapy. Table 50-1 depicts the classification of acute renal injuries recently developed by the Organ Injury Scaling Committee of the American Association for Surgery of Trauma.[1] Some traditionalists continue to advocate liberal use of excretory urography in emergency room facilities.[1] Others, including the authors, recommend bypassing this and proceeding directly to a more informative evaluation with computed tomography (CT) in stable patients and angiography in unstable patients while reserving urography for patients going directly to emergency surgery.[3] Fortunately, the majority of renal artery injuries are minor (75–80 percent) and represent contusions or superficial lacerations that can be managed conservatively. Major renal injuries (grade V) are uncommon (5 percent) and are usually surgical emergencies. The remaining 10 percent are generally serious injuries,[4] and it is here that interventional radiologists can play a significant role. Furthermore, the current trend toward more conservative (nonsurgical) management of renal trauma[1] may increase the use of interventional techniques.

Mechanism of Injury

The traditional division of renal injuries into blunt or penetrating has some descriptive shortcomings, and we prefer to categorize trauma as wide impact or tract injuries and narrow tract injuries.

Wide Impact or Tract Injuries

Injuries by street trauma, firearms, or surgery can potentially damage a broad volume or "wide tract" in the kidney or even involve its entire volume. Superficial or deep lacerations with intrarenal or perinephric hematomas or even renal rupture can occur. Wide tract blunt trauma, as in deceleration, can result in avulsion of main renal arteries or intimal disruption. Because the kidneys are relatively mobile, the more securely anchored vessels are stretched to the point of injury.[5] Wide tract injuries may need debridement, particularly in higher-category injuries, as indicated in Table 50-1 and Figure 50-1, and unstable patients may therefore go directly to the operating theater. A few may have an overriding indication for emergent angiography and embolization as a primary mode of treatment before or even in the place of surgery (Fig. 50-2).[6] Most stable patients, however, should be evaluated with CT for staging before further clinical decisions regarding conservative versus surgical management. Interventional procedures may be applicable at this time as well as in the postoperative patient with persistent or recurrent hematuria.[6–9]

Narrow Tract Injuries

Injuries from street assaults, biopsies, and nephrostomies predictably leave a more narrow, sharply defined residual wound tract. The potential for arterial injury is very high, especially with street assaults, and there is a propensity for false aneurysm formation with or without an associated arterial venous fistula.[6,10,11] Typically patients have persistent gross hematuria, severe enough in some to cause shock. The surgical evaluation of a narrow wound tract has its limitations because it does not allow proper assessment of the depth of the injury. The exact location of vessel damage is

Table 50-1. Angiography and Embolotherapy of Renal Artery Injuries: Renal Injury Scale[a]

Grade[b]		Injury Description[c]
I.	Contusion	Microscopic or gross hematuria; urologic studies normal
	Hematoma	Subcapsular, nonexpanding without parenchymal laceration
II.	Hematoma	Nonexpanding perirenal hematoma confined to renal retroperitoneum
	Laceration	<1.0-cm parenchymal depth of renal cortex without urinary extravasation
III.	Laceration	>1.0-cm parenchymal depth of renal cortex with collecting system rupture or urinary extravasation
IV.	Laceration	Parenchymal laceration extending through the renal cortex, medulla, and collection system
	Vascular	Main renal artery or vein injury with contained hemorrhage
V.	Laceration	Completely shattered kidney
	Vascular	Avulsion of renal hilum which devascularizes kidney

[a]This classification scheme for acute renal injuries has been devised by the Organ Injury Scaling Committee of the American Association for Surgery of Trauma. (From McAnich JW. Genitourinary trauma. In: Moore EE, Mattox KL, Feliciano DV, eds. Trauma. 2nd ed. Norwalk: Appleton & Lange, 1991: 575. Used with permission.)
[b]Advance one grade for multiple injuries to the same organ.
[c]Based on most accurate assessment at autopsy, laparotomy, or radiologic study.

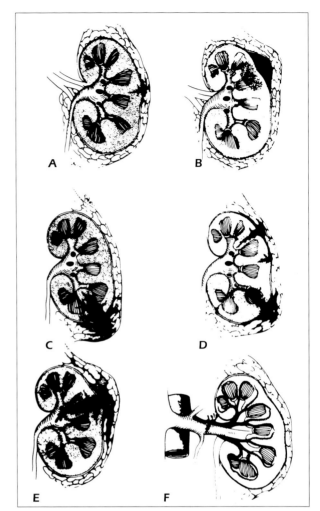

Figure 50-1. Renal injury classification. (A and B) Minor injuries: superficial lacerations, subcapsular hematomas, and contusions. (C to E) Major parenchymal injuries: extended deep into the medulla and/or the collecting system, causing extravasation. (F) Vascular injuries: involve the central renal artery and vein. (From McAnich JW. Genitourinary trauma. In: Moore EE, Mattox KL, Feliciano DV, eds. Trauma. 2nd ed. Norwalk: Appleton & Lange, 1991: 576. Used with permission.)

best determined with angiography except in those cases with penetrating vascular pedicle injuries, which require immediate surgical control.[1] CT assessment for narrow tract penetrating trauma can be helpful, but direct angiographic evaluation is more likely to be definitive and also provides the route for therapy.

Renal vascular injuries from biopsy or nephrostomy may be destabilizing, requiring immediate angiographic diagnosis and prompt treatment.[12] However, most heal spontaneously. If hematuria should persist for 2 to 3 days, angiographic investigation and possible embolization are warranted.[10,13] On the other hand, a few injuries may remain clinically silent and present with hematuria and/or hypertension months to years later as the result of an undiagnosed arteriovenous fistula (AVF).[4]

An additional iatrogenic injury that somewhat defies classification is vessel occlusion or rupture due to angioplasty. Fortunately, this is an uncommon complication and one that generally requires immediate surgical intervention. However, there is at least one instance of successful management of an angioplasty-induced renal artery rupture using a balloon occlusion catheter (Medi-Tech).[14]

Angiographic Evaluation

Renal Arterial Injuries

A variety of arterial injuries can result from trauma, including main renal artery intimal disruption (Fig. 50-3) or avulsion (Fig. 50-4), renal artery branch transection without (Fig. 50-5) or with extravasation (Fig. 50-6), false aneurysm formation (Fig. 50-7), and AVF with (Fig. 50-8) or without (Fig. 50-9) a recognizable false aneurysm. Multiple injuries are also possible (Fig. 50-10).

Text continues on page 1236

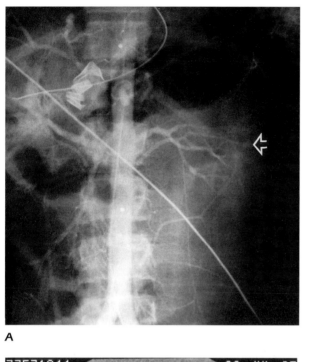

A

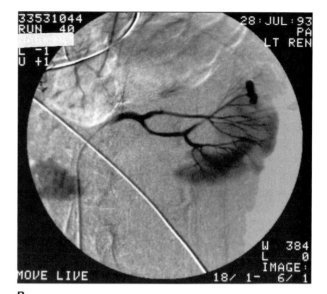

B

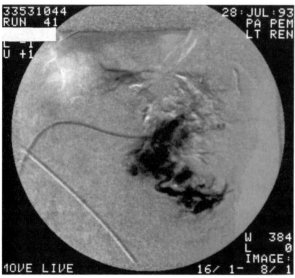

C

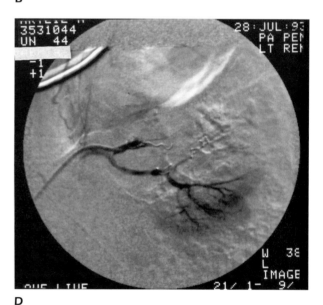

D

Figure 50-2. Sixteen-year-old boy who fell 50 feet from a bridge. CT revealed a large left retroperitoneal hematoma. A trauma angiographic survey (arch, abdomen, pelvis) revealed an intact aortic arch and normal pelvic vessels. (A) Abdominal aortogram demonstrates two left renal arteries and a subtle false aneurysm in the left upper pole (*arrow*).

(B) Selection of the upper renal artery shows the false aneurysm arising from a branch vessel. (C) Subselection and hand injection produced massive extravasation (not uncommon in the authors' experience with trauma patients). (D) This was promptly controlled with embolization with two Gelfoam strips and five 3-mm, 2-cm-long steel coils.

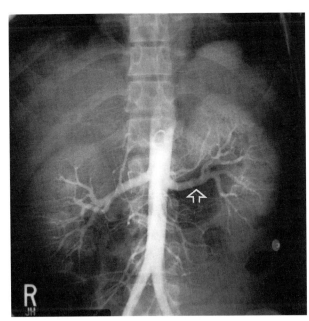

Figure 50-3. Thirty-one-year-old man who jumped from the fifth floor of a building while fleeing an assailant and suffered multiple fractures of the lower extremities. An abdominal aortogram revealed a subtle intimal tear in the left renal artery (*arrow*). Follow-up angiography 11 days later showed persistence of the intimal tear, which was then surgically repaired.

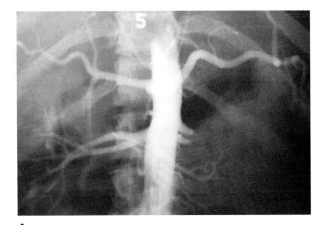

A

B

Figure 50-4. Twenty-year-old motor vehicle accident victim with hemoperitoneum as determined by peritoneal lavage. Aortography revealed (A) an unexpected left pedicle injury with amputation of duplicate renal arteries and (B) extravasation in the spleen (*arrows*) indicative of splenic rupture. Both injuries were repaired surgically.

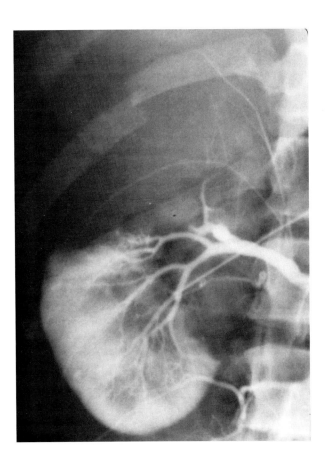

Figure 50-5. Twenty-one-year-old man who was involved in an auto–pedestrian accident and had gross hematuria. Selective right renal arteriogram demonstrates a major branch transection with devascularization of over half of the kidney.

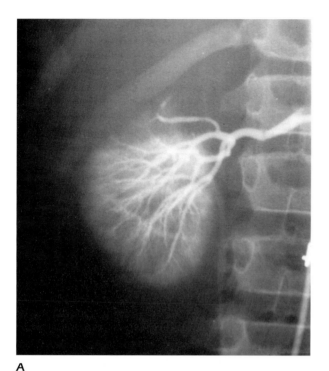

A

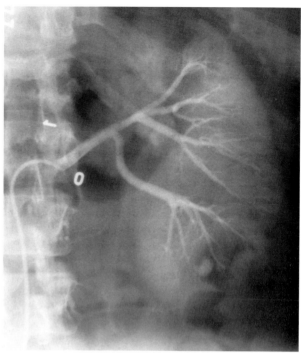

Figure 50-7. Fifty-one-year-old woman with persistent hematuria following percutaneous renal biopsy. Selective left renal arteriography shows a false aneurysm in the lower pole.

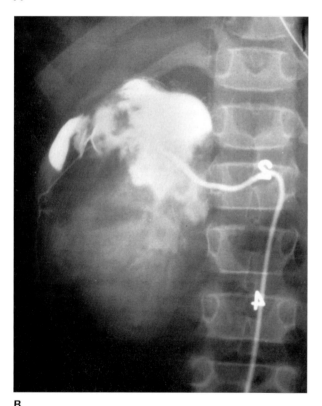

B

Figure 50-6. Ten-year-old boy with a history of blunt trauma to the abdomen. (A) Selective right renal arteriogram displays occlusion of a segmental artery branch and no opacification of the upper pole. (B) Selection of an additional vessel just above the right renal artery, presumed to be an accessory renal artery. The injection "blew out" the clot in this lacerated vessel, and major extravasation occurred. (This artery did not fill on prior aortography.) Emergency heminephrectomy was done (preembolization era).

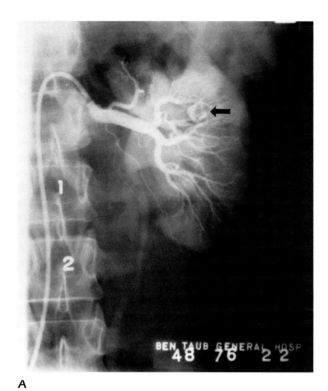

A

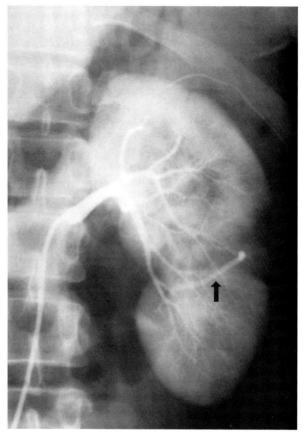

Figure 50-9. Thirty-four-year-old man with a history of blunt trauma. Selective left renal arteriogram shows a defect across the lower kidney representing a laceration and an associated AVF (*arrow*).

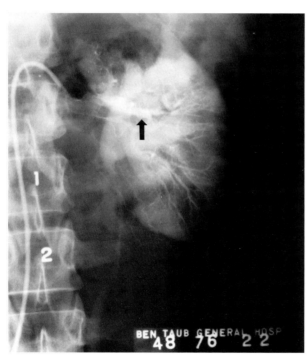

B

Figure 50-8. Twenty-four-year-old man with a history of a stab wound to the left flank. Selective left renal arteriography displays (A) a false aneurysm (*arrow*) in the upper kidney and (B) an associated AVF (*arrow*).

Figure 50-10. Thirty-two-year-old man who was a victim of a bicycle–auto accident. Aortography reveals bilateral circumferential renal artery intimal injuries (*arrows*). These were repaired surgically with primary anastomosis being done on either side.

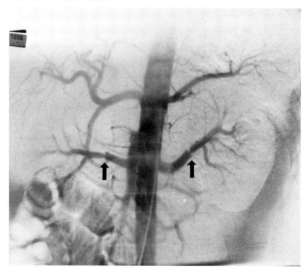

The angiographic evaluation of renal vascular injuries typically begins with an abdominal aortogram, usually by way of a femoral artery approach, to assess the location and number of renal arteries and to determine the presence or absence of main renal artery injuries (Fig. 50-11; see also Fig. 50-4). This may also demonstrate intrarenal lesions (Fig. 50-12), but selective arteriography is necessary for a more exact localization and potential embolization (Fig. 50-13). The authors generally prefer the cut-film technique for survey aortographic and selective imaging, reserving the more expedient but less detailed digital imaging for guidance during subselective angiography and/or embolization.

A variety of catheter shapes (cobras, double renal curves, Simmons, etc.) (Cook, Inc.) are available for use, as well as a selection of guidewires (J's, movable cores, Benson, etc.) (Cook, Inc.). More recently, hydrophilic "slippery" guidewires (Medi-Tech) have greatly assisted selective techniques, and coaxial catheter systems have been particularly helpful in difficult subselection circumstances.[15]

Timing of Angiography and Embolization

Angiography is valuable in both narrow and wide tract injuries for definitive diagnosis. In wide tract blunt trauma, prompt and accurate diagnosis of main renal artery injuries is essential. A high index of suspicion

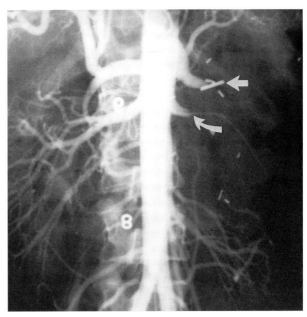

Figure 50-11. Twenty-eight-year-old woman who was involved in a severe motor vehicle accident. Aortography demonstrates surgical amputation of the splenic artery (*straight arrow*) and left renal artery (*curved arrow*), with the latter representing a typical pedicle injury (not appreciated during surgery).

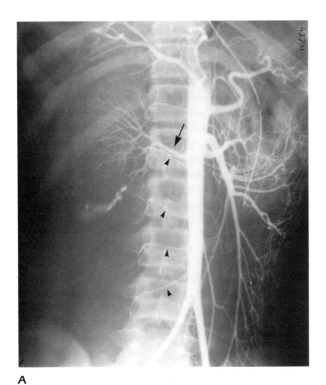

A

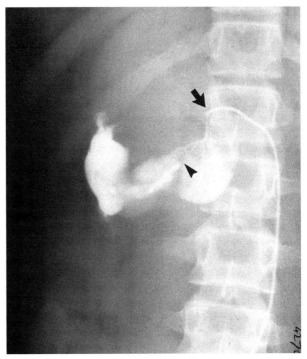

B

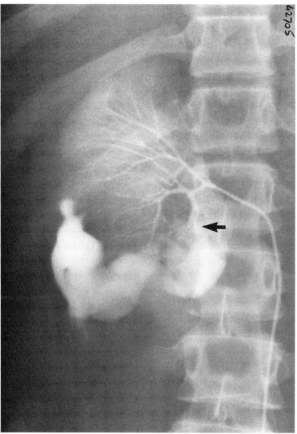

C

Figure 50-12. Thirty-five-year-old man who hemorrhaged following a right kidney biopsy. Hemorrhage continued despite multiple transfusions. Ultimately arteriography and embolization were requested. (A) An abdominal aortogram demonstrates intrarenal hemorrhage and marked displacement of the liver, bowel, and aorta by a huge hematoma with stretching of the renal artery (*arrow*) and lumbar arteries (*arrowheads*). (B) Selection of the bleeding branch (*large arrow*) was hampered by the distorted anatomy but ultimately showed marked extravasation (*arrowhead*). (C) Follow-up renal arteriogram shows the vessel occluded with a single Gelfoam plug (*arrow*). Extravasation from preembolization injection is still visible. (From Fisher RG, Ben-Menachem Y, Whigham C. Stab wounds of the renal artery branches: angiographic diagnosis and treatment by embolization. AJR 1989;152:1231–1235. Used with permission.)

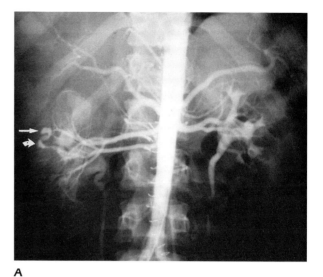

A

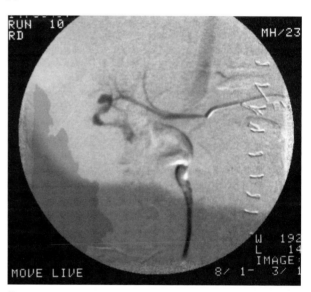

B

Figure 50-13. Twenty-three-year-old man who was stabbed in the left flank. (A) Abdominal aortogram shows duplicate right renal arteries, a false aneurysm (*straight arrow*), and an AVF (*curved arrow*). (B) Selective renal arteriography documents that the false aneurysm and AVF arise from the upper right renal artery. Note the opacification of the inferior vena cava. (From Fisher RG, Ben-Menachem Y, Whigham C. Stab wounds of the renal artery branches: angiographic diagnosis and treatment by embolization. AJR 1989;152:1231–1235. Used with permission.)

and aggressive investigation with angiography are necessary for early diagnosis and subsequent expedient surgery to obtain maximum preservation of renal tissue.[5] If renal ischemia persists for 3 hours or more, it is likely to result in severe tubular necrosis and dysfunction.[1] Unfortunately, some of these injuries can be relatively silent clinically and may therefore escape early detection (Fig. 50-14). They may also be overlooked during emergency celiotomy for other solid

visceral intraperitoneal injuries unless they are suspected clinically and/or demonstrated angiographically before surgery. The authors have personal experience with at least three cases in which renal artery injuries were not recognized during surgery (see Fig. 50-11).

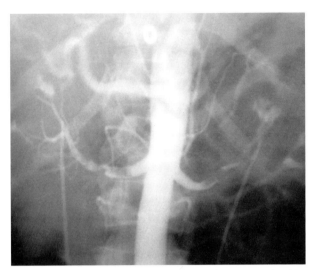

Figure 50-14. Forty-five-year-old man who was involved in an auto–pedestrian accident in 1976. The initial emergency room evaluation was considered unremarkable. The patient returned 3 days later with a history of back pain, left upper quadrant pain, and oliguria. Peritoneal lavage was "positive" for blood, and a splenectomy was done. Bilateral retrograde pyelograms were done seeking bilateral ureteral injuries and were normal. A subsequent aortogram revealed bilateral renal artery injuries with associated intraluminal clot and partial occlusion of both renal arteries.

Embolotherapy is more likely to be used in the treatment of narrow tract vascular injuries. Patient stability and the absence of suspected concomitant bowel injury are essential considerations in selecting patients for interventional management. However, emergency angiography and embolization could potentially stabilize a patient with poorly controlled shock and decrease the risk of subsequent exploratory surgery. In the authors' opinion, interventional procedures should be encouraged as a viable alternative to surgery in selected patients (Fig. 50-15), particularly in those with narrow tract street trauma,[11] since most reported cases of successful embolization of these specific injuries have been in patients in which surgery had failed to achieve permanent hemostasis.[10,11] Alternatively, most injuries resulting from biopsy or nephrostomy have been treated primarily with embolization, thus avoiding surgery.[10,13,15] However, these injuries tend to be less urgent and typically involve only the kidney. Furthermore, hemorrhage from renal biopsies may only be pursued after 2 to 3 days of persistent or recurrent hematuria because most stop bleeding spontaneously.

Figure 50-15. Fifty-four-year-old man with a history of blunt trauma to the abdomen. CT showed a laceration of the spleen and a laceration of the left kidney. (A) Selective left renal arteriography revealed a large false aneurysm (*arrow*) and a cortical defect from the laceration. The renal artery branch feeding the false aneurysm was subselected, and the false aneurysm was embolized with Gelfoam strips (torpedoes). (B) Postembolization arteriogram shows absence of the false aneurysm and of the large feeding artery.

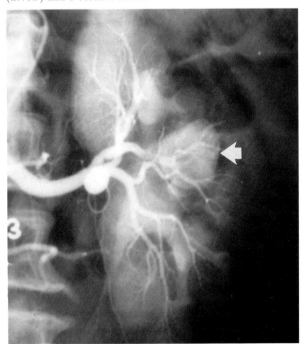

A

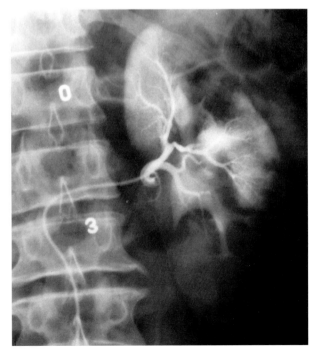

B

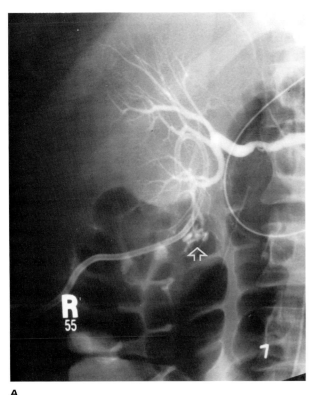

A

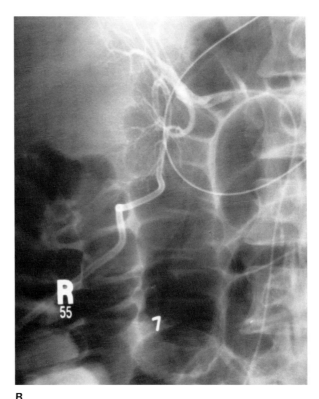

B

Figure 50-16. Forty-five-year-old man with a history of bilateral nephrostomy tube placement to relieve bilateral ureteral obstruction. Forty-eight hours later the patient's hematocrit dropped significantly, and CT demonstrated a large right perirenal hematoma. (A) Selective right renal arteriogram reveals extravasation of contrast material (*arrow*) in the lower pole indicative of active hemorrhage. The bleeding branch was selected and embolized with Gelfoam strips (torpedoes). (B) Postembolization arteriogram shows no further extravasation.

Embolization

Indications

The criteria for embolization begin with clinical findings of posttraumatic hematuria and/or a dropping hematocrit or the demonstrated presence of a large intrarenal or perinephric hematoma by CT. As indicated earlier, patients must be sufficiently stable to permit an angiographic investigation. Extravasation (Fig. 50-16), false aneurysms (see Fig. 50-2), AVFs (Fig. 50-17), and arterial caliceal fistulas (Fig. 50-18), occurring individually or in combination, are potentially controllable with embolization.[6,7,10,11] On occasion, one also may consider empirically embolizing a large transected renal artery branch to avoid a future unexpected hemorrhage that may require management in less controlled circumstances.

Techniques

Specific selection of the injured renal artery branch is ideal before embolizations because some degree of renal infarction usually occurs.[6] Occasionally this is not technically possible and embolization particles or objects may be "flow-directed" to the lesion (Fig. 50-19).[10]

Gelfoam has been used most commonly for embolization because of its utility (one can shape different-size particles quickly) and its absorbability. Larger vessel injuries or fast-flowing AVFs require a more aggressive approach, necessitating the use of steel coils (Cook, Inc.)[6,10] or detachable balloons[9] for occlusion (see Figs. 50-2, 50-17, and 50-19).

Alternatively, the use of coaxial catheter systems for precise subselection and embolization of peripheral lesions with microcoils or small Gelfoam particles has been recently demonstrated.[15]

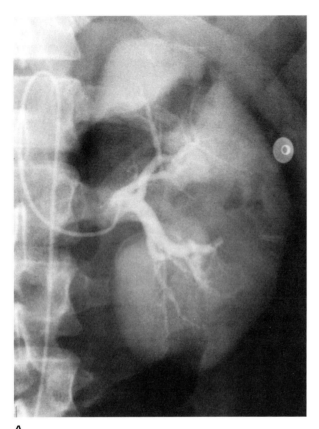

A

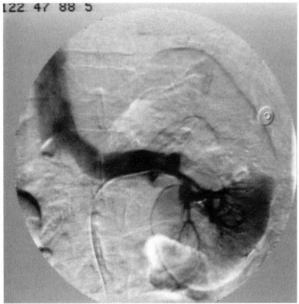

B

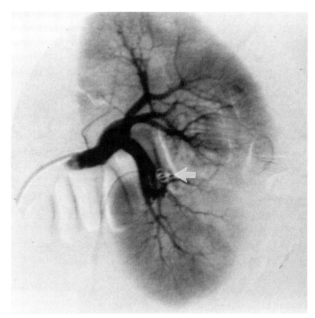

C

Figure 50-17. Twenty-one-year-old man with a history of multiple stab wounds. Exploratory laparotomy was done. In addition to other repairs, a left renal laceration was oversewn. Four weeks later he developed gross hematuria. An intravenous pyelogram revealed a large blood cast in the left renal pelvis. (A) Selective left renal arteriography does not show an obvious abnormality, but an AVF was suspected during fluoroscopically guided test injections. (B) Subselective digital arteriogram shows a large, fast-flowing AVF arising from the lower pole. (C) Renal arteriogram following occlusion with a single 3-mm steel coil (*arrow*) shows absence of the AVF and relatively normal renal vascular anatomy. (From Fisher RG, Ben-Menachem Y, Whigham C. Stab wounds of the renal artery branches: angiographic diagnosis and treatment by embolization. AJR 1989;152:1231–1235. Used with permission.)

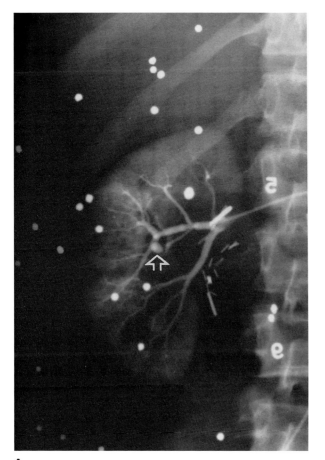

A

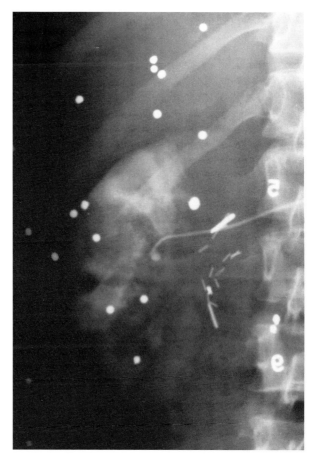

B

Figure 50-18. Twenty-seven-year-old man with a history of shotgun injury to the abdomen. Exploratory laparotomy discovered multiple colon and right renal puncture wounds. A segment of colon was resected, and the renal punctures were oversewn. Four days later the patient developed gross hematuria, and (A) selective right renal arteriography showed a small false aneurysm arising from a segmental artery (*arrow*). Test injections during fluoroscopy showed immediate but transient opacification of the calices, indicating an arterial caliceal fistula. (B) The catheter was positioned immediately adjacent to the false aneurysm, and a 3-mm stainless steel coil was introduced and conveniently coiled in the false aneurysm, occluding it. (C) Follow-up of renal arteriogram shows the coil (*arrow*) and no false aneurysm. Bleeding ceased. (From Fisher RG, Ben-Menachem Y. Embolization procedures in trauma: the abdomen—extraperitoneal. Semin Intervent Radiol 1985;2:148–157. Used with permission.)

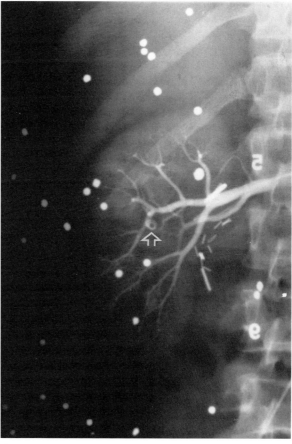

C

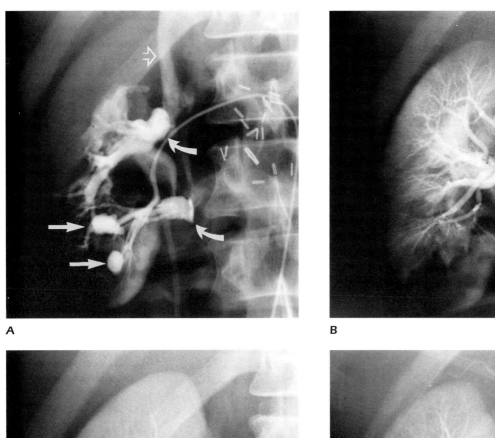

A

B

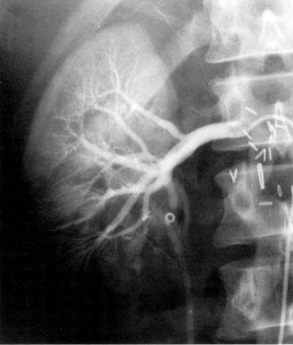

C

D

Figure 50-19. Thirty-year-old man who was stabbed in the right flank, sustaining injuries to the duodenum and the right kidney. Both were repaired surgically, and 5 days later the patient developed gross hematuria. (A) A difficult subselective arteriogram of the right lower renal artery vessels shows two large false aneurysms (*straight arrows*) in the lower pole and two large AVFs (*curved arrows*) with opacification of the inferior vena cava (*hollow arrow*). (B) Renal arteriogram following embolization with large Gelfoam torpedoes shows occlusion of the lower pole branch, the false aneurysms, and the AVFs. Three days later (8 days after the operation), the patient began to develop gross hematuria. (C) Repeat right renal arteriogram shows a recurrent, large, multilobulated false aneurysm. Repeat selection of the injured artery was not successful. Flow-directed Gelfoam embolization was ineffective. (D) A single 3-mm steel coil was then inserted which flow-directed to the injured branch, occluding it and the false aneurysm. No further bleeding occurred.

Successes and Failures

In most reported larger series, embolization was successful in all cases.[4,7,10,15] Heyns and van Vollenhoven[11] were also successful in 9 of 11 patients with renal branch injuries from street stabbings. Hemorrhage recurred in 2, 1 of which was successfully controlled with reembolization. A heminephrectomy was necessary in the other. They also described a patient with a giant AVF diagnosed 18 months after the injury that was considered too large to be safely embolized.

A delay in diagnosis can also complicate angiography and embolization. Deformity of the kidney by a large intrarenal hematoma can occur with stretching of vessels, which in turn may prevent subselection and necessitate a more proximal embolization with more tissue loss due to infarction (see Fig. 50-12).[3]

Complications

Potential complications of renal embolotherapy include those at the puncture site, such as hemorrhage or potential vessel occlusion.[4] "Reactions" to the contrast material may also occur but are uncommon with intraarterial injections. Perhaps of greatest concern is nontarget embolization,[4] with materials inadvertently distributing to alternate areas of the kidney or to other locations "downstream" in the aorta. Furthermore, the actual placement of steel coils may displace the catheter and result in a more central occlusion, producing a larger area of infarction.[10] Postembolic hypertension, although feared, is uncommon and will generally be self-limiting even with large-volume infarctions.[10] Postembolic infection has not been a factor, but application of good sterile technique continues to be essential in any embolization procedure. Finally, the postembolization infarction syndrome (pain, leukocytosis, and transient low-grade fever) is also, fortunately, uncommon.[4]

References

1. McAnich JW. Genitourinary trauma. In: Moore EE, Mattox KL, Feliciano DV, eds. Trauma. 2nd ed. Norwalk: Appleton & Lange, 1991:571–586.
2. Ivatury RA, Zubowski R, Stahl WM. Penetrating renal vascular trauma. J Trauma 1989;29:1620–1623.
3. Ben-Menachem Y. Bleeding from trauma. In: Dondelinger RF, Rossi P, Kurdziel JC, Wallace S, eds. Interventional radiology. Stuttgart: George Thieme Verlag, 1990:378–395.
4. Larsen DW, Pentecost MJ. Embolotherapy in renal trauma. Semin Intervent Radiol 1992;9:13–18.
5. Tisnado J, Bezirdjian DR. Angiographic evaluation of main renal artery injury secondary to blunt trauma. Semin Intervent Radiol 1990;7:93–107.
6. Sclafani SJA, Ben-Menachem Y. Embolotherapy in abdominal trauma. In: Neal MP Jr, Tisnado J, Cho S, eds. Emergency interventional radiology. Boston: Little, Brown, 1989:53–77.
7. Fisher RG, Ben-Menachem Y. Embolization procedures in trauma: the abdomen—extraperitoneal. Sem Intervent Radiol 1985;2:148–157.
8. Pilla TJ, Tantana S, Shields JB. Cardiovascular interventional radiology. 1987;10:153–156.
9. Teigen CL, Venbrux AC, Quinlan DV, Jeffs RD. Late massive hematuria as a complication of conservative management of blunt renal trauma in children. J Urol 1992;147:1333–1336.
10. Fisher RG, Ben-Menachem Y, Whigham C. Stab wounds of the renal artery branches: angiographic diagnosis and treatment by embolization. AJR 1989;152:1231–1235.
11. Heyns CF, van Vollenhoven P. Increasing role of angiography in segmental artery embolization in the management of renal stab wounds. J Urol 1992;147:1231–1234.
12. Low RN, Brooke-Jeffrey R Jr. Intraperitoneal hemorrhage after renal biopsy: a great prognostic sign. AJR 1988;151:113–114.
13. Cope C, Zeit RM. Pseudoaneurysms after nephrostomy. AJR 1982;139:255–261.
14. Ashenburg RG, Blair RJ, Rivera FJ, Weigele JB. Renal arterial rupture complicating transluminal angioplasty: successful conservative management. Radiology 1990;174:983–985.
15. DeSouza NM, Reidy JF, Koffman CJ. Arterial venous fistulas complicating biopsy of renal allografts: treatment of bleeding with super selective embolization. AJR 1991;156:507–510.

51

Renal Arteriography in Hypertension

HERBERT L. ABRAMS
CLEMENT J. GRASSI

Renal arteriography has clarified many of the underlying renal vascular changes in patients with hypertension and is considered to be a "gold standard" for the identification of patients with renovascular disease. The primary focus of this chapter is on renovascular hypertension; the chapter also reviews the alterations found in essential and malignant hypertension and in several other renal lesions associated with high blood pressure.

The relationship between hypertension and renal disease, suspected for many decades, was established by Goldblatt et al.'s report in 1933 that dogs subjected to nephrectomy and narrowing of the contralateral renal artery developed significant elevation of the blood pressure.[1] The renin-angiotensin system, studied for many years, has progressively been elucidated, with understanding of its precise role in the hypertension associated with unilateral renal arterial disease in humans. What is clearly known is that renin acts on renin substrate to produce angiotensin I, which is metabolized by converting enzyme to angiotensin II in the lungs and other organs. Angiotensin II raises blood pressure, both because of its direct vasoconstrictive effect and because it stimulates aldosterone production by the adrenal cortex. Aldosterone, in turn, raises blood pressure by increasing sodium reabsorption, with resultant elevation of blood volume.

It has been well established that unilateral elevation of renal venous renin activity is associated with a high likelihood of cure of hypertension when renal artery stenosis is present.[2] In the past, the enthusiasm for surgery for all patients with hypertension and demonstrated renal arterial disease has waxed and waned. The morbidity and mortality associated with such surgery are recognized, and investigators have provided unequivocal evidence that renal artery stenosis per se need not cause hypertension. In arteriographic studies of normotensive and hypertensive adults, Eyler et al. found all types of major renal arterial stenosis in both the normotensive and the hypertensive groups.[3] Holley demonstrated that renal artery stenosis was present at autopsy in a significant percentage of patients who had been normotensive during life.[4] Except on rare occasions, therefore, the arteriogram should not be the sole determinant of whether an intervention is undertaken: supporting physiologic data and renin assays are essential, particularly in regard to patients whose hypertension can be controlled on drug therapy without important side effects. Nevertheless, renal arteriography is indicated for all patients under the age of 35 who have persistent hypertension even if the hypertension is controlled by medication. Today, in addition to surgery, balloon angioplasty and renal artery stenting can be offered as effective therapy.[5–8]

The incidence of renovascular hypertension (RVH) in the general population is approximately 1 percent[9]; however, it is higher at referral centers, varying 4.3 to 33.0 percent.[10] This discrepancy is due, at least in part, to the prior absence of a generally accepted definition of the disease. For some the definition is arteriographic; for others, functional. Although a significant number of stenotic arterial lesions are found in hypertensive patients, renovascular disease can be found in 32 to 49 percent of normotensive elderly patients with atherosclerosis.[3,4] Historically, the test of a purely renal etiology rested on one parameter: diastolic normotension 1 year after surgery in the patient with previously established diastolic hypertension. Such a definition was by no means inclusive: it did not account for individuals with operable lesions in whom reconstructive vascular surgery was technically inadequate, and it excluded patients with a significant lesion whose kidneys are the site of small-vessel disease so profound as to preclude any benefit from intervention. Today, the diagnosis of RVH can be made only after normalization of blood pressure after nephrectomy or after reestablishment of renal blood flow by surgery, angioplasty, or arterial stenting.

Angiography is the most precise method of demonstrating renal artery anatomy and the presence of stenosis of the renal artery or its branches before therapy. Although arteriography is sometimes less than 100 percent reliable in assessing the significance of such a lesion, it is a necessary preliminary to any more intensive search to define treatable patients. In addition, captopril renal scintigraphy has been an important advance in the detection of RVH patients following work by Majd et al.[11]

This chapter includes the findings from an analysis of 340 arteriograms in hypertensive patients.[12] An additional 250 arteriograms of hypertensive patients have been reviewed. Xenon washout studies on many of these patients have permitted a comparison of flow studies with the appearance of the renal vascular bed.

Normal Renal Arteriogram

The position of the kidney is variable. In adults in the supine position, the upper pole is at the T12 vertebra and the lower pole is at T3. The kidney drops about one vertebral body when the upright position is assumed[13]; it is not unusual to have considerably more mobility, especially in women. A useful centering point for the examination is a point halfway between the umbilicus and the xiphoid process. Usually the central ray will be just under the origin of the renal arteries.

The renal arteries, although described as dorsal branches, are usually lateral in origin and arise from the aorta at, slightly above, or slightly below the interspace between L1 and L2 (Figs. 51-1 and 51-2) (see Chapter 45). Seventy-two percent of cadavers have single vessels bilaterally of approximately equal size.[14] The right renal artery may originate slightly anterior to the coronal plane. The inferior supplemental branches tend to originate somewhat anteriorly, especially on the right.

Occasionally the single main renal artery arises as high as the inferior aspect of T12 and as low as L2. The right renal artery may be either slightly higher or slightly lower than the left renal artery. This is in contrast to the usually lower position of the right kidney. The right renal artery generally follows a somewhat more caudal course than the left.

Accessory renal vessels pose a problem on selective angiography because they are time-consuming to find and to film, and, if they are small, they may easily be obstructed by the catheter tip. Their range of origin is wide, from T11 down to the iliac vessels (see Figs.

Figure 51-1. Normal renal arteriogram. (A) Expiration. The vessels arborize normally. There is minimal irregularity of the right renal artery. (B) Valsalva maneuver. The kidneys are now far more caudal than during the initial study. The renal arteries are stretched and uncoiled. The minimal fibromuscular hyperplasia of the right renal artery is of no dynamic significance. Split-function studies demonstrated equivalent renal plasma flows on both sides.

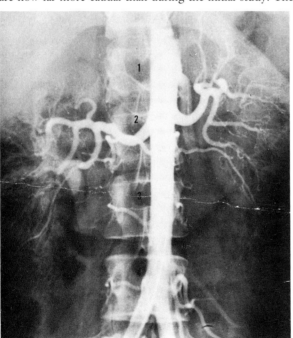

A

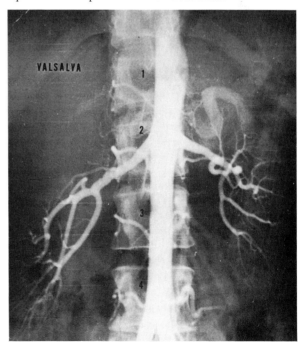

B

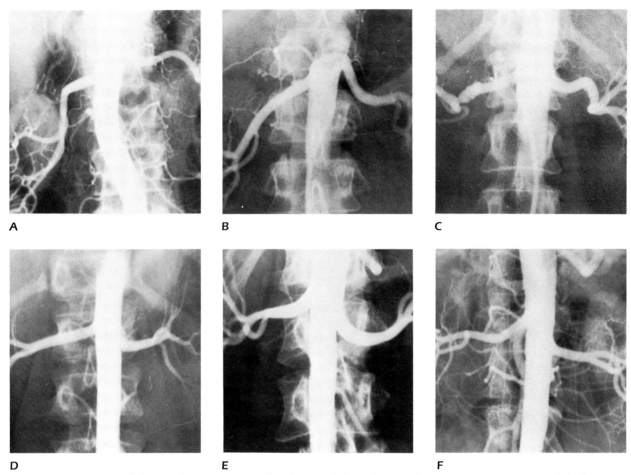

Figure 51-2. Origin of the renal arteries. Normally, the right renal artery arises at a level somewhat lower than the left, and the right kidney is more caudal. The position is variable, however, and it is essential that these variations in anatomy be fully understood. (A and B) A higher origin of the left renal artery, the more common situation. (C) The origin of both right and left arteries at the same level. (D to F) A more caudal origin of the left renal artery than of the right renal artery. In (E) and (F), the left kidney is lower than the right kidney, in contrast to the usual situation.

51-2, 51-21, and 51-29). Rarely, accessory branches arise from visceral aortic branches.[15]

The kidney may be divided into dorsal and ventral segments, and the arteries to these segments may be identified. Graves divides the kidney into five segments, recognizing two anterior and one posterior position in the middle of the kidney, a small apical segment, and a larger caudal segment.[16] The orientation of the kidney is such that the dorsal arteries are medial and the dorsal segments and subsegments are not border-forming at the lateral margin of the kidney in the true anteroposterior projection.[17] The ventral arteries are lateral, and the ventral subsegments are border-forming along the lateral aspect of the kidney. The lower pole is usually supplied by the ventral vessel, and the dorsal vessel extends cephalad to supply a variable part of the superior pole.

A careful analysis of the normal arborization of distal renal vessels demonstrates a reproducible, even, and regular progression to smaller and smaller vessels that have a straight or mildly curved course. Normal vessels taper uniformly and evenly (Figs. 51-3 and 51-4). The interlobar arteries branch repeatedly until they give rise to the arcuate arteries. The interlobular arteries of the cortex arise from the arcuate vessels, extend into the cortex in a more or less parallel fashion (see Fig. 51-4), and may be defined with good-quality magnification angiography.[18] As the cortex opacifies, it develops a granular pattern, thought to be produced by overlapping glomeruli.[18]

In general, the nephrogram reflects the volume of flow to the kidney and is well visualized within a few seconds after injection. With catheter injection into the abdominal aorta, however, the nephrogram frequently may reflect laminar flow rather than the total mixing of the contrast agent. Under these circum-

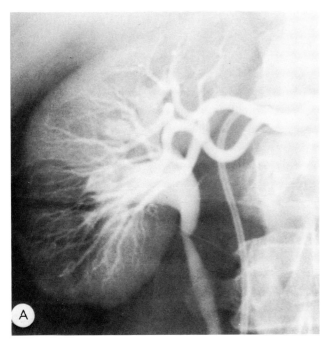

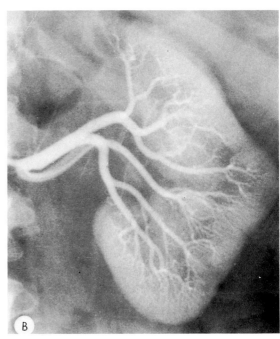

Figure 51-3. Normal selective renal arteriogram. (A) Right kidney. The cortex is well defined in the upper pole. There is an even, regular progression to smaller vessels, which have a straight or a mildly curved course. The tapering is uniform. (B) Left kidney. The catheter tip has been placed beyond the bifurcation of the main renal artery. As a consequence, there has been only flash filling of the dorsal renal arterial branch; the ventral renal artery is well filled. The artifactual lack of opacification of the central medial portion of the kidney and the upper pole might have been interpreted as representing a large area of infarction.

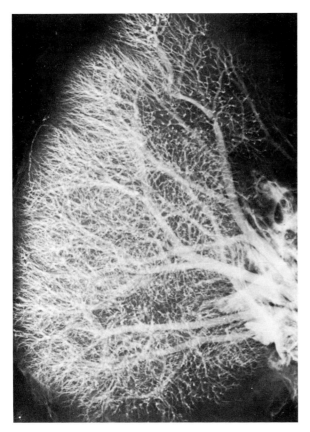

A

Figure 51-4. Normal renal vascular bed. (A) An injected specimen at autopsy. Note the progressive gradual tapering of the vessels and the multiple interlobular branches that arise from the arcuate arteries to enter the cortex of the kidney. (B) Diagrammatic representation of the renal arteries.

stances, a diminished nephrogram may be found in the absence of renal artery stenosis, and a relatively augmented nephrogram may be found in its presence. During the nephrographic phase, contrast material is present in the capillaries and in the renal excretory tissue. There is a general increase in density, although the cortex is usually well defined—and its width measurable—as a dense, homogeneous band around the kidney that is about 5 to 8 mm thick. The nephrogram is most useful when it demonstrates a local area of ischemia (see Figs. 51-21, 51-22, and 51-30). Normally, the contrast-filled arteries have a smooth, even appearance throughout their course (see Fig. 51-2). Occasionally during aortography or selective arteriography, "standing waves" may be observed—regular, periodic, localized, symmetric indentations of the vessel wall thought to be caused by spasm (Fig. 51-5). Standing waves are important because they may be mistaken for dysplastic disease of the renal artery.

Another important finding to be recognized and understood is renal spasm during angiography (Fig. 51-6). Various types of spasm are visible: (1) concentric short-segment stenosis, which may resemble fixed stenosis; (2) long-segment fusiform narrowing; and (3) multiple small perfusion defects during the nephrographic phase of the angiogram, suggestive of renal parenchymal disease (see Fig. 51-6B and C).[19] Such confusing appearances may be better evaluated after the use of acetylcholine, which eliminates them, or sometimes simply by abdominal aortography without a selective study.

Renovascular Hypertension

Diagnosis

Perhaps the most important single clinical reference point is the patient's age: renovascular hypertension is frequently a disease of young adults. On *physical examination,* aside from high blood pressure and, at times, cardiac enlargement and ocular examination changes, the most conspicuous finding may be a bruit in the epigastrium. Although it has been claimed that bruits are heard in a high percentage of patients with renovascular hypertension, the figures are variable. In the presence of stenosis above 50 percent, bruits are ab-

Figure 51-5. Standing waves in the renal arteries. (A) Main renal artery. Multiple serrated indentations are visible in the main renal artery (*arrow*), symmetrically distributed and at evenly spaced intervals. They have the characteristic appearance of "standing waves"; these have no pathologic significance and may represent a form of spasm. (B) Main and branch renal arteries. The standing waves in this patient extend from the main renal artery (*arrow, right*) to multiple interlobar branches (*arrows, left*) within the kidney. The appearance is characteristic of standing waves.

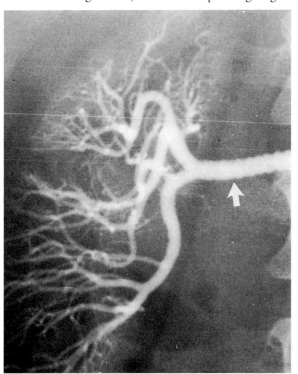

A

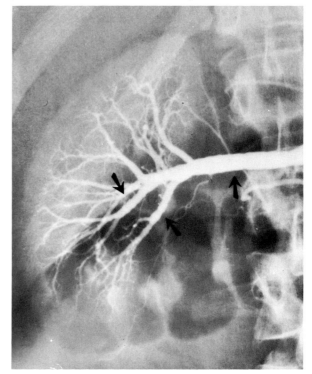

B

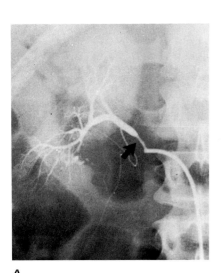 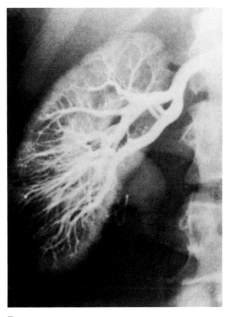 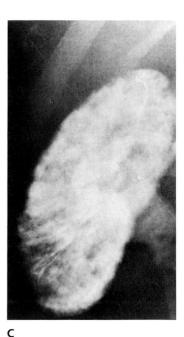

A   **B**   **C**

Figure 51-6. Renal artery spasm. (A) Localized. Precisely at the site of the catheter tip, the renal artery is profoundly narrowed (*arrow*). Removal of the catheter from the renal artery and an intraaortic injection demonstrated that the caliber of the renal artery was normal. (B and C) Spasm of the small renal arteries. Many distal vessels are narrowed in association with the selective injection. The nephrogram (C) demonstrates multiple lucent areas in the cortex, all of which disappeared following an intraaortic bolus injection. (Courtesy of David Levin, M.D.)

sent as often as they are present. In about 10 percent of patients, such bruits are heard in the absence of renal artery stenosis: this phenomenon may be related to aortic arteriosclerosis or to involvement of any of the other branch vessels of the aorta.

The most significant *urographic findings* that accompany a strongly positive arteriogram are disparities in size, appearance time, and concentration of the contrast agent in the collecting system.[20] In approximately 20 percent of patients with renovascular hypertension, these signs may be absent (and the study results false negative), and, conversely, these signs may be present in 10 percent of patients with essential hypertension (and the study results false positive).

Pathologically the kidney may demonstrate various degrees of nephrosclerosis as well as atrophic changes in the tubules. The juxtaglomerular apparatus is frequently increased in number, and its cellularity may be augmented. Although the ischemic kidney may have less arteriolar change than the nonischemic diseased kidney, the changes of arteriolar nephrosclerosis may be bilateral in a significant percentage of cases.

What is significant arterial stenosis? When the diameter of the vessel is reduced to 20 percent or less of its original size, the stenosis has a high chance of being causally related to hypertension known to be present. In practice, this implies a reduction in the diameter of the lumen to 1.0 to 1.5 mm.[21] The presence of stenosis, however, is not enough to guarantee the presence of hypertension,[3] nor its causative role if hypertension is present. A well-developed collateral circulation is an important ancillary sign of the hemodynamic significance of arterial stenosis. Another laboratory test of significant stenosis lies in the renal vein renin assays. Lateralization of high levels of renin secretion to the underperfused kidney is associated with a 93 percent benefit rate after surgical correction.[21,22] Even in the absence of lateralization, however, 50 percent of patients with renal artery stenosis and hypertension may respond to surgery,[22] indicating that renin assays have a high false-negative rate. Renal vein renins have not been sufficiently reliable in predicting the response to revascularization in patients with hypertension.[23]

In patients cured of renovascular hypertension, the preoperative arteriogram almost invariably shows an apparently significant lesion. Nevertheless, in the past many patients with abnormal arteriograms have not been cured by surgery because the lesion is not causative, contralateral disease is profound, surgery is inadequate, or operative death occurs.[24]

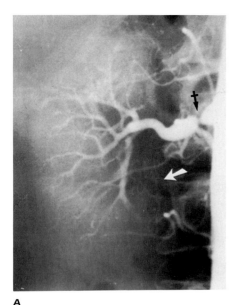

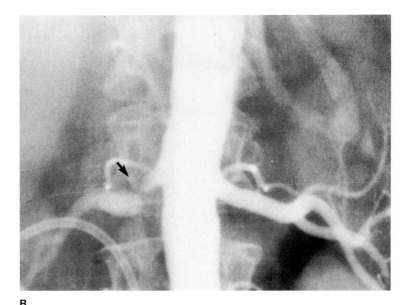

A   **B**

Figure 51-7. Arteriosclerotic stenosis of the renal artery. (A) Concentric stenosis. This 58-year-old man had a blood pressure of 180/110 mmHg. Arteriography demonstrates a discrete zone of stenosis about 8 mm beyond the origin of the right renal artery, with circumferential narrowing and only minimal eccentricity (*barred arrow*). Poststenotic dilatation is visible. Both the radioactive renogram and the split-func- tion studies were also abnormal. The appearance is typical of arteriosclerotic stenosis. Small collateral vessels are visible (*white arrow*). (B) Eccentric stenosis. Significant eccentric narrowing of the renal artery within the proximal third of the vessel strongly suggests the arteriosclerotic etiology. The lumen is no more than 1 mm in diameter (*arrow*). Note the dilatation beyond the stenosis.

Arteriosclerosis

Arteriosclerosis is the most common cause of narrowing of the renal arterial lumen. It is usually observed in patients over 40 years of age and is more common in males. Because plaques develop most frequently at the origins or bifurcations of vessels, it is not surprising that renal artery stenosis due to arteriosclerosis usually is orificial or is located in the proximal one-third of the artery (Fig. 51-7). Furthermore, atherosclerotic involvement of the renal artery is frequently accompanied by aortic disease (Figs. 51-8 and 51-9; see also Fig. 51-47).[25] Aortic plaques may cause stenosis or occlusion at the ostia of the renal artery.

Arteriosclerotic narrowing may be of any degree—from a small plaque to complete occlusion (see Figs. 51-8 and 51-9). It is frequently localized (see Fig. 51-7), and it may be eccentric (see Figs. 51-7B and 51-8) or circumferential (see Fig. 51-7A), but usually irregularly so. The lesions may be single or multiple. In 30 to 50 percent of the cases, the lesions are bilateral (see Fig. 51-7A), with one side more severely affected.[12,25] Immediately beyond the stenosis, marked poststenotic dilatation may be observed (see Fig. 51-7).

Renal Artery Dysplasia

This condition (also known as fibroplasia and fibromuscular hyperplasia) occurs predominantly in females,[26] although the authors have seen many cases in young males as well. The female-male incidence is approximately 4:1 or 5:1.[27] The youngest patient in our series was 6 months old. Most patients were in their thirties, forties, and fifties. The disease is not localized to the renal arteries, and other visceral branches as well as the carotid arteries may be involved.[26–28] There is also an association with cerebral aneurysms.

Histologically, there may be focal areas of intimal proliferation, possibly secondary to organized mural thrombi. The media is most often involved, usually by fibrous thickening, less commonly by muscular hyperplasia.[29] In some cases, there are two distinct medial layers: an inner muscular coat and an outer circular fibrous coat, distinct from the longitudinal adventitial investment of the vessel. A variable increase in the polysaccharide content of the media is present. The muscle cells are plump with decreased eosinophilia, and they may be difficult to differentiate from fibroblasts. Disruption and duplication of the elastic fibers are also identified.

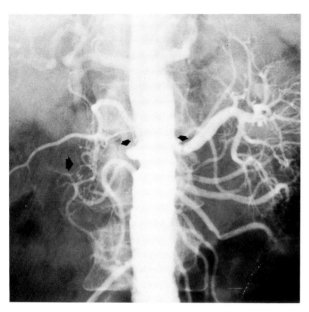

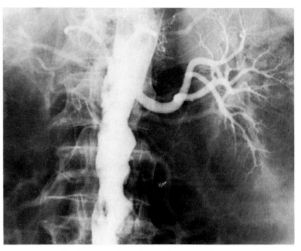

Figure 51-8. Arteriosclerotic stenosis and occlusion of the renal artery. This 56-year-old man had a 7-year history of hypertension (blood pressure of 228/100 mmHg). A bruit was heard in the epigastrium, and there was hypertensive retinopathy. There is complete occlusion of the right renal artery approximately 8 mm beyond its origin (*right central arrow*). On the right, profuse collateral vessels fill from the lumbar arteries (*right lateral arrow*). Moderate renal artery stenosis is present in the left renal artery (*left central arrow*), and multiple irregularities indicate the presence of arteriosclerosis of the remainder of the main renal artery. Arteriosclerosis of the aorta is also visible, and there are large plaques immediately adjacent to the origin of the right renal artery.

Figure 51-9. Arteriosclerotic occlusion of the renal artery. Bolus aortography demonstrates the left renal artery with normal bifurcations and multiple arteriosclerotic plaques in the aorta. The origin of the right renal artery is totally occluded by arteriosclerotic plaques.

The classification of dysplastic lesions of the renal artery has been a focus of controversy for many years. Three histologic varieties have been delineated—intimal, medial, and periadventitial dysplasia.[30] On the basis of the studies of McCormack and colleagues,[29,31] as well as those of Kincaid et al.,[32,33] together with the case series of Abrams, the following classification is described, which combines the pathologic and angiographic characteristics of these lesions. (Figure 51-10 delineates the angiographic findings of the different types of dysplastic disease.)

1. *Intimal fibroplasia.* The intima is thickened by fibrous tissue. These lesions may be localized (Fig. 51-11), or they may involve a long segment of the

Figure 51-10. Dysplastic lesions of the renal artery. (Modified from McCormack LJ, et al. Am Heart J 1966;72:188; McCormack LJ, et al. Semin Roentgenol 1967;2:126; and Kincaid OW. Renal angiography. Chicago: Year Book, 1966.)

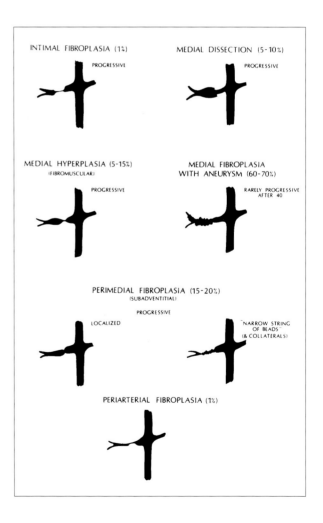

INTIMAL FIBROPLASIA (1%) PROGRESSIVE

MEDIAL DISSECTION (5-10%) PROGRESSIVE

MEDIAL HYPERPLASIA (5-15%) (FIBROMUSCULAR) PROGRESSIVE

MEDIAL FIBROPLASIA WITH ANEURYSM (60-70%) RARELY PROGRESSIVE AFTER 40

PERIMEDIAL FIBROPLASIA (15-20%) (SUBADVENTITIAL) PROGRESSIVE LOCALIZED NARROW STRING OF BEADS (& COLLATERALS)

PERIARTERIAL FIBROPLASIA (1%)

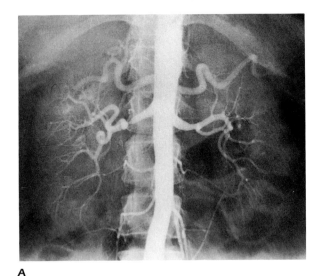

A

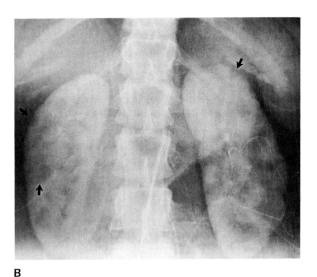

B

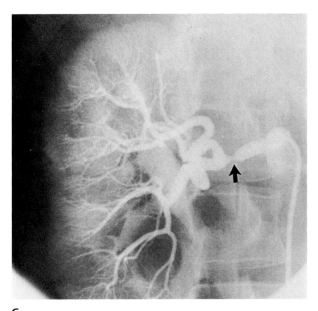

C

Figure 51-11. Renal artery dysplasia, intimal fibroplasia. (A) Aortogram. A discrete area of narrowing in the midportion of the right renal artery is visible, about 1 cm in length, with no other abnormalities of the main renal artery. Note that bilaterally the kidneys are large and the vessels appear somewhat spread. (B) Nephrographic phase. Multiple lucent areas are seen in both kidneys (*arrows*), representing small to moderate-sized cysts. The patient had polycystic disease coexisting with renal artery dysplasia. (C) Selective renal arteriogram, left posterior oblique projection. The single area of involvement (*arrow*) is symmetric and concentric in its appearance.

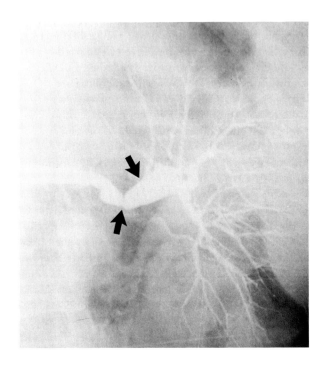

renal artery. They account for a relatively small number of the total group of patients with fibroplastic disease.

2. *Medial dissection.* This lesion also is characterized by the accumulation of collagen within the internal elastic lamina. It appears most frequently in the younger age group and is accompanied by fibroplasia of the intima and media, with degeneration of the media. As it progresses, a hematoma develops in the weakened media, and a communication between the lumen of the vessel and the media occurs because of the alterations in intima and media. The classic histologic and angiographic appearance of dissection may then be observed (Fig. 51-12).[34,35] This occurs in approximately 5 to 10 percent of all patients with fibroplastic disease.

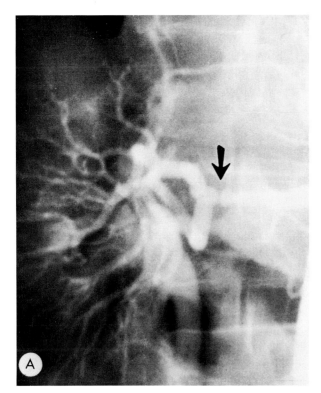

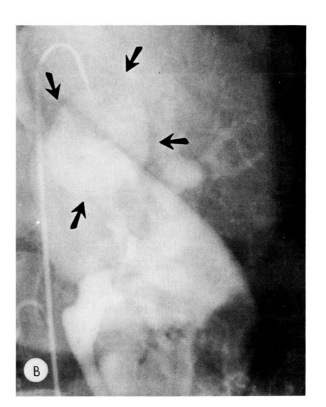

Figure 51-13. Renal artery dysplasia, medial hyperplasia (fibromuscular). (A) Right side. The classic appearance of fibromuscular hyperplasia with an area of apparently significant stenosis (*arrow*) is visible. Despite this, there was no reduction of the blood flow to the right kidney. (B) Left side. A pheochromocytoma is well defined in the adrenal area (*arrows*), coexisting with the right renal artery stenosis. (C) Medial (fibromuscular) hyperplasia (*arrow*). The involvement is somewhat more tubular in character and is less localized.

3. *Medial hyperplasia.* Uncomplicated medial hyperplasia actually represents fibromuscular hyperplasia, with muscular as well as fibrous elements involved. The narrowing is frequently localized (Fig. 51-13) and sometimes tubular and involves the middle and distal thirds of the renal artery. It occurs in no more than 5 to 15 percent of patients with dysplastic disease.

◀ **Figure 51-12.** Renal artery dysplasia, medial dissection. A selective left renal arteriogram demonstrates a normal proximal renal artery, a localized aneurysmal bulge just proximal to a stenotic area (*lower arrow*), and apparent dilatation of the vessel beyond (*upper arrow*). This dilatation extends into some of the branch arteries. Although the arteriographic change is not necessarily specific, it is suggestive. The false lumen represented by the dilated area is located in the media, which is markedly altered by the fibroplastic process. Disruption of the internal elastic lamina is also present, and intimal fibroplasia coexists. Compression of the normal lumen by the dissection produces renal ischemia, which may cause renin-dependent hypertension to develop.

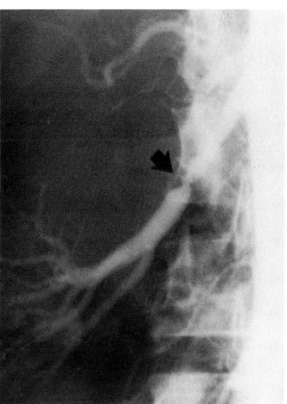

C

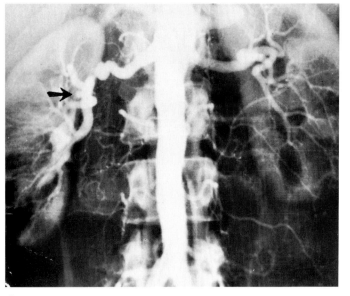

A

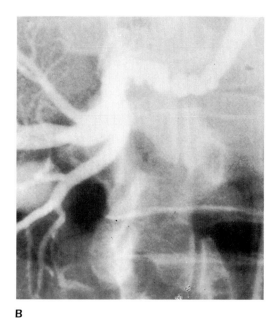

B

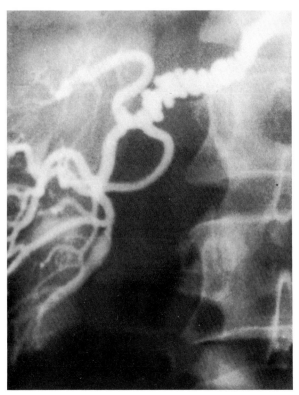

C

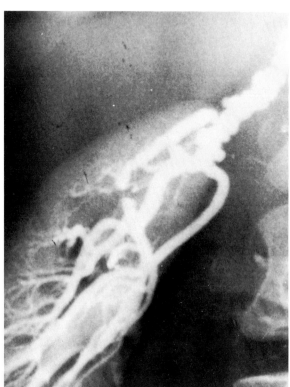

D

Figure 51-14. Renal artery dysplasia, medial fibroplasia with aneurysms. (A) Aortogram. This 46-year-old woman had hypertension of 5 years' duration (blood pressure of 200/110 mmHg). A bruit was heard in the midepigastrium. Split-function studies showed hyperconcentration on the right associated with a decreased urine output. At operation, there was a gradient of 50 mmHg. Multiple asymmetric areas of narrowing are noted in the right main artery, about 2.5 cm beyond its origin and extending to the bifurcation. There is an aneurysm of the main renal artery. Just inferior to the branch to the right upper pole, there is a small aneurysmal dilatation (*arrow*). The findings are those of medial fibro-plasia with aneurysms. (B) A selective renal arteriogram of a 33-year-old woman with hypertension. There is a peculiar corrugated appearance, the "string-of-beads" pattern characteristic of medial fibroplasia with aneurysms. The internal elastic membrane and the muscle layers are thinned, with associated aneurysmal dilatation in some areas. In other areas, there is thickening of the media, with replacement of muscle tissue by collagen. (C and D) Anteroposterior and oblique selective renal arteriograms of a 35-year-old woman with hypertension. Alternative areas of narrowing and aneurysm formation involve the middle and distal thirds of the main renal artery and extend into the branches.

4. *Medial fibroplasia with aneurysm.* Areas of thickened, fibrotic media alternate with thinned areas, the typical string-of-beads appearance that reflects the multiple concentric rings produced by the hyperplastic changes in the wall interspersed with local aneurysm formation at the site of elastic and muscle tissue degeneration in the media. The most common type of fibroplasia, it occurs in 60 to 70 percent of all patients with dysplastic disease. It is found in all age groups, and the angiographic appearance is quite characteristic (Fig. 51-14). It usually affects the renal artery in the middle and distal thirds to a variable degree, with localized constrictions alternating with aneurysmal dilatations. In contrast to perimedial fibroplasia, the aneurysms bulge beyond the expected diameter of the renal artery and appear to represent true aneurysms. This lesion is of particular importance because, in contrast to the others, it is relatively stable and rarely progressive after the age of 40. Hence the definition of the type of fibroplastic disease has important prognostic connotations. Conversely, medial hyperplasia with aneurysms has been shown to develop in individuals with angiographically normal renal arteries examined during adult life, strongly supporting the concept of renal artery dysplasia as an acquired disease.[36]

5. *Perimedial fibroplasia, localized type.* These lesions characteristically have a collagen collar of variable thickness between the media and the adventitia. When localized (Fig. 51-15), they are indistinguishable either from medial hyperplasia or from intimal fibroplasia.

6. *Perimedial fibroplasia, diffuse type* (Figs. 51-16 and 51-17). This type of lesion sometimes resembles medial fibroplasia with aneurysm and has been called the narrow string-of-beads. Characteristically, the dilatations are smaller in caliber than the portions of the renal artery that are uninvolved, and therefore the appearance is distinctive from that of medial fibroplasia with aneurysm.

7. *Periarterial fibroplasia.* Fibrous thickening of the adventitia with cicatrix formation produces a relatively localized or (sometimes) diffuse area of narrowing in the main renal artery (Fig. 51-18), usually in the middle or distal thirds. This is a rare type

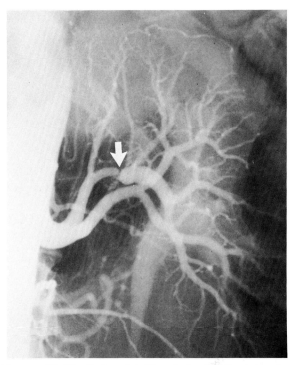

Figure 51-15. Perimedial fibroplasia, localized involvement. Aortography, performed in this young woman with hypertension, demonstrates an early bifurcation of the left renal artery, with tight stenosis in the dorsal renal branch (*arrow*). This appearance represents the localized form of perimedial fibroplasia, in which a thick collagen collar surrounds the media and occupies the area between the media and the adventitia. The appearance may be similar to that in localized intimal fibroplasia, or so-called medial hyperplasia (fibromuscular hyperplasia).

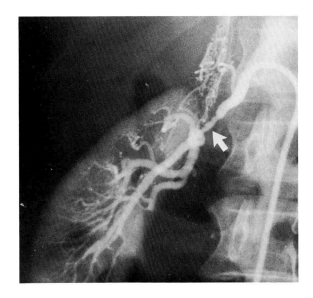

Figure 51-16. Perimedial fibroplasia. The distal third of the right renal artery (up to the point of bifurcation) is irregularly narrowed, with alternating areas of narrowing and dilatation well within the projected size of the proximal renal artery (*arrow*). The superior capsular-adrenal artery fills a florid coiled network of vessels, which represent part of the collateral circulation.

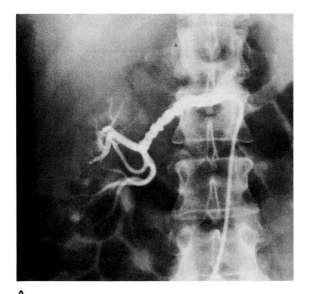

A

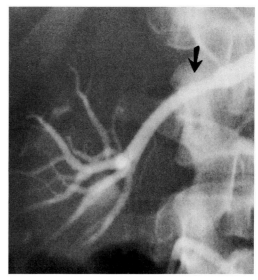

Figure 51-18. Periarterial fibroplasia. This 20-year-old woman had a 3-month history of hypertension (blood pressure of 220/140 mmHg). The electrocardiogram showed left ventricular hypertrophy, and the hypertension ran a malignant course. The arteriogram demonstrates an area of smooth symmetric narrowing of the main renal artery beginning about 1.5 cm beyond its orifice (*arrow*). The tunnel-like constriction of the main renal artery is characteristic of one form of periarterial fibroplasia.

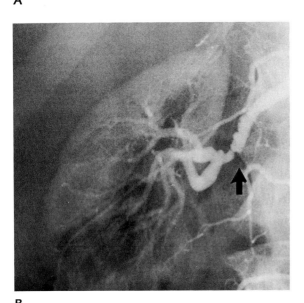

B

Figure 51-17. Perimedial fibroplasia, diffuse involvement. (A) Right selective renal arteriogram in a 29-year-old man with hypertension. Beginning in the middle third of the right renal artery, there are areas of corrugation (the "narrow string of beads"). These corrugations are not true aneurysms and do not extend beyond the projected area of the renal artery, judging from its proximal third. The appearance is that of classic perimedial fibroplasia. (B) Right renal arteriogram. The appearance is that of the narrow string of beads, but there is also a more sharply localized high-degree stenosis just proximal to the bifurcation of the renal artery into its dorsal and ventral branches (*arrow*).

of dysplastic disease but is equally capable of causing hypertension because of renal ischemia.

Thus the localized lesions of intimal fibroplasia, medial hyperplasia (or fibromuscular hyperplasia), and perimedial fibroplasia are difficult to distinguish from each other angiographically, and they have the capacity for being progressive. In contrast, the most common single type of fibroplastic disease, medial fibroplasia with aneurysm, is rarely progressive after the age of 40. In 21 of 125 patients studied with fibroplastic disease, mixed lesions were noted that could not be categorized explicitly into a single pathologic type.[32]

The proximal one-third of the main renal artery is usually spared in dysplastic disease, but the middle and distal thirds are typically involved (see Figs. 51-11 through 51-18). Much of the main renal artery and the interlobar branches may be the site of disease (see Figs. 51-15 through 51-17). When the process extends into the secondary branches, it may produce complete occlusion of vessels to the upper or lower pole, so that the total blood supply to the kidney segment may be derived from the collateral circulation. In about 40 to 70 percent of cases, the lesions are bilateral.[27,32,37] When unilateral, renal artery dysplasia is far more common on the right than on the left.[24] When the lesions are localized and nonrepetitive, and particularly if they are located in the proximal one-third of the artery, they may be difficult to distinguish from arteriosclerotic disease. The periarterial adventitial lesions may involve a long segment of the vessel, with a segment of smooth, tubular narrowing (see Fig. 51-18).

Renal artery dysplasia has been demonstrated in the absence of hypertension and need not be causative of hypertension even when hypertension is present. Figure 51-13A illustrates the case of a young woman with hypertension and fibromuscular hyperplasia of the right renal artery. The Regitine test was positive, and urinary catecholamine levels were elevated. The split-function studies demonstrated equal blood flow to both kidneys. The patient's hypertension was cured when her pheochromocytoma was removed (see Fig. 51-13B). Aberrant pheochromocytoma may also involve the renal artery, and it may produce renal artery stenosis resembling dysplastic disease.[38]

When renovascular hypertension is caused by renal artery dysplasia, a favorable response to percutaneous balloon angioplasty may be anticipated with a cumulative 5-year patency rate of 89 percent. For this reason, percutaneous transluminal angioplasty (PTA) is the treatment of choice for patients with fibromuscular dysplasia.[5]

Neurofibromatosis

A rare but important cause of renal artery stenosis is found in patients with neurofibromatosis.[39,40] In most cases, the narrowing of the renal arteries is the direct effect of fibrous proliferation of the intima or the media. In other cases, neurofibromatous tissue has been demonstrated within the adventitia of the artery, producing periarterial fibrosis of a high degree indistinguishable from that caused by the intimal lesions. In most patients, the site of stenosis is near the origin of the artery, and these lesions may be bilateral.

Angiographically, there is a smooth stenotic segment usually at the orifice of the artery, with a tubular segment of dilatation beyond (Fig. 51-19). Thus the appearance is different from that in dysplastic disease of the renal artery. The funnel-shaped appearance of poststenotic dilatation may be due to diffuse involvement of the arterial wall with thickening, disorganization, and/or atrophy of the media and fibrosis of the adventitia.[39] The renal artery stenosis may be unilateral or bilateral, and it may be accompanied by renal artery aneurysm and occasionally by coarctation of the abdominal aorta as well. Rarely, iliac artery stenosis may be found. When aneurysms are present, it is because of localized fragmentation and atrophy of the media.[39]

Hypertension in patients with neurofibromatosis

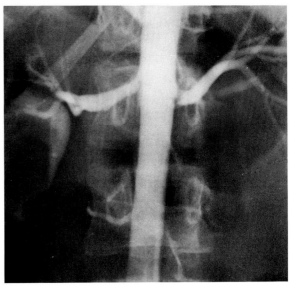

A

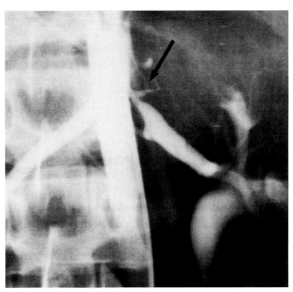

B

Figure 51-19. Renal artery stenosis, neurofibromatosis. (A) Anteroposterior projection. (B) Left posterior oblique projection. Both renal arteries are involved, predominantly at the orifice but also extending for about 1 to 2 cm beyond the orifice (*arrow*). The distal portion of the renal artery looks entirely smooth and normal. This appearance may be due either to a desmoplastic fibrotic involvement of the wall of the artery or to the actual presence of neurofibromatous tissue within the adventitia of the vessel, producing periarterial fibrosis. (Courtesy of Joseph Bookstein, M.D.)

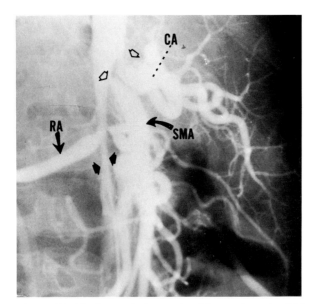

Figure 51-20. Congenital stenosis of the renal arteries. This 6-year-old girl had high blood pressure in the upper extremities (180/110 mmHg) and lower blood pressure in the lower extremities (120/100 mmHg). A thoracotomy had been done to look for coarctation, but none was found. A transfemoral abdominal aortogram demonstrates marked abdominal aortic narrowing beginning at the level of the celiac artery (*CA*). There is further reduction of the lumen (*black arrows*) at and below the origin of the superior mesenteric artery (*SMA*). The origins of these arteries (*open arrows*) are considerably narrowed. Both renal arteries (*RA*) are stenotic, with poststenotic dilatation.

may also be associated with pheochromocytoma. In patients below the age of 18, renal artery stenosis is a more common cause, whereas in patients over the age of 18, pheochromocytoma is the predominant factor.[41]

Congenital Stenosis

Congenital stenosis, so-called coarctation of the renal artery, is a rare lesion that is assumed to be congenital because of its discovery in early life. The stenosis is relatively localized in the main renal artery.[25] It may coexist with coarctation of the abdominal aorta (Fig. 51-20), although some of these cases are probably the result of arteritis of the aorta. Other cases may demonstrate the classic pathologic findings of renal artery dysplasia or neurofibromatosis.[39,40]

Branch Stenosis

Branch stenosis may be due to arteriosclerosis, renal artery dysplasia, thrombus, embolus, or arteritis. In the authors' experience, branch stenosis has been seen relatively commonly with fibroplastic disease although

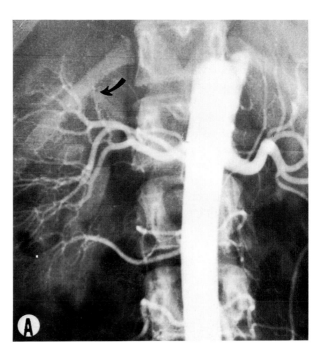

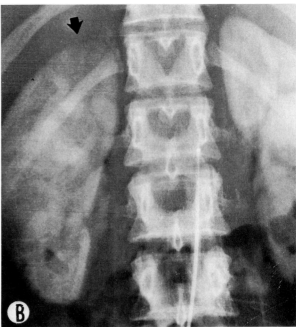

Figure 51-21. Renal artery branch stenosis. This 26-year-old woman had known hypertension of 4 years' duration. (A) Abdominal aortogram. Three renal arteries are visible on the right, and an occlusion of a small, somewhat tortuous branch to the right upper pole is seen (*arrow*). The peripheral small branches to the upper pole are not adequately defined. (B) Nephrographic phase. The absence of contrast density in the upper pole of the right kidney reflects the segmental disease of the artery (*arrow*). The localized area of occlusion was caused by arteritis.

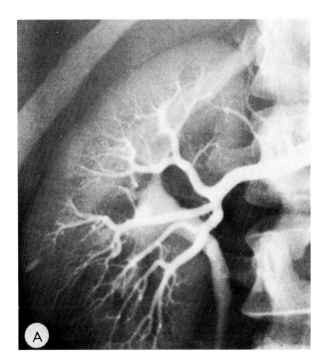

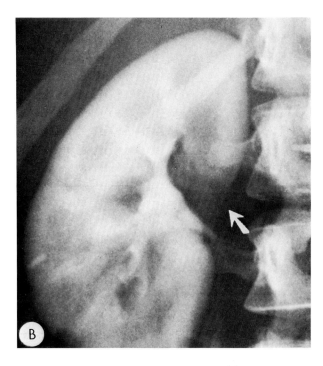

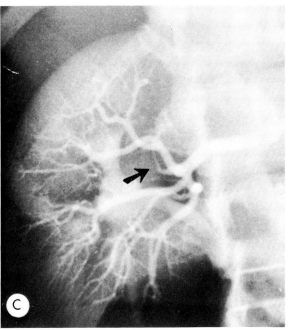

Figure 51-22. Renal artery branch stenosis. This 31-year-old woman had an episode of right flank pain about 3 months before her admission to the hospital. Increasing hypertension was then discovered; her blood pressure reached 220/140 mmHg. Split-function data showed a 25 percent decrease in urine output on the right. A translumbar aortogram performed in another hospital was considered normal. (A) Selective renal arteriogram. The right kidney demonstrates a lack of the usual crossing vessels characteristically found in the normal arteriogram. A paucity of dorsal branches is apparent. This was also present, although not originally described, on the aortogram. (B) Nephrographic phase. There is decreased density in the medial, central aspect of the kidney (*arrow*). (C) Selective renal arteriogram, left posterior oblique view. A small, blind-end channel represents the proximal portion of the occluded dorsal arterial branch (*arrow*). At operation, a large area of infarction was found on the dorsal aspect of the kidney. Histologic examination demonstrated periarteritis nodosa.

not necessarily as an isolated lesion. The importance of the isolated branch stenosis lies in the occasional difficulty of its detection on the conventional arteriogram, although aortography may at times be valuable (Fig. 51-21A). It is essential to study both the arteriographic phase and the nephrographic phase because the latter may reveal ischemic areas with great clarity (see Fig. 51-21B). If there is any question as to

the presence of branch stenosis, the proper approach is a selective renal arteriogram. Multiple views may be required before the branch stenosis is detected (Fig. 51-22).

Essential Hypertension

In patients with essential hypertension of relatively short duration, there is no detectable alteration in the appearance of the major renal arteries or the intrarenal arterial branches. With the passage of time, mild-to-moderate changes in the appearance of the arterial bed

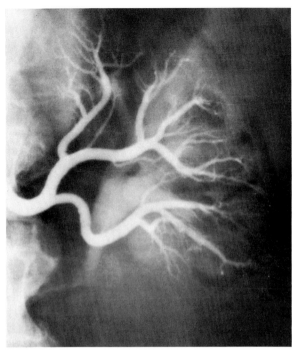

Figure 51-23. Mild arteriolar nephrosclerosis. Selective renal arteriography. Contrast material has been injected into one of the two vessels to the kidney. The interlobular and arcuate arteries are slightly tortuous, and there is diminished filling of the interlobular vessels.

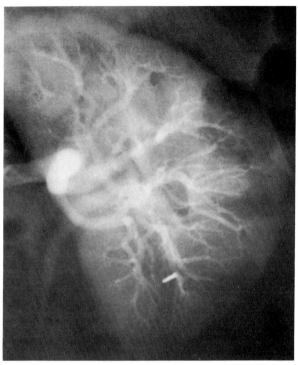

Figure 51-24. Slight to moderate arteriolar nephrosclerosis. There is more marked tortuosity of the arcuate vessels and, to a lesser extent, of the interlobar vessels. Diminished filling of the interlobular vessels is apparent. The metallic clip in the lower pole of the kidney represents the site of biopsy, which demonstrated arteriolar nephrosclerosis.

appear, and these changes seem to be related to the mean renal blood flow.[42] In these selective arteriograms, the increasing tortuosity, irregularity, and narrowing of the arteries are related to the stage of the disease, the alterations in renal hemodynamics, and the mean renal blood flow (Figs. 51-23 and 51-24). These findings may progress to those described in the following discussion.

Arteriolar Nephrosclerosis

Selective arteriography is usually necessary to obtain adequate detail of the small-vessel pattern of the kidney. In mild cases of nephrosclerosis, the arteriogram may be normal. As the disease progresses, histologically there is hyperplastic intimal proliferation in the small arteries and arterioles, with a reduction in luminal size. This is associated with a necrotizing arteriolitis and fibrinoid necrosis of the arteriolar wall.[43] Angiographically the main renal artery may be normal in size or even larger than usual, but the interlobar and arcuate vessels are reduced in caliber and have a curled or gnarled appearance, with irregularities and beading along their course (Fig. 51-25; see also Fig. 51-24).

Normally these small vessels are smooth in outline and curve gently without tortuosity or narrowing; bifurcation in the periphery usually occurs with narrow angles. With disease, the gradual curvature is replaced by sharp angulations and tortuosity. Contrast flow into the periphery is delayed and results in an irregular pattern of small-vessel filling. Because of a decrease in the size and number of fine vessels opacified, the classic "pruned-tree" appearance is produced. Perhaps because the kidney size is reduced secondary to cortical atrophy, the subsegmental vessels bifurcate with broader angles, and the interlobar and arcuate arteries appear tortuous.[44]

Hollenberg et al.[42] attempted to distinguish patients with essential hypertension from those with accelerated hypertension on the basis of the arteriographic findings. The arteriograms were graded 0 to 4. In the grade 4 arteriogram, there were few cortical vessels visible, marked tortuosity, abnormal vascular tapering, vessel irregularity with filling defects in the lumen, and a prolonged vascular transit time of contrast material (Fig. 51-26). These patients had a mean blood flow well below the lower limit of normal, and the cortical flow, as evaluated on the xenon washout,

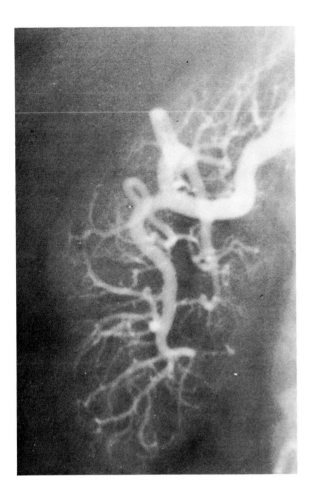

◄ **Figure 51-25.** Severe arteriolar nephrosclerosis. This 47-year-old man entered the hospital because of right flank pain and hypertension. An intravenous urogram showed poor concentration and poor filling bilaterally. Selective renal arteriography demonstrates a slightly enlarged main renal artery. The interlobar and arcuate vessels are tortuous and irregular. They are somewhat diminished in caliber and have a curled or gnarled appearance. Sharp angulations of the small arteries are present. The peripheral vessels do not fill normally, and the cortex is thin and irregular. The angiographic features are those of arteriolar nephrosclerosis. (Courtesy of Aaron J. Fink, M.D.)

was decreased. Transit time of the isotope, like that of the contrast material, was prolonged. Thus the arteriogram accurately reflected significant decreases in the renal blood flow and alterations in the distribution of the intrarenal blood flow. In uncomplicated essential hypertension, the renin secretion is low, whereas in the presence of accelerated hypertension and small-artery disease, the renin secretion is significantly increased.[45]

Figure 51-26. End-stage arteriolar nephrosclerosis. Selective renal arteriography. (A) Early phase. The main renal artery and the large branches are filled. The branches are strikingly thin. (B) Later phase. The intrarenal arteries are uniformly narrowed, and the distal terminations are tortuous. No filling of the interlobular vessels is apparent. A protracted transit time was observed. The nephrographic phase was very faint, and the cortex was markedly thin. The patient was uremic at the time of the study. Subsequently, bilateral nephrectomy and renal transplantation were done. An examination of the excised kidneys showed far-advanced nephrosclerosis.

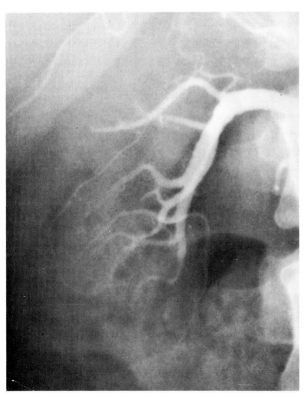

A

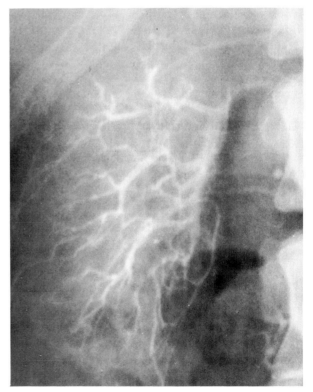

B

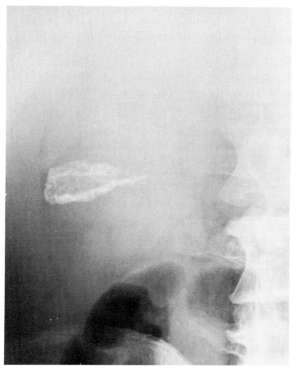

Figure 51-27. Renal infarction. A wedge-shaped area of calcification is visible on the plain film, with an indentation of the surface of the kidney precisely at the site of the calcification. The indentation represents a wedge-shaped infarction following arterial embolism in which the necrotic tissue has become heavily calcified.

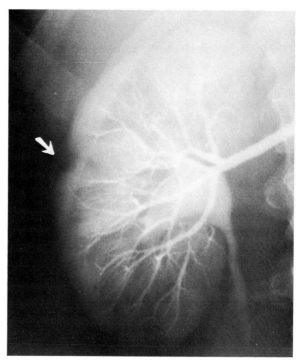

Figure 51-28. Renal infarction. Selective renal arteriogram. A localized area of underperfusion is visible adjacent to the surface of the kidney (*arrow*). The vessel to this area has been occluded, with consequent infarction, fibrosis, and retraction of renal tissue. This woman had hypertension, which was relieved by wedge resection of the area of infarction.

Renal Hypertension Without Main Renal Arterial Stenosis

It has been shown that occasional cures of hypertension may be effected by nephrectomy when the kidney is small and contracted even though the main renal artery shows no evidence of stenosis. McDonald, in a series of patients without renal artery stenosis, used only the split-function data of diminished urine volume associated with an elevated paraaminohippuric acid concentration as an indication for surgery.[46] Of 18 patients with a small kidney and an ischemic functional pattern, 15 were cured of hypertension. Interestingly, among 10 patients who had a kidney that was 1 cm shorter than the other kidney and no ischemic functional pattern and who were treated with nephrectomy, 3 became normotensive. It must be inferred that the group of patients with a small kidney and the ischemic functional pattern had small-vessel disease serious enough to cause local areas of ischemia.

Infarction of the Kidney

Infarction may result from embolism or thrombosis. Thrombosis, in turn, may be secondary to severe stenosis, arteritis, trauma, polycythemia, or aneurysm.

Initially the plain film shows a normal or a slightly enlarged kidney. The enlargement is due to severe edema. Nonspecific ileus may also be seen with various degrees of obliteration of the renal outline and psoas shadows. In chronic segmental renal infarction, a wedge-shaped area of calcification may sometimes be observed (Fig. 51-27).

The intravenous pyelogram may show normal or small calices, or lack of function. The local calix in segmental disease may be only faintly opacified. After infarction, the kidney becomes smaller, with indentations reflecting areas with a loss of volume. The local calix may become distorted, similar to that in focal pyelonephritis, except that the loss of renal tissue appears excessive when compared to the degree of caliceal distortion. When the whole kidney is infarcted, there is a general decrease in size, and the kidney may resemble a congenitally hypoplastic kidney.

Angiography is helpful: cutoff or absence of normal vessels is visible and is associated with defects in the arteriogram and the nephrogram (Figs. 51-28 through 51-30). These defects may represent the infarcted tissue or the scar that has replaced it. Local increase in the circulation time can be seen. The disease is bilateral in half of the cases, and so both kidneys should be studied.

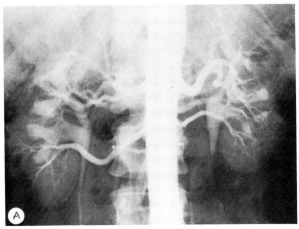

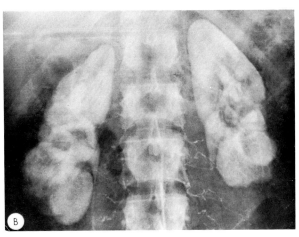

Figure 51-29. Renal infarction. This 39-year-old woman had mitral stenosis, a long history of atrial fibrillation, and multiple renal embolic episodes with recurrent bouts of flank pain and hematuria. (A) Aortogram. Double renal arteries are present bilaterally. The intrarenal branches demonstrate decreased arborization. The vessels to the midportion of the right kidney are truncated, as are those in the middle and lower portions of the left kidney. Incidentally noted is blunting of the calices bilaterally, resembling the appearance in pyelonephritis. (B) Nephrographic phase. The left side shows gross loss of cortex and marked irregularity in the lower part of the kidney. On the right side, similar findings are visible on the lateral aspect of the kidney and in the upper pole.

Figure 51-30. Renal embolism and infarction. Selective renal arteriography. (A) Arterial phase. Multiple emboli have occluded some of the small interlobar arteries (*arrows*). (B) Nephrographic phase. Localized areas of ischemia are visible (*arrows*) at the site of occlusion of the renal artery subserving these areas. These represent sites of infarction.

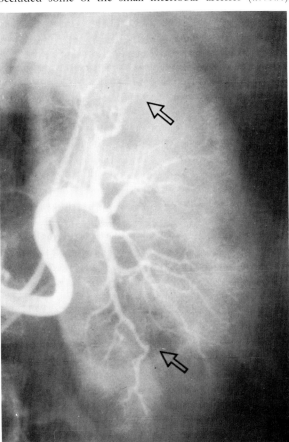

A

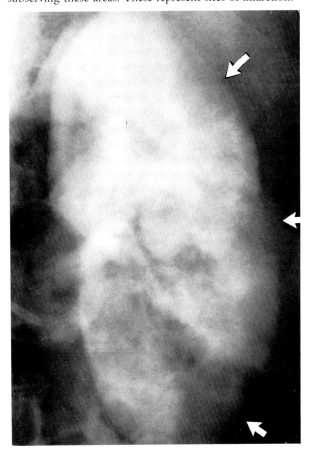

B

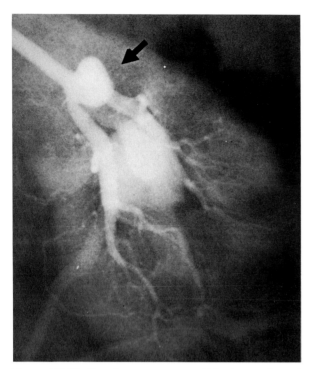

Figure 51-31. Renal artery aneurysm. Selective renal arteriography demonstrates a large localized sac filling with contrast agent just at the bifurcation of the main renal artery into dorsal and ventral renal branches (*arrow*). The patient had no evidence of a dysplastic disease of the renal arteries, nor was there clinical evidence of a mycotic or false aneurysm. It was assumed that the aneurysm was congenital.

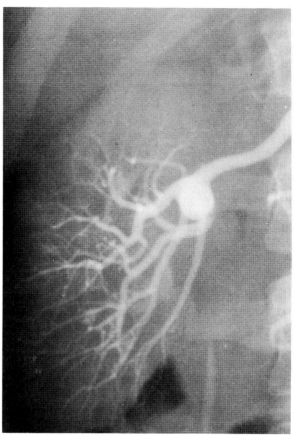

Figure 51-32. Renal artery aneurysm. Selective right renal arteriogram. As in Figure 51-31, an aneurysm is present almost exactly at the bifurcation of the main renal artery into its dorsal and ventral branches. The patient was mildly hypertensive, and only the renal artery aneurysm was demonstrated as an abnormality in the renal vascular bed.

Embolism with consequent infarction may result in hypertension. Embolism of a single renal artery that leads to infarction of the entire kidney need not produce hypertension. An accessory renal artery or a collateral blood supply, however, commonly furnishes enough circulation to prevent the complete necrosis of the kidney; the ischemic kidney may then cause hypertension. Similarly, if an embolus passes into a small secondary branch, only part of the kidney will be infarcted, and hypertension may well develop (see Fig. 51-30). Pathologically, the source of the emboli is demonstrated at necropsy in 76 percent of the cases.[47] Clinically, the abrupt onset of constant flank pain with microscopic hematuria is typical of renal embolism. When renal embolism causes incomplete infarction and hypertension or when segmental renal artery stenosis is associated with hypertension, transcatheter therapeutic embolism may result in the infarction of the remaining viable tissue and so control hypertension.[48]

Renal Artery Aneurysm

The true aneurysm is defined as a localized dilatation of the renal artery retaining one or more of the original layers of the vessel wall (Figs. 51-31 and 51-32). The pathologic process is weakening of the arterial wall due to degenerative changes, particularly in the elastic tissue of the media. This weakening may be congenital, traumatic, inflammatory, or degenerative in origin; the process is accelerated by the pulsatile arterial pressure. Aneurysms are usually unilateral but may also be found bilaterally. They may occur in children but are most often found in patients between 50 and 70 years of age and are frequently associated with degenerative atherosclerosis. The exception is renal artery dysplasia, in which aneurysms are frequently found in the fourth and fifth decades of life (Fig. 51-33).

Clinically, aneurysms are often asymptomatic. They may cause pain and hematuria.

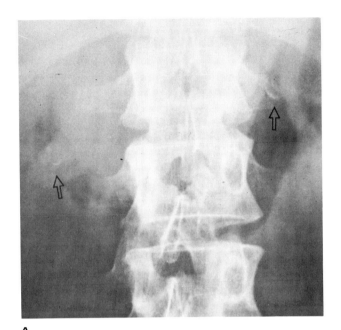

A

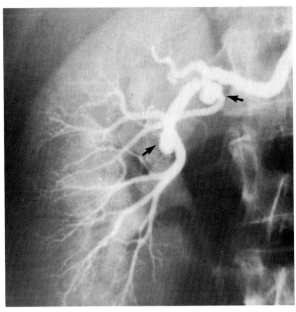

B

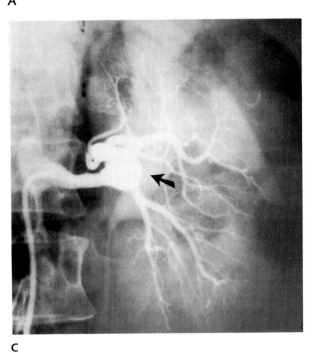

C

Figure 51-33. Renal artery aneurysm. This 47-year-old woman had hypertension of 15 years' duration. Her blood pressure was 190/130 mmHg. An intravenous urogram was normal. (A) Plain film of the abdomen. Curvilinear calcific densities are visible in the region of the renal artery on the right and the left (*arrows*). (B) Selective renal arteriography. Renal artery dysplasia is present, with an aneurysm at the bifurcation of the main renal artery (*upper arrow*) and a second smaller aneurysm (*lower arrow*) at the division of the ventral renal arterial branch. It is this second aneurysm that is calcified. (C) Selective left renal arteriogram. A large aneurysm at the bifurcation of the left main renal artery is visible precisely at the site (*arrow*) where calcification was apparent on the plain films. On both sides there is early evidence of arteriolar nephrosclerosis, with cortical narrowing and tortuosity of the peripheral branches.

Boijsen and Köhler[49] found that hypertension accompanied renal aneurysms in about 15 percent of cases. The hypertension is presumably due to the decreased renal blood flow that may follow compression due to aneurysm. The reduction in blood flow may be segmental in location.[50]

About 33 to 50 percent of renal artery aneurysms contain some calcium in their walls (see Fig. 51-33), and recognition may be possible on plain radiographs of the abdomen. The increased incidence of renal aneurysm rupture during pregnancy has been described by Burt et al.[51]

Angiographically, an aneurysm is either saccular (characterized by an outpouching from the artery, with an area of communication of variable width; see Figs. 51-31 through 51-33) or fusiform (with circumferential and rather uniform dilatation of the arterial lumen over a variable distance). The fusiform type is more likely to be secondary to localized arteriosclerotic stenosis or renal artery dysplasia and occurs as a region of poststenotic dilatation also known as a jet aneurysm. The circulation time of contrast material within the aneurysm tends to be retarded, particularly in the saccular type, whereas the general circulation throughout the rest of the kidneys is often normal.

The association of hypertension and renal artery

aneurysms has been well reviewed by Harrow and Sloane,[52] Boijsen and Köhler,[49] and Kincaid.[33] The best evidence suggests that cure of hypertension when aneurysms are present occurs only when renal artery stenosis and the physiologic stigmata of renovascular hypertension are present.[53]

Renal Arteriovenous Fistula

Renal arteriovenous fistulas are now being identified with increasing frequency. They are thought to be a cause of renovascular hypertension because localized renal ischemia is produced by the "steal" of arterial blood shunted directly to the renal venous system. One of the characteristics of this lesion on physical examination is a continuous bruit over the upper abdomen. It should be noted, however, that there are numerous other causes of a continuous upper abdominal bruit.

Love et al.[54] offer the following classification of arteriovenous fistulas:

1. Congenital fistula due to arteriovenous malformation
2. Acquired fistula
   a. Fistula following rupture of an arterial aneurysm
   b. Traumatic arteriovenous fistula resulting from penetrating trauma or trauma of the renal tissue in association with nephrolithotomy, partial

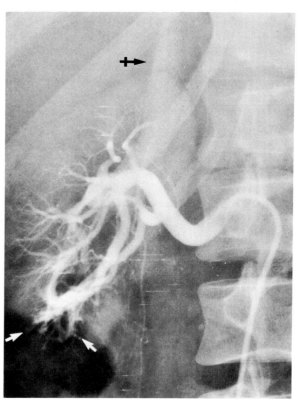

Figure 51-35. Renal arteriovenous malformation. Selective right renal arteriogram. A cluster of small and large vessels in the lower pole of the right kidney is apparent (*white arrows*), with immediate venous opacification. Note that the inferior vena cava is opacified (*black arrow*).

nephrectomy, or percutaneous needle biopsy of the kidney
   c. Arteriovenous fistula in renal carcinoma, particularly where tumor has eroded the vein
   d. Stump fistula after nephrectomy

Routine radiographic studies of the abdomen usually show no abnormalities; on occasion calcification may be visible. The intravenous urogram may show some caliceal distortion, but differentiation from tumor or cyst is frequently impossible.

It is important to establish the diagnosis via angiography because there may eventually be cardiac complications due to hypertension or high output cardiac failure. There is often physiologic evidence of increased cardiac output and blood volume and a decrease in the overall circulation time. The subject has been reviewed by Maldonado et al.,[55] Boijsen and Köhler,[56] and Love et al.[54]

Renal arteriovenous fistulas received increasing attention with the more widespread use of renal biopsy a few decades ago. Meng and Elkin demonstrated by arteriography immediately following percutaneous

Figure 51-34. Renal arteriovenous fistula. Bolus aortogram. Simultaneous with opacification of the renal arteries is visualization of the renal vein (*black arrow*). An arteriovenous communication is readily defined in the lower pole (*white arrow*) as the source of immediate venous opacification.

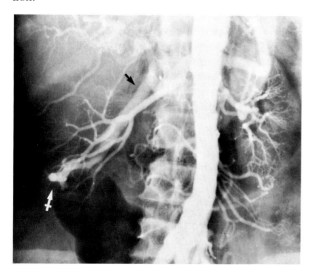

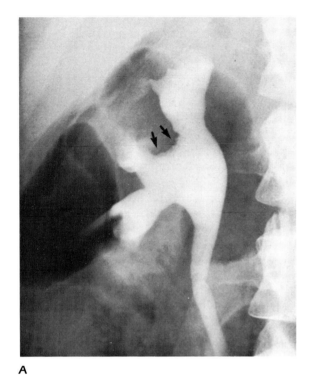

A

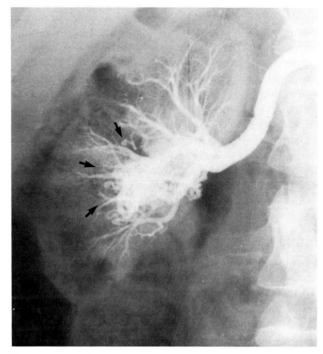

B

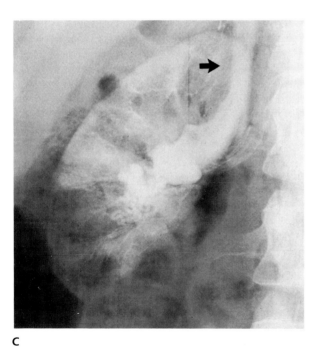

C

Figure 51-36. Renal arteriovenous fistula. The patient entered the hospital for evaluation of hematuria and hypertension. (A) Intravenous urogram. The collecting system appears normal, except for an irregular serration of the lateral aspect of the pelvis between the upper and middle pole calices (*arrows*). The appearance suggests a papillary tumor of the pelvis, extrinsic pressure on the pelvis from an intrarenal mass, or possibly a vascular impression. (B) Selective renal arteriography. "Stationary waves" are visible in the distal third of the renal artery. A large cluster of vessels in and adjacent to the hilus of the kidney is opacified (*arrows*). (C) Nephrographic phase (4 seconds). There is early dense filling of the renal vein and the inferior vena cava (*arrow*) while some of the renal artery branches are still opacified. Note the absence of a nephrogram in the lower pole. Double renal arteries were present. The hypertension in this patient was thought to be associated with ischemia of the lower pole of the right kidney associated with the "steal" provoked by the direct arteriovenous communication.

needle biopsy that the needle tract could be visualized, that perirenal extravasation occurred commonly, that arteriovenous communication was present in about 10 percent of patients, and that arterial occlusion, thrombus, or spasm was present in about 20 percent of patients.[57] In other series, the incidence of arteriovenous fistulas following renal biopsy has varied from 11 to 18 percent.[58-61]

Angiographically, the renal artery and the renal vein may be normal in size or wider than normal. Rapid passage of contrast material directly from the artery to a vein can be visualized at the site of the arteriovenous communication (Figs. 51-34 through 51-36). Rapid passage of contrast material into the inferior vena cava may also be noted on serial angiography (see Fig. 51-35). When the arteriovenous fistula is smaller and more localized, one may note enlargement and a serpentine appearance of the segmental arterial vessel and its branches. Vascularity of the renal parenchyma in the area adjacent to large fistulas is usually diminished. It may be difficult to differentiate numerous arteriovenous malformations from the arteriovenous shunts that occur in renal carcinoma, because wide, tortuous vessels and localized areas with rapid shunting to the venous system may be noted in each. In arteriovenous malformations, however, there are no pathologic vessels or displacement of vessels.

Chronic Pyelonephritis

In mild cases of chronic pyelonephritis, no angiographic abnormality may be noted. With the destruction and subsequent fibrosis of renal tissue, the diameter of the main renal arteries tends to shrink, usually in proportion to the decrease in kidney size and function. Because the renal volume is diminished, the interlobar and arcuate vessels become crowded and tortuous (Fig. 51-37). There may be localized areas of reduced vascularity, and scar formation may so distort the vascular pattern that a mottled, irregular nephrogram is produced. The renal cortex is frequently irregular in

outline, but the nephrogram may be disproportionately dense due to crowding of the vasculature secondary to a loss of interstitial renal tissue. The intrarenal vessels are small, and the cortex is thin (Fig. 51-38). Anastomoses between the parenchymal and capsular vessels may be demonstrated.[44] In addition, the renal veins may be visualized before the usual 6 to 12 seconds after contrast injection.[43]

If renal size is reduced and there is atrophy of the renal artery, it may be difficult to differentiate between chronic atrophic pyelonephritis and congenital hypoplasia of the kidney. Some authors feel that differentiation is impossible, but others conclude that in a majority of cases small kidneys, particularly in young people, are the result of early infantile pyelonephritis and that congenital hypoplasia of the kidney is rare. It is generally felt that pyelonephritis is often superimposed on congenital hypoplasia.[62] In the few cases of true congenital renal hypoplasia in which angiographic material is available, the arteries are smaller than normal, but the main vessels and branches retain the usual pro-

Figure 51-37. Pyelonephritis. This 31-year-old man had poor renal function and a history of pyeloncphritis. (A) Renal arteriogram. The major renal artery is normal. The small branches are tortuous and irregular, and some are crowded together. Marked narrowing of the peripheral vessels is present. (B) Nephrographic phase. The kidney is small, and there is premature venous filling. The nephrogram is relatively dense but irregular. The cortex is grossly thin, particularly over the lower pole and the middle segment of the kidney laterally. The contour is deformed because of fibrosis secondary to chronic infection.

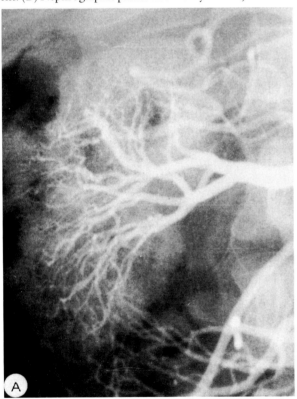

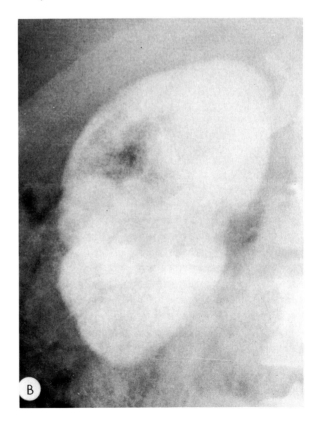

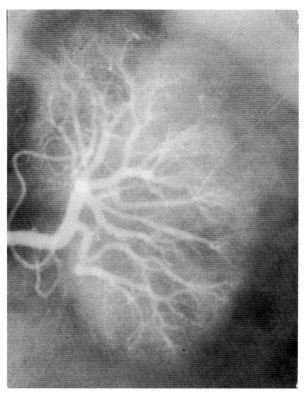

Figure 51-38. Chronic pyelonephritis. The kidney is small in association with a small main renal artery and small intrarenal branches. The arcuate vessels can be defined and reach virtually to the edge of the kidney. They are moderately tortuous. There is a striking decrease in cortical tissue, which is somewhat more uniform than is usually seen in chronic pyelonephritis. The vessels are tortuous, and there are local areas of ischemia.

portions and taper smoothly into the periphery. The flow of contrast material through the hypoplastic kidney is usually diminished, and opacification is less marked than in the normal kidney.

Chronic Glomerulonephritis

It may be difficult in the end stages to differentiate arteriolar nephrosclerosis from chronic glomerulonephritis or chronic pyelonephritis.[63] Examination of the nephrographic phase and the extent of overall involvement may be helpful. In glomerulonephritis, involvement is usually symmetric bilaterally. There is prolonged opacification and abrupt attenuation of the larger vessels, whereas opacification of the smaller vessels in the periphery may be markedly reduced. The nephrogram is usually homogeneous and relatively faint, but the cortical margin is smooth. The cortex is significantly thinned. Considerable tortuosity and ir-

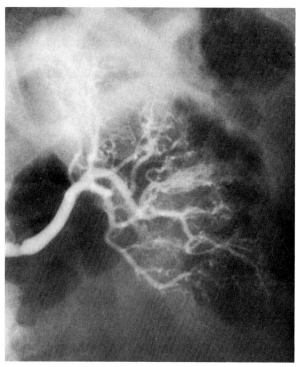

Figure 51-39. Chronic glomerulonephritis. Selective renal arteriogram. The main renal artery is small. A local area of narrowing, caused by spasm, is visible near its origin. The intrarenal branches are attenuated, and there is marked tortuosity of the interlobular and arcuate vessels. The cortex is uniformly thin. The subsequent nephrographic phase was very faint, and the cortical edge appeared relatively smooth.

regularity of the vascular lumen are important features (Fig. 51-39). In acute glomerulonephritis, the kidney, rather than being small, is frequently large, and the vessels are narrow but significantly separated from each other. At times, some of the vessels may appear to be crowded, depending on the uniformity of disease throughout the kidney.

Extrinsic Compression of the Renal Artery

On rare occasions, the main renal artery may be compressed locally by a fibrous musculotendinous band, resulting in renal ischemia and hypertension that may be cured by appropriate surgery. This entity has been described in a small number of patients by D'Abreau and Strickland,[64] Kincaid,[33] and Lampe.[65] Musculotendinous fibers of the psoas minor muscle or of the diaphragmatic crura are responsible for the renal artery compression. Compression by the crura of the diaphragm usually occurs when its insertion is abnormal and particularly when the renal artery takes off at a slightly higher position than normal. In all the cases reported, a normal blood pressure was restored after surgery. These lesions presumably are present from birth, with hypertension developing in adult life.

Angiographically, it may be very difficult to differentiate this lesion from a localized stenosis due to an intrinsic abnormality of the renal artery. There is usually a very short segmental constriction near the renal artery origin, and the remaining renal vessels may be free of atheromatous disease. The bandlike area of stenosis may lie just lateral to the vertebral margin, an observation of potential diagnostic importance.[66] In some patients, the hypertension may be labile, and angiography may be required in varying positions (supine and prone and with full inspiration and expiration). The effect of position and diaphragmatic contraction on the presence and degree of arterial narrowing and contrast filling of the renal vasculature can then be evaluated.[64]

Extrinsic renal artery compression may also be produced by tumor. Lampe reported a case in which a hilar adenocarcinoma produced extrinsic pressure on the renal pedicle and impaired the renal blood flow.[65] The resulting hypertension was reversed by removing the affected kidney. In another case, acceleration of preexisting hypertension occurred secondary to renal artery compression from a metastatic implant of a carcinoma of the colon. Other causes of pressure on the renal artery include lymphosarcoma, hydatid cysts, and abdominal aortic aneurysms.

Dissecting Aneurysm of the Renal Artery

In an analysis of the literature on primary renal artery dissecting aneurysm, Rao and Blaivas found that hypertension was present in 89 percent of cases.[35] When angiography was performed, the diagnosis was usually made correctly. Following nephrectomy, most patients had a prompt remission of their hypertension. In one-fifth of cases, the dissection was bilateral, and, as a consequence, nephrectomy was thought to be a hazardous procedure. The typical appearance is demonstrated in Figure 51-40, in which the compression

Figure 51-40. Renal artery dissection. Selective renal arteriography. (A) Early phase. There is compression of the proximal renal artery, with a curvilinear band extending across the vessel (*arrow*), representing the intima of the artery. Beyond the intimal flap, an irregular broad-based accumulation of contrast material is visible in the media, representing the dissection. Vessels to the midportion of the kidney are compressed. (B) Later phase. Contrast material persists in the false lumen of the main renal artery for a protracted period of time. Portions of the upper pole of the kidney are well perfused, but there is virtually complete obstruction to branches to the midportion of the kidney. (Courtesy of Christos A. Athanosoulis, M.D.) In most patients, the dissection occurs in the media. The intramural hematoma collects between the media and the external elastic lamina. Renal infarction is a common accompaniment of dissection.

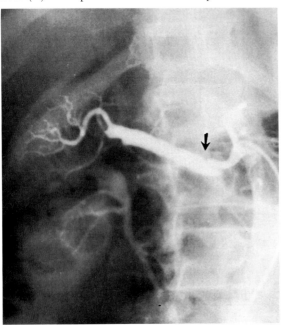

A

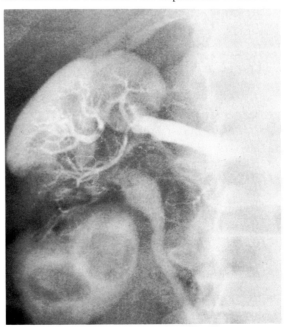

B

of the main renal artery, the intimal flap, and the contrast material in the dissection itself are vividly demonstrated. This case also illustrates the impaired renal perfusion that may occur when dissection is present.

An important cause of renal artery dissection is dysplastic disease of the renal artery (see Fig. 51-12).[34] Dissection has also been reported in association with angiomatous malformation in the subadventitial layer of the renal artery.[67]

Renal Trauma

Hypertension as a sequel of renal trauma, particularly of blunt trauma, has been reported.[68,69] The mechanism by which hypertension results is probably varied: (1) compression of the kidney by subcapsular and perirenal hematoma may occur, with eventual fibrous thickening of the capsule; (2) thrombosis, spasm, or stenosis of the renal artery or the development of an arteriovenous aneurysm may be involved; (3) posttraumatic pyelonephritis, infection, nephrolithiasis, and stasis may occur[63]; or (4) large or small parts of the kidney parenchyma may be torn off without stopping the blood supply and thus remain vital but ischemic.[70] Retroperitoneal hematoma may produce localized constriction of the main renal artery with ensuing hypertension.

The history of a fall or impact is usually elicited, and the physical examination shows flank tenderness and sometimes an obvious mass with tenderness. The kidney may suffer contusion, laceration, or rupture.[71]

A plain film of the abdomen may demonstrate rib fractures, obscured renal and psoas outlines, evidence of a soft tissue mass, and various degrees of localized and generalized ileus. The urogram generally shows a decrease or a lack of contrast on the affected side and possibly extravasation. Crowding and displacement of the entire involved kidney and blood clots with filling defects in the kidney pelvis may be seen.

Figure 51-41. Renal trauma. This 51-year-old woman had fallen on her right flank, and pain and hematuria ensued. The plain film demonstrated a fracture of the right 10th rib and loss of the right psoas and kidney margin. The intravenous pyelogram showed poor opacification of the lower pole, with compression and distortion of the pelvis. (A) Selective renal arteriogram. The vessels are displaced around an area of intrarenal hemorrhage (*arrows*). The spotty areas of increased density may be caused by leakage of contrast material. (B) Nephrographic phase. An area of decreased opacification is visible (*arrow*). Its borders are irregular and extend to the lateral margin of the kidney. The appearance is that of a large intrarenal hemorrhage. (Courtesy of James McCort, M.D.)

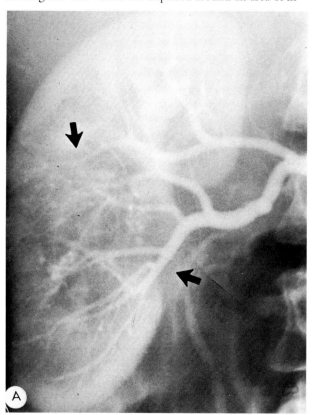

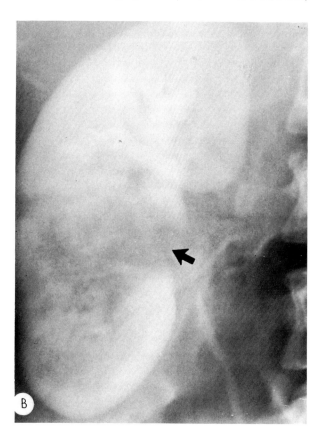

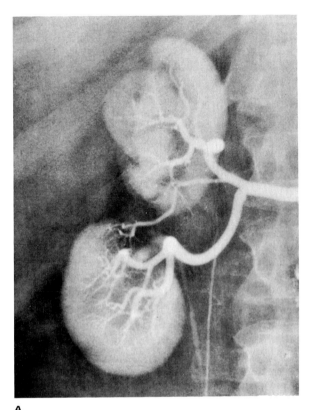

A

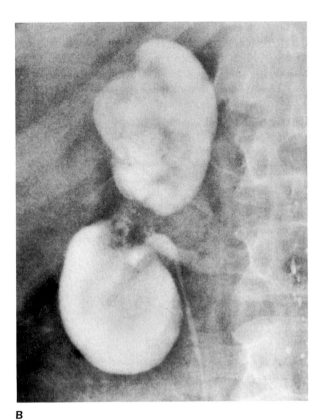

B

Figure 51-42. Renal trauma. This patient entered the hospital because of hypertension. Three years before, he had been in an automobile accident and thereafter had had a great deal of right flank pain. (A) Selective renal arteriogram. A fracture through the midportion of the right kidney is apparent. Although the visible portions of the kidney are subserved by branches of the renal arteries, there is gross distortion of the upper pole and a large area of dead tissue, which is not opacified. (B) Nephrogram. On the nephrogram, the distortion is apparent, and some areas in the midportion of the kidney, which seem lacking in vascular supply, appear to be faintly mottled, indicating that some contrast medium and therefore blood is reaching this ischemic segment.

The renal arteriogram may disclose the following conditions[72]: (1) subcapsular hematoma (see Fig. 51-44); (2) intrarenal hematoma (Fig. 51-41); (3) rupture of the renal artery branches; (4) disrupted continuity of the renal outline, with abnormal straining of the traumatized tissue; and (5) so-called fractured kidney (Fig. 51-42). Displacement of the vessels is particularly common in the presence of intrarenal hematoma (see Fig. 51-41); the hematoma usually appears as an "avascular" site in the kidney in the absence of continued bleeding.

Arteritis

Periarteritis nodosa is a relatively rare cause of renovascular hypertension, and only a few angiographic descriptions of this disease have been reported.[73–76] The renal vessels are involved in about 80 percent of cases, and the pathologic lesion, a necrotizing inflammatory process, primarily involves the arterioles and the smaller intrarenal branches of the renal artery. The intravascular inflammatory process eventually results in the formation of granulation tissue and fibrosis intermixed with areas of vessel-wall destruction. Hemorrhage, thrombosis, and aneurysm formation, which is characteristic of the disease, result.

Angiographically, the demonstration of multiple aneurysms in the small and medium-sized arteries is highly suggestive (Fig. 51-43), although the authors have seen the same appearance in lupus erythematosus. These aneurysms are most often of various sizes and shapes and are distributed throughout the renal parenchyma bilaterally. In addition, the medium and smaller intrarenal arteries may be stretched, attenuated, and diminished in number (probably as a result of thrombosis with secondary recanalization). This rather diffuse small-vessel thrombosis results in variable degrees of cortical ischemia and in an irregular renal outline during the nephrographic phase due to scattered renal

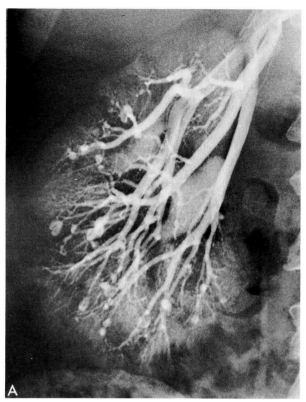

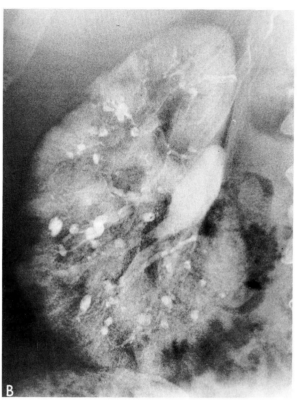

Figure 51-43. Periarteritis nodosa. The findings in the kidney are characteristic, with multiple renal artery aneurysms distributed throughout many segments of the kidney and affecting many branches of the renal artery. (A) Selective renal arteriogram. (B) Nephrographic phase. Note that in the nephrographic phase the aneurysms retain contrast agent and remain opacified long after the arteries have lost their contrast agent. Although this finding is characteristic of periarteritis nodosa, it has also been seen in Wegener granulomatosis, drug abuse patients, and disseminated lupus erythematosus. (Courtesy of Victor Millan, M.D.)

infarction (see Fig. 51-43B). Abdominal aortography may show numerous small aneurysms in the splenic, hepatic, and other visceral vessels.

There are numerous types of vasculitis in which the renal vascular bed may be involved.[75,77] Drug abuse, ergot, and serum sickness may all produce similar renal blood vessel abnormalities.

Wegener granulomatosis is associated with a destructive arteritis of blood vessels and granuloma formation. When it involves the kidney, it usually produces a focal necrotizing glomerulonephritis, with uncommon involvement of the large arteries.[78] At times, however, it may produce disruption of the arterial wall and pseudoaneurysms (Fig. 51-44). Intrarenal or subcapsular hematomas may then develop, and hypertension may be due to the presence of a "Page" kidney, with constriction and compression of the renal parenchyma.[79]

Arteritis may affect multiple vessels and produce an appearance in the renal arteries that is similar to that in renal artery dysplasia (Fig. 51-45). Together with aneurysm formation due to destruction of the media, fibrosis and cicatrix develop; there may be profound narrowing or vascular occlusion. The disease is similar to Takayasu disease and to giant-cell aortitis and arteritis of the Bantu type. The aorta may be involved, as well as the celiac artery (see Fig. 51-45D), the superior mesenteric artery, and many other aortic branches.

Unilateral Irradiation Damage

The deleterious effect of x-irradiation on the vascular system is well known and has been summarized by Asscher.[80] Crummy et al. have reported a case of unilateral irradiation damage that resulted in hypertension 24 years later and that was relieved by nephrectomy.[81] The average dose to the left kidney was 3900 rem, and to the right kidney, 2300 rem. After surgery, the patient's blood pressure fell gradually to normotensive levels.

The production of renal artery stenosis by irradia-

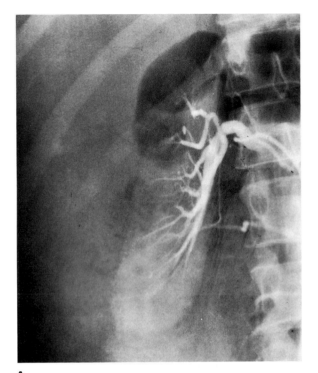

A

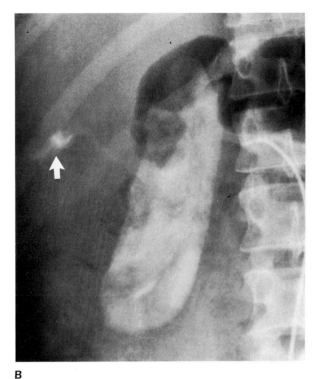

B

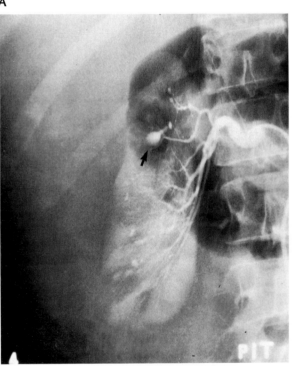

C

Figure 51-44. Wegener granulomatosis. Involvement of the renal vessels. The patient entered with pain in the right flank and a falling hematocrit. Urography suggested the presence of a mass at the lateral aspect of the right kidney. (A) Selective renal arteriogram. There is obvious compression of the intrarenal vessels, which fill poorly. The kidney appears to be displaced medially by a large mass that extends to the lateral abdominal wall. (B) Nephrogram. The distorted appearance of the lateral aspect of the right kidney is clearly related to compression by a large collection of subcapsular fluid. Contrast agent has extravasated in a small tract into the center of the subcapsular hematoma (*arrow*). (C) Arteriogram following the administration of pitressin. The pitressin has produced narrowing of virtually all the intrarenal arterial branches. At the same time, local areas of extravasation are now delineated far better than on the conventional arteriogram, and there is a well-defined pseudoaneurysm in the upper portion of the kidney (*arrow*).

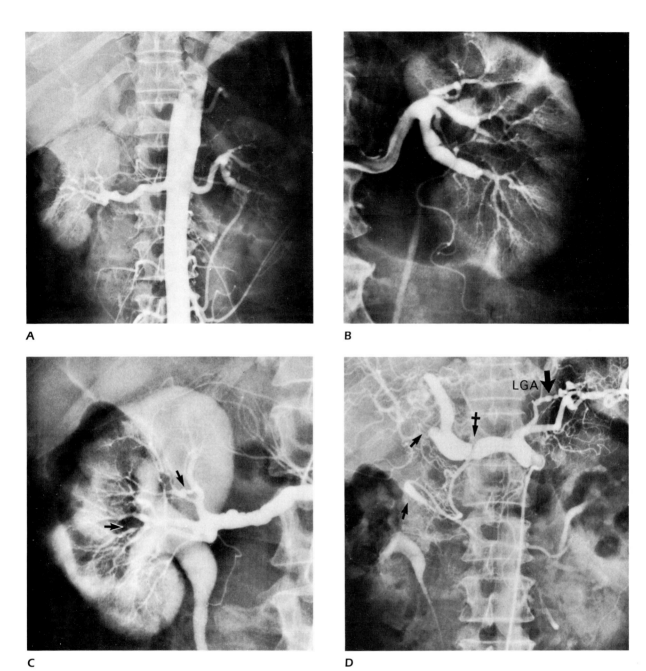

A

B

C

D

Figure 51-45. Arteritis involving the renal arteries and multiple other vessels. (A) Bolus arteriogram. Irregularity of the right main renal artery and its branches, together with localized areas of dilatation of the ventral branch of the left renal artery, is apparent. (B) Selective left renal arteriogram. Both main branches of the left renal artery at the hilus demonstrate localized areas of narrowing and dilatation and wall irregularity. (C) Selective right renal arteriogram. The appearance of the main renal artery resembles the appearance in renal artery dysplasia, with extension into multiple intrarenal arterial branches of localized areas of narrowing and dilatation (*arrows*). (D) Celiac arteriogram. There is a striking degree of stenosis in the common hepatic artery (*barred arrow*). In addition, areas of narrowing and dilatation (*large arrow*) are visible in the left gastric artery (*LGA*) and the right gastroepiploic artery (*arrows*). Complete occlusion of a branch of the right hepatic artery is apparent. (Courtesy of R. Freeman, M.D.)

tion is understandable. Changes of arterial damage occur, including thickening of the vascular wall and damage with consequent fibrosis in the intima, media, and adventitia.[82,83]

Other Renal Causes of Hypertension

The following factors have been associated with renal hypertension:

1. *Oral contraceptives.* A case report of hypertension thought to be caused by oral contraceptives described occlusion of two renal arteries on the right side as well as other arterial occlusions. No embolic source was discovered, and the hypertension was cured by nephrectomy.[84]
2. *Umbilical artery catheterization.* In six neonates with hypertension and elevated peripheral renin levels, renal artery stenosis or occlusion was shown in all. All these patients had had umbilical artery catheterization because of respiratory distress.[85] They became normotensive on conservative therapy.
3. *Dissecting aortic aneurysm repair.* Although it is well known that acute hypertension may accompany dissection with compromise of the renal blood flow, one report describes surgical repair of a type I dissection in which hypertension developed with demonstrated stenosis of the left renal artery and a small left kidney. The surgical repair of the aneurysm had established a compromised flow through the left renal artery that had resulted in hypertension, whereas a complete absence of blood flow before repair was consistent with normotension. Gelfoam embolization of both branches of the left renal artery was associated with the recovery of normal blood pressure.[86]
4. *Solitary cyst.* Most patients with solitary cysts are asymptomatic. Rarely, a large renal cyst may produce unilaterally increased plasma renin activity with elevation of the blood pressure. In one recent report, a patient was described in whom hypertension and a cyst coexisted, with left renal vein renin activity four times as high as that of the right. Aspiration of the cyst was accompanied by a return to normal blood pressure. Subsequently, a reaccumulation of fluid in the cyst was associated with hypertension. When the cyst was evacuated percutaneously a second time, the patient became normotensive.[87]
5. *Polycystic disease.* Hypertension is an important and known concomitant of adult polycystic disease. In relatively few patients has there been documentation of elevation of renin levels, although the

mechanism is thought to be ischemia due to compression by the multiple cysts.[88]
6. *Renal cell carcinoma.* Hypertension is found in a significant percentage of patients with renal tumors, including both renal cell carcinoma and Wilms tumor. The mechanism in some patients is thought to be renal artery compression, in others arteriovenous shunting, and in rare cases actual release of renin from the tumor.[89] The hypertension can be the symptom that brings the patient to clinical attention.[90]
7. *Page kidney.* It has been shown that external renal compression may produce hypertension in the laboratory animal as well as in humans. A number of patients have been described in whom there was a causal relationship between hypertension and subcapsular hematomas with compression of renal parenchyma both by the hematoma and by the thickened capsule and subcapsular scar. Evacuation of the hematoma in one patient and nephrectomy in another patient were accompanied by cure of the hypertension.[79]
8. Other less common causes include hydronephrosis, renal tuberculosis, xanthogranulomatous polynephritis, and renal vein thrombosis.

Collateral Circulation in Renal Ischemia

Some years ago, Abrams et al. studied the collateral channels in 24 patients with renal artery stenosis.[91] This study is the basis for the discussion that follows.

The origin and termination of the collateral channels were found to be as indicated in Table 51-1. The first three lumbar arteries were the most common source of the collateral vessels to the ischemic kidney. Flow from the contralateral side was never demonstrated. The branches from the lumbar arteries coiled in wormlike fashion and entered the peripelvic (Figs. 51-46B, 51-47A, 51-48C, 51-49B, 51-50B), periureteric (see Figs. 51-46B, 51-47A, 51-48D, 51-49C), or capsular branches of the kidney (see Figs. 51-46, 51-47). Most often, they communicated with the plexus of peripelvic vessels, but there were many capsular and periureteric anastomoses as well. Although the first, second, and third lumbar arteries communicated with both the superior and inferior capsular branches, the fourth lumbar artery branches were directed only to the inferior capsular collateral vessels. The course of these vessels was sometimes labyrinthine, but flow into the intrarenal branches could be demonstrated during the later phases of the angiography in many cases.

Table 51-1. Origins and Communications of Collateral Vessels in 24 Cases with Renal Artery Stenosis or Occlusion

| | Vessels Supplied | | | | | |
| | Capsular Arteries | | | | | |
Origin of Collaterals	Superior	Inferior	Lateral	Peripelvic	Periureteric	Total
1st lumbar artery	2	2	2	6	—	12
2nd lumbar artery	4	1	—	5	4	14
3rd lumbar artery	4	3	—	6	6	19
4th lumbar artery	—	5	—	—	5	10
Aorta	—	—	—	7	3	10
Internal iliac artery	—	2	1	—	7	10
Testicular or ovarian artery	—	—	—	2	3	5
Intercostal artery	1	—	2	—	—	3
Inferior adrenal artery	3	—	3	4	—	10
Total	14	13	8	30	28	

From Abrams HL, Cornell SH. Patterns of collateral flow in renal ischemia. Radiology 1965;84:1001. Used with permission.

Vessels arising directly from the aorta and communicating with the peripelvic or periureteric channels were often observed (see Fig. 51-47). In five instances, branches from the most proximal capsular artery, particularly the superior capsular vessel shortly after its origin from the renal artery, connected directly with peripelvic vessels and also bridged the gap to the main renal artery distal to the stenosis (Fig. 51-51). The inferior adrenal artery filled the capsular vessels and the peripelvic vessels in a significant number of cases (see Fig. 51-46). Collateral channels arising from

Text continues on page 1283

Figure 51-46. Renal collateral circulation. A 23-year-old woman with hypertension of 1 year's duration (blood pressure of 240/160 mmHg). (A) Renal arteriogram at 1.5 seconds. There is profound narrowing of the main renal artery (*middle arrow*) and stenosis of the supplementary artery to the lower pole (*lower arrow*). The inferior adrenal branch, arising from the main renal artery, is opacified (*upper arrow*).

(B) At 4 seconds, a periureteric collateral vessel fills from the internal iliac artery and anastomoses with peripelvic collateral vessels (*medial arrows*). The capsular collateral vessels that filled in part from the inferior adrenal artery (*lateral arrow*) empty into tortuous vessels that cross the midportion of the kidney.

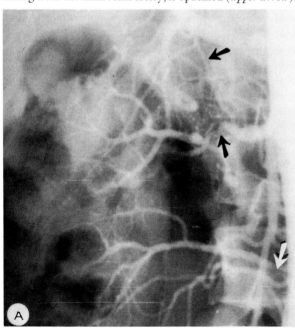

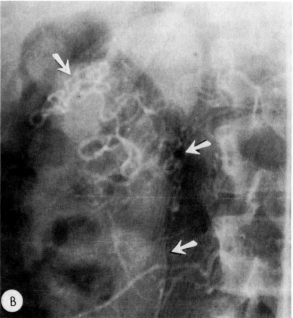

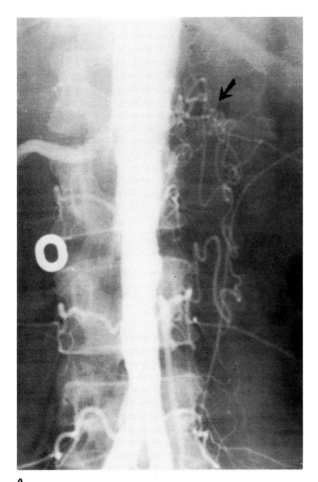

A

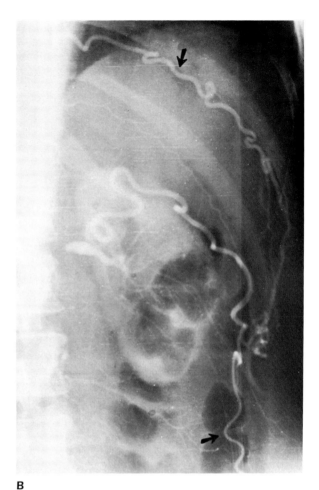

B

Figure 51-47. Renal collateral circulation. This 37-year-old woman had known hypertension for 3 years (blood pressure of 260/150 mmHg). (A) Renal arteriogram 2 seconds after injection. There is complete occlusion of the left renal artery due to arteriosclerotic disease (*arrow*). Peripelvic and peri-ureteric collateral vessels arise directly from the aorta, the adrenal artery, and the lumbar vessels. (B) At 18 seconds after injection, a tortuous collateral artery along the left flank (*lower arrow*) is visible anastomosing with a branch of the 10th intercostal artery (*upper arrow*). These two vessels join the dilated superior capsular artery and drain in a retrograde direction into the renal artery, which is reconstituted 1 cm to the left of the spine. A left nephrectomy was following by profound lowering of the blood pressure but not to completely normal levels.

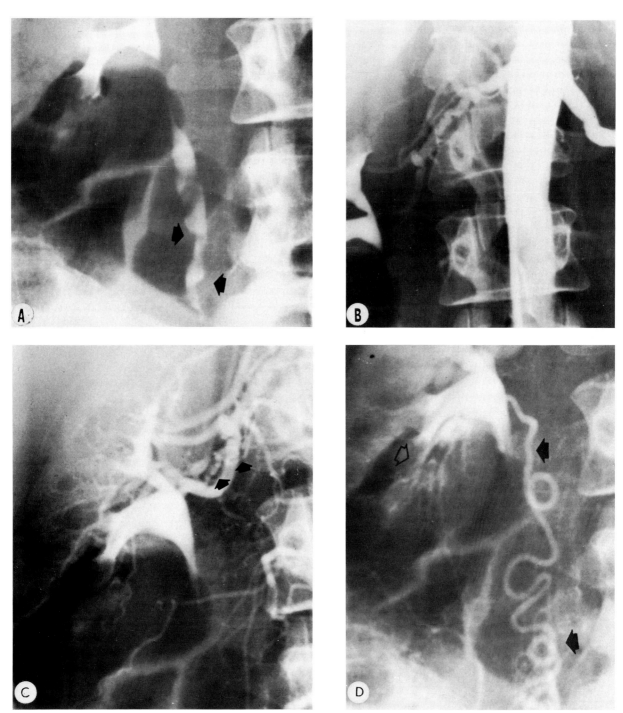

Figure 51-48. Renal artery dysplasia. Perimedial fibroplasia with florid renal collateral circulation. This 43-year-old woman had hypertension of 4 years' duration (blood pressure of 210/120 mmHg). (A) Intravenous urogram shows hyperconcentration and gross scalloping of the ureter (*arrows*). (B) Renal arteriogram, 0.5 second after injection. Both renal arteries show irregular narrowing, much more extensive on the right. (C) At 2 seconds, tortuous peripelvic collateral vessels are visible (*arrows*). No arterial branches are visible in the lower pole. (D) At 5 seconds, a dilated periureteric vessel (*black arrows*) is visible ascending in tortuous fashion and communicating with lower pole branches (*open arrow*). It impinges on the pelvis and the ureter, causing the shallow notching seen in (A). The pathologic lesion is perimedial fibroplasia.

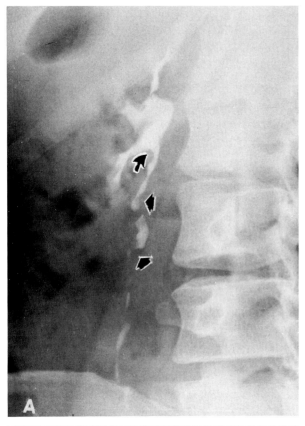

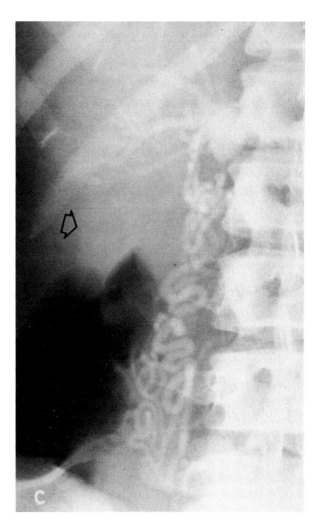

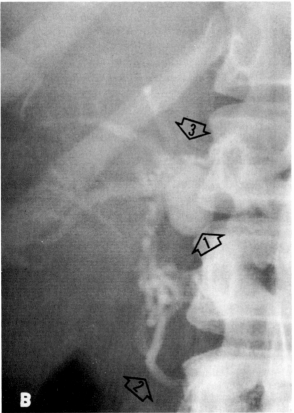

Figure 51-49. The collateral circulation in a renal artery aneurysm. A 24-year-old woman with known hypertension for 6 years (blood pressure of 160/110 mmHg). (A) Intravenous urogram. An oblique 20-minute film shows extensive ureteral notching (*lower arrows*). A small notch in the caudal aspect of the renal pelvis is also seen (*upper arrow*). (B) Renal arteriogram, 1.5 seconds after injection. A large aneurysm of the right renal artery is opacified (*1*). A large collateral trunk arising from the aorta feeds the upper periureteric complex (*2*). A small branch of the proximal renal artery (*3*) gives rise to peripelvic collateral vessels. (C) Film, 5 seconds. Many tortuous, dilated periureteric collateral vessels arise from the lumbar and ovarian arteries. No lower pole intrarenal vessels are visible (*arrow*). These vessels filled later via a retrograde flow from the periureteric collateral chain. (From Abrams HL, Cornell SH. Patterns of collateral flow in renal ischemia. Radiology 1965;84:1001. Used with permission.)

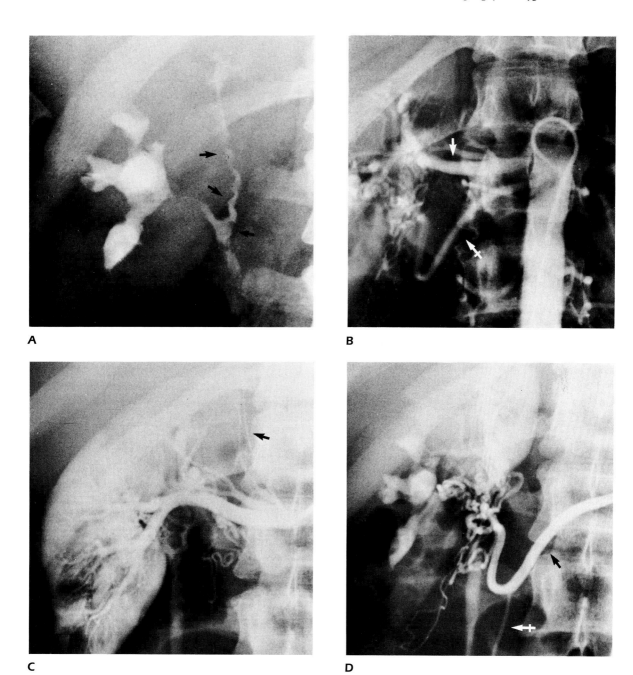

Figure 51-50. Renal collateral circulation. This young man entered the hospital because of hypertension. (A) Intravenous urogram. A bifid renal pelvis is present, with gross irregularity and notching of the pelvis to the upper pole of the kidney (*two upper arrows*) but notching as well of the renal pelvis (*lower arrow*). (B) Bolus aortogram. The main renal artery is visualized (*upper arrow*), and caudal to it a vessel of relatively large size is also opacified (*lower arrow*). Multiple peripelvic collateral vessels are visualized. (C) Selective right renal arteriogram. A normal distribution of vessels to the lower and middle portions of the kidney is apparent, with a striking absence of branches to the upper pole. The adrenal-capsular branches are well visualized (*arrow*). Tortuous collateral vessels are seen adjacent to the spine. (D) Injection of the large caudally located arterial trunk to the kidney demonstrates that it is in fact the proximal portion of the gonadal artery (*black arrow*). This vessel supplies virtually all the blood to the upper pole of the kidney, produces a dense nephrogram, and is accompanied by multiple small collateral channels. Note that the normal gonadal artery (*white arrow*) extends caudally into the pelvis.

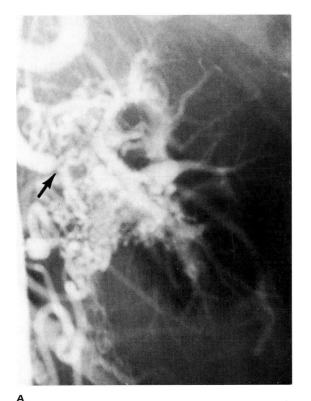

A

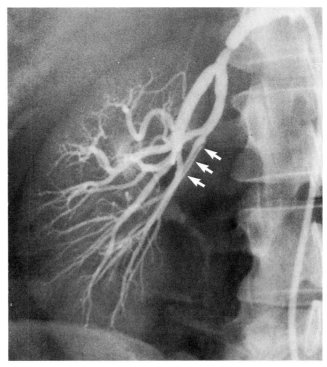

B

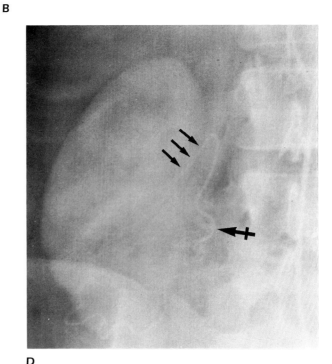

C

D

Figure 51-51. Renal collateral circulation. (A) This 20-year-old woman was studied because of hypertension. Arteriography demonstrates irregularity of the proximal renal artery, due to perimedial fibroplasia, with complete occlusion of the artery (*arrow*). An enormous cluster of peripelvic and periureteric collateral channels is opacified. The collateral pathways have carried the contrast agent into the renal artery beyond the area of occlusion so that the intrarenal branches are opacified. The appearance resembles that in an arteriovenous malformation. (B to D) Reversal of the flow in a collateral channel. Medial hyperplasia. (B) A localized zone of nar-rowing produced by medial (fibromuscular) hyperplasia is visible in the right renal artery. In addition, a linear lucent band (*arrows*) is seen in a dorsal branch to the lower pole. This represents nonopaque blood entering the branch beyond the stenotic zone because of lower pressure. (C) With injection pressure at its height, the communication is revealed by contrast at its insertion (*arrow*), and a "dilution" defect is no longer apparent. (D) Late phase of an aortogram. A periureteric vessel (*lower arrow*), filling retrogradely, supplies the collateral branch visible in (B) and (C), after turning in a caudal direction (*three upper arrows*).

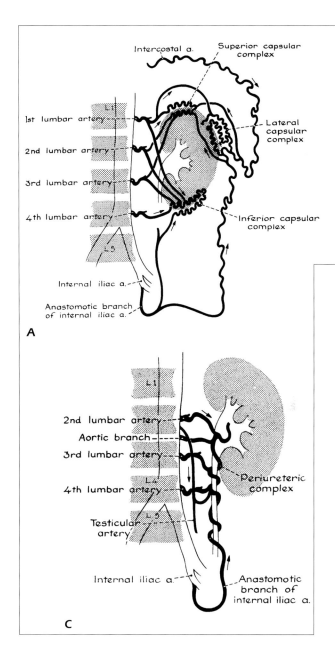

Figure 51-52. Diagrams of renal collateral circulation. (A) The capsular system. The first four lumbar arteries, branches of the internal iliac and the intercostal arteries, contribute significantly to the capsular complex. In addition (not pictured here), the inferior adrenal and capsular branches proximal to the stenosis also make major contributions. Note that a separate lateral capsular complex has been indicated; it represents a continuation of the superior capsular system but has been designated lateral because of its location and mode of filling. (B) The peripelvic system. The aorta, inferior adrenal, first three lumbar, and testicular (or ovarian) arteries each supply branches to the peripelvic system. Other important pathways are the direct capsular branches from the renal artery proximal to the stenosis. (C) The periureteric system. The internal iliac artery is the single most common source of periureteric collateral vessels. The second, third, and fourth lumbar branches, the testicular branches, and the direct aortic branches are also large and important components of this collateral pathway.

the intercostal arteries, communicating with the capsular branches of the kidney (see Fig. 51-47), were also observed. The major flow to the periureteric circulation arose from the hypogastric artery in seven instances and ascended from the pelvis into the paraspinal area (see Fig. 51-48D). In some instances, the testicular or the ovarian artery was also a major source of collateral flow to the periureteric channels and the capsular arteries (see Fig. 51-50).

The width and length of many of the collateral channels were striking. In a number of instances, segmental occlusion had occurred, and the intrarenal branches to a particular part of the kidney that had

failed to fill initially were opacified late in the study from the collateral circulation (see Fig. 51-48).

Figure 51-52 is a diagrammatic sketch of the total collateral renal blood flow in humans. Both Table 51-1 and Figure 51-52 fail to include the bridging collateral vessels directly from the proximal to the distal main renal artery. The proximal renal artery was also an occasional source of direct peripelvic collateral vessels. Stenosis was located in the middle third of the main renal artery in two-thirds of these patients.

The literature on the collateral circulation of the kidney is sparse, even though in 1906 ligation of the renal artery was found to be compatible with life in the dog if the renal capsule had previously been removed.[92] In 1940 Mason et al., in the course of experiments on hypertension in dogs, discovered a large periureteric branch of the ovarian artery that supplied the kidney in one animal.[93] Flasher et al., in a study of renal collateral blood flow in rabbits, emphasized that the collateral vessels represented dilatation of preexisting, nonfunctioning channels and that the initiation of collateral flow was related to the presence of renal ischemia.[94] More recently, attention has been focused on the periureteric collateral vessels because of the scalloped imprint that they produce on the ureter.[36,44,95]

The vessels in humans that supply the renal collateral vessels are largely the lumbar, internal iliac, testicular or ovarian, inferior adrenal, renal capsular, and intercostal arteries, as well as the aorta itself. Of all these vessels, the third lumbar artery is the most common source of anastomotic flow to the kidney. Although it seems reasonable that the connections between the lumbar arteries and the renal circulation represent pathways already present, these anastomoses have not been demonstrated in postmortem injections in humans in the absence of renal ischemia. Nevertheless, it is difficult to conceive of the development of such a multiplicity of vessels de novo.

The collateral channels are coiled, tortuous, and enormously lengthened in comparison with the normal. They are also conspicuously dilated. Although it is relatively easy to understand why thin-walled venous channels become grossly distended, as in the collateral system in portal hypertension or superficial leg varices, it is somewhat more difficult to explain why all collateral arterial beds have the serpiginous elongated appearance so well demonstrated in coarctation of the aorta. The relatively thick walled arteries should be able to distend without elongating but obviously do not. Instead, a striking increase in length is denoted by the multiple coils that are visible (see Fig. 51-51A). Because blood flow through an arterial collateral bed always requires, at some point in the delivery system, the reversal of the normal direction, it is possible that retrograde flow may partially account for the elongation of the collateral vascular channels.

A well-developed collateral circulation on angiography implies a significant arterial lesion, although significant stenosis need not be accompanied by visible collateral vessels.[91] Pharmacoangiographic methods have been employed and advocated for defining collateral vessels more. Epinephrine diminishes pressure gradients by producing distal vasoconstrictions; collateral flow is thus reduced, and the angiographic injection may then opacify collateral vessels not previously visible by retrograde flow. Conversely, vasodilatation produced by such drugs as acetylcholine augments the gradient, increases collateral flow, reduces retrograde collateral visualization during angiography, and may afford demonstration of nonopaque streams produced by collateral filling (see Fig. 51-51B through D).[96] Sometimes a collateral circulation may develop that is sufficient to reduce renal ischemia, with a striking remission of hypertension in the presence of complete renal artery occlusion.[97]

Angiography After Surgery in Renovascular Hypertension

Angiography is most often performed in the postsurgical patient with renal artery stenosis because hypertension either has persisted or, having responded to surgery, has recurred. It is not surprising, therefore, that changes are observed in the grafts in a large number of patients. Ekelund et al. studied the postoperative appearance in 128 patients and found that with saphenous-vein bypass grafts there were 30 dilated grafts, 29 stenoses, 9 occlusions, 2 aneurysms, and 2 infarctions. When repeat angiograms were performed on patients with dilatation, progressive enlargement was usually found.[59,98]

In 19 patients with Dacron grafts, there were no abnormalities in 9, stenosis of the distal anastomosis in 6, and total occlusion in 4. In 13 patients with endarterectomies, 11 appeared normal, and stenosis appeared in 1 and dilatation in another.[98]

In one study, the postsurgical results in 35 patients with complete occlusion of the main renal artery were analyzed. Among these, nephrectomy was required in 14, and there were two deaths; in the remainder, the hypertension disappeared or improved. Follow-up studies in 20 patients showed continued patency of all revascularizations.[99]

The ideal result is a widely patent graft or prosthesis that fully perfuses the kidney (Fig. 51-53). Unfortunately, even when the saphenous vein graft is dilated, stenosis may be present at the anastomotic junction with the renal artery (Fig. 51-54). Occasionally bilateral renal artery stenosis requires bypass grafting with Teflon prostheses (Fig. 51-55). An alternative approach is to anastomose the splenic artery to the obstructed renal artery (Fig. 51-56). With vein grafts, stenosis need not occur at the anastomotic site itself but may actually develop within the body of the vein (Fig. 51-57). Multiple projections and selective studies may be required before the anatomy can be unfolded completely (see Fig. 51-57, which shows that 9 months after the initial study not only had the major visualized stenosis in the body of the vein graft become more profound but also there was a distal stenotic lesion at the site of the saphenous vein anastomosis to the renal artery). If thrombosis occurs after vein bypass, the native circulation may become occluded (Fig. 51-58), so that the patient may end up with a total absence of perfusion. Finally, it should be emphasized that even in patients who have had renal artery reconstructive

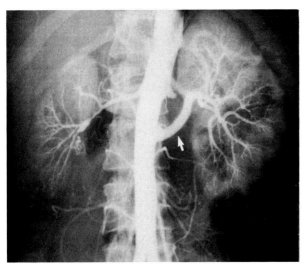

Figure 51-53. Renal artery bypass in renal artery stenosis. The bypass (*arrow*) is functioning well, with a good-sized kidney, large intrarenal interlobar vessels, and excellent filling of the cortex. Note the widespread disease of the right main renal artery and some of the branches.

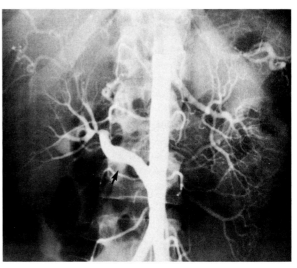

Figure 51-54. Renal artery bypass. Contrast material fills the intrarenal vessels, but there is stenosis at the site of anastomosis with the renal artery (*arrow*). Blood flow to the kidney is diminished, and the intrarenal branches are small.

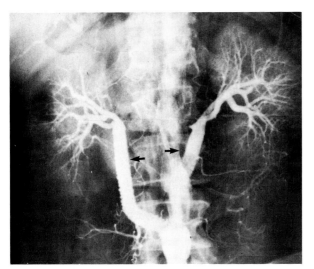

Figure 51-55. Bilateral renal artery bypass (*arrows*). Teflon prostheses are functioning very well to provide blood supply to the kidneys in the presence of bilateral renal artery stenosis.

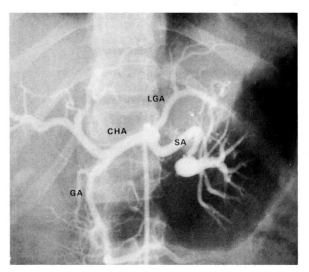

Figure 51-56. Renal artery stenosis after a splenic renal artery anastomosis. The catheter is in the celiac renal artery. The splenic artery (*SA*) has been anastomosed to the left renal artery beyond the area of renal artery occlusion. Although there is narrowing of the anastomotic site, good filling of the intrarenal arterial branches is demonstrated. Note the usual trifurcation of the celiac artery into the common hepatic artery (*CHA*) (with the gastroduodenal artery, *GA*, arising from it), the left gastric artery (*LGA*), and the splenic artery (*SA*).

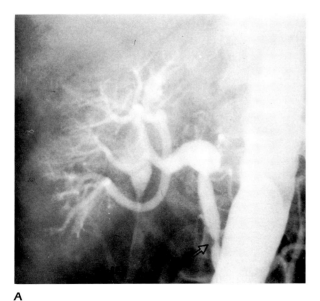

A

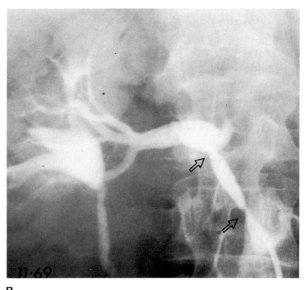

B

Figure 51-57. Arteriosclerotic occlusion of the renal artery. Vein bypass. (A) Aortogram, February. The renal artery on the right is occluded. The bypass extends from the level of the third lumbar vertebra to the dilated main renal artery. An area of narrowing is visible in the bypass (*arrow*). (B) Selective renal arteriogram, November. Stenoses of the by-pass adjacent to the aorta (*medial arrow*) and at the anastomosis with the renal artery (*lateral arrow*) are now visible. The distal graft stenosis was obscured in the aortographic study of February. The patient's hypertension responded well to surgery initially but then recurred later, probably in association with the narrowing of the saphenous vein bypass.

Figure 51-58. Renal artery vein bypass with subsequent occlusion of the renal artery and the bypass. (A) Aortogram. Bilateral renal artery dysplasia is visible, with involvement of both main renal arteries by perimedial fibroplasia. There is marked stenosis of the right renal artery (*arrow*). (B) Aortogram, 4 months after surgery. Venous bypass surgery was done to increase the renal blood flow. The bypass is occluded (*lower arrow*), and the main renal artery has now developed complete occlusion as well (*upper arrow*). Occlusion of the native circulation following bypass surgery may occur, with dominant flow moving through the bypass and with thrombosis of the aortic artery.

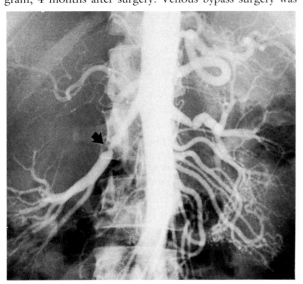

A

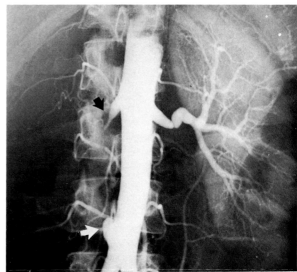

B

surgery with persistent improvement, restenosis or new lesions in the involved kidney may develop.[100]

Interventional Radiology in Hypertension

Because the angiographic catheter has become so important a part of medical diagnosis, its application to medical therapy has been an expected advance. Thus transcatheter thromboembolectomy with aspiration of emboli has been employed to treat acute renal artery obstruction, with successful application to uncontrollable hypertension.[101] Because it is possible to occlude arteriovenous fistulas using such materials as cyanoacrylate,[102] patients with hypertension associated with renal arteriovenous fistulas may be treated by this nonsurgical method.

Similarly, because surgical revascularization is a major operation with significant morbidity and mortality, it was natural that percutaneous transluminal angioplasty would be extended. PTA has been used successfully in atherosclerotic and other lesions, and is the procedure of choice for the treatment of renal fibromuscular dysplasia.[5] In addition, advances in the use of metallic stents have been promising and are being applied to the renal arteries, using the Palmaz,[6] Strecker,[7] and Wallstent endoprostheses.[8]

Acknowledgments

Several of the illustrations in this chapter are reproduced with permission from Abrams HL, Marshall WH, Kupric EA. The renal vascular bed in hypertension. Semin Roentgenol 1967;2:157.

References

1. Goldblatt H, Lynch J, Hanzal RF. The production of persistent hypertension in dogs. Am J Pathol 1933;9:942.
2. Amsterdam EA, Couch NP, Christlieb AR. Renal vein renin activity in the prognosis of surgery for renovascular hypertension. Am J Med 1969;47:860.
3. Eyler WR, Clark MD, Garman JE. Angiography of the renal areas including a comparative study of renal arterial stenoses in patients with or without hypertension. Radiology 1962;78:879.
4. Holley KE, Hunt JC, Brown AL Jr, et al. Renal artery stenosis: a clinical-pathologic study in normotensive and hypertensive patients. Am J Med 1964;37:14.
5. Klinge J, Willem PT, Puijilaert CB, Geyskes GG, Becking WB, Feldberg MA. Percutaneous transluminal renal angioplasty: initial and long-term results. Radiology 1989;171:501–506.
6. Rees CR, et al. Palmaz stent in atherosclerotic stenoses involving the ostia of the renal arteries: preliminary report of a multicenter study. Radiology 1991;181:507.
7. Kuhn FP, Kutkuhn B, Torsello G, Modder U. Renal artery stenosis: preliminary results of treatment with the Strecker stent. Radiology 1991;180:367.
8. Wilms GE, et al. Renal artery stent placement with use of the Wallstent endoprosthesis. Radiology 1991;179:457.
9. Baldwin DS, Van den Broeck H, Harnes JR, et al. Renovascular hypertension in unselected patients. Arch Intern Med 1967;120:176–179.
10. Dean RH. Renovascular hypertension. Curr Probl Surg 1985;22:6–67.
11. Majd M, Potter BM, Guzzetta PC, et al. Effect of captopril on efficiency of renal scintigraphy in detection of renal artery stenosis. J Nucl Med 1983;24:23.
12. Abrams HL, Marshall WH, Kupic EA. The renal vascular bed in hypertension. Semin Roentgenol 1967;2:157.
13. Moody RO, Van Nyys RG. The position and mobility of the kidneys in healthy young men and women. Anat Rec 1940;76:111.
14. Merklin RJ, Michels NA. The variant renal and suprarenal blood supply with data on the inferior phrenic, ureteral and gonadal arteries. J Intern Coll Surg 1958;29:41.
15. Gruntzig A. Treatment of renovascular hypertension with percutaneous dilatation of a renal artery stenosis. Lancet 1978;1:801.
16. Graves F. The anatomy of the intrarenal arteries and its application to segmental resection of the kidney. Br J Surg 1954;42:132.
17. Boijsen E. Angiographic studies of the anatomy of single and multiple renal arteries. Acta Radiol (Stockh) 1959;Suppl 183.
18. Bookstein JJ, Clark R. Renal microvascular disease. Boston: Little, Brown, 1980.
19. Spriggs DW, Brantley RE. Recognition of renal artery spasm during renal angiography. Radiology 1978;127:363.
20. Bookstein JJ, Abrams HL, Buenger RE, et al. Radiologic aspects of renovascular hypertension: II. The role of urography in unilateral renovascular disease. JAMA 1972;220:1225.
21. Bookstein JJ. Appraisal of arteriography in estimating the hemodynamic significance of renal artery stenoses. Invest Radiol 1966;1:281.
22. Kaufman JJ. Renovascular hypertension: the UCLA experience. J Urol 1979;121:139.
23. Roubidoux MA, Dunnick NR, Klatman PE, Newman GE, Cohen RH, Kadir S, Svetkey LP. Renal vein renins: inability to predict response to revascularization in patients with hypertension. Radiology 1991;178:819–822.
24. Bookstein JJ, Abrams HL, Buenger RE, et al. Radiologic aspects of renovascular hypertension: III. Appraisal of arteriography. JAMA 1972;221:368.
25. Halpern M, Finby N, Evans JA. Percutaneous transfemoral renal arteriography in hypertension. Radiology 1961;77:25.
26. Palubinskas AJ, Wylie EJ. Roentgen diagnosis of fibromuscular hyperplasia of the renal arteries. Radiology 1961;76:634.
27. Ekelund L, Gerlock J Jr, Molin J, Smith C. Roentgenologic appearance of fibromuscular dysplasia. Acta Radiol 1977;19:433.
28. Perry MO. Fibromuscular disease of carotid artery. Surg Gynecol Obstet 1972;134:57.
29. McCormack LJ, Poutasse EF, Meaney TF. A pathologic-arteriographic correlation of renal arterial disease. Am Heart J 1966;72:188.
30. Harrison EG, McCormack LJ. Pathologic classification of renal arterial disease in renovascular hypertension. Mayo Clin Proc 1971;46:161–167.
31. McCormack LJ, Dustan HP, Meaney TF. Selected pathology of the renal artery. Semin Roentgenol 1967;2:126.
32. Kincaid OW, Davis GD, Hallerman FJ, et al. Fibromuscular dysplasia of the renal arteries: arteriographic features, classification, and observations on natural history of the disease. AJR 1968;104:271.
33. Kincaid OW. Renal angiography. Chicago: Year Book, 1966.
34. Meyers DS, Grim CE, Keltze WF. Fibromuscular dysplasia of the renal artery with medial dissection: a case simulating polyarteritis nodosa. Am J Med 1974;56:412.
35. Rao CN, Blaivas JG. Primary renal artery dissecting aneurysm: a review. J Urol 1977;118:716.

36. Aurell M. Fibromuscular dysplasia of the renal arteries. Br Med J 1979;1:1180.
37. Gill WM Jr, Meaney TF. Medial fibroplasia of the renal artery. Radiology 1969;92:861.
38. Alvestrand A, Bergstrom J, Wehle B. Pheochromocytoma and renovascular hypertension: a case report and review of the literature. Acta Med Scand 1977;202:231.
39. Itzchak Y, Katznelson D, Boichis H, Jonas A, et al. Angiographic features of arterial lesions in neurofibromatosis. AJR 1974;122:643.
40. Schurch W, Messerl FH, Genest J, et al. Arterial hypertension and neurofibromatosis: renal artery stenosis and coarctation of abdominal aorta. Can Med Assoc J 1975;113:879.
41. Black HR, Glickman MG, Schiff M Jr, et al. Renovascular hypertension: pathophysiology, diagnosis, and treatment. Yale J Biol Med 1978;51:635.
42. Hollenberg NK, Epstein N, Basch RI, et al. "No man's land" of the renal vasculature: an arteriographic and hemodynamic assessment of the interlobar and arcuate arteries in essential and accelerated hypertension. Am J Med 1969;47:845.
43. Foster RS, Shuford WH, Weens HS. Selective renal arteriography in medical diseases of the kidney. AJR 1965;95:291.
44. Bookstein JJ, Stewart BH. The current status of renal arteriography. Radiol Clin North Am 1964;2:461.
45. Hollenberg NK, Epstein N, Basch I, et al. Renin secretions in essential and accelerated hypertension. Am J Med 1969; 47:855.
46. McDonald DF. Renal hypertension without main arterial stenosis: function tests predict cure. JAMA 1968;203:932.
47. Hoxie HJ, Coggin CB. Renal infarction: a statistical study of 205 cases and detailed report of an unusual case. Arch Intern Med 1940;65:587.
48. Reuter SR, Pomeroy PR, Chuang VP, et al. Embolic control of hypertension caused by segmental renal artery stenosis. AJR 1976;127:389.
49. Boijsen E, Köhler R. Renal artery aneurysms. Acta Radiol 1963;1:1077.
50. Dodds WJ, Noyes WE, Hinman F Jr. Renal artery aneurysm: the cause of segmental alteration in renal blood flow and hypertension. AJR 1968;104:302.
51. Burt RL, Johnston FR, Silverthorne RG. Ruptured renal artery aneurysm in pregnancy: report of a case with survival. Obstet Gynecol 1956;7:229.
52. Harrow BR, Sloane JA. Aneurysm of renal artery: report of five cases. J Urol 1959;81:35.
53. Cummings KB, Lecky JW, Kaufman JJ. Renal artery aneurysms and hypertension. J Urol 1973;109:144.
54. Love L, Moncada R, Lescher AJ. Renal arteriovenous fistulae. AJR 1965;95:364.
55. Maldonado JE, Sheps SG, Bernatz PE, et al. Renal arteriovenous fistula: a reversible cause of hypertension and heart failure. Am J Med 1964;37:499.
56. Boijsen E, Kohler R. Renal arteriovenous fistulae. Acta Radiol 1962;57:433.
57. Meng CH, Elkin M. Immediate angiographic manifestations of iatrogenic renal injury due to percutaneous needle biopsy. Radiology 1971;100:335.
58. Bennett AR, Wiener SN. Intrarenal arteriovenous fistula and aneurysm. AJR 1975;95:372.
59. Ekelund L, Lindholm T. Arteriovenous fistulae following percutaneous renal biopsy. Acta Radiol (Stockh) 1972;Suppl 321.
60. Kohler R, Edgren J. Angiographic abnormalities following percutaneous needle biopsy of the kidney. Acta Radiol 1974; 15:514.
61. Lundstrom B. Angiographic abnormalities following percutaneous needle biopsy of the kidney. Acta Radiol (Stockh) 1972;Suppl321.
62. Kittredge RD, Hemley SD, Kanick V, et al. The atrophic renal artery. AJR 1964;92:309.
63. Friedenberg MJ, Eisen S, Kissane J. Renal angiography in pyelonephritis glomerulonephritis and arteriolar nephrosclerosis. AJR 1965;95:349.
64. D'Abreau F, Strickland B. Developmental renal artery stenosis. Lancet 1962;2:517.
65. Lampe WT II. Renovascular hypertension: a review of reversible causes due to extrinsic pressure on the renal artery and report of three unusual cases. Angiology 1965;16:677.
66. Sutton D, Brunton FJ, Foot EC, et al. Fibromuscular, fibrous, and nonatheromatous renal artery stenosis and hypertension. Clin Radiol 1963;14:381.
67. Acconcia A, Manganelli A. Dissecting aneurysm of renal artery owing to subadventitial angioma. J Urol 1978;119:268.
68. Downs RA, Hewett AL. Hypertension due to subcapsular renal hematoma. J Urol 1962;88:22.
69. Hemley SD, Finby N. Renal trauma: a concept of injury to the renal artery. Radiology 1962;79:816.
70. Olsson O, Lunderquist A. Angiography in renal trauma. Acta Radiol 1963;1:1.
71. Forsythe WE, Persky L. Comparison of ureteral and renal injuries. Am J Surg 1959;97:558.
72. Marenta VE, Schnauder A. Angiographie und Nierentrauma. Schweiz Med Wochenschr 1964;94:1484.
73. Bron KM, Strott CA, Shapiro AP. The diagnostic value of angiographic observations in polyarteritis nodosa. Arch Intern Med 1965;116:450.
74. Fleming RJ, Stern LZ. Multiple intraparenchymal renal aneurysms in polyarteritis nodosa. Radiology 1965;84:100.
75. Halpern M, Citron BP. Necrotizing angiitis associated with drug abuse. AJR 1971;111:663.
76. Robins JM, Bookstein J. Percutaneous transcaval biopsy technique in the evaluation of inferior vena cava occlusion. Radiology 1972;105:451.
77. Christian CL, Sargent JS. Vasculitis syndromes: clinical and experimental models. Am J Med 1976;3:385.
78. Reidbord HE, McCormack LJ, O'Duffy JD, et al. Necrotizing angiitis: II. Findings at autopsy in twenty-seven cases. Cleve Clin J Med 1965;32:191.
79. Marshall WH Jr, Castellino RA. Hypertension produced by constricting capsular renal lesions ("Page" kidney). Radiology 1971;101:561.
80. Asscher AW. The delayed effects of renal irradiation. Clin Radiol 1964;15:320.
81. Crummy AB Jr, Heliman S, Stansel HC Jr, et al. Renal hypertension secondary to unilateral radiation damage relieved by nephrectomy. Radiology 1965;84:108.
82. Staab GE, Tegtmeyer CJ, Constable WC. Radiation-induced renovascular hypertension. AJR 1976;126:634.
83. Thomas E, Forbus WD. Irradiation injury to aorta and lung. Arch Pathol 1959;67:256.
84. Delin K, Aurell M, Claes GT, et al. Multiple arterial occlusions and hypertension probably caused by an oral contraceptive: a patient in whom the development of renovascular hypertension has been followed. Clin Nephrol 1976;6:453.
85. Merten DF, Vogel JM, Adelman RD, et al. Renovascular hypertension as a complication of umbilical arterial catheterization. Radiology 1978;126:751.
86. Rose EA, McNicholas KW, Bethea MC, et al. Renovascular hypertension following surgical repair of dissecting aneurysm of the thoracic aorta. Surgery 1978;83:235.
87. Mang HYL, Markovic PR, Chow S, et al. Solitary intrarenal cyst causing hypertension: with plasma renin activity study before and after cyst aspiration. NY State J Med 1978;78:654.
88. Hatfield PM, Pfester RC. Adult polycystic disease of the kidneys. JAMA 1972;222:1527.
89. Conn JW, Bookstein JJ, Cohen EL. Renin-secreting juxtaglomerular cell adenoma. Radiology 1973;106:543.
90. Abrams HL. Renal tumor versus renal cyst: I and II. Cardiovasc Radiol 1978;1:125.
91. Abrams HL, Cornell SH. Patterns of collateral flow in renal ischemia. Radiology 1965;84:1001.
92. Martini E. Ueber die Möglichkeit der Niere einen neuen col-

lateralen Blutzufluss zu schaffen. Arch Klin Chir 1906;78:
619.

93. Mason MF, Robinson CS, Blalock A. Studies on the renal
arterial blood pressure and the metabolism of kidney tissue in
experimental hypertension. J Exp Med 1940;72:289.

94. Flasher J, Drury DR, Jacobson G. Experimental arterial stenosis: post stenotic dilatation and collateral blood flow. Angiology 1951;2:60.

95. Halpern M, Evans JA. Coarctation of the renal artery with
"notching" of the ureter: a roentgenologic sign of unilateral
renal disease as a cause of hypertension. AJR 1962;88:159.

96. Bookstein JJ, Walter JF, Stanley JC. Pharmacoangiographic
manipulation of renal collateral blood flow. Circulation 1976;
54:328.

97. Dobrzinsky SJ, Voegeli E, Grant H, et al. Spontaneous reestablishment of renal function after complete occlusion of a
renal artery. Arch Intern Med 1971;128:266.

98. Ekelund L, Gerlock J Jr, Goncharenko V. Angiographic findings following surgical treatment for renovascular hypertension. Radiology 1978;126:345.

99. Lawson JD, Hollifield JH, Foster JH, et al. Hypertension secondary to complete occlusion of the renal artery. Am Surg
1978;136:648.

100. Ekestrom S, Liljeqvist L, Nordhus O. Persisting hypertension
after renal artery reconstruction: a follow-up study. Scand J
Urol Nephrol 1979;13:83.

101. Millan VG, Sher MH, Deterring RA Jr, et al. Transcatheter
thromboembolectomy of acute renal artery occlusion. Arch
Surg 1978;113:1086.

102. Kerber CW, Freeny PC, Cromwell L, et al. Cyanoacrylate occlusion of a renal arteriovenous fistula. AJR 1977;128:663.

52

Renal Venography

HERBERT L. ABRAMS
BENJAMIN B. FAITELSON

*I*n the past, renal vein catheterization has been employed in both physiologic and radiologic studies. Within recent years its usefulness has been especially emphasized in the study of renal vein thrombosis in patients whose clinical and laboratory examinations are suggestive of that diagnosis. It has also been applied extensively to the investigation of patients with malignant disease of the kidney, and it has been helpful in confirming the presumptive diagnosis of renal agenesis, the presence of renal vein abnormalities in transplantation patients, and the likelihood of closure of splenorenal shunts. It has been used in essential hematuria to search for renal vein varices and has played an important role in the determination of renin levels in the renal venous effluent. A relatively simple procedure technically, it may be highly rewarding when properly performed in selected cases.

Technique

A flexible, radiopaque catheter (Fig. 52-1A) large enough to permit a sufficiently rapid injection (e.g., a 5 or 6 French catheter with multiple side holes) is passed percutaneously into the right femoral vein and advanced to the level of the renal vein. The catheter tip should be bent 130 degrees. The bent tip should be about 5 cm long on the right catheter and about 10 cm long on the left catheter; however, the right catheter can be used for both sides if a guidance system is used for placement into the distal left renal vein. Alternatively, a catheter with less curvature (e.g., an abdominal visceral catheter) may be introduced into both renal veins with a controllable guidewire. The catheter should have two side holes within 1 cm of its tip. For selective catheterization of segmental veins, the tip may be deflected downward an additional 30 degrees. With different degrees of rotation, various portions of the intrarenal venous system may be catheterized. A coaxial catheter system or a controllable tip guidewire facilitates some examinations.[1]

Total sustained opacification of the renal venous bed is best obtained with deliberate slowing of the renal blood flow by injecting 10 μg of epinephrine into the renal artery through a selectively placed arterial catheter.[2] Because tumor vessels are less responsive than normal vessels, epinephrine is often not useful in improving the visualization of the veins draining renal carcinomas.[3] Transient balloon occlusion of the corresponding renal artery achieves a similar result[4,5] and may be an alternative if epinephrine is contraindicated, as it is in patients with arrhythmias. Excellent renal vein opacification is obtained by selective occlusive renal phlebography.[5,6] In this method, a double-lumen catheter with distal side holes and a proximal balloon for occlusion of the renal vein are employed during selective venous injection, in addition to intraarterial epinephrine administration. If visualization of only the main renal vein is desired, epinephrine venography is not necessarily required; forceful countercurrent injection may be adequate.

The volume of contrast agent may be varied, depending on the reason for the examination. If good depiction of the intrarenal venous bed and the small veins is desired, 30 ml of a contrast agent with 76 percent iodine concentration should be injected in 2 seconds, with the catheter tip placed in the renal hilus. If thrombus is suspected, 20 ml in 2 seconds may be injected. In renal carcinoma, the inferior vena cava (IVC) should be studied first to rule out tumor thrombus extending into the IVC. The catheter tip is then positioned in the mouth of the renal vein, and a low-pressure hand injection of 15 ml is made. With small peripheral lesions, the catheter is placed more distally, and epinephrine-aided venography at 20 ml in 2 seconds is performed.[7] Generally the volume of contrast material used should be based on a preliminary test injection and the assessment of the renal venous flow. Although the standard has been the use of cut-film venography, digital subtraction venography, for the diagnosis of renal vein thrombosis, has also been reported.[8]

1290

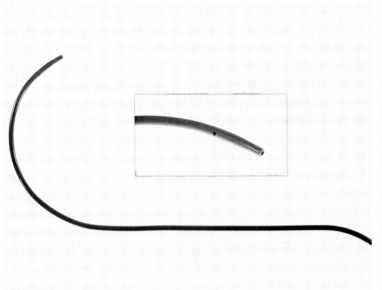

A

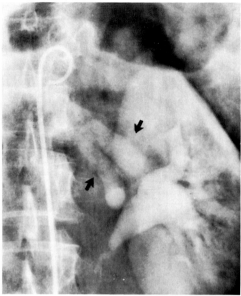

B

Figure 52-1. Technique of renal venography. (A) Renal vein catheter. The catheter has a curve of about 130 degrees, with two side holes 1 cm from the end. (B) Renal vein opaci-

fication during arteriography. Visualization is adequate but not optimal. Two renal veins (*arrows*) unite medial to the kidney to form a single preaortic vein.

Sometimes the renal vein valves may interfere with venography and impede satisfactory visualization. In such a case, venography should be repeated with adequate slowing of the renal blood flow; a normal renal venous bed may thus be displayed. The occasional failure to catheterize the renal vein and its branches selectively may well be explained by the presence of competent renal vein valves.[9]

If the femoral vein cannot be used for catheter entry (because of IVC thrombosis), in an alternative method a catheter is passed from the antecubital vein, into the superior vena cava, through the right atrium, and into the IVC.

The renal veins may be visualized during arteriography, depending on the presence or absence of renal disease and on the amount of contrast material used (see Fig. 52-1B). Usually opacification is not adequate for diagnostic purposes. Once a carcinoma has been demonstrated and a nephrectomy is anticipated, a larger than usual volume of contrast material (25 ml or more) may be injected into the renal artery with a reasonable likelihood that the renal vein will be visualized if it is not occluded.[10] Nonvisualization of the renal veins and even demonstration of collateral vessels, however, do not necessarily mean tumor invasion; selective renal venography is usually required[11,12] for optimal visualization of renal vein invasion.

Complications

There are very few reported complications. Takaro et al.[5] described a case of renal vein thrombosis that followed renal venography. A single case of intimal dissection without untoward sequelae to the patient has also been reported.[13] In a series of 132 consecutive renal venograms there were no complications.[1]

Renal Vein Anatomy

Variations of the right and left renal veins can best be understood by reviewing their development (Fig. 52-2). In the embryo, three pairs of longitudinal veins provide drainage for the lower part of the body.[14–16] Posterior cardinal veins appear first, soon atrophy, and then are replaced by the anteromedially situated subcardinal veins. Subsequently, by 8 weeks, the supracardinal veins have appeared posterolateral to the aorta. The ringlike anastomoses at the renal level between the subcardinal and supracardinal veins form the circumaortic venous ring (see Fig. 52-2A).[15] Two renal veins on each side connect the kidneys with these anastomoses. The definitive right-sided IVC is then formed largely from portions of the right supracardinal vein, together with some elements of the right subcar-

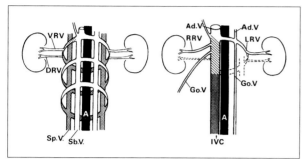

Figure 52-2. Development of the renal veins and the superior vena cava. Schematic drawing. (A) Patterns at the eighth week of fetal life. The posterior cardinal veins have already atrophied, and the venous drainage of the lower body is provided by the paired subcardinal and supracardinal veins, which are interconnected by venous rings. The venous ring at the renal level is called a renal collar. *VRV*, ventral renal vein; *DRV*, dorsal renal vein; *Sp.V*, supracardinal vein; *Sb.V*, subcardinal vein; *A*, aorta. (B) Adult pattern. The inferior vena cava develops out of the right supracardinal vein (*crosshatching*), the right supracardinal anastomosis (*diagonal lines*), and portions of the intersubcardinal anastomosis and right subcardinal vein (*white areas*). Both the adrenal and the gonadal veins are derived from the subcardinal veins. *Go.V*, gonadal vein; *Ad.V*, adrenal vein; *A*, aorta; *IVC*, inferior vena cava; *RRV*, right renal vein; *LRV*, left renal vein.

dinal veins (see Fig. 52-2B). Normally, these veins atrophy on the left. On the right, one renal vein also atrophies, and the remaining vein connects directly with the future IVC. On the left, the retroaortic segment of the venous ring, together with the dorsal renal vein, which is closely connected to the left lumbar-hemiazygos system, normally atrophies. A single preaortic vein remains, formed from an anastomosis between the anterior subcardinal veins. This anastomosis receives the ventral embryonic renal vein and the adrenal and gonadal veins. Variations in the development of these venous channels are common and account for the different renal venous patterns encountered on renal venography.[15,17]

Intrarenal Veins

The intrarenal veins are larger than the arteries, but their distribution is similar (Fig. 52-3A and B). Small interlobular vessels drain the renal cortex (see Fig. 52-3C) and join medullary veins to form the arcuate veins, which run along the corticomedullary junction. The arcuate veins communicate with each other and drain into the interlobar vessels, which in turn form three or four lobar veins. These veins unite anterior to the renal pelvis to form the main renal vein. In contrast to the arteries, there are multiple communications be-

tween the segmental interlobar veins and the arcuate veins (Figs. 52-3 through 52-5).[18]

Right Renal Vein

The variations in the right renal vein are described in Table 52-1. The right renal vein varies in length from 20 to 45 mm[26]; the average is 32 mm. The course of the vein is anterior and superior to the right renal artery.[27] It is single in 85 percent of people; in 4 percent of people the single renal vein splits before joining the IVC. The spermatic artery may course through the hiatus formed by this split.[19] From two to four entirely separate renal veins are found in 15 percent of people. There is no correlation between the number of veins and the number of arteries.[19] In about 6 percent of people the renal vein is joined by the right gonadal vein; valves have been reported in the gonadal vein in 77 percent of men and 94 percent of women.[28] It may also be joined by an accessory branch of the adrenal vein (in 31 percent of people).[23] Retroperitoneal veins join the renal vein in about 3 percent of people (see Table 52-1). Ureteric and capsular veins join the renal vein in the hilar region.

The radiographic anatomy of the right renal vein is given in Table 52-2. Because of its anteriorly oriented course, the right renal vein appears foreshortened, and the angle of entry into the IVC varies with the degree of expiration. In a large series the average length of the right renal vein was 26 mm (range 4–51 mm), and the average diameter was 14 mm (range 17–23 mm).[1] The right renal vein entered the IVC at the level of the lowest third of L1 (the range was the middle third of D12 to the interspace of L2 and L3) and formed an angle of 59 degrees with the intrarenal IVC (range 20–120 degrees). A single vein was found in 40 (72 percent) of 56 patients (see Fig. 52-4A), and in 15 patients it was formed by anastomoses of intrarenal venous branches outside the renal hilus. Two veins were found in 23 percent of patients and three veins were found in 5 percent of patients (see Fig. 52-4B to D), each with a separate caval entry. Usually there is one large vein with smaller accessory veins, but occasionally all are of equal size.

The gonadal vein joined the right renal vein in 7 percent of patients. Rarely, there was filling of the adrenal vein, which joined at the superior point of the junction of the renal vein and the IVC. In 12 percent of patients, capsular and subcapsular veins were visualized that drained either through the renal cortex or to the renal hilus to join the main renal vein. This happens more frequently when the catheter is wedged in a small renal vein branch. In 4 percent of patients, the

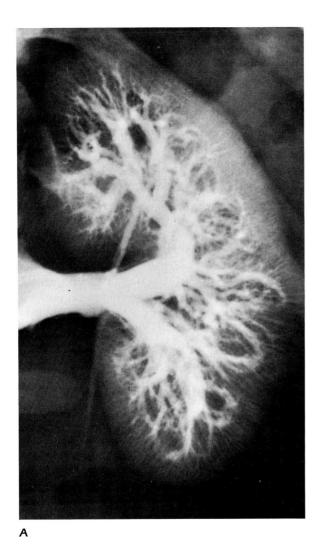

A

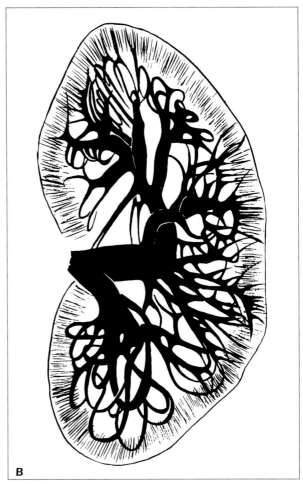

B

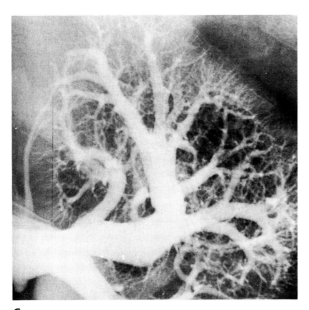

C

Figure 52-3. Intrarenal venous anatomy. (A) Normal left renal venogram. (B) Schematic drawing. The intrarenal veins, which are larger than the arteries, show multiple communications between segmental interlobar and, especially, arcuate veins. There is a single left renal vein in a typical location. (C) Normal magnification venogram showing the fine detail of the interlobular venous anatomy.

ureteric vein was opacified. The incidence of multiple renal veins was twice as high in this series[1] as in other reported analyses (see Table 52-2).[29,30]

Left Renal Vein

The more complex embryology of the left renal vein compared to the right is associated with more anatomic variations (Table 52-3). The left renal vein, which is longer than the right, varies from 60 to 110 mm in length; the average is 84 mm.[26] After crossing the aorta ventrally, it enters the IVC at about a 90-degree angle. Posteriorly it is near the third portion of the duodenum and the pancreas. A single preaortic left renal vein is seen in 86 percent of people,[19-21] and a

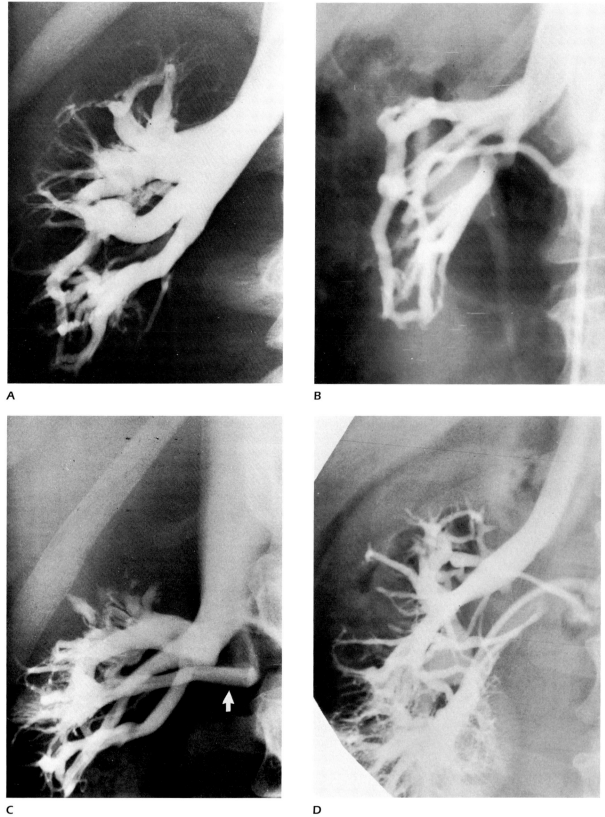

A

B

C

D

Figure 52-4. Variations of renal vein anatomy. (A) Single renal vein. Multiple branches communicate with larger interlobar veins. (B) Double renal veins. A small caudal vein enters the IVC at the level of L2, well below the major vein entry. Note the plexoid configuration of the veins. (C) Double renal veins. A caudal vein (*arrow*) enters the IVC at virtually the same level as the major vein. (D) Triple renal veins. Three separate veins join the IVC.

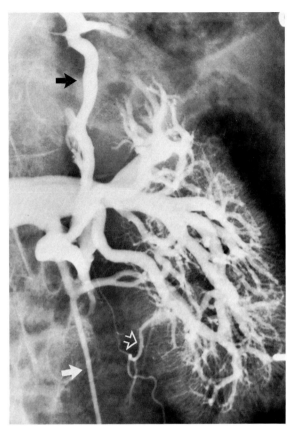

Figure 52-5. Left renal vein with a hemiazygos connection. There is confluence of the lobar veins outside the renal hilus. Both the gonadal vein (*solid white arrow*) and the hemiazygos vein (*black arrow*) communicate with the left main renal vein. In addition, a capsular vein (*open white arrow*) is seen extending from the intrarenal branches into the renal capsule.

single retroaortic vein is described in 2.4 percent.[19–21] Multiple renal veins with separate renal origin and separate caval entry are rare (1 percent of people) on the left side.[19,20]

A circumaortic vein is found in 7 percent of people.[19,20,31] The renal vein splits in these people to form a preaortic component in the usual location and a retroaortic component that runs caudally to enter the IVC in the lower lumbar region. The preaortic and the postaortic components of the ring are frequently equal in size.[31] The retroaortic portion may receive lumbar veins[32] and may also split before entering the IVC. The hiatus formed by such a split may contain the left gonadal artery.[19]

The adrenal vein, usually joined by the inferior phrenic and capsular veins, enters the left renal vein superiorly, just lateral to the lumbar spine. The gonadal vein joins inferiorly, lateral to the adrenal vein[19,20,24,32]; if there is a circumaortic venous ring, it joins either the preaortic portion or the unsplit renal vein trunk. Multiple gonadal veins occur in about 15 percent of people[19] but rarely number more than two. Gonadal vein valves have been described in 60 percent of men and 86 percent of women.[28]

In addition, the left renal vein communicates with the retroperitoneal veins (e.g., the lumbar, ascending lumbar, and hemiazygos veins) in 75 percent of people (see Table 52-3).[19,25,33] Communications occur directly through lumbar veins joining posteriorly or indirectly through the gonadal veins.[32,34] The intrahilar portion of the left renal vein receives the ureteric vein.[34] The capsular veins drain into the adrenal and gonadal veins or directly into the renal vein.[32,34] A left-sided IVC occurs in less than 1 percent of people[19,20,22]; the left gonadal vein then enters the left IVC directly.

In a study of 76 consecutive left renal venograms at Brigham and Women's Hospital, the average length of the left renal vein was found to be 68 mm (range 35–100 mm) (Table 52-4). In the preaortic portion, the average diameter was 19 mm (range 11–25 mm), and in the hilar portion, it was 13 mm (range 7–16 mm). Entrance into the IVC was typically at the interspace between L1 and L2 (the range was the middle

Table 52-1. Variations of Right Renal Vein (Anatomic Literature)

Variation	Number of Positive Cases	Total Number Examined	Percentage Positive	Percentage Range	References
Single RRV[a]	762	897	85.0	73–89	19–21
Multiple RRV[a]	135	897	15.0	11–28	19–21
Split of RRV[a] at IVC[b] entry	28	694	4.0	1.6–10.0	19, 20
Gonadal vein connected to RRV[a]	49	764	6.4	3–15	19, 20, 22
Accessory adrenal vein connected to RRV[a]	5	16	31.0	31	23
Retroperitoneal connections	7	258	2.7	2.7	24, 25

[a]RRV = right renal vein.
[b]IVC = inferior vena cava.

Table 52-2. Radiographic Anatomy of the Right Renal Vein

Parameter	Present Series* (56 patients)	Previous Series (72 patients)[29,30]
Average length (range)	26 mm (4–51 mm)	22 mm (5–62 mm)
Number of renal veins		
1	72%	86%
2	23%	14%
3	5%	
Extrarenal confluence of lobar veins	27%	25%
Average diameter (range)	14 mm (7–23 mm)	15 mm (10–20 mm)
Angle to IVC[a] (range)	59° (20–120°)	45° (15–85°)
Ureteric vein	4%	—
Demonstration of capsular and subcapsular veins	12%	—
Demonstration of gonadal vein connected to RRV[b]	7%	9%
Demonstration of adrenal vein	4%	—
Usual site of entry into IVC[a]	Lowest third of L1	Lowest third of L1
Variation in site of entry into IVC[a]	Middle third of D12 to L2-L3 interspace	Upper third of L1 to mid L2

*Brigham & Women's Hospital series.
[a]IVC = inferior vena cava.
[b]RRV = right renal vein.

Table 52-3. Variations of Left Renal Vein (Anatomic Literature)

Parameter	Number of Positive Cases	Total Number Examined	Percentage Positive	Percentage Range	References
Single preaortic LRV[a]	613	702	86.0	79–91	19, 20
Multiple LRV[a]	6	694	1.0	0.8–1.0	19, 20
Circumaortic LRV[a]	68	972	7.0	1.5–16.8	19, 20, 31
Retroaortic single LRV[a]	24	972	2.4	1.8–3.4	19, 20, 31
Gonadal vein draining into IVC[b] (all left-sided IVC[b])	5	765	0.7	0.4–1.2	19, 20, 22
Multiple gonadal veins	28	181	15.4	15.4	19
Adrenal vein draining into LRV[a]	291	291	100.0	100	23, 26, 32
Persistent left-sided IVC[b]	35	1820	1.8	1.0–2.4	17, 19, 20, 22
Retroperitoneal venous connections	339	455	75.0	59–88	19, 25, 33

[a]LRV = left renal vein.
[b]IVC = inferior vena cava.

third of T12 to the upper third of L3) with an angle of 74 degrees to the infrarenal IVC (range 25–105 degrees).

There was a single preaortic vein in 89 percent of patients (see Fig. 52-3); in 14 percent of patients it was formed by a confluence of renal veins outside the renal hilus (see Fig. 52-5; see also Fig. 52-13A). Rarely, a single retroaortic vein was observed (Fig. 52-6). In 11 percent of the patients, there was a circumaortic venous ring—that is, a preaortic vein in a typical location and a retroaortic limb that was always smaller and that entered the IVC in the low lumbar region (Figs. 52-7 through 52-9). In one instance, the retroaortic portion split before entering the IVC (see Fig. 52-9). In six of eight patients, the retroaortic limb arose from an unsplit main renal vein trunk within 2

cm of the renal hilus (see Fig. 52-9). In two patients, the bifurcation occurred within the renal hilus (see Figs. 52-7 and 52-8) or at the confluence of the lobar veins, and the retroaortic vein seemed to drain parts of the lower pole preferentially. No patients had multiple renal veins. Computed tomography (CT) has been used to define circumaortic renal vein and other renal vein and caval anomalies.[36,37]

The adrenal vein was demonstrated in 57 percent of patients (see Fig. 52-8), and one or two gonadal veins were filled in 83 percent of patients (Fig. 52-10; see also Fig. 52-5). Filling varied, probably depending on the presence of competent venous valves. In 55 percent of patients, lumbar, hemiazygos, or ascending lumbar veins (retroperitoneal veins) were demonstrated (see Figs. 52-5 and 52-10). In 34 percent of

Table 52-4. Radiographic Anatomy of the Left Renal Vein

Parameter	Present Series* (76 patients)	Previous Series (197 patients)[29,30,35]
Average length (range)	68 mm (35–100 mm)	77 mm (55–120 mm)
Single preaortic vein	89%	91%
Extrarenal confluence of lobar veins	14%	2.5%
Periaortic venous ring	11%	9%
Single retroaortic vein	1%	1%
Average preaortic diameter		
Preaortic portion (range)	19 mm (11–25 mm)	—
Hilar portion (range)	13 mm (7–16)	—
Average angle to IVC (range)	74° (25–105°)	78° (50–90°)
Demonstration of adrenal veins	57%	49%
Demonstration of gonadal vein	83%	70%
Demonstration of retroperitoneal branches	55%	40%
Demonstration of capsular or subcapsular veins	34%	5%
Usual site of entry into IVC	L1-L2 interspace	L1-L2 interspace
Variation of site of entry into IVC (range)	Middle third of D12 to upper third of L3	Lowest third of D12 to lowest third of L2
Persistent left-sided IVC	None	2%

*Brigham & Women's Hospital series.

Figure 52-6. Solitary retroaortic renal vein. (A) The vein originates at the interspace between L1 and L2 and extends caudally from the kidney to enter the inferior vena cava in the region of L3. (B) In this case, the vein originates at the interspace between L2 and L3 and descends to the interspace of L3 and L4.

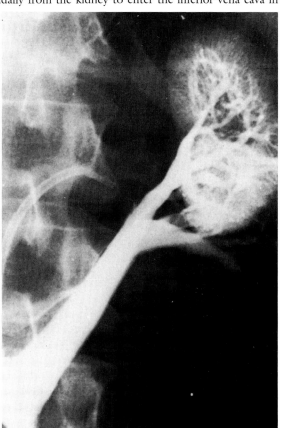

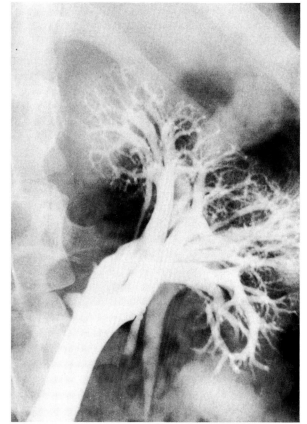

A   B

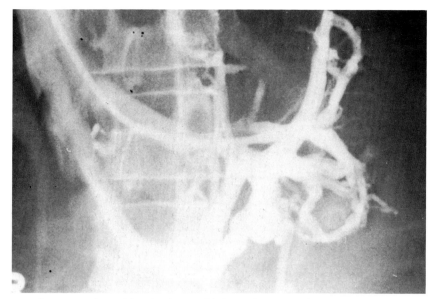

Figure 52-7. Circumaortic venous ring arising in the renal hilus. The veins of the lower pole drain preferentially into the retroaortic vein.

Figure 52-9. Circumaortic venous ring. The inferior vena cavogram demonstrates three communications of the ring with the vena cava. The retroaortic vein arises from an unsplit main renal trunk and splits before joining the inferior vena cava.

Figure 52-8. Circumaortic venous ring. Both the preaortic and the retroaortic renal veins (*open white arrow*) arise in the renal hilus. The latter vein seems to drain the lower pole preferentially. The adrenal vein (*solid white arrow*) joins the preaortic renal vein in the typical location. Note the valve of the preaortic vein (*black arrows*).

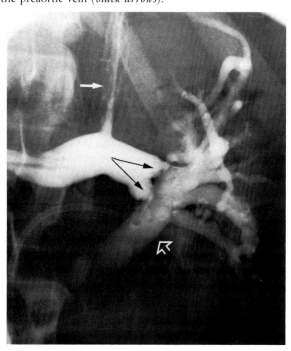

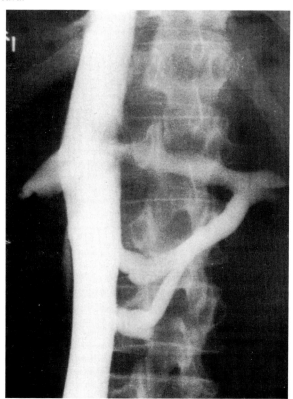

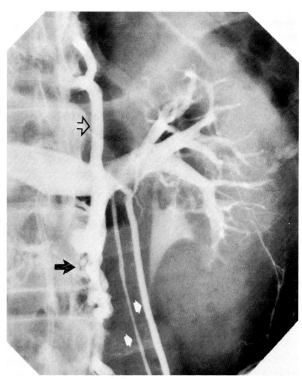

Figure 52-10. Azygos vein and gonadal vein opacification. Normal left renal venogram in a renal donor. Two left spermatic veins (*solid white arrows*) are opacified. Note the communications between the left main renal vein and the ascending lumbar vein (*black arrow*) and the hemiazygos vein (*open black arrow*).

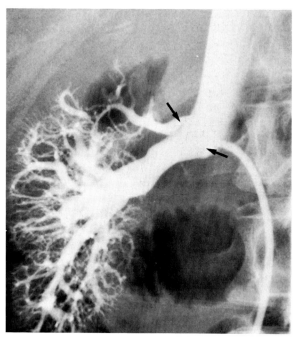

Figure 52-11. Right renal vein valves. The valves are clearly defined (*arrows*) close to the entry of the renal vein into the inferior vena cava.

patients, capsular or subcapsular veins (see Fig. 52-5) joined intrarenal branches through the renal cortex or directly joined the adrenal vein, the gonadal vein, or the intrahilar portion of the renal vein.

These findings, with some exceptions, were similar to those of other authors.[29,30,35]

Renal Vein Valves

Filling of side branches and demonstration of valves depend on the position of the catheter, the injection rate, and the blood flow. Autopsy studies have demonstrated renal vein valves in 28 to 70 percent of right renal veins and in 4 to 36 percent of left renal veins.[5,22]

In an analysis of renal venograms, valves were visualized in 16 percent on the right. They can be located anywhere from the renal hilus to the IVC confluence (Figs. 52-11 and 52-12). On the left, valves were detected in 15 percent. Most valves were located in the main renal vein (Fig. 52-13A) or at the renal hilus (Fig. 52-13B and C).[1]

Angiographically, renal vein valves appeared as thin, weblike structures that may block passage of the catheter or contrast material and hence cause poor venographic filling (see Figs. 52-11 through 52-13). There was a 12 to 31 percent higher incidence of inadequate venograms when valves were present. This inadequacy occurred more commonly when the renal blood flow was not slowed; the effect of the valve is then coupled with dilution of contrast by the normal antegrade flow of unopacified blood. Rarely, valves produced total obstruction to the retrograde flow of contrast material (Fig. 52-14), in which case they had to be distinguished from renal vein thrombus or neoplastic involvement.

Applications

Carcinoma of the Kidney

Preoperative radiologic evaluation of the renal vein is needed for detection of congenital variants, surgical planning,[38] and tumor staging. Renal vein invasion occurs in approximately one-third of patients with resectable renal cell carcinoma, and a number of studies, many based on autopsy, show an association between extension into the renal vein and relative decreased survival rates at 5 and 10 years compared to those without renal vein involvement (Table 52-5).[39-47] A

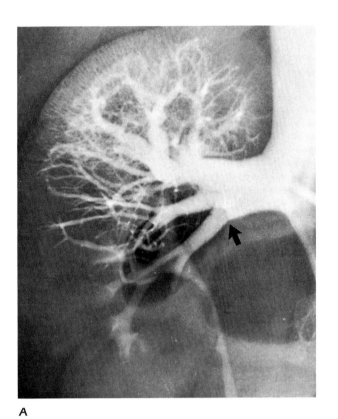
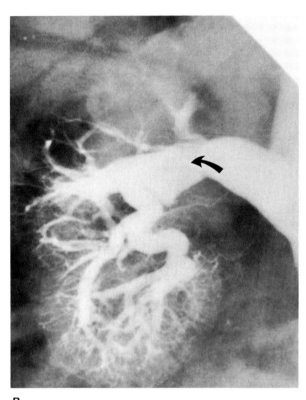

A
B

Figure 52-12. Right renal vein valves. These valves are located in the renal hilus. (A) The valve (*arrow*) has impaired the filling of the lower pole veins. (B) The valve (*arrow*) has impaired the filling of the upper pole veins.

Table 52-5. Renal Vein Invasion and Survival in Renal Cell Carcinoma

Author	Year	Number of Patients with Renal Vein Invasion/Total Number	Percentage with Renal Vein Invasion	5-Year Survival			
				With Invasion		Without Invasion	
				Number/ Total Number	%	Number/ Total Number	%
Hand and Broders[42]	1932	38/193	20	—	—	—	—
McDonald and Priestley[48]	1943	275/509	54	60/207	29	103/186	55
Griffiths and Thackray[41]	1949	23/80	29	2/10	20	13/26	50
Riches et al.[47]	1951	199/816	24	17/90	19	114/308	37
Riches[45]	1963	41/110	37	7/26	27	35/60	58
Riches[46]	1964	—	—	—	—	—	—
Arner et al.[39]	1965	51/172	30	15/51	29	62/121	51
Myers et al.[43]	1968	228/508	50	78/228	34	179/280	64
Crocker[40]	1975	31/84	37	—	—	—	—
Total		886/2472	36	179/612	29	506/981	52

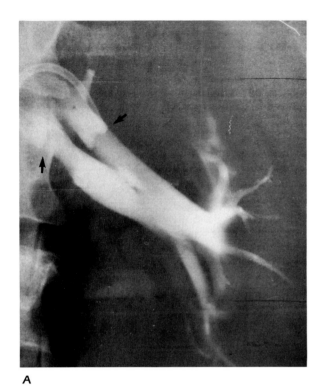

A

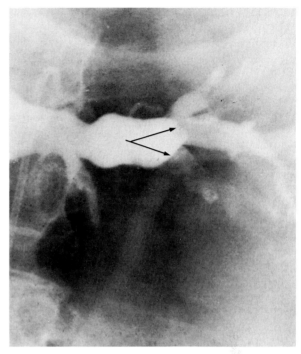

B

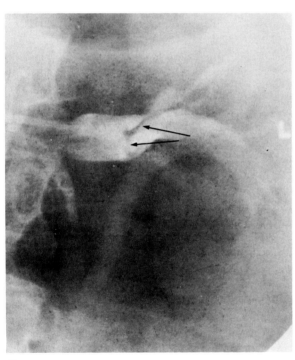

C

Figure 52-13. Left renal vein valves. (A) Two left renal veins, each with a valve (*arrows*), join ventral to the aorta. These valves may cause incomplete filling of the intrarenal branches. (B) The renal vein at the hilus (*arrows*) impedes renal venous filling. (C) Same as (B). With the termination of injection, the valve leaflets (*arrows*) are clearly delineated.

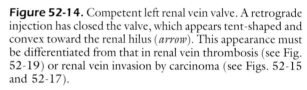

Figure 52-14. Competent left renal vein valve. A retrograde injection has closed the valve, which appears tent-shaped and convex toward the renal hilus (*arrow*). This appearance must be differentiated from that in renal vein thrombosis (see Fig. 52-19) or renal vein invasion by carcinoma (see Figs. 52-15 and 52-17).

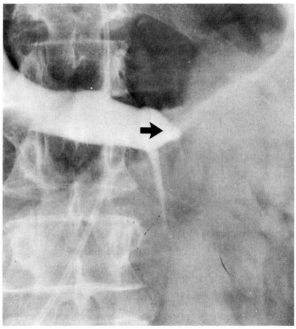

Table 52-6. Renal Vein Invasion and Survival in Carcinoma of the Renal Pelvis

| | | | | 5-Year Survival | | |
| | | | | With Invasion | | Without Invasion |
Author	Year	Number of Patients with Renal Vein Invasion/Total Number	Percentage with Renal Vein Invasion	Number/ Total Number	%	Number/ Total Number
McDonald and Priestley[48]	1943	31/76	40	1/21	5	15/35
Crocker[40]	1975	1/12	8	—	—	—
Total		32/88	36			

Table 52-7. Renal Vein Invasion and Survival in Wilms Tumor and Sarcoma of the Kidney

| | | | | 3-Year Survival | | |
| | | | | With Invasion | | Without Invasion |
Author	Year	Number of Patients with Renal Vein Invasion/Total Number	Percentage with Renal Vein Involvement	Number/ Total Number	%	Number/ Total Number
Wilms tumor						
McDonald and Priestley[48]	1943	31/31	42	—	—	—
Riches et al.[47]	1951	9/110	8	—	—	—
Perez et al.[44]	1973	17/40	42	4/17	24	16/23
Total		39/181	22			
Sarcoma						
McDonald and Priestley[48]	1943	2/20	10	—	—	—

similar effect on prognosis occurs with carcinoma of the renal pelvis and Wilms tumor (Tables 52-6 and 52-7).

Because CT scanning and MRI can accurately evaluate the renal vein and IVC[49-53] and also provide information regarding local invasion and lymphadenopathy, the role of renal venography is best restricted to equivocal or difficult cases.[54] Widespread use of CT scanning has resulted in detection of small renal masses, cysts, and incidental carcinomas, many of which can present challenging management and radiologic problems.[55] With the growing interest in renal-sparing surgery, a new role for renal venography, where meticulous analysis of tributary veins can help suggest malignancy, has been proposed.[56]

Renal venography may also be helpful in establishing the diagnosis in infiltrating avascular renal cell carcinoma[57-59] and transitional cell carcinoma.[4,57-59] In these patients, the absence of typical arteriographic findings or the presence of only small abnormal arterial branches contrasts often with the striking abnormalities on the venogram (Fig. 52-15). At times, segmental renal vein involvement may be visualized (Fig. 52-16).

Preoperatively it is important to know the extent of the tumor and whether it is operable. Instead of the traditional lateral incision, some authors[60-62] favor a transperitoneal approach in patients with renal vein invasion to enable early inspection of the renal vein and its medial clamping and to prevent tumor embolization during surgical manipulation.

When the arteriogram does not allow differentiation between a renal tumor and an adrenal tumor, the renal venogram may show the drainage of the tumor veins either into the intrarenal veins (renal tumor) or into the adrenal veins (adrenal tumor), provided there is no proximal occlusion.

Because of the valuable information renal venography affords, most authors[4,7,11,57-59,61,63] feel that, when the procedure is indicated, its usefulness outweighs the risk of tumor embolization during it. An inferior vena cavogram should be the first step to rule out tumor thrombus extending into the IVC,[11,58] particularly with the advent of caval resection in such patients.[64] Invasion of the IVC is usually accompanied by a persistent, sharply margined and sometimes lobular filling defect originating from the renal vein.[65,66] Tumor thrombus and bland thrombus are not always distinguishable,[66] however, unless actual tumor vascularity is demonstrated in the thrombus on selective renal arte-

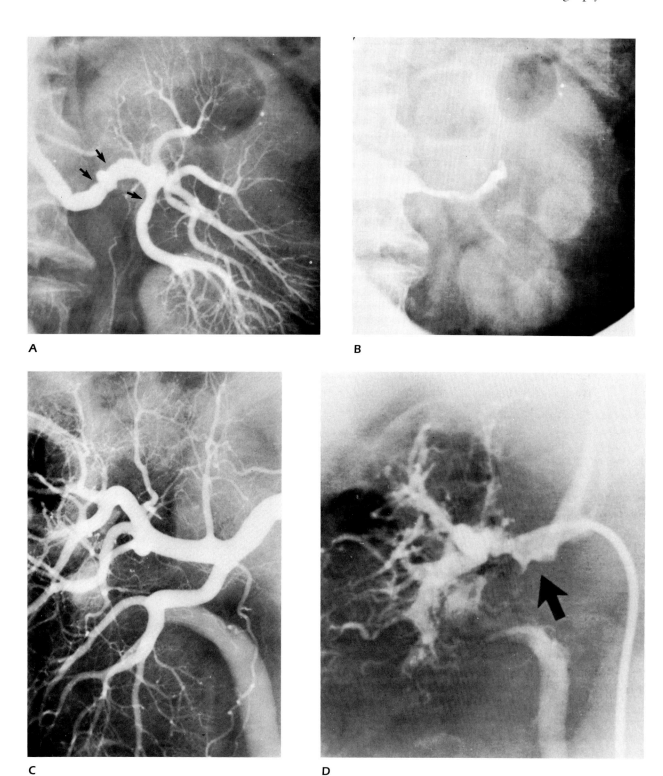

A

B

C

D

Figure 52-15. Renal vein invasion in carcinoma, discrepancy between arteriographic and venographic findings. (A) Transitional cell carcinoma of the left kidney. Arteriogram shows minimal encasement of the central renal arteries (*arrows*) but a striking absence of neovascularity. (B) Venogram, same patient as (A). The left renal vein is occluded by a tumor. The irregularity of contour reflects a malignant invasion. (C) Transitional cell carcinoma. Arteriogram shows thin but definite tumor vessels close to the renal hilus but no major vessel involvement. (D) Venogram, same patient as in (C), shows gross tumor invasion (*arrow*).

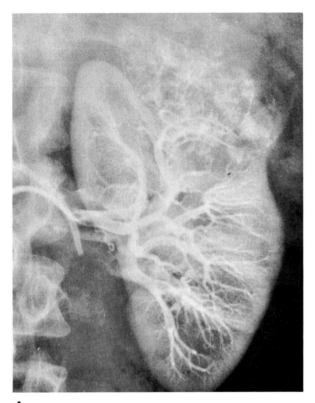

A

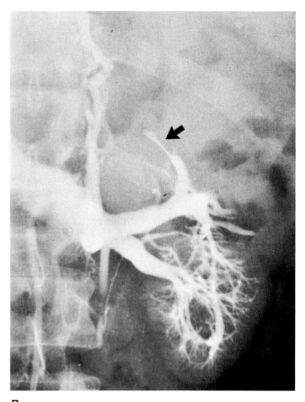

B

Figure 52-16. Renal cell carcinoma with segmental vein involvement. (A) Arteriogram shows that the area of neovascularity is confined to the upper pole. (B) Venogram shows poor opacification of the upper pole branches. Note the narrowing, displacement, and occlusion of the upper pole branch (*arrow*) by the tumor.

riography (Fig. 52-17).[67,68] At times the IVC may be indented by metastatic nodes.[68]

A normal inferior vena cavogram should be followed by a selective renal venogram. Typical findings indicating invasion of the renal vein include irregular narrowing (see Fig. 52-15B), abrupt vessel termination (see Figs. 52-15B and D, 52-16B), indentations of the vessel wall, differences of contrast density, and filling defects within the renal veins (see Fig. 52-17).[58] In hypervascular tumors, however, flow artifact secondary to venous washout may be observed, especially in smaller veins.[58] These can be indistinguishable from those secondary to tumorous extension into the venous system, and a positive diagnosis of renal vein invasion should be made only if the main renal vein or its major tributaries are involved.[58]

Retroperitoneal Tumors

In contrast to the right renal vein, the left renal vein may be an important vessel in the evaluation and staging of retroperitoneal disease.[38] The left renal vein runs a course directly anterior to the pancreas and is located close to periaortic, mesenteric, and renal lymph nodes. Therefore, this vessel often shows early involvement in retroperitoneal tumors. The typical findings on venography include splaying and smooth narrowing of the vein when nodes or a mass is impinging on but not invading the renal vein and segmental irregular narrowing when there is malignant invasion. Cope and Isard[69] found significant distortion of the left renal vein in 60 percent of patients in a series of 17 proved retroperitoneal tumors. In 9 patients with cancer of the pancreas, 7 had invasion of the renal vein. Among these 7, 3 had little or no arteriographic evidence of malignancy.

Renovascular Hypertension

Although arteriography can easily demonstrate a stenosis in the renal arteries, the functional significance of the stenosis may be uncertain unless collateral vessels are present.[70,71]

The renal venous washout time has been shown to reflect the rate of blood flow through the kidney and to be related to the renal plasma flow and to the pres-

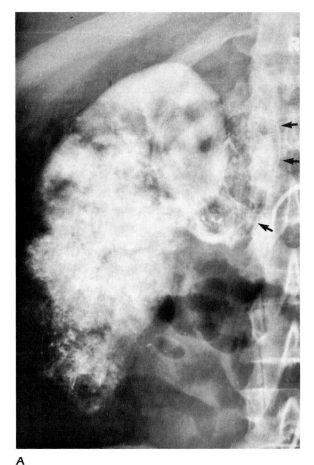

A

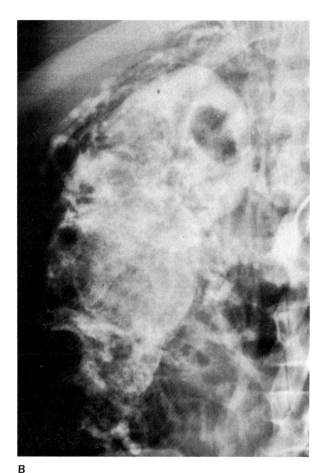

B

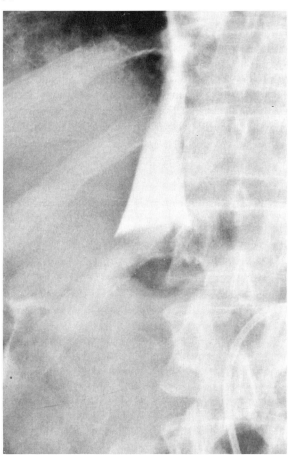

C

Figure 52-17. Renal vein and inferior vena cava invasion by renal cell carcinoma. (A) The late arterial phase film shows a large tumor of the lower half of the right kidney and an area of tumor vascularity in the region of the right renal vein and the inferior vena cava (*arrows*). (B) The venous phase film demonstrates multiple retroperitoneal collateral vessels. (C) An inferior vena cavogram demonstrates the upper extent of the caval occlusion, correlating with the tumor thrombus as seen on the arteriogram.

ence of significant renal artery stenosis.[29] In the method used, contrast material was injected into the renal veins and the washout time was determined cineangiographically. With this method, both kidneys could be evaluated and compared. With significant renal artery stenosis and reduction in the renal blood flow, the washout time was usually prolonged.

Renal Vein Renin Determination

The functional significance of arteriographically proven anatomic lesions and their potential surgical curability are commonly evaluated in the light of renal vein renin activity.[72-78] Renin, secreted in response to stimuli that compromise kidney perfusion, increases plasma angiotensin, which stimulates aldosterone secretion.[79] Vascular tone is regulated by an interaction between angiotensin levels and the available intravascular sodium ions. The two hormones, angiotensin and aldosterone, thus restore the sodium balance and the arterial pressure, thereby reducing renin release. Sealey et al.[80] showed that under steady-state circumstances each kidney adds 24 percent more renin to the renal artery renin. They concluded that, if the normal kidney is suppressed by high blood pressure, all the renin should be coming from the diseased kidney, which then will add at least 48 percent more renin to the renal artery level. The renal vein renin of the normal kidney should equal the renal artery renin. This line of reasoning supports the clinically established criteria used in diagnosing renovascular hypertension and predicting surgical curability:

1. Increased renin production of the suspect kidney: $V - A/A > 0.48$ (V = venous renin activity; A = arterial renal activity).[78,81] This is the Vaughan formula.[79,82]
2. Suppression of renin secretion on the contralateral, normal side: $V - A \sim 0$.[81,82]
3. A renal vein renin ratio of $1.5 : 1.0$ or more between the involved kidney and the uninvolved kidney.[72,76,77,81,82]
4. Elevated plasma renin activity.[81]

The sensitivity and specificity of the test will vary depending on which criteria are used; the Vaughan formula is considered most accurate.[83]

The renin-angiotensin-aldosterone system is easily influenced by many factors in both normal patients and hypertensive patients. *Upright posture* leads to increased renin production.[84] In renovascular hypertension, Michelakis et al.[84,85] found that the kidney with the stenotic artery produced excess renin, which led to a marked disparity in the renal vein renin concentrations between the involved side and the uninvolved side. If such a patient changes from an upright position to a recumbent one, exaggerated renin production is only stimulated after some time because of the high baseline concentration. As a result, the renal vein ratio between the involved kidney and the uninvolved kidney approaches unity and briefly loses its diagnostic usefulness.[84,85]

Salt depletion induced by diuretics or a low dietary intake of sodium increases the renin activity. The stimulus to increased renin production affects the involved kidney more than the contralateral kidney, leading to an exaggerated renin ratio.[86]

Antihypertensive drugs[79,87] influence renin release in both directions (Table 52-8). These drugs may increase renin release either by directly lowering the blood pressure or by their diuretic effect, with conse-

Table 52-8. Antihypertensive Drug Effect on Renin Release

Renin Inhibitors	Renin Stimulators
Propranolol	Aldosterone antagonists
Clonidine	Diuretics
Methyldopa	Vasodilators
Reserpine	Nitroprusside
Ganglionic blockers	Diazoxide
Guanethidine	Hydralazine

Adapted from Laragh JH, Baer L, Brunner HR, et al. Renin, angiotensin and aldosterone system in pathogenesis and management of hypertensive vascular disease. Am J Med 1972;52:633.

quent decrease in the blood pressure.[87] The kidney with significant renal artery stenosis secretes disproportionately more renin than does the uninvolved kidney.[88] Other drugs suppress the plasma renin activity, probably by directly interfering with the physiologic pathways of renin release.[87]

Technique of Venous Sampling for Renin Assay

The same catheter used for renal venography may be employed for renin sampling. For segmental vein sampling, an additional downward deflection of 30 degrees should be incorporated in the catheter tip. Alternatively, a 5 French visceral catheter (e.g., C-2 catheter) with one or two side holes cut close to the tip, can be used. Samples are taken from the main right renal vein, the main left renal vein peripheral to the entry of the gonadal vein, and the IVC above and below the renal veins. The lower caval sample value is interchangeable with the renal artery renin concentration.[78] Correct localization of the catheter tip is essential for proper sampling (Fig. 52-18A and B).[89] In the presence of a left circumaortic renal vein, the retroaortic vein can preferentially drain the lower poles (see Fig. 52-18C and D); therefore samples should be taken from both veins. In branch stenosis or local infarction, the sample must be obtained from the draining renal vein branch, because venous blood from the nonischemic portions of the kidney may dilute the main renal vein renin and lead to false-normal values (see Fig. 52-18A).[75,89,90] The same holds true in those rare cases of locally circumscribed, renin-producing tumors of juxtaglomerular origin[91] or of a renal cyst compressing renal parenchyma and thereby creating focal ischemia. Care should be taken to catheterize both branches in the duplicated renal venous system, which occurs on the right side frequently. Samples should be drawn slowly to prevent aspiration from side branches.[75,89] Simultaneous sampling of renal veins is unnecessary.[92]

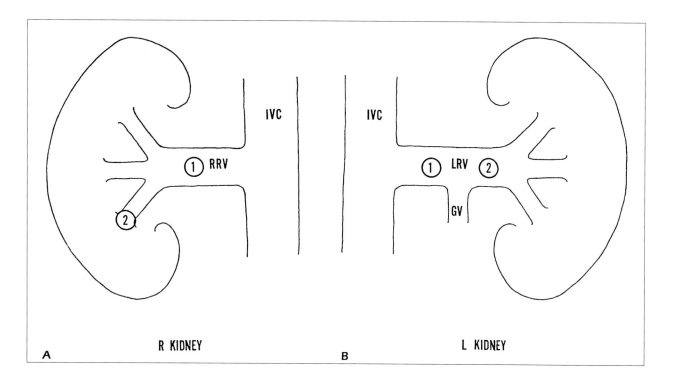

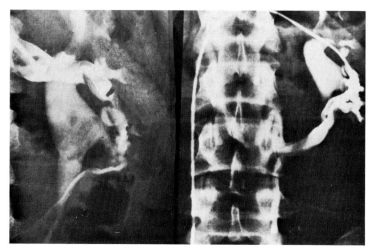

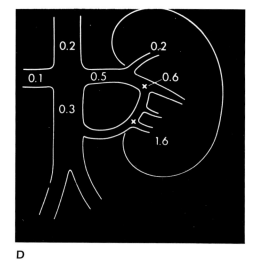

Figure 52-18. Renal vein renin determination. Importance of the catheter site. (A) Diagram of the right kidney in a 33-year-old woman with hypertension following surgical amputation of the right lower pole renal artery. Sampling showed lower renin values (3636 ng/100 ml) at site 1 (the main renal vein) than at site 2 (the lower pole segmental vein) (4916 ng/100 ml). This difference was due to dilution from the middle and upper pole veins at site 1. *IVC,* inferior vena cava; *RRV,* right renal vein. (B) Diagram of the left kidney in a 54-year-old man with hypertension following embolic occlusion of the left renal artery. Sampling showed lower renin values (2381 ng/100 ml) at site 1 (the proximal renal vein) than at site 2 (the distal renal vein) (14,815 ng/100 ml). This difference was due to dilution from the gonadal vein at site 1. *IVC,* inferior vena cava; *LRV,* left renal vein; *GV,* gonadal vein. (C) Left renal venogram in a 16-year-old boy with posttraumatic hypertension and obstruction of a lower pole renal artery. A circumaortic venous ring is present. When the catheter was advanced through the preaortic vein, injection of contrast material into the lower pole vein showed preferential drainage into the retroaortic vein. (Courtesy of Christos A. Athanasoulis, M.D.) (D) Renin sampling. Samples from the retroaortic vein localize the ischemic focus to the lower pole.

A rigid protocol should be followed for renin sampling. Samples should be obtained in hypertensive patients only after arteriographic demonstration of renal artery stenosis. This may follow abdominal aortography; Harrington et al.[92] found no significant change of renal vein renin activity 10 minutes after aortography in a series of 56 patients. Other authors, however, have found an increase of renin secretion after selective renal arteriography or renal venography.[93,94] It is desirable, therefore, to obtain renin samples within 15 minutes of arteriography. These patients should have no signs or symptoms of congestive heart failure and should preferably have received no diuretics or antihypertensive drugs.[73] Under standard conditions of recumbency and normal sodium intake, venous samples may then be drawn.

Although there is no consensus on its necessity, renin secretion can be stimulated by various methods:

1. Upright posture for 20 minutes[84] to 4 hours[73]
2. Sodium depletion by 3 days of severe sodium restriction at 10 mEq per day or administration of furosemide[73,84]
3. Controlled hypotension[88]
4. Administration of angiotensin-converting enzyme inhibitors[83]

Accuracy of Renin Assay

As a predictive index of the outcome of surgery in hypertensive patients with renal artery stenosis, the accuracy of renin activity varies between 70 and 95 percent.[72,73,76-78] The variability may be explained by the different criteria used and by the difference in how the patients are prepared. If the renal vein renin ratio between the involved kidney and the uninvolved kidney is used alone, the accuracy is approximately 85 percent (Table 52-9). The ratios between the two sides do not take into account the occult hypersecretion of renin (although to a lesser degree) on the presumably uninvolved side.[81] Such a finding suggests a nephrosclerotic kidney, and surgery might therefore be contraindicated. The additional demonstration of suppressed renin release or of an abnormally high peripheral plasma renin activity in relation to sodium excretion (indicating increased renin release) may increase the accuracy of predicting the surgical outcome to 95 percent.[78,81]

It is important to emphasize that absence of lateralization does not preclude a successful result from surgery; 21 percent of such patients with renovascular disease experience amelioration of hypertension.[72]

Renal Vein Thrombosis

Renal vein thrombosis in adults differs from that in children.[95] In children, it is almost exclusively found in the presence of diarrhea and dehydration, and the prognosis is grave. In adults, renal vein thrombosis is often associated with underlying renal disease, including both systemic diseases, such as lupus erythematosus and amyloidosis, and primary renal diseases, such as nephrosclerosis, chronic glomerulonephritis, pyelonephritis, and membranous glomerulonephritis.[96-99] Whether renal vein thrombosis is the cause or is an effect of membranous glomerulonephritis is not fully established; many authors consider it a consequence of the disease.[100-102] Patients with the nephrotic syndrome have a hypercoagulable state[103] that may account for a high incidence of peripheral thrombophlebitis, renal vein thrombosis, and pulmonary embolism (Table 52-10). Renal vein thrombosis may occur as an extension of thrombus within the IVC,[104] or it may be associated with extrinsic pressure on the renal vein from an adjacent mass, such as a tumor or an aneurysm.[96] Trauma is a rare cause.[105-107]

The response of the kidney to renal vein thrombosis depends on the rapidity and completeness of the occlusion and on the availability of collateral pathways.[108-110] If the occlusion is rapid and complete, hemorrhagic infarction may occur. If the occlusion is gradual, collateral vessels may develop. The balance between the speed with which this collateral system develops and the rapidity of the occlusion determines the outcome. If the collateral system cannot accommodate the renal blood flow, the kidneys become enlarged and congested; later they may atrophy. Ligation

Table 52-9. Accuracy of Lateralizing Renal Vein Renin Ratios (1.5:1.0 or Higher) in Predicting Cure of Hypertension in Unilateral Renal Artery Stenosis

Author	Year	Total Number of Patients	Number Cured	Percentage Cured
Bourgoignie et al.[72]	1970	124	107	85
Simmons and Michelakis[77]	1970	21	19	90
Stockigt et al.[82]	1972	22	19	86
Schaeffer and Fair[76]	1974	17	12	71
Total		184	157	85

Table 52-10. Pulmonary and Sex Distribution in Patients with Renal Vein Thrombosis

Author	Total Number of Patients	Female-Male Ratio	Number with Pulmonary Embolism
Llach et al.[101]	12	4:8	4
O'Dea et al.[123]	11	3:8	3
Chait et al.[105]	6	2:4	2
McCarthy et al.*[104]	38	10:28	14
Rosenmann et al.[95]	15	8:7	7
Present series†	7	1:6	1
Total	89	26:61 (31%:69%)	31 (35%)

*Autopsy series.
†Brigham and Women's Hospital series.

of the left renal vein may be accomplished with no long-term effects because of the collateral venous drainage, although temporary renal dysfunction may be observed.[111]

Renal vein thrombosis is twice as common in males as in females (see Table 52-10). Clinically it is associated with the nephrotic syndrome and frequently with hematuria.[107] In addition, a third of these patients may develop pulmonary embolism (see Table 52-10); at times, this may be the presenting symptom.[107] Patients with traumatic renal vein thrombosis and associated arterial occlusion do not exhibit the nephrotic syndrome but may present with recurrent pulmonary embolism.[107] Autopsy examination of patients with renal vein thrombosis has shown associated IVC thrombosis in 24 percent and iliofemoral vein thrombosis in 29 percent.[104]

Among patients with the nephrotic syndrome examined by renal venography, renal vein thrombosis is seldom found.

Urography may be negative; when it is positive, it is most often nonspecific. In the acute stage, the involved kidney is typically enlarged, with a moderate to marked reduction in function. Later, ureteral collateral vessels may produce notching of the renal pelvis and ureter. In the end stage, the kidney may be small and shrunken. These findings, either alone or together, are present in about one-third of patients; two-thirds have entirely normal urograms (Table 52-11).

Sectional imaging methods can succeed in diagnosing renal vein thrombosis. In children, especially neonates, ultrasonography is the initial method of choice,[112-114] although the contrast dose required for renal venography can be significantly reduced when examining children by using digital subtraction venography.[8] After renal transplantation, routine ultrasonographic monitoring of the allograft provides an opportunity to detect acute venous thrombosis.[115-117]

In adults, experience in evaluation of renal cell carcinoma has shown that the renal veins are frequently difficult to visualize, especially on the left side.[118] Both CT scanning and MRI have merit in diagnosing bland venous thrombosis,[119,120] but a prospective study comparing these modalities to renal venography has not been reported.

Renal arteriography demonstrates stretching of the intrarenal arteries in the acute stage. During the venous phase, the main renal vein fails to opacify, and in total renal vein occlusion retroperitoneal collateral vessels may be filled.[109,121] These findings, although

Table 52-11. Radiologic Findings in Patients with Renal Vein Thrombosis

Author	Number of Patients with Thrombosis	Renal Vein Thrombus on Venography			Number of Patients Studied	Normal Urogram	Abnormal Urogram
		Right	Left	Bilateral			
Llach et al.[101]	12	2	3	7	12	5	7
O'Dea et al.[123]	14	3	8	3	14	14	0
Rosenmann et al.[95]	10	0	2	8	14	9	5
Barclay et al.[97]	34	5	5	24	—	—	—
Present series*	7	1	4	2	7	3	4
Total	77 (100%)	11 (14%)	22 (29%)	44 (57%)	47 (100%)	31 (66%)	16 (34%)

*Brigham and Women's Hospital series.

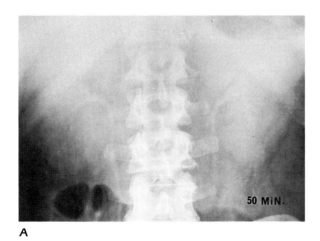

A

Figure 52-19. Renal vein thrombosis. (A) Intravenous urogram. At 50 minutes, the concentration of the contrast agent in the collecting system and ureters remains sharply decreased and the kidneys appear swollen. (B) Arteriogram at 3 seconds. The arterial branches are normal in caliber and appearance. (C) Arteriogram at 6 seconds. The transit time is markedly prolonged. (D) Arteriogram at 13 seconds. The main renal vein is not opacified. Capsular collateral veins are visualized (*arrows*). (E) Inferior vena cavogram. No thrombus is seen in the inferior vena cava. The usual dilution defects, visible at the points of union with the renal veins, are absent, suggesting renal vein thrombosis. (F) Right renal venogram. Chronic renal vein thrombosis with synechiae formation is apparent. A periureteric collateral vein fills. (G) Left renal venogram. Chronic left renal vein thrombosis is present.

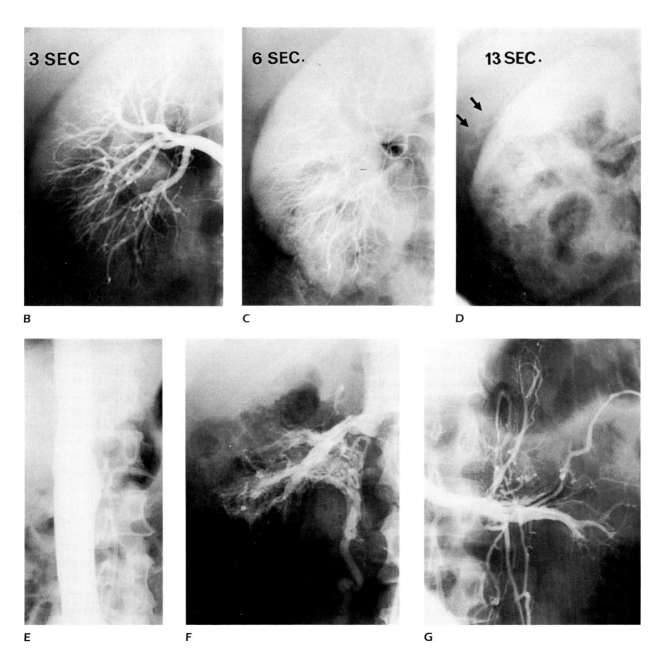

B

C

D

E

F

G

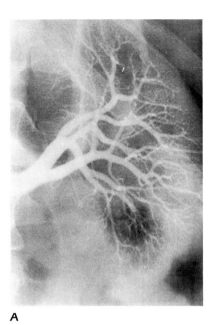
A

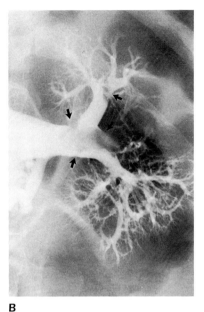
B

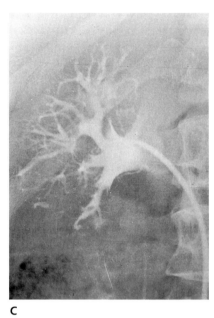
C

Figure 52-20. Bilateral renal vein thrombosis. (A) Left renal arteriogram. Stretching of branches is present in a moderately swollen kidney. (B) Left renal venogram demonstrating multiple thrombi (*arrows*). (C) Right renal venogram.

Multiple partially occlusive intraluminal filling defects are visible in both the main renal vein and the intrarenal branches.

highly suggestive, are not diagnostic; they may be found in the absence of demonstrable renal vein thrombosis.[39,122]

An accurate diagnosis can be made by direct visualization of an intravascular thrombus at renal venography. One kidney is involved almost as often as both, the left kidney more commonly (see Table 52-11). Both sides, therefore, should always be examined (Figs. 52-19 and 52-20). The renal vein may be totally occluded near the entry to the IVC or adjacent to the kidney and thus prevent opacification of the intrarenal branches (Fig. 52-21A). In contrast to neoplastic invasion (see Fig. 52-15A and B), the thrombosed renal veins are distended and the central portion of the clot has a margin convex toward the IVC (see Fig. 52-21A).[9] In some cases, the clot produces only partial obstruction and is seen as an intraluminal filling defect in the main renal vein (see Fig. 52-20B) or in intrarenal branches (see Figs. 52-21B and 52-29A). Chronic or organized renal vein thrombus may be recognized by the demonstration of a narrow renal vein lumen with ill-defined outlines, linear bands representing synechiae, and peripheral occlusion (see Figs. 52-21C and 52-19). In the transplanted kidney, oliguria, although most commonly caused by rejection, may also be associated with acute tubular necrosis, recurrence of glomerular nephritis, arterial stenosis or occlusion, renal vein thrombosis, and other causes. Venography is one method of detecting renal vein thrombosis (Fig.

52-22). The early diagnosis of renal vein thrombosis is important; with appropriate anticoagulation therapy, pulmonary embolism may be prevented.[100,123]

The risk of dislodging thrombus by the manipulation of a selective renal vein catheter is low, and pulmonary embolism after renal venography is rare.[1,123] This low risk is amply justified if initial or repeated pulmonary embolism can be prevented.

Although standard therapies have been anticoagulation or surgical thrombectomy, acute renal venous thrombosis can also be treated with thrombolytic drug administration into the selectively catheterized renal vein.[124,125] Intravenous thrombolysis has been performed for unilateral or bilateral disease[126] in adults and children[127,128] using urokinase or streptokinase. Successful thrombolysis occurred in both native and transplanted kidneys.[122,129] There is also a case report of caval filter insertion in a patient with recurrent pulmonary emboli.[130]

Renal Vein Varices

Pelviureteric varices are well-documented sequelae of renal vein thrombosis.[131,132] Although there are few reports of idiopathic renal vein varices,[133] they were found in eight (6 percent) patients in one series. All were in the left renal venous system and consisted of either a solitary varix of the left renal vein (Fig. 52-23A) or a network of veins (varicosities) adjacent to

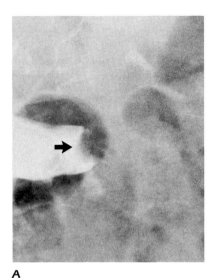

A

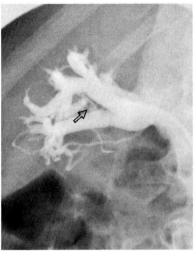

B

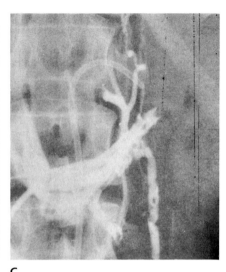

C

Figure 52-21. Renal vein thrombosis. (A) Total occlusion. This patient had membranous glomerulonephritis. The thrombus within the main renal vein prevents opacification of the intrarenal branches. In contrast to competent renal vein valves (see Fig. 52-14), the thrombus is convex toward the inferior vena cava (*arrow*). (B) Segmental thrombus. This patient had biopsy-proven membranous glomerulonephritis. Bilateral renal venography revealed only one small segmental thrombus (*arrow*) in the right kidney. (C) Organized thrombus. This 29-year-old woman with a 12-year history of systemic lupus erythematosus and a 4-year history of nephrotic syndrome. The left renal venogram shows peripheral occlusion. There are irregularly shaped filling defects in the central portion of the main renal vein, representing partially recanalized thrombus. This appearance is typical of chronic renal vein thrombosis.

Figure 52-22. Renal transplant with renal vein thrombosis. This patient had marked oliguria in association with rejection. (A) Arteriogram. The intrarenal branches were profoundly narrowed, failed to fill adequately, and demonstrated a protracted transit time. (B) Common iliac venogram. Complete thrombosis of the common iliac vein adjacent to its anastomosis with the renal vein was present. A nephrectomy demonstrated the pathologic changes of both rejection and renal vein thrombosis extending into the common iliac vein.

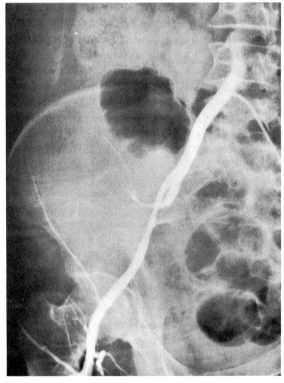

A

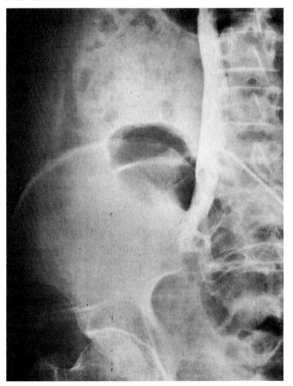

B

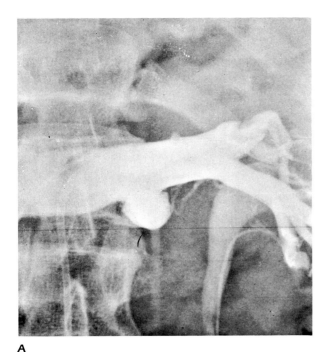

A

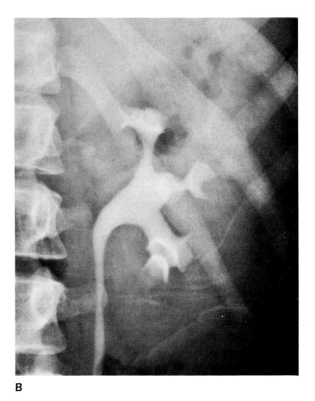

B

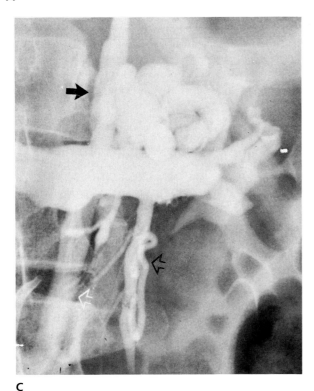

C

Figure 52-23. Renal vein varices. (A) Left renal venogram in an asymptomatic potential renal donor. There is a solitary varix at the entry of the spermatic vein. (B) Asymptomatic potential renal donor. An intravenous pyelogram shows a normal left collecting system. (C) Left renal venogram. A typical retroaortic vein (*open white arrow*) is seen arising from an unsplit main renal vein trunk. Note the network of varicose veins adjacent to the renal pelvis; there is opacification of the hemiazygos vein (*solid black arrow*) and of the ovarian vein (*open black arrow*).

may be normal, even in cases in which varices are the source of bleeding.[135,136]

Nonfunctioning Kidney

In hypertensive patients, the differentiation of renal agenesis from a nonfunctioning hypoplastic kidney or a small, contracted kidney is clinically important. Diagnostic methods, such as abdominal aortography, cystoscopy, and retrograde pyelography, may be inconclusive and even misleading in these patients.[137,138] Aortography may show the absence of a renal artery in both renal agenesis and small, shrunken kidneys.[135] In addition, the presence of a ureteral orifice on cystoscopy need not imply the presence of a kidney on that side.[139]

On the other hand, the absence of a renal vein on venography is pathognomonic of agenesis of the kidney.[137,138,140] On the left side, the central portion of the

the renal pelvis (see Fig. 52-23B and C). Renal vein varices are also formed in portal hypertension (Fig. 52-23D and E).[134] Varices are probably more common than was previously reported, and the majority of the patients who have varices are free of symptoms. Rarely, varices may cause bleeding (Fig. 52-24). The urogram

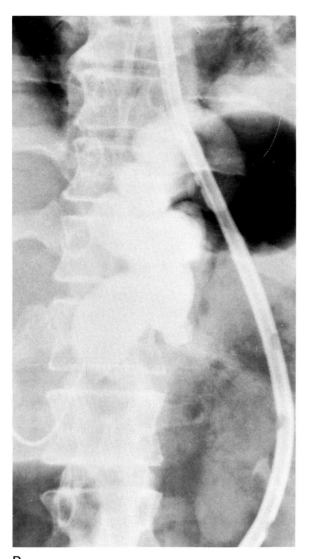

D

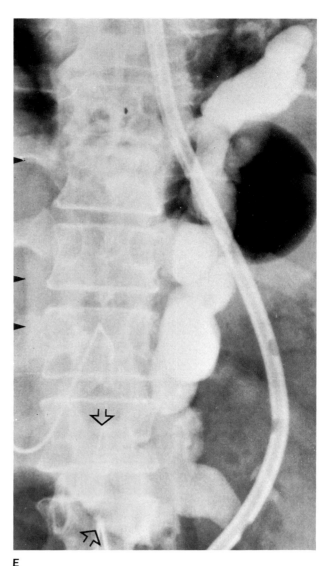

E

Figure 52-23 (continued). (D) Spontaneous portal vein–renal vein communication and varices in a patient with cirrhosis and portal hypertension, studied by transhepatic portography. Early phase film of a selective coronary vein injection shows large gastric varices. (E) Late phase film shows large varices in the region of the inferior phrenic and left adrenal veins that drain via the left renal vein (*open black arrows*) into the inferior vena cava (*arrowheads*).

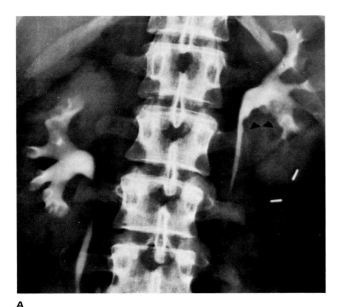
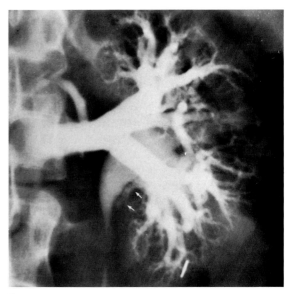

A   **B**

Figure 52-24. Renal vein varices. This 19-year-old woman had a history of recurrent hematuria. During prior surgery, varices had been ligated. (A) Intravenous pyelogram shows notching of the renal pelvis. (B) Left renal venogram shows a tortuous vein that notches the pelvis and ureter (*arrows*).

renal vein (embryologically, the preaortic portion of the renal collar) is still present, but it drains only the adrenal and the gonadal veins, thus creating a characteristic appearance on venography (Fig. 52-25). On the right side, if the kidney does not develop, there is no renal vein to catheterize.

The demonstration of a main renal vein with its lobar tributaries rules out renal agenesis. In contrast, in acquired diseases (e.g., shrunken kidneys), the main renal vein is of either normal size or only slightly diminished size, and the lobar veins are crowded and tortuous.[138,140] In congenital hypoplasia, the main renal vein is small, and the intrarenal veins show an otherwise normal distribution.[138] In renal dysplasia,[137,138] venography shows the presence of a disordered venous architecture.

Preoperative and Postoperative Evaluation of the Renal Veins

Prior knowledge of renal venous variations is important when retroperitoneal surgery is planned.[38] A left circumaortic venous ring constitutes an instantaneous collateral pathway immediately after caval interruption (Fig. 52-26)[141]; multiple right renal veins can serve as an alternative collateral route if the cava has been interrupted between these veins.[142] Therefore, a careful search for these frequent anatomic variations should be made by preoperative renal venography. If multiple right renal veins or a left circumaortic venous ring is

found, the caval interruption must be below the orifice of these veins in the lower lumbar region.

During retroperitoneal surgery, the surgeon may visualize a preaortic vein but may be unaware of an additional retroaortic component and thus may involuntarily tear it while mobilizing the kidney or clamping the aorta.[143] Warren et al.[144,145] have stressed the importance of preoperative angiographic evaluation of the left renal vein in preparation for splenorenal shunts for portal hypertension. Prior knowledge of the location, appearance, and possible variations of the left renal vein allows the procedure to be tailored to the needs of each patient and therefore results in less tissue manipulation at the operating table, to the advantage of the patients, who often are critically ill. Postoperatively, venography is important in evaluating the patency of these shunts. Even in the presence of occlusion of the left renal vein, however, these shunts might still be patent and drain into retroperitoneal collateral vessels.[146]

Benign Renal Parenchymal Disease

Selective renal venography can be a useful but nonspecific method of evaluating diseases of the renal parenchyma.

In acute glomerulonephritis, the renal venogram is normal; however, in chronic glomerulonephritis there may be diffuse loss of cortex as documented by the distance between the arcuate veins and the renal

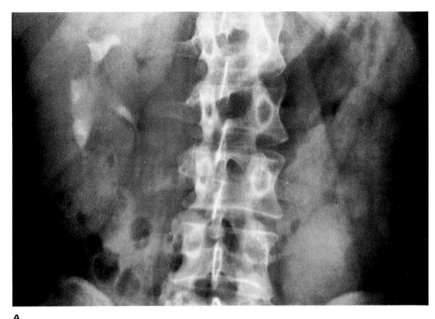

A

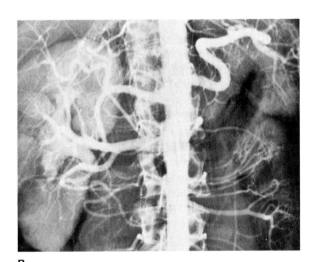

B

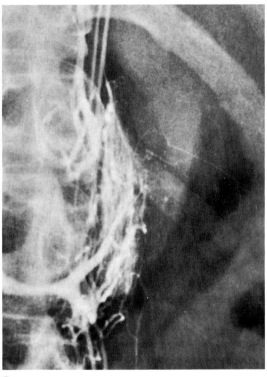

C

Figure 52-25. Agenesis of the left kidney. This patient had essential hypertension. (A) An intravenous pyelogram shows a large right kidney but no evidence of a left kidney. (B) On abdominal aortography, no left renal artery is seen. (C) Left renal venogram. In the expected location of the left renal vein, a small vein is seen draining both the left adrenal and the gonadal veins. The peripheral portion of the left renal vein, however, is absent. This appearance is pathognomonic for renal agenesis. (Courtesy of R.R. Freeman, M.D.)

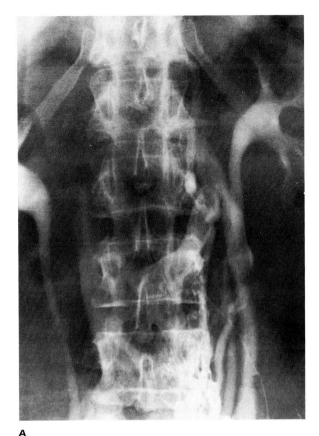

A

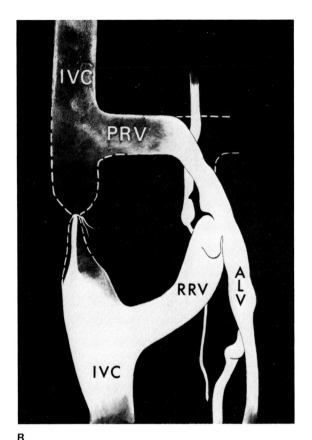

B

Figure 52-26. Caval ligation in a patient with a circumaortic venous ring. (A) Inferior vena cavogram after the injection of contrast material into both iliac veins. (B) Explanatory drawing. The inferior vena cava (*IVC*) is occluded in the region of L11. Opacified blood drains via the retroaortic renal vein (*RRV*) into the preaortic renal vein (*PRV*). *ALV,* ascending lumbar vein.

surface. Similar diffuse findings may be seen in shrunken nephrosclerotic kidneys.[3,58]

Localized abnormalities are characteristic of pyelonephritis. Areas of closely approximated veins are found in pyelonephritic scars.[3] Pyelonephritic pseudotumors may produce displacement of both interlobar and arcuate veins.[135,147]

In hydronephrosis (Figs. 52-27 and 52-28), there is spreading of the central veins, which appear narrowed, stretched, and curved,[58] and the arcuate veins are irregularly filled and stretched. Rarely, anomalous renal veins may produce hydronephrosis.[148] In polycystic disease (Fig. 52-29), the interlobar veins primarily are stretched, narrowed, and curved around the centrally located cysts. Typically, however, the deformed veins have smooth outlines.[58]

Renal fibrolipomatosis (Fig. 52-30) represents fatty

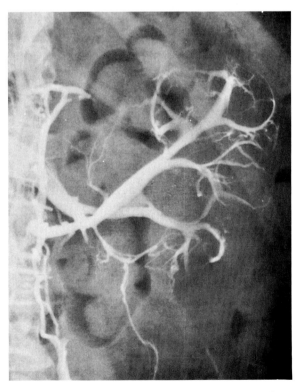

Figure 52-27. Venography in hydronephrosis. There is spreading and narrowing of the central veins, which are curved around the dilated renal calices. In contrast to intrarenal cysts (see Fig. 52-29), these veins are curved convex toward the periphery.

1317

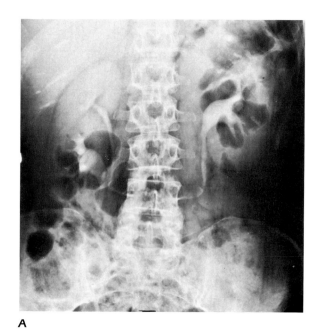

A

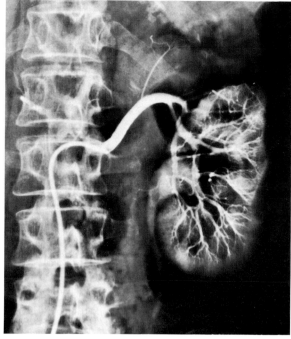

B

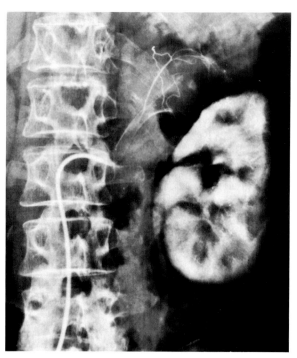

C

Figure 52-28. Venography in hydronephrosis of the upper pole of a double kidney. (A) Intravenous urogram. On the right, a bifid kidney is visible. On the left, the collecting system is normal insofar as it is visualized. No collecting system is visualized in the upper pole, which was thought to represent a mass. (B and C) Selective left renal arteriogram. Normal branches and nephrogram in the midsegment and the lower segment of the left kidney are apparent. An adrenal-capsular branch appears to supply the hypovascular upper pole. (D) Left renal venogram. The intrarenal veins in the midsegment and the lower pole appear normal. There is an unusual network of veins, including the adrenal vein, supplying the upper pole. The presence of an adrenal mass cannot be excluded on the basis of this study alone. (E) Selective upper pole renal venogram. Following injection, a network of veins is visible arising from the renal vein and draped around the avascular "mass" in the pole of the kidney. It strongly suggests the renal origin of the apparent mass lesion. (F) Percutaneous puncture of the upper pole. A contrast injection demonstrates a hydronephrotic upper pole of a bifid collecting system, with gross hydroureter, which indicates obstruction in the distal ureter. (Courtesy of R. Hooshmand, M.D.)

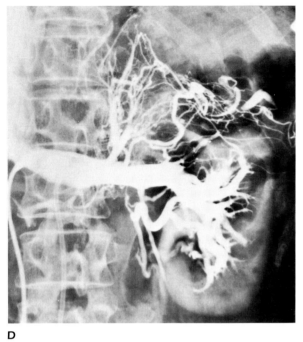

D

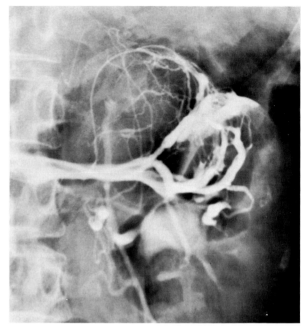

E

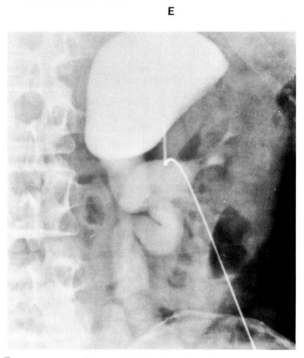

F

Figure 52-58 (continued).

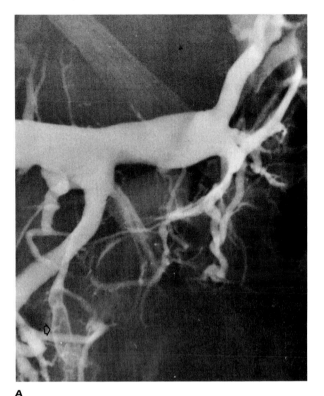

A

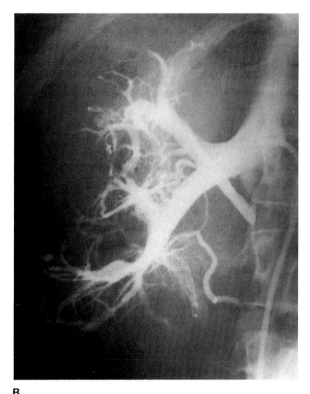

B

Figure 52-29. Polycystic disease. Bilateral renal venogram obtained because of suspected renal vein thrombosis in patients with known polycystic disease. (A) Left renal venogram. (B) Right renal venogram. The intrarenal veins are stretched and curved around the large intrarenal cysts in a fashion convex toward the renal hilus. Note the presence of two right renal veins and a capsular vein communicating with a lumbar branch. In (A), a small intravascular thrombus (*arrow*) is seen in the lower pole branch.

replacement of destroyed or atrophic renal parenchyma. The venogram may demonstrate a relatively normal distribution of venous tributaries when the urogram and the arteriogram are equivocal or suggestive of cysts or other mass lesions.

Renal venography is not required to establish the diagnosis of hydronephrosis, polycystic disease, or fibrolipomatosis. Nevertheless, when venography is indicated for other reasons (e.g., unexplained hematuria), familiarity with the venographic findings in these patients is important if the correct interpretation is to be made.

Acknowledgments

Some of the illustrations and text in this chapter are reproduced with permission from Beckmann CF, Abrams HL. Renal venography: anatomy, technique, applications, analysis of 132 venograms, and a review of the literature. Cardiovasc Intervent Radiol 1980;3:45.

References

1. Beckmann CF, Abrams HL. Renal venography: anatomy, technique, applications, analysis of 132 venograms, and a review of the literature. Cardiovasc Intervent Radiol 1980;3:45.
2. Olin TB, Reuter SR. A pharmacoangiographic method for improving nephrophlebography. Radiology 1965;85:1036.
3. Kahn PC. Selective venography in renal parenchymal disease. Radiology 1960;92:345.
4. Georgi M, Marberger M, Gunther R, et al. Retrograde Nierenphlebographie bei Ballonverschluss der Nierenarterie. ROEFO 1975;123:341.
5. Takaro T, Dow JA, Kishew S. Selective occlusive renal phlebography in man. Radiology 1970;94:589.
6. Novak D. Selective renal occlusion phlebography with a balloon catheter. Br J Radiol 1976;49:589.
7. Kahn PC, Wise HM, Robbins AH. Complete angiographic evaluation of renal cancer. JAMA 1968;204:753.
8. Said R, Hamzeh Y. Digital subtraction venography in the diagnosis of renal vein thrombosis. Am J Nephrol 1991;11:305–308.
9. Beckmann CF, Abrams HL. Renal vein valves: incidence and significance. Radiology 1978;127:351.
10. Boijsen E, Folin J. Angiography in the diagnosis of renal carcinoma. Radiologe 1961;1:173.
11. Lang EK. Arteriographic assessment and staging of renal-cell carcinoma. Radiology 1971;101:17.
12. Whitley NO, Kinkhabwala M, Whitley JE. The collateral vein

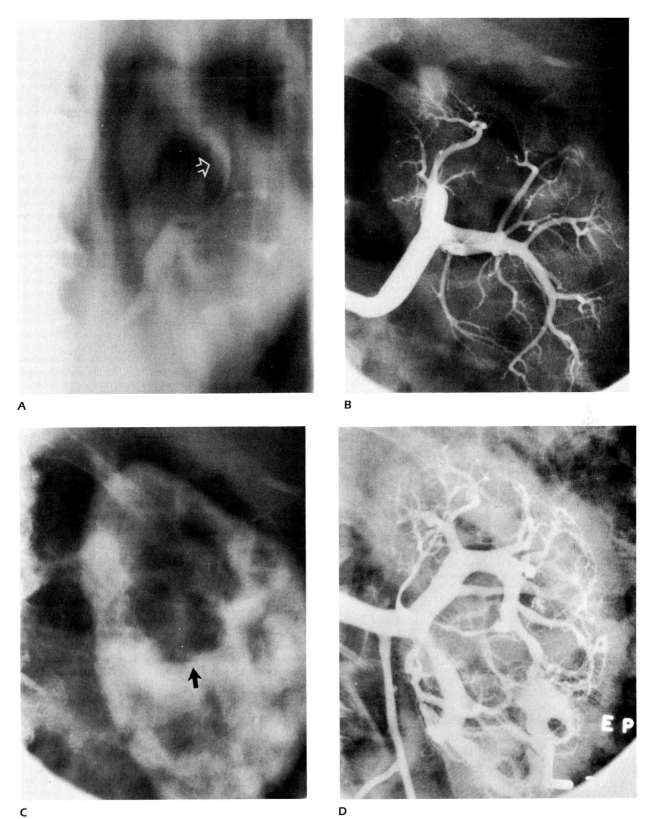

A

B

C

D

Figure 52-30. Renal fibrolipomatosis. (A) A tomographic section of the intravenous pyelogram suggests an upper pole mass indenting the upper pole infundibulum (*arrow*). The kidney of the peri-infundibular areas suggests a lipomatous infiltration. Early phase (B) and late phase (C) film of a selec-tive renal arteriogram again suggest the presence of a cystic avascular mass lesion of the upper pole (*arrow*, C). (D) The left renal venogram, however, shows a normal distribution of intrarenal venous branches, ruling out a mass lesion and supporting the diagnosis of renal fibrolipomatosis.

sign, a fallible sign in the staging of renal cancer. AJR 1974; 120:660.

13. Anatkow J, Kumanow C. Selective nephro-phlebography. In: L Diethelm, ed. Symposium of the European Association of Radiology. Mainz: Springer, 1972.

14. Chuang VP, Mena CE, Hoskins PA. Congenital anomalies of the inferior vena cava: review of embryogenesis and presentation of a simplified classification. Br J Radiol 1974;47:214.

15. Field S, Saxton H. Venous anomalies complicating left adrenal catheterization. Br J Radiol 1974;47:219.

16. Hamilton WJ, Mossman HW. Human embryology. 4th ed. Baltimore: Williams & Wilkins, 1972:192–195.

17. Adachi B. Cited by Reis RH, Esenther G. Variations in the pattern of renal vessels and their relation to the type of posterior vena cava in man. Am J Anat 1959;104:295.

18. Dow JA, Takaro T. Anomalous tributary of the left renal vein diagnosed by selective renal phlebography: case report. J Urol 1967;98:150.

19. Pick JW, Anson BJ. The renal vascular pedicle. J Urol 1940; 44:411.

20. Reis RH, Esenther G. Variations in the pattern of renal vessels and their relation to the type of posterior vena cava in man. Am J Anat 1959;104:295.

21. Weinstein BB, Countiss EH, Derber VS. Renal vessels in 203 cadavers. Urol Cutan Rev 1940;44:137.

22. Ahlberg NE, Bartley O, Chidekel N. Occurrence of valves in the main trunk of the renal vein. Acta Radiol 1968;7:431.

23. Clark K. The blood vessels of the adrenal gland. J R Coll Surg 1959;4:257.

24. Fagarasanu I. Recherches anatomiques sur la veine renale gauche et ses collaterales; leurs rapports avec la pathogenie du variococele essential et des varices du ligament large (demonstrations experimentales). Ann Anat Pathol 1938;15:9.

25. Notkovich H. Variations of the testicular and ovarian arteries in relation to the renal pedicle. Surg Gynecol Obstet 1956; 103:487.

26. Anson BJ, Daseler EH. Common variations in renal anatomy, affecting blood supply, form, and topography. Surg Gynecol Obstet 1961;112:439.

27. Hollinshead WH. Renovascular anatomy. Postgrad Med 1966;40:241.

28. Ahlberg NE, Bartley O, Chidekel N. Right and left gonadal veins, an anatomical and statistical study. Acta Radiol 1966; 4:593.

29. Abrams HL, Baum S, Stamey T. Renal venous washout time in renovascular hypertension. Radiology 1964;83:597.

30. Kahn PC. Selective venography of the branches. In: Ferris E, ed. Venography of the inferior vena cava and its branches. Baltimore: Williams & Wilkins, 1969:154–224.

31. Davis CJ, Lundberg GD. Retroaortic left renal vein. Am J Clin Pathol 1968;50:700.

32. Anson BJ, Pick JW, Cauldwell EW, et al. The anatomy of the pararenal system of veins, with comments on the renal arteries. J Urol 1948;60:714.

33. Lejar RC. Cited by Pick JW, Anson BJ. The renal vascular pedicle. J Urol 1940;44:411.

34. Hollinshead WH, McFarland JA. The collateral venous drainage from the kidney following occlusion of the renal vein in the dog. Surg Gynecol Obstet 1953;97:213.

35. Lien HH, Kolbensrvedt A. Phlebographic appearances of the left renal and left testicular veins. Acta Radiol 1977;18:3211.

36. Turner RJ, Young SW, Castellino RA. Dynamic continuous computed tomography: study of retroaortic left renal vein. J Comput Assist Tomogr 1980;4:109.

37. Royal SA, Callen PW. CT evaluation of anomalies of the inferior vena cava and left renal vein. AJR 1979;132:759.

38. Hoeltl W, Houby W, Aharinejad S. Renal vein anatomy and its implications for retroperitoneal surgery. J Urol 1990;143: 1108–1114.

39. Arner O, Blank C, Schreeb TB. Analysis with references to malignancy grading and special morphological features. Acta Chir Scand 1965;346(Suppl):1.

40. Crocker DW. Renal tumors. In: Sommers SC, ed. Kidney pathology decennial 1966–1975. New York: Appleton-Century-Crofts, 1975.

41. Griffiths JH, Thackray AC. Parenchymal carcinoma of the kidney. Br J Urol 1949;21:128.

42. Hand JP, Broders AC. Carcinoma of kidney. J Urol 1932;28: 199.

43. Myers GH, Fehrenbaker LG, Kelalis PP. Prognostic significance of renal vein invasion by hypernephroma. J Urol 1968; 100:420.

44. Perez CA, Kaiman HA, Keith J, et al. Treatment of Wilms' tumor and factors affecting prognosis. Cancer 1973;32:609.

45. Riches E. On carcinoma of the kidney. Ann R Coll Surg 1963; 32:201.

46. Riches EW. Analysis of patients with adenocarcinoma in a personal series. In: Riches EW, ed. Tumors of the kidney and ureter: neoplastic disease at various sites. Baltimore: Williams & Wilkins, 1964; vol. 5.

47. Riches EW, Griffiths IH, Thackray AC. New growths of the kidney and ureter. Br J Urol 1951;23:297.

48. McDonald JR, Priestley JT. Malignant tumors of the kidney. Surg Gynecol Obstet 1943;77:295.

49. Lang EK. Comparison of dynamic and conventional computed tomography, angiography, and ultrasonography in the staging of renal cell carcinoma. Cancer 1984;54:2205–2214.

50. Hricak H, Thoeni RF, Carroll PR, Demas BE, et al. Detection and staging of renal neoplasms: a reassessment of MRI. Radiology 1988;166:643–649.

51. Horan JJ, Robertson CN, Choyke PL, et al. The detection of renal carcinoma and extension into the renal vein and IVC: a prospective comparison of venacavography and magnetic resonance imaging. J Urol 1989;142:943–947.

52. Roubidoux MA, Dunnick NR, Sostman HD, Leder RA. Renal carcinoma: detection of venous extension with gradient-echo MRI. Radiology 1992;182:269–272.

53. Fritzscha PJ, Millar C. Multimodality approach to staging renal cell carcinoma. Urol Radiol 1992;14:3–7.

54. Levine E. Malignant renal parenchymal tumors in adults. In: Pollack HM, ed. Clinical urography. Philadelphia: Saunders, 1990;2:1260.

55. Bosniak M. The small (<3.0 cm) renal parenchymal: detection, diagnosis and controversies. Radiology 1991;179:307–317.

56. L'orente C, Linares R, Rodriguez J, Vicioso L, Varela JA. Incidental carcinoma of the kidney with renal vein thrombosis. Actas Urol Esp 1990;14:231–232.

57. Braedel HU, Haage H, Moeller JF, et al. Differential diagnostic importance in cases of unusual ectasia and renal pelvic deformity. Radiology 1976;119:65.

58. Rösch J, Antonovic R, Goldman ML, et al. Epinephrine renal venography. ROEFO 1975;126:501.

59. Smith JC, Rösch J, Athanasoulis C, et al. Renal venography in the evaluation of poorly vascularized neoplasms of the kidney. AJR 1975;123:552.

60. Ahlberg NE, Bartley O, Chidekel N, et al. An anatomic and roentgenographic study of the communications of the renal vein in patients with and without renal carcinoma. Scand J Urol Nephrol 1967;1:43.

61. Dorr RP, Cerny JC, Hoskins PA. Inferior venacavograms and renal venograms in the management of renal tumors. J Urol 1973;110:280.

62. Duckett JW, Lifland JH, Peters PC. Resection of the inferior vena cava for adjacent malignant disease. Surg Gynecol Obstet 1973;136:711.

63. Simpson A, Baron MG, Mitty HA. Angiographic patterns of venous extension of hypernephroma. J Urol 1974;111:441.

64. McCullough DL, Gittes RF. Vena cava resection for renal cell carcinoma. Urol 1974;112:162.

65. Petasnick JP, Patel SK. Angiographic evaluation of the nonvisualizing kidney. AJR 1973;119:757.

66. Watson RC, Fleming RJ, Evans JA. Arteriography in the diagnosis of renal carcinoma. Radiology 1968;91:888.

67. Ferris EJ, Bosniak MA, O'Connor JF. An angiographic sign demonstrating extension of renal carcinoma into the renal vein and vena cava. AJR 1968;102:384.

68. Palmer J, Barry B, Williams R, et al. Diagnosis of venous extension in renal cell carcinoma: the value of routine inferior venacavography. Australas Radiol 1975;19:265.

69. Cope C, Isard HJ. Left renal vein entrapment. Radiology 1969;92:867.

70. Bookstein JJ. Appraisal of arteriography in estimating the hemodynamic significance of renal artery stenosis. Invest Radiol 1966;1:281.

71. Ernst CB, Bookstein JJ, Moutie J. Renal vein renin ratios and collateral vessels in renovascular hypertension. Arch Surg 1972;104:496.

72. Bourgoignie J, Kurz S, Catanzaro FJ, et al. Renal venous renin in hypertension. Am J Med 1970;48:332.

73. Genest J, Boucher R. The renin-angiotensin system in human renal hypertension. In: Onesti G, ed. Hypertension: mechanism and management. New York: Grune & Stratton, 1971: 411–420.

74. Hunt JC, Strong CG. Renovascular hypertension. Am J Cardiol 1973;32:562.

75. Korobkin M, Glickman MG, Schambelan M. Segmental renal vein sampling for renin. Radiology 1976;118:307.

76. Schaeffer AJ, Fair WR. Comparison of split function ratios with renal vein renin ratios in patients with curable hypertension caused by unilateral renal artery stenosis. J Urol 1974; 112:697.

77. Simmons JL, Michelakis AM. Renovascular hypertension: the diagnostic value of renal vein renin ratios. J Urol 1970;104: 497.

78. Vaughan ED, Buhler FR, Laragh JH, et al. Renovascular hypertension: renin measurements to indicate hypersecretion and contralateral suppression, estimate renal plasma flow and score for surgical curability. Am J Med 1973;55:402.

79. Laragh JH, Baer L, Brunner HR, et al. Renin, angiotensin and aldosterone system in pathogenesis and management of hypertensive vascular disease. Am J Med 1972;52:633.

80. Sealey JE, Buhler FR, Laragh JH, et al. The physiology of renin secretion in essential hypertension: estimation of renin secretion rate and renal plasma flow from peripheral and renal vein renin levels. Am Med 1973;55:391.

81. Vaughan ED. Renin sampling: collection and interpretation. N Engl J Med 1974;290:1195.

82. Stockigt JR, Noakes CA, Collins RD, et al. Renal-vein renin in various forms of renal hypertension. Lancet 1972;1:1194.

83. Sos TA, Pickering TG. Percutaneous transluminal angioplasty in renal artery stenosis. In: Pollack HM, ed. Clinical Urology. Philadelphia: Saunders, 1990:3036.

84. Michelakis AM, Simmons J. Effect of posture on renal vein renin activity in hypertension. JAMA 1969;208:659.

85. Michelakis AM, Woods JW, Liddle GW, et al. A predictable error in use of renal vein renin in diagnosing hypertension. Arch Intern Med 1969;123:359.

86. Vermillion SE, Sheps SG, Strong CG, et al. Effect of sodium depletion on renin activity of renal venous plasma in renovascular hypertension. JAMA 1969;208:2303.

87. Kuchel O, Genest J. Effect of antihypertensive drugs on renin release. In: Onesti G, ed. Hypertension: mechanism and management. New York: Grune & Stratton, 1971:411–420.

88. Kaneko Y, Ikeda T, Takeda T, et al. Renin release during acute reduction of arterial pressure in normotensive subjects and patients with renovascular hypertension. J Clin Invest 1967;46: 705.

89. Paster S, Adams DF, Abrams HL. Errors in renal vein renin collections. AJR 1974;122:804.

90. Stockigt JR, Hertz P, Schambelan M. Segmental renal-vein renin sampling for segmental renal infarction. Ann Intern Med 1973;79:67.

91. Schambelan M, Howes EL, Stockigt JR, et al. Role of renin and aldosterone in hypertension due to a renin-secreting tumor. Am J Med 1973;55:86.

92. Harrington DP, White RI, Kaufman SL, et al. Determination of optimum methods of renal venous renin sampling in suspected renovascular hypertension. Invest Radiol 1975;10:45.

93. Katzberg RW, Morris TW, Burgener FA, et al. Renal renin and hemodynamic responses to selective renal artery catheterization and angiography. Invest Radiol 1977;12:381.

94. Mazo EB, Akopian AS, Koriakin MV, Kuznetsova BA. The effect of renal arteriography and phlebography on the function of the renin-angiotensin and hypophyseal-adrenal systems. Urol Nefrol (Mosk) 1990;1:22–27.

95. Rosenmann E, Pollack VE, Pirani CL. Renal vein thrombosis in the adult: a clinical and pathologic study based on renal biopsies. Medicine 1968;47:269.

96. Renert WA, Rudin LJ, Casarella WJ. Renal vein thrombosis in carcinoma of the renal pelvis. AJR 1972;114:735.

97. Barclay GP, Cameron HM, Loughridge LW. Amyloid disease of the kidney and renal vein thrombosis. Q J Med 1960;29: 137.

98. Hamilton CR, Tumulty PA. Thrombosis of renal veins and inferior vena cava complicating lupus nephritis. JAMA 1968; 206:2315.

99. Janower ML. Nephrotic syndrome secondary to renal vein thrombosis. AJR 1962;79:911.

100. Appel GB, Williams GS, Meltzer JJ, et al. Renal vein thrombosis, nephrotic syndrome and systemic lupus erythematosus. Ann Intern Med 1966;85:310.

101. Llach F, Arieff AJ, Massey SG. Renal vein thrombosis and nephrotic syndrome: a prospective study of 36 adult patients. Ann Intern Med 1975;83:8.

102. Susin M, Mailloux L, Becker C. Renal vein thrombosis in patients with membranous glomerulonephritis. Kidney Int 1974;6:103A.

103. Kendall AG, Lohmann RC, Dossetor JB. Nephrotic syndrome. Arch Intern Med 1971;127:1021.

104. McCarthy LJ, Titus JL, Daugherty GW. Bilateral renal vein thrombosis and the nephrotic syndrome in adults. Ann Intern Med 1963;58:837.

105. Chait A, Stoane L, Moskowitz H, et al. Renal vein thrombosis. Radiology 1968;90:886.

106. March TL, Halpern M. Renal vein thrombosis demonstrated by selective renal phlebography. Radiology 1963;81:958.

107. Stables DP, Thatcher GN. Traumatic renal vein thrombosis associated with renal artery occlusion. Br J Radiol 1973;46: 64.

108. Hipona FA, Crummy AB. The roentgen diagnosis of renal vein thrombosis. Clinical aspects. AJR 1966;98:122.

109. Koehier PR, Bowles WT, McAlister WH. Renal arteriography in experimental renal vein occlusion. Radiology 1966;86:851.

110. Wegner GP, Crummy AB, Flaherty TT, et al. Renal vein thrombosis, a roentgenographic diagnosis. JAMA 1969;209: 1661.

111. McCullough DL, Gittes RF. Ligation of the renal vein in the solitary kidney: effects on renal function. J Urol 1975;113: 295.

112. Rosenberg ER, Trought WS, Kirks DR, Sumner TE, Gross H. Ultrasonic diagnosis of renal vein thrombosis in neonates. AJR 1980;134:35–38.

113. Wiggelinkhuizen J, Oleszczuk-Raszke K, Nagel FO. Renal venous thrombosis in infancy. S Afr Med J 1989;75:413–416.

114. Trattnig S, Frenzel K, Eilenberger M, Khoss A, Schwaighofer B. Acute renal vein thrombosis in children: early detection with duplex and color-coded Doppler ultrasound. Ultraschall Med 1993;14:40–43.

115. Reuther G, Wanjura D, Bauer H. Acute renal vein thrombosis in renal allografts: detection with duplex Doppler US. Radiology 1989;170:557–558.

116. Baxter GM, Morley P, Dall B. Acute renal vein thrombosis in renal allografts: new Doppler ultrasonic findings. Clin Radiol 1991;43:125–127.

117. Duckett T, Bretan PN Jr, Cocharan ST, Rajfer J, Rosenthal JT. Noninvasive radiological diagnosis of renal vein thrombosis in renal transplantation. J Urol 1991;146:403–406.

118. Schwerk WB, Schwerk WN, Rodeck G. Venous renal tumor extension: a prospective ultrasound evaluation. Radiology 1985;156:491–495.

119. Glazer GM, Francis IR, Gross BH, Amendola MA. Computed tomography of renal vein thrombosis. J Comput Assist Tomogr 1984;8:288–290.

120. Tempany CM, Morton RA, Marshall FF. MRI of the renal veins: assessment of non-neoplastic venous thrombosis. J Comput Assist Tomogr 1992;16:929–934.

121. Itzchak Y, Deutsch V, Adar R, Mozes M. Angiography of renal capsular complex in normal and pathological conditions and its diagnostic implications. Crit Rev Diagn Imaging 1974; 5:111.

122. Schwieger J, Reiss R, Cohen JL, Adler L, Makoff D. Acute renal allograft dysfunction in the setting of deep venous thrombosis: a case of successful urokinase thrombolysis and a review of the literature. Am J Kidney Dis 1993;22:345–350.

123. O'Dea MJ, Malel RS, Tucker RM, et al. Renal vein thrombosis. J Urol 1976;116:410.

124. Rowe JM, Rasmussen RL, Mader SL, Dimarco PL, Cockett AT, Marfer VJ. Successful thrombolytic therapy in two patients with renal vein thrombosis. Am J Med 1984;77:1111–1114.

125. Dimarco PL, Sheinfeld J, Gutierrez OH, Cockett AT. Direct fibrinolytic therapy for renal vein thrombosis: radiographic followup. J Urol 1984;132:966–968.

126. Crowley JP, Matarese RA, Quevedo SF, Garella S. Fibrinolytic therapy for bilateral renal vein thrombosis. Arch Intern Med 1984;144:159–160.

127. Vogelzang RL, Moel DI, Cohn RA, Donaldson JS, Langman CB, Nemcek AA Jr. Acute renal vein thrombosis: successful treatment with intraarterial urokinase. Radiology 1988;169:681–682.

128. Bromberg WD, Firlit CF. Fibrinolytic therapy for renal vein thrombosis in the child. J Urol 1990;143:86–88.

129. Robinson JM, Cockrell CH, Tisnado J, Beachley MC, Posner MP, Tracy TF. Selective low-dose streptokinase infusion in the treatment of acute transplant renal vein thrombosis. Cardiovasc Intervent Radiol 1986;9:86–89.

130. O'Brien AA, O'Donnell JP, Keogh JA. Renal vein thrombosis with recurrent pulmonary emboli in the nephrotic syndrome: use of the Greenfield filter. Postgrad Med J 1986;62:223–225.

131. Elsen S, Friedenberg MJ, Kjahr S. Bilateral ureteral notching and selective renal phlebography in the nephrotic syndrome due to renal vein thrombosis. J Urol 1965;93:343.

132. Weiner PL, Lim MS, Knudson DH. Retrograde pyelography in renal vein thrombosis. Radiology 1974;111:77.

133. Blaivas JG, Previte SR, Pais VM. Idiopathic pelvic ureteric varices. J Urol 1977;9:207.

134. Keshin JG, Joffe A. Varices of the upper urinary tract and their relationship to portal hypertension. J Urol 1956;76:350.

135. Jonsson K. Renal angiography in patients with hematuria. AJR 1972;116:758.

136. Mitty HA, Goldman H. Angiography in unilateral renal bleeding with a negative urogram. AJR 1974;121:508.

137. Athanasoulis CA, Brown B, Baum S. Selective renal venography in differentiation between congenitally absent and small contracted kidney. Radiology 1973;108:301.

138. Itzchak Y, Adar R, Mozes M, et al. Renal venography in the diagnosis of agenesis and small contracted kidney. Clin Radiol 1974;25:379.

139. Ney C, Friedenberg RM. Radiographic atlas of the genitourinary system. Philadelphia: Lippincott, 1966.

140. Braedel HU, Schindier E, Mociler JF, et al. Renal phlebography: an aid in the diagnosis of the absent or non-functioning kidney. J Urol 1976;116:703.

141. Beckmann CF, Abrams HL. Circumaortic venous ring: incidence and significance. AJR 1979;132:561.

142. Greweldinger J, Coomaraswamy R, Luftschein S, et al. Collateral circulation through the kidney after inferior vena cava ligation. N Engl J Med 1969;281:541.

143. Mitty HA. Circumaortic renal collar: a potentially hazardous anomaly of the left renal vein. AJR 1975;125:307.

144. Warren WD, Salam AA, Faislalo A. End renal vein-to-splenic vein shunts for total or selective portal decompression. Surgery 1972;72:995.

145. Warren WD, Salam AA, Hutson D. Selective distal splenorenal shunt. Arch Surg 1974;108:306.

146. Sones PJ, Rude JC, Berg DJ. Evaluation of the left renal vein in candidates for splenorenal shunts. Radiology 1978;127:357.

147. Sorby WA. Renal phlebography. Clin Radiol 1969;20:166.

148. Gilsanz V, Rabadan M, Leiva Galvis O, et al. A singular case of hydronephrosis produced by inferior left lobar renal vein demonstrated by transparietal renal phlebography. Angiology 1972;23:311.

53

Renal Transplantation

RICHARD D. SHLANSKY-GOLDBERG

Renal transplantation is the definitive therapy for end-stage renal disease and has especially flourished in the postcyclosporine era. Rarely, renal autotransplantation is performed for other reasons, such as for trauma resulting in bilateral renal artery thrombosis.[1] Historically, angiography has been performed for evaluating allograft rejection, delineating donor anatomy prior to surgery, and investigating the failing renal allograft after transplantation. Today, renal biopsy and noninvasive imaging, primarily with ultrasound and nuclear medicine, have replaced the use of potentially nephrotoxic contrast angiography for most renal transplantation evaluations. Newer modalities such as magnetic resonance angiography and carbon dioxide digital subtraction angiography are being explored. Screening angiography is performed prior to transplantation to evaluate the donor kidney anatomy, and limited studies are made after the transplant for specific problems. At the author's institution, the posttransplant angiographic evaluation is usually performed to evaluate hypertension suspected to be caused by renal artery stenosis or vascular complications usually associated with renal allograft biopsy.

Surgical Technique

Whether the transplant kidney is from a living relative or a cadaver, the renal artery is anastomosed to the internal iliac artery as an end-to-end anastomosis or to the external iliac artery as an end-to-side anastomosis.[2,3] The kidney is surgically implanted in either iliac fossa from a retroperitoneal approach via an oblique incision extending from the midline 3 to 4 cm from the inguinal ligament to a point just above the anterior superior iliac spine.[4] When there are multiple vessels in a cadaver donor, a Carrel patch of aorta is used (Fig. 53-1).[5] With living related donors, multiple renal arteries are a surgical challenge because a patch of aorta containing the additional vessels cannot be obtained. If the additional vessel is small and perfuses only a small segment of kidney, it may be ligated. Larger ac-

cessory vessels may be anastomosed end to side to the main renal artery, although this anastomosis may encroach on the main renal artery lumen. Two or more renal arteries can be anastomosed together side to side to create a "double-barrel anastomosis" that preserves the lumen of each vessel.[6] Other authors have suggested performing separate anastomoses to either the recipient internal or external iliac arteries or one renal branch to each (Fig. 53-2). Another surgical option is to use the recipient's inferior epigastric artery for the accessory vessel.[7] Pediatric cadaveric donors may have both kidneys with a segment of aorta transplanted en bloc with an anastomosis to the recipient iliac artery (see Fig. 53-1D).[8]

The renal vein is usually anastomosed to a mobilized recipient iliac vein in an end-to-side fashion.[2] When two or more renal veins are present, the smaller veins are typically ligated, resulting in a single anastomosis of the larger vein with drainage through intrarenal venous anastomoses.[4] When the veins are similar in size, the smaller of the two is first clamped to test for adequate venous collaterals.[5] When the artery or vein is too short, grafting may be performed, usually with saphenous vein or occasionally a gonadal vein.[9] When significant vascular arterial or venous pathology is present, such as inferior vena cava (IVC) agenesis, unusual surgical anastomoses may be needed.[10] In children, the renal artery and vein may be anastomosed to the lower aorta and IVC, respectively. Three types of anastomoses are usually performed to create urinary continuity. The most common is the ureteroneocystostomy, which has the lowest incidence of extravasation. Recently, more involved transplant surgeries have been performed in diabetics using both kidney and pancreatic allografts.[11]

Renal Donor Angiography

Arteriography of kidneys is a standard presurgical examination in all possible living related donors. Donor angiography has four objectives.[12] The first is to deter-

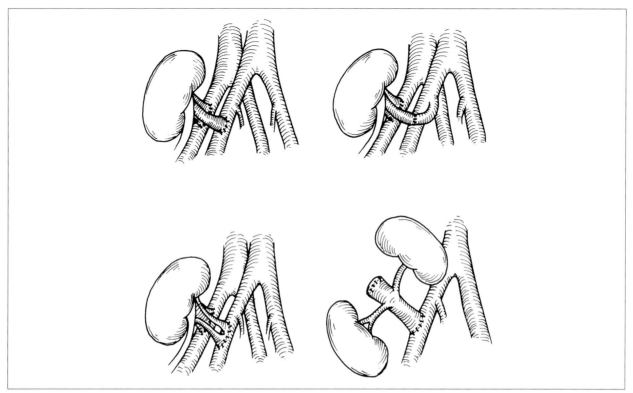

Figure 53-1. Different surgical techniques for transplant vascular anastomoses. (A) End-to-side renal artery to external iliac artery and end-to-side renal vein to external iliac vein. (B) End-to-end renal artery to internal iliac artery. (C) Cadaver donor Carrel patch for multiple renal arteries. (D) En bloc anastomosis of paired pediatric kidneys with a portion of aorta. (From Hanto D, Simmons R. Renal transplantation: clinical considerations. Radiol Clin North Am 1987;25:239–248. Used with permission.)

mine the number of renal arteries. This determines which kidney is harvested so that one can optimize reimplantation of the donor kidney into the recipient and ensure that the remaining kidney is free from major abnormalities. The number of renal arteries per kidney is identified, since more than one increases the difficulty of the surgical reconstruction. Multiple renal arteries are found in 24 to 28 percent of the population.[13,14] The second important objective is to demonstrate the length of the main renal artery, and the third is to exclude aortic or renal arterial disease, such as atherosclerosis or fibromuscular dysplasia, which may preclude transplantation. The incidence of fibromuscular dysplasia, atheromatous disease, and renal arterial aneurysms in the renal donor population is 6 percent.[14] The last reason is to exclude parenchymal diseases that may have gone undetected by a previous intravenous urogram.

There has been considerable debate as to the utility of conventional aortography versus intravenous digital subtraction (IV-DSA) and intraarterial digital subtraction angiography (IA-DSA). Conventional angiography has been considered the gold standard, and IA-DSA has been shown to be more accurate than IV-DSA.[15]

The advantages of conventional angiography are better spatial resolution and possible improved detection of the polar branch arteries of the kidney. The main advantages of IA-DSA are the reduction in contrast load and the time it takes to perform the study.[16] As the resolution of digital systems improves, the advantage of conventional angiography is reduced. Although the touted advantage of IV-DSA is that it is less invasive than an intraarterial study, it is no longer used because of its poor resolution and the increased requirement for intravenous contrast compared to IA-DSA.

At the author's institution we generally perform IA-DSA studies with a large, 40-cm image intensifier and a 1024 × 1024 imaging matrix. We use a 4 or 5 French pigtail catheter with the tip placed just above the renal arteries to reduce reflux into the superior mesenteric and celiac arteries. Ionic contrast, 43 percent iodine, or nonionic contrast, dilute 300 mg iodine per milliliter, is injected at a rate of 20 ml per second for 2 seconds with filming of three images per

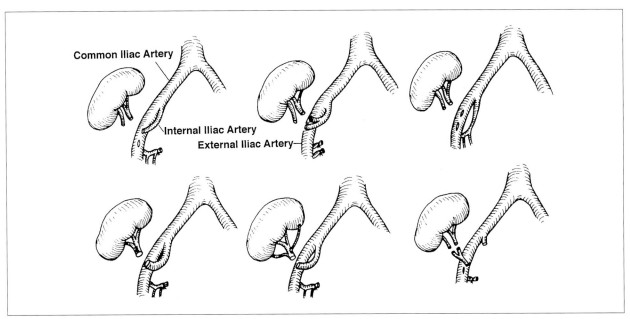

Figure 53-2. Several techniques for managing multiple renal arteries from living related donors. (From Hanto D, Simmons R. Renal transplantation: clinical considerations. Radiol Clin North Am 1987;25:239–248. Used with permission.)

second for a IA-DSA examination. If there is doubt as to the number of renal arteries, an additional view, usually 10- to 20-degree right posterior oblique, is performed, which will throw the overlying intercostal or jejunal branches off the kidney. The catheter can also be repositioned to reduce filling of the celiac or superior mesenteric vessels.[17] Selective injections of the renal vessels may be necessary in about 20 percent of patients to better define possible vascular or parenchymal diseases.[17]

Renal Transplant Angiography

Early angiography was performed with serial cut-film radiography using direct two- to fourfold magnification and a 0.1- to 0.3-mm focal spot to obtain clear definition of cortical vascular structures in order to differentiate different intraparenchymal disease processes.[18-20] With the decreasing need to visualize intrarenal parenchymal anatomy to diagnose problems such as rejection and acute tubular necrosis (ATN), intraarterial digital subtraction angiography began being used to successfully image renal transplants, typically for vascular complications such as arterial occlusions or stenoses.[21] Because of technological improvements in equipment, including digital systems with a 1024 × 1024 imaging matrix with rapid acquisition, digital angiography has replaced film-screen imaging in many interventional clinical laboratories.[22]

Because of the risk of nephrotoxicity associated with iodinated contrast media, angiographic technique should be carefully tailored to the clinical question, with careful consideration of the vascular anatomy, clinical scenario, and possible therapeutic intervention.[8] Catheter and wire manipulation near the anastomosis or donor transplant renal artery should be kept to a minimum, especially when the transplant has been recently performed. Consideration should be given to the use of nonionic contrast because of its possible reduced nephrotoxicity, although this remains controversial.[23]

Angiography is usually performed from the contralateral common femoral artery when the anastomosis is end to end to the internal iliac artery. The ipsilateral or contralateral common femoral artery can be used when an end-to-side anastomosis is performed to the external iliac artery. A cobra configuration of catheter works well when performing a contralateral approach. Another useful catheter for a diagnostic nonselective arteriogram is the Cope minivascular set (Cook, Inc.), which includes a 4 French straight multi-side-hole catheter with a 0.018-inch taper. The catheter is available in two lengths, a 20-cm version that can be used for ipsilateral iliac injections near the anastomosis or a 65-cm version that can be used to perform an aortogram and then pulled into the ipsilateral iliac artery (Fig. 53-3). The catheter is introduced using a 21-gauge needle to minimize arterial trauma. It performs like a tip occluder catheter because it is tapered to 0.18 inch, making it excellent for nonselective procedures.

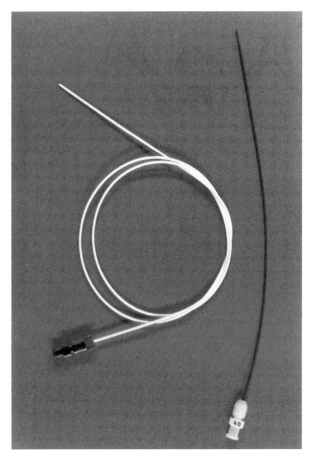

Figure 53-3. Straight minivascular catheter, 4 French (Cook, Inc.), in 20-cm and 65-cm lengths. Both lengths are tapered to 0.018 inch and have multiple side holes at the tip. The catheter performs like a tip occluder catheter for nonselective injections of contrast.

If necessary, this system is easily converted to a conventional 0.038-inch wire system with a 5 French coaxial "5.01" exchange catheter (Cook, Inc.). Examination of the distal aorta and common iliac arteries should be considered in hypertensive patients because atherosclerosis or clamp injuries can cause an inflow stenosis.[24]

During conventional angiography, filming should be initially rapid to adequately image the arterial phase and then slower for the parenchymal and venous phases. Imaging should be performed with two images per second for 3 seconds, then one film per second for 3 seconds, followed by an additional three films in 6 seconds (one film every other second).[17,20,25] Filming rates should be higher when the digital technique is used.[21] Contrast injection rates depend on the location of the catheter tip and should be guided by fluoroscopic hand injections. As with donor angiography, conventional filming generally requires full-strength

ionic or nonionic contrast, and digital filming requires contrast diluted to 20 to 50 percent with saline. Common iliac artery injections are performed at a rate of 7 to 15 ml per second for a total of 12 to 30 ml, and internal iliac artery injections are performed at 5 ml per second for a total of 7 ml, depending on the type of imaging technique used (Fig. 53-4). Selective injection into the renal artery is generally not required.[25] Initial films can be obtained in the 30-degree left or right posterior oblique projection for the left- or right-sided transplant, respectively, unless a test injection dictates a different view. Multiple projections such as steep obliques or even a lateral view are generally required to adequately image the course of the arteries and to visualize the in-profile anastomosis, which is typically placed anterior on the vessel. On average, three views are required to adequately image the transplant, although as many as six images may be required because of vessel overlap (Fig. 53-5).[17,21] Hand injections during fluoroscopic observation may be helpful in determining which oblique view demonstrates the

Figure 53-4. Nonselective injection of the ipsilateral common iliac artery using a minivascular catheter demonstrates a normal-appearing anastomosis and transplant.

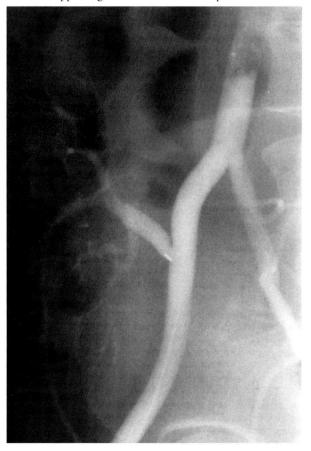

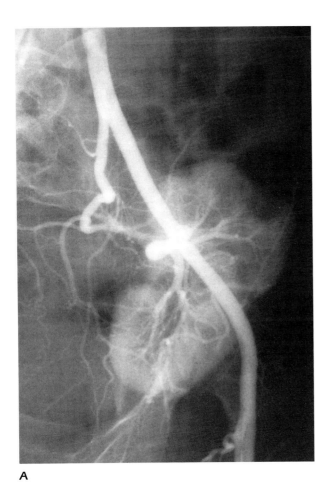
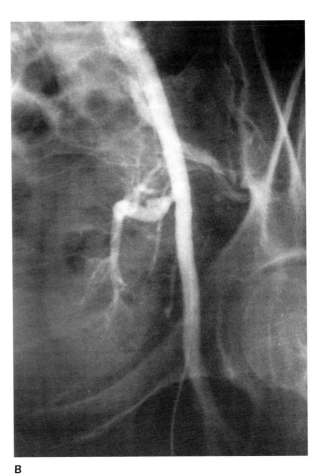

A   B

Figure 53-5. Normal arteriogram demonstrating the need for the proper obliquity. (A) The anteroposterior view obscures the end-to-side anastomosis. (B) The oblique view demonstrates the anastomosis.

anastomosis best. Compression of the ipsilateral common femoral artery to prevent runoff into the leg may improve opacification of the renal artery and anastomosis.[26] An occlusion balloon can also be used in the ipsilateral external iliac artery below the anastomosis in conjunction with rotational cineangiography to obtain retrograde filling of the vessels and the anastomosis in various projections.[8]

The angiographic appearance of a normal functioning transplant is similar to a normal native kidney, but its size may vary (Figs. 53-6 and 53-7). The size of a normal transplant may measure up to 16×9 cm and increases 10 percent in the first month and 1 percent a month for the first year.[27,28] Complications associated with renal transplant angiography are typical of other similar diagnostic and interventional angiographic procedures. The risk of vascular injury is related to the risk and difficulty of the procedure, and contrast nephrotoxicity is related to underlying impairment of renal function.[23]

If the renal transplant is poorly functioning with an elevated creatinine level and contrast angiography is being considered, carbon dioxide angiography may be used to confirm or exclude a diagnosis of a vascular abnormality. Carbon dioxide acts as a negative contrast when combined with IA-DSA and is cleared by the lungs rather than the kidneys.[29] Since it is not nephrotoxic, it can be used in patients with impaired renal function.[29] Carbon dioxide has not been shown to significantly change renal function with selective injections.[30] In addition, it works well with renal transplants because the vessels are anteriorly located and the gas rises into the graft, giving good visualization.[30] The potential for gas trapping in the renal artery is eliminated if the minimal volumes for imaging are injected 1 to 2 minutes apart.[29] Percutaneous intervention can be performed with carbon dioxide; however, this is more difficult because imaging is dependent on digital subtraction acquisition.

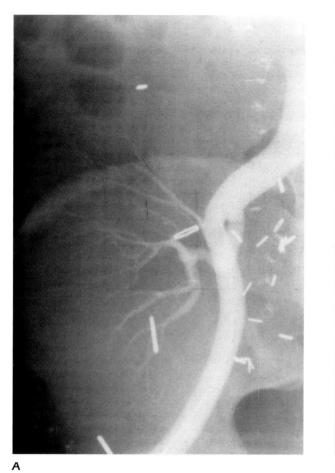

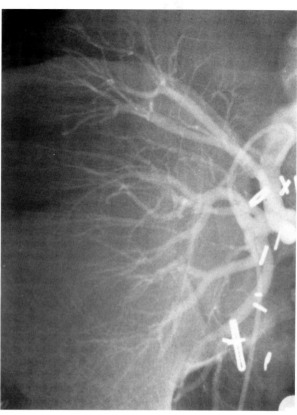

A

B

Figure 53-6. Internal iliac anastomosis to a normal kidney allograft. (A) Arterial phase with normal intrarenal branches. (B) 3× geometric magnification.

Venous Angiography

Renal vein catheterization is typically performed on the ipsilateral side when evaluating venous drainage such as measuring renin levels or evaluating the venous anastomosis. If there is concern about thrombosis of the iliac vein on the side of the transplant, the contralateral or jugular approach may be indicated. A 5 or 6 French catheter is adequate with an injection of 5 to 10 ml per second for a total injection of 10 to 20 ml for evaluating the iliac vein. Selective injection of the segmental veins may be indicated if renal vein thrombosis is suspected and is necessary for local infusion of a thrombolytic drug. Renal renin sampling should be performed below the kidney, within the renal vein and in the IVC. If there is concern about renin production from the native kidney, sampling of both native kidneys and upper IVC is also recommended.

Historical Review

In the 1960s and 1970s renal transplant angiography was performed for several reasons, including the need to evaluate renal transplants for intrarenal diseases associated with acute and chronic transplant dysfunction and rejection.[18,19] Oliguria or anuria after transplant was not infrequent and typically resulted from the different types of acute rejection (hyperacute, accelerated, or acute) or acute tubular necrosis.[31] Differentiation was difficult on clinical grounds, and the fine needle biopsy material was generally insufficient for an adequate determination, so that angiography was advocated to aid in making the diagnosis.[32] Renal transplant angiography was used to differentiate acute rejection from ischemic acute tubular necrosis.

During the acute forms of rejection, angiographically the kidney is enlarged and swollen with stenotic

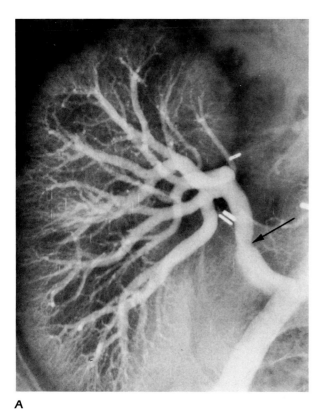

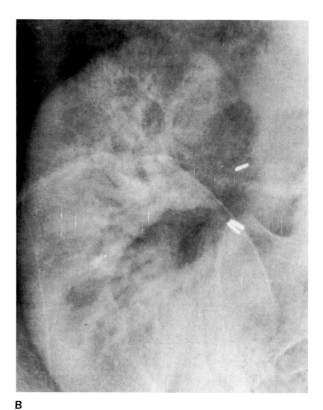

A   B

Figure 53-7. Angiogram of a normally functioning transplant. (A) Arterial phase with slight narrowing at the anastomosis (*arrow*). (B) Venous phase.

or obliterated vessels with prolonged arterial washout. Perfusion to the cortex and nephrogram is poor. Little contrast is seen in the renal vein, although simultaneous filling of the artery and vein may be seen with arteriovenous shunting. The total renal blood flow as determined by arterial washout may be normal because of this shunting.[20,33] Other findings associated with acute rejection include a large vessel vasculitis, prolonged arterial washout time, poor cortical vessel filling, ill-defined corticomedullary junction with a poor nephrogram, and arteriovenous (AV) shunting (Fig. 53-8).

Acute tubular necrosis is due to allograft ischemia after harvest and is the most common form of transplant dysfunction. It is usually demonstrated by anuria within the first few days after surgery without evidence of a hyperacute rejection. It is less often seen with donor-related transplants because there is less ischemic

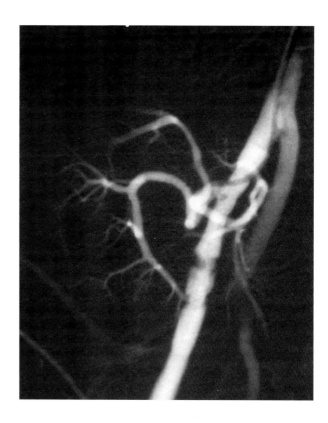

Figure 53-8. Acute renal transplant rejection. Arteriogram performed 36 hours after transplant, arterial phase, shows irregular, tapering vessels with little parenchymal staining. The irregularity below the anastomosis is most likely related to surgical clamps.

time than with cadaveric transplants.[32] Angiographically it is difficult to distinguish between acute rejection and tubular necrosis, since cortical ischemia due to vasoconstriction develops in both disease entities.[19] Vasculitis is usually not seen, and the arteriogram may be normal or near normal without excretion of contrast.[20] Kaude et al. graded their angiographic findings to give a prognostic outcome of the transplant after immunosuppressive therapy. The grading scale suggested reversible disease with three or less angiographic abnormalities.[34]

Chronic rejection, which is due to an ongoing humoral injury, demonstrates a normal-size to small kidney and may have postinfarct scarring with narrowed and fewer vessels due to fibrosis and scarring. Angiographically, arterial washout time is normal or minimally prolonged, with excretion of contrast depending on the functioning of the kidney (Figs. 53-9 through 53-11).[18,19] Findings of acute rejection may be superimposed on findings of chronic rejection (Fig. 53-12).[20] Other parenchymal abnormalities of renal transplants may be seen, such as acute glomerulonephritis. As in a nontransplanted kidney, the allograft may be enlarged, with dilated arteries and poor cortical perfusion with edema.[35] Renal papillary necrosis may also

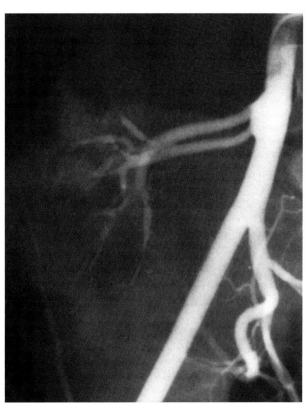

Figure 53-9. Chronic renal transplant rejection. Arterial phase shows that all the arteries are narrow and have several occlusions and stenoses. There is irregular parenchymal staining. Note the Carrel patch used to anastomose two renal arteries to the external iliac artery and the standing waves in the upper renal artery.

Figure 53-10. Chronic rejection with occlusion of the upper pole artery (*arrow*) and several peripheral interlobar branches. The lower pole continues to have some residual function. (A) Arterial and (B) late arterial-capillary phase with 3× geometric magnification. *C,* contrast medium in ilial conduit.

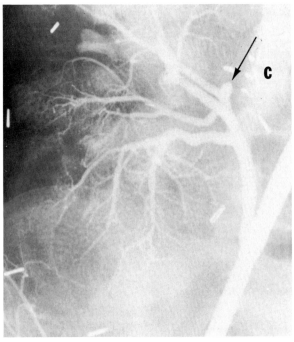

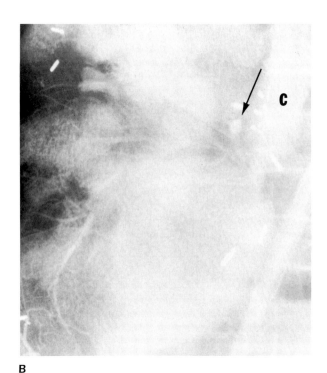

A

B

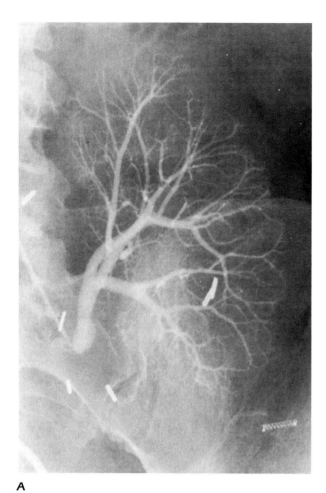

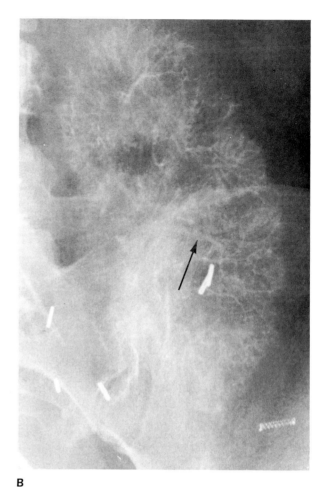

A

B

Figure 53-11. (A) Arterial phase showing severely stenotic constricted arteries throughout the kidney and total ischemia of the cortex. (B) Delayed arterial washout with simultaneous venous filling (*arrow*). These findings represent severe acute rejection with cortical necrosis.

be seen, due to ischemia from episodes of rejection. It appears as avascular areas next to the calices, which are dilated and clubbed because of the necrotic papillae.[36]

Current Evaluation of Transplant Dysfunction

Renal allograft dysfunction may be due to several causes, including surgical vascular and urologic complications, acute and chronic forms of rejection, cyclosporine toxicity, recurrent disease, and acute tubular necrosis.[37] The initial assessment of renal allograft dysfunction is usually performed with ultrasound and radioisotope imaging. Ultrasound imaging is use-

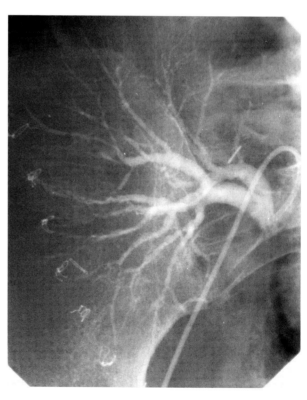

Figure 53-12. Acute rejection superimposed on chronic rejection. The patient's clinical course was typical for acute rejection with angiographic findings of chronic rejection. There are diffusely irregular vessels with multiple stenoses and occlusions.

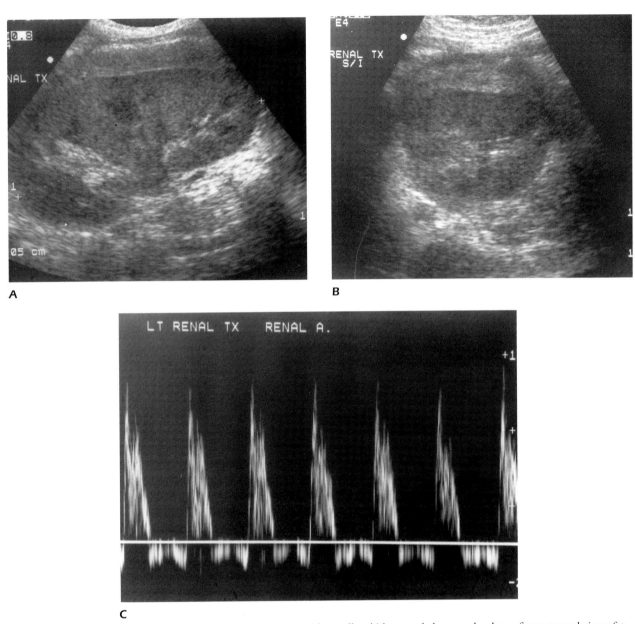

Figure 53-13. Ultrasound demonstrating acute rejection with swollen kidney and decreased echoes from central sinus fat. (A) Longitudinal. (B) Transverse. Note the hyperechoic collection related to a previous biopsy. (C) Doppler demonstrates reversed diastolic flow, which correlated with acute rejection.

ful to evaluate for perinephric collections or hydronephrosis.[38,39] In addition, it can give dimensions and volume of the kidney.[39,40] Acute rejection is often accompanied by an increase in renal size and prominence of the pyramids as well as a decrease in the echoes from the central sinus fat (Figs. 53-13 and 53-14).[39,40] Doppler imaging has furthered ultrasound's ability to screen for arterial or venous abnormalities, including renal artery stenosis.[41–48] In addition, color-coded Doppler ultrasound has become more valuable in detecting vascular abnormalities than duplex sonography

alone.[49] Several researchers have attempted to use Doppler to differentiate acute rejection from the other types of renal dysfunction, such as acute tubular necrosis and cyclosporine toxicity, using resistive and pulsativity indices in addition to intrarenal flow velocities. Reversed arterial flow during diastole has been associated with rejection, ATN, and renal vein thrombosis, whereas low arterial resistance flow and turbulent or "arterialized" vein signals are characteristic of an arterial venous fistula.[48,50,51]

Renal scintigraphy can evaluate renal transplant

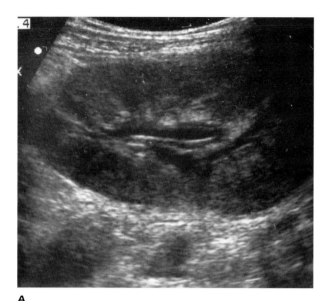
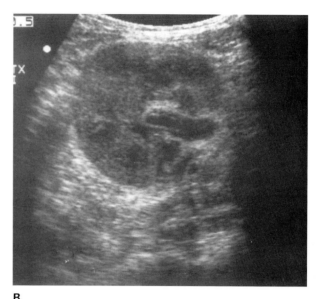

A   B

Figure 53-14. Ultrasound of renal transplant with chronic rejection demonstrating thickening of renal pelvis. (A) Longitudinal. (B) Transverse.

dysfunction. Renal perfusion using ^{99m}Tc-DTPA and tubular function using ^{131}I-Hippuran can be assessed. Interval deterioration of perfusion in the presence of a maintained or declining tubular function suggests acute rejection, and a deterioration in tubular function with preserved renal perfusion suggests acute tubular necrosis (Fig. 53-15). With ^{131}I-Hippuran, the delay in time of peak activity and/or prolonged clearance half-time of the isotope, called *delay washout,* represents tubular necrosis. Nuclear medicine does not readily distinguish cyclosporine toxicity from changes of acute rejection and acute tubular necrosis.[52] Radionuclide angiography can detect abnormalities in perfusion due to vascular abnormalities such as renal arterial and venous occlusions and stenoses. A newer single agent, ^{99m}Tc-MAG3, a technetium-labeled Hippuran analogue, may replace the combination of ^{99m}Tc-DTPA and ^{131}I-Hippuran, since it combines the biologic properties of Hippuran without the undesirable effects of ^{131}I and can be used for flow studies.[53] ^{99m}Tc-DTPA with captopril, which is an angiotensin-converting enzyme (ACE) inhibitor, has been demonstrated to be a physiologic test to diagnose hypertension due to transplant renal artery stenosis by causing a diagnostic acute rise in serum creatinine.[54]

Conventional CT may detect morphologic abnormalities in the renal allograft such as fluid collections due to infection or urinary leak or possible vascular abnormalities such as pseudoaneurysm.[55] It has little value in detecting rejection except for demonstrating renal size or other associated abnormalities. Newer spiral computed tomography, with its ability to quickly

acquire images properly timed to a contrast bolus and to produce three-dimensional reconstruction, allows for excellent visualization and demonstration of three-dimensional vascular anatomy and may have a role in detecting vascular abnormalities, including renal artery stenoses.[56]

Newer investigations with magnetic resonance angiography (MRA) provide new noninvasive imaging techniques to detect vascular abnormalities.[57] In one study by Holland et al., MRA had 100 percent specificity in detecting renal artery stenoses compared to conventional angiograms; however, the lesions were overestimated by 15 to 20 percent.[58] In another study, MRA had a sensitivity of 83 percent and a specificity of 97 percent compared to intraarterial digital subtraction angiography when all images were graded for severity of transplant stenoses (Fig. 53-16).[59] The value of MRI and spectroscopy in differentiating acute rejection from acute tubular necrosis remains to be determined.[60-62]

Among the multiple noninvasive modalities to diagnose renal allograft dysfunction, ultrasound-guided percutaneous biopsy remains the gold standard for determining the etiology of a dysfunctional graft. The major drawback in percutaneous biopsy is that rejection may not be distributed uniformly throughout the kidney. Fine-needle aspiration biopsy may be used because it has a low complication rate and may be obtained often.[63] However, fine-needle biopsy has several disadvantages, since it is based on cytologic information rather than histologic tissue.[63,64] At the present time large-core biopsy remains the most accurate way

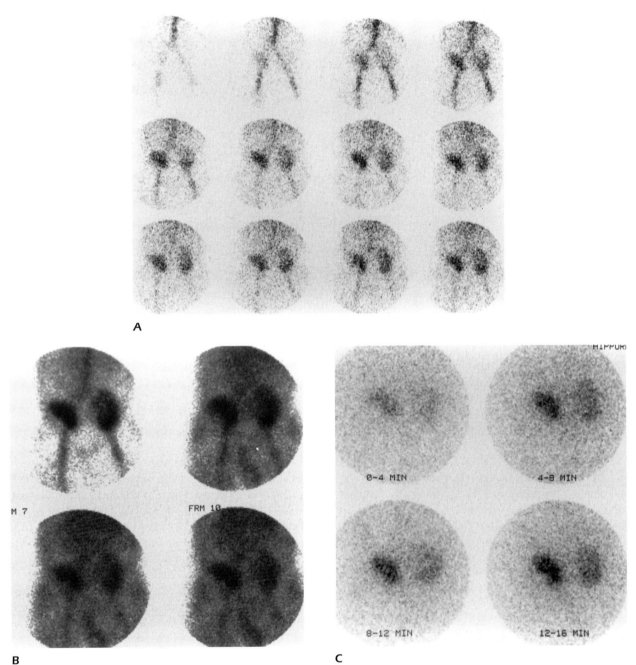

Figure 53-15. Patient with failed renal transplant in right pelvis due to chronic rejection and a failing new transplant in the left pelvis due to acute rejection. (A) ^{99m}Tc-DTPA angiogram demonstrates poor perfusion and function in both kidneys, worse on the left than on the right. (B) ^{99m}Tc-DTPA delayed images demonstrate poor function with no excretion, with a small right kidney and an enlarged edematous left kidney. (C) ^{131}I-Hippuran reveals a significantly decreased function on the left and diminished function on the right.

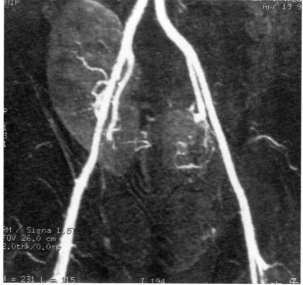

A

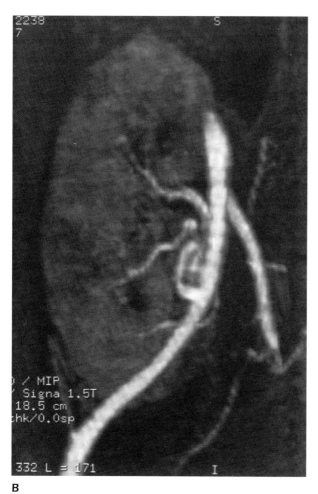

B

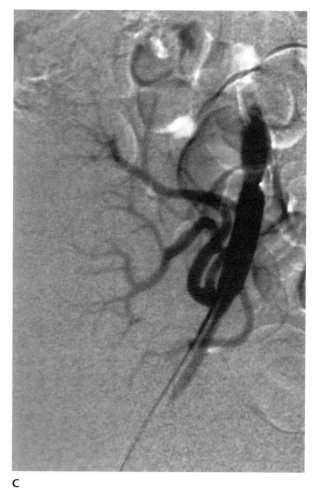

C

Figure 53-16. Three-dimensional time-of-flight MR angiogram (repetition time [TR]/echo time [TE] 5.4/1.1 milliseconds) after gadolinium injection in a patient suspected of having a renal vascular abnormality. (A) Pelvic MRA image demonstrates normal iliac vessels and multiple renal arteries. (B) MRA image demonstrates two normal renal arteries. (C) Arteriogram of same patient for comparison.

to differentiate the etiology of renal allograft dysfunction. Larger tissue samples allow one to evaluate the glomeruli, vascular tree, and parenchymal architecture so that one may separate acute rejection from other complications.[63-66] However, large-core renal biopsy carries several risks, including bleeding from the biopsy site, hematuria, perirenal hematoma, kidney rupture, pseudoaneurysm, and arteriovenous fistula. The complication rate for these procedures is 1 to 10 percent, with hematuria being the most common complication.[64,65,67,68] These complications have been reduced by the use of noninvasive tests prior to biopsy and the use of spring-loaded devices to reduce the size of the needle and number of passes needed to acquire a satisfactory specimen.[68-70]

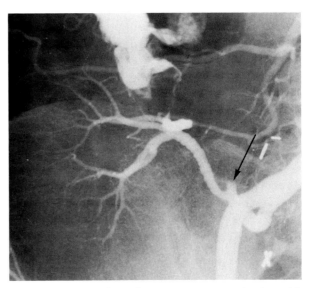

Figure 53-17. Findings due to severe acute rejection with occlusion of the upper pole renal artery (*arrow*). Standing waves are seen in the middle and lower pole renal artery, with occlusion of the distal branches of the interlobar arteries and no cortical perfusion.

Angiographic Evaluation of Renal Transplant Dysfunction and Complications

After noninvasive imaging and biopsy of a failing allograft have been done, several abnormalities or complications require diagnostic angiographic evaluation and possible intervention.

Renal Artery Thrombosis

The incidence of renal artery thrombosis of the transplanted kidney varies from 0.8 to 3.5 percent.[71-73] The risk is particularly significant in the pediatric population of patients, in which the donor and recipient vessels are smaller.[74] Arterial thrombosis usually occurs within a month after transplant, with predisposing factors being multiple renal arteries, surgical technique, torsion or kinking of vessels, hemodynamic events perioperatively, rejection, renal artery atherosclerosis or stenosis, and membranous glomerulopathy (Fig. 53-17).[75-77] Latter thrombosis may occur and usually is related to rejection, technical problems occurring at surgery, or renal artery stenosis.[78] In a review of 2500 transplants, there was an overall incidence of 1.8 percent, with 80 percent of the thromboses occurring within 1 month of transplant and 93 percent within the first year.[78] Rarely, late thrombosis may occur without rejection in a well-functioning graft.[78]

Another controversial cause of arterial thrombosis is related to the use of the immunosuppressive drug cyclosporine. Cyclosporine has several effects on the arterial wall, including a reversible dose-dependent arteriolar vasoconstriction, resulting in decreased renal blood flow; an angiopathy caused by proteinaceous deposition, resulting in intimal narrowing; and a de-

creased production of prostacyclin by the vascular endothelial cells, resulting in platelet aggregation.[79] One report demonstrated a 1.8 percent rate of thrombosis of patients taking cyclosporine, whereas none of the patients taking other forms of immunosuppressive medication (azathioprine and prednisone), experienced arterial thrombosis.[80] Another study demonstrated a 7 percent rate of arterial thrombosis with cyclosporine, with a 1 percent rate on conventional immunosuppressive therapy.[81] Since renal artery thrombosis has not been described in nonrenal transplant patients on cyclosporine, other factors are thought to be involved, such as the number of renal arteries in their allograft.[76]

Arterial thrombosis usually leads to loss of the graft; however, there also may be segmental arterial thromboses, which may not infarct the whole kidney. In a review of the literature, 92 percent of the patients required nephrectomy after arterial thrombosis.[78] Rare cases of successful recanalization of a thrombosed renal artery have been performed up to 12 hours after thrombosis, including a case of percutaneous thrombolysis using intraarterial streptokinase.[82] Embolization to the transplant kidney may also be seen from remote sites such as the heart or thoracic aorta (Fig. 53-18). The diagnosis of renal artery thrombosis should be considered in any patient developing acute anuria, and the diagnosis should be made quickly so that therapy can be initiated because graft salvage is unlikely after several hours of ischemia.

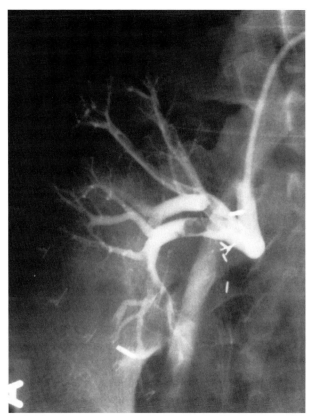

Figure 53-18. Saddle embolus with extension of thrombus into the upper pole. The thrombus is also seen in the lower pole artery.

Renal Artery Stenosis

The incidence of transplant renal artery stenosis, which can cause renal dysfunction and hypertension, is 0.6 to 25.0 percent.[83–86] Before the use of cyclosporine, approximately 50 percent of transplant patients were hypertensive. Although the incidence of rejection has decreased after the introduction of cyclosporine, the incidence of hypertension has increased.[87] Hypertension is associated with poor graft survival and cardiovascular mortality. Although it is the most common long-term complication of renal transplantation, renal artery stenosis is the etiology of elevated blood pressure in only 3 to 12 percent of the hypertensive patients.[83,88] Hypertension can be caused by several mechanisms. The transplant kidney itself can cause hypertension from renin production due to the ischemia caused by chronic rejection, by renal artery stenosis, or by recurrent renal disease.[89–91] Native kidneys can mediate hypertension by renin production, which can be treated by ACE inhibitors, bilateral native nephrectomy, or native renal artery embolization.[90,92–94] Antirejection medications also cause an elevation in blood pressure. Corticosteroids, through their mineralocor-

ticoid effect, cause salt and fluid retention.[90,92–94] Cyclosporine also causes a sodium-dependent rise in blood pressure unrelated to the production of renin.[87] More than one etiology of the hypertension can be superimposed on the others, such as chronic rejection and renal artery stenosis. Thus it can often be difficult to differentiate the cause of hypertension. Renin sampling can be helpful; however, production from the transplant kidney may be due to chronic rejection rather than renal artery stenosis.[95] In addition, the native kidneys may also produce elevated renins, which may confuse the values obtained from the transplant renal vein. Elevated values from the native kidneys with normal values from the transplant may suggest the native kidneys to be the culprit; however, since the values of both the transplant and the native kidneys may be elevated, the renin levels may not be a reliable indicator.[89,96]

The clinical manifestations of renal artery stenosis are usually hypertension refractory to medication and rising creatinine levels, usually developing during the first year after transplantation with or without an abdominal bruit.[71,97] Stenoses are more common in cadaver grafts from young donors than from living related donors.[97–99] Several locations can develop stenoses. An arterial stenosis may be (1) preanastomotic, usually due to atherosclerosis or a clamp injury; (2) at the anastomosis, usually due to a technical problem related to surgery; (3) just distal to the anastomosis, usually due to immune reactions or hemodynamic turbulence from the anastomosis causing an intimal hyperplasia; or (4) intrarenal, due to chronic rejection.[5,8,96] Postanastomotic strictures tend to be more severe and associated with end-to-side anastomoses as compared to end-to-end anastomosis, which tend to be at the anastomosis (Figs. 53-19 through 53-21).[84,96]

Although a renal artery stenosis can be suggested from Doppler studies and captopril stimulation tests, angiography remains the gold standard. Angiography has been reported to have a 41 percent false-positive rate in one retrospective review of 950 transplant arteriograms.[100] Because of the potential of a false-positive angiogram, Roberts et al. suggest that an angiographic stenosis should demonstrate some physiologic significance before an intervention is performed, such as a captopril-associated rise in creatinine or a large pressure gradient.[101]

Patients with significant renal artery stenoses that result in uncontrollable hypertension or graft dysfunction may be treated with percutaneous transluminal angioplasty (PTA) with balloons or surgery. PTA is now generally considered the treatment of choice, although some investigators have had high complication rates with low clinical response rates and advocate

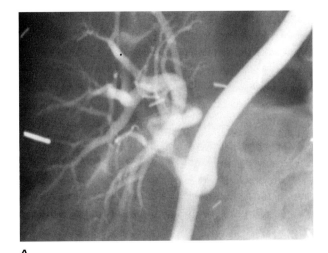

A

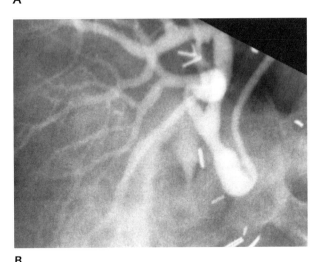

B

Figure 53-19. Renal artery stenosis in a hypertensive patient. (A) Predilatation. (B) Postdilatation.

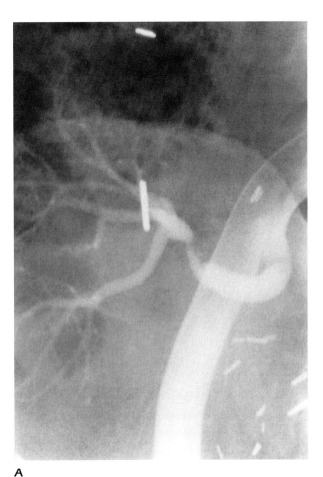

A

Figure 53-20. Stricture at the anastomosis of the internal iliac to the renal artery. (A) Predilatation. (B) Postdilatation.

surgery.[101,102] The initial technical success of PTA has been reported to be approximately 58 to 88 percent, and clinical success is approximately 74 to 87 percent.[84,103,104] The long-term clinical success is between 53 and 67 percent at 1 year.[103,105] Complication rates are generally low, with the rate of graft loss lower for PTA than for surgery[84,95,96,103,104,106]; however, Roberts et al. report that their loss after PTA is as high as 13 percent, higher than their surgical rate (Fig. 53-22).[101]

PTA of an end-to-side anastomosis can be performed either from the contralateral or ipsilateral side, depending on the angle of the anastomosis. An end-to-end anastomosis, which is generally to the hypogastric artery, is performed from the contralateral side. Serious complications that may lead to graft loss include acute thrombosis, arterial dissection, renal artery rupture, branch occlusion, distal embolization, and contrast-induced renal failure. As with any renal artery an-

gioplasty, complications can be reduced by using adequate heparinization, vasodilators, minimal wire manipulations, proper balloon sizing, and proper inflation pressures. Surgical standby during angioplasty is recommended, although the warm ischemic time may reduce the chances of salvaging the transplant. Newer techniques such as renal artery stenting, which have high technical success rates with good patency rates, may improve outcome, but their success depends on adequate stent expansion.[107]

Other arterial causes of renal transplant hypertension and dysfunction include inflow stenoses or dissections involving common, external, or internal iliac arteries (Figs. 53-23 and 53-24).[24,108] In addition, the Page kidney phenomenon, which causes renal dysfunction and hypertension, has been linked to peritransplant hematomas and lymphoceles compressing the artery or ureter.[95,109,110]

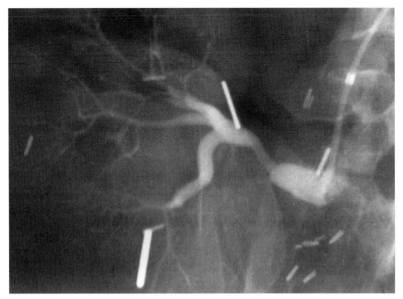

B   **Figure 53-20** (continued).

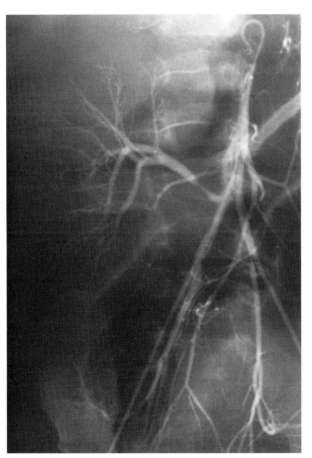

A

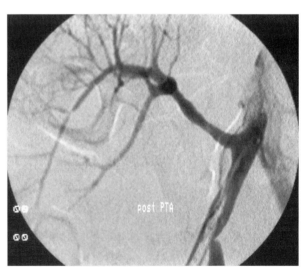

B

Figure 53-21. Pediatric transplant patient with anastomosis near the aortic bifurcation. (A) Renal artery stenosis. Note the small caliber of the vessels due to the small size of the patient and accompanying spasm. (B) Postangioplasty result.

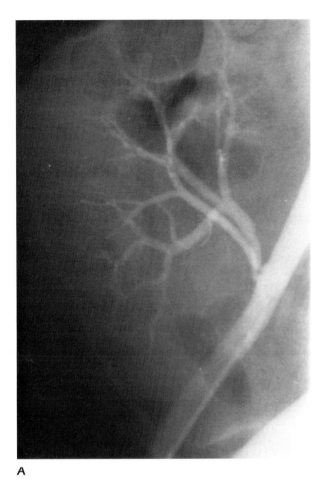

A

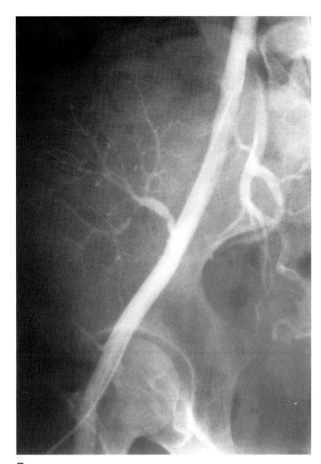

B

Figure 53-22. Postangioplasty complication. (A) Preangioplasty arteriogram demonstrates a Carrel patch at the external iliac artery with two renal arteries. Both arteries were individually dilated with an adequate result. (B) Follow-up film several months later when the patient's hypertension returned. The lower pole branch is occluded. Note the areas of stenoses distally in the upper pole branch, most likely representing rejection.

Renal Vein Abnormalities

Renal vein thrombosis, a rare complication of renal transplantation, usually occurs within a few days of transplantation but may present after several weeks.[72] It occurs in 1.1 to 7.6 percent of renal allographs.[111] Renal vein thrombosis usually results in nephrectomy because of the delay in diagnosis. The clinical symptoms are nonspecific, with pain, hematuria, proteinuria, and sudden decrease in urine output. Diagnostic studies are often nonspecific and more often represent acute rejection. Angiography is usually not initially performed, and the diagnosis is made by radioisotope study or ultrasound. The multiple causes of venous thrombosis include a short renal vein anastomosed un-

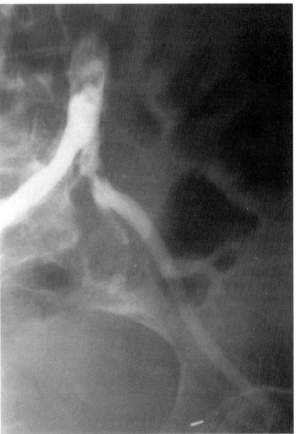

Figure 53-23. Inflow common iliac stenosis causing hypertension.

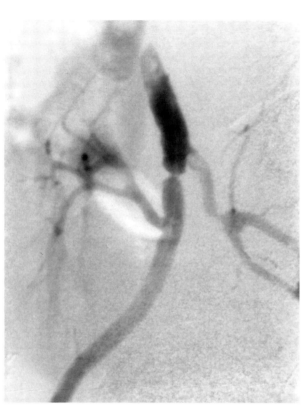

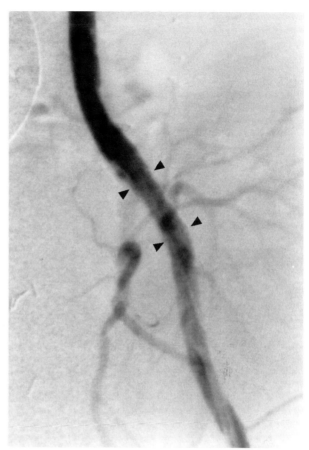

Figure 53-24. Inflow external iliac stenosis treated with a Palmaz stent. (A) Almost lateral view demonstrating the inflow stenosis just above the renal artery anastomosis, which appears widely patent. (B) Post–Palmaz stent placement with elimination of the stenosis. The *arrowheads* delineate the position of the stent, which is subtracted out of the image by the IA-DSA technique.

der tension, hypovolemia, acute rejection, immune complex–associated glomerulonephritis, platelet dysfunction, immunosuppression with cyclosporine, extension of lower extremity venous thrombosis and renal vein compression by hematoma, urinoma, lymphocele, or abscess.[47,72,111–114] If two renal veins are present, typically the smaller one is ligated, and outflow is provided by the larger vein. Rarely, renal infarction can happen if the two are nearly equal in size and only one vein is anastomosed.[113] In the pediatric population, because of the discrepant size of the kidney to the recipient, cases of compression of the renal vein in the iliac fossa resulting in thrombosis have been reported.[114] With renal vein thrombosis, angiography demonstrates delayed contrast clearance, a poor nephrogram, and poor venous opacification (Fig. 53-25). Since these findings are similar to those of acute rejection, the diagnosis should be confirmed with venography by retrograde catheterization of the allograft vein. Rarely, renal vein thrombosis can lead to allograft rupture, which is a life-threatening surgical emergency.[115] Most of the cases of venous thrombosis are made at surgery, and thrombectomy is rarely successful. Potential alternative therapies include the low-dose local intravenous infusion of thrombolytic agents to salvage the transplant after renal vein thrombosis.[116]

Renal vein stenoses are rare complications of transplant and may also be due to problems at harvest, transportation, or implantation. Olliff et al. reported a series of eight patients diagnosed by angiography or duplex sonography.[117] Five of these patients had associated arteriovenous fistulas, which may have contributed to the development of the stenosis because of the increased turbulent flow and resulting injury to the vein. Venoplasty was attempted in four of the patients, with limited success. Some have speculated that possibly longer balloon inflations, or the larger balloon diameters or inflation pressures typically used in dialysis grafts, might improve the outcome of these venous abnormalities.[118]

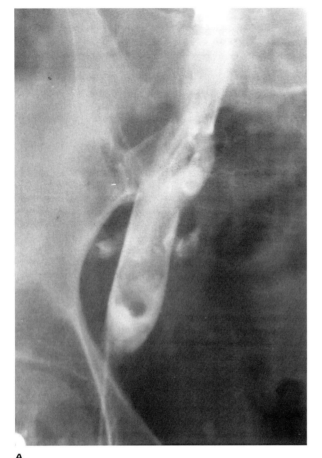

A

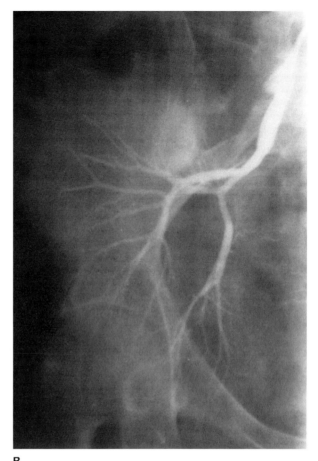

B

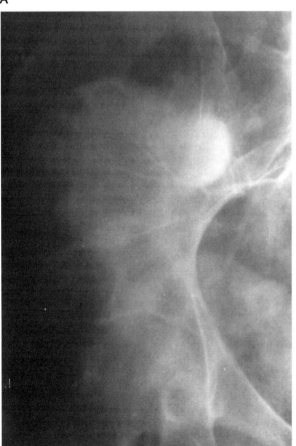

C

Figure 53-25. Iliac vein thrombosis with renal vein involvement causing renal dysfunction. (A) Ipsilateral common femoral venogram demonstrating a clot in the external iliac vein extending into the common iliac vein. (B) Arteriogram demonstrating poor parenchymal perfusion with small-caliber vessels. (C) Late arterial film demonstrating no parenchymal filling due to venous infarction.

Renal Artery Aneurysms, Pseudoaneurysms, and Arteriovenous Fistulas

Small arterial aneurysms in the interlobar branches of the renal artery have been demonstrated to be associated with chronic rejection.[119] Intrarenal aneurysms may rupture into the collecting system or perinephric space, causing a hematuria or a hematoma, respectively. Rupture may also result in renal loss. Intrarenal pseudoaneurysms may be found after percutaneous biopsy for the evaluation of rejection or after other percutaneous procedures.[41,120–122]

Extrarenal aneurysms are caused by infection and are usually associated with a perinephric abscess, wound infection, or urinary tract infection. Transplant patients are particularly at risk for infection because of their compromised immune system. Reports of mycotic aneurysms and renal artery rupture due to infections from organisms such as *Candida* have been

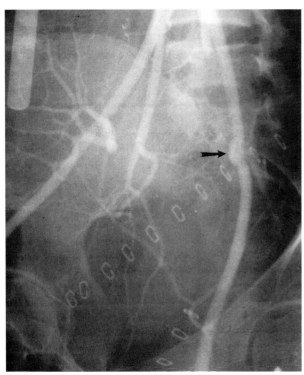

Figure 53-26. Left external iliac artery demonstrating a pseudoaneurysm due to a previous transplant (*arrow*). A right renal transplant is present.

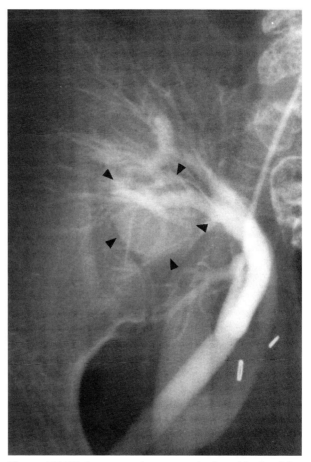

Figure 53-27. Larger renal aneurysm in the midpole of the kidney (*arrowheads*).

documented.[123,124] Extrarenal pseudoaneurysms are generally found at the arterial anastomosis and are due to problems with surgical reconstruction or infection (Fig. 53-26).[125,126] They can also be caused by biopsy or other percutaneous procedures such as percutaneous nephrostomy.[120,121]

There is an approximate 2 percent incidence of pseudoaneurysm formation after biopsy.[49] These pseudoaneurysms are generally asymptomatic when small and usually thrombose spontaneously.[48,49,127] Typically, they are incidentally diagnosed with Doppler ultrasound during or immediately after biopsy.[48] When symptomatic, they may present as a pulsatile mass in the pelvis, produce renal dysfunction from compression or shunting of blood when associated with an arteriovenous fistula, or rupture with bleeding. Angiographically, aneurysms and pseudoaneurysms appear as a localized segment of arterial dilatation that may appear smooth or irregular, depending on the chronicity and the amount of associated thrombus (Fig. 53-27).

Arteriovenous fistulas within the kidney are almost always complications of percutaneous needle biopsy or an interventional procedure. The fistula is caused by a laceration of an artery and adjacent vein, in contrast

to a pseudoaneurysm, which is caused by a laceration of only the artery. The fistula may also communicate with the collecting system, creating an arteriocaliceal fistula. The incidence of an arteriovenous fistula is 0 to 17.5 percent after biopsy.[128,129] The patient may present with hypotension, abdominal bruit, or macroscopic hematuria if the fistula communicates with the collecting system. It may or may not also be associated with a pseudoaneurysm. Usually 70 to 95 percent of arteriovenous fistulas due to renal biopsies resolve.[130,131] Angiographically there is early filling of the vein simultaneously with the artery. If the fistula is chronic, the artery and vein may dilate because of the increased flow. There may be extravasation of contrast into the collecting system if an arteriocaliceal fistula is present (Figs. 53-28 through 53-30).

Arteriography may be performed to confirm the diagnosis and to perform therapeutic embolization (Fig. 53-31).[66,122,132] Embolization should be performed as distally as possible with coaxial subselective catheters such as a Tracker-18 (Target Therapeutics) to reduce the size of intrarenal infarction.[133] Usually the neck of

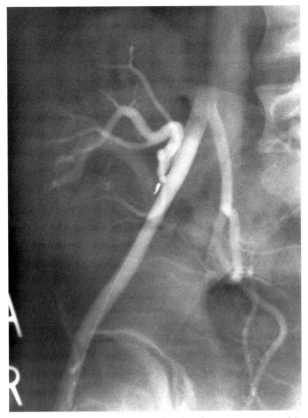

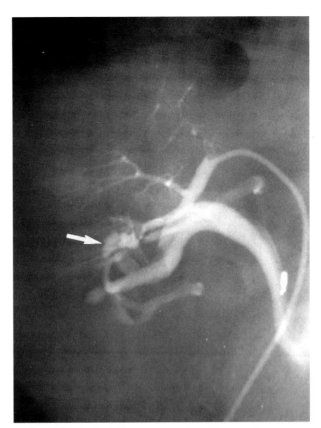

Figure 53-28. Arteriovenous fistula after percutaneous biopsy with simultaneous filling of the artery and vein without evidence of an accompanying pseudoaneurysm.

Figure 53-29. Arteriovenous fistula with a small accompanying pseudoaneurysm (*arrow*).

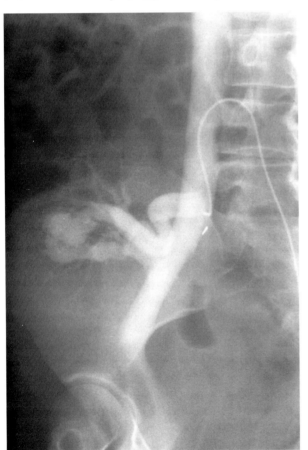

the pseudoaneurysm or the inflow and outflow portion of the feeding vessel is embolized.[132] In a report by deSouza et al., who used selective embolization, none of the patients experienced a worsening in renal function by nuclear medicine study or had a procedurally related complication from the embolization.[133] When access to the feeding vessel is not possible, percutaneous transcapsular embolization of the pseudoaneurysm may be performed.[122]

Parenchymal Masses Within Renal Allografts

Because of immunosuppression, the risk of neoplasm is elevated in the transplant patient. Malignancies may initially be seen on ultrasound, CT, or scintigraphy but may need further evaluation angiographically. Renal malignancies within transplant allographs may become more common as the age of the cadaver donors increases because of the decreasing availability of younger donors. Previous reports document de novo development of renal cell carcinoma and lym-

Figure 53-30. Chronic arteriovenous fistula that has caused hypertrophy of the renal artery and vein. There is simultaneous filling of the artery with the renal vein and IVC.

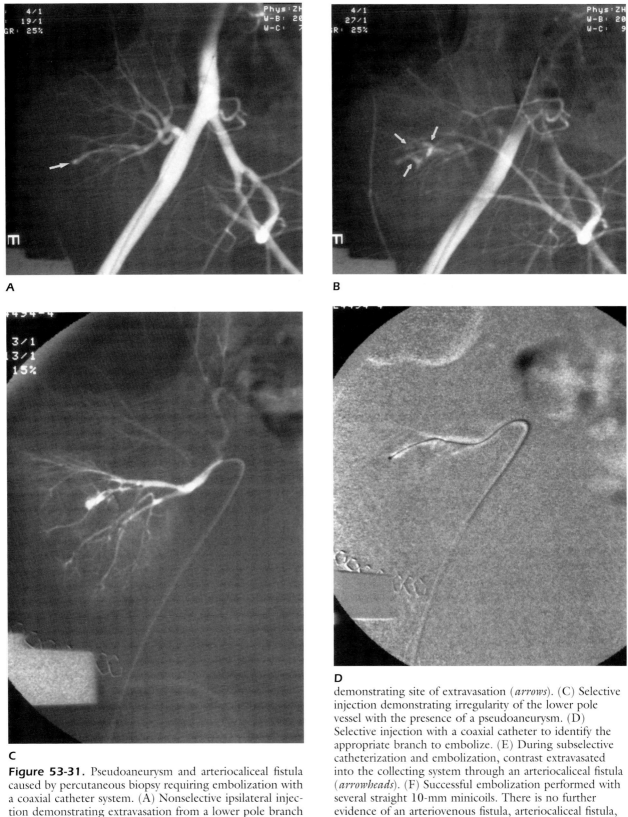

A

B

C

D

Figure 53-31. Pseudoaneurysm and arteriocaliceal fistula caused by percutaneous biopsy requiring embolization with a coaxial catheter system. (A) Nonselective ipsilateral injection demonstrating extravasation from a lower pole branch artery (*arrow*). (B) Longer during the nonselective injection demonstrating site of extravasation (*arrows*). (C) Selective injection demonstrating irregularity of the lower pole vessel with the presence of a pseudoaneurysm. (D) Selective injection with a coaxial catheter to identify the appropriate branch to embolize. (E) During subselective catheterization and embolization, contrast extravasated into the collecting system through an arteriocaliceal fistula (*arrowheads*). (F) Successful embolization performed with several straight 10-mm minicoils. There is no further evidence of an arteriovenous fistula, arteriocaliceal fistula, or pseudoaneurysm.

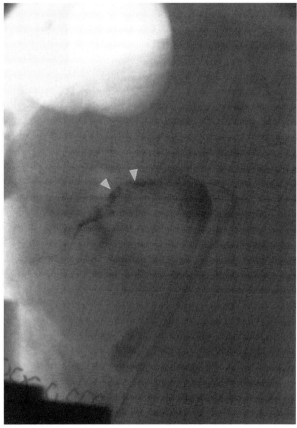

E

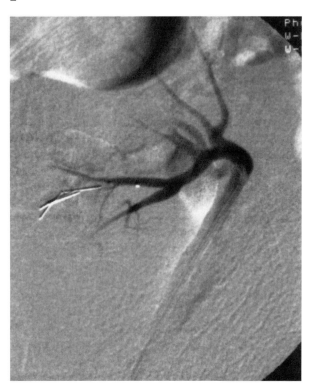

F

Figure 53-31 (continued).

phoma.[134-136] The incidence of carcinoma in transplant recipients has been 4.8 percent, which is greater than twice the normal rate. Eleven percent of these carcinomas developed within the kidney allograft.[135] Angiographically the malignancy may be difficult to diagnose because of the superimposed arterial changes associated with transplantation, such as chronic rejection. The graft may also contain cysts, abscesses, hematomas, or areas of necrosis that are hypovascular and difficult to differentiate angiographically.

Acknowledgments

I would like to thank many of my coworkers for their contribution to the text and illustrations: Constantin Cope, M.D., Michael C. Soulen, M.D., Ziv J. Haskal, M.D., and George A. Holland, M.D.

References

1. Brunetti DR, Sasaki TM, Friedlander G, et al. Successful renal autotransplantation in a patient with bilateral renal artery thrombosis. Urology 1994;43:235–237.
2. Hanto D, Simmons R. Renal transplantation: clinical considerations. Radiol Clin North Am 1987;25:239–248.
3. Flye MW. Renal transplantation. In: Flye MW, ed. Principles of organ transplantation. Philadelphia: Saunders, 1989:264–293.
4. Lee H. Surgical techniques of renal transplantation. In: Morris P, ed. Kidney transplantation. 3rd ed. Philadelphia: Saunders, 1988:215–234.
5. Belzer F, Glass N, Sollinger H. Technical complications after renal transplantation. In: Morris P, ed. Kidney transplantation. 3rd ed. Philadelphia: Saunders, 1988:511–532.
6. Guerra EE, Didone EC, Zanotelli ML, et al. Renal transplants with multiple arteries. Transplant Proc 1992;24:1868.
7. Ganesan KS, Huilgol AK, Sundar S, et al. Management of multiple arteries in renal transplantation. Transplant Proc 1994;26:2101–2102.
8. Crain MR, Ditmanson PM, Finlay DE. Vascular complications of renal transplantation: angiographic diagnosis and intervention. Semin Intervent Radiol 1992;9:235–245.
9. Nghiem DD. Spiral gonadal vein graft extension of right renal vein in living renal transplantation. J Urol 1989;142:1525.
10. Talbot-Wright R, Carretero P, Alcaraz A, et al. Complex renal transplant for vascular reasons. Transplant Proc 1992;24:1865–1866.
11. Boudeaux JP, Nealon WH, Carson RC, et al. Pancreas transplantation. Am Surg 1991;57:114–117.
12. Strauser G, Staples D, Weil R. Optimal technique of renal arteriography in living renal transplant donors. AJR 1978;131:813–816.
13. Boijsen E. Angiographic studies of the anatomy of single and multiple renal arteries. Acta Radiol Suppl (Stockh) 1959;183:1–135.
14. Spring D, Salvatierra O, Palubinskas A, et al. Results and significance of angiography in potential renal donors. Radiology 1979;133:45–47.
15. Shokeir A, El-Diasty T, Nabeeh A, et al. Digital subtraction angiography in potential live-kidney donors: a study of 1,000 cases. Abdom Imaging 1994;19:461–465.
16. Petty W, Spigos D, Abejo R, et al. Arterial digital angiography in the evaluation of potential renal donors. Invest Radiol 1986;21:122–124.

17. Gedroyc WMW, Reidy JF, Saxton HM. Arteriography of renal transplantation. Clin Radiol 1987;38:239–243.
18. Vinik M, Smellie WA, Freed TA, et al. Angiographic evaluation of the human homotransplant kidney. Radiology 1969; 92:873–879.
19. Foley WD, Bookstein JJ, Tweist M, et al. Arteriography of renal transplants. Radiology 1975;116:271–277.
20. Kaude JV, Hawkins IF. Angiography of renal transplant. Radiol Clin North Am 1976;14:295–308.
21. Picus D, Neeley JP, McClennan BL, et al. Intraarterial digital subtraction angiography of renal transplants. AJR 1985;145: 93–96.
22. Katzen B. Current status of digital angiography in vascular imaging. Radiol Clin North Am 1995;33:1–14.
23. McClennan B, Stolberg H. Intravascular contrast media: ionic versus nonionic. Current status. Radiol Clin North Am 1991; 29:437–454.
24. Weigele JB. Iliac artery stenosis causing renal allograft–mediated hypertension: angiographic diagnosis and treatment. AJR 1991;157:513–515.
25. Thomsen HS, Dorph S, Mygind T, et al. The transplanted kidney: diagnostic and interventional radiology. Acta Radiol 1985;26:353–367.
26. Lerona PT. Angiography of renal transplant using ipsilateral femoral artery compression. Radiology 1975;114:737.
27. Fletcher E, Lecky J. The radiological size of renal transplants: a retrospective study. Br J Radiol 1969;42:892–898.
28. Burgener F, Schabel S. The radiographic size of renal transplants. Radiology 1975;117:547–550.
29. Kerns S, Hawkins IJ, Sabatelli F. Current status of carbon dioxide angiography. Radiol Clin North Am 1995;33:15–29.
30. Harward T, Smith S, Hawkins I, et al. Follow-up evaluation after renal artery bypass surgery with use of carbon dioxide arteriography and color-flow duplex scanning. J Vasc Surg 1993;18:23–30.
31. Tilney N. The early course of a patient with a kidney transplant. In: Morris P, ed. Kidney transplantation. 3rd ed. Philadelphia: Saunders, 1988:263–284.
32. Kaude J, Slusher DH, Pfaff WW, et al. Angiographic diagnosis of rejection and tubular necrosis in human kidney allografts. Acta Radiol Diag 1970;10:476–488.
33. Lingardh G, Lundstom B. Renal blood flow determined by angiography. Acta Radiol Diag 1974;15:529–538.
34. Kaude J, Fuller J, Hawkins I, et al. Prognostic value of angiography in management of severe acute renal transplant rejection. ROFO 1977;127:119–123.
35. Ekelund L, Kaude J, Lindolm T. Angiography in glomerular disease of the kidney. AJR 1973;119:739–747.
36. Kaude JV, Stone M, Fuller TJ, et al. Papillary necrosis in kidney transplant patients. Radiology 1976;120:69–74.
37. Becker J. The role of radiology in evaluation of the failing renal transplantation. Radiol Clin North Am 1991;29:511–526.
38. Irving H, Kashi S. Complications of renal transplantation and the role of interventional radiology. J Clin Ultrasound 1992; 20:545–552.
39. Pozniak M, Dodd G, Kelcz F. Ultrasonographic evaluation of renal transplantation. Radiol Clin North Am 1992;30:1053–1066.
40. Griffin J, McNicholas M. Morphological appearance of renal allografts in transplant failure. J Clin Ultrasound 1992;20: 529–537.
41. Weissman J, Giyanani V, Landreneau M, et al. Postbiopsy arterial pseudoaneurysms in a renal allograft. J Ultrasound Med 1988;7:515–518.
42. Middleton W, Kellman G, Melson G, et al. Postbiopsy renal transplant arteriovenous fistulas: color Doppler US characteristics. Radiology 1989;171:253–257.
43. Morton M, Charboneau J. Arteriovenous fistula after biopsy of renal transplant: detection and monitoring with color flow and duplex ultrasonography. Mayo Clin Proc 1989;64:531–534.
44. Snider J, Hunter D, Moradian G, et al. Transplant renal artery stenosis: evaluation with duplex sonography. Radiology 1989;172:1027–1030.
45. Grenier N, Douws C, Morel D, et al. Detection of vascular complications in renal allografts with color Doppler flow imaging. Radiology 1991;178:217–223.
46. Maia CR, Bittar AE, Goldani JC, et al. Doppler ultrasonography for the detection of renal artery stenosis in transplanted kidneys. Hypertension 1992;19(Suppl II):207–209.
47. Plainfosse MC, Calonge VM, Beyloune-Mainardi C, et al. Vascular complications in the adult kidney transplant recipient. J Clin Ultrasound 1992;20:517–527.
48. Bach A, Merton D, Burke J, et al. Sonographic diagnosis of arteriovenous fistula and pseudoaneurysm after biopsy of a transplanted kidney. J Ultrasound Med 1993;12:545–547.
49. Hubsch P, Mostbeck G, Barton P, et al. Evaluation of arteriovenous fistulas and pseudoaneurysms in renal allografts following percutaneous needle biopsy. J Ultrasound Med 1990; 9:95–100.
50. Kaveggia L, Perrell R, Grant E, et al. Duplex Doppler sonography in renal allografts: the significance of reversed flow in diastole. AJR 1990;155:295–298.
51. Baxter G, Morley P, Dall B. Acute renal vein thrombosis in renal allografts: new Doppler ultrasonic findings. Clin Radiol 1991;43:125–127.
52. Kim E, Pjura G, Lowry P, et al. Cyclosporin-A nephrotoxicity and acute cellular rejection in renal transplant recipients: correlation between radionuclide and histologic findings. Radiology 1986;159:443–446.
53. Pouteil-Noble C, Yatim A, Najem R, et al. Diagnostic value of [99mTc]MAG-3 imaging in the oligoanuria of the renal transplant patient in the first month after transplantation. Transplant Proc 1994;26:303–304.
54. Curtis J, Luke R, Whelchel J. Inhibition of angiotensin-converting enzyme in renal transplant recipients with hypertension. N Engl J Med 1983;308:377–381.
55. Tobben P, Zajko A, Sumkin J, et al. Pseudoaneurysms complicating organ transplantation: roles of CT, duplex sonography, and angiography. Radiology 1988;169:65–70.
56. Mell MW, Alfrey EJ, Rubin GD, et al. Use of spiral computed tomography in the diagnosis of transplant renal artery stenosis. Transplantation 1994;57:746–748.
57. Holland GA, Baum RA, Danhey E, et al. MR angiography of the aortoiliac system: prospective comparison of contrast-enhanced 3D and 2D time-of-flight techniques. J Vasc Intervent Radiol 1995;6:4–5.
58. Holland GA, Baum RA, Owen R, et al. MR angiographic evaluation of the vasculature of transplanted kidneys. SMRM Book of Abstracts 1992;2:3104.
59. Gedroyc W, Negus R, al-Kutoubi A, et al. Magnetic resonance angiography of renal transplants. Lancet 1992;339: 789–791.
60. Hanna S, Helenon O, Legendre C, et al. MR imaging of renal transplant rejection. Acta Radiol 1991;32:42–46.
61. Liou J, Lee J, Heiken J, et al. Renal transplants: can acute rejection and acute tubular necrosis be differentiated with MR imaging? Radiology 1991;179:61–65.
62. Foxall P, Mellotte G, Bending M, et al. NMR spectroscopy as a novel approach to the monitoring of renal transplant function. Kidney Int 1993;43:234–245.
63. Danovitch G, Nast C, Wilkinson A, et al. Evaluation of fine-needle aspiration biopsy in the diagnosis of renal transplant dysfunction. Am J Kidney Dis 1991;17:206–210.
64. Waltzer W, Miller F, Argnold A, et al. Value of percutaneous core needle biopsy in the differential diagnosis of renal transplant dysfunction. J Urol 1987;137:1117–1121.
65. Wilczek H. Percutaneous needle biopsy of the renal allograft. Transplantation 1990;50:790–797.
66. Boschiero LB, Saggin P, Galante O, et al. Renal needle biopsy of the transplant kidney: vascular and urologic complications. Urol Int 1992;48:130–133.
67. Pillay V, Kurtzman N. Percutaneous biopsy of the transplanted kidney. JAMA 1973;226:1561–1562.

68. Bogan M, Kopecky K, Kraft J, et al. Needle biopsy of renal allografts: comparison of two techniques. Radiology 1990; 174:273–275.

69. Wahlberg J, Andersson T, Busch C, et al. The Biopty biopsy technique: a major advance in the monitoring of renal transplant recipients. Transplant Proc 1988;20:419–420.

70. Merkel FK, Silver B. Automated biopsy device for renal transplant monitoring. Transplant Proc 1992;24:1882–1885.

71. Palleschi J, Novick AC, Braun WE, et al. Vascular complications of renal transplantation. J Urol 1980;16:61–67.

72. Jordan ML, Cook GT, Cardella CJ. Ten years of experience with vascular complications in renal transplantation. J Urol 1982;128:689–692.

73. Jones RM, Murie JA, Ting A, et al. Renal vascular thrombosis of cadaveric renal allografts in patients receiving cyclosporine, azathioprine and prednisolone triple therapy. Clin Transplant 1988;2:122–126.

74. Harmon WE, Stablein D, Alexander SR, et al. Graft thrombosis in pediatric renal transplant recipients. Transplantation 1991;51:406–412.

75. Abbitt P, Chevalier R, Rodgers B, et al. Acute torsion of a renal transplant: cause of organ loss. Pediatr Nephrol 1990; 4:174–175.

76. Dodhia N, Rodby RA, Jensik SC, et al. Renal transplant arterial thrombosis: association with cyclosporine. Am J Kidney Dis 1991;17:532–536.

77. Frauchiger B, Bock A, Spoendlin M, et al. Early renal transplant dysfunction due to arterial kinking stenosis. Nephrol Dial Transplant 1994;9:76–79.

78. Groggel GC. Acute thrombosis of the renal transplant artery: a case report and review of the literature. Clin Nephrol 1991; 36:42–45.

79. Kahan BD. Cyclosporine nephrotoxicity: pathogenesis, prophylaxis, therapy and prognosis. Am J Kidney Dis 1986;8: 323–331.

80. Rigotti P, Flexhner SM, Buren CTV, et al. Increased incidence of renal allograft thrombosis under cyclosporine immunosuppression. Int Surg 1986;71:38–41.

81. The Canadian Multicentre Transplant Study Group. A randomized clinical trial of cyclosporine in cadaveric renal transplantation. New Engl J Med 1983;309:809–815.

82. Zajko AB, McLean GK, Grossman RA. Percutaneous transluminal angioplasty and fibrinolytic therapy for renal allograft arterial stenosis and thrombosis. Transplantation 1982;33: 447–450.

83. Munda R, Alexander JW, Miller S, et al. Renal allograft artery stenosis. Am J Surg 1977;134:400–403.

84. Grossman R, Dafoe D, Shoenfeld R, et al. Percutaneous transluminal angioplasty treatment of renal transplant artery stenosis. Transplantation 1982;34:339–343.

85. Feinstein EI, Campese VM, Fink E, et al. Hypertension in a renal transplant recipient. Am J Nephrol 1984;4:262–271.

86. Greenstein S, Verstandig A, McLean G, et al. Percutaneous transluminal angioplasty. Transplantation 1987;43:29–32.

87. Curtis JJ. Cyclosporine and hypertension. Clin Transplant 1990;4:337–340.

88. Smith R, Cosimi A, Lordon R, et al. Diagnosis and management of arterial stenosis causing hypertension after successful renal transplantation. J Urol 1976;115:639–642.

89. Popvtzer M, Pinnggera W, Katz F, et al. Variations in arterial blood pressure after kidney transplantation: relation to renal function, plasma renin activity, and the dose of prednisone. Circulation 1973;47:1297–1305.

90. Waltzer W, Turner S, Frohnert P, et al. Etiology and pathogenesis of hypertension following renal transplantation. Nephron 1986;42:102–109.

91. Dubovsky E, Russell C. Diagnosis of renovascular hypertension after renal transplantation. AJH 1991;4:724S–730S.

92. Shu KH, Lian JD, Lu YS, et al. Hypertension following successful renal transplantation. Transplant Proc 1992;24:1583–1584.

93. First MR, Neylan JF, Rocher LL, et al. Hypertension after renal transplantation. J Am Soc Nephrol 1994;4:S30–S36.

94. Ponticelli C, Montagnino G, Tarantino A, et al. Hypertension in renal transplantation. Contrib Nephrol 1994;106:190–192.

95. Ricotta J, Schaff H, Williams G, et al. Renal artery stenosis following transplantation: etiology, diagnosis, and prevention. Surgery 1978;84:595–602.

96. Sniderman K, Sprayregen S, Sos T, et al. Percutaneous transluminal dilation in renal transplant arterial stenosis. Transplantation 1980;30:440–444.

97. Rijksen J, Koolen M, Walaszewski J, et al. Vascular complications in 400 consecutive renal allotransplants. J Cardiovasc Surg 1982;23:91–98.

98. Stanley P, Malekzadeh M, Diament M. Posttransplant renal artery stenosis: angiographic study in 32 children. AJR 1987; 148:487–490.

99. Henning P, Bewick M, Reidy J, et al. Increased incidence of renal transplant arterial stenosis in children. Nephrol Dial Transplant 1989;4:575–580.

100. Henriksson C, Nilson A, Thoren O. Artery stenosis in renal transplantation. Scand J Urol Nephrol 1975;29(Suppl):89–90.

101. Roberts J, Ascher N, Fryd D, et al. Transplant renal artery stenosis. Transplantation 1989;48:580–583.

102. Chandrasoma P, Aberele A. Anastomotic line renal artery stenosis after transplantation. J Urol 1986;135:1159–1162.

103. Raynaud A, Bedrossain J, Remy P, et al. Percutaneous transluminal angioplasty of renal transplant arterial stenoses. AJR 1986;146:853–857.

104. Matalon TA, Thompson MJ, Patel SK, et al. Percutaneous transluminal angioplasty for transplant renal artery stenosis. J Vasc Intervent Radiol 1992;3:55–58.

105. Benoit G, Moukarzel M, Hiesse C. Transplant renal artery stenosis: experience and comparative results between surgery and angioplasty. Transplant Int 1990;3:137–140.

106. Merkus JW, Huysmans FT, Hoitsma AJ, et al. Renal allograft artery stenosis: results of medical treatment and intervention. A retrospective analysis. Transplant Int 1993;6:111–115.

107. Rees C, Snead D, Niblett R. Multicenter study of Palmaz-Schatz in the renal arterial. J Vasc Intervent Radiol 1995;6: 60.

108. Merkus JW, Dun GC, Reinaerts HH, et al. Iliac artery dissection after renal transplantation. Nephrol Dial Transplant 1992;7:1242–1245.

109. Yussim A, Shmuely D, Levy L, et al. Page kidney phenomenon in kidney allograft following pretransplant lymphocele. Urology 1988;31:512–514.

110. Nguyen BD, Nghiem DD, Adatepe MH. Page kidney phenomenon in allograft transplant. Clin Nucl Med 1994;19: 361–363.

111. Merion R, Calne R. Allograft renal vein thrombosis. Transplant Proc 1985;17:1746–1750.

112. Clark RA, Colley D. Radiological evaluation of renal vein thrombosis. CRC Crit Rev Diagn Imaging 1980;13:337–388.

113. Hilfiker ML, Feddersen RM, Gibel LJ, et al. Allograft renal vein thrombosis in a kidney with two veins. Transplantation 1992;54:738–739.

114. Borowicz MR, Hanevold CD, Cofer JB, et al. Extrinsic compression in the iliac fossa can cause renal vein occlusion in pediatric kidney recipients but graft loss can be prevented. Transplant Proc 1994;26:119–120.

115. Richardson AJ, Higgins R, Jaskowski A, et al. Renal allograft rupture and renal vein thrombosis. Transplant Proc 1990;22: 1419.

116. Robinson J, Cockrell C, Tisnado J, et al. Selective low-dose streptokinase infusion in the treatment of acute transplant renal vein thrombosis. Cardiovasc Intervent Radiol 1986;9:86–89.

117. Olliff S, Negus R, Deane C, et al. Renal transplant vein stenosis: demonstration and percutaneous venoplasty of a new vas-

cular complication in the transplant kidney. Clin Radiol 1991; 43:42–46.

118. Saeed M, Newman G, McCann R, et al. Stenoses in dialysis fistulas: treatment with percutaneous angioplasty. Radiology 1987;164:693–697.

119. Castañeda-Zuñiga W, Sibley R, Zollikofer C, et al. Renal artery aneurysms: an angiographic sign of transplant rejection. Radiology 1980;136:333–335.

120. Cope C, Zeit RM. Pseudoaneurysms after nephrostomy. AJR 1982;139:255–261.

121. Gavant M, Gold R, Church J. Delayed rupture of renal pseudoaneurysms: complications of percutaneous nephrostomy. AJR 1982;138:948–949.

122. Sennett CA, Messersmith R, Yousefzadeh D, et al. Percapsular and percutaneous embolization of renal transplant pseudoaneurysm and AV fistula: case report. Cardiovasc Intervent Radiol 1989;12:270–273.

123. Benoit G, Icard P, LeBaleur A, et al. Mycotic aneurysm and renal transplant. Urology 1988;31:63–65.

124. Pluemecke G, Williams J, Elliott D, et al. Renal transplant artery rupture secondary to *Candida* infection. Nephron 1992;61:98–101.

125. Renigers S, Spigos D. Pseudoaneurysm of the arterial anastomosis in a renal transplant. AJR 1978;131:525–526.

126. Mulderije E, Berden J, Buskens F, et al. False and true aneurysms of the renal artery after kidney transplantation: a report of two cases. Br J Radiol 1985;58:896–899.

127. Bennet A, Weiner S. Intrarenal arteriovenous fistula and aneurysms. AJR 1965;95:372–382.

128. Diaz-Buxo J, Kopen D, Donadio J. Renal allograft arteriovenous fistula following percutaneous biopsy. J Urol 1974;112:577–580.

129. Deane C, Cowan N, Giles J, et al. Arteriovenous fistulas in renal transplants: color Doppler ultrasound observations. Urol Radiol 1992;13:211–217.

130. Messing E, Kessler R, Kavaney P. Renal arteriovenous fistulas. Urology 1976;8:101–107.

131. Wickre C, Golper T. Complications of percutaneous needle biopsy of the kidney. Am J Nephrol 1982;2:173–178.

132. Benoit G, Charpentier B, Roche A, et al. Arteriocalyceal fistula after grafted kidney biopsy: successful management by selective embolization. Urology 1984;24:487–490.

133. deSouza N, Reidy J, Koffman C. Arteriovenous fistulas complicating biopsy of renal allografts: treatment of bleeding with superselective embolization. AJR 1991;156:507–510.

134. Olcott E, Goldstein R, Salvatierra O. Lymphoma presenting as allograft hematoma in a renal transplant recipient. J Ultrasound Med 1990;9:239–241.

135. Feldman JD, Jacobs SC. Late development of renal carcinoma in allograft kidney. J Urol 1992;148:395–397.

136. Lawrence SK, Van Buren DH, MacDonell RC Jr, et al. Carcinoma in a transplanted kidney detected with MAG3 scintigraphy. J Nucl Med 1993;34:2185–2187.

54

The Roles of Angiography in Adrenal Disease

STEVEN B. OGLEVIE
JOSEPH J. BOOKSTEIN

*M*ost diseases of the adrenal gland are associated with endocrine dysfunction and produce relatively characteristic clinical and biochemical abnormalities. Diagnosis of the basic disease process, therefore, is usually accomplished clinically, and diagnostic imaging or angiography is generally reserved for localizing an adrenal or extraadrenal tumor, or for differentiating adrenal tumor from hyperplasia. A few adrenal diseases are not associated with endocrine dysfunction; in these circumstances, imaging methods are ordinarily intended to reveal the presence of an adrenal mass, such as a cyst or carcinoma.

Over the past two decades, techniques for adrenal vascular catheterization have been considerably refined and currently enable safe and reliable evaluation by arteriographic, venographic, or sampling methods. More recently, alternative noninvasive diagnostic techniques, such as ultrasound, computed tomography, isotope scintigraphy, and magnetic resonance imaging have also undergone remarkable development. Thus, while diagnostic potential has advanced rapidly across a broad front, the relative roles of each diagnostic modality have fluctuated with time and with regionally available expertise.

In general, the role of angiography in the evaluation of adrenal disease has been diminished by the advances in noninvasive imaging. However, angiography remains a valuable diagnostic tool for evaluating certain specific adrenal diseases. The exact role of angiography as opposed to noninvasive methods must be individually assessed in each adrenal disease or condition. The conditions to be separately considered in this chapter include (1) the normal adrenal gland, (2) aldosteronism, (3) Cushing disease, (4) virilizing syndromes, (5) pheochromocytoma and Sipple syndrome, (6) nonfunctioning adrenal tumors, (7) adrenal cysts, (8) hyperfunction after adrenalectomy due to remnants, (9) adrenal carcinoma, (10) Addison disease, (11) miscellaneous diseases, and (12) transcatheter adrenal ablation. For each condition, the exact role of adrenal catheterization in the diagnostic algorithm will be discussed.

The continuing, albeit limited, role for vascular catheterization requires that one maintain a high degree of catheter expertise. However, as this procedure is performed less frequently, expertise wanes proportionally. It is therefore appropriate to emphasize the technical considerations that enable adrenal arteriography, venography, and venous sampling to be consistently performed in a safe and effective fashion.

Vascular Anatomy

Each adrenal gland has three sources of arterial supply (Fig. 54-1): a superior adrenal artery that arises from the inferior phrenic artery, a middle adrenal artery that arises from the lateral aspect of the aorta at a level between the celiac and renal arteries, and an inferior adrenal artery that arises from the superior aspect of the ipsilateral renal artery. Each arterial trunk then breaks up into 10 to 20 smaller branches that ramify and intercommunicate over the outer aspect of the gland. The smaller branches terminate as perforating arteries that pass perpendicularly through the cortex into the medulla. No direct arterial supply to the adrenal medulla seems to be present.

The perforating arteries gradually assume the histologic characteristics of veins as they pass centripetally into the medulla, and no other direct cortical venous supply is present. When these venules reach the central portion of the medulla, they join a central vein at right

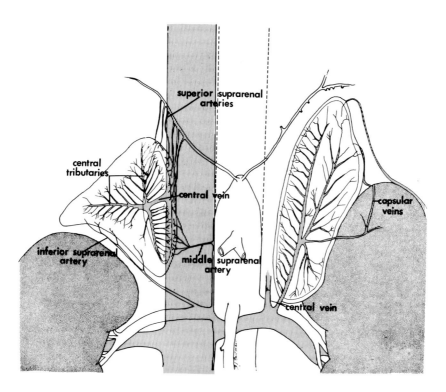

Figure 54-1. Artist's representation of the arterial and venous anatomy of the adrenal gland. Note the three different sources of the arterial supply—the superior, middle, and inferior adrenal arteries. There is one central vein on each side; the right arises from the posterolateral aspect of the inferior vena cava, and the left from the superior aspect of the left renal vein.

angles. The junction of the perforating and central veins is deficient in medial musculature[1] and probably constitutes a site of predilection for rupture during adrenal venography.[2]

On the left side the venous anatomy is constant. The central vein is valveless, usually solitary, and passes down the entire long axis of the gland. It generally joins an inferior phrenic vein just above the left renal vein, and then joins the left renal vein as a phrenicoadrenal trunk. The junction of the phrenicoadrenal trunk and the left renal vein usually occurs within 1 cm of the lateral margin of the vertebral column. The phrenic vein is medial to the adrenal vein and generally contains a competent terminal valve. During left adrenal venography and sampling, special manipulations or catheter shapes are sometimes required to direct the catheter from the inferior phrenic vein toward the central adrenal vein.

The central vein usually communicates, via large emissary veins, with an adrenal capsular vein, particularly via perforators at the apex of the gland. The adrenal capsular veins in turn communicate with renal capsular veins. Observation of these communications during adrenal venography may be helpful in confirming proper catheter position.

On the right, three central tributaries are generally present, one from the superior aspect of the gland, another from the inferior aspect, and a third from the posterior aspect. These three tributaries join to form a short central trunk that passes forward to join the right posterolateral aspect of the inferior vena cava. In about 10 percent of individuals, the right adrenal vein joins the posterior aspect of a hepatic vein near the inferior vena cava, rather than the inferior vena cava directly. Such an anatomic arrangement does not preclude successful right adrenal vein catheterization. Rarely, the right adrenal vein may drain into the right renal vein.

Angiographic Techniques

Arteriography

Complete arteriographic depiction of both adrenal glands is likely to require selective injections of six arteries, three on each side. The minor communications that exist over the surface of the gland between the major arterial branches are not usually large enough to allow opacification of the entire gland from a single selective injection. To facilitate localization of the major adrenal arteries, an aortogram is first obtained. For large or hypervascular tumors, aortography alone may provide sufficient information. If selective arteriography is to be performed, the aortogram catheter is exchanged for a 5 French "shepherd's crook" catheter (Fig. 54-2).

The catheter is initially passed above the celiac artery, and the correct reversed configuration within the aorta is obtained. The anterior aorta is then explored just above the origin of the celiac artery, and the inferior phrenic arteries are engaged from the aorta or proximal celiac artery by exerting traction on the catheter. From 4 to 6 ml of Hexabrix or nonionic contrast material is injected at a rate of 1 to 3 ml per second with sequential filming at two images per second for 3 seconds, and then one image per second for 3 seconds.

The catheter is then disengaged from the inferior phrenic artery while the downward angulation of the tip is maintained, and the lateral aspect of the aorta above the renal arteries is explored. When the middle adrenal artery is engaged, filming is performed as just

discussed, except that the amount of contrast medium and rate of injection are reduced in proportion to the usual small size of this artery. Injection of contrast medium into the adrenal gland may be associated with a fair amount of pain. This may be minimized with the use of Hexabrix.

To catheterize the inferior adrenal artery, the operator disengages the catheter from the middle adrenal artery, maintaining the downward angulation of the tip, and then withdraws the catheter until the tip enters the renal artery. Continued withdrawal will then direct the tip superiorly. As the tip is withdrawn medially toward the origin of the renal artery, small injections of contrast medium will indicate the point at which the inferior adrenal artery has been engaged. Injection and filming are the same as for the middle adrenal artery.

At times, selective adrenal arteriography may not be possible. Selective renal arteriography, after administration of 3 to 5 μg of epinephrine, may provide an acceptable alternative. The epinephrine causes disproportionate constriction of renal microvasculature, diverting contrast material preferentially into the inferior adrenal artery.

Venography

Adrenal venography offers two distinct advantages over adrenal arteriography. First, in contrast to the multiple adrenal arteries, adrenal venous drainage is singular, so that the entire gland can be delineated angiographically by retrograde injection into one vessel. Second and more importantly, selective blood samples can be obtained, permitting measurement of hormonal concentrations, localization of functional adrenal tumors, and differentiation of adrenal tumors and hyperplasia.

The ideal catheter shapes for right and left adrenal venography are demonstrated in Figure 54-2B and C, respectively. Two tiny side holes are punched in the distal portion of the right adrenal vein catheter within 5 mm of the tip to facilitate aspiration of blood. At the authors' institution we prefer to catheterize the right adrenal vein initially. The search begins on the posterolateral aspect of the inferior vena cava, at the anticipated level of the center of the gland just above the upper pole of the kidney. When minor advances and withdrawals at the shaft do not produce comparable motions at the tip, a test injection is performed to determine whether the adrenal vein has been entered. Considerable experience is required to recognize that the right adrenal veins have indeed been properly engaged. One looks for the typical stellate appearance, produced by two or three central tributaries opacifying

Figure 54-2. Catheters for adrenal angiography. *A,* Catheter shape for engaging superior, middle, or inferior adrenal arteries; *B,* right adrenal venous configuration; *C,* left adrenal venous configuration.

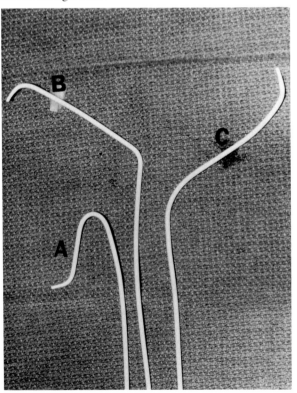

from the short main trunk. Small accessory hepatic veins are often encountered in the same region but may be distinguished from adrenal veins by observing the following:

1. Injection into the adrenal gland is often somewhat painful, whereas injection into a hepatic vein is usually painless.
2. Injection into a hepatic vein often produces a homogeneous persistent blush, whereas a blush does not usually occur after a small adrenal venous injection.
3. Downward-coursing adrenal and renal capsular veins are often opacified after adrenal injections, whereas upward-curving hepatic veins may be well visualized after hepatic vein injections.

The catheter is not infrequently somewhat unstable in its position within the right adrenal vein. Minor adjustments in rotation, shallow respiration, slight adjustments in catheter shape, and conduction of the examination with alacrity are maneuvers that help maintain proper catheter position. Often during fluoroscopy, it may be observed that the intraadrenal veins are much better opacified during one phase of respiration, and *that* respiratory phase should be selected for filming.

In experienced hands, the right adrenal vein can be successfully catheterized in 90 to 95 percent of cases.[3] Difficulty is often due to entrance of the adrenal vein into the origin of a hepatic vein rather than directly into the inferior vena cava. This problem can be overcome by elongating the distal tip of the catheter so that it will reach through the hepatic vein to the adrenal vein. Alternatively, the shepherd's crook catheter can be used.

If adrenal venous sampling is to be performed, it must be accomplished before definitive injections of contrast medium are made, inasmuch as the injections may affect the concentration of metabolites.

To minimize the incidence of intraadrenal hemorrhage, gentle technique is required. The amount of contrast to be injected varies greatly and is best determined by noting the point at which the patient experiences the pain of glandular distention. We perform the injections by hand and generally have about 6 ml of contrast in the syringe. The patient is asked to hold his or her clenched fist in a visible position, usually near the ear, and to extend one finger when discomfort is noted. The injection is then begun slowly, during filming, and the injection rate gradually increased until the finger snaps open. At this point the injection is stopped. In most patients about 3 or 4 ml is injected,

with the final injection rate often being about 2 ml per second. Sometimes, however, a much greater or lesser volume or rate is required. Filming is at the rate of two films per second for 3 seconds and one film per second for 3 seconds. Anteroposterior projections are used, usually with magnification technique; repeat injections or projections are performed infrequently to minimize the incidence of extravasation.

After right adrenal venous catheterization is completed, the right adrenal catheter is passed into the left renal vein. A guidewire is advanced far into the peripheral renal venous bed, and a catheter shaped as shown in Figure 54-2C is exchanged. The catheter is then slowly withdrawn while the tip is directed superiorly until a sudden visible cephalic motion indicates entrance into the phrenicoadrenal trunk. Entrance into this trunk usually occurs within a centimeter of the left lateral vertebral margin. After engagement of the phrenicoadrenal trunk, test injection should show most of the contrast medium passing toward the central adrenal vein; if toward the phrenic vein, adjustment of the catheter shape or position may be necessary. Blood samples are then drawn, if indicated. Venography is performed in a manner similar to that described for the right adrenal vein. Often slightly larger amounts of contrast medium are required on the left before the discomfort of glandular distention is indicated by the patient.

Venous Sampling

Venous sampling remains the most accurate method for evaluating adrenal cortical and medullary function and for localizing sites of excessive hormonal production. Despite satisfactory catheterization of the adrenal veins, it may be difficult to aspirate the amounts of blood required for radioimmunoassay (about 5 ml at the authors' institution). The problem is usually due to obturation of the catheter end holes by the venous wall and is much more frequent on the right side. Small side holes near the top of the right catheter are usually, but not always, helpful. Changes in respiration, or the Valsalva maneuver, are sometimes effective. Excessive force of aspiration on the syringe can be avoided by introducing 5 cc of air into the syringe, or by collecting the blood with gravity drainage. If all else fails, the adrenal vein wall can be displaced away from the catheter tip by passing a narrow guidewire (outer diameter 0.020 inch) through and a little beyond the catheter tip, while a side-armed gasket adapter around the externally protruding end of the guidewire prevents leakage and allows continued aspiration from the adrenal vein.

Complications

Complications of adrenal arteriography are most common in patients with unsuspected pheochromocytomas.[4] In these patients an unexpected, life-threatening hypertensive crisis may be precipitated by arterial and much less commonly by venous injections of contrast material. Management of an acute hypertensive crisis is complex and involves the intravenous administration of nitroprusside or phentolamine. Physicians capable of managing this complication should be in attendance during the procedure. Any patient suspected of having a pheochromocytoma should be pretreated with an alpha-adrenergic blocker such as phenoxybenzamine. Generally 1 to 2 mg/kg per day is divided into four equal doses and administered for several days before the procedure. With pretreatment and continuous blood pressure monitoring in the angiography suite, the risk of such complications has been significantly decreased.[4,5]

The major risk of adrenal vein catheterization is intraadrenal extravasation of contrast material or blood. In experienced hands, this complication occurs in up to 4 percent of cases.[6] It is more prevalent in patients with aldosteronism or Cushing disease, in whom the adrenal veins, as well as other systemic veins, are more fragile.[7,8] Actual extravasation of contrast material is evident in the minority of cases. More frequently, the films are normal, but the patient will complain of persistent pain after the injection that increases in intensity for 30 to 60 minutes. The pain may eventually become excruciating, requiring large doses of narcotic analgesics. Pain and fever usually persist for 24 to 36 hours and then subside. This sequence of events indicates intraadrenal hemorrhage and is almost invariably associated with complete and permanent destruction of glandular function. In this fashion, hormonally active tumors within these injured glands may be temporarily or permanently ablated.[9-13] Radionuclide adrenal scans obtained days or months later generally demonstrate total lack of uptake in the involved gland. If extravasation is bilateral, Addison disease develops. Thus extravasation occurring on one side is virtually an absolute contraindication to performance of adrenal venography on the other side, unless transcatheter adrenal ablation is the desired goal. Clinicians should be alerted to this potential complication and must be prepared to recognize and manage an acute Addisonian crisis in any patient who has undergone adrenal vein catheterization.

Minimal extravasation of contrast material from extraadrenal venules is occasionally observed during the course of the study. This complication is of little clinical significance and is accompanied by only minimal transient discomfort. Adrenal dysfunction does not follow. Differentiation from intraadrenal extravasation is accomplished by noting the extraadrenal location of contrast deposition.

Shortly after the introduction of adrenal venography, experienced surgeons began to note adhesions or edema around the glands, which they had not observed previously. These changes occurred despite lack of venographic or clinical evidence of extravasation at the time of the study.[6] Occult rupture of tiny paraadrenal venules during the venographic examination is presumed to be the responsible factor.

The Normal Angiogram

Normal adrenal arteriograms are demonstrated in Figure 54-3. Note that the gland is not usually entirely opacified after injection of any one artery. The parallel folds of the cortex produce a characteristic double density resembling railroad tracks. Each cortical tract measures about 2 mm in thickness. The medulla is not distinctly opacified. Because only a portion of the gland is visualized with each injection, the overall appearance of the gland can only be appreciated by mental summation of separate injections or by using the sophisticated addition of photographic images.

Figure 54-4A illustrates the normal left adrenal venogram. Note the single central venule and the clear demonstration of the normal size, contour, and position of the left adrenal gland. The pinnate branching pattern of the central vein is particularly evident. The phrenic vein is seen medial to the adrenal vein. Because the venules lie within the medulla, the cortex is infrequently opacified. Communications between adrenal venules and renal capsular venules are frequently present.

A normal right adrenal venogram is illustrated in Figure 54-4B. Note two or three diverging branches from the short central vein. The pinnate branching pattern of the central venous tributaries is evident.

Other Methods of Adrenal Imaging

Brief descriptions of adrenal scintigraphy, computed tomography (CT), magnetic resonance imaging (MRI), and ultrasound (US) are in order.

Adrenal Scintigraphy

The techniques for adrenal cortical and medullary scintigraphy were developed and evaluated primarily by Beierwaltes and his group at the University of Michigan.[14-18] Scintigraphy reflects adrenal function and morphology, and may make possible tumor localiza-

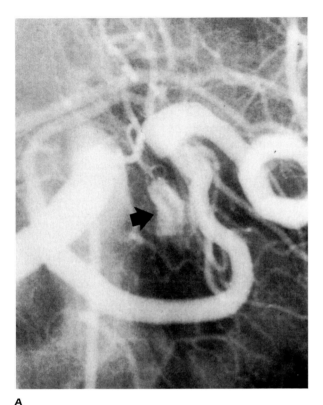

A

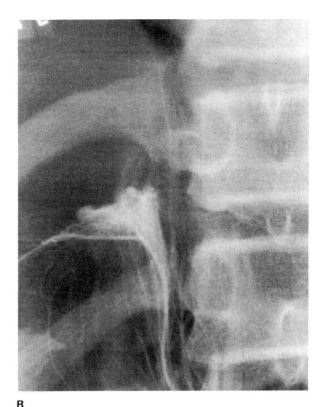

B

Figure 54-3. Arteriographic demonstration of normal adrenal glands. (A) Stain of superior pole of the left adrenal gland (*arrow*) after celiac arteriography, with preferential injection into the left inferior phrenic artery. Note that only the superior portion of the gland is opacified, reaffirming the need to inject all adrenal arterial sources to opacify a normal gland completely. Also note the characteristic short parallel streaks, reflecting segments of cortical folds. (B) Selective inferior adrenal arteriogram of a normal right adrenal gland. Again, only the inferior portion of the gland is opacified.

tion when purely morphologic modalities are normal or inconclusive. The whole body may be scanned to evaluate extraadrenal or metastatic disease. The main limitations of these techniques are spatial resolution and availability.

For adrenal cortical scintigraphy, NP-59 ([131]iodine-labeled iodomethyl norcholesterol) has proven to be the agent of choice.[19] Dexamethasone suppression is usually carried out for 7 days before administration of NP-59, and continued during the 5- to 6-day scanning period. One to 2 mCi of ^{131}I NP-59 is injected intravenously, and nuclear imaging is performed on the third and fifth days after the injection. The sensitivity of adrenal cortical scanning with NP-59 is about 89 percent, specificity is about 96 percent, and overall accuracy is about 90 percent.[19] Despite the fairly high accuracy, the technique has several drawbacks. The radiation dose absorbed by the adrenal gland is high (about 25 rad/mCi). The procedure takes 5 to 6 days and requires nearly a 2-week period of dexamethasone administration. There may be significant drug interactions, and, again, NP-59 is not widely available.

For adrenal medullary scintigraphy, MIBG (meta-iodobenzylguanidine) has proven to be the agent of choice.[16-18] The usual dose is 0.5 to 1.0 mCi of ^{131}I-labeled MIBG given intravenously. The patient is scanned at 48 and 72 hours. If available, ^{123}I-labeled MIBG may be advantageous because of its approximately 100 times less absorbed dose to the adrenals and slightly improved accuracy. The sensitivity of ^{131}I-labeled MIBG is reported to be from 80 to 89 percent, and the specificity is from 94 to 99 percent.[19] Again, the procedure is not widely available, and its cost-efficacy relative to CT for evaluation of suspected pheochromocytoma has been questioned.[20]

Computed Tomography

CT has emerged as the imaging modality of choice for evaluation of most adrenal tumors.[20-23] Nearly all tumors greater than 1 cm in diameter can be depicted with CT. In one series of 121 patients, the sensitivity of CT for demonstration of adrenal tumors was 98 percent.[22] However, specificity remains a problem.

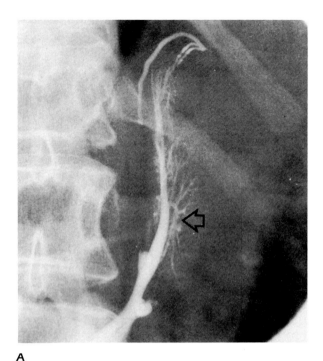

A

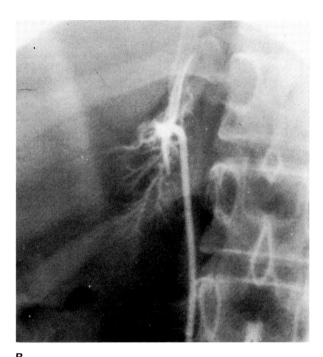

B

Figure 54-4. Normal adrenal venograms. (A) Normal left adrenal venogram. Note the single central vein, a recurrent vein to the lower pole (*arrow*), and communications with adrenal and capsular veins. (B) Normal right adrenal veno-gram. Note the posterior origin of the central vein from the inferior vena cava and its division into branches to the apex and the lower pole. The posterior branch is obscured in this case.

Only adrenal cysts and myelolipomas have distinctive CT characteristics. Lesion size usually permits distinction of adrenal carcinoma from adenoma but is not helpful in distinguishing metastatic disease from adrenal adenoma. Hence, for definitive distinction of adenomas, carcinomas, metastases, pheochromocytomas, and neuroblastomas, correlation with clinical and biochemical features is required. CT enables one to distinguish unilateral disease (adenoma) from bilateral disease (hyperplasia) in the majority of cases of aldosteronism or Cushing syndrome. Adrenal venous sampling is more accurate for this distinction, however.[8] Note also that patients with macronodular hyperplasia may be falsely assumed to have unilateral disease (an adenoma) because of asymmetric involvement. "Incidentalomas" (nonfunctioning adenomas) evident on CT may be erroneously assumed to be the cause of hyperendocrine states. Functional studies, especially venous sampling, can prevent such diagnostic errors. The advantages of CT include its universal availability and, relative to MRI, lower cost, better spatial resolution, and less motion sensitivity.

Magnetic Resonance Imaging

The utility of MRI for evaluation of the adrenal glands has been intensely evaluated over the past decade.[24–28]

Although the spatial resolution of MRI is slightly less than that of CT, it was hoped that the tissue characterization afforded by MRI would permit the distinction of adrenal masses. Although these hopes have not been fully realized, a comparative evaluation of numerous techniques[28] showed that the chemical shift imaging technique (Fig. 54-5) and the T2*-weighted sequence provided fairly accurate differentiation of adrenal adenomas from metastases and pheochromocytomas. Although these techniques enabled the statistical separation of groups of lesions, the accuracy in individual cases was insufficient for reliable clinical application. The wide variety of histologic appearances and varying amounts of cytoplasmic fat may account for the difficulty in distinguishing adrenal adenomas from metastases or pheochromocytomas using MRI.[26,28]

Although adrenal MRI has not provided consistent tissue-specific diagnoses, the technique has several advantages. The absence of ionizing radiation makes it attractive for children and pregnant women. The multiplanar imaging capabilities facilitate the distinction of adrenal masses from renal, hepatic, and pancreatic masses. Vascular involvement is depicted to a better degree than with other noninvasive techniques. MRI has proven to be more accurate than CT or US for demonstrating hepatic metastatic disease.

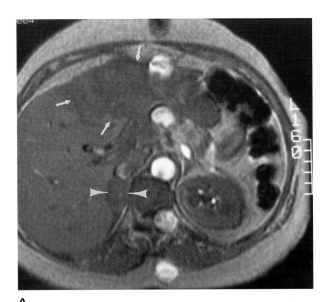

A

Figure 54-5. Nonfunctioning right adrenal adenoma on chemical shift MR imaging. This 56-year-old woman had adenocarcinoma of unknown primary origin involving the left hepatic lobe, and an incidentally detected right adrenal mass. (A) In-phase image (echo time 4.2 milliseconds) shows a large left hepatic mass (*arrows*) and 2- to 3-cm right adrenal mass (*arrowheads*). Note that the signal of the adrenal mass is slightly less than liver and about equal to kidney.

B

(B) Opposed-phase image (echo time 6.3 milliseconds) shows dramatic loss of signal in the adrenal mass (*arrowheads*) relative to both liver and kidney. This indicates that the adrenal mass has a homogeneous mixture of fat and water and probably represents a nonfunctioning adenoma rather than a primary or metastatic malignant neoplasm. (Courtesy of R. O'Laoide, M.B.)

Ultrasound

The utility of US in evaluating the adrenal glands is limited. The echogenic retroperitoneal fat surrounding the glands makes their evaluation challenging in most adults, although the paucity of fat in children facilitates the examination (Fig. 54-6). The sensitivity of US for demonstrating known adrenal tumors is only 71 percent, whereas the sensitivity for CT is up to 98 percent.[22] The technique is particularly well suited for characterizing adrenal cysts. Myelolipomas, large carcinomas, or metastases may also be well evaluated with US. The absence of ionizing radiation is an advantage, particularly in children.

Specific Adrenal Entities

Aldosteronism

Aldosterone is the principal mineralocorticoid secreted by the outer adrenal cortex, the zona glomerulosa. The major clinical manifestations of aldosteronism (hyperaldosteronism) are hypertension, hypokalemia, metabolic alkalosis, and increased serum and urine concentrations of aldosterone. Aldosteronism may be secondary to renal disease or to primary adrenal disease. Secondary aldosteronism is classically associated

Figure 54-6. US of normal right adrenal gland in neonate. The adrenal cortex is hypoechoic (*arrows*), and the medulla is more echogenic (*arrowheads*). However, in older children and adults, the presence of echogenic retroperitoneal fat precludes satisfactory US imaging of the adrenal glands. (Courtesy of G. Leopold, M.D.)

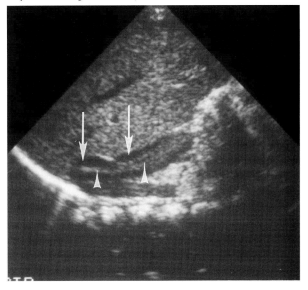

Figure 54-7. Aldosteronomas. (A) Typical 1-cm lesion in the inferolateral portion of the left gland (*arrows*). The adjacent adrenal veins are displaced in a parenthetic configuration and are slightly enlarged. (B) Typical aldosteronoma in upper portion of left adrenal gland (*open arrows*). (C) Ovoid right aldosteronoma, measuring about 1 × 2 cm on magnification venography. (D) Photograph of gross specimen of (C). Note the excellent correlation between the tumor size on venography and gross examination.

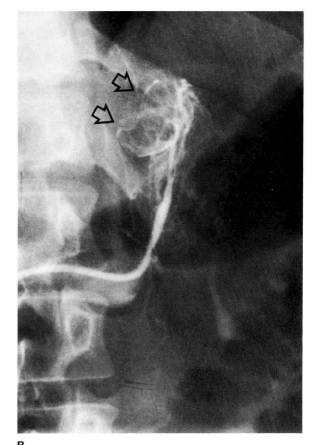

B

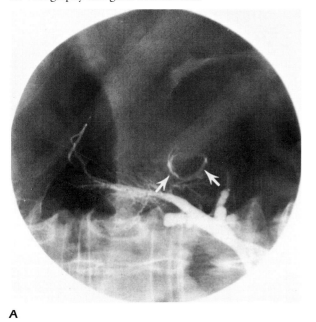

A

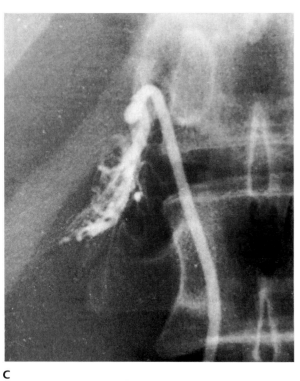

C

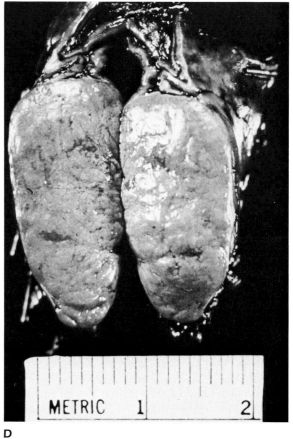

D

with elevated serum renin levels, whereas renin levels are depressed in the primary form. Thus, in evaluating the cause of aldosteronism, serum renin determinations play a major role in directing investigation toward the kidney when renin levels are high, or toward the adrenal gland when they are low. Secondary aldosteronism is usually due to renal artery stenosis, or rarely to reninoma or other renal conditions, and will not be further considered here.

The primary form of aldosteronism is due to adrenal adenoma in about 75 percent of cases. Bilateral multinodular adrenal hyperplasia accounts for 20 to 25 percent of cases, and less than 1 percent are due to adrenal carcinoma.[29-31] The adenomas are relatively small; the mean size reported in two series was 1.6 to 1.8 cm.[32,33] Some series have shown a slight preponderance of left-sided involvement.

Treatment of primary aldosteronism is usually required because of hypertension. In those patients with solitary adrenal adenomas, resection of the diseased gland is curative. Hypertension secondary to multinodular hyperplasia, however, responds poorly to adrenalectomy, and medical treatment with aldosterone antagonists (spironolactone) is the treatment of choice. Thus the distinction between adenoma and hyperplasia is critical in determining therapy, and this distinction usually cannot be made on clinical grounds alone.

High-resolution CT should be the first radiologic procedure performed in patients with clinically diagnosed aldosteronism.[8,30-33] Differentiation of adenoma from hyperplasia and localization of adenoma may be accomplished with CT as the only radiologic study performed. However, because of their small size, adenomas have been missed in 20 to 40 percent of cases.[8,31] The adenomas missed on CT have usually been 1.0 to 1.2 cm in diameter.[33] Even with the current generation of scanners, the sensitivity of CT for aldosteronomas is only 80 percent.[34] When CT is equivocal or negative, venography with venous sampling is usually indicated.[3,8,11,29,31,35,36]

Solitary adenomas are indicated venographically by arcuate displacement of one or more intraadrenal venules (Fig. 54-7). Rarely, contrast material refluxes into, and directly opacifies, the tumor itself (Fig. 54-8). Tumors as small as 0.3 and 0.5 cm have been visualized,[8,37] but most tumors detected venographically are 1.0 to 1.5 cm in diameter. Because the tumors are not hypervascular, the veins draining from and displaced by the tumors are usually of normal caliber or only slightly enlarged.

Venography will demonstrate the adenoma in 75 to

Figure 54-8. Aldosteronoma with retrograde tumor stain. (A) Early film shows normal venographic anatomy of the right gland, except for minimal opacification within the tumor. (B) Later film shows retrograde stain of a bilobate tumor (*arrows*). Retrograde tumor stain is not infrequent.

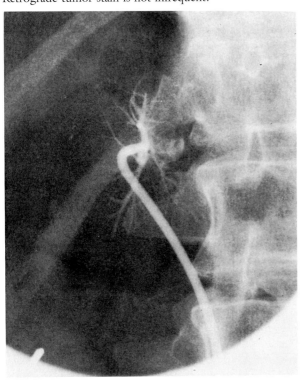

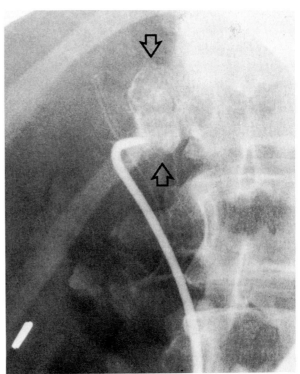

A

B

93 percent of cases.[29,36,38] In two studies that the authors performed, good-quality magnification venograms (frontal projection only) were negative in proven cases. In two of the false-negative venograms, the normal venogram was explained by a central cylindrical adenoma in one case and by a very flattened one in a second. These cases and the less than perfect accuracy of venography underscore the importance of concomitant venous sampling.

In multinodular hyperplasia, venography is usually near normal. Occasionally there are multiple areas of mild curvilinear venous displacement, or the gland may be diffusely enlarged (Fig. 54-9).

In at least four cases, intraadrenal extravasation of contrast material has infarcted the gland harboring an aldosteronoma and cured the disease.[10–13]

Sampling of venous effluent is particularly rewarding in unilateral adenoma, and should precede venography. Differences in the concentration of aldosterone are usually great because of increased produc-

tion on one side with decreased production on the contralateral side. Activity ratios of 20, 50, or even 100 to 1 are frequent,[3,36] so that positive results are usually obtained even when adrenal vein and caval blood are admixed. To overcome the problem of sample dilution due to technique or anatomic differences between the two sides, simultaneous determination of cortisol levels with calculation of an aldosterone-cortisol (A/C) ratio is advocated.[35] The side harboring the adenoma has an A/C ratio at least five times the contralateral side. Some authors also emphasize the value of presampling stimulation with intravenous corticotropin (ACTH) to minimize false negatives secondary to episodic secretion of steroids.[35] The accuracy of the localization of unilateral adenomas using venous sampling techniques is consistently over 90 percent.[3,8,30,35,38]

CT and venography with sampling are mutually complementary studies. In cases that demonstrate bilateral adrenal masses on CT, venous sampling is particularly important (Fig. 54-10). The patient may have

Figure 54-9. Aldosteronism due to bilateral adrenal hyperplasia in a 39-year-old woman with hypertension, hypokalemia, and elevated aldosterone excretion. Sampling from both adrenal veins indicated aldosterone levels more than twice maximal upper normal levels. (A) The right adrenal gland is enlarged, and the intraadrenal venules are increased in caliber. The typical convergence of three veins to form the central vein is well shown. One vein leads inferiorly, another is arched posteriorly, and a small one drains the upper portion of the gland. (B) The left gland is not so well opacified, but still demonstrates enlarged venules and a rounded external contour.

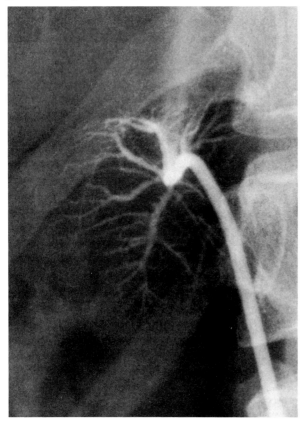

A

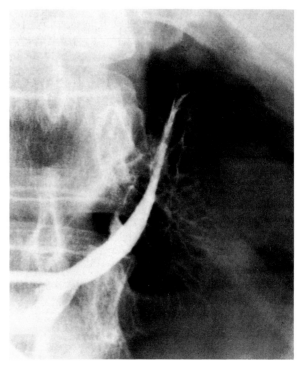

B

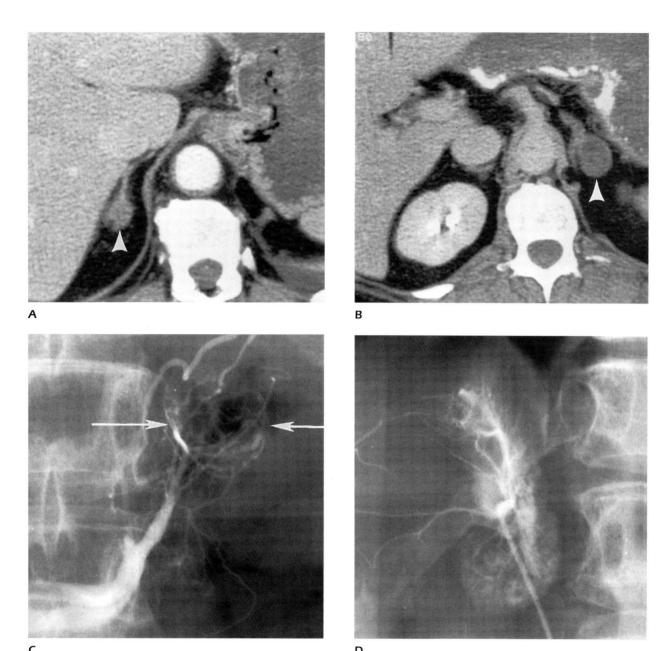

A

B

C

D

Figure 54-10. Bilateral adrenal masses in a 55-year-old female with aldosteronism. (A) CT scan showing 2-cm round lesion in superior portion of right adrenal (*arrowhead*). (B) CT scan showing 2.5-cm low-density lesion in left adrenal (*arrowhead*). The peripheral venous aldosterone level was elevated at 86 (4–31 ng/dl), and the cortisol level was 9 (6–24 μg/dl). Bilateral adrenal venous sampling revealed markedly elevated aldosterone levels on the left (aldosterone 4700 ng/dl, cortisol 60 μg/dl, ratio ≈ 78) and normal aldosterone levels on the right (aldosterone 65 ng/dl, cortisol 55 μg/dl, ratio ≈ 1.2). (C) Left adrenal venography show-ing aldosteronoma (*arrows*) in midportion of gland with circumferential displacement of adrenal veins. (D) Right adrenal venography confirming satisfactory catheter position and showing communication with renal capsular veins but no evidence of adrenal tumor. The left adrenal was resected and the aldosteronism resolved. The left adenoma was pathologically proven. After resection the aldosterone level was less than 1 ng/dl. The right-sided lesion is thought to be a nonfunctioning adenoma or "incidentaloma." This case underscores the need for sampling and venography in cases of primary aldosteronism and bilateral adrenal masses.

a functioning adenoma on one side and an incidental nonfunctioning adenoma or myelolipoma on the contralateral side. It is imperative to not mistake this situation for bilateral nodular hyperplasia and thus miss the opportunity for appropriate surgical therapy. Likewise, it is important not to confuse markedly asymmetric bilateral macronodular hyperplasia with a unilateral functioning adenoma. This diagnostic error would inappropriately suggest surgical resection rather than spironolactone therapy, and can be avoided by venous sampling.

On the other hand, venous sampling is also fallible. In bilateral multinodular hyperplasia, elevated aldosterone concentrations are typically present in the effluent from both adrenal glands, but the ratios may occasionally mimic unilateral adenoma.[30] Hence, in this small minority of cases, venous assay does not invariably distinguish unilateral adenoma from bilateral hyperplasia.

Adrenal arteriography has occasionally demonstrated a stain of adenoma[11,39] or the stain of multinodular hyperplasia.[40] Because venography is fairly accurate and also allows biochemical assay, arteriography is almost never performed in aldosteronism, and the true incidence of positive arteriograms is unknown.

Adrenal cortical scintigraphy using NP-59 is an alternative method for localizing an aldosteronoma. The accuracy of this technique is enhanced by dexamethasone suppression and at 90 percent[19] may be slightly superior to CT. MRI has not proven to be as valuable for evaluation of aldosteronism as CT.[28] Because most aldosterone-producing tumors are small, ultrasound examination of the adrenal glands has been relatively insensitive in the diagnosis of aldosteronism.[38]

In summary, the differentiation of adenoma from nodular hyperplasia is often inconclusive by CT alone, and adrenal venography and sampling are indicated in a large percentage, perhaps a majority, of cases of primary aldosteronism.

Cushing Syndrome

Cushing syndrome is characterized clinically by truncal obesity, abdominal striae, hypertension, hirsutism, diabetes, purpura, muscular wasting, and psychosis. It is the result of excess glucocorticoids from either exogenous or endogenous sources. Exogenous Cushing syndrome is seen in patients being treated with large doses of steroids and will not be considered further here. Endogenous Cushing syndrome is caused by bilateral adrenal cortical hyperplasia due to excessive corticotropin (ACTH) in about 70 percent of cases. In about 20 percent of cases the syndrome is caused by an adrenal adenoma and in about 10 percent of cases by an adrenal carcinoma. In cases with elevated ACTH, the source of ACTH is a pituitary adenoma in 90 percent of cases (Cushing disease) and ectopic in about 10 percent. The ectopic sources include bronchial carcinoid, pheochromocytoma (Fig. 54-11), islet cell tumor of the pancreas, thymic carcinoid, oat cell carcinoma, medullary carcinoma of the thyroid, and ovarian carcinoma. Adrenal cortical hyperplasia is usually smooth but may be micro- or macronodular. The rare macronodular variety may be difficult to distinguish from adrenal adenoma when involvement is asymmetric.

The diagnosis is usually suspected on the basis of characteristic clinical findings. Biochemical evaluation reveals elevated cortisol and increased urinary excretion of 17-hydroxy-corticoids. A negative dexamethasone suppression test may help distinguish adrenal tumors from hyperplasia. If the biochemical evaluation unequivocally indicates ACTH-dependent Cushing syndrome (elevated ACTH and positive dexamethasone suppression test), then no adrenal imaging is necessary. If the biochemical evaluation shows ACTH-independent Cushing syndrome (low ACTH and negative dexamethasone suppression test) or is equivocal, then radiologic evaluation is indicated. The role of the radiologist is to confirm the presence of hyperplasia or, if neoplasia is present, to lateralize the tumor and determine its extent.

CT should be the first imaging modality employed in the evaluation of Cushing syndrome.[23,31] If CT shows an adenoma or carcinoma, surgical resection is the treatment of choice. CT is particularly well suited for evaluation of adrenals in Cushing syndrome because the abundant fat enhances the conspicuity of these retroperitoneal glands. Hyperplasia results in bilaterally thickened or elongated adrenal limbs, particularly in cases due to ectopic ACTH. Adrenal adenomas responsible for Cushing syndrome are usually easily detected because their average size is 2.0 to 2.5 cm and the contralateral adrenal gland may appear atrophic. Adrenal carcinoma is suggested if a mass larger than 4 cm is demonstrated. If CT is normal or equivocal, adrenal cortical scintigraphy using NP-59 should be carried out, if available. Bilateral uptake indicates hyperplasia, unilateral uptake indicates adenoma, and nonimaging is worrisome for adrenal carcinoma. If adrenal scintigraphy is unavailable or inconclusive, adrenal venous sampling and venography should follow.

Although not commonly required, venous sampling and venography have nearly perfect accuracy for distinguishing between the various causes of Cushing syndrome.[8,41] Adrenal venous samples show elevation of cortisol bilaterally in hyperplasia and unilaterally in functioning adrenal adenomas or carcinomas. On venography, 50 percent of cases of adrenal hyperplasia show enlarged, rounded adrenal glands with enlarged

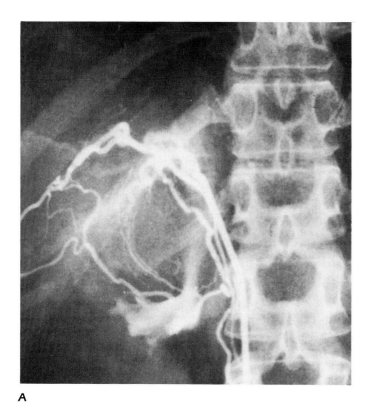

A

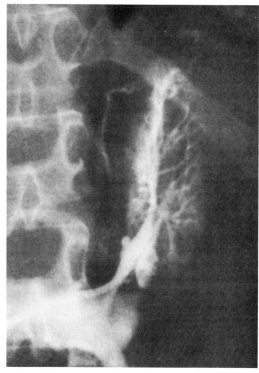

B

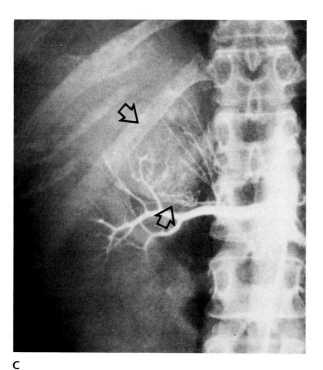

C

Figure 54-11. Cushing disease and hyperpigmentation due to ectopic ACTH and beta-MSH production by a pheochromocytoma. (A) Right adrenal venogram demonstrates arcuate displacement of adrenal venules around a large mass. Sampling from this side revealed high concentrations of ACTH and beta-MSH. (B) Left adrenal venogram demonstrates a slightly enlarged and rounded gland with enlarged intraadrenal venules. The absence of atrophy on this side was an important clue to the fact that the contralateral tumor was not cortisol-producing. The cortisol concentration was seven times as great on the left as on the right. (C) Selective right renal arteriography, after intrarenal administration of 7 μg epinephrine, demonstrates a mildly hypervascular adrenal tumor (*arrows*). An ACTH-producing right pheochromocytoma was pathologically proven.

venules (Fig. 54-12)[36,42]; the remainder appear normal venographically. Hyperplasia may assume a nodular character, but this is made apparent only occasionally by venography (Fig. 54-13). Adenomas, usually 2 to 5 cm in diameter, are indicated by the presence of displaced and enlarged adrenal veins (Fig. 54-14), and occasionally by the stain of the tumor. Contralateral adrenal atrophy is almost invariably present, reflected venographically by the decreased size of the gland and the decreased caliber of the individual adrenal venules (see Fig. 54-14C). Because the adenomas producing Cushing syndrome are relatively large, venography has invariably been positive in the authors' experience when technically successful. In the presence of adrenal

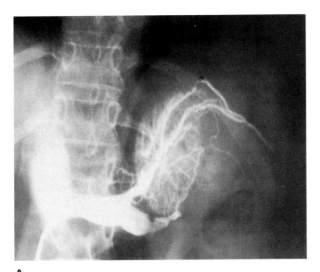

A

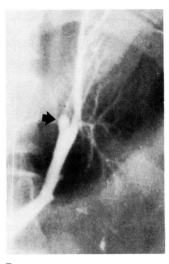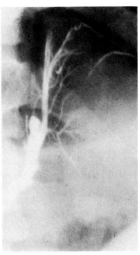

B

Figure 54-12. Cushing disease due to bilateral adrenal hyperplasia. (A) Markedly hypertrophied, enlarged left adrenal gland. Note the abundant number and generous size of the intraadrenal venules. The gland has an excessively round contour. (B) Left adrenal venogram demonstrating adrenal hyperplasia in another patient with Cushing disease (*left*). Note the valve of the inferior phrenic vein (*arrow*). Regression of hyperplasia is noted following pituitary irradiation (*right*).

Figure 54-13. Cushing disease due to rare bilateral macronodular hyperplasia. Bilateral tumors were evident on CT and venography. Adjacent portions of each gland, however, did not demonstrate the usual secondary atrophy. Venous sampling showed a markedly elevated cortisol level bilaterally. (A) Right adrenal venogram demonstrating 1.5-cm nodule in the inferior portion and sizable venules elsewhere (*arrows*). (B) Left gland showing a 3-cm nodule and sizable venules elsewhere (*arrows*). At operation, the cortices contained the two large tumors shown, plus multiple 1- to 2-cm nodules elsewhere. The cortices were thickened throughout both glands.

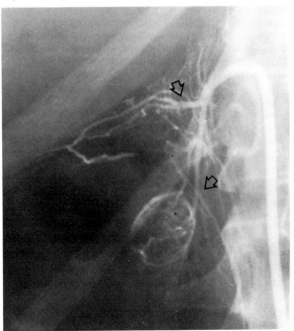

A

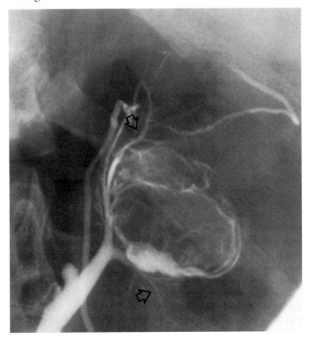

B

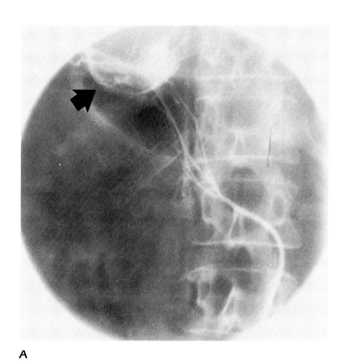

A

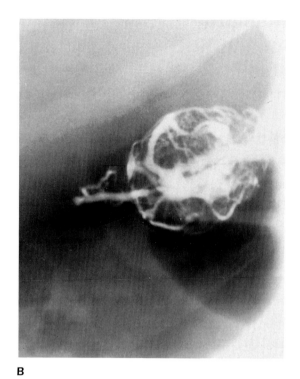

B

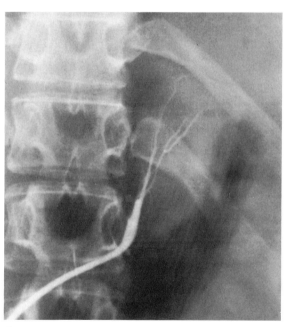

C

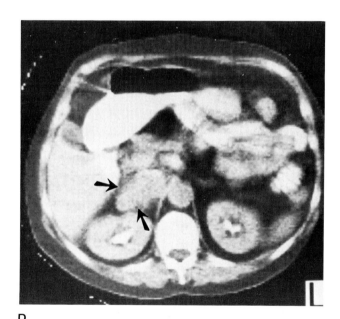

D

Figure 54-14. Cushing disease secondary to right adrenal adenoma. (A) Inferior adrenal arteriogram shows portion of right adrenal adenoma (*arrow*). (B) Right adrenal venogram outlines a 5-cm tumor. As illustrated in this case, the cortisol-producing adenomas are usually larger than those producing aldosterone. (C) Left adrenal venogram shows glandular atrophy. Note the reduced size and number of intraadrenal venules and the reduced overall area occupied by the gland. Glandular atrophy contralateral to an adenoma indicates cortisol production and secondary depression of ACTH. In the authors' experience, such contralateral atrophy occurs invariably in Cushing disease and is not usually seen in aldosteronomas. (D) CT scan from another patient with Cushing disease due to a large right adrenal adenoma (*arrows*).

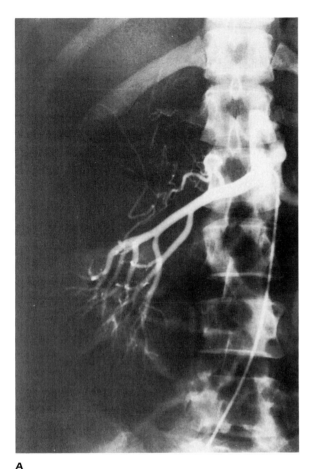

A

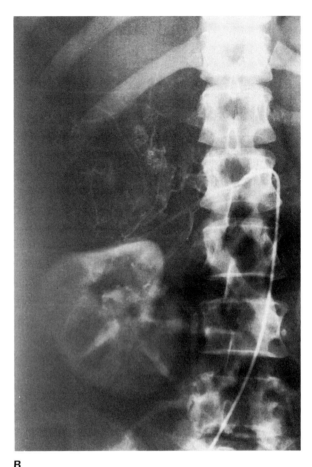

B

Figure 54-15. Cushing disease due to adrenal cortical carcinoma. (A) Selective right renal arteriography demonstrates enlargement of the right inferior adrenal artery, which supplies much of the moderately vascular carcinoma. (B) Nephrogram phase shows the inferior and lateral displacement of the kidney, the impression upon the superior renal pole, and the typical inhomogeneous whorled arterial pattern in adrenocortical carcinoma. Note also the characteristic large tumor size. (Courtesy of L.B. Talner, M.D.)

carcinoma, adrenal venography may partially demonstrate a large mass. More frequently, the adrenal veins are invaded and obstructed by tumor, so the carcinoma is poorly demonstrated by venography. The contralateral gland is atrophic.

Adrenal arteriography is usually diagnostic but now very rarely required for evaluation of Cushing syndrome. Hyperplastic glands are often hypervascular, and their size and vascularity can be appreciated arteriographically in about 50 percent of cases.[43] Adenomas are sufficiently large and vascular to be visualized even if all appropriate adrenal arteries are not injected (see Fig. 54-14A). Adrenal carcinomas are moderately hypervascular, as a rule, and tend to be much larger than adenomas (Fig. 54-15). Consequently, arteriography almost always indicates a large mass in patients with adrenal carcinoma and may aid in the distinction of adrenal carcinoma from renal cell carcinoma or retroperitoneal sarcoma.

In summary, despite the reliability of angiographic evaluation of Cushing syndrome, noninvasive investigation with CT and scintigraphy is usually sufficient for diagnosis.

Adrenogenital Syndromes

Virilizing or femininizing disorders may be caused by an adrenal abnormality (hyperplasia, adenoma, carcinoma), a gonadal tumor, or a corticotropin- or gonadotropin-producing tumor. In the congenital adrenogenital syndrome, a deficiency in the enzyme 11β- or 22-hydroxylase results in defective cortisols. This, in turn, results in insufficient ACTH suppression, cortical hyperplasia, and incidental overproduction of androgens. This syndrome is usually diagnosed clinically in newborns and infants. US is preferable to CT for confirming the diagnosis because periadrenal fat in these young patients is insufficient for reliable CT visualization of the adrenal glands. The glands are usually symmetrically enlarged and thickened and may even develop adenomas if diagnosis is delayed.[31]

Postpubertal masculinization or femininization is more commonly due to adrenal adenoma, adrenal carcinoma, or gonadal tumors. CT is the initial imaging modality of choice used to evaluate these patients. Because the adrenal tumors are usually several centimeters in diameter, they will usually be evident on CT. However, retroperitoneal fat is less abundant than in Cushing disease, and it is not uncommon for CT to be inconclusive. If an adrenal adenoma or carcinoma is evident, surgical intervention is indicated. If CT shows symmetrical enlargement or is equivocal, adrenal cortical scintigraphy using NP-59 should be performed, if available. If this shows unilateral visualization, an adenoma is diagnosed and surgical intervention should follow. If there is bilateral visualization, hyperplasia is diagnosed and medical therapy may be initiated.

If NP-59 scintigraphy is not available or is equivocal, adrenal venous sampling and venography may be indicated. Adrenal venography is reliable in demonstrating the presence of adrenal tumor and may also demonstrate hyperplasia in many members of this older group (Fig. 54-16). The gonadal veins should also be sampled to detect gonadal tumors.[44] The angiographic findings of adrenal disorders causing adrenogenital syndrome are indistinguishable from those observed in Cushing syndrome.[7,37,43] Contralateral adrenal atrophy is seen in about 30 percent of virilizing adrenal tumors.[45] Adrenal arteriography is not indicated for the evaluation of adrenogenital syndrome.

Pheochromocytomas

Pheochromocytomas are rare chromaffin tissue tumors that produce epinephrine and norepinephrine. Clinical manifestations of pheochromocytoma include (1) paroxysmal symptoms (palpitations, headache, sweating, and pallor), (2) hypertension (labile, accelerated, or in

Figure 54-16. Virilization in a 25-year-old woman. Ovarian tumor was suspected, but adrenal venography, as well as adrenal and ovarian venous sampling, indicated adrenal hyperplasia. (A) Left adrenal venography shows a slightly enlarged gland and intraadrenal venules. (B) Both ovarian veins were catheterized for sampling. The venograms were obtained to document proper catheter position.

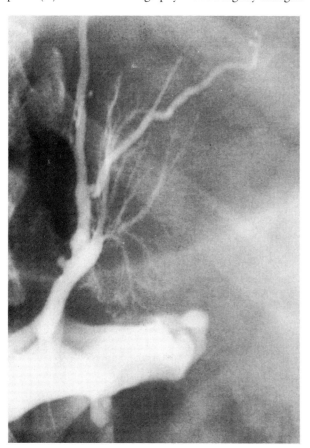

A

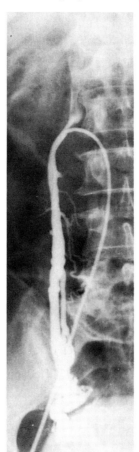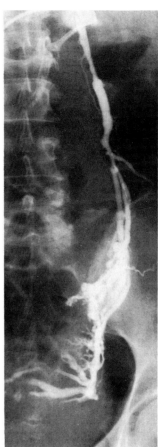

B

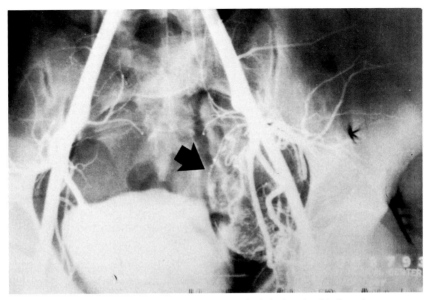

Figure 54-17. Arteriography showing pelvic paraganglioma (*arrow*). A lesion in this location cannot, of course, be shown by adrenal venography. Arteriography or noninvasive imaging with CT, US, or MRI would be required for localization.

response to pharmacologic agents), (3) hyperglycemia, and (4) suprarenal or midline abdominal masses. Although the vast majority (approximately 90 percent) of these tumors are intraadrenal, they may appear anywhere along the sympathetic chain in the chest, abdomen, or pelvis. In adults, about 10 percent are extraadrenal in location, and are called paragangliomas. Common sites outside the adrenal gland include the renal hilus, around the origin of the inferior mesenteric artery (organ of Zuckerkandl), or adjacent to the bladder (Fig. 54-17). In about 10 percent of cases of sporadic pheochromocytoma, multiple tumors are present. Pheochromocytomas may also occur in association with familial syndromes, such as multiple endocrine neoplasia or MEN-IIA (Sipple syndrome), von Hippel–Lindau disease, tuberous sclerosis, neurofibromatosis, and familial pheochromocytomas. When located within the adrenal gland they ordinarily secrete epinephrine and norepinephrine, whereas extraadrenal tumors generally secrete norepinephrine only. At least 10 percent of pheochromocytomas are malignant, and extraadrenal tumors are more likely to be malignant than those arising from the adrenal medulla.

The clinical diagnosis is confirmed with biochemical testing. These tests show increased urinary excretion of catecholamines (epinephrine or norepinephrine) or their metabolites (metanephrines and/or vanillylmandelic acid) or increased plasma concentrations of the catecholamines.

Once the diagnosis is confirmed biochemically, pre-operative localization and staging are of paramount importance. CT has emerged as the imaging modality of choice for localizing pheochromocytomas.[20,23] The accuracy of CT is about 94 percent for intraadrenal pheochromocytoma and about 82 percent for extraadrenal lesions.[20] Intravenous contrast is rarely required because the lesions are usually sufficiently large to be detected without contrast. If intravenous contrast is to be used, pretreatment with an alpha-adrenergic blocking agent is suggested to prevent precipitation of a hypertensive crisis. The accuracy of MRI for evaluating suspected pheochromocytoma is similar to that of CT. The superior tissue characterization of MRI in comparison to CT is offset by the slightly decreased spatial resolution and the cost and time required to obtain MRI sequences from the chest through the pelvis. If available, scintigraphy using [131]I- or ^{123}I-MIBG is also useful for localizing pheochromocytomas. The overall accuracy of MIBG is similar to that of CT and MRI, but scintigraphy has several advantages. With a single injection of radionuclide, the entire body can be scanned. This is particularly useful in cases of extraadrenal tumors, metastatic tumors, or recurrent tumors. Unfortunately, once grossly localized with MIBG, the lesions detected usually require more precise imaging with CT to demonstrate the relationship of the tumor to adjacent organs and vascular structures. For this reason, CT remains the imaging modality of choice for localizing these tumors.

Although angiographic techniques for the evalua-

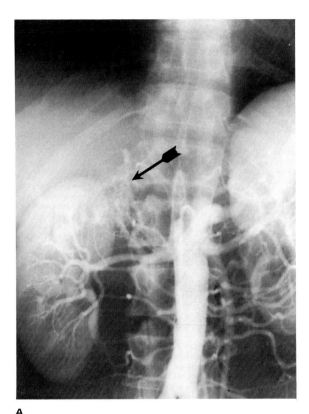

A

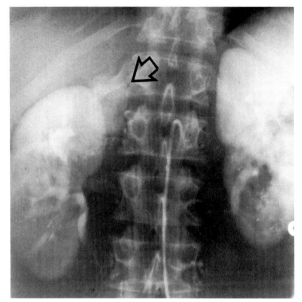

B

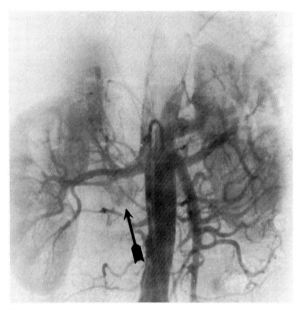

C

Figure 54-18. Pheochromocytoma, with multiple tumors demonstrated with subtraction techniques. (A) Aortogram showing some increased vascularity in the right adrenal region (*arrow*). (B) Capillary phase showing faint opacification of a right adrenal pheochromocytoma (open arrow). (C) Subtraction film, now showing an additional tumor adjacent to the right renal artery (*arrow*). (Courtesy of S. Reuter, M.D., and L.B. Talner, M.D.)

tion of pheochromocytoma are reasonably safe and highly accurate, the advancements in noninvasive imaging techniques have rendered adrenal arteriography, venography, and sampling practically obsolete for this condition. Arteriography is now indicated when noninvasive imaging is negative, when concurrent renal artery stenosis is suspected, or when a preoperative vascular road map is desired. Aortography is ordinarily performed initially as a survey procedure of the entire abdomen and pelvis. Subtraction techniques should be used because the tumor stain is often faint and easily overlooked (Fig. 54-18).[46] Two series of exposures are usually required, one to include the upper abdominal and adrenal regions and the other to include the pelvis. Subsequently, depending on aortographic observations, selective studies are performed. Selective renal or adrenal arteriography will frequently demonstrate tumors missed by aortography. The tumors are typi-

cally only moderately hypervascular. The adrenal arteries are somewhat enlarged, and a fine network of arteries surrounds the tumor.[47] The tumor usually stains homogeneously in the capillary phase. Central relative hypovascularity is common, however, and often reflects central necrosis.[48] The diagnosis of malignancy cannot be made angiographically unless metastases, local tumor invasion, or tumor where no chromaffin tissue is present can be identified. In various series, 85 to 100 percent of pheochromocytomas have been detected by arteriography.[4,5,7,39,48,49] Pheochromocytomas that occur adjacent to major renal arteries frequently

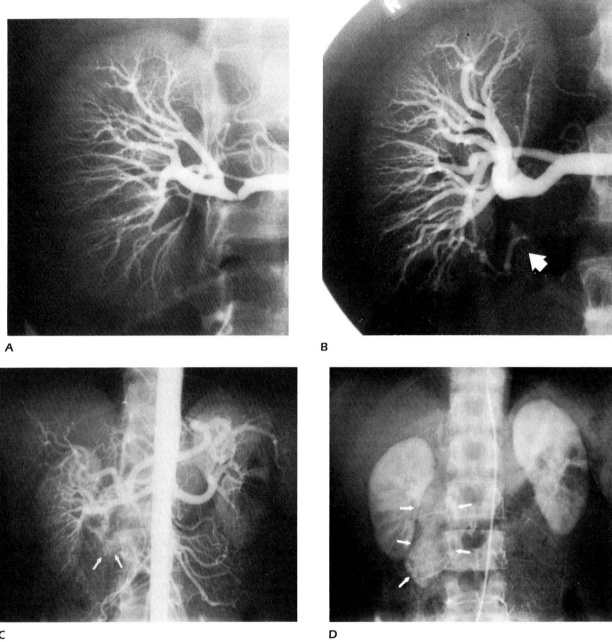

A

B

C

D

Figure 54-19. Pheochromocytoma demonstrating usual moderate hypervascularity and associated renal artery spasm that was relieved by phenoxybenzamine. (A) Selective renal arteriogram shows segmental renal arterial constrictions. (B) Subsequent arteriogram, after administration of the alpha-blocking agent phenoxybenzamine, shows that the stenoses have almost completely disappeared, and a few tumor vessels are now evident (*arrow*). (C) Early phase of the aortogram shows a few fine tumor vessels in the region of the pheochromocytoma (*arrows*). (D) Late aortogram shows the typical stain of a large bilobulated pheochromocytoma (*arrows*). (From Velick WT, Bookstein JJ, Talner LB. Pheochromocytoma with reversible renal artery stenosis. AJR 1978;131:1069. Used with permission.)

produce focal functional arterial constrictions (Fig. 54-19).[50] The combination of systemic hypertension and renal artery stenosis is then easily misinterpreted as renovascular hypertension.

It must be remembered that pheochromocytomas may be associated with tumors of the brown fat, so-called hibernomas.[51] Hibernomas may occur in the retroperitoneum around the adrenal glands or kidneys and, because of their usual moderate hypervascularity, may simulate pheochromocytomas angiographically.

In the authors' experience, adrenal venography is more sensitive in detecting small intraadrenal pheochromocytomas than is arteriography. In fact, we are unaware of any false-negative adrenal venograms in intraadrenal pheochromocytoma, and a negative adrenal venogram serves effectively to exclude the adrenal gland as the tumor site.[49] However, because venography is applicable to intraadrenal tumors only, it is usually used as a complement to, rather than instead of, arteriography. Thus adrenal venography is usually part of the angiographic workup in pheochromocytoma and is generally applied only to those adrenal glands that do not demonstrate a tumor arteriographically. In the presence of pheochromocytoma, the adrenal veins are ordinarily somewhat enlarged, reflecting the usual moderate hypervascularity of the tumor (Fig. 54-20). Intraadrenal venules are displaced around the tumor.[52] Because of the possibility of multiple (sometimes more than half a dozen) pheochromocytomas in any given patient, both arteriography and venography are usually employed. Even so, there is no assurance that all tumors have been detected preoperatively, and the surgeon too must perform a search for additional lesions at the time of operation. The possibility of multiple pheochromocytomas also underscores the value of preoperative nuclear imaging with MIBG.

Venous Sampling for Catecholamine Levels

Most laboratories now have the capacity to determine catecholamine levels in serum. Thus catecholamine assay of selective blood samples may be used to localize the side and level of chromaffin tumor. In the absence of imaging or angiographic evidence of tumor, caval catheterization with sampling from multiple positions in the chest and abdomen have proved reliable in indicating the level of tumor, but less reliable in indicating laterality.[49,53,54]

Patient Preparation

There is always some risk of precipitating a hypertensive crisis through diagnostic angiographic procedures.[4] Indeed, in the absence of alpha-adrenergic blockade, mere aortography regularly causes significant rise in arterial pressure, apparently secondary to

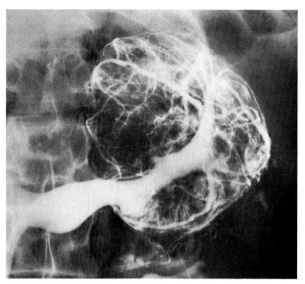

Figure 54-20. Large hypervascular left pheochromocytoma, shown by venography.

release of hormones from the tumor.[55] Hypertensive crises and rarely death have occurred after arteriography; crisis but no death to the authors' knowledge has occurred after venography.[56] Proper premedication of the patient is therefore mandatory. Furthermore, a physician capable of managing a hypertensive reaction should be readily available during the procedure.

Pretreatment should be given to any patient suspected of having a pheochromocytoma and usually consists of alpha-adrenergic blockade. The patient is generally given phenoxybenzamine, 1 to 2 mg/kg per day, divided into four equal doses and administered for several days before the procedure. During the procedure, phentolamine is kept readily available in case of a reaction despite premedication. Nitroprusside is also helpful in managing an acute hypertensive crisis. With pretreatment and continuous blood pressure monitoring in the angiography suite, the risk of such complications has been significantly decreased.[4,5]

Nonfunctioning Tumors of the Adrenal Gland

Most adrenal tumors appear clinically with hormonal dysfunction. Those that do not are considered nonfunctioning adrenal tumors and include hemangiomas, myelolipomas, nonfunctioning adenomas, neuroblastomas, ganglioneuromas, adrenal carcinomas, metastases, and lymphomas. Some, such as neuroblastomas, are not regularly associated with clinically apparent hormonal derangements, even though they may produce hormonal precursors. Other tumors, such as myelolipomas, almost never cause clinical manifestations unless associated with hemorrhage. Others, such as adrenal carcinoma, characteristically present late with symptoms due to mass effect, tumor necrosis, hemorrhage, or hormonal effects.

Because of the advancements in noninvasive imaging with CT, MRI, and US, the role of angiography for evaluating these nonfunctioning adrenal tumors has been diminished. The arteriographic and venographic features of most of these lesions are generally nonspecific. In hemangioma, arteriography may show characteristic punctate accumulations of contrast material, often arranged in C- or O-shaped clusters, that retain contrast material for prolonged periods.[57] The pattern is identical to that seen in liver hemangioma. Myelolipomas tend to be moderately hypervascular with predominantly peripheral vascularity and very little tumor stain.[40] However, the characteristic CT and US findings for myelolipoma (Fig. 54-21) should virtually eliminate the need for angiography in this setting unless an actively bleeding lesion is to be embolized in a nonoperative candidate. Neuroblastoma, adrenal carcinoma, and pheochromocytoma all demonstrate a noncharacteristic hypervascular arteriographic pattern, which are described and illustrated in other sections of this chapter.

As has been stated, the major use of venography for nonfunctioning tumors is in the patient with hormonal dysfunction and bilateral tumors on CT, when venous sampling will enable distinction of the functional from the inert tumor.

Adrenal metastases are very frequent in patients who are dying of malignancy. In 1000 consecutive autopsies of patients with carcinoma, Abrams et al. found adrenal metastases in 27 percent[58]; in patients with carcinoma of the breast or lung the incidence was 54 and 36 percent, respectively. Renal cell carcinoma and melanoma are also frequent primary sources (Fig. 54-22). Noninvasive imaging with MRI or CT has replaced angiography for the evaluation of suspected adrenal metastases. Nevertheless, metastases are sometimes discovered during angiography of a retroperitoneal mass[59,60] and may easily be confused with a primary tumor. Unfortunately, there are no angiographic features of adrenal metastases that allow them to be distinguished from other adrenal tumors. MRI appears to hold a promising future for distinguishing adrenal metastases from other nonfunctioning adrenal tumors (see Fig. 54-5), although at the present time the overlap of adrenal metastases with nonfunctioning adenomas is large enough that application to an individual patient is problematic.[26,28] Knowledge of a primary tumor elsewhere should suggest the likelihood that the

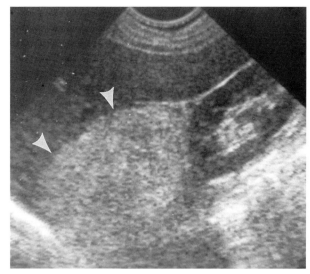

A

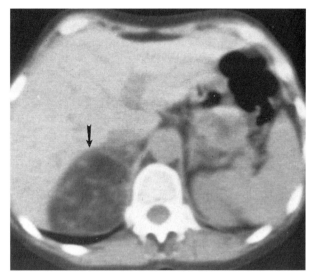

B

Figure 54-21. Myelolipoma. (A) US shows bulky right adrenal mass (*arrowheads*) with characteristic homogeneously high echogenicity of a myelolipoma. (B) CT scan reveals that the right adrenal mass is of fat density (*arrow*), confirming the diagnosis of myelolipoma. (Courtesy of G. Leopold, M.D.)

adrenal mass is metastatic. However, because of the high incidence of adrenal adenomas in the normal population (about 3 percent), even in the presence of a known primary, the most likely cause of an incidentally identified adrenal mass remains adrenal adenoma.[61] Percutaneous aspiration biopsy remains the most definitive method to confirm or exclude adrenal metastasis in this difficult group of patients, with a reported accuracy of 80 to 100 percent (Fig. 54-23).[23]

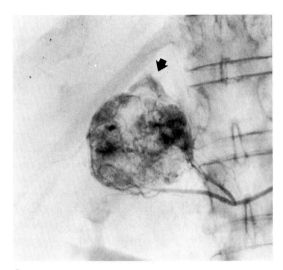
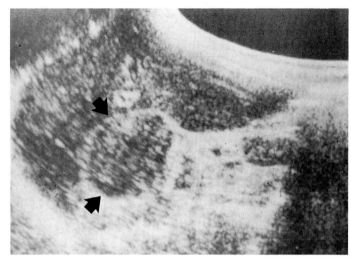

A   **B**

Figure 54-22. Adrenal metastasis from renal cell carcinoma. Overlying the metastasis is a normal adrenal remnant (*arrow, A* and *B*), exemplifying the usual persistence of functional adrenal tissue in metastatic disease and the infrequency of clinically evident Addison disease. (Courtesy of L. Ekelund, M.D.)

Adrenal Cysts

Adrenal cysts are uncommon, with less than 300 cases currently reported.[62-65] They are more frequent in women than in men and are most commonly discovered between the third and fifth decades. In the series by Kearney and Mahoney,[62] adrenal cysts were classified as follows:

Parasitic cysts (7 percent)
Epithelial cysts (9 percent)
   True glandular cysts
   Cystic adenomas
Endothelial cysts (45 percent)
   Lymphangiomatous
   Angiomatous
Hemorrhagic pseudocysts (39 percent)

Differentiating simple adrenal cyst from solid, cystic, or necrotic adrenal tumor is of obvious clinical importance. US is the imaging modality of choice for making this distinction because of the well-established sonographic characteristics of a simple renal cyst. However, unlike renal cysts, adrenal cysts may demonstrate a thick wall, and hemorrhagic adrenal pseudocysts may show internal septations.[23] In these situations, if a soft tissue masslike component is present, percutaneous biopsy or surgical resection should be performed. The CT appearance of an adrenal cyst is also characteristic and permits distinction from pancreatic or renal cysts.

There is currently no indication for angiography in

Figure 54-23. Percutaneous biopsy of right adrenal mass in patient undergoing staging of newly diagnosed bronchogenic carcinoma. Note the use of the decubitus patient positioning to reduce risk of pneumothorax. The biopsy proved to be positive for metastasis, precluding curative resection of lung primary. (Courtesy of H.B. D'Agostino, M.D.)

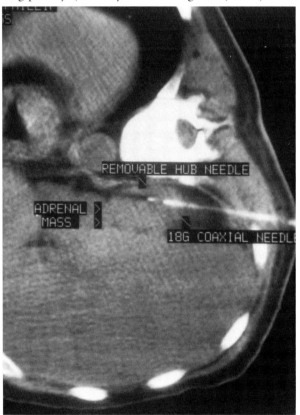

the evaluation of adrenal cysts because the findings are both less sensitive and specific than those afforded with US and CT. Arteriography will demonstrate an avascular mass in the adrenal region with displacement of the adrenal arteries. Adrenal venography is typically very suggestive, demonstrating smooth, arcuate displacement of normal-sized adrenal venules, without any veins within the mass (Fig. 54-24). When the distinction of a simple adrenal cyst from a cystic malignancy is equivocal, diagnostic cyst aspiration and opacification may be helpful if the fluid is clear and the cytology is benign.[65] Cyst aspiration has also been shown to be a safe and effective alternative to surgical resection for symptomatic adrenal cysts (see Fig. 54-24D).[65]

Neuroblastomas and Ganglioneuromas

Neuroblastomas are the second most common solid tumor of infancy and childhood, following cerebral tumors in this age group.[66,67] They are tumors of primitive sympathoblast cells and may arise anywhere along the sympathetic chain, with 20 to 40 percent arising from the adrenal glands. The clinical presentation is usually prompted by an abdominal mass. The tumors commonly secrete catecholamine precursors or metabolites, but hypertension develops only rarely. Elevated serum vanillylmandelic acid is detected in about 80 percent of cases. Because of the usually large size of the tumor at the time of presentation, a mass in the adrenal region is usually apparent on plain radiographs of the abdomen. CT, US, and MRI are all useful in showing the tumor, localizing it to the adrenal glands, and staging the extent of disease.

Although angiography is now rarely performed, it may be advantageous as a preoperative procedure because it (1) provides a vascular road map, (2) defines the source and degree of vascularity, and (3) may demonstrate signs of nonresectability not seen on other imaging studies. Angiographically, neuroblastomas are moderately hypervascular (Fig. 54-25). The adrenal arteries are usually enlarged, and there is a dense tumor stain during the capillary phase.

Ganglioneuromas are benign tumors that may arise anywhere along the sympathetic chain; 60 percent of them appear in children or adolescents under the age of 20.[68] About 20 percent arise from the adrenal glands (medullary portion). Histologically they consist of mature nerve cells and fibers. A continuum exists between the immature cells of neuroblastomas, the intermediate maturity of ganglioneuroblastomas, and the mature cells of ganglioneuromas. Ganglioneuromas are commonly small and are often discovered as incidental findings because of calcification apparent on plain films. Like neuroblastomas, ganglioneuromas usually produce catecholamine precursors.[69] In patients with ganglioneuromas, the catecholamine precursors may cause an intractable watery diarrhea syndrome clinically indistinguishable from that due to islet cell tumor of the pancreas.[70] Rarely, hypertension may also develop secondary to catecholamine excess. Neuroblastomas may undergo maturation and convert to ganglioneuromas.[71] Arteriographically, ganglioneuromas appear as hypovascular to moderately vascular masses.

Localization of Adrenal Remnants

Occasionally after bilateral adrenalectomy for Cushing disease, there is recurrent ACTH-responsive adrenal cortisol hyperproduction. Localization of the adrenal residua can be a vexing problem. In the past, attempts at localizing the residual adrenal tissue with venography and venous sampling have been fraught with difficulty and inaccuracy. The clearly superior method in this clinical scenario is nuclear scintigraphy using NP-59. Beierwaltes and colleagues reported 11 patients with recurrent hyperadrenalism after bilateral adrenalectomy.[72] With adrenal scintigraphy, adrenal remnants were localized in 9. Most commonly the remnant was thought to represent the upper tail of the gland, which is easily separated from the excised gland when surgical manipulation is vigorous or exposure is imperfect. On the right, this tail may retract superiorly and be lost behind the liver; on the left it may retract onto the diaphragm.

Adrenal Cortical Carcinoma

Adrenal cortical carcinoma is an uncommon malignancy that comprises about 0.1 percent of human cancers.[73] It occurs with a frequency of approximately one case per million people and affects men and women about equally. The median age at presentation is the fifth decade, although patients with adrenal cortical carcinoma have been reported from 1 to 80 years old.[23] There seems to be two peak periods of incidence, childhood and middle age.[74] The most common presentation of patients with adrenocortical carcinoma is abdominal pain or a palpable mass. These tumors are typically large (6–15 cm) at presentation, although a tumor as small as 1 cm has been reported.[23] About half of these tumors are functional and may be detected by manifestations of excess hormone production.[73,75] Cushing syndrome is most frequent, followed by virilization and femininization. Hyperaldosteronism is rarely due to carcinoma.[23] Adrenocortical carcinoma occurs more commonly in the left adrenal gland and is bilateral in up to 10 percent of cases.

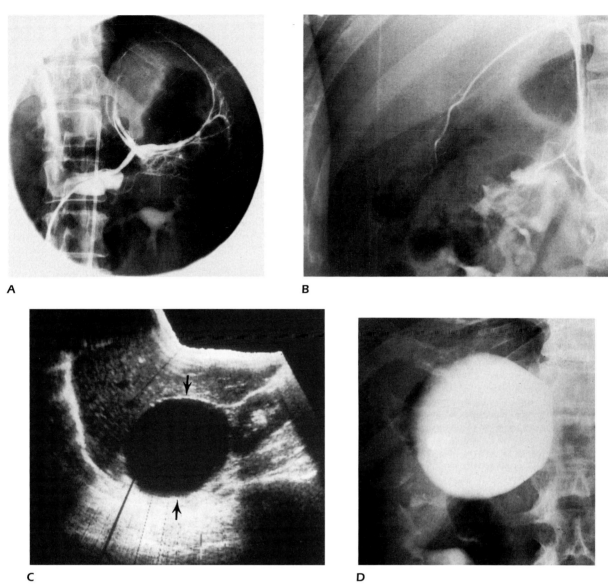

Figure 54-24. Adrenal cysts. (A) Multicystic adrenal gland. A mass was discovered above the left kidney during intravenous urography. The patient had no evidence of hormonal dysfunction. Arteriography had shown an avascular mass in the adrenal gland. The venogram shows smooth arcuate displacement of adrenal venules above the central vein, suggesting a large adrenal cyst. Displacement of venules below the central vein reflects the association of several smaller cysts. (B) Selective arteriography from another patient with adrenal cyst. Note the displacement of small adrenal arteries from the region of an avascular mass. (C) US examination of the right adrenal cyst (*arrows*). (Courtesy of G. Leopold, M.D.) (D) Right adrenal cyst puncture, aspiration, and opacification. (Courtesy of H. Rosenkrantz, M.D.)

Because of the typically large size at presentation, these tumors may be easily detected with noninvasive imaging modalities, including plain films of the abdomen, urography, CT, US, and MRI. CT suffices in the majority of cases, but occasionally has problems distinguishing the organ of origin of these large masses.[76] Additionally, detection of direct hepatic invasion is difficult with CT. Because of the multiplanar imaging potential afforded by MRI, there tends to be less difficulty in visualizing direct hepatic or renal invasion and in distinguishing masses of adrenal origin from those of renal origin. MRI is also able to demonstrate venous extension using limited flip angle techniques.

Adrenal angiography maintains several distinct advantages over noninvasive imaging techniques.[76] The intraadrenal origin of the tumor can be most reliably defined arteriographically. In addition, venous and caval extension can be accurately assessed and a preoper-

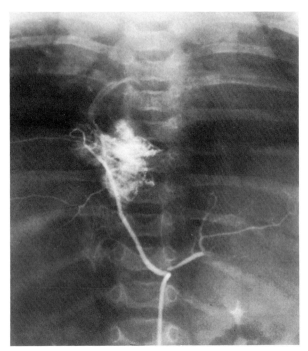

Figure 54-25. Neuroblastoma on right inferior phrenic arteriogram. The tumor arises along the sympathetic chain above the right adrenal gland and is markedly hypervascular. Venous drainage was via a pulmonary vein.

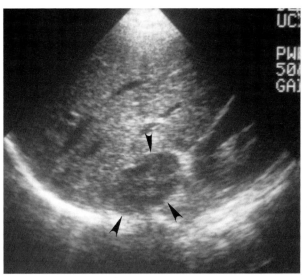

Figure 54-26. Addison disease secondary to histoplasmosis. The patient developed clinically apparent adrenal insufficiency at the time of histoplasmosis dissemination. US shows an enlarged, lobulated right adrenal gland (*arrowheads*).

ative vascular road map is provided. There are typically numerous tortuous arterial feeders extending over the surface of the tumor, and the mass itself demonstrates moderate neovascularity (see Fig. 54-15). The tumor stain is likely to be inhomogeneous, with areas of hypovascularity probably reflecting necrosis. The extent of tumor is demonstrated, and invasion of the kidney or liver, extension into renal veins or IVC, or hepatic metastases are frequently evident.[68] Because the carcinomas are usually large, venography is not generally necessary. When occasionally performed, it usually demonstrates only a portion of the large intraadrenal mass. Renal venography and inferior vena cavography are simple, safe techniques that accurately demonstrate venous extension invisible on noninvasive imaging.

Adrenal arterial embolization has been reported for four adrenocortical carcinomas and five metastatic adrenal lesions.[77] The goals were to reduce tumor bulk, suppress hormonal function, relieve pain, and reduce tumor vascularity before surgical resection. These goals were achieved in the majority of cases. As in renal embolization, the most common complications were pain and low-grade fever lasting less than 48 hours. One patient had a hypertensive episode. The authors conclude that adrenal arterial embolization is safe and effective in the management of inoperable adrenal

neoplasms. Certainly, larger series are needed to confirm these data.

Addison Disease

Primary adrenal insufficiency, or Addison disease, occurs after 90 percent or more of the adrenal cortex has been destroyed. The most common cause in the United States is idiopathic adrenal atrophy, which accounts for 60 to 70 percent of cases and is most likely an autoimmune phenomenon. The other common cause of Addison disease is destruction of the adrenal glands by granulomatous diseases, including tuberculosis, sarcoidosis, histoplasmosis, blastomycosis, and coccidioidomycosis (Fig. 54-26). Rare causes include adrenal hemorrhage secondary to anticoagulants or coagulation disorders, sepsis, shock, metastatic disease, iatrogenesis (adrenal venography or surgery), and amyloidosis. Adrenal insufficiency can also be secondary to pituitary disease.

CT is the most useful imaging modality for the evaluation of Addison disease. In idiopathic Addison disease, cortical atrophy is so severe that the adrenal glands may be difficult to detect.[78] Granulomatous involvement by either tuberculosis or histoplasmosis is bilateral, with calcification occurring commonly. The glands are enlarged but usually maintain a normal configuration.[79]

Because of the accuracy of CT for the evaluation of Addison disease, angiography is probably no longer

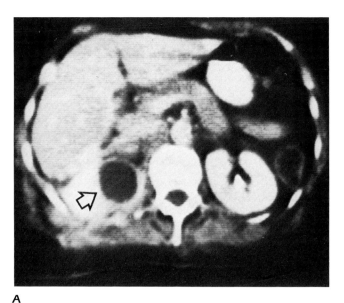

A

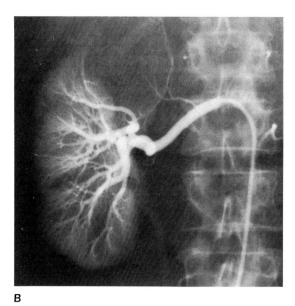

B

Figure 54-27. Adrenal abscess secondary to *Escherichia coli* in a 62-year-old woman with fever and back pain of 3 weeks' duration. (A) CT scan reveals a fluid collection in the right adrenal gland (*arrow*). (B) Arteriography indicates a hypovascular mass supplied primarily from the inferior adrenal artery, and possibly from very small renal branches.

indicated. In previously performed angiograms for idiopathic adrenal atrophy or adrenal atrophy secondary to pituitary disease, the glands were noted to be small and to have narrow intraadrenal venules. Except for its bilaterality, this appearance is indistinguishable from the atrophy seen contralaterally to a cortisol-producing adenoma. If the glands have been destroyed by inflammatory disease, venous distortion and truncation are seen on venography.

Miscellaneous Conditions

Infectious processes of the adrenal glands may be acute or chronic. As indicated in the previous section, chronic tuberculous infection and histoplasmosis of the adrenal gland are relatively common causes of Addison disease. Acute infections are much more rare. The authors have performed angiography in two cases of acute suppurative adrenal infection secondary to *Escherichia coli*. In one case, marked enlargement of the gland and diffuse capillary blush were present. The other, a subacute abscess, resembled an adrenal neoplasm angiographically but was relatively low attenuation on CT (Fig. 54-27). We have successfully performed percutaneous drainage for adrenal abscess.

Adrenal hemorrhage is not an uncommon condition which may develop spontaneously or secondary to trauma or anticoagulation.[23] Spontaneous adrenal hemorrhage occurs with septicemia, hypertension, renal vein thrombosis, or adrenal disease such as a tu-

mor. The hemorrhage may be unilateral or bilateral. When bilateral, it more commonly involves the right side. Adrenal hemorrhage is more common in neonates than in older children or adults. It is usually due to the trauma of delivery, asphyxia, septicemia, or abnormal clotting factors.[80] If the hemorrhage is large, a palpable mass, anemia, or prolonged jaundice may occur. Most adrenal hematomas will be resorbed, but some may liquefy and persist as an adrenal pseudocyst. In the neonate, adrenal insufficiency develops rarely secondary to adrenal hemorrhage.

In the older child or adult, adrenal hemorrhage is usually due to trauma, systemic illness, or anticoagulation. When related to anticoagulation, it usually occurs in the first 3 weeks of treatment.[81] However, it is not thought to be due to excessive anticoagulation because associated hemorrhage does not occur elsewhere. The hematoma is usually located in the adrenal medulla, with stretching of the surrounding cortex.[23]

CT is the most reliable method of identifying adrenal hemorrhage. The hematoma is initially noted to be high density, 50 to 90 Hounsfield units. Sonography is often used to detect adrenal hemorrhage in children. An anechoic mass is usually identified, and its relationship to the kidney is well seen. Occasionally, sufficient echogenicity is present to suggest a solid mass. MRI has also been used to evaluate adrenal hemorrhage[81] and shows the evolution of hemoglobin breakdown. Angiography for adrenal hemorrhage is practically never indicated. If, despite correction of any predisposing factors, ongoing hemorrhage is suspected in a nonoperative patient, adrenal angiography and embolization might be considered, but this condition has not as yet been reported to our knowledge.

Transcatheter Adrenal Ablation

On the basis of a few early cases that developed unilateral or bilateral adrenal atrophy (Addison disease) after adrenal venography, the possibility of intentional transcatheter adrenal ablation was considered. A few small series[82,83] described results after injecting nitrogen mustards via the adrenal venous catheter into the adrenal gland harboring metastatic disease. There was evidence of adrenal suppression in about two-thirds of cases and some regression of metastatic disease in about half. In one study, adrenal infarction was attempted using forceful injections of contrast material alone into the adrenal vein.[84] Five attempts were made in four glands, and in none was satisfactory adrenal suppression achieved. Theoretically, injection of ethanol seemed more promising. Retrograde venous injection of ethanol was used to ablate the adrenal glands in five monkeys.[85] These injections resulted in severe hypertensive crises, and postmortem studies showed residual viable tissue. The authors concluded that this procedure, although technically feasible, was neither safe nor effective. Thus, because of the potential for the release of large and potentially fatal amounts of catecholamines, adrenal alcohol injections are contraindicated.

In a small clinical series of nine patients, adrenal arterial embolization appeared to be a safe and effective treatment for the management of primary and secondary neoplasms.[77] Larger series are needed to confirm these data.

Summary

Over the past quarter-century, angiography has been displaced as the primary imaging method for adrenal disease. CT is now the primary imaging modality in most instances. But despite the advancements in CT, MRI, US, and scintigraphy, a definite, albeit limited, role for adrenal vascular catheterization remains. Adrenal venography and sampling are still indicated for the majority of patients with primary aldosteronism. Arteriography, venography, and/or venous sampling are occasionally indicated in selected patients with Cushing disease, adrenogenital syndrome, pheochromocytoma, and adrenal cortical carcinoma.

The materials and techniques for adrenal vascular catheterization, opacification, and sampling have

evolved as well. Despite the decreased frequency with which these procedures are being performed, familiarity with adrenal vascular anatomy and meticulous attention to technical details enable adrenal vascular catheterization, opacification, and sampling to be consistently carried out with a high degree of safety and accuracy.

References

1. Dobbie JW, Symington T. The human adrenal gland with special reference to the vasculature. J Endocrinol 1966;34:479.
2. Mikaelsson CG. The adrenal glands after epinephrophlebography. Acta Radiol 1970;10:1.
3. Horton R, Finck E. Diagnosis and localization in primary aldosteronism. Ann Intern Med 1972;76:885.
4. Rossi P, Young IS, Panke WF. Techniques, usefulness, and hazards of arteriography of pheochromocytoma: a review of 99 cases. JAMA 1968;205:547–553.
5. Zelch JV, Meaney TF, Belhobek GH. Radiologic approach to the patient with suspected pheochromocytoma. Radiology 1974;111:279–284.
6. Bookstein JJ, Conn J, Reuter SR. Intra-adrenal hemorrhage as a complication of adrenal venography in primary aldosteronism. Radiology 1968;90:778.
7. Lecky JW, Wolfman NT, Modic CW. Current concepts of adrenal angiography. Radiol Clin North Am 1976;14:309–332.
8. Dedrick CG. Adrenal arteriography and venography. Urol Clin North Am 1989;16:515–526.
9. Eagan RT, Page MI. Adrenal insufficiency following bilateral adrenal venography. JAMA 1971;215:115.
10. Fisher CE, Turner FA, Horton R. Remission of primary hyperaldosteronism after adrenal venography. N Engl J Med 1971; 285:334.
11. Kahn PC, Kelleher MD, Egdahl RH, Melby JC. Adrenal arteriography and venography in primary aldosteronism. Radiology 1971;101:71.
12. Taylor HC, Sachs CR, Bravo EL. Primary aldosteronism: remission and development of adrenal insufficiency after adrenal venography. Ann Intern Med 1976;85:207.
13. Teixeira PE, Dwyer DE, Voil GW. Remission of primary hyperaldosteronism consequent on adrenal venography. Can Med Assoc J 1977;117:789.
14. Beierwaltes WH, Lieberman LM, Ansari AN, Nishiyama H. Visualization of human adrenal gland in vivo by scintillation scanning. JAMA 1971;216:275–277.
15. Basmadjian GP, Hetzel KR, Ice RD, Beierwaltes WH. Synthesis of a new adrenal cortex scanning agent 6β-^{131}I-iodomethyl-19-nor-cholest-5(10)-EN-3β-OL (NP-59). J Labelled Compd Radiopharm 1975;11:427–434.
16. Wieland DM, Swanson DP, Brown LE, Beierwaltes WH. Imaging the adrenal medulla with an I-131-labeled antiadrenergic agent. J Nucl Med 1979;20:155–158.
17. Sisson JC, Frager MS, Valk TW, Gross MD, Swanson DP, Wieland DM, Tobss MC, Beierwaltes WH, Thompson NW. Scintigraphy localization of pheochromocytoma. N Engl J Med 1981;305:12–17.
18. Shapiro B, Copp JE, Sisson JC, Eyer PL, Beierwaltes WH. Iodine-131 metaiodobenzylguanidine for the locating of suspected pheochromocytoma: experience in 400 cases. J Nucl Med 1985;26:576–585.
19. Lamki LM, Haynie TP. Role of adrenal imaging in surgical management. J Surg Oncol 1990;43:139–147.
20. Whalen RK, Althausen AF, Daniels GH. Extra-adrenal pheochromocytoma. J Urol 1992;147:1–10.
21. Bretan PN, Lorig R. Adrenal imaging: computed tomographic

scanning and magnetic resonance imaging. Urol Clin North Am 1989;16:505–513.

22. Schwarz RJ, Schmidt N. Efficient management of adrenal tumors. Am J Surg 1991;161:576–579.
23. Dunnick NR. Adrenal imaging: current status. AJR 1990;154: 927–936.
24. Reinig JW, Doppman JL, Dwyer AJ, Johnson AR, Knop RH. Distinction between adrenal adenomas and adrenal metastases using MR imaging. J Comput Assist Tomogr 1985;9:898–901.
25. Mitchell DG, Crovello M, Matteucci T, Peterson RO, Miettinen MM. Benign adrenocortical masses: diagnosis with chemical shift MR imaging. Radiology 1992;185:345–351.
26. Reinig JW. MR imaging differentiation of adrenal masses: has the time finally come? Radiology 1992;185:339–340.
27. Tsushima Y, Ishizaka H, Matsumoto M. Adrenal masses: differentiation with chemical shift, fast low-angle shot MR imaging. Radiology 1993;186:705–709.
28. Reinig JW, Stutley JE, Leonhardt CM, Spicer KM, Margolis M, Caldwell CB. Differentiation of adrenal masses with MR imaging: comparison of techniques. Radiology 1994;192:41–46.
29. Seabold JE, Cohen EL, Beierwaltes WH, Hinerman DL, Nishiyama RH, Bookstein JJ, Ice RD. Adrenal imaging with [131]I-19-iodocholesterol in the diagnostic evaluation of patients with aldosteronism. J Clin Endocrinol Metab 1976;42:41.
30. Weinberger MH, et al. Primary aldosteronism. Ann Intern Med 1979;90:386.
31. Francis IR, Gross MD, Shapiro B, Korobkin M, Quint LE. Integrated imaging of adrenal disease. Radiology 1992;184:1–13.
32. Dunnick NR, Doppman JL, Gill JR Jr, et al. Localization of functional adrenal tumors by computed tomography and adrenal venous sampling. Radiology 1982;142:429–433.
33. Geisinger MA, Zelch MG, Bravo EL, et al. Primary hyperaldosteronism: comparison of CT, adrenal venography and venous sampling. AJR 1983;141:299–302.
34. Ikeda DM, Francis IR, Glazer GM, et al. The detection of adrenal tumors and hyperplasia in patients with primary hyperaldosteronism: comparison of scintigraphy, CT and MR imaging. AJR 1989;153:301–306.
35. Dunnick NR, Doppman JL, Mills SR, Gill JR Jr. Preoperative diagnosis and localization of aldosteronomas by measurement of corticosteroids in adrenal venous blood. Radiology 1979; 133:331–333.
36. Mitty HA, Gabrilove JL, Nicolis GL. Nontumorous adrenal hyperfunction: problems in angiographic-clinical correlation. Radiology 1977;122:89.
37. Mitty HA, Nicolis GL, Gabrilove JL. Adrenal venography: clinical-roentgenographic correlation in 80 patients. AJR 1973; 119:564.
38. Hogan MJ, McRae J, Schambelan M, Biglieri EG. Location of aldosterone producing adenomas with [131]I-19-iodocholesterol. N Engl J Med 1976;294:410.
39. Alfidi RJ, Gill WM, Klein HJ. Arteriography of adrenal neoplasms. AJR 1969;106:635.
40. Costello P, Clouse ME, Kane RA, Paris A. Problems in the diagnosis of adrenal tumors. Radiology 1977;125:335.
41. David R, Shirkhoda A, Fisher RG. The adrenal glands: plain film, excretory urographic, and angiographic findings. Semin Roentgenol 1988;23:259–270.
42. Reuter SR, Blair AJ, Schteingart DE, Bookstein JJ. Adrenal venography. Radiology 1967;89:805.
43. Lee KR, Lin F, Sibala J. Adrenal adenoma and hyperplasia: importance of arteriographic differential diagnosis. AJR 1973; 119:796.
44. Weiland AJ, Bookstein JJ, Cleary RE, Judd HL. Preoperative localization of virilizing tumors by selective venous sampling. Am J Obstet Gynecol 1978;131:797.
45. Weinberg T. Contralateral adrenal atrophy associated with cortical adrenal neoplasms. N Y State J Med 1941;41:884.
46. Reuter SR, Talner LB, Atkin T. The importance of subtraction

in the angiographic evaluation of extra-adrenal pheochromocytomas. AJR 1973;117:128.
47. Rossi P. Arteriography in adrenal tumors. Br J Radiol 1968; 41:81.
48. Zelch JV, Meaney TF, Belhobek GH. Radiologic approach to the patient with suspected pheochromocytoma. Radiology 1974;111:279.
49. Kadir S, Robinette C. Accuracy of angiography in the localization of pheochromocytoma. J Urol 1981;126:789–793.
50. Velick WT, Bookstein JJ, Talner LB. Pheochromocytoma with reversible renal artery stenosis. AJR 1978;131:1069.
51. English JT, Patel SK, Flanagan MJ. Association of pheochromocytomas with brown fat tumors. Radiology 1973;107:279.
52. Christenson R, Smith CW, Burko H. Arteriographic manifestations of pheochromocytoma. AJR 1976;126:567–575.
53. Harrison TS, Frier DT. Pitfalls in the technique and interpretation of regional venous sampling for localizing pheochromocytoma. Surg Clin North Am 1974;54:339.
54. Harrison TS, Seaton JF, Cerny JC, Bookstein JJ, Bartlett JD. Localization of pheochromocytoma by caval catheterization. Arch Surg 1967;95:339.
55. Meaney TF, Buonocore E. Selective arteriography as a localizing and provocative test in the diagnosis of pheochromocytoma. Radiology 1966;87:309.
56. Gold RE, Wisinger BM, Geraci AR, Heinz LM. Hypertensive crisis as a result of adrenal venography in a patient with pheochromocytoma. Radiology 1972;102:579.
57. Rothberg M, Bastidas J, Mattey WE, Bernas E. Adrenal hemangiomas: angiographic appearance of a rare tumor. Radiology 1978;126:341.
58. Abrams HL, Spiro R, Goldstein N. Metastases in carcinoma: analysis of 1000 autopsied cases. Cancer 1950;3:74.
59. Hoevels J, Ekelund L. Angiographic findings in adrenal masses. Acta Radiol 1979;20:337.
60. Reuter SR. Demonstration of adrenal metastases by adrenal venography. N Engl J Med 1968;278:1423.
61. Glazer GM, Francis IR, Quint L. Imaging of the adrenal glands. Invest Radiol 1988;23:3–11.
62. Kearney GP, Mahoney EM. Adrenal cysts. Urol Clin North Am 1977;4:273.
63. Chemma P, Cartegna R, Staubitz W. Adrenal cysts: diagnosis and treatment. J Urol 1981;126:396–399.
64. Ghandur-Mnaymneh L, Slim M, Muakassa K. Adrenal cysts: pathogenesis and histological identification with a report of 6 cases. J Urol 1979;122:87–91.
65. Tung GA, Pfister RC, Papanicolaou N, Yoder IC. Adrenal cysts: imaging and percutaneous aspiration. Radiology 1989; 173:107–110.
66. Duckett JW, Koop CE. Neuroblastoma. Urol Clin North Am 1977;4:285.
67. Wilson LM, Draper GJ. Neuroblastoma, its natural history and prognosis. A study of 487 cases. Br Med J 1974;3:301.
68. Lecky JW, Wolfman NT, Modic CW. Current concepts of adrenal angiography. Radiol Clin North Am 1976;14:309.
69. Greer M, Anta AA, Williams CM, Echevarria RA. Tumors of neural crest origin. Arch Neurol 1965;13:139.
70. Trump DC, Livingston JW, Baylis SB. Watery diarrhea syndrome in an adult with ganglioneuroma-pheochromocytoma. Cancer 1977;117:789.
71. Fox F, Davidson J, Thomas LB. Maturation of sympathicoblastoma into ganglioneuroma. Cancer 1959;12:108.
72. Freitas JE, Herwig KR, Cerny JC, Beierwaltes WH. Preoperative localization of adrenal remnants. Surg Gynecol Obstet 1977;145:705.
73. Hutter AM, Kayhoe DE. Adrenal cortical carcinoma. Am J Med 1966;41:572.
74. Lewinsky BS, Grigor KM, Symington T, Neville AM. The clinical and pathologic features of "non-hormonal" adrenocortical tumors. Cancer 1974;33:778.
75. Bodie B, Novick AC, Pontes JE, et al. The Cleveland Clinic experience with adrenal cortical carcinoma. J Urol 1989;141: 257–260.

76. Kolmannskog F, Kolbenstvedt A, Brekke IB. CT and angiography in adrenocortical carcinoma. Acta Radiol 1992;33:45–49.
77. O'Keefe FN, Carrasco CH, Charnsangavej C, et al. Arterial embolization of adrenal tumors: results in nine cases. AJR 1988; 151:819–822.
78. Eason RJ, Croxson MS, Perry MC, Somerfield SD. Addison disease, adrenal autoantibodies and computerized adrenal tomography. N Z Med J 1982;95:569–573.
79. Wilson DA, Muchmore HG, Tisdal RG, et al. Histoplasmosis of the adrenal glands studied by CT. Radiology 1984;150: 779–783.
80. Khuri FJ, Alton DJ, Hardy BE, et al. Adrenal hemorrhage in neonates: report of 5 cases and review of the literature. J Urol 1980;124:684–687.
81. Itoh K, Yamashita K, Satoh Y, Sawada H. MR imaging of bilateral adrenal hemorrhage. J Comput Assist Tomogr 1988;12: 1054–1056.
82. Zimmerman CE, Eisenberg H, Rosoff CB. Transvenous adrenal destruction: clinical trials in patients with metastatic malignancy. Surgery 1974;75:550.
83. Jablonski RD, Meaney TF, Schumacher OP. Transcatheter adrenal ablation for metastatic carcinoma of the breast. Cleve Clin Q 1977;44:57.
84. Dunnick NR, Doppman JL, Gill JR Jr, et al. Failure to ablate the adrenal gland by injection of contrast material. Radiology 1982;142:67–69.
85. Doppman JL, Girton M. Adrenal ablation by retrograde venous ethanol injection: an ineffective and dangerous procedure. Radiology 1984;150:667–672.

55

Pancreatic Angiography

ERIK BOIJSEN

*I*n 1956, a few years after Seldinger's percutaneous angiographic technique was introduced, Ödman presented his method for selective angiography of the main branches of the abdominal aorta.[1] Already in 1951 Bierman et al.[2] had performed intraarterial catheterization of visceral branches after exploration of the femoral and brachial arteries. However, it was not until the percutaneous technique and the radiopaque catheters became available that a giant step forward took place in abdominal visceral angiography. Ödman documented his experience in several reports on both celiac angiography and pancreatic angiography, the latter as a chapter in the first edition of *Angiography*.[3–5] During the 1960s angiography of the pancreas became a well-established, safe, and reliable method for diagnosing pancreatic disease, as is documented in the second edition.[6] Technical improvements, including superselective catheterization of pancreatic arteries, pharmacoangiography, and magnification, increased the diagnostic accuracy, as reported in the third edition.[7] Therefore, angiography was the most reliable diagnostic method also in the 1970s. During this decade, however, new techniques have entered the competition: endoscopic retrograde cholangiopancreatography (ERCP), radionuclide imaging, ultrasonography, and computed tomography (CT). With the exception of radionuclide imaging, these methods eventually took over as primary imaging methods during the 1980s, and comparative prospective studies definitely showed that angiography was no longer the best diagnostic study to diagnose pancreatic disease.

The technical improvements in the 1980s, including duplex and color Doppler, incremental dynamic CT, and magnetic resonance imaging (MRI), have almost completely, but not entirely, replaced pancreatic angiography. Not only is improved information about the parenchyma obtained, but also the vessels around the pancreas can be analyzed with these noninvasive techniques. Thus, despite the improvements in angio-graphic technique—increased contrast resolution in digital subtraction angiography (DSA) with better contrast media and with less trauma due to smaller catheters and guidewires—the noninvasive methods, with few exceptions, give better information about pancreatic disease.

For the radiologist, however, it is still important to be aware of what angiography can add in information regarding vascular anatomy and pathology. No imaging method can compete with the high resolution obtained at angiography, and there are still many situations when pancreatic angiography is the ultimate method that can solve a difficult clinical problem.

Vascular Anatomy

Arteries

Dissection studies of the pancreatic vasculature by Pierson,[8] Woodburne and Olsen,[9] Michels,[10] and others form the basis of roentgenologic angiographic anatomy (Fig. 55-1). The following description of the pancreatic arterial pattern is based on reports on angiographic studies in vivo and on specimens.[3,5,11–17] Unlike other organs, the pancreas has no hilus and no main artery supplying it. It is encircled by arteries originating from the celiac axis and superior mesenteric arteries. The splenic and common hepatic arteries are in close contact with the upper border of the organ; the gastroduodenal artery and the pancreaticoduodenal arcades form an incomplete lateral and inferior border of the head of the pancreas; and the transverse pancreatic artery follows the inferior margin of the body and tail of the pancreas. Large anatomic variations exist, but these arteries can usually be defined if contrast medium is injected into both the celiac axis and the superior mesenteric artery (Fig. 55-2).

From cadaver specimens it is obvious that the pan-

1383

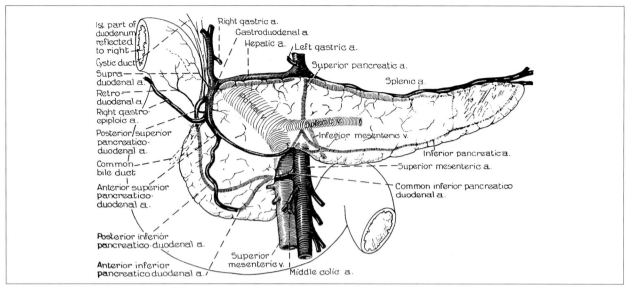

Figure 55-1. The arterial supply of the pancreas, anterior view. (From Pierson JM. The arterial blood supply of the pancreas. Surg Gynecol Obstet 1943;77:426. Used with permission.)

creas has a rich vascular network with large interarterial anastomoses. In the pancreatic tail, however, the anastomoses may be absent—an important consideration when ligation of the splenic artery is performed for splenectomy.[12,16] The small ramifications of the intrapancreatic arteries preclude the use of lumbar aortography for demonstration of this vasculature.[11,13,15] Only high-quality celiac and superior mesenteric angiography gives acceptable information about the pancreatic arteries, and sometimes even superselective injection of contrast medium into hepatic, splenic, or pancreatic arteries is the only method by which to obtain the necessary information (Figs. 55-2 and 55-3).

To demonstrate the complete pancreatic arterial supply by angiography, the arteries described here should be well defined because they are usually involved in pancreatic disease.

Celiac Axis

Best observed in the lateral view, the celiac axis has a varying course in the anterior direction[3,13,18] (Fig. 55-4).

Splenic Artery

The splenic artery usually arises from the celiac axis, but occasionally it stems from the aorta or superior mesenteric artery. Great variations occur in the course of this vessel because of its inconstant degree of tortuosity. According to Kupic et al.,[15] it can be divided into four main segments: the suprapancreatic, which is the first 1 to 3 cm of the vessel; the pancreatic, which is usually the most tortuous and lies on the dorsal surface of the pancreas; the prepancreatic, which runs on the anterior surface of the tail of the pancreas; and the prehilar, which courses between the pancreas and the spleen.

Common Hepatic Artery

The common hepatic artery has a variable course along the cranial border of the body and head of the pancreas, and tortuosity is usually not observed. Anatomic variation is common. Most often this occurs as an aberrant right hepatic artery, which can traverse the pancreatic head during its passage from the superior mesenteric artery to the liver and give off branches to the pancreas. Also, the common hepatic artery may arise from the superior mesenteric artery and traverse the pancreas.[19] These anatomic variations are particularly important to define prior to pancreaticoduodenectomy or pancreatic resection.[20,21]

Gastroduodenal Artery

The gastroduodenal artery arises from the common hepatic artery in most cases but may take its origin from an aberrant right or left hepatic artery. It has a variable course in a caudal direction that depends largely on the degree of filling of the stomach and on the size and position of the liver and gallbladder.

Pancreaticoduodenal Arcades

The pancreaticoduodenal arcades are represented by the superior and inferior pancreaticoduodenal arteries with wide interconnections via posterior and anterior branches forming single or double arcades on the

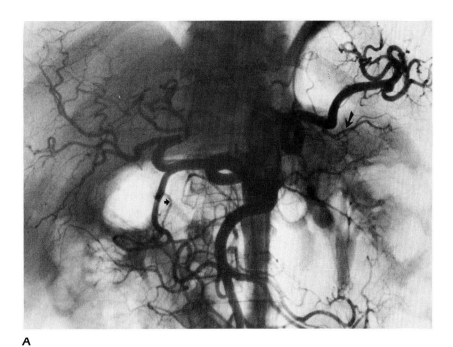

A

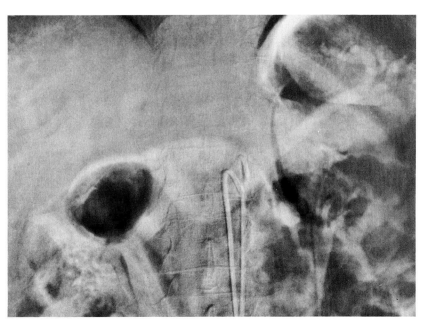

B

Figure 55-2. Normal pancreas. Simultaneous injection of contrast medium into celiac and superior mesenteric arteries. Arterial (A) and venous (B, subtraction) phase in frontal projection without drugs; in right posterior oblique projection (C and D) after injection of 25 mg tolazoline into the superior mesenteric artery. The superior mesenteric vein is best observed in the latter series. All pancreatic arteries are demonstrated by these two series but are far better outlined after injection of contrast medium into the gastroduodenal artery (E, subtraction). The catheter deforms the gastroduodenal artery. Observe the increased width of the pancreatic arteries with the exception of the superior posterior pancreaticoduodenal artery (*short arrow*, E, A). This artery is not distended because the tip of the catheter is positioned distal to the origin. The transverse pancreatic artery (*long arrowhead*, E) arises from the gastroduodenal artery and communicates with the dorsal pancreatic artery (*short arrowhead*, E) and the artery of the pancreatic tail. The pancreatic magna artery (*long arrow*, E) is observed only at celiac injection (A–C).

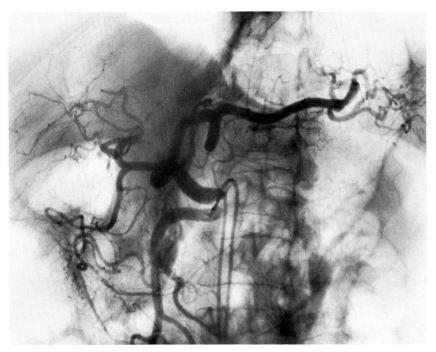

C

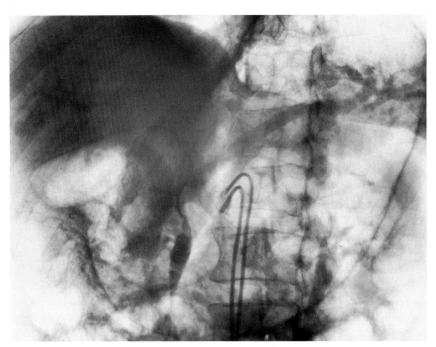

D   **Figure 55-2** (continued).

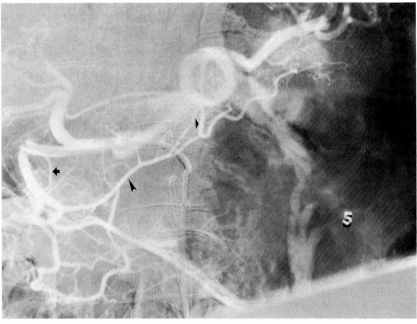

E   **Figure 55-2** (continued).

posterior and anterior aspects of the pancreas. The superior arteries arise separately from the gastroduodenal artery; the posterior artery is consistently the first branch, and the anterior artery arises a few centimeters further distally. The inferior arteries arise as a common branch directly from the posterior aspect of the superior mesenteric artery or, more often, from the first branch of the jejunal artery passing behind the superior mesenteric artery (see Fig. 55-4).

Arterial anastomoses between the pancreaticoduodenal arteries and the dorsal pancreatic artery are regularly observed. Often, direct anastomoses with the transverse pancreatic artery are also noted (Fig. 55-5; see also Fig. 55-2).

Dorsal Pancreatic Artery

The dorsal pancreatic artery usually arises from the hepatic or splenic artery, but an origin from the superior mesenteric artery is not uncommon. Branches to the uncinate process and the superior pancreaticoduodenal arteries are frequently observed. The transverse pancreatic artery usually takes its origin from this vessel (see Figs. 55-3 through 55-5). Wide communication with the superior mesenteric artery is sometimes shown. The middle colic or left colic arteries may originate from the dorsal pancreatic artery.

Transverse Pancreatic Artery

Although not regularly observed, probably because it is too small,[13] the transverse pancreatic artery usually originates from the dorsal pancreatic artery. Other common origins are from the superior mesenteric or the gastroduodenal artery. When arising from the latter, the vessel may be wide and may not anastomose with arteries in the tail of the pancreas coming from the splenic artery. This feature is important to note when a right-sided pancreatic resection is contemplated.[17]

Splenic Branches to the Body and Tail of the Pancreas

These branches vary in appearance and are often the most difficult to define on the angiogram. Usually the largest one is called the *pancreatic magna artery* (see Fig. 55-2). In addition, numerous small branches originate from the splenic artery. They run in a more or less vertical direction and can be the only vessels demonstrated to the left part of the body and the tail of the pancreas. One more constant branch is the caudal pancreatic artery, which arises from the splenic artery in the hilus of the spleen or from the left gastroepiploic artery.

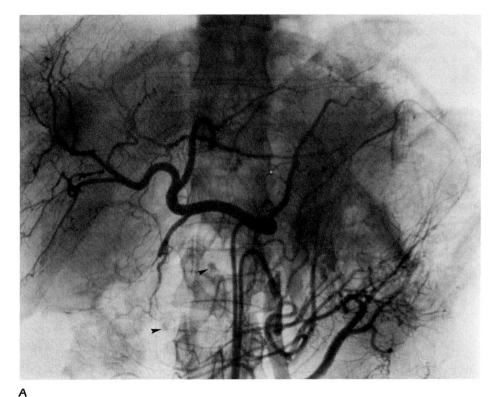

A

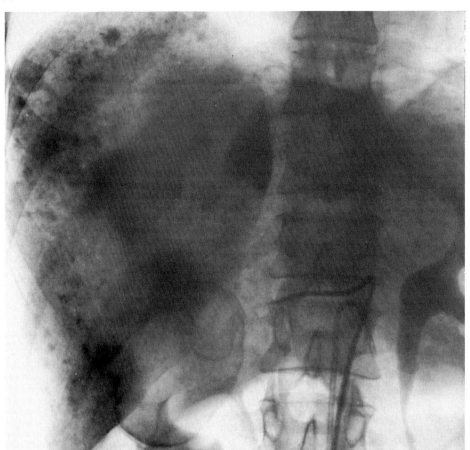

B

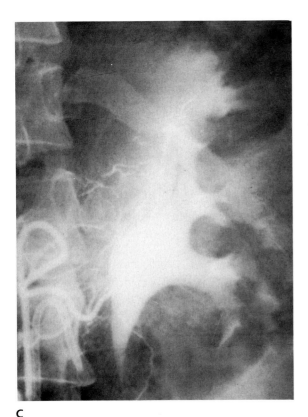

C

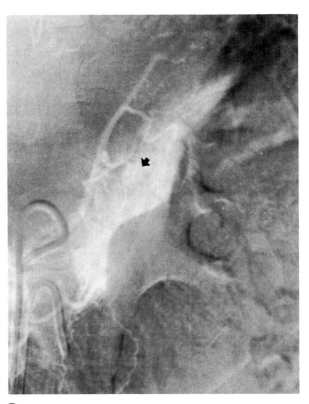

D

Figure 55-3. Multiple malignant gastrinomas in the pancreas and hepatic metastases in a patient with previous operation for hyperparathyroidism and the Zollinger-Ellison syndrome. Gastrectomy, splenectomy, and enucleation of a gastrinoma in the head of the pancreas had been performed previously. At celiac and superior mesenteric angiography (A) two 4-mm tumors (*arrowheads*) are observed in the head of the pancreas, and one 6-mm tumor was suspected in the tail of the pancreas (*arrow*). The richly vascularized small hepatic metastases were not observed until hepatic artery injection of contrast medium was performed (B). Selective injection of contrast medium into the dorsal pancreatic artery (C and D) shows that the transverse pancreatic and small pancreatic tail arteries communicate with the small splenic artery, and in late arterial phase a small tumor in the tail of the pancreas is verified (*arrow*, D).

Superior Mesenteric Artery

The superior mesenteric artery arises from the aorta posterior to the body of the pancreas. Its first part is usually not shown with the commonly employed angiographic procedures because of its course, which is almost perpendicular to the central ray. For complete information a lateral view is necessary (see Fig. 55-4).

Veins

The pancreatic veins are normally not observed at celiac and superior mesenteric angiography. Because veins adjacent to the pancreas are liable to change in pancreatic disease, the angiographic study should clearly demonstrate and outline the splenic, portal, and superior mesenteric veins (see Fig. 55-2). Pharmacoangiography is therefore recommended as an additional procedure to the more conventional celiac and superior mesenteric arteriogram.[22]

Technique

Various methods are recommended for pancreatic angiography. The original cutdown technique of the brachial artery, including antegrade catheterization of the splanchnic arteries,[2,23–25] has been replaced by the percutaneous femoral retrograde[1,3] or the axillary antegrade approach.[26,27]

The radiopaque polyethylene catheters introduced by Ödman for percutaneous use facilitated the procedure and reduced the complications.[4] The retrograde technique became the routine procedure and is still regarded as the method of choice. The technique of retrograde catheterization has not changed since the report in the first edition of this book, except for minor modifications (see Chapters 57 and 60 for a discussion of the technique of celiac arteriography). Boijsen and Olin[28] recommended using one of the renal arteries to reverse the tip of the catheter to enter the splanchnic

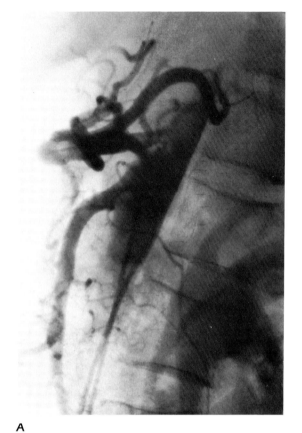

A

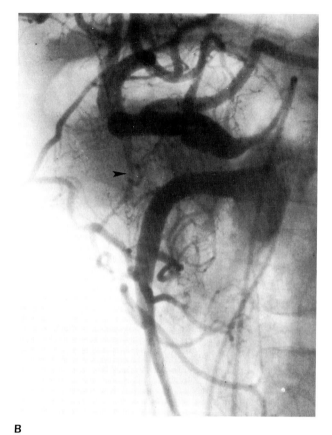

B

Figure 55-4. Lateral view of combined celiac and superior mesenteric arteries after 0.5 IU vasopressin (Pitressin) and then 20 ml of contrast medium were selectively injected into each artery. (A) Normal course of vessels in a thin patient. (B) Stenosis of celiac axis at origin by atherosclerosis. Infiltration of gastroduodenal artery (*arrowhead*) by carcinoma of the head of the pancreas. (C) Infiltration of the celiac and superior mesenteric arteries by carcinoma of the body of the pancreas. Observe that the inferior pancreaticoduodenal arcade arises from the posterior aspect of the superior mesenteric artery.

C

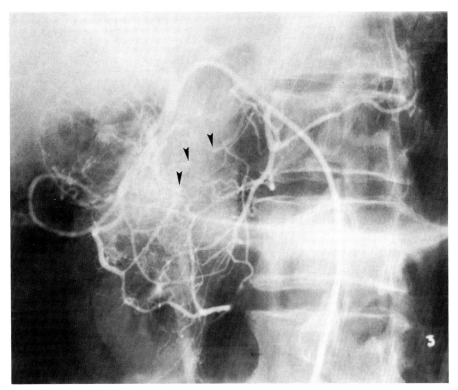

Figure 55-5. Gastroduodenal angiography in a patient with carcinoma of the head of the pancreas causing jaundice and intra- and extrahepatic bile duct dilatation. At operation the tumor was believed to have a diameter of about 5 cm, but pathologic examination of specimen proved the tumor to have a diameter of less than 1 cm. Angiography reveals several abrupt arterial occlusions within a small area (*arrowheads*), the site of the tumor. Marked hypervascularization around the tumor is a secondary reaction due to ductal obstruction. Dorsal and transverse pancreatic arteries communicate with anterior superior arcades.

arteries when direct catheterization proved difficult. It has been shown on dogs that the reversal of the catheter in the renal arteries involves an increased risk of aortic or renal intimal lesions and subintimal bleeding with possible consequent renal infarctions.[29] The original technique recommended by Ödman caused the same complications to a lesser degree except that no renal complications were observed.[3] The aortic intima of the dog as well as that of young patients is more vulnerable than the aortic wall in patients with atherosclerosis. Because the problems of splanchnic artery catheterization occur in the older age group, the risks with the reversal technique using the renal arteries seem small. Although no complications of this kind have been observed in vivo, the increased risk should be recognized during angiography.

To reduce the complication rate, a smaller catheter than that originally recommended by Ödman should be used. With the development of image amplification, thin-walled catheters are now recommended.

Simultaneous and Sequential Approaches

Because the pancreas is supplied from both celiac and superior mesenteric arteries, most authors agree that angiography of both arteries should be performed. The use of two catheters, previously introduced through bilateral femoral artery punctures with injection of contrast medium simultaneously into the celiac and superior mesenteric arteries through a Y connection, has been recommended.[13,28,30–32] Nevertheless, most authors prefer sequential catheterization of the arteries with one catheter.[33–37] Proponents of the sequential technique suggest that there is less trauma to the femoral arteries because only one vessel is punctured and that the delineation is better because there are fewer superimposed contrast-filled arteries in the pancreatic area. Gastric insufflation,[3,13] stereoscopic filming, and vasoconstrictive drugs, however, reduce these problems when the simultaneous technique is employed.[38] Both methods are acceptable and should be regarded as screening procedures.

Routine Technique

As mentioned previously, there are many variations in the routine technique, depending on the policy of the institution and the experience of the angiographer. But the routine technique also varies with indications, which have changed over the years. Angiography is today seldom used as a diagnostic method because ultrasonography, CT, MRI, percutaneous transhepatic cholangiography (PTC), and ERCP have high diagnostic accuracy in pancreatic disease. One or several of these methods should be used before angiography is contemplated. During the last few years, duplex and/or color Doppler, bolus-dynamic CT, and MR angiography (MRA) have improved to such an extent that also the large vessels around the pancreas can be observed, further reducing the indications for pancreatic angiography.[39–44] It is therefore only in exceptional cases that the superselective technique is required, as in patients suspected of having islet cell tumors of the pancreas. This does not mean that the quality of the angiographic examination should be inferior; it means that the procedure can be carried out faster and with fewer complications.

Anteroposterior (AP) Projection

With the simultaneous technique, a total of 60 ml of contrast medium containing 300 to 350 mg iodine/ml is injected at a rate of 20 ml per second simultaneously into the celiac and superior mesenteric arteries (30 ml at a rate of 10 ml/sec into each artery). Exposures are made at a rate of two per second for 5 seconds, one per second for 5 seconds, and then one every other second for 10 seconds (10/5, 5/5, 5/10) (see Fig. 55-2A and B).

Right Posterior Oblique (RPO) Projection

A second series always follows in the RPO projection after injection of a vasodilating substance into the superior mesenteric artery (bradykinin 5–10 μg[22]; tolazoline 25–50 mg[45]); 80 to 100 ml of the contrast medium is injected simultaneously at a rate of 25 ml per second (10/5, 10/20). The patient is turned only slightly to the right in order to have maximum information on the venous system (see Fig. 55-2C and D).

If the expected information is obtained with the AP and RPO views, no further injections are made and the examination is concluded. On the other hand, if the information is not in agreement with other diagnostic data or if there is clinical reason to suspect an islet cell tumor, or if the two series mentioned give incomplete or inadequate information, pharmacoangiographic methods and/or superselective angiography should be employed at the same time.

Pharmacoangiography

Vasoconstricting Drugs

Injection of small doses of vasoconstrictors into the celiac and superior mesenteric arteries before the injection of contrast medium will usually improve the visualization of the pancreatic arteries. Epinephrine (5–10 μg), norepinephrine (5–10 μg), and vasopressin (0.5–1.0 IU) are those most extensively used.[38,46–50] These drugs, when injected intraarterially in small doses, cause a marked constriction of all splanchnic arteries, but the effect is different on different vascular beds, and the main stems of the celiac and superior mesenteric arteries are not influenced. Thus the pancreatic vasculature reacts less than the gastric and splenic vasculatures. The density of the contrast medium therefore increases in the pancreatic arteries, and previously superimposed gastric arteries are eliminated. Because of the higher density of the contrast medium in the arteries and probably also because neoplastic and collateral vessels do not constrict, the scanty tumor vessels of pancreatic carcinoma or the collateral arteries around infiltrated or occluded arteries are better observed (Fig. 55-6). In patients with obstructive jaundice a reverse flow is often observed in the gastroduodenal artery because of an increased arterial supply to the liver. Regular celiac angiography will then not fill the pancreaticoduodenal arteries (see Fig. 55-6). Arterial collaterals are not affected by the vasoconstrictive drug; therefore, far better demonstration of the pancreatic arteries is obtained in those cases after injection of vasoconstrictors.

Because of the improvement in angiographic technique (superselectivity, magnification), pharmacoangiography is now rarely performed to obtain diagnostic information about the pancreas. However, vasoconstrictors are often of great support in the evaluation of the first parts of the celiac and superior mesenteric arteries in a lateral view (see Fig. 55-4). This method is used in patients with an angiographically normal pancreas who have upper abdominal pain but otherwise normal pancreatic tests. Stenosis or infiltration of the arteries is best observed in this view, which therefore may show that the cause of the upper abdominal pain is abdominal angina.

Vasodilating Drugs

Experimental and in vivo angiographic studies have been performed after intraarterial injection of vasodilating substances employed to increase pancreatic blood flow and enhance the accumulation of contrast medium in the pancreas. Priscoline, bradykinin, papaverine, trypsin, histamine, acetylcholine, secretin, and cholecystokinin have given somewhat varying results

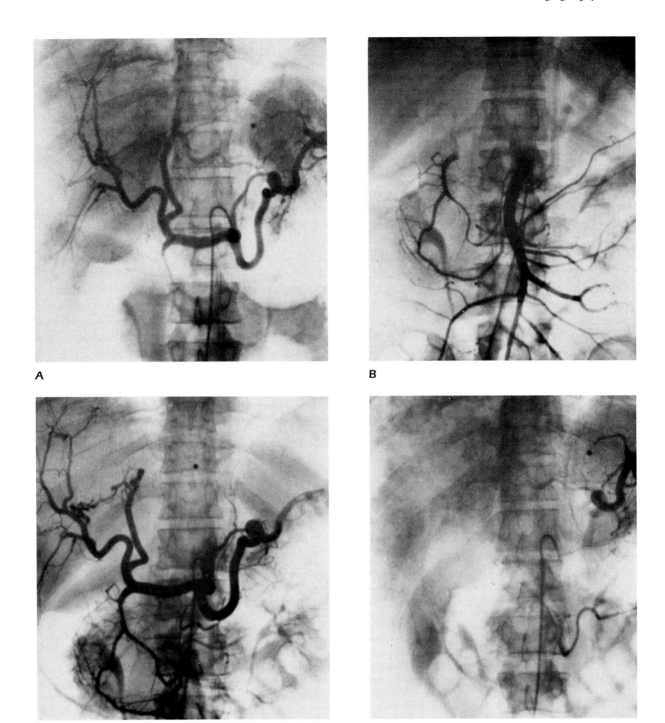

A

B

C

D

Figure 55-6. Cystic carcinoma of the head of the pancreas with nodular lesions within the liver proved to be abscesses. (A and B) Sequential celiac and superior mesenteric angiography performed without any previous drug. (C and D) Celiac angiography after 1 IU of vasopressin was injected. Increased vascular supply of the liver secondary to bile stasis and abscesses caused a reversal of flow in the gastroduodenal artery; tumor of the head of the pancreas was therefore not demonstrated in the control study. Decreased flow in the hepatic artery after injection of vasopressin permitted complete filling of gastroduodenal and pancreatic arteries, and the tumor is well demonstrated. Displacement of pancreatic arteries and tumor vessels is observed, but there is no infiltration of the arteries. In the capillary phase abscess formation was demonstrated after vasopressin injection (D) but not in the control study. At superior mesenteric angiography, the tumor is demonstrated by reverse flow through the pancreaticoduodenal arteries (B).

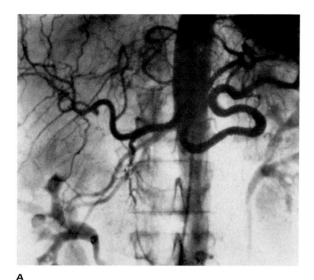

A

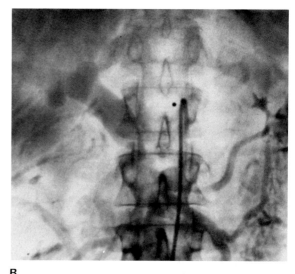

B

Figure 55-7. (A) Carcinoma of the head of the pancreas. At celiac angiography the gastroduodenal, superior anterior, and posterior pancreaticoduodenal arteries and the first part of the gastroepiploic artery are seen to be infiltrated by tumor. Abnormal tumor vessels. (B) Venous phase of superior mesenteric angiography. Compression of the vein at the level of the tumor is demonstrated. The high density of the contrast medium in the vein was obtained by injecting 10 μg of bradykinin immediately before the contrast medium injection.

in terms of their usefulness for demonstrating the pancreas and pancreatic lesions.[5,22,51–59] So far the most promising results have been obtained with secretin injected in high doses intraarterially or intravenously, but the results are not consistent. Injection of these substances in the superior mesenteric artery increases the circulation through the bowel and results in better filling of the superior mesenteric vein (Fig. 55-7; see also Fig. 55-2). In this respect bradykinin, tolazoline, secretin, prostaglandin E_1 and F_2-alpha have been found useful without causing any complications.[22,45,57,60,61] For angiographic demonstration of the splenic vein, an increased dose of contrast medium in the celiac artery is usually sufficient,[34,62] but it has been shown that a combination of alpha-blocking and beta-stimulating drugs improves opacification of the portal venous system.[63] From a diagnostic point of view, superselective injection of tolazoline has been found to give the best information about the pancreas and its arteries.[64,65]

Combined Vasodilating and Vasoconstricting Drugs

A combination of vasodilating and vasoconstricting drugs has also been tested with good results, from a diagnostic point of view, in celiac angiography. Thus Udén[66] combined secretin and epinephrine and improved the technical quality.

Superselective Angiography

Superselective pancreatic angiography is a selective catheterization of splenic, common hepatic, gastroduodenal, or separate pancreatic arteries. In 1958 Morino et al.,[67] using the cutdown brachial antegrade technique, demonstrated its great potential. Later investigations[27,34,62,64,65,68–81] have proved that better information is obtained about the pancreatic vasculature with this technique. Reuter[71] showed in a large series that this technique can be performed consistently with relative ease, is safe, and adds minimally to the time required for conventional pancreatic angiography. The method should first of all not be used if the conventional technique has shown a pancreatic abnormality, unless there is an islet cell tumor. In the latter case, more than one endocrine tumor may be present, and therefore superselective angiography should be performed (see Fig. 55-3). Superselectivity does indeed increase accuracy in the diagnosis of pancreatic carcinoma to more than 94 percent.[64,77,79] Pharmacoangiography increases information about pancreatic vasculature, and so does magnification technique.[64,65,77,80,81] Because of its high resolution, the magnification technique can in fact replace the superselective one in most instances[82] (Fig. 55-8). No doubt, in experienced hands the superselective technique is a satisfactory method, but often the examination time and conse-

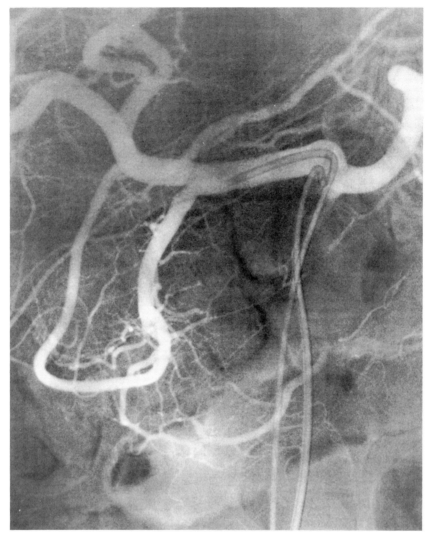

Figure 55-8. Carcinoma of the head of the pancreas. Magnification angiography shows infiltration and abrupt occlusion of branches of the posterosuperior pancreaticoduodenal artery.

quently the complications are unduly high with this technique. It is therefore recommended only on specific indications, as in patients with endocrine tumors. It should also be stated that a normal pancreatic angiogram of the highest quality does not rule out a pancreatic lesion.

To have complete filling of all pancreatic arteries, injection into gastroduodenal, dorsal pancreatic, and splenic arteries is required, but this is only occasionally feasible.[71] When it is impossible to reach the pancreatic arteries by superselective technique, modification of the pancreatic blood flow may be obtained by balloon catheters with consequent improvement in the density of the pancreatic arteries.[83] Further developments in guidewires and catheters have made catheterization of

small arterial branches easier and less traumatic. The catheters are thinner (outer diameter 1.4–1.7 mm) and more flexible. The guidewires are smaller and more flexible and yet have better torque control.[84-86] The digital radiographic technique with "road-mapping" and DSA has completely replaced the conventional amplification fluoroscopy and the full-sized film changers.[87-89] Because of the increased contrast resolution with DSA, increased information is also obtained in small vascular lesions such as islet cell tumors.[90,91]

Contrast Material and Filming

The amount and type of contrast medium used for pancreatic angiography vary. The most commonly used medium has been a sodium methylglucamine salt of diatrizoate, metrizoate, or iothalamate acid, administered in a 76 percent solution when given into main stems. These high-osmolar contrast agents have been almost completely replaced by the low-osmolar ionic (ioxaglate) or nonionic (iohexol, iopamidol) contrast media because they have a lower general toxicity and cause less reaction during injection. The medium amount and injection rates used in conventional technique are the same as for the high-osmolar media but are reduced for superselective techniques. In DSA, contrast medium is injected at a lower dose and in lower concentration. The amount and rate of contrast medium injection in specific pharmacoangiographic studies, superselective studies, or combinations thereof, vary. There is a tendency to use larger amounts and higher rates because no complications caused by the contrast medium per se have been observed. The total amount of about 300 ml of contrast medium is well tolerated by an adult patient who is well hydrated and has normal renal function.[92] The procedure usually takes about 1 hour. If the procedure is prolonged, up to 500 ml can be used.[64]

The film series should cover the various phases of the angiogram. The transit of the contrast medium through the arteries to the capillary bed should be followed at a rate of two frames per second unless the circulation is slowed down by a vasoconstrictor or balloon. The appearance of contrast in the portal system varies, and therefore the whole series must cover about 20 seconds; during the capillary phase one frame per second is adequate, followed later by one frame every other second. The pancreatic veins are sometimes observed after administration of secretin or a combination of secretin and epinephrine in celiac angiography[52,66] but are even better observed after administration of secretin in superselective angiography.[64] In most cases the main interest is to image the maximum density of the portal venous system, which will be obtained after vasodilating drugs have been given according to the regimen previously mentioned.

Complications

Acute pancreatitis has been observed after injection of contrast medium at translumbar aortography.[93,94] The contrast media used were more toxic than those now employed and were the probable cause of this complication. Dogs with normal pancreases and with experimentally induced pancreatitis were found not to have any histopathologic changes after contrast medium injection into the celiac axis and superior mesenteric artery.[29] The amounts and concentration of medium

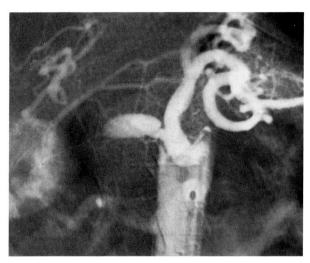

Figure 55-9. Subintimal dissection of the common hepatic artery after attempts to catheterize the vessel. Collateral circulation to the liver is observed via the left gastric artery.

were comparable to those used in vivo. Extensive experience with pancreatic angiography gives the same impression that the method does not cause any complications as far as the pancreas is concerned. At first there was some hesitance at the superselective injection of pancreatic arteries, but later experience showed that even 20 to 50 ml of contrast medium may be injected at a high rate (up to 10 ml/sec), especially after vasodilation with tolazoline (12.5 mg).

Intimal and subintimal lesions in the aorta and the visceral arteries can be kept at a minimum with adequate technique.[71] However, in a prospective study of a consecutive series such lesions were found to occur more often than expected.[95,96] Nevertheless, they are rarely of any significance within the branches of the celiac artery because of the collateral circulation (Fig. 55-9).

Complications at the puncture site are unusual with good technique and with the small catheters recommended.

Angiography in Pancreatic Disease

Pancreatic Carcinoma

Diagnosis

Selective angiography in carcinoma of the pancreas (Fig. 55-10; see also Figs. 55-4 through 55-8) became a frequently used method soon after the new technique with radiopaque catheters became established.[3]

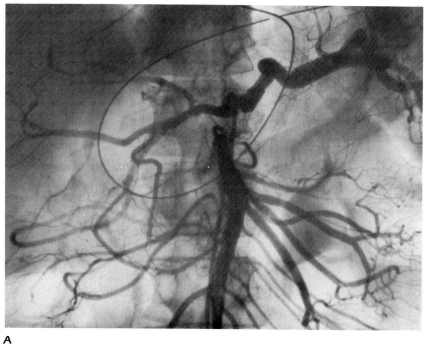

A

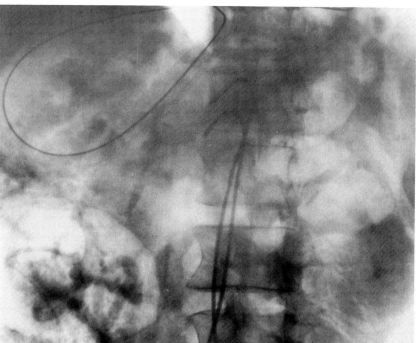

B

Figure 55-10. (A) Inoperable carcinoma of the body of the pancreas with typical infiltration of the common hepatic, splenic, and superior mesenteric arteries observed in simultaneous celiac and superior mesenteric angiography. Infiltration of celiac and superior mesenteric arteries is best ob-served in lateral projection (see Fig. 55-4C). (B) In the venous phase, after administration of tolazoline, occlusion of superior mesenteric, splenic, and portal veins is observed with collateral circulation to the intrahepatic portal system via the veins of the gallbladder and stomach.

In the following years a few case reports appeared on the angiographic findings[28,97–101] but it was not until 1965 that the real breakthrough occurred. Lunderquist[13] presented a series of 26 patients with pancreatic carcinoma who had had angiography with the simultaneous technique. Abnormal angiograms were observed in retrospect in 92 percent of the cases. Numerous reports during the next decade dealt with various aspects of diagnostic importance in angiography of pancreatic carcinoma.[15,26,27,32,34–36,78,79,102–120]

During this period the superselective technique for diagnosis of pancreatic carcinoma was developed and proved to be a remarkable improvement in the diagnosis of this lesion,[64,65,68,70,77–79] as was pharmacoangiography, with special emphasis on arterial and venous contrast medium enhancement.[33,38,45,47,55] At the same time the value of angiography as a method for predicting resectability and prognosis increased.[121–127] Although some negative reports on the accuracy of pancreatic angiography as a method for diagnosis of pancreatic carcinoma were published in the first years of this period, it became apparent that experience and high quality gave a sensitivity better than what Lunderquist reported in his retrospective analysis.[64,77,79,126] It is not to be inferred that routine preoperative angiography in pancreatic disease reached these high levels of accuracy in all institutions. In a review of preoperative reports in 116 patients with pancreatic carcinoma, Tylén[118] found a correct diagnosis noted in 68 percent. Mackie et al.[20] found a sensitivity of 72 percent and a specificity of 71 percent in a series of 103 patients, including 40 with carcinoma. The high rate of false-positive findings in their material was due partly to the fact that periampullary and other tumors were included as false-positive results, a procedure that is not usually followed. Nevertheless, false-positive diagnoses of pancreatic carcinoma are not rare and result mainly from misinterpretation of vascular changes caused by pancreatitis or pseudocysts.[128,129]

In the middle of the 1970s, new diagnostic methods reduced the importance of angiography as a diagnostic tool. It is true that the combination of angiography and other diagnostic methods (PTC, cytology, pancreatic function tests, pancreatic scintigraphy) were used before this time.[130–133] ERCP became the first serious alternative to angiography, but in most reports where both methods were used it became obvious that ERCP and angiography were complementary.[134–138] To rely entirely on ERCP as a way to diagnose pancreatic carcinoma seemed impossible after a study of observer variation and error in interpretation of the pancreatogram.[139] By the end of the 1970s and during the following few years ERCP and the noninvasive imaging methods were compared with angiography,

most often in retrospective studies, but a number of controlled and prospective evaluations were also performed to test the "new" methods in patients with pancreatic carcinoma.[80,81,128,140–145] Ultrasonography and ERCP were found to have a higher sensitivity than angiography, in both resectable and nonresectable carcinoma.[81] Soon, however, it became obvious that well-performed CT had a higher sensitivity than ultrasonography[141,145] and ERCP.[145] Therefore, during the 1980s CT became the most dominating and reliable method in patients with suspected pancreatic carcinoma. Thus Freeny et al.[146] found with incremental bolus-dynamic CT in a prospective series of 174 patients that a correct diagnosis of adenocarcinoma was made in 91 percent with only two false-negative diagnoses. Megibow[147] reported similar results and convincingly showed the importance of the new CT technology in the late 1980s compared with the technique in the early 1980s.

Despite the high accuracy of CT, ultrasonography is not outdated in pancreatic imaging. During the last decade, improvements in resolution as well as duplex and color Doppler imaging have increased the diagnostic accuracy of both parenchymal lesions and of peripancreatic extension. Particularly in patients with suspected obstructive jaundice, ultrasonography is the first imaging method because the etiology as well as the site of the obstruction can be reliably defined.[148] In those cases, ultrasonography will greatly support the CT findings, and a definite diagnosis is obtained if either of these methods is combined with fine-needle aspiration biopsy.[146,149,150]

MRI of pancreatic ductal carcinoma has continuously improved since 1982, when Smith et al.[151] first reported on the potentialities of this technique. Recent reports give the impression that MRI of the pancreas in carcinoma is as good or even better than CT in defining the mass lesion.[152–155] The technical advances with echo-planar MRI and with intravenous and oral contrast agents have further improved the information of the pancreatic parenchyma.[156–159]

A short stricture of the pancreatic duct observed on ERCP could be a benign stricture or a small ductal carcinoma.[137] Previously, angiography with a superselective technique and magnification could rule out the presence of a carcinoma, but today dynamic CT and MRI with contrast enhancement, short echo times, and fat suppression are the methods of choice for correct diagnosis.

The typical angiographic findings in a patient with pancreatic carcinoma are irregular stenosis or occlusions of arteries within or adjacent to the pancreas (see Figs. 55-5, 55-7, and 55-10). Stenoses of arteries adjacent to the pancreas may also be observed in athero-

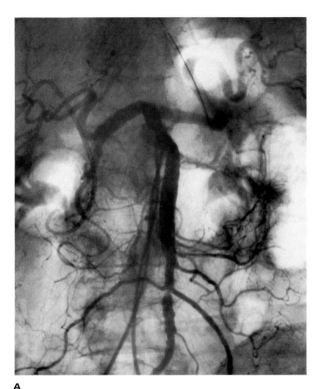

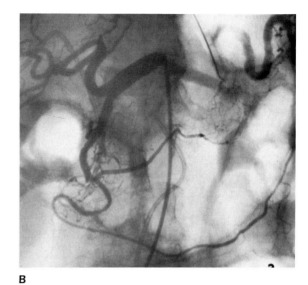

B

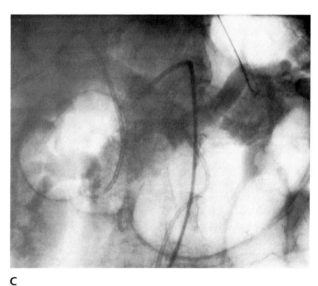

C

A

Figure 55-11. Arteritis or severe arteriosclerosis in splanchnic arteries in a 76-year-old patient with silent jaundice and known temporal arteritis. At PTC, stones were seen to be present in the common bile duct. Pancreatic angiography (A) reveals marked irregularities in the arteries surrounding the pancreas. The superior mesenteric artery is severely stenosed at its origin and in its distal part. (Drainage catheter in common bile duct after PTC.) Gastroduodenal angiography (B and C) also shows marked narrowing in small pancreatic arteries, and the pancreas is hypervascularized. The splenic and portal veins are intact.

sclerosis, chronic pancreatitis, arteritis, and fibromuscular dysplasia[17,36,160–162] (Fig. 55-11). These changes may simulate tumor encasement, but in atherosclerosis and chronic pancreatitis the arterial wall usually has a different appearance, with single-plaque formation in the former and a smooth outline in the latter. Nevertheless, these changes may at times be impossible to differentiate from carcinoma (Figs. 55-12 and 55-13).

Displacement of vessels in and around the pancreas may occur in carcinoma but usually cannot be appreciated because of the frequent congenital variations. When it is present, there will often be an abrupt change of direction different from the arc-shaped displacement observed in pancreatitis and other tumors. There are, however, exceptions to this rule (see Fig. 55-6).

Accumulation of contrast medium within the carci-

noma may occur but is not a reliable finding with current methods. On the contrary, in superselective pharmacoangiography, tumors of about 1 cm in diameter are observed as filling defects in the parenchyma, and often there are no vascular abnormalities at all. Tumor vessels have been observed in as many as 60 percent of the cases of pancreatic carcinoma.[13] These abnormal vessels are probably not of the same type as observed in richly vascularized malignancies like renal carcinoma. The scirrhous carcinoma is almost avascular and infiltrates or occludes vessels. The abnormal vessels observed are therefore probably infiltrated arteries or collateral arteries caused by occlusion. This situation may also explain the improved filling of these vessels after administration of vasoconstrictive drugs because collateral arteries are not influenced by vasoconstrictors.

Compression or occlusion of veins is commonly

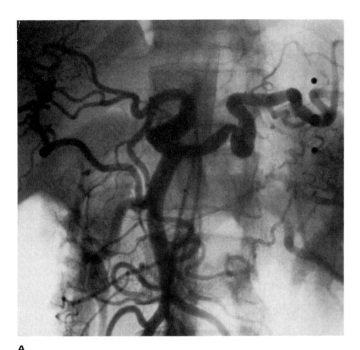
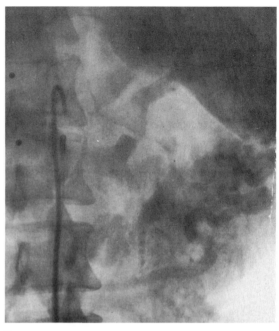

A **B**

Figure 55-12. (A) Chronic pancreatitis with marked irregular changes in splenic, transverse pancreatic, and middle colic arteries observed in arterial phase. (B) Venous phase showing splenic vein compressed by the tortuous splenic artery; collaterals noted over the gastroepiploic veins.

seen[115,163] and should, if present, be demonstrated by angiography (see Figs. 55-7 and 55-10).

Resectability and Operability

Extension beyond the capsule means that the tumor is not resectable. With high-quality angiographic technique, arterial wall changes close to the carcinoma, as well as in arteries surrounding the pancreas, will be detected earlier than with any other techniques.

With few exceptions,[20] it is agreed that if no vascular abnormalities are observed in a patient with pancreatic carcinoma there are good prognostic signs of resectability. Local resectability is particularly well defined by angiography, because smaller artery branches cannot be defined as well with any other method.[6,20,69,115,121,122,124,125,127,163] As has been pointed out by Suzuki et al.,[138] lesions that cause ductal abnormalities but have small or no vascular changes have a better prognosis for resectability because the lesions are in the center of the gland. Most of the pancreatic arteries we observe at routine angiography are located on the surface of the gland; thus if any of them are infiltrated, the carcinoma has probably passed through the capsule. Consequently, although only one of the pancreaticoduodenal arcades is infiltrated, the tumor may have passed the resectable stage, particularly if the

tumor is positioned on the posterior aspect of the head of the pancreas.[124,127] With increasing numbers of vessels infiltrated, the chance of resectability is decreased and, if the tumor is nevertheless resectable, the possibility of recurrence rises. Veins should always be well demonstrated. Even if the tumor can be resected when the mesenteric or portal veins are deformed by the tumor, the risk of recurrence is high. The possibility of predicting survival time from the angiographic findings has been another reason for showing the local extent of tumor by angiography.[123,125]

With noninvasive imaging, the tumor extension beyond the pancreatic capsule is noted as abnormalities in the fat and in vessels surrounding the pancreas.[39,43,44,146,147,149,164-169] The vascular inner wall is not observed as well as with angiography. On the other hand, perivascular adventitial changes of the celiac axis and superior mesenteric artery will be observed, and these will not necessarily deform the vessel lumen. Originally the periarterial cuff and the infiltrative changes in the fat were considered pathognomonic for pancreatic carcinoma at CT.[170] However, later analyses have shown that similar changes are also, but rarely, found in chronic pancreatitis[147,171,172] and in malignant lesions other than pancreatic engaging the lymph nodes.[173] Peripheral artery lesions of the common

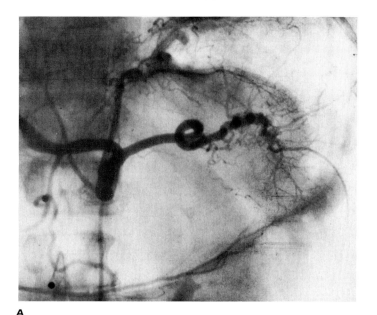

A

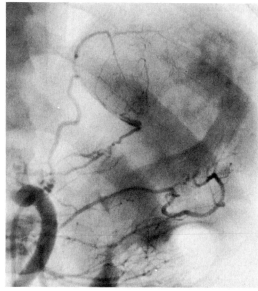

B

Figure 55-13. Chronic pancreatitis with pseudocyst in the tail of the pancreas with irregular stenoses and tortuosity of pancreatic and peripancreatic arteries noted at celiac (A) and superior mesenteric (B) angiography. The cyst extends lateral to the spleen, displacing the latter medially. Beading of the distal part of the splenic artery is observed.

hepatic and splenic arteries will be observed with MRA, and certainly venous abnormalities will be better observed with this technique (Fig. 55-14).

Because of the diagnostic information provided by noninvasive technology, there is hardly any advantage to performing angiography to prove the extension of a carcinoma beyond the capsule in a patient in whom high-quality dynamic CT has shown that a tumor is situated exclusively in the pancreas.[146,147]

Operability in a patient with proven pancreatic carcinoma depends partly on whether there are metastases in the liver. Noninvasive imaging is the preferred method, and thus there is no reason to perform hepatic angiography in pancreatic carcinoma.

The main indication for angiography in ductal carcinoma of the pancreas is preoperative "mapping" in those few cases who have resectable tumors and are considered operable. It is most important for the surgeon to know whether there is a vascular anomaly. This can of course be searched for during operation, but sometimes the pulsations in an accessory right hepatic artery passing over or through the head of the pancreas are impossible to palpate.[19,21] Some 25 percent of the patients have an anomaly of the celiac and superior mesenteric vessels, and in about 90 percent of these the arteries supplying the liver are involved. This is of importance because, as has been noted by Mackie et al.[20]: "In our experience ligation of a major

hepatic artery, in the presence of jaundice, uniformly leads to fatal hepatic necrosis." Also, in patients with complete celiac stenosis, ligation of collateral arteries of the superior mesenteric artery is hazardous.[6] With the development of duplex and color Doppler imaging and MRA, this last reason to perform conventional angiography (i.e., to exclude stenosis of the main stems) will be eliminated in attempted pancreatic resection.

Islet Cell Tumors

More than a hundred different peptides are produced and released from the neuroendocrine cell system, to which the islet cells of the pancreas belong along with cells in the pituitary, gastrointestinal tract, thyroid, adrenal medulla, lungs, urogenital tract, and carotid body. These endocrine cells are closely related to the autonomic nervous system in that amines and regulatory peptides are present and released from both nerves and endocrine cells. Tumors may arise from these cells and produce biogenic amines and regulatory peptides in excess of what is normal and cause a number of different syndromes. In tumors of the islet cells of the pancreas at least five different syndromes are recognized in which different hormones are produced: (1) the hypoglycemic syndrome (insulinoma); (2) the Zollinger-Ellison syndrome (gastrinoma); (3) the Verner-Morrison or watery diarrhea, hypokalemia,

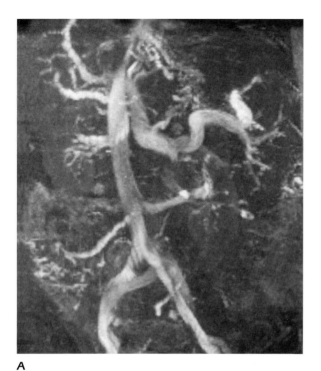

A

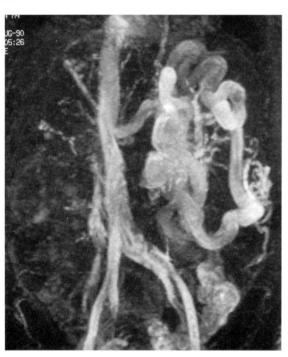

C

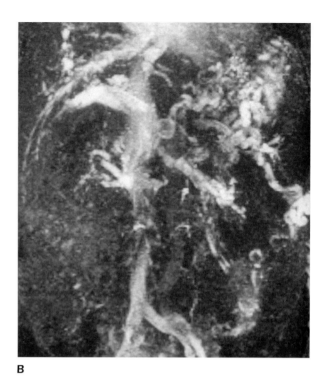

B

Figure 55-14. MR projection angiograms using gradient-echo pulse sequences based on time-of-flight effect and sequential two-dimensional technique. (A) Patent splenic and portal veins in a patient with cirrhosis, portal hypertension, and gastric varices. (B) Occlusion of the portal vein due to carcinoma of the head of the pancreas with mesenteric and hemorrhoidal venous collaterals. (C) Chronic pancreatitis with splenic vein thrombosis and venous collateral changes around the spleen. (Courtesy of Professor Dr. Med. Ingolf Arlart, Stuttgart, Germany.)

Endocrine tumors are slowly growing lesions that may transform to malignant neoplasms. The tumors of the islet cells may be single or multiple, and they may be associated with tumors in other parts of the neuroendocrine system (MEN-1-syndrome).

Islet cell tumors of the pancreas (see Figs. 55-14, 55-17, and 55-18) may produce hormones in excess of what is normally produced in islet cells of the adult pancreas (insulinoma, glucagonoma, somatostatinoma) or in glands in the fetal pancreas or in the gastrointestinal system (gastrinoma, VIPoma, carcinoids). The tumors may produce not only one hormone or peptide but several, and the produced peptides may not necessarily cause any specific symptoms.[174–180]

The clinical diagnosis of an active, hormone-producing islet cell tumor is made by radioimmunoassays of regulatory peptides, which are synthesized as large precursor molecules. These are cleaved to smaller active forms of metabolites by specific enzymes.[174] The clinical diagnosis is thus not primarily

achlorhydria (WDHA) syndrome (VIPoma); (4) the glucagonoma syndrome; and (5) the somatostatinoma syndrome. Diagnosis is made by measuring the regular peptides and amines in blood or urine. This is also the case with so-called nonfunctioning endocrine tumors, from which the produced peptides do not give rise to characteristic symptoms.[174]

based on radiologic imaging. When operation is contemplated, the radiologic investigation starts and the size, site, number, and extension of the lesion(s) are defined. The hormone-producing tumor may be very small (<5 mm). Sometimes no tumor can be observed, and then the condition is often called *diffuse hyperplasia* or *microadenomatosis*[181] (occult adenoma). A tumor may also be present in the wall of the duodenum as microgastrinoma.[182] Islet cell tumors may therefore be impossible to identify by any imaging method. Without previous identification it is a hopeless task for the surgeon to find the lesions, and, if one lesion is found, a second and third adenoma may be present in other sites. The recent use of intraoperative ultrasonography has improved the localization of islet cell tumors not detected preoperatively or by palpation during operation.[183,184]

Insulinoma and Gastrinoma

The symptoms caused by hypoglycemia and in the Zollinger-Ellison syndrome are produced by insulinoma and gastrinoma, respectively. These tumors are the most common and the smallest neoplasms of the endocrine pancreatic tumors. Therefore, when considering the detectability of hormone-producing pancreatic tumors with various imaging techniques, it is important to consider the insulinomas and gastrinomas separately from other tumors, which usually have reached a considerable size before they are examined with imaging methods.[91] Certain hormone-producing tumors reach a substantial size before symptoms are observed.

Real-time ultrasonography is usually the initial method to reveal hormone-producing islet cell tumors. However, the method has a rather low sensitivity (20 to 60 percent), depending on the size and the site of the tumor.[90,183–187] Preoperative localization with dynamic CT of insulinomas and gastrinomas has been obtained in 45 to 60 percent of cases, again depending on the size and site of the tumors.[90,91,183–187] The experience with MRI in islet cell tumors is not extensive enough to define its position. Frucht et al.[186] found that MRI had a low sensitivity in primary extrahepatic gastrinoma (20 percent) and a somewhat better sensitivity in metastatic liver gastrinoma (43 percent). MRI detected no tumors smaller than 1 cm. That MRI nevertheless has a potential in detecting insulinomas is exemplified in a case report by Mitchell et al.[188]: CT and angiography each detected one solitary lesion, whereas MRI with contrast enhancement revealed seven lesions in the pancreas.

Angiography of the pancreas is still the method of choice in patients supposed to have an endocrine neoplasm. Since 1963, when Olsson[189] reported on the first insulinoma detected at angiography, there has been a continuous debate regarding the detectability of insulinoma with this technique. Detection rates between 20 and 90 percent are on record.[90,91,183–187,190–200] The great differences observed both in sensitivity and specificity over the years depend on a number of factors. The frequency of small-sized tumors in the different materials is important, but the most decisive factor is the quality of the angiographic technique. Today, pancreatic angiography is not just celiac and superior mesenteric angiography. Selective techniques with injection of contrast medium into the common hepatic, splenic, gastroduodenal, dorsal pancreatic, and pancreaticoduodenal arteries should be attempted in all patients with islet cell tumors. DSA will probably further improve the accuracy[90,183] because it is particularly the local contrast enhancement that gives the correct information. Thus a meticulous angiographic technique and high-quality radiographs are prerequisites for adequate pancreatic angiography. Pharmacoangiography has been used[185,196] but is usually not necessary if adequate superselective technique is performed.[91,192,193,195,199] Magnification, if available, should be used.

The angiographic findings in a small (<2-cm) insulinoma or gastrinoma are a dense, well-delineated accumulation of contrast medium that can be observed a few seconds after the start of the injection of the contrast agent (Fig. 55-15). The accumulation of contrast medium increases for another 4 to 5 seconds and then slowly fades away. A tumor accumulation of contrast medium will usually be observed for about 15 seconds. Tumor vessels may be observed in these small tumors but are seen more often in larger lesions, which are usually malignant. Some of the insulomas are cystic, but contrast medium is accumulated in the wall.[90,181] Early-draining veins are frequent findings.

Differential diagnostic problems may occur. Thus, an accessory spleen,[192,201,202] metastatic nodes close to the pancreas,[201,203] bleeding into pancreatic pseudocysts,[201] or angioma of the pancreas[202–204] (Figs. 55-16 and 55-17) may simulate an insulinoma. Superselective injection into the splenic artery or pancreatic branches[192,205] may simulate an insulinoma of the tail of the pancreas.

The insulin- and gastrin-producing tumors have a similar angiographic appearance but a different localization. The insulinomas are almost exclusively found in the pancreas, and when malignant, richly vascularized metastases may be observed in the liver. The gastrinomas may be localized only to the pancreas, but just as often no tumor is found in the pancreas, but

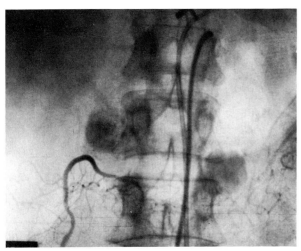

Figure 55-15. Two insulinomas, 1.5 and 2.0 cm in diameter, in the head and uncinate process of the pancreas, respectively. The latter was not seen or palpated during operation until incision of the parenchyma was made.

only richly vascularized small tumors are present in the liver or liver hilum. The gastrinomas may also be present in the duodenum or the gastric antrum and are then often very small.[182] At angiography they may be hidden by the accumulated contrast medium in the mucosa.[206] Previously pancreatic gastrinomas were considered more difficult to identify by angiography than insulinomas,[206–208] but this is not supported in recent studies.[91,185,186,192,202,203]

In the preoperative evaluation of endocrine pancreatic tumors hepatic angiography is always included because the richly vascularized metastases are particularly well observed with this technique.[186,187,209] It has been convincingly shown that a combination of noninvasive methods, including MRI and MRA, gives the best results in detecting both the primary endocrine tumors and the hepatic metastases.[90,91,185–187]

Despite the many imaging techniques, the very small (<15-mm) endocrine neoplasms are usually impossible to find (occult islet cell tumors), as mentioned previously. Percutaneous transhepatic catheterization of pancreatic veins and venous sampling for hormone assays will in these cases usually localize the small islet cell tumors (see Chapter 52). However, the technique is traumatic, and another method has recently proved successful and promising. Doppman et al.[210,211] selectively catheterized the hepatic, splenic, gastroduodenal, and superior mesenteric arteries. They injected secretin sequentially into these arteries in patients with gastrinoma and calcium in patients with insulinoma to stimulate increased production of the hormones. With the less traumatic catheterization of hepatic veins, they

Figure 55-16. Splenic angiography in a patient with Rendu-Osler-Weber disease. Multiple angiomatous lesions are present in the tail of the pancreas. Shunting to the splenic vein is noted (subtraction).

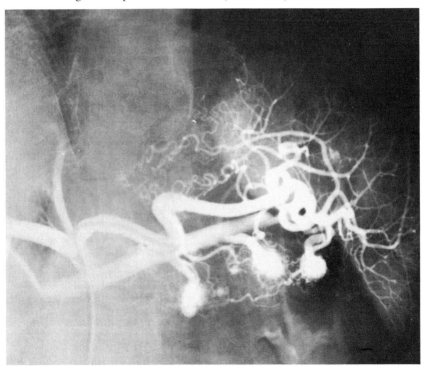

could register the increased levels of hormones and thereby locate the tumors.

Other Endocrine Pancreatic Tumors

VIPomas, glucagonomas, somatostatinomas, PP-omas, and carcinoid tumors are rare endocrine tumors that may cause syndromes.[177,179,212,213] They are often large and malignant and have the same rich vascular supply as the large malignant insulinomas.[176,214–218] They usually grow slowly and give symptoms late and therefore come for radiologic examination when they have a substantial size (Fig. 55-18). The inactive islet cell tumors (Fig. 55-19), which in some series represent close to 50 percent of all endocrine pancreatic tumors,[218] behave angiographically like the large hormone-producing tumors.[192,193,215,219–222] They also frequently grow through the pancreatic capsule and invade arteries and veins[222] in a way similar to adenocarcinoma. The hepatic metastases are richly vascularized, but the malignant tumors may be calcified and avascular.[219] Discrete and nodular calcifications in an islet cell tumor suggest malignancy.[223]

With the richly vascularized tumors, differentiation between cystadenoma and rare peritoneal tumors such as leiomyosarcoma is not always possible by angiographic technique.

Cystic Neoplasms

Cystic tumors of the pancreas are rare. The main types are serous cystadenoma and the mucin-containing tumor. With noninvasive imaging more of these lesions

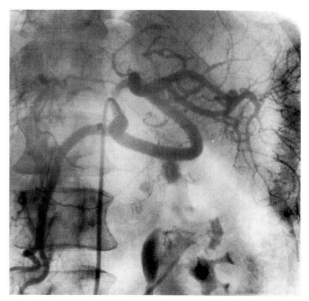

Figure 55-17. Metastases of a renal carcinoma to the tail of the pancreas.

are observed today than previously.[224] The serous cystadenoma or microcystic adenoma is built up of a large number of small cysts, whereas the mucinous tumor consists of only one or a few large cysts (>3 cm). Whereas the microcystic neoplasms are always benign, the slow-growing mucinous tumors are both benign and malignant. The chance of the tumor being malignant increases with its size. In verified series the benign mucinous cystadenomas dominate.[225]

Benign as well as malignant cystic neoplasms have a rich or moderate vascular supply with neovascularity

Figure 55-18. Arterial (A) and late arterial (B) angiography of a moderately vascularized glucagonoma with a diameter of 3 cm in the tail of the pancreas. Adjacent to the tumor is an accessory spleen (*arrowheads,* B).

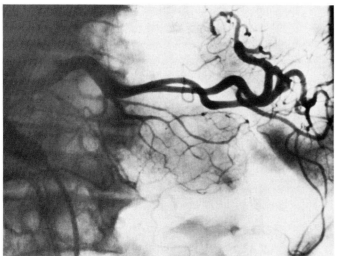

A

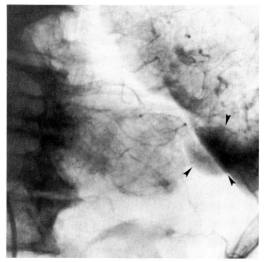

B

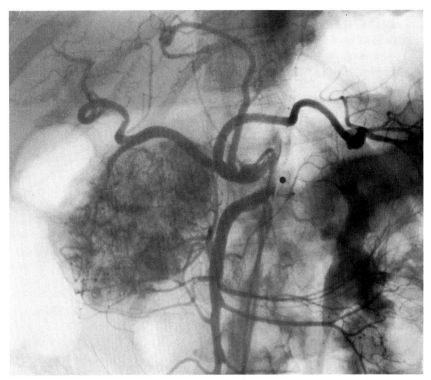

Figure 55-19. Nonactive malignant insulinoma of the head of the pancreas. The highly vascularized, well-circumscribed, large tumor is a characteristic finding.

and irregular contrast accumulation in the tumor at angiography (Figs. 55-6, 55-20, and 55-21).[225-228] If malignant, arteries as well as veins may be observed infiltrated or occluded by the tumor. Otherwise it is not possible to distinguish by angiography whether the neoplasm is benign or malignant unless metastases are observed. Irregular uptake of the contrast medium, which is often observed, causes a heterogeneous appearance of the tumor corresponding to the cystic and solid tissue components in the tumor. Compression or occlusion of the portal venous system is often noticed. This type of lesion may be difficult or impossible to distinguish from nonactive endocrine tumors of the pancreas or leiomyosarcoma originating in or infiltrating the gland.

A low grade of vascularization has been observed in benign tumors[227] as well as in cystadenocarcinomas.[224,227] In this situation the tumors will be difficult to distinguish from pancreatic pseudocysts or even cystic adenocarcinoma (see Figs. 55-6 and 55-21). Ultrasonography or CT including biopsy will, however, give the necessary information about the lesion. Cystic islet tumors are rare, but a cystic transformation has been observed both in insulinomas and gastrinomas.[90,181]

Uncommon Tumors

Angiomatous lesions of different types occur in the pancreas: telangiectasia of the hereditary type as a manifestation of Rendu-Osler-Weber disease, true hemangiomas, or an unspecific type of angiodysplasia.[35,137,202,204,229-233] From a differential point of view these lesions, when small and well circumscribed, may have an appearance similar to that of an insulinoma, but the draining veins are observed earlier and better in the angiomatous lesions (see Fig. 55-16). In their more diffuse form the lesions may resemble the hypervascular types of pancreatitis.[234-236]

Leiomyosarcoma,[28,225] reticulum cell sarcoma,[237-239] and other retroperitoneal tumors[14,34] may invade the pancreas and cause angiographic abnormalities. Primary pancreatic lymphoma with a local or diffuse mass may be associated with local adenopathy. At angiography some of these tumors may simulate cystadenocarcinoma; at other times they infiltrate arteries as in adenocarcinoma. Usually, however, they cause more prominent changes than the scirrhous ductal carcinoma. Also, invasion from gastric cancer[35,240] or metastatic nodes[112,241] may produce abnormalities, as in

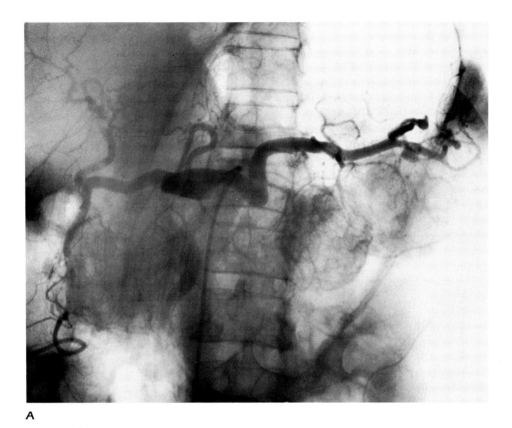

A

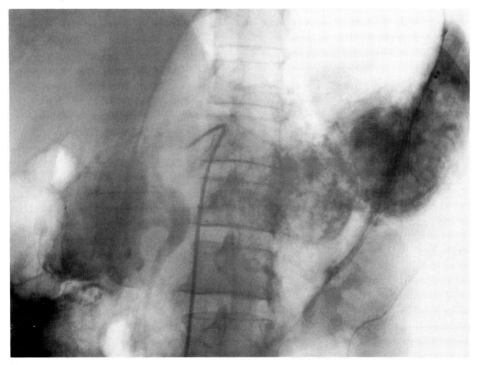

B

Figure 55-20. (A and B) Multiple benign cystadenomas of the pancreas. At celiac angiography multiple richly vascularized tumors with cystic components are found in the body and tail of the pancreas. Additional tumors were present in the head and body of the pancreas, supplied from the common hepatic and superior mesenteric arteries.

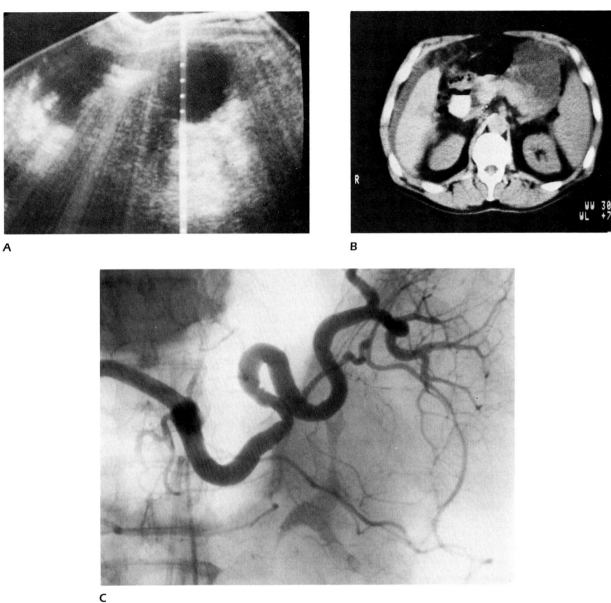

A

B

C

Figure 55-21. (A) Palpable mass thought to represent a pancreatic pseudocyst at ultrasonography. (B) CT proved the lesion to have an irregular attachment to the tail of the pancreas. (C) At celiac angiography a poorly vascularized lesion was observed. The splenic artery has a local constriction. Percutaneous biopsy verified a malignant lesion, which proved to be a cystadenocarcinoma.

ductal cancer. Lymphomatous abnormalities usually cause only displacement of vessels.[237,238] The combination of ultrasonography or CT and biopsy has made angiography less important in the diagnosis of these lesions.[242,243]

Pancreatitis

By the end of the 1970s angiography was replaced by ERCP, ultrasonography, and CT but was still regarded as a valuable method in the diagnosis of pancreatitis (Figs. 55-22 through 55-26; see also Figs. 55-12 and 55-13) when characteristic, although not pathognomonic, abnormalities could be observed in the pancreatic vasculature. These vascular abnormalities occurred often in both acute and chronic pancreatitis but were most prominent in patients who had had the disease for more than 2 years.[244,245] Particularly ERCP, but also ultrasonography, CT, and MRI have since then drastically reduced the indications for angiography in pancreatitis and its sequelae. Nevertheless, there is still reason to be aware of the vascular changes that can be observed. Destruction of vessel walls by pancreatic enzymes with secondary hemorrhage or thrombosis cannot always be detected with the noninvasive imaging methods. It is therefore important to be aware of the detailed information that can be obtained by the high-resolution angiographic technique.

Acute Pancreatitis

In the uncomplicated form of acute pancreatitis the angiogram usually appears normal, but a widening and stretching of the pancreatic arteries due to edema may be observed.[244-246] If angiography is performed after the acute attack has subsided, tortuosity and arterial irregularities may be seen as well as venous compression or occlusion.[245] Also, aneurysms of the splenic or gastroduodenal arteries have been observed after an acute attack of pancreatitis.

In the severe forms of acute pancreatitis (i.e., pancreatic necrosis and infected pancreatic necrosis), the extent of the lesion can be determined with bolus-dynamic CT because areas of necrosis fail to enhance.[247] Angiography is not performed in this severe form of pancreatitis unless life-threatening hemorrhage is present, and then only to embolize vessels[40,248] in patients who do not require emergency surgery.

Most cases of acute pancreatitis, excluding the life-threatening forms, are first explored by ultrasonography to establish a clinical diagnosis, to define pancreatic or peripancreatic phlegmons or acute fluid collections, and to reveal vascular compromise of arteries and veins.[249] Further information is obtained with

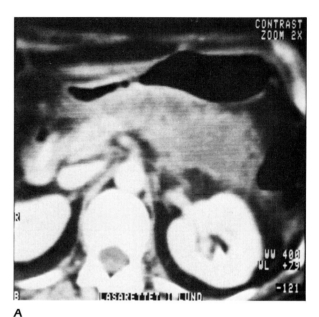

A

Figure 55-22. Abscess of the tail of the pancreas following blunt trauma in a patient with chronic alcoholism. (A) CT showing tail of pancreas expanded by a poorly outlined lesion. (*Figure continues on page 1410.*)

CT, particularly in the more advanced cases of cysts and abscesses, and then not only for diagnosis but also for staging and prognosis.[250,251] Also, MRI with or without contrast enhancement gives information in acute pancreatitis that may be superior to that of other noninvasive techniques.[153,154] The most important vascular lesions found in acute pancreatitis are venous thrombosis, which is best demonstrated with noninvasive imaging methods,[39,43,44,164,165,167] and aneurysm formation, which may be observed at Doppler ultrasonography.[39,249] MRA[41,42] has also a potential to show pseudoaneurysms. Conventional angiography is used to confirm the findings at noninvasive imaging and, further, to show aneurysms and bleeding sites before interventional radiography or surgery is contemplated.

Recurrent Acute or Chronic Pancreatitis

Recurrent acute or chronic pancreatitis (relapsing pancreatitis) almost always shows vascular abnormalities of the same kind as previously described. There is a continuous progression of the vascular changes depending on how long the disease has been present and on the severity of the attacks. Sequelae, such as pseudocysts and abscesses, can cause marked vascular displacement and venous compression or occlusion (see Figs. 55-12, 55-13, and 55-22). Hypervascularization of the pancreas may be present but is not regularly observed (see Fig. 55-23).

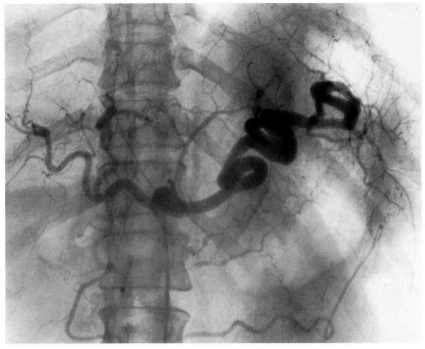

B

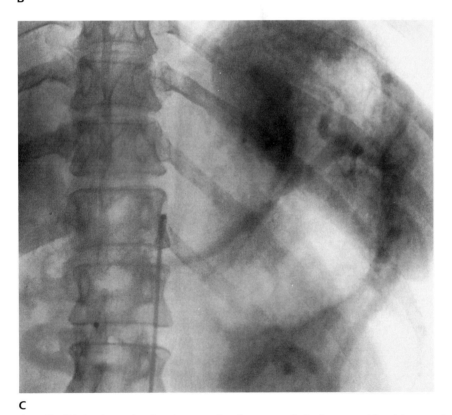

C

Figure 55-22 (continued). (B) Angiography showing vascular changes typical of pancreatitis with smooth narrowing of the distal part of the splenic artery. (C) Venous phase showing splenic vein compressed by pancreatic abscess and venous collaterals.

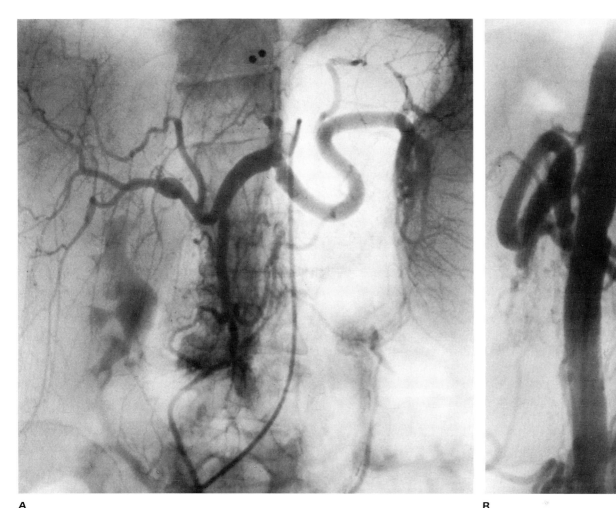

A
B

Figure 55-23. Chronic recurrent calcifying pancreatitis. At celiac angiography (A) and lumbar aortography (*lateral view,* B) marked stenosis of the celiac axis and occlusion of the superior mesenteric artery are observed. Local short con-striction typical of pancreatitis is seen in the splenic artery. Marked hypervascularization and irregular, tortuous pancreatic arteries are other typical findings.

Chronic Pancreatitis

The characteristic finding, first described by Reuter et al.,[244] is the beaded appearance of smaller pancreatic arteries, with short dilated segments alternating with stenosed parts. Short diaphragmlike stenoses are frequently observed in the larger arteries.[14,231] Smooth regular stenoses of arteries surrounding the pancreas are typical in a high percentage of cases. Changes resembling fibromuscular dysplasia may also be noted (see Fig. 55-13). Stenoses of the celiac and/or superior mesenteric arteries are often encountered.[245,252] Arterial aneurysms may be observed in the spleen and in the hepatic, gastroduodenal, and jejunal arteries. Displacement of arteries sometimes occurs with pseudocysts or abscesses but is also due to retraction secondary to peripancreatic fibrosis.[245,253] The vascularization of the pancreas varies from markedly in-creased[235,236] to markedly decreased.[14,231] Occlusion or compression of the splenic, superior mesenteric, or portal veins is a common finding.

It appears obvious that the vascular changes observed in the various forms of pancreatitis depend largely on when the angiographic procedure is performed and also on the intensity of the disease and whether pseudocysts or abscesses have occurred. It is likewise clear that in chronic pancreatitis the duration of the disease is of importance.[236,244,245] This may explain the somewhat contradictory reports of findings in chronic pancreatitis, ranging from an increased vascular supply to hypovascularization, from normal arteries to various forms of arterial stenoses, tortuosity, beading, displacement, and so forth.[28,32,34–36,53,113,161,236,252,254]

Celiac and/or superior mesenteric arterial stenosis

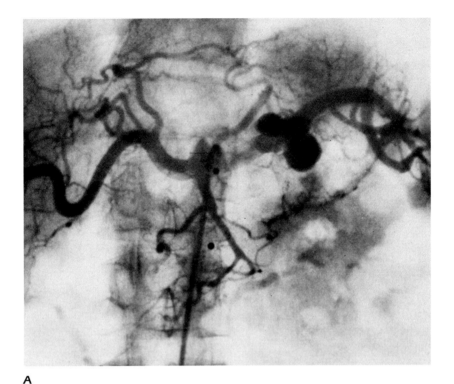

A

B

Figure 55-24. Chronic pancreatitis with aneurysm of the splenic artery rupturing into the pancreatic duct with gastrointestinal bleeding. (A) Celiac angiography showing a 16-mm aneurysm of the splenic artery penetrating the pancreas with hypervascularization of the tail of the pancreas.

(B) Marked constriction of the portal vein due to peripancreatic fibrosis is observed in the venous phase of superior mesenteric angiography. Bradykinin was used to increase the flow rate.

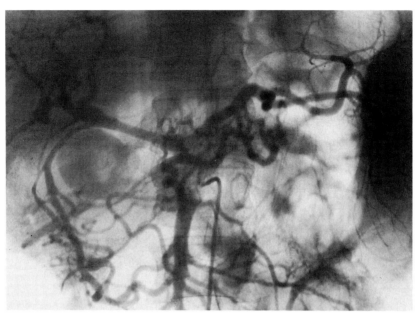

Figure 55-25. Recurrent chronic pancreatitis with complete occlusion of celiac axis and a blood cyst in the head of the pancreas. Because there was no severe bleeding in the gastrointestinal tract, no operation was performed. At control angiography 6 months later the aneurysm had disappeared.

is found more often in patients with pancreatitis[113,245,252] than in unselected series of patients examined with angiography.[255] Arteriosclerosis or compression from the crura may cause the constriction.[256–258] It is, however, conceivable that the close relationship of these vessels to the pancreas is of importance and could explain the increased frequency of abnormalities (see Fig. 55-23).

The most important angiographic observation in patients with pancreatitis is aneurysms, which in collected series are found in approximately 10 percent of patients.[245,253,259] Numerous reports of single or a few cases of multiple aneurysms that have ruptured and caused gastrointestinal hemorrhage, ordinarily in combination with cysts or abscesses, have appeared.[40,259–267] Most aneurysms occur in the splenic or gastroduodenal arteries, but aneurysms have been observed in other arteries as well, such as the jejunal and left gastric arteries (see Fig. 55-24). One can expect that in a patient with severe pancreatitis the enzymes will first attack the arteries within or close to the pancreas.

The so-called blood cysts of the pancreas are probably the result of destroyed small intrapancreatic arteries (see Fig. 55-25). Later on, when the pancreatic enzymes pass out into the "mesenteric planes,"[268] destruction of more peripherally situated arteries can be expected (see Fig. 55-26). Aneurysms in these areas can of course have other etiologies than pancreatitis.[263,269] Tylén did not find any aneurysms in patients with calcifying chronic pancreatitis,[245] and he thought the explanation lay in the fact that peripancreatitis is not so prominent in this type of disease. A bleeding arterial aneurysm has, however, been found even in calcifying pancreatitis.[264,270,271] In severe attacks of pancreatitis, both arterial wall destruction and thrombosis, with consequent bowel infarction, may occur.[272]

Another important and frequent sequela of pancreatitis is venous compression or occlusion by thrombosis. Like other vascular structures in or around the pancreas, the veins showed progression of the disease when they were later followed up by repeat angiography.[253]

Vascular abnormalities may thus occur both in carcinoma of the pancreas and in pancreatitis. In most cases high-quality angiography can distinguish between these two entities,[109,112,119] but there are clearly cases in which it is not possible to make a distinction between them. Most often the angiographic changes caused by chronic pancreatitis are said to be the result of a carcinoma, but the opposite error also occurs.

Since noninvasive imaging methods are the techniques of choice in evaluating chronic pancreatitis, the marked vascular changes do not dominate the information as they did when pancreatic angiography was the prominent diagnostic method. Ultrasonography and CT are the primary methods, and when combined with biopsy in cases of focal lesions, a reliable differen-

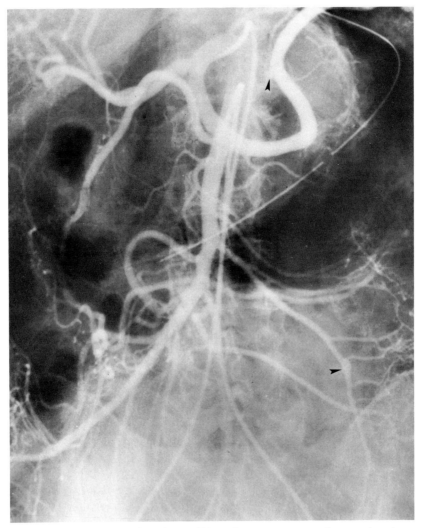

Figure 55-26. Pseudocyst in the lesser sac and in the small bowel mesentery secondary to chronic pancreatitis. Aneurysms are present in the splenic and jejunal arteries (*arrowheads*).

tiation between ductal adenocarcinoma and chronic pancreatitis is obtained.[150,273,274]

Perivascular infiltration as a reliable differential diagnostic sign observed on CT has been debated, and the circumferential thickening of the superior mesenteric artery[147,170–173] seems to be an almost reliable diagnosis of carcinoma. In a recent prospective study, MRI gave good information in a few cases of chronic pancreatitis, but in one out of five cases both MRI and CT missed a focal lesion due to carcinoma.[155] Venous compression or thrombosis with collateral circulation is well demonstrated with MRA (see Fig. 55-14).

Pseudocysts and Abscesses

Ultrasonography and CT are more reliable methods than angiography for disclosing pseudocysts and abscesses (see Figs. 55-13, 55-22, 55-25, and 55-26), but it is in patients with this condition that angiography is particularly important, mainly because of the severe vascular complications that often occur. Thus there is every reason to follow the patients closely if operation or intraarterial therapy is not contemplated (see Fig. 55-25).

Another reason for angiography is the fact that the

pseudocysts may be secondary to pancreatic carcinoma obstructing the duct. Neither CT nor ultrasonography may show the true cause for the cyst formation, and therefore ERCP and/or angiography should give complementary information.

In cases of cystadenoma, ultrasonography and CT may not reveal the true lesion but only suggest the presence of a cystic tumor. Abundant tumor vessels may disclose the true nature, but it should be emphasized that the hypovascular cystadenoma might simulate a pseudocyst or an abscess. In one case we observed, CT and percutaneous biopsy gave reliable information whereas ultrasonography and angiography gave the impression of a pseudocyst (see Fig. 55-21).

Extrahepatic portal hypertension is frequently observed in pseudocysts and abscesses. This is always shown by angiography, but the noninvasive imaging methods also give adequate information about venous occlusion and collateral circulation in these cases (Fig. 55-14). The interventional procedures in case of hemorrhage, pseudocyst, and abscesses are dealt with in Chapter 55 in *Abrams' Angiography: Interventional Radiology.*

Trauma

Direct contusion of the pancreas by a steering wheel or in bicycle accidents is not rare. The close relationship of the pancreas and the spine forms the anatomic basis for blunt traumatic lesions of the gland (see Fig. 55-22). Occlusion of pancreatic arteries and impaired circulation of the organ are common angiographic findings in the acute phase. Displacement of arteries adjacent to the pancreas and spleen occurs when hematoma is present.[275,276] Rupture of the splenic artery with extravasation has also been observed.[277] Compression or occlusion of the portal venous system as well as displacement secondary to hematoma formation may be observed. Portal venous thrombosis is a known complication of pancreatic trauma.[278]

The most frequent complication of pancreatic trauma is pseudocyst or abscess formation, which may appear within a few weeks. The lesions of posttraumatic pancreatitis and pseudocysts are the same as in other types of pancreatitis.

Pancreatic Transplants

Transplantation of the pancreas has become a realistic option to prevent complications in patients with type I diabetes. Rejections, acute or chronic, and vascular complications occur frequently and may eventually re-

sult in transplant removal. It is important to distinguish between rejection and primary vascular complication because the therapy differs. Percutaneous biopsy of the pancreatic allograft is not as useful as it is in renal allografts. Angiography and scintigraphy became the first methods used in the early days of transplantation[279] to define whether vascular complications such as arterial and venous thrombosis, anastomosis-leak, aneurysms, or arteriovenous fistulas were present. However, arterial and venous abnormalities with deterioration of blood flow were also observed in graft rejection, and scintigraphy was not specific.

In addition to radionuclides and angiography, a variety of noninvasive imaging modalities have over the years been used to define the presence of rejection (ultrasonography, CT, and MRI).[280–283] In an extensive, partly prospective study, Snider et al.[284] found that scintigraphy was a valuable screening method in suspected graft thrombosis because a normal scintigram eliminates a diagnosis of vascular occlusion. They also found that nonenhanced CT and ultrasonography were sensitive to show graft abnormalities, but not specific for thrombosis. Bolus-dynamic CT might give more information in this respect,[285] as well as color Doppler imaging.[284] MRI also appears to be of value in early pancreas allograft rejection,[283] but experience is limited. MRA has not been used to clarify vascular abnormalities in pancreatic allografts but has definite potential. Therefore, "currently, definite evaluation of graft thromboses and other vascular lesions remains dependent on arteriography or surgical exploration."[284]

References

1. Ödman P. Percutaneous selective angiography of the main branches of the aorta. Acta Radiol 1956;45:1.
2. Bierman HR, Miller ER, Byron RL Jr, Dod KS, Kelly KH, Black DH. Intra-arterial catheterization of viscera in man. AJR 1951;66:555.
3. Ödman P. Percutaneous selective angiography of coeliac artery. Acta Radiol Suppl (Stockh) 1958;159:1.
4. Ödman P. The radiopaque polythene catheter. Acta Radiol 1959;52:52.
5. Ödman P. Pancreatic angiography. In: Abrams HL, ed. Angiography. Boston: Little, Brown, 1961.
6. Boijsen E. Pancreatic angiography. In: Abrams HL, ed. Angiography. 2nd ed. Boston: Little, Brown, 1971.
7. Boijsen E. Pancreatic angiography. In: Abrams HL, ed. Abrams angiography: vascular and interventional radiology, 3rd ed. Boston: Little, Brown, 1983.
8. Pierson JM. The arterial blood supply of the pancreas. Surg Gynecol Obstet 1943;77:426.
9. Woodburne RT, Olsen LL. The arteries of the pancreas. Anat Rec 1951;111:255.
10. Michels NA. Blood supply and anatomy of the upper abdominal organs, with a descriptive atlas. Philadelphia: Lippincott, 1955.

11. Moretti S. Studio-anatomo-radiografico del circolo arterioso pancreatico. Radiol Med (Torino) 1965;51:16.
12. Hentschel M. Pankreas-Anatomie. Langenbecks Arch Chir 1965;313:233.
13. Lunderquist A. Angiography in carcinoma of the pancreas. Acta Radiol Suppl (Stockh) 1965;235:1.
14. Chérigié E, Mellière D, Bennet J, Doyon D, Chenard JC. Anatomie radiologique de la vascularisation du pancréas. J Radiol Electrol Med Nucl 1967;48:346.
15. Kupic EA, Marshall WH, Abrams HL. Splenic arterial patterns: angiographic analysis and review. Invest Radiol 1967;2:70.
16. Hentschel M. Die Oberbauch-Chirurgie im lichte neurer anatomischer Untersuchungen. Fortsch Prax Fortbild 1967;18:647.
17. Hepp J, Hernandez C, Moreaux J, Bismuth H. L'artériographie dans les affections chirurgicales du foie, du pancréas et de la rate. Paris: Masson, 1968.
18. Boijsen E. Angiography in pancreatic disease. In: Forell MM, ed. Handbuch der inneren Medizin, III/6. Berlin, Heidelberg, New York: Springer-Verlag, 1976.
19. Braasch JW, Gray BN. Technique of radical pancreatoduodenectomy with consideration of hepatic arterial relationships. Surg Clin North Am 1976;56:631.
20. Mackie CR, Lu CT, Noble HG, Cooper MB, Collins P, Block GE, Moossa AR. Prospective evaluation of angiography in the diagnosis and management of patients suspected of having pancreatic cancer. Ann Surg 1979;189:11.
21. Moossa AR, Lewis MH, Mackie CR. Surgical treatment of pancreatic cancer. Mayo Clin Proc 1979;54:468.
22. Boijsen E, Redman HC. Effects of bradykinin on celiac and superior mesenteric angiography. Invest Radiol 1966;1:422.
23. Morino F, Tarquini A. Cateterismo attraverso l'arteria omerale per l'arteriografia dei rami collaterali dell'aorta addominale. Minerva Med 1956;47:935.
24. Morino F, Tarquini A, Olivero S. Artériographie abdominale sélective par le cathétérisme de l'artère humérale. Presse Med 1956;64:1944.
25. Morino F, Tarquini A, Quaglia C. Unsere Erfahrungen mit einer neuen Methode der selektiven abdominellen Arteriographie. Chirurg 1957;28:152.
26. Roy P. Percutaneous catheterization via the axillary artery: a new approach to some technical roadblocks in selective arteriography. AJR 1965;94:1.
27. Boijsen E. Selective visceral angiography using a percutaneous axillary technique. Br J Radiol 1966;39:414.
28. Boijsen E, Olin T. Zöliakographie und Angiographie der Arteria mesenterica superior. In: Schinz HR, Glauner G, Rüttiman A, eds. Ergebnisse der medizinische Strahlenforschung Neue Folge. Stuttgart: Thieme, 1964.
29. Weyer KH van de, Kössling FK, Habighorst LV, Albers P. Experimentelle Untersuchungen zu Technik und Risiko der Pankreasangiographie. ROEFO 1968;108:733.
30. Olsson O. Angiographie bei Pankreastumoren. Radiologe 1965;5:281.
31. Olsson O, Boijsen E, Olin T. Portography by simultaneous catheterization of the celiac and superior mesenteric arteries. In: X. International Congress book of abstracts, Montreal, 1962.
32. Ranniger K, Saldino RM. Arteriographic diagnosis of pancreatic lesions. Radiology 1966;86:470.
33. Hernandez C, Morin G, Ecarlat B. L'embole pulsé en artériographie sélective digestive. Presse Med 1965;73:2889.
34. Rösch J, Bret J. Arteriography of the pancreas. AJR 1965;94:182.
35. Nebesar RA, Pollard JJ. A critical evaluation of selective celiac and superior mesenteric angiography in the diagnosis of pancreatic diseases, particularly malignant tumor: facts and "artefacts." Radiology 1967;89:1017.
36. Sammons BP, Neal MP Jr, Armstrong RH Jr, Hager HG. Ten years experience with celiac and upper abdominal superior mesenteric arteriography. AJR 1967;101:345.
37. van Voorthuisen AE. Ervaringen met Selectieve Arteriografie van de Arteria Coeliaca en de Arteria Mesenterica Superior. Leiden: Stafleu's Wetenschappelijke Uitgeversmaatschappij N.V., 1967.
38. Boijsen E, Redman HC. Effect of epinephrine on celiac and superior mesenteric angiography. Invest Radiol 1967;2:184.
39. Scoutt LM, Zawin ML, Taylor KJW. Doppler US: Part II. Clinical applications. Radiology 1990;174:309.
40. Vujic I. Vascular complications of pancreatitis. Radiol Clin North Am 1989;27:81.
41. Vock P, Terrier F, Wegmüller H, et al. Magnetic resonance angiography of abdominal vessels: early experience using the three-dimensional phase-contrast technique. Br J Radiol 1991;64:10.
42. Lewin JS, Laub G, Hausmann R. Three-dimensional time-of-flight MR-angiography: applications in the abdomen and thorax. Radiology 1991;179:261.
43. Vogelzang RL, Gore RM, Anschuetz SL et al. Thrombosis of the splanchnic veins: CT diagnosis. AJR 1988;150:93.
44. Mori H, McGrath FP, Malone DE, et al. The gastrocolic trunk and its tributaries: CT evaluation. Radiology 1992;182:871.
45. Redman HC, Reuter SR, Miller WJ. Improvement of superior mesenteric and portal vein visualization with tolazoline. Invest Radiol 1969;4:24.
46. Aronsen K-F, Nylander G. Angiographic studies of the action of vasopressin in the dog. Vasc Dis 1964;1:127.
47. Kahn PC, Frates WJ, Paul RE. The epinephrine effect in angiography of gastrointestinal tract tumors. Radiology 1967;88:686.
48. Nylander G. Vascular response to vasopressin as reflected in angiography: an experimental study in the dog. Acta Radiol Suppl (Stockh) 1967;266:1.
49. Cen M, Rosenbusch G. Zöliakographie mit Adrenalin. Möglichkeiten der Pharmakoangiographie in der Pankreasdiagnostik. ROEFO 1970;111:82.
50. Boijsen E, Göthlin J. Abdominal angiography after intraarterial injection of vasopressin. Acta Radiol 1980;21:523.
51. Kahn PC, Callow AD. Selective vasodilatation as an aid to angiography. AJR 1965;94:213.
52. Taylor DA, Macken KL, Fiore AS. Angiographic visualization of the secretin-stimulated pancreas. Radiology 1966;87:525.
53. Lewicki AM, Kupic EA, Kohatsu S. Selective visceral canine angiography for pancreatic visualization: use of pharmacodynamic agents. Invest Radiol 1967;2:119.
54. Bennet J, Chérigié E, Caroli J, Doyon D, Economopoulos P, Plessier J, Stoopen M. La pancréatographie après stimulation par la sécrétin intra-artérielle (à propos de 33 cas). Ann Radiol (Paris) 1967;10:617.
55. Lenarduzzi G, Romani S, Zacchi C. La stimulazione farmacologica della funzione esocrina nella contrastografia opaca del pancreas. Radiol Med (Torino) 1968;54:97.
56. Rosenbusch G, Cen M. Zöliakographie mit Sekretin. Möglichkeiten der Pharmakoangiographie in der Pankreasdiagnostik. ROEFO 1969;110:639.
57. Udén R. Effect of secretin in celiac and superior mesenteric angiography. Acta Radiol 1969;8:497.
58. Schmarsow R. Angiography of the pancreas following the administration of secretin, trypsin and histamine. Acta Radiol 1972;12:175.
59. Udén R. Cholecystokinin-pancreozymin in celiac and superior mesenteric angiography. Acta Radiol 1972;12:363.
60. Davis LJ, Anderson JH, Wallace S, Gianturco C, Jacobson ED. The use of prostaglandin E$_1$ to enhance the angiographic visualization of the splanchnic circulation. Radiology 1975;114:281.
61. Dencker H, Göthlin J, Hedner P, Lunderquist A, Norryd C, Tylén U. Superior mesenteric angiography and blood flow following intra-arterial injection of prostaglandin F$_{2\alpha}$. AJR 1975;125:111.
62. Nebesar RA, Pollard JJ. Advances in abdominal angiography. Postgrad Med 1965;37:504.

63. Van Heertum RL, Cioffi CM, Ruzicka FF. The use of alpha blocking and beta stimulating drugs in combination to improve opacification of the portal venous system. Radiology 1971;100:679.

64. Hawkins IF, Kaude JV, MacGregor A. Priscoline and epinephrine in selective pancreatic angiography: a comparison study using high-pressure injection, Valsalva maneuver and geometric magnification. Radiology 1975;116:311.

65. MacGregor AMC, Hawkins IF Jr. Selective pharmacodynamic angiography in the diagnosis of carcinoma of the pancreas. Surg Gynecol Obstet 1973;137:917.

66. Udén R. Secretin and epinephrine combined in celiac angiography. Acta Radiol 1976;17:17.

67. Morino F, Olivero S, Tarquini A. Arteriografia selettiva del tronco celiaco e delle sue branche. (Studio-anatomo-morfolgico). Minerva Chir 1958;13(Suppl):279.

68. Paul RE Jr, Miller HH, Kahn PC, Callow AD, Edwards TL Jr, Patterson JF. Pancreatic angiography, with application of subselective angiography of the celiac and superior mesenteric artery to the diagnosis of carcinoma of the pancreas. N Engl J Med 1965;272:283.

69. Almén T. A steering device for selective angiography and some vascular and enzymatic reactions observed in its clinical application. Acta Radiol Suppl (Stockh) 1966;260.

70. Boijsen E. Selective pancreatic angiography. Br J Radiol 1966;39:481.

71. Reuter SR. Superselective pancreatic angiography. Radiology 1969;92:74.

72. Rösch J, Grollman JH Jr. Superselective arteriography in the diagnosis of abdominal pathology: technical considerations. Radiology 1969;92:1008.

73. Takashima T, Yamamoto I, Mitani I, Shin M. Transfemoral superselective celiac angiography. AJR 1970;110:813.

74. Takashima T, Shin M. Transfemoral superselective celiac catheterization. Technical considerations. AJR 1971;113:280.

75. Bücheler E, Thelen M. Angiographie der Äste des Truncus coeliacus. Roentgenblaetter 1971;24:11.

76. Tavernier J, Delorme G, Fagola M. L'artériographie "superselective" du pancréas. Ann Radiol (Paris) 1971;14:555.

77. Eisenberg H. Angiography of the pancreas. In: Hilal SK, ed. Small vessel angiography. Imaging, morphology, physiology, and clinical applications. St. Louis: Mosby, 1973.

78. Ariyama J, Shirakabe H, Ikenobe H, Kurosawa A, Sumida M. Angiographic diagnosis of pancreatic carcinoma. Stomach and Intestine 1976;11:1605.

79. Ariyama J, Shirakabe H, Ikenobe H, Kurosawa A, Owman T. The diagnosis of the small resectable pancreatic carcinoma. Clin Radiol 1977;28:437.

80. Freeny PC, Ball TJ, Ryan J. Impact of new diagnostic imaging methods on pancreatic angiography. AJR 1979;133:619.

81. Mackie CR, Blackstone MO, Dhorajiwala J, Bowie J, Moossa AR. Value of new diagnostic aids in relation to the disease process in pancreatic cancer. Lancet 1979;2:385.

82. Boijsen E, Maly P. Vergrösserungstechnik in der abdominellen Angiographie. Radiologe 1978;18:167.

83. Reuter SR. Modification of pancreatic blood flow with balloon catheters: a new approach to pancreatic angiography. Radiology 1970;95:57.

84. Sos TA, Cohn DJ, Srur M, et al. A new open-ended guidewire/catheter. Radiology 1985;154:817.

85. Meyerovitz MF, Levin DC, Boxt LM. Superselective catheterization of small-caliber arteries with a new high-visibility steerable guide wire. AJR 1985;144:785.

86. Okazaki M, Higashihara H, Koganemaru F, et al. Emergent embolization for control of massive hemorrhage from a splanchnic artery with a new coaxial catheter system. Acta Radiol 1992;32:57.

87. Crummy AB, Stieghorst MF, Turski PA, et al. Digital subtraction angiography: current status and use of intraarterial injection. Radiology 1982;145:303.

88. Foley WD, Stewart ET, Milbrath JR, et al. Digital subtraction angiography of the portal venous system. AJR 1983;140:497.

89. Katzen BT. Peripheral, abdominal, and interventional applications of DSA. Radiol Clin North Am 1985;23:227.

90. Päivänsalo M, Mäkäräinen H, Siniluoto T, et al. Ultrasound compared with computed tomography and pancreatic angiography in the detection of endocrine tumours of the pancreas. Eur J Radiol 1989;9:173.

91. Rossi P, Allison DJ, Bezzi M, et al. Endocrine tumors of the pancreas. Radiol Clin North Am 1989;27:129.

92. Doust BD, Redman HC. The myth of 1 ml/kg in angiography. Radiology 1972;104:551.

93. McAfee JG. A survey of complications of abdominal aortography. Radiology 1957;68:825.

94. Robinson AS. Acute pancreatitis following translumbar aortography: case report with autopsy findings seven weeks following aortogram. Arch Surg 1956;72:290.

95. Jonsson K, Lunderquist A, Pettersson H, Sigstedt B. Subintimal injection of contrast medium as a complication of selective abdominal angiography. Acta Radiol 1977;18:55.

96. Sigstedt B, Lunderquist A. Complications of angiographic examinations. AJR 1978;130:455.

97. Pirker E. Angiographische Röntgendiagnostik der Oberbauchorgane. Radiol Austria 1961;12:79.

98. Cortesini R. L'arteriografia selettiva del tripode celiaco e delle arterie renali. Policlinico [Prat.] 1963;70:817.

99. Meaney TF, Winkelman EI, Sullivan BH, Brown CH. Selective splanchnic arteriography in the diagnosis of pancreatic tumors. Cleve Clin J Med 1963;30:193.

100. Glenn F, Evans JA, Halpern M, Thorbjarnarson B. Selective celiac and superior mesenteric arteriography. Surg Gynecol Obstet 1964;118:93.

101. Nebesar RA, Pollard JJ, Edmunds LH Jr, McKahn CF. Indications for selective celiac and superior mesenteric angiography: experience with 128 cases. AJR 1964;92:1100.

102. Baum S, Roy R, Finkelstein AK, Blakemore WS. Clinical application of selective celiac and superior mesenteric arteriography. Radiology 1965;84:279.

103. Meaney TF, Buonocore E. Arteriographic manifestations of pancreatic neoplasm. AJR 1965;95:720.

104. Baron MG. Carcinoma of the pancreas demonstrated by selective celiac angiography. Mt Sinai J Med (N.Y.) 1966;33:97.

105. Lang EK. Angiographic demonstration of carcinoma of the tail of the pancreas. J Indiana State Med Assoc 1966;59:252.

106. Weissleder H, Baumeister L, Fischer P, Renemann H. Die selektive Darstellung der Arteria coeliaca und mesenterica superior in der abdominalen Diagnostik. ROEFO 1966;104:137.

107. Ludin H, Fahrländer HJ, Maurer W. Arteriographische Diagnostik von Karzinomen des Pancreaskörpers und schwanzes. Schweiz Med Wochenschr 1966;96:871.

108. Baron MG, Mitty HA, Wolf BS. The arteriographic appearance of carcinoma of the uncinate process of the pancreas. AJR 1967;101:649.

109. Bookstein JJ, Reuter SR, Martel W. Angiographic evaluation of pancreatic carcinoma. Radiology 1969;93:757.

110. Fredens M, Egeblad M, Holst-Nielsen F. The value of selective angiography in the diagnosis of tumors in pancreas and liver. Radiology 1969;93:765.

111. Lechner G, Pokieser H, Zaunbauer W, Brücke P. Zur angiographischen Diagnose des Pankreaskarzinoms. ROEFO 1970;113:340.

112. Reuter SR, Redman HC, Bookstein JJ. Differential problems in the angiographic diagnosis of carcinoma of the pancreas. Radiology 1970;96:93.

113. Bücheler E, Boldt I, Frommhold H, Käufer C. Die angiographische Diagnostik der Pankreastumoren und der Pankreatitis. ROEFO 1971;115:726.

114. Pokieser H. Angiographie bei Pankreaserkrankungen. Roentgenblaetter 1971;24:281.

115. Buranasiri S, Baum S. The significance of the venous phase of celiac and superior mesenteric arteriography in evaluating pancreatic carcinoma. Radiology 1972;102:11.

116. Olsson O, Tylén U. Angiography in carcinoma at the papilla of Vater. Acta Radiol 1972;12:375.

117. Suzuki T, Kuratsuka H, Uchida K, Matsumoto Y, Honjo I. Carcinoma of the pancreas arising in the region of the uncinate process. Cancer 1972;30:796.

118. Tylén U. Accuracy of angiography in the diagnosis of carcinoma of the pancreas. Acta Radiol 1973;14:449.

119. Tylén U. Angiographic differentiation between inflammatory disease and carcinoma of the pancreas. Acta Radiol 1973;14:257.

120. Anacker H. Pankreas-Karzinom—Angiographische Diagnostik. Langenbecks Arch Chir 1975;339:239.

121. Sato T, Saito Y, Koyama K, Watanabe K. Preoperative determination of operability in carcinomas of the pancreas and the periampullary region. Ann Surg 1968;168:876.

122. Suzuki T, Kawabe K, Nakayasu A, Takeda H, Kobayashi K, Kubota N, Honjo I. Selective arteriography in cancer of the pancreas at a resectable stage. Am J Surg 1971;122:402.

123. Suzuki T, Kawabe K, Imamura M, Honjo I. Survival of patients with cancer of the pancreas in relation to findings on arteriography. Ann Surg 1972;176:37.

124. Suzuki T, Kuratsuka H, Uchida K, et al. Correlation between clinical aspects and location of lesions in carcinoma of the head of the pancreas. Am J Surg 1973;125:546.

125. Tylén U, Arnesjö B. Resectability and prognosis of carcinoma of the pancreas evaluated by angiography. Scand J Gastroenterol 1973;8:691.

126. Goldstein HM, Neiman HL, Bookstein JJ. Angiographic evaluation of pancreatic disease: a further appraisal. Radiology 1974;112:275.

127. Suzuki T, Tani T, Honjo I. Appraisal of arteriography for assessment of operability in periampullary cancer. Ann Surg 1975;182:66.

128. Fitzgerald PJ, Fartner JG, Watson RC, et al. The value of diagnostic aids in detecting pancreas cancer. Cancer 1978;41:868.

129. Sigstedt B, Lunderquist A, Tylén U, Boijsen E. Angiography in pancreatic disease revisited: a prospective and blind evaluation. Acta Radiol 1981;22:235.

130. Boijsen E, Lundh G, Stormby N. Roentgenologic, secretoric and cytologic diagnosis of cancer of the pancreas. Acta Chir Scand 1965;332(Suppl):104.

131. Boijsen E, Reuter SR. Combined percutaneous transhepatic cholangiography and angiography in the evaluation of obstructive jaundice. AJR 1967;99:153.

132. Eaton SB, Fleischli DJ, Pollard JJ, Nebesar RA, Potsaid MS. Comparison of current radiologic approaches to the diagnosis of pancreatic disease. N Engl J Med 1968;279:389.

133. Göthlin J, Mansoor M, Tranberg K-G. Combined percutaneous transhepatic cholangiography (PTC) and selective visceral angiography (SVA) in obstructive jaundice. AJR 1973;117:419.

134. Classen M, Koch H, Rösch W. Duodenoskopische Diagnose des Pankreaskarzinoms. Leber Magen Darm 1974;4:222.

135. Clouse ME, Gregg JA, Sedgwick CE. Angiography vs pancreatography in diagnosis of carcinoma of the pancreas. Radiology 1975;114:605.

136. Triller J, Voegeli E, Halter F, Witzel L, Wanger F. Die selektive Pankreas-Angiographie und retrograde Pankreas-Cholangiographie als Kombinationsuntersuchung. ROEFO 1975;122:138.

137. Ariyama J, Shirakabe H, Sumida M, Bartram CI. Angiographic evaluation of the abnormal endoscopic pancreatogram. Gastrointest Radiol 1979;4:231.

138. Suzuki T, Imamura M, Tamura K, Sumiyoshi A, Sakanashi S, Nishimura Y, Tobe T. Correlative evaluation of angiography and pancreatoductography in relation to surgery for cancer of the pancreas. Surgery 1979;85:644.

139. Reuben A, Johnson AL, Cotton PB. Is pancreatogram interpretation reliable? A study of observer variation and error. Br J Radiol 1978;51:956.

140. Mackie CR, Cooper MJ, Lewis MH, Moossa AR. Non-operative differentiation between pancreatic cancer and chronic pancreatitis. Ann Surg 1979;189:480.

141. Schmarsow R, Kiefer H, Linhart P, Gruner HJ, Hammes PH. Sonographie und Pharmakoangiographie des Pankreas. ROEFO 1979;131:392.

142. Lee JKT, Stanley RJ, Nelson GL, Sagel SS. Pancreatic imaging by ultrasound and computed tomography: a general review. Radiol Clin North Am 1979;17:105.

143. Hessel S, Siegelman SS, Adams DF, et al. Prospective analysis of computed tomography and ultrasound in evaluating the pancreas. Presented at the Radiological Society of North America meeting in Atlanta, November, 1979.

144. Karp W, Lunderquist A, Tylén U, Ihse I. Angiography and ultrasonography in the evaluation of pancreatic lesion. Acta Radiol 1980;21:169.

145. Freeny PC, Marks WM, Ball TJ. Impact of high-resolution computed tomography of the pancreas on utilization of endoscopic retrograde cholangiopancreatography and angiography. Radiology 1982;142:35.

146. Freeny PC, Marks WM, Ryan JA, et al. Pancreatic ductal adenocarcinoma: diagnosis and staging with dynamic CT. Radiology 1988;166:125.

147. Megibow AJ. Pancreatic adenocarcinoma: designing the examination to evaluate the clinical questions. Radiology 1992;183:297.

148. Laing FC, Jeffrey RB Jr, Wing VW, et al. Biliary dilatation: defining the level and cause by real-time US. Radiology 1986;160:39.

149. Freeny PC. Radiologic diagnosis and staging of pancreatic ductal adenocarcinoma. Radiol Clin North Am 1989;27:121.

150. DelMaschio A, Vanzulli A, Sironi S, et al. Pancreatic cancer versus chronic pancreatitis: diagnosis with CA 19-9 assessment, US, CT, and CT-guided fine needle biopsy. Radiology 1991;178:95.

151. Smith FW, Reid A, Hutchinson JMS, et al. Nuclear magnetic resonance imaging of the pancreas. Radiology 1982;142:677.

152. Smith FW, Bayliss AP, Hussey JK, et al. Low-field (0.08 T) magnetic resonance imaging of the pancreas: comparison with computed tomography and ultrasound. Br J Radiol 1989;62:796.

153. Tscholakoff D, Hricak H, Thoeni R, et al. MR imaging in the diagnosis of pancreatic disease. AJR 1987;148:703.

154. Semelka RC, Kroeker MA, Shoenut JP, et al. Pancreatic disease: prospective comparison of CT, ERCP, and 1.5-T MR imaging with dynamic gadolinium enhancement and fat suppression. Radiology 1991;181:785.

155. Vellet AD, Romano W, Bach DB, et al. Adenocarcinoma of the pancreatic ducts: comparative evaluation with CT and MR imaging at 1.5 T. Radiology 1992;183:87.

156. Gehl H-B, Vorwerk D, Klose K-C, et al. Pancreatic enhancement after low-dose infusion of Mn-DPDP. Radiology 1991;180:337.

157. Reimer P, Saini S, Hahn PF, et al. Technique for high-resolution echo-planar MR imaging of the pancreas. Radiology 1992;182:175.

158. Hamed MM, Hamm B, Ibrahim ME, et al. Dynamic MR imaging of the abdomen with gadopentetate dimeglumine: normal enhancement patterns of the liver, spleen, stomach, and pancreas. AJR 1992;158:303.

159. Mitchell DG, Vinitski S, Saponaro S, et al. Liver and pancreas: improved spin-echo T1 contrast by shorter echo time and fat suppression at 1.5 T. Radiology 1991;178:67.

160. Palubinskas AJ, Ripley HR. Fibromuscular hyperplasia in external arteries. Radiology 1964;82:451.

161. Baum S, Kuroda K, Roy RH. The value of special angiographic techniques in the management of patients with abdominal neoplasms. Radiol Clin North Am 1965;3:583.

162. Kincaid OW, Davis GD, Hallermann FJ, Hunt JC. Fibromuscular dysplasia of the renal arteries: arteriographic features, classification and observations on natural history of the disease. AJR 1968;104:271.

163. Serebro H. A diagnostic sign of carcinoma of the body of the pancreas. Lancet 1965;1:85.

164. Gehl H-B, Bohndorf K, Klose K-C, et al. Two-dimensional MR angiography in the evaluation of abdominal veins with

gradient refocused sequences. J Comp Asst Tomogr 1990;14: 619.

165. Marn CS, Glazer GM, Williams DM, et al. CT-angiographic correlation of collateral venous pathways in isolated splenic vein occlusion: new observations. Radiology 1990;175:375.

166. Zerin JM, DiPietro MA. Mesenteric vascular anatomy at CT: normal and abnormal appearances. Radiology 1991;179: 739.

167. Arrivé L, Menu Y, Dessarts I, et al. Diagnosis of abdominal venous thrombosis by means of spin-echo and gradient-echo MR imaging: analysis with receiver operating characteristic curves. Radiology 1991;181:661.

168. Arlart IP, Guhl L, Fauser L, et al. MR-Angiographie (MRA) der Abdominalvenen. Radiologe 1991;31:192.

169. Arlart IP, Guhl L, Edelman RR, et al. Magnetic resonance angiography of the abdominal arteries and veins: assessment of the 2D and 3D technique. Electromedica 1992;60:58.

170. Megibow AJ, Bosniak MA, Ambos MA, et al. Thickening of the celiac axis and/or superior mesenteric artery: a sign of pancreatic carcinoma on computed tomography. Radiology 1981;141:449.

171. Luetmer PH, Stephens DH, Fischer AP. Obliteration of peri-arterial retropancreatic fat on CT in pancreatitis: an exception to the rule. AJR 1989;153:63.

172. Schulte SJ, Baron RL, Freeny PC, et al. Root of the superior mesenteric artery in pancreatitis and pancreatic carcinoma: evaluation with CT. Radiology 1991;180:659.

173. Baker ME. Pancreatic adenocarcinoma: are there pathogno-monic changes in the fat surrounding the superior mesenteric artery? Radiology 1991;180:613.

174. Theodorsson E. Regulatory peptides as tumour markers. Acta Oncol 1989;28:319.

175. Breidahl HD, Priestly JT, Rynearson EH. Hyperinsulinism: surgical aspects and results. Ann Surg 1955;142:698.

176. Goulon M, Rapin M, Charleux H, Baguet J-C, Kuntziger H, Nouailhat F, Barois A, Breteau M. Diarrhée aqueuse et hypokaliémie associées à une tumeur langerhansienne non insulino-sécrétante: discussion nosologique de ce syndrome avec celui de Zollinger et Ellison. Presse Med 1966;74:2345.

177. McGavran NH, Unger RH, Recant L, Polk HC, Kilo C, Levin ME. A glucagon-secreting alpha-cell carcinoma of the pancreas. N Engl J Med 1966;274:1408.

178. Zollinger RM, Moore FT. Zollinger-Ellison syndrome comes of age. JAMA 1968;204:361.

179. Bloom SR, Polak JM, Pearse AGE. Vasoactive intestinal pep-tide and watery-diarrhoea syndrome. Lancet 1973;2:14.

180. Zollinger RM. Islet cell tumors and the alimentary tract. AJR 1976;126:933.

181. Pogany AC, Kerlan RK Jr, Karam JH, et al. Cystic insulinoma. AJR 1984;142:951.

182. Thompson NW, Vinik AI, Eckhauser FE. Microgastrinomas of the duodenum: a cause of failed operations for the Zol-linger-Ellison syndrome. Ann Surg 1989;209:396.

183. Günther RW, Klose KJ, Rückert K, et al. Localization of small islet-cell tumors: preoperative and intraoperative ultrasound, computed tomography, arteriography, digital subtraction an-giography, and pancreatic venous sampling. Gastroint Ra-diol 1985;10:143.

184. Galiber AK, Reading CC, Charboneau JW, et al. Localization of pancreatic insulinoma: comparison of pre- and intraopera-tive US with CT and angiography. Radiology 1988;166:405.

185. Dunnick NR, Long JA Jr, Krudy A, et al. Localizing insulino-mas with combined radiographic methods. AJR 1980;135: 747.

186. Frucht H, Doppman JL, Norton JA, et al. Gastrinomas: com-parison of MR imaging with CT, angiography, and US. Radi-ology 1989;171:713.

187. London JF, Shawker TH, Doppman JL, et al. Zollinger-Ellison syndrome: prospective assessment of abdominal US in the localization of gastrinomas. Radiology 1991;178:763.

188. Mitchell DG, Cruvella M, Eschelman DJ, et al. MRI of pan-creatic gastrinomas. J Comp Asst Tomogr 1992;16:583.

189. Olsson O. Angiographic diagnosis of an islet cell tumor of the pancreas. Acta Chir Scand 1963;126:346.

190. Madsen B. Demonstration of pancreatic insulomas by angiog-raphy. Br J Radiol 1966;39:488.

191. Bookstein J, Oberman HA. Appraisal of selective angiography in localizing islet-cell tumors of the pancreas. Radiology 1966;86:682.

192. Boijsen E, Samuelsson L. Angiographic diagnosis of tumors arising from the pancreatic islets. Acta Radiol 1970;10:161.

193. Gray RK, Rösch J, Grollman JH Jr. Arteriography in the diag-nosis of islet cell tumors. Radiology 1970;97:39.

194. Skjoldborg H, Madsen B. Selective angiography in surgical management of pancreatic insulomas. Acta Chir Scand 1971; 137:169.

195. Alfidi RJ, Bhyun DS, Crile G Jr, Hawk W. Arteriography and hypoglycemia. Surg Gynecol Obstet 1971;133:447.

196. Robins JM, Bookstein JJ, Oberman HA, Fajans SS. Selective angiography in localizing islet-cell tumors of the pancreas. Ra-diology 1973;106:525.

197. Fujii K, Yamagata S, Sasaki R, Ohneda A, Shoji T, Suzuki J. Arteriography in insuloma. AJR 1974;120:634.

198. Fulton RE, Sheedy PF II, McIlrath DC, Ferris DO. Preopera-tive angiographic localization of insulin-producing tumors of the pancreas. AJR 1975;123:367.

199. Clouse ME, Costello P, Legg MA, Soeldner SJ, Cady B. Sub-selective angiography in localizing insulomas of the pancreas. AJR 1977;128:741.

200. Hernandez C. Angiographie des hypoglycémies organique. Ann Gastroenterol Hepatol 1977;13:145.

201. Korobkin MT, Palubinskas AJ, Glickman MG. Pitfalls in arte-riography of islet cell tumors of the pancreas. Radiology 1971; 100:319.

202. Reuter SR, Redman HC. Gastrointestinal angiography. 2nd ed. Philadelphia: Saunders, 1977.

203. Deutsch V, Adar R, Jacob ET, Bank H, Mozes M. Angio-graphic diagnosis and differential diagnosis of islet-cell tu-mors. AJR 1973;119:121.

204. Nyman U. Angiography in hereditary hemorrhagic telangiec-tasia. Acta Radiol 1977;18:581.

205. Reuter SR. Potential overdiagnosis of pancreatic islet cell ade-nomas. J Can Assoc Radiol 1971;22:184.

206. Mills SR, Doppman JL, Dunnick NR, McCarthy DM. Evalua-tion of angiography in Zollinger-Ellison syndrome. Radiol-ogy 1979;131:317.

207. Rosenbusch G, Lamers CBH, van Tongeren JHM, Boetes C, Snel P, Lubbers EJC. Röntgendiagnostik beim Zollinger-Ellison-Syndrom. ROEFO 1978;129:168.

208. Ludin H, Enderlin F, Fahrländer HJ, Scheidegger S. Failure to diagnose Zollinger-Ellison syndrome by pancreatic arteri-ography. Br J Radiol 1966;39:494.

209. Andersson T, Eriksson B, Hemmingsson A, et al. Angio-graphy, computed tomography, magnetic resonance im-aging and ultrasonography in detection of liver metastases from endocrine gastrointestinal tumours. Acta Radiol 1987; 28:535.

210. Doppman JL, Miller DL, Chang R, et al. Gastrinomas: local-ization by means of selective intraarterial injection of secretin. Radiology 1990;174:25.

211. Doppman JL, Miller DL, Chang R, et al. Insulinomas: local-ization with selective intraarterial injection of calcium. Radiol-ogy 1991;178:237.

212. Mallinson CN, Bloom SR, Warin AP, Salmon PR, Cox B. A glucagonoma syndrome. Lancet 1974;2:1.

213. Eriksson B, Öberg K, Skogseid B. Neuroendocrine pancreatic tumors: clinical findings in a prospective study of 84 patients. Acta Oncol 1989;28:373.

214. Andersson H, Dotevall G, Fagerberg G, et al. Pancreatic tu-mor with diarrhea, hypokalemia and hypochlorhydria. Acta Chir Scand 1972;138:102.

215. Auerbach RC, Koehler PR. The many faces of islet cell tu-mors. AJR 1973;119:133.

216. Gold RP, Black TJ, Rotterdam H, Casarella WJ. Radiologic

and pathologic characteristics of the WDHA syndrome. AJR 1976;127:397.

217. Thomas ML, Lamb GHR, Barraclough MA. Angiographic demonstration of a pancreatic "Vipoma" in the WDHA syndrome. AJR 1976;127:1037.

218. Thompson GB, van Heerden JA, Grant CS, et al. Islet cell carcinomas of the pancreas: a twenty-year experience. Surgery 1988;104:1011.

219. Boijsen E. Inactive malignant endocrine tumors of the pancreas. Radiologe 1975;15:177.

220. Baghery S, Alfidi RJ, Zelch MG. Angiography of non-functioning islet cell tumors of the pancreas. Radiology 1976;120:57.

221. Adler O, Kaftori JK, Rosenberger A, Ben Arieh J. Non-functioning islet cell tumors of the pancreas: a review of radiological literature and a report of two cases. ROEFO 1977;127:559.

222. Bok EJ, Cho KJ, Williams DM, et al. Venous involvement in islet cell tumors of the pancreas. AJR 1984;142:319.

223. Imhoff I, Frank P. Pancreatic calcifications in malignant islet cell tumors. Radiology 1977;122:333.

224. Mathieu D, Guigui B, Valette PJ, et al. Pancreatic cystic neoplasms. Radiol Clin North Am 1989;27:163.

225. Freeny PC, Weinstein CJ, Taft DA, Allen FH. Cystic neoplasms of the pancreas: new angiographic and ultrasonographic findings. AJR 1978;131:795.

226. Bieber WP, Albo RJ. Cystadenoma of the pancreas: its arteriographic diagnosis. Radiology 1963;80:776.

227. Abrams RM, Berenbaum ER, Berenbaum SL, Ngo NL. Angiographic studies of benign and malignant cystadenoma of the pancreas. Radiology 1967;89:1028.

228. Hawkins IF Jr, Kaude JV. Angiographic findings in some rare pancreatic tumors. ROEFO 1976;125:521.

229. Couinaud, Jouan, Prot, Chalut, Schneider. Hémo-lymphangiome de la tête du pancréas. Mem Acad Chir (Paris) 1966;92:152.

230. Halpern M, Turner AF, Citron BP. Hereditary hemorrhagic telangiectasia: an angiographic study of abdominal visceral angiodysplasia associated with gastrointestinal hemorrhage. Radiology 1968;90:1143.

231. Hernandez C, Ecarlat B, Bismuth V. L'artérioportographie des affections pancréatiques. J Radiol Electrol Med Nucl 1967;48:327.

232. Lande A, Bedford A, Schechter LS. The spectrum of angiographic findings in Osler-Weber-Rendu disease. Angiology 1976;27:223.

233. Chuang VP, Pulmano CM, Walter JF, Cho KJ. Angiography of pancreatic arteriovenous malformation. AJR 1977;129:1015.

234. Legre J, Guien C, Clément JP, Piétri H. Tumeurs pancréatiques a caractère angiomateux revelées par angiographie sélective. J Radiol Electrol Med Nucl 1969;50:229.

235. Bennet J, Bigot R, Monnier JP, Goldlust M, Doyon D. Les hypervascularisations pancréatiques. J Radiol Electrol Med Nucl 1971;52:485.

236. Roe M, Greenough WG. Marked hypervascularity and arteriovenous shunting in acute pancreatitis. Radiology 1974;113:47.

237. Neiman HL, Goldstein HM, Silverman PJ, Bookstein JJ. Angiographic features of peripancreatic malignant lymphoma. Radiology 1975;115:389.

238. Tylén U. Angiography in disease of the peripancreatic lymph nodes. Acta Radiol 1975;16:625.

239. Albrechtsson U, Tylén U. Angiography in reticulum cell sarcoma. Acta Radiol 1977;18:210.

240. Boijsen E, Wallace S, Kanter IE. Angiography in tumors of the stomach. Acta Radiol 1966;4:306.

241. Bron KM, Sherman L. Arteriography in evaluating retroperitoneal mass lesions. NY State J Med 1967;67:1875.

242. Wilson TE, Korobkin M, Francis IR. Pancreatic plasmocytoma: CT findings. AJR 1989;152:1227.

243. Webb TH, Lillemoe KD, Pitt HA, et al. Pancreatic

244. Reuter SR, Redman HC, Joseph RR. Angiographic findings in pancreatitis. AJR 1969;107:56.

245. Tylén U, Arnesjö B. Angiographic diagnosis of inflammatory disease of the pancreas. Acta Radiol 1973;14:215.

246. Aakhus T, Hofsli M, Vestad E. Angiography in acute pancreatitis. Acta Radiol 1969;8:119.

247. Kivisaari L, Sopmer K, Standertskjöld-Nordenstam CG, et al. Early detection of acute fulminant pancreatitis by contrast enhanced computed tomography. Scand J Gastroenterol 1983;18:39.

248. Waltman AC, Luers PR, Athanasoulis CA, et al. Massive arterial hemorrhage in patients with pancreatitis: complementary roles of surgery and transcatheter occlusive techniques. Arch Surg 1986;121:439.

249. Jeffrey RB Jr. Sonography in acute pancreatitis. Radiol Clin North Am 1989;27:5.

250. Balthazar EJ. CT diagnosis and staging of acute pancreatitis. Radiol Clin North Am 1989;27:19.

251. Balthazar EJ, Robinson DL, Megibow AJ, et al. Acute pancreatitis: value of CT in establishing prognosis. Radiology 1990;174:331.

252. Lechner G, Pokieser H. Ergebnisse angiographischer Untersuchungen bei Pankreatitis. ROEFO 1971;114:49.

253. Boijsen E, Tylén U. Vascular changes in chronic pancreatitis. Acta Radiol 1972;12:34.

254. Moskowitz H, Chait A, Mellins HZ. "Tumor encasement" of the celiac axis due to chronic pancreatitis. AJR 1968;104:641.

255. Bron KM, Redman HC. Splanchnic artery stenosis and occlusion: incidence; arteriographic and clinical manifestations. Radiology 1969;92:323.

256. Reuter SR, Olin T. Stenosis of the celiac artery. Radiology 1965;85:617.

257. Dunbar JD, Molnar W, Beman FF, Marable SA. Compression of the celiac trunk and abdominal angina: preliminary report of 15 cases. AJR 1965;95:731.

258. Drapanas T, Bron KM. Stenosis of the celiac artery. Ann Surg 1966;164:1085.

259. White AF, Baum S, Buranasiri S. Aneurysms secondary to pancreatitis. AJR 1976;127:393.

260. Sheps SG, Spittel JA Jr, Fairbairn JF II, Edwards JE. Aneurysms of the splenic artery with special reference to blind aneurysms. Mayo Clin Proc 1958;33:381.

261. Baum S, Greenstein RH, Nusbaum M, Blakemore W. Diagnosis of ruptured noncalcified splenic artery aneurysm by selective celiac arteriography. Arch Surg 1965;91:1026.

262. Boijsen E, Efsing H-O. Aneurysm of the splenic artery. Acta Radiol 1969;8:29.

263. Boijsen E, Göthlin J, Hallböök T, Sandblom P. Preoperative angiographic diagnosis of bleeding aneurysms of abdominal visceral arteries. Radiology 1969;93:781.

264. Greenstein A, deMaio EF, Nabseth DC. Acute hemorrhage associated with pancreatic pseudocysts. Surgery 1971;69:56.

265. L'Herminé C, Gautier-Benoit C, Vankemmel M, Lemaitre G. Les érosions artérielles des pseudokystes pancréatiques. Etude angiographique de six observations. Ann Radiol (Paris) 1971;14:55.

266. Francillon J, Grandjean JP, Vignal J, Tissot E, Moulay A. Hemorrhagie artérielle dans l'évolution des pseudokystes pancréatiques. Lyon Chir 1974;70/3:192.

267. Levin DC, Eisenberg H, Wilson R. The role of arteriography in the evaluation of pancreatic pseudocysts. AJR 1977;129:243.

268. Meyers MA, Evans JA. Effect of pancreatitis on the small bowel and colon: spread along mesenteric planes. AJR 1973;119:151.

269. Harris RD, Anderson JE, Coel MN. Aneurysms of the small pancreatic arteries: a cause of upper abdominal pain and intestinal bleeding. Radiology 1975;115:17.

270. Chermet J, Bigot J-M, Monnier J-P. Les hémorrhagies diges-

tives par érosions artérielles au cours des pancréatites: diagnostic pré-opératoire par l'artériographie en urgence. J Radiol Electrol Med Nucl 1974;55:117.

271. Schechter LM, Gordon HE, Passaro E Jr. Massive hemorrhage from the celiac axis in pancreatitis. Am J Surg 1974; 128:301.

272. Tylén U, Dencker H. Roentgenologic diagnosis of pancreatic abscess. Acta Radiol 1973;14:9.

273. Bolondi L, Bassi SL, Gaiani S, et al. Sonography in chronic pancreatitis. Radiol Clin North Am 1989;27:815.

274. Luetmer PH, Stephens DH, Ward EM. Chronic pancreatitis: reassessment with current CT. Radiology 1989;171:353.

275. Bléry M, Etienne J, Farah A, Bismuth V. Le traumatisme du pancréas. Intérêt de l'artériographie sélective. Sem Hop Paris 1972;48:473.

276. Haertel M, Fuchs WA. Angiography in pancreatic trauma. Br J Radiol 1974;47:641.

277. Geindre M, Marty F, Fournet J, Baudain Ph, Champetier M. Aspects angiographiques des contusions du pancréas. Ann Radiol 1973;16:341.

278. Chvojka J. Ein Beitrag der gezielten Angiographie zur Diagnostik der Pankreasverletzungen. ROEFO 1970;113:336.

279. Svahn T, Lewander R, Hårdstedt C, et al. Angiography and scintigraphy of human pancreatic allografts. Acta Radiol 1978;19:297.

280. Toledo-Pereyra LH, Kristen KT, Mittal VK. Scintigraphy of pancreatic transplants. AJR 1982;138:621.

281. Maile CW, Crass JR, Frick MP, et al. CT of pancreas transplantation. Invest Radiol 1985;20:609.

282. Letourneau JG, Maile CW, Sutherland DER, et al. Ultrasound and computed tomography in the evaluation of pancreatic transplantation. Radiol Clin North Am 1987;25:345.

283. Yuh WTC, Hunsicker LG, Nghiem DD, et al. Pancreatic transplants: evaluation with MR imaging. Radiology 1989; 170:171.

284. Snider JF, Hunter DW, Kuni CC, et al. Pancreatic transplantation: radiologic evaluation of vascular complications. Radiology 1991;178:749.

285. Bradley EL, Murphy F, Ferguson C. Prediction of pancreatic necrosis by dynamic pancreatography. Ann Surg 1989;210: 495.

56

Portal and Pancreatic Venography

ANDERS LUNDERQUIST
KRASSI IVANCEV

Direct Portal Venography

From the mid-1970s to the early 1980s percutaneous portography was used to investigate the portal venous system in patients with portal hypertension. The direct access to the portal venous system in comparison with splenoportography made it possible to catheterize specific branches and led to the presumption that bleeding esophageal varices might be treated by occlusion.

Occlusion was performed in several different ways, with injection of Gelfoam and Sotradecol,[1] cyanoacrylate,[2] absolute alcohol, or Gianturco coils.[3,4] It was soon realized that this kind of treatment only temporarily stopped the bleeding, and new collaterals rapidly developed. The treatment could prevent an emergency portosystemic shunt operation but was rarely used.

At the same time endoscopic sclerotherapy of esophageal varices was developed and rapidly took over the therapy of the patient bleeding from portal hypertension and esophageal varices. This new technique had fewer complications than direct portal venography. Furthermore, it was demonstrated that patients treated percutaneously rebled earlier than patients who had received endoscopic treatment.[5,6]

Transhepatic treatment of esophageal varices is used infrequently. In patients who do not respond to endoscopic treatment, portosystemic shunts are made surgically or, more recently, by percutaneous transjugular techniques (TIPS) (see Chapter 33 in *Abrams' Angiography: Interventional Radiology*). During the years that percutaneous portography was performed, important knowledge was collected about portal venous anatomy and collateral pathways in portal hypertension. An investigation by Hoevels et al.[7] demonstrated that the most common portosystemic collaterals were esophageal varices (88 percent) (Fig. 56-1), followed by the inferior mesenteric vein (59 percent) (Fig. 56-2), short gastric veins (58 percent) (Fig. 56-3), paraesophageal veins (29 percent), and umbilical-paraumbilical veins (29 percent) (Fig. 56-4). In addition, a large number of retroperitoneal portosystemic collaterals could be mapped running from the splenic hilum veins to the renal veins (Fig. 56-5), pancreatic veins, and diaphragmatic veins. It was found that the size and number of collaterals did not correlate to the portal pressure in portal hypertensive patients.[8] This signified that large collaterals did not reduce the risk of gastrointestinal hemorrhage or reduce the portal pressure.

Anatomy of the Portal Vein

The splenic and the superior mesenteric vein join behind the head of the pancreas to form the portal vein, which runs in a craniolateral direction to the hilum of the liver. Variations are seen in the branching of the portal vein into the right and left lobe (Fig. 56-6). In about 80 percent of cases[9] it divides into two right and one left branch. The right branches supply the anterior segment and the posterior segment of the right lobe. The branch to the right posterior segment may be seen to take off directly from the portal trunk in 5 to 6 percent of cases, and the branch to the anterior segment of the right lobe is a branch of the left portal vein in 3 to 4 percent of cases (Fig. 56-7).[10,11] The horizontal segment of the left portal vein may be missing (Fig. 56-8), and there might be a complete absence of the right portal vein. In these cases the right lobe of the liver is smaller than normal and supplied from the left portal vein.

As a single trunk the left branch of the portal vein turns transversely to the left between the quadrate and caudate lobes. After 1 to 5 cm it reaches the fissure for the ligamentum teres, where it turns ventrally as the pars umbilicalis. At the turn it gives off the branch to the dorsolateral segment, then the branch to the ventrolateral segment. At this level and from the right side of the pars umbilicalis two to four branches leave to the medial segment of the left lobe. The pars umbilicalis ends ventrally as the recessus umbilicalis with the entrance of the umbilical vein.[11,12]

Portal branches to the caudate lobe leave from the transverse portion of the left portal vein, from the first

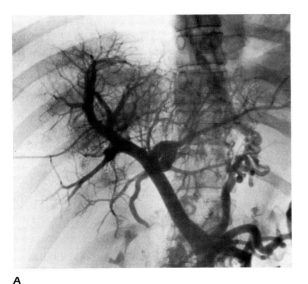

A

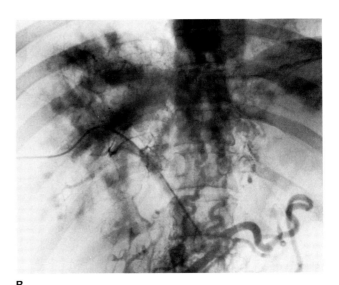

B

Figure 56-1. Transhepatic portal venography in a patient with liver cirrhosis and portal hypertension. Retrograde flow is seen in the left gastric veins to the esophageal varices.

part of the right portal vein, or directly from the portal trunk.

In less than 1 percent of cases the transverse segment of the portal vein is absent and the left lobe is supplied by the right anterior segmental branch. A rare anomaly, but nevertheless of great surgical importance, is the preduodenal position of the portal vein. Coming from behind the head of the pancreas, the portal vein turns ventrally to the duodenal cap toward the hilum of the liver. The hepatic artery and the bile duct remain in normal position.[13,14]

In adults, the diameter of the portal vein after its confluence has been reported to be 9 to 11 mm as measured by ultrasound.[15,16] Interestingly, the diameter increases when the patient is examined in the left lateral decubitus position as compared with the supine position, probably because of the reduced outflow from the hepatic veins; in a similar way, inspiration can completely interrupt hepatic vein outflow.[17]

The relationship between the portal vein and the intrahepatic bile ducts might be of importance in percutaneous transhepatic procedures. It is generally accepted that the bile duct lies anterior to the portal vein. This is almost always correct in the porta hepatis. In an examination of 17 cadaver livers, Bret et al.[18] found the bile ducts anterior in 10, posterior in 1, and tortuous in 5; 1 case could not be interpreted. Intrahepatic

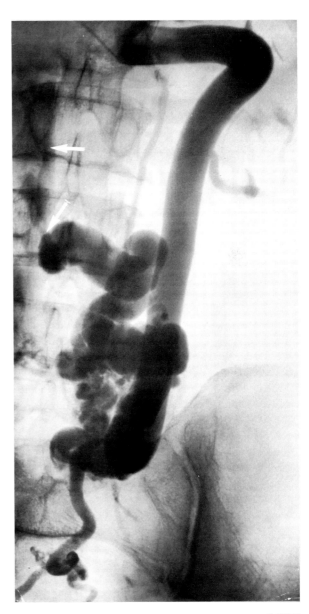

Figure 56-2. Transhepatic catheterization of markedly enlarged inferior mesenteric vein in a patient with portal hypertension. There is hepatofugal flow via retroperitoneal collaterals to the inferior vena cava (*upper arrow*). The portosystemic anastomosis (*lower arrow*) is very narrow in comparison to the feeding collateral vein.

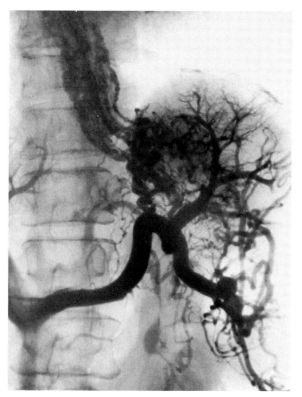

Figure 56-3. Transhepatic portal venography in a patient with portal hypertension. Selective injection of contrast medium into the splenic vein near hilus of spleen. There is hepatofugal flow via short gastric and capsular veins of the spleen to esophageal varices.

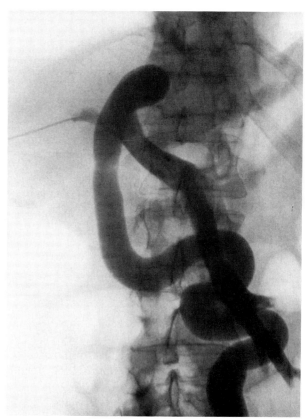

Figure 56-4. Transhepatic portography in a patient with portal hypertension. There is total hepatofugal intrahepatic portal vein flow despite hepatopetal flow in the main stem of portal vein. A wide umbilical vein serves as a portosystemic collateral.

Figure 56-5. Transhepatic catheterization of a spontaneous splenorenal shunt. The portosystemic anastomosis (*arrow*) is narrower than the feeding collateral.

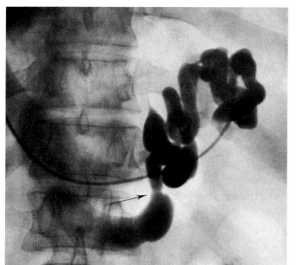

bile ducts were seen posterior to the portal vein in about the same number of cases as they were seen anterior.[18,19]

Percutaneous Approach to the Portal Vein

Transhepatic Approach

Under local anesthesia a puncture is made with a 0.9-mm needle in the right axillary line.[4] Puncture is performed well below the visible costophrenic angle during normal respiration and as straight as possible toward a position slightly above the anticipated liver hilum. Frequently the needle with this approach will transverse the obliterated pleural sinus, but when ascites is not present no complications will occur. The needle is slowly retracted during continuous contrast injection. When contrast is seen to flow into a branch of the portal vein a slightly curved platinum-tipped guidewire is introduced through the needle and its tip is manipulated through the portal vein branch into the main stem of the portal vein. With the platinum-tipped

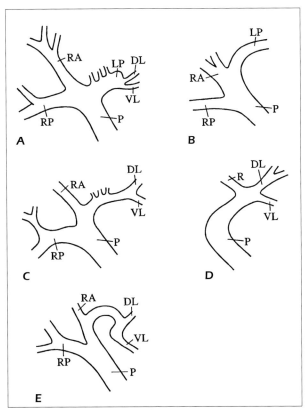

Figure 56-6. Schematic drawing of portal vein anomalies. *P*, main stem of portal vein; *RP*, right posterior segmental branch; *RA*, right anterior segmental branch; *LP*, left portal vein; *DL*, left dorsolateral segmental branch; *VL*, left ventrolateral segmental branch. (A) Trifurcation is seen in 80 percent of cases. (B) The right posterior segmental branch takes off directly from the main stem of the portal vein (5–6 percent). (C) The right anterior segmental branch takes off from the left portal vein (3–4 percent). (D) Complete absence of right portal vein. A small right lobe is supplied from the left portal vein. (E) The horizontal segment of the left portal vein is missing.

guidewire in this position, the needle is removed and replaced by a 5 French polyethylene catheter, which is advanced over the guidewire together with a 3 French coaxial catheter to reduce resistance. With the 5 French polyethylene catheter in the portal vein, the platinum-tipped guidewire and the 3 French catheter are removed. A curved 0.035-inch guidewire can be used to assist in catheterization of desired branches.

Complications. Bleeding is the most feared complication, especially in patients with portal hypertension and coagulopathy. In these patients the incidence has been reported to be 1.5 to 7.0 percent.[1,4,20] Portal vein thrombosis (2–8 percent) has been reported only in patients with portal hypertension and when obliteration of varices has been performed. In some patients the injected sclerosing material has been the cause of

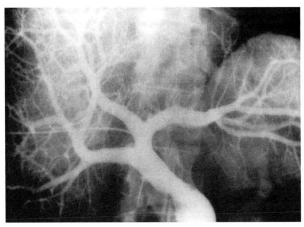

Figure 56-7. Transhepatic portography. The right anterior segment takes off from the left portal vein.

thrombosis; in others changes in flow pattern caused by the obliteration are thought to be responsible.

Transjugular Approach

Transjugular catheterization of the bile ducts has been performed, and the same approach has been used for liver biopsy. The transjugular technique for entering the portal venous system, introduced by Rösch et al.,[21] has found wide acceptance.

The right jugular vein is punctured under local anesthesia, and a 0.035-inch guidewire is introduced for further manipulation into the superior vena cava. A 6.5 French polyethylene catheter with a slightly curved tip is advanced over the guidewire and manipulated into the right hepatic vein. With the guidewire in the hepatic vein, the catheter is removed and a long 9 French vascular sheath with introducer is manipulated into the right hepatic vein. The introducer is removed and a

Figure 56-8. Transhepatic portography in a patient with portal hypertension. The horizontal segment of the left portal vein is missing.

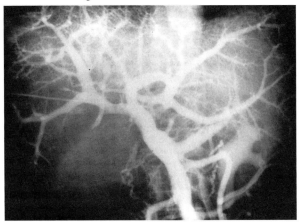

curved transjugular needle (Cook, Inc.) is advanced through the sheath until it is end to end with the sheath. A puncture is performed in an anterior direction toward the right portal vein. When blood can be aspirated and injection of contrast confirms the position in the portal vein, a 0.035-inch guidewire is passed into the portal vein and further down into the superior mesenteric vein. After the needle has been removed, an angiographic catheter is advanced over the guidewire into the superior mesenteric vein, from which position further catheterizations can be performed.

Complications. Because transperitoneal passage and puncture of the liver capsule is not performed, the likelihood of hemorrhage is almost eliminated. Unintended puncture through the liver parenchyma into the peritoneal cavity has been reported with hemorrhage as a consequence. Portal vein thrombosis is a complication seen only in patients with portal hypertension.

Umbilical Vein Approach

Under local anesthesia an incision is made in the midline 5 cm above the umbilicus.[22,23] The umbilical cord is isolated and a small incision is made to find the obliterated lumen. A blunt probe can usually be advanced without resistance through the umbilical vein until its entrance into the left portal vein branch, where a moderate resistance is felt. Under a slight increase in pressure the probe moves quickly into the portal vein. The probe is then removed and an angiographic catheter can be advanced into the portal vein. As soon as the catheter has entered the vein, a curved guidewire is used to manipulate the catheter through the left portal vein and into the main stem of the portal vein.

Complications. Complications are mainly seen when the catheter has been left in place for several days. Among the complications reported are wound infection (1.2 percent), bleeding from the surgical wound (1.3 percent), and thrombosis of the portal vein or its branches (0.9 percent).[22]

Pancreatic Venography

Little attention was paid to the pancreatic veins until it became obvious that blood sampling from these veins could facilitate localization of pancreatic endocrine tumors.[24] Selective sampling from the veins of the pancreas has shown to be more accurate than both CT and angiography.[25] When venous sampling is to be performed, a thorough knowledge of the anatomy is necessary.

Anatomy

The anatomy of the pancreatic veins has been carefully investigated by Petrén,[26] Falconer and Griffiths,[27] and Reichardt and Cameron.[28] The pancreatic head is mainly drained by two veins, the posterior superior pancreaticoduodenal vein (PSPD) and the anterior superior pancreaticoduodenal vein (ASPD) (Fig. 56-9). The PSPD (Fig. 59-10) enters directly into the dorsocaudal circumference of the portal vein 1 to 3 cm from its confluence with the superior mesenteric vein. In most cases the PSPD runs on the posterior surface of the pancreatic head and receives a large number of small veins from the pancreas and from the adjacent part of the duodenum. An additional vein may be found in this region, but it is draining the ventrocranial part of the pancreatic head and enters the portal vein close to the PSPD.

The PSPD may form an arcade together with the posterior inferior pancreaticoduodenal vein (PIPD) running in the dorsal groove between the pancreatic head and duodenum and receiving branches from the pancreas as well as from the duodenum. The PIPD usually drains into the first jejunal vein close to the superior mesenteric vein (SMV) but can also be seen to drain into the second jejunal vein or directly into the SMV. Shortly before the PIPD enters a jejunal vein

Figure 56-9. Venous anatomy of the pancreas, schematic. *PV*, portal vein; *SV*, splenic vein; *SMV*, superior mesenteric vein; *IMV*, inferior mesenteric vein; *PSPD*, posterior superior pancreaticoduodenal vein; *ASPD*, anterior superior pancreaticoduodenal vein; *PIPD*, posterior inferior pancreaticoduodenal vein; *AIPD*, anterior inferior pancreaticoduodenal vein; *TP*, transverse pancreatic vein; *DP*, dorsal pancreatic vein; *CV*, coronary vein. The dotted veins are anterior, the striped veins posterior, to the pancreas. (From Reichardt W, Ingemansson S. Selective vein catheterization for hormone assay in endocrine tumors of the pancreas: technique and results. Acta Radiol 1980;21:177. Used with permission.)

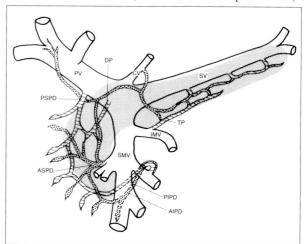

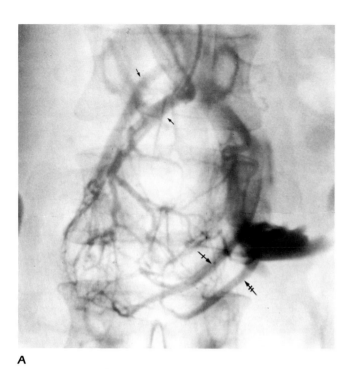

A

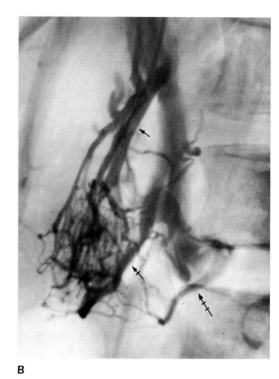

B

Figure 56-10. Selective injection of contrast into the PSPD. (A) Anteroposterior view. (B) Lateral view. Two PSPDs are demonstrated (*arrows*). Over collaterals the anterior superior (*barred arrows*) and posterior inferior pancreaticoduodenal veins (*double-barred arrows*) are filled.

or the SMV it often receives a tributary from the anterior inferior pancreaticoduodenal vein (AIPD). This vein follows the ventral groove between the anterior aspect of the pancreatic head and the duodenum, receiving branches from the pancreas as well as from the duodenum before it passes through the parenchyma of the pancreas to join the PIPD.

The ASPD (Fig. 56-11), which drains the anterior part of the head of the pancreas, consists of several small branches that drain separately or with a common stem into the gastrocolic trunk. Sometimes the ASPD forms an anterior arcade together with the AIPD.

The dorsal pancreatic vein (DP), which drains the dorsomedial part of the head and body of the pancreas, enters the confluence of the splenic vein, SMV, and portal vein in its dorsal wall. The DP has anastomoses to the PSPD and often to the coronary vein.

The left part of the body and the tail of the pancreas are drained into the splenic vein by a large number of veins of varying sizes. Several of these veins make anastomoses with the transverse pancreatic (TP) vein (Fig. 56-12) running along the inferior border of the body and tail of the pancreas. The TP drains into the upper part of the inferior mesenteric vein, the SMV, and the left part of the splenic vein, or into the confluence of the splenic, SMV, and portal vein.

Figure 56-11. Injection of contrast into the ASPD (*straight arrow*). Over collaterals the AIPD (*double-barred arrow*), gastrocolic trunk (*curved arrow*), and two branches of the PSPD (*barred arrows*) are demonstrated.

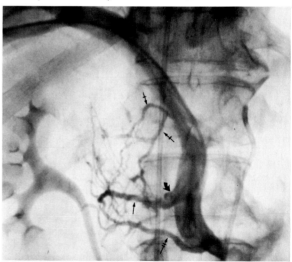

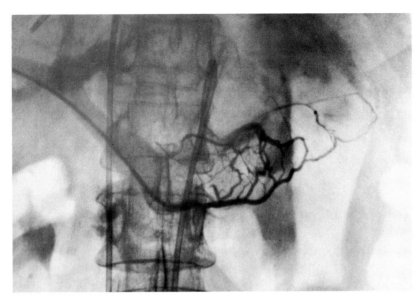

Figure 56-12. Injection of contrast into transverse pancreatic vein. Over collaterals a faint filling of the splenic vein is received. (From Reichardt W, Cameron R. Anatomy of the pancreatic veins: a post mortem and clinical phlebographic investigation. Acta Radiol 1980;21:33–41. Used with permission.)

Technique of Pancreatic Vein Catheterization

The technique of portal vein catheterization has been described in the previous section on direct portal venography. The transhepatic approach is preferred when pancreatic veins are to be catheterized. This shorter distance makes manipulation of guidewire and catheter easier when small pancreatic veins are to be found. After the portal vein has been entered, a 5 French radiopaque polyethylene catheter with a side hole close to its tip is introduced into the portal vein and manipulated to the left part of the splenic vein, where a contrast injection is performed for rough anatomic interpretation. After this a curved 0.035-inch guidewire is used to localize the different pancreatic veins. The 5 French catheter is carefully advanced over the guidewire into the vein that is found, and when the guidewire has been removed a slow contrast injection is used to identify the vein. This is followed by slow aspiration of blood for hormone assay.

Catheterization of the pancreatic veins can be facilitated by using a Tracker catheter (Target Therapeutics) or Micro Ferret catheter (Cook Europe A/S) through the 5 French polyethylene catheter. The high torque control of their 0.018-inch guidewires makes the finding of small branches much easier.

If catheterization of pancreatic vein branches is unsuccessful, multiple blood samples should be taken in the splenic vein, the upper part of the SMV, and the main stem of the portal vein. Care should be taken in interpreting these samples because lamellar flow in large veins may give false results.[29]

Indications for Pancreatic Vein Catheterization

With the new imaging techniques now available, the only indication for pancreatic vein catheterization is venous sampling in endocrine tumors of the pancreas. In a recent review of 50 patients with insulinomas, CT showed an accuracy of 26 percent, angiography 44 percent, and transhepatic venous sampling 94 percent in localizing the tumors.[25] Even here indications have been reduced because of the success with intraoperative ultrasound, endoscopic ultrasound (US),[30] and MRI of the pancreas.[31]

When external US, CT, and angiography, as well as endoscopic US and MRI, are negative, pancreatic venous sampling still has a place, but should be used as the last option before laparotomy and intraoperative US.

Pancreatic venography has no place in the imaging of pancreatitis or pancreatic tumors, with the exception of the endocrine tumors. Although pancreatic phlebography will demonstrate abnormalities in these lesions of the pancreas (Figs. 56-13 and 56-14), this is not an indication for its use.

Complications

There are few complications from pancreatic phlebography, and they are rarely serious. The most common complication is pain, reported in 16 percent of cases.[32] As always, when puncture through the liver parenchyma is performed, an arteriovenous fistula (2 percent) or hemobilia (1 percent) may occur. An asymp-

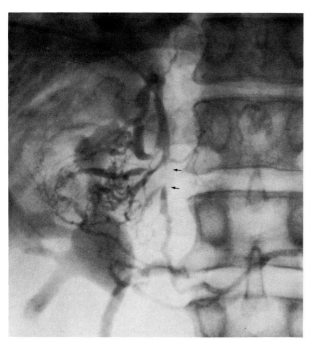

Figure 56-13. Nonresectable carcinoma. Injection into the PSPD. Main branches are obstructed (*arrows*).

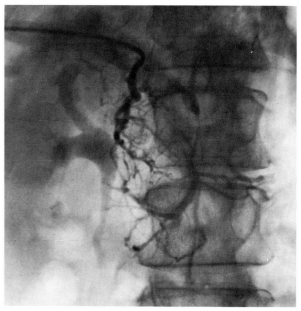

Figure 56-14. Chronic pancreatitis. Irregular intrapancreatic veins but patent collaterals between PSPD and ASPD. (From Reichardt W. Selective phlebography in pancreatic and peripancreatic disease. Acta Radiol 1980;21:513. Used with permission.)

tomatic superior mesenteric vein occlusion has also been reported.[32]

Endocrine Tumors

The insulin-producing adenoma is the most common endocrine tumor of the pancreas. Since it is usually less than 3 cm in size, it cannot be demonstrated by morphologic changes at pancreatic phlebography.[33]

In patients with rare endocrine tumors such as glucagonomas, vipomas, and somatostatinomas, the diagnosis is often established late and the detected tumors are larger. If the tumor exceeds 4 cm in diameter, an expanding lesion with displacement of the veins can be found at phlebography (Fig. 56-15). In smaller tumors no venous changes are seen.[33] Selective pancreatic phlebography is therefore not a useful way to localize endocrine pancreatic tumors.

On the other hand, catheterization of pancreatic veins is essential if blood sampling and hormone assay for localization of endocrine pancreatic tumors are performed (Table 56-1).[24,34–36] Blood sampling in the main portal vein tributaries only does not allow a correct localization of all endocrine tumors (Table 56-2).[37] Selective phlebography has to be performed because the venous anatomy varies considerably and must be investigated individually. The sites for blood sampling have to be documented to obtain a proper interpretation of hormone analyses regarding tumor localization (Fig. 56-16). For this purpose, too, selec-

Figure 56-15. Islet cell tumor in the head of the pancreas, 5 cm in diameter. Only displacement of the PSPD (*arrow*) is found at phlebography. (From Reichardt W. Selective phlebography in pancreatic and peripancreatic disease. Acta Radiol 1980;21:513. Used with permission.)

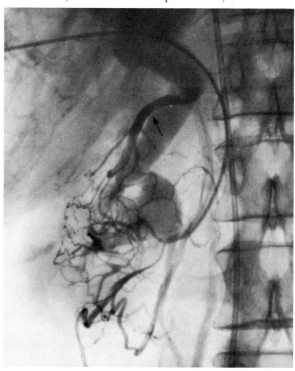

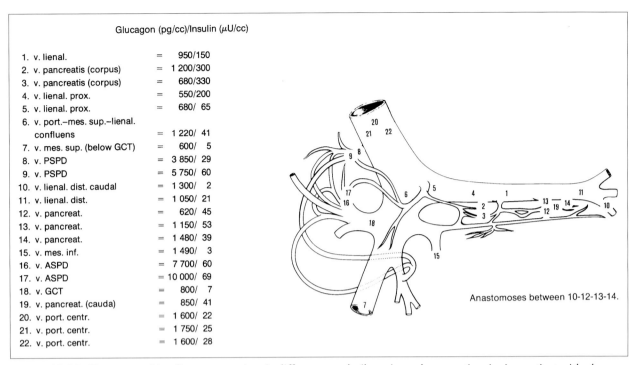

Glucagon (pg/cc)/Insulin (μU/cc)

1. v. lienal.	=	950/150
2. v. pancreatis (corpus)	=	1 200/300
3. v. pancreatis (corpus)	=	680/330
4. v. lienal. prox.	=	550/200
5. v. lienal. prox.	=	680/ 65
6. v. port.–mes. sup.–lienal. confluens	=	1 220/ 41
7. v. mes. sup. (below GCT)	=	600/ 5
8. v. PSPD	=	3 850/ 29
9. v. PSPD	=	5 750/ 60
10. v. lienal. dist. caudal	=	1 300/ 2
11. v. lienal. dist.	=	1 050/ 21
12. v. pancreat.	=	620/ 45
13. v. pancreat.	=	1 150/ 53
14. v. pancreat.	=	1 480/ 39
15. v. mes. inf.	=	1 490/ 3
16. v. ASPD	=	7 700/ 60
17. v. ASPD	=	10 000/ 69
18. v. GCT	=	800/ 7
19. v. pancreat. (cauda)	=	850/ 41
20. v. port. centr.	=	1 600/ 22
21. v. port. centr.	=	1 750/ 25
22. v. port. centr.	=	1 600/ 28

Anastomoses between 10-12-13-14.

Figure 56-16. Glucagon and insulin concentrations in different portal tributaries and pancreatic veins in a patient with glucagonoma of the head of the pancreas, mainly drained by the ASPD (*samples 16, 17*).

Table 56-1. Patients with Islet Cell Tumors or Islet Cell Hyperplasia Examined with Angiography and Selective Pancreatic Catheterization for Hormone Assay— University Hospital, Lund, Sweden, Series

Patient Number	Angiography	Hormone Assay	Final Diagnosis
1	+	+	Insulinoma
2	—	+	B-cell hyperplasia
3	—	+	B-cell hyperplasia
4	+	+	Insulinoma
5	—	+	Insulinoma
6	—	+	Insulinoma
7	—	—[a]	Insulinoma
8	+	+	Glucagonoma
9	(+)[b]	+	Glucagonoma
10	+	+	Tumor-producing glucagon, insulin, and serotonin
11	+	(+)[b]	Somatostatinoma
12	+	—	D-cell tumor
13	(+)[c]	(+)[d]	Multiple gastrinomas
14	(+)[c]	(+)[d]	Multiple gastrinomas
15		(+)[d]	Multiple gastrinomas
16	+	+	Gastrinoma, not verified

+ = correct localization.
[a] Venous abnormality.
[b] Found retrospectively.
[c] One of multiple tumors demonstrated.
[d] Generally elevated gastrin concentration. No distinct localization of tumors possible.

Table 56-2. Hormone Concentrations in Tumor-Draining Veins Compared with Main Portal Vein Tributary Outside the Tumor-Draining Veins

Tumors	In Tumor-Draining Vein	In Main Portal Vein Tributary at Tumor Level	Range of Concentrations in Main Portal Vein Tributaries
		(μU/ml)	
Insulinomas			
1	—	865	93–260
2	600	300	13–58
3*	1130	45	11–165
4*	245	14	11–68
5	6200	179	14–28
6	974	95	95–230
		(pg/ml)	
Glucagonomas			
1	24,000	2900	1320–2400
2	10,000	800	600–1750
3	10,650	?	856–2213

*B-cell hyperplasia.

tive phlebography is necessary. Because the main pancreatic veins are to be found on the surface of the organ, the veins can be dissected and located during operation, and the phlebographic anatomy can be identified. Using the results from the hormone assay, the surgeon thus can find even nonpalpable adenomas or islet cell hyperplasia by following the tumor-draining vein.[37]

Gastrinomas are often multiple. In these cases a generally elevated gastrin concentration in all the veins may indicate multiplicity of gastrin-releasing tumors but does not allow a distinct localization of the tumors.[35] If the gastrin-producing tissue is limited to one part of the pancreas, a curative resection may be possible.[38]

References

1. Widrich WC, Robbins AH, Nabseth DC. Transhepatic embolization of varices. Cardiovasc Intervent Radiol 1980;3:298–307.
2. Lunderquist A, Börjesson B, Owman T, Bengmark S. Isobutyl 2-cyanoacrylate (Bucrylate) obliteration of gastric coronary vein and esophageal varices. AJR 1978;130:1–6.
3. Yune HY, Klatte EC, Richmond BD, Rabe FE. Absolute ethanol thrombotherapy of bleeding esophageal varices. AJR 1982;138:1137–1141.
4. L'Herminé C, Chastanet P, Delemazure O, et al. Percutaneous transhepatic embolization of gastroesophageal varices: results in 400 patients. AJR 1989;152:755–760.
5. O'Connor KW, Lehman G, Yune H, et al. Comparison of three nonsurgical treatments for bleeding esophageal varices. Gastroenterology 1989;96:899–906.
6. Terabayashi H, Ohnishi K, Tsunoda T, et al. Prospective controlled trial of elective endoscopic sclerotherapy in comparison with percutaneous transhepatic obliteration of esophageal varices in patients with nonalcoholic cirrhosis. Gastroenterology 1987;93:1205–1209.
7. Hoevels J, Lunderquist A, Tylén U, Simert G. Porto-systemic collaterals in cirrhosis of the liver. Acta Radiol 1979;20:865–877.
8. Simert G, Lunderquist A, Tylén U, Vang J. Correlation between percutaneous transhepatic portography and clinical findings in 56 patients with portal hypertension. Acta Chir Scand 1978;144:27–34.
9. Yamane T, Mori K, Sakamoto K, et al. Intrahepatic ramification of the portal vein in the right and caudate lobes of the liver. Acta Anat 1988;133:162–172.
10. Atri M, Bret PM, Fraser-Hill MA. Intrahepatic portal venous variations: prevalence with US. Radiology 1992;184:157–158.
11. Inoue T, Kinoshita H, Hirohashi K, et al. Ramification of the intrahepatic portal vein identified by percutaneous transhepatic portography. World J Surg 1986;10:287–293.
12. Gupta SC, Gupta CD, Arora AK. Intrahepatic branching patterns of portal vein: a study by corrosion cast. Gastroenterology 1977;72:621–624.
13. Stevens JC, Morton D, McElvee R, Hamit HF. Preduodenal portal vein: two cases with differing presentation. Arch Surg 1978;113:311–313.
14. Davis JM. Preduodenal portal vein. NY State J Med 1976;76:2038.
15. Rahim N, Adam EJ. Ultrasound demonstration of variations in normal portal vein diameter with posture. Br J Radiol 1985;58:313–314.
16. Weinreb J, Kumari S, Phillips G, Pochaczevsky R. Portal vein measurements by real-time sonography. AJR 1982;139:497–499.
17. Moreno AH, Burchell AR. Respiratory regulation of splanchnic and systemic venous return in normal subjects and in patients with hepatic cirrhosis. Surgery 1982;154:257–267.
18. Bret PM, de Stempel JV, Atri M, et al. Intrahepatic bile duct and portal vein anatomy revisited. Radiology 1988;169:405–407.
19. Lim JH, Ryu KN, Ko YT, Lee DH. Anatomic relationship of

intrahepatic bile ducts to portal veins. J Ultrasound Med 1990; 9:137–143.

20. Bengmark S, Börjesson B, Hoevels J, et al. Obliteration of esophageal varices by percutaneous transhepatic embolization: a follow-up of 43 patients. Ann Surg 1979;190:549–554.

21. Rösch J, Antonovic R, Dotter CT. Transjugular approach to the liver biliary system and portal circulation. AJR 1975;125: 602–608.

22. Everth S, Angelin B. Cannulation of the umbilical vein in adult man: a review of surgical techniques, possible complications and clinical applications. Acta Chir Scand 1980;500(Suppl): 75–78.

23. Göthlin J, Dencker H, Tranberg K-G. Technique and complications of transumbilical catheterization of the portal vein and its tributaries. AJR 1975;125:431–436.

24. Ingemansson S, Holst J, Larsson LI, Lunderquist A. Localization of glucagonomas by catheterization of the pancreatic veins and with glucagon assay. Surg Gynecol Obstet 1977;145:509–516.

25. Pasieka JL, McLeod M, Thompson NW, Burney RE. Surgical approach to insulinomas: assessing the need for preoperative localization. Arch Surg 1992;127:442–447.

26. Petrén T. Die Arterien und Venen des Duodenums und des Pankreaskopfes beim Menschen. Zeit f d ges Anat 1929;90: 234–277.

27. Falconer A, Griffiths E. The anatomy of the blood-vessels in the region of the pancreas. Br J Surg 1950;37:334–344.

28. Reichardt W, Cameron R. Anatomy of the pancreatic veins: a post mortem and clinical phlebographic investigation. Acta Radiol 1980;21:33–41.

29. Roche A, Raisonnier A, Gillon-Savouret M-C. Pancreatic venous sampling in localizing insulinomas and gastrinomas: procedure and results in 55 cases. Radiology 1982;145:621–627.

30. Rösch T, Lightdale CJ, Botet JF, et al. Localization of pancreatic endocrine tumors by endoscopic ultrasonography. N Engl J Med 1992;326:1721–1726.

31. Mitchell DG, Cruvella M, Eschelman DJ, et al. MRI of pancreatic gastrinomas. J Comput Assist Tomogr 1992;16:583–585.

32. Miller DL, Doppman JL, Metz DC, et al. Zollinger-Ellison syndrome: technique, results, and complications of portal venous sampling. Radiology 1992;182:235–241.

33. Reichardt W. Selective phlebography in pancreatic and peripancreatic disease. Acta Radiol 1980;21:513.

34. Ingemansson S, Kühl C, Larsson LI, Lunderquist A, Lundquist I. Localization of insulinomas and islet hyperplasia by pancreatic vein catheterization and insulin assay. Surg Gynecol Obstet 1978;146:725.

35. Ingemansson S, Larsson LI, Lunderquist A, Stadil F. Pancreatic vein catheterization with gastrin assay in normal patients and in patients with the Zollinger-Ellison syndrome. Am J Surg 1977; 134:558.

36. Lunderquist A, Eriksson M, Ingemansson S, Larsson LI, Reichardt W. Selective pancreatic vein catheterization for hormone assay in endocrine tumors of the pancreas. Cardiovasc Radiol 1978;1:117.

37. Reichardt W, Ingemansson S. Selective vein catheterization for hormone assay in endocrine tumors of the pancreas: technique and results. Acta Radiol 1980;21:177.

38. Burcharth F, Stage JG, Stadil F, Jensen LI, Fischermann K. Localization of gastrinomas by transhepatic portal catheterization and gastrin assay. Gastroenterology 1979;77:444.

57

Hepatic Arteriography

STANLEY BAUM

Although the in vivo arterial pattern of the liver had been demonstrated with percutaneous translumbar aortography, it remained for Bierman et al. in 1951[1] first to describe the technique of selective hepatic arteriography. The examination was performed by injecting contrast material directly into the hepatic artery during intraarterial catheterization or laparotomy. This procedure, however, did not become widely accepted as a diagnostic aid because of the many technical problems involved in the surgical exposure of the brachial artery for the passage of the intraarterial catheters and the relatively toxic nature of the contrast material available at the time. The introduction in 1953 of the Seldinger catheter replacement technique,[2] serial film changers, automatic injectors, and safe water-soluble contrast agents was essential for the development of hepatic arteriography.

In 1958 Ödman published a monograph on percutaneous selective arteriography of the celiac artery that demonstrated the ease with which the celiac and superior mesenteric arteries could be selectively catheterized and injected.[3] Although computed tomography (CT), magnetic resonance imaging (MRI), and ultrasound (US) examinations have assumed an increasingly important role in the evaluation of disease of the liver,[4-7] selective hepatic arteriography remains an important diagnostic tool in the diagnosis of liver disease. Hepatic arteriography has also provided insights into many pathophysiologic states.

Technique

Celiac arteriography is performed in most angiographic laboratories by the same technique described by Ödman. A preshaped radiopaque catheter is percutaneously inserted into either the femoral or the axillary artery, and, by means of image-intensification fluoroscopy preferably with television monitoring, the celiac axis is selectively catheterized. In most patients the celiac axis arises as an anterior branch of the aorta at the T12-L1 interspace. Orientation can usually be

obtained by identifying the last rib and counting the vertebral bodies. The superior mesenteric artery generally arises from the anterior portion of the abdominal aorta at the bottom of the midportion of the first lumbar vertebral body. The renal arteries are generally posterolateral branches of the aorta at the level of L1-L2. At times it is helpful to turn the patient to a sharp left posterior oblique position during the catheter manipulation to clearly identify the anterior portion of the abdominal aorta. After the tip of the catheter is securely in place in the celiac trunk, approximately 0.5 to 0.75 ml per kilogram of body weight of a water-soluble diatrizoate contrast material is injected by automatic injector at a rate of 4 to 8 ml per second. Filming begins with the injection of the contrast material and continues during the arterial, capillary, and venous phases (spanning a total of 24 to 28 seconds after the start of the injection). During the arterial phase of the study, exposures are made every 0.5 second. Then films are taken every second, and finally one every third second. The hepatic arteriogram can be divided into an arterial phase, a capillary hepatogram phase, and a portal hepatogram phase.

In keeping with the current trend in vascular opacification studies of introducing the catheter as close as possible to the organ being studied, the hepatic artery is frequently catheterized directly by passing the catheter more peripherally after its insertion into the celiac trunk. This superselective injection technique provides excellent visualization of the intrahepatic arterial branches. The technique also avoids superimposition of extraneous vessels, such as the left gastric, gastroepiploic, and splenic arteries. It has the disadvantage that it does not afford evaluation of the portal hepatogram phase, since there is no contrast returning from the spleen. The performance of superselective arteriography of the hepatic artery requires more experience with catheter manipulation than does celiac arteriography. The techniques currently employed for superselective catheterization include the use of catheter manipulators, coaxial catheter methods, and specially shaped catheters and guidewires. Prior to superselective hepatic arteriography it is useful to have a celiac arteriogram, since this affords an arterial road map of the arterial blood flow to the liver. When the injection of contrast material is made directly into the hepatic artery, the volume used in the average adult is 20 to 40 ml (depending on the size of the liver) injected at a rate of 4 to 6 ml per second. This is generally accompanied by a sensation of warmth in the right upper quadrant.

The use of direct serial magnification techniques with fractional focal-spot x-ray tubes and air gap radiography has greatly increased the resolution obtained during arteriography. Vessels of approximately 100 μ in diameter can readily be seen.

Normal Anatomy

Because of the great frequency of anatomic variation in the arterial blood supply to the liver, only half the patients will have the entire hepatic arterial supply demonstrated after the injection into a common hepatic artery. The remaining 40 to 50 percent of patients have significant anatomic variations in the celiac and superior mesenteric arteries and, as Michels has pointed out,[8] these variations occur most often in the origins of the hepatic artery. The most common of them are the following:

1. Right hepatic and middle hepatic arteries arising from the celiac axis with the left hepatic artery arising from the left gastric artery (approximately 10–12 percent) (Figs. 57-1, 57-2).

2. Left hepatic and middle hepatic arteries arising from the celiac common hepatic artery with the right hepatic artery arising from the superior mesenteric artery (approximately 14 percent) (Fig. 57-3).

3. Right, left, and middle hepatic arteries arising from the celiac common hepatic with an accessory left hepatic artery from the left gastric artery (8 percent).

4. Right, middle, and left hepatic arteries arising from the celiac common trunk with an accessory right hepatic artery arising from the superior mesenteric artery (6 percent).

5. The entire common hepatic artery arising from the superior mesenteric artery and no hepatic artery originating from the celiac axis (2.5 percent).

Additional, less frequent variations such as hepatic-lienal-mesenteric trunks have also been reported (Fig. 57-4). Almost all the major variations described by Michels in his dissection of the arterial trees of cadavers have also been noted in vivo during visceral angiography.

Corrosion casts of human livers by Healey and Schroy[9] have shown that it is the internal distribution of the arteries, bile ducts, and portal veins rather than the external morphology that determines the surgically significant divisions. The morphologic plane of division of the liver, therefore, is the lobar fissure and not

Figure 57-1. Left hepatic artery originating from a left gastric artery. *a*, left hepatic artery; *b*, left gastric artery; *c*, common hepatic artery.

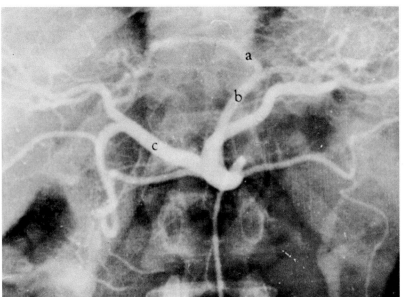

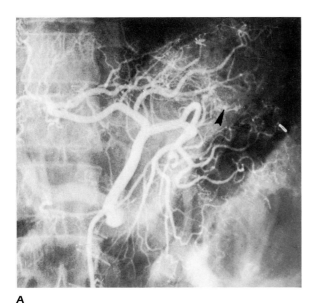

A

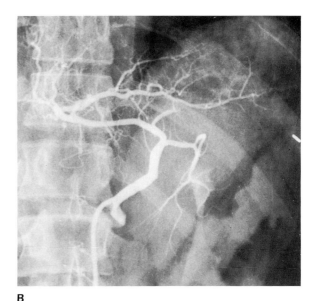

B

Figure 57-2. Selective left gastric–left hepatic arteriogram. (A) Selective arteriography of a common left gastric–left hepatic trunk demonstrates site of bleeding stress ulcer in the stomach (*arrowhead*). (B) Infusion of vasopressin selectively into the common trunk demonstrates marked vasoconstriction of the left gastric portion of the vessel with little effect on the caliber of the left hepatic branches. The infusion of vasopressin continued for 2 days, and there was complete control of the patient's bleeding without any evidence of injury to the liver.

the falciform ligament, left sagittal fossa, or ligamentum venosum. The lobar fissure is a parasagittal plane through the liver corresponding to a line extending from the gallbladder anteroinferiorly to the fossa of the inferior vena cava on the posterior surface of the liver. This fissure is characterized by the absence of hepatic arteries, portal veins, and bile ducts. No significant branches of the bile ducts, hepatic arteries, or portal veins cross the main lobar fissure, and thus it is a surgically safe plane for hepatic incisions and partial or complete lobectomies.

Nebesar et al.[10] pointed out that the bifurcation of the common hepatic artery, even when it arises from the celiac axis itself, may be atypical. Examples of a very proximal bifurcation of a common hepatic artery into a right hepatic and a middle hepaticogastroduo-

Figure 57-3. Selective celiac and superior mesenteric arteriography performed by injecting two catheters simultaneously, one positioned in the celiac axis and the other in the superior mesenteric artery. The right hepatic artery takes origin from the superior mesenteric artery (*arrow*). The celiac axis gives origin to the middle and left hepatic arteries, and the gastroduodenal artery is a branch of the left hepatic artery.

Figure 57-4. Common hepatic-lienal-mesenteric trunk.

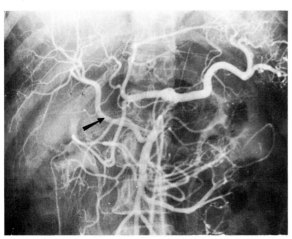

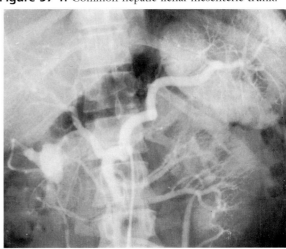

denal trunk have been seen. Other unusual bifurcations of the common hepatic artery are also encountered on occasion. All of these are important surgically because they may cause considerable confusion if they are not appreciated.

Because of the frequency of anatomic variations in the arterial supply of the liver, hepatic arteriography has proved to be a valuable procedure prior to major hepatic surgery. Since displacement and occasional thrombosis of the hepatic artery occur in the presence of neoplastic disease, arteriography is a prerequisite to hepatic arterial cannulation in cancer chemotherapeutic infusions.[11]

Cirrhosis

The arteriographic appearance of the cirrhotic liver depends on the amount of volume loss of the liver itself. In the fibrotic, contracted, cirrhotic liver, the intrahepatic branches of the hepatic artery exhibit a characteristic corkscrew tortuosity (Fig. 57-5).[12,13] This correlates very well with the disorganization of the vascular tree as seen in corrosion studies of the hepatic artery of cirrhotic livers. Such tortuosity, however, is not

Figure 57-5. Cirrhosis. Selective hepatic arteriography demonstrates characteristic intrahepatic arterial tortuosity due to fibrosis in a contracted, cirrhotic liver.

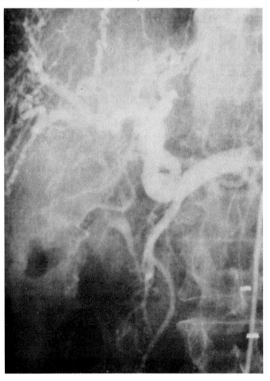

present until substantial loss in liver parenchyma has occurred. In the early stages of cirrhosis, therefore, the arterial changes are not at all obvious.

There is considerable evidence to indicate that in cirrhosis an increased blood flow through the hepatic artery occurs, and this itself has caused intrahepatic vascular changes, including telangiectasis and aneurysms.[14] Hepatic arterial–portal venous shunting has long been postulated in cirrhotic patients, and on occasion it can be demonstrated during hepatic arteriography (Fig. 57-6).

In the presence of portal hypertension, selective celiac and superior mesenteric arteriography has proved to be a valuable technique for evaluating the portal venous system and for demonstrating venous collaterals.

In the normal patient, the hepatic artery accounts for only 20 to 25 percent of the total hepatic blood flow, with the remainder coming from the portal vein. There appears to be a sensitive reciprocal nature to the blood flow to the liver, so that a reduction of flow in one vessel causes an almost immediate increase in the other. Angiographically, this reciprocity can be readily demonstrated during the selective hepatic arterial infusion of vasopressin. Initially there is a decrease in the hepatic arterial blood flow. However, a rise in the systemic level of vasopressin causes a decrease in superior mesenteric blood flow and hence a decrease in the amount of portal venous return. The hepatic artery then appears to break free of the vasoconstricting effect of the vasopressin, and there is a reciprocal increase of hepatic arterial flow.[15]

Around the periphery of the hepatic lobule are portal spaces containing branches of the hepatic artery, portal vein, bile duct, and lymphatics. As pointed out by Reuter and Redman,[16] the terminal arterioles of the hepatic artery and the terminal radicles of the portal vein empty into a common sinusoid. This mixed hepatic arterial and portal venous blood flows through the sinusoid, in contact with the hepatocytes, and finally drains via the central vein into the hepatic veins. Some of the angiographic features seen in cirrhosis are related to the drainage of the hepatic artery and portal venous radicles into a common sinusoidal space.[17]

In early cirrhosis, when the amount of portal venous flow is normal, the hepatic arterial changes are minimal. If fatty infiltration exists within the liver, the small hepatic arterial branches appear stretched, and not infrequently there is a peculiar mottled appearance during the parenchymal phase of the study. When the cirrhosis is moderate to severe, there tends to be reduction in the portal venous return to the liver and therefore an increase in hepatic artery blood flow.[18,19] The peripheral branches of the hepatic artery exhibit

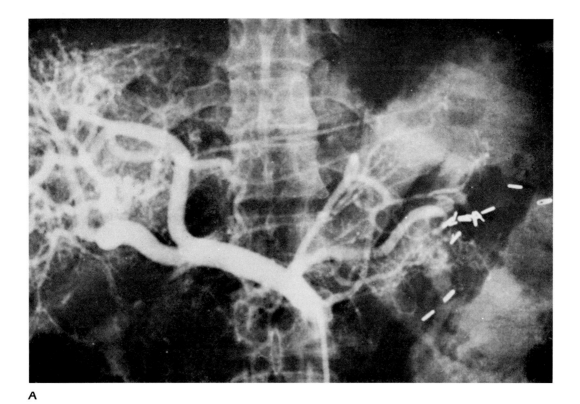

A

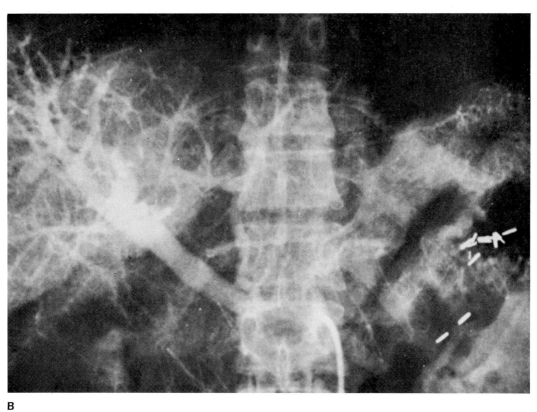

B

Figure 57-6. Hepatic arterial–portal venous shunt in a patient with portal hypertension and cirrhosis. (A) Selective celiac arteriography demonstrates large intrahepatic arterial branches and marked tortuosity of the smaller vessels due to a contracted, fibrotic liver. The splenic artery had been tied off as part of the patient's splenorenal shunt. (B) During the late arterial phase of the examination, prompt filling of the portal vein can be seen. (C) Several seconds later there is reversal of flow within the portal system with filling of gastric collaterals. The splenorenal shunt is nonfunctioning. (Courtesy of K. Kuroda, M.D.)

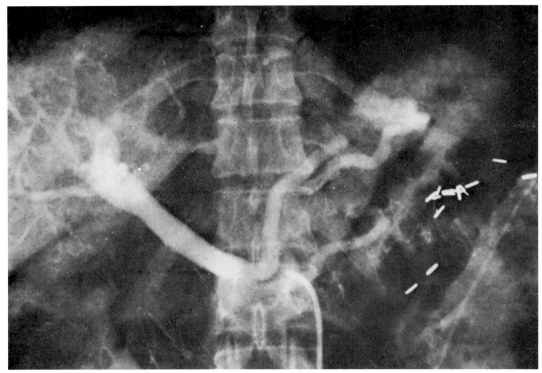

C   **Figure 57-6** (continued).

a characteristic corkscrew appearance as fibrosis becomes a prominent feature of the disease.

One must always be alert to the possibility of a hepatoma superimposed on a cirrhotic liver. Because of the hepatic arterial changes that are present in cirrhosis, the diagnosis of a hepatoma can be difficult to make, especially since both cirrhosis and hepatomas tend to exhibit hepatic arterial–portal venous shunting. The presence of regenerating nodules in cirrhosis causes further confusion, since these may often be confused with hepatomas (Fig. 57-7). The regenerating nodule has fewer hepatic arterial branches than does the adjacent liver, but because of the mass effect of the nodule, the arteries appear stretched and on occasion distorted.[20] Regenerating nodules usually do not show the hypervascularity of hepatomas, nor does one see the hepatic arterial–portal venous shunting.

Inflammatory Disease

Inflammatory disease of the liver generally takes the form of either a diffuse process involving all of the organ (as in cholangitis, serum hepatitis, and infectious hepatitis) or hepatic abscesses, which may be solitary or multifocal.

Cholangitis, Serum Hepatitis, and Infectious Hepatitis

The arteriographic findings in these diseases are not characteristic. In the few cases that have been reported, the findings have ranged from normal arteriograms to diffuse hypervascularity. Evans[13] has described an attenuated spastic appearance of the intrahepatic branches (Fig. 57-8). This angiographic appearance is probably due to the stretching of the vessels in the swollen and inflamed liver. It certainly does not appear to be pathognomonic, and a similar arteriographic configuration is seen in cholangitis and the fatty infiltration that frequently accompanies cirrhosis.

Hepatic Abscess

The arteriographic appearance of a hepatic abscess is very much like the appearance of abscess cavities anywhere in the body. If the abscess cavity is large, the arteriogram will reflect a relatively avascular mass with increased vascularity within the wall (Fig. 57-9). This is also the angiographic appearance of echinococcus (Fig. 57-10)[21,22] and ameba cysts.[23] Obviously, the clinical history is of great importance in making the diagnosis and in differentiating widespread abscess cavities in the liver from metastatic disease.

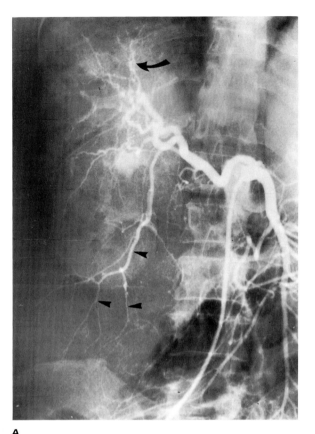

A

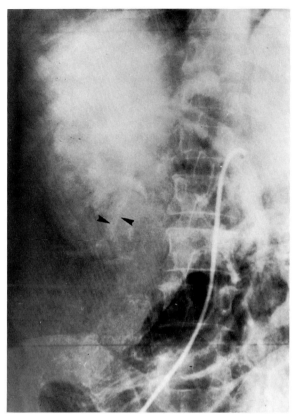

B

Figure 57-7. Large regenerating nodule in the right lobe of the liver in a patient with advanced cirrhosis. (A) Selective hepatic arteriography demonstrates a large mass extending down from the inferior portion of the right lobe of the liver. The vessel supplying the nodule appears stretched (*arrowheads*). The peripheral branches of the remaining portion of the hepatic artery exhibit the characteristic changes of advanced cirrhosis (*curved arrow*). (B) The venous phase of a superior mesenteric arteriogram demonstrates an elongated branch of the portal vein (*arrowheads*). (Courtesy of Josh Becker, M.D.)

Benign Hepatic Tumors

Cavernous Hemangiomas

Cavernous hemangiomas are the most common of the benign hepatic tumors and are usually very characteristic in their angiographic features as well as in their appearance by MRI.[5,24–26] Some pathologists question whether they should be considered true neoplasms or hamartomatous malformations. These lesions are

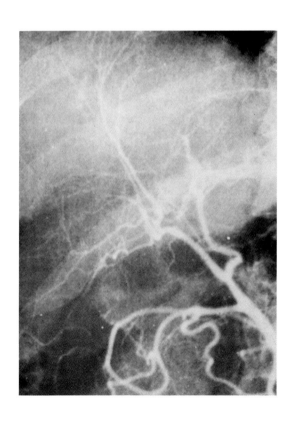

Figure 57-8. Viral hepatitis. Selective celiac arteriography demonstrates thin, spastic intrahepatic branches of the hepatic artery. The capillary hepatogram phase of the study was less dense than normal.

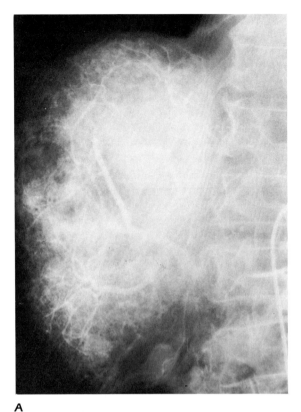

A

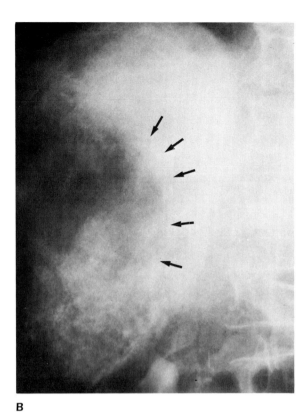

B

Figure 57-9. Hepatic abscess. (A) Arterial phase of the selective arteriogram shows displacement of peripheral branches of the hepatic artery. (B) Various-sized radiolucent defects are seen during the capillary phase of the study. In addition, the walls of the abscess cavity exhibit increased vascularity (*arrows*).

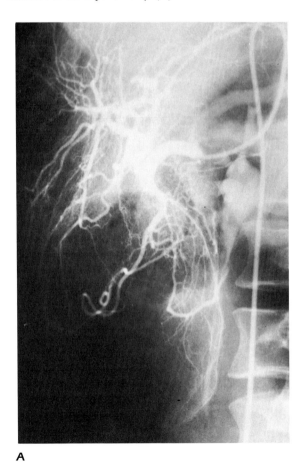

A

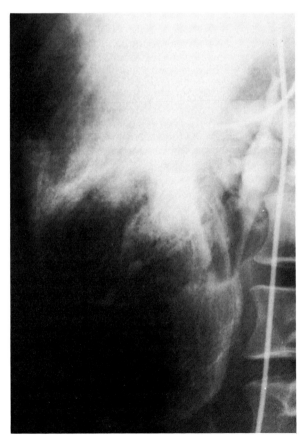

B

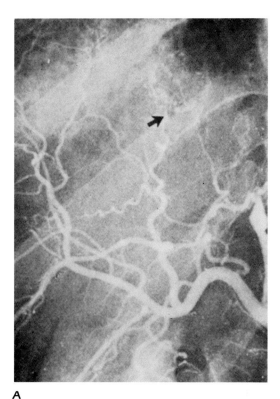

A

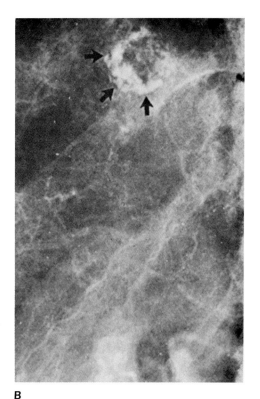

B

Figure 57-11. Cavernous hemangioma. (A) Selective hepatic arteriogram demonstrates a round vascular mass being fed by branches of the hepatic artery (*arrow*). (B) During the capillary phase of the study a spherical vascular stain is identified associated with pooling of contrast material without any evidence of arterial shunting (*arrows*).

usually no larger than 3 cm in diameter (Figs. 57-11, 57-12), although occasionally they may be quite big and occupy large areas of the liver (Fig. 57-13). Histologically the vascular spaces are lined by endothelium and in most cases can be seen extending from one or more arterial branches. On the arteriogram, the contrast-containing vascular spaces are usually orderly in their configuration, and the opaque material persists well into the venous phase of the study because of the extremely slow blood flow. Often these contrast-filled spaces are curvilinear. Arteriovenous shunting, which is so typical of primary hepatocellular carcinoma, is not seen.

The vascular pattern of hemangioendothelioma,[27] the other form of hepatic angioma, frequently mimics malignant disease and can be difficult to diagnose angiographically (Fig. 57-14).

Focal Nodular Hyperplasia

This lesion is benign, generally innocuous, and of uncertain pathogenesis.[28] Because of its multicellular nature, some pathologists have called it hepatic hamartoma,[29] parenchymal hamartoma,[30] focal nodular cirrhosis,[31] and even minimal deviation hepatoma.[32] When possible, such lesions should be differentiated from hepatic adenomas, which have a different pathogenesis and prognosis.

Focal nodular hyperplasia tends to be well circumscribed, subcapsular, occasionally pedunculated, and, in approximately 20 percent of cases, multiple.[33] Pathologically the tumor is white and hard and has a central scar out of which radiate fibrous bands. Histologically these fibrous septa separate normal-appearing liver tissue. There are many blood vessels and bile

◄ **Figure 57-10.** Echinococcus cyst. (A) The arterial phase of the study demonstrates a 10-ml avascular mass extending from the inferior margin of the right lobe of the liver. Because the patient was in a right posterior oblique position during the filming, the gastroduodenal and right gastro-epiploic arteries as well as the pancreatic arcades are superimposed on the superior portion of the cyst. (B) During the capillary phase of the study, the wall of the cyst appears hypervascular and thickened.

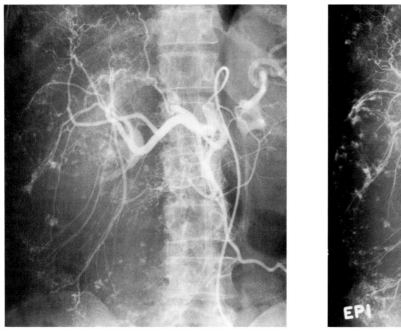

A

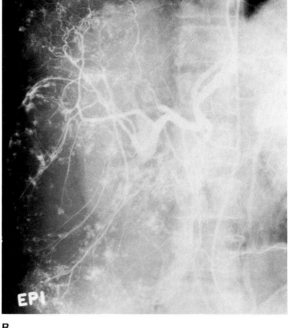

B

Figure 57-12. Enhanced visualization of multiple hepatic hemangiomas. (A) Nonenhanced hepatic arteriogram showing multiple hemangioma. (B) Thirty seconds following the intraarterial injection of 10 µg of epinephrine.

Figure 57-13. Cavernous hemangioma involving a large portion of the right lobe of the liver. (A) Selective hepatic arteriography demonstrates a large vascular mass deriving its blood supply from the right and middle hepatic arteries. (B)

Contrast material persists within large vascular spaces of the cavernous hemangioma well into the venous phase of the examination.

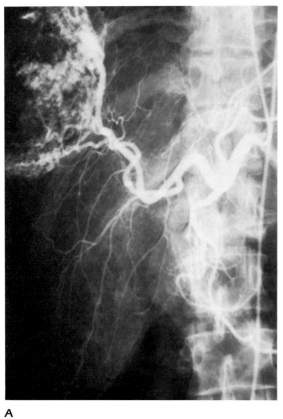

A

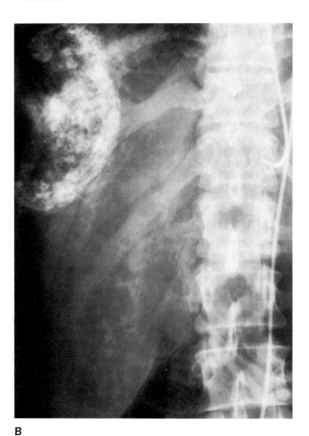

B

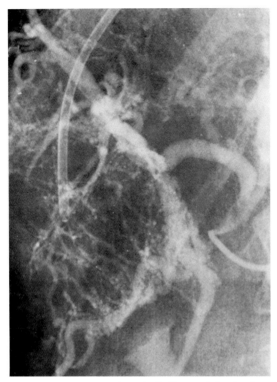

Figure 57-14. Hemangioendothelioma. Selective hepatic arteriogram demonstrates markedly increased vascularity in the right lobe of the liver associated with saccular dilatation of many intrahepatic arterial branches. During the capillary phase there was an intense tumor blush. No arteriovenous shunting was visible.

lesions, a dilated branch of the hepatic artery penetrates the mass and in the center of the lesion divides into small, fine branches that seem to radiate like spokes on a wheel (Figs. 57-15 to 57-17). There is an absence of arteriovenous shunting, and during the hepatographic phase the lesion looks granular or nodular. In smaller tumors, large penetrating arteries are not visible; however, there is a diffuse hypervascularity caused by small branches that penetrate the lesion, resulting in a reticular pattern during the hepatographic phase.

The pathogenesis of focal nodular hyperplasia remains obscure. It is probably not related to the ingestion of oral contraceptives, nor does it appear to be hormone-dependent. After an extensive literature review, Casarella et al.[34] concluded that there is no association between focal nodular hyperplasia and hepatocellular carcinoma. No deaths have been reported as being due to the natural history of the disease, but several deaths have occurred during attempted surgical resections. Although focal nodular hyperplasia has been seen in young children as well as in the elderly, in whom it is found as an incidental finding at autopsy, Knowles and Wolff[33] found 86 percent of patients with this lesion to be female with a mean age of 39 years. Because of the presence of Kupffer cells in focal nodular hyperplasia, some patients have normal uptake of labeled colloid on radionuclide scans.

Hepatic Adenomas

Liver cell adenomas tend to be solitary, encapsulated tumors that differ both macroscopically and microscopically from focal nodular hyperplasia.[35] Adenomas are likely to be larger than the lesions in focal nodular

ducts interspersed among the normal hepatocytes, and one can usually identify Kupffer cells. Angiographically focal nodular hyperplasia tends to be hypervascular and associated with dense capillary blushing. In large

Figure 57-15. Focal nodular hyperplasia. (A) Hypervascular mass in the left lobe of the liver is supplied by a dilated left hepatic artery. As the artery penetrates the mass, it divides into small, fine branches. (B) During the capillary phase of the study, the tumor shows an intense, homogeneous, granular blush.

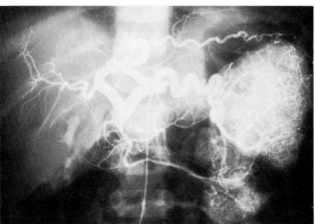

A

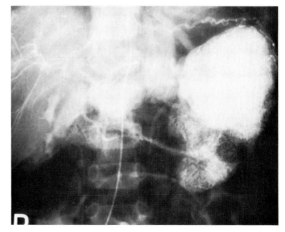

B

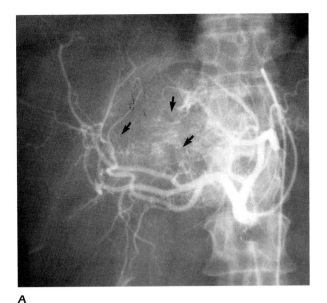

A

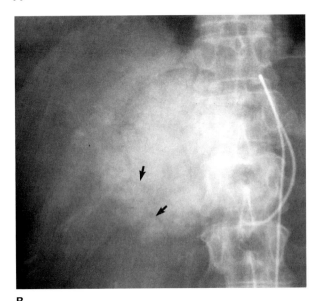

B

Figure 57-16. Focal nodular hyperplasia. A 39-year-old woman with abnormal liver function studies noted during workup prior to hysterectomy. (A) Arterial phase of a selective hepatic arteriogram shows irregular tumor vessels that appear to radiate from the periphery to the center of the tumor (*arrows*). (B) Capillary phase of the study shows an intense tumor blush with internal septations (*arrows*).

hyperplasia and when cut do not have the characteristic radiating scar of focal nodular hyperplasia. Also, areas of hemorrhage, necrosis, and bile stasis are often seen. Histologically adenomas are composed of atypical hepatocytes without any evidence of bile ducts or Kupffer cells. As pointed out by Phillips et al.,[29] the hepatocytes are very uniform and show an abnormally simplified ultrastructure. In 1973 Baum et al.[36] reported an association between adenomas and the in-

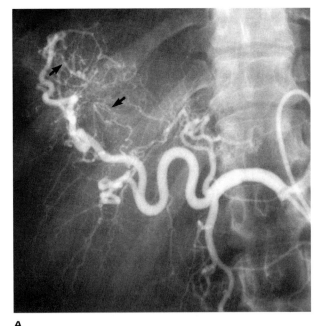

A

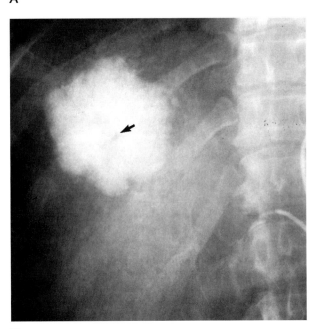

B

Figure 57-17. Focal nodular hyperplasia. A 36-year-old woman with right upper abdominal pain. (A) Arterial phase of a selective hepatic arteriogram shows characteristic "spokewheel" arteries penetrating from the periphery to the center of the tumor (*arrows*). (B) Capillary phase of the study demonstrates "central stellate scar" (*arrow*). (Courtesy of Dr. Ziv Haskal.)

gestion of oral contraceptives. Unlike focal nodular hyperplasia, with its innocuous natural history, hepatic adenomas have the potential for spontaneous intra-abdominal hemorrhage. The exact frequency of these

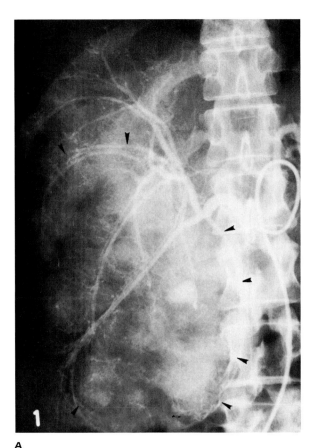

A

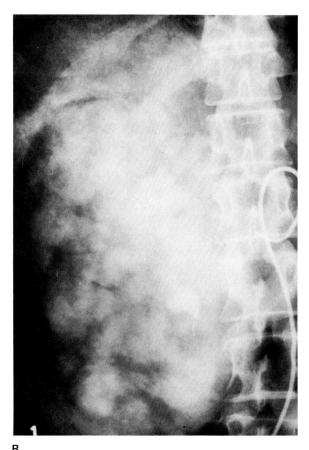

B

Figure 57-18. Hepatic adenoma. After taking oral contraceptives for several years a 45-year-old female presented with a palpable right upper quadrant mass. (A) Selective hepatic arteriography demonstrates a hypervascular 18-cm mass occupying the right lobe of the liver (*arrows*). (B) During the capillary phase of the examination the staining of the mass is not homogeneous but exhibits areas of radiolucency, due presumably either to necrosis or to small areas of hemorrhage. This hepatic adenoma was successfully resected.

tumors is unknown, since they are asymptomatic and come to attention only incidentally during laparotomy or angiography or when they cause massive hemorrhage.

Angiographically adenomas have a wide spectrum of appearances. Although some may be as, or even more, vascular than focal nodular hyperplasia, cases are also seen in which the tumors appear hypovascular. The angiographic picture may be further complicated by areas of necrosis and hemorrhage. In general, the vascularity of adenomas is not as fine and orderly as the pattern seen in focal nodular hyperplasia (Fig. 57-18), nor does one usually see the septa within the tumor. The tumor staining also tends to be more homogeneous than in hyperplasia. At times, however, the arteriogram can be quite difficult to differentiate from that obtained in hyperplasia, and in these cases radionuclide scans can be helpful. Since adenomas do not have any Kupffer cells, they do not take up labeled colloid.

Whether adenomas have a malignant potential is not altogether clear, especially since histologically it can be difficult at times to differentiate an adenoma from a hepatocellular carcinoma. Because of the chance of malignancy plus the risk of life-threatening hemorrhage, many hepatic adenomas are surgically removed.

Hamartomas and Other Rare Tumors

Hepatic hamartomas are rare, and their angiographic appearance varies greatly, depending on the primary cell type involved in the tumor mass.[37] These lesions frequently undergo cystic degeneration, and when this occurs, they may resemble benign cysts. Other benign tumors of the liver are very rare, and although biliary adenomas, cystadenomas, and leiomyomas have been reported, characteristic arteriographic findings in these tumors have not been described.

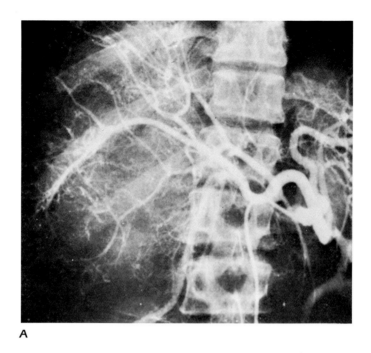

A

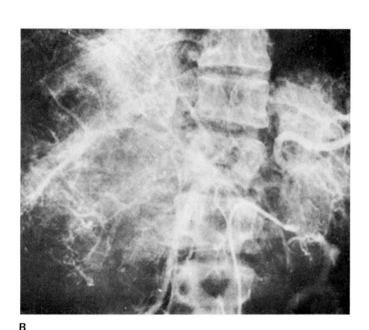

B

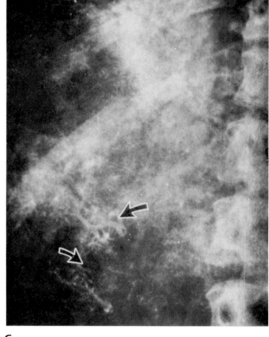

C

Figure 57-19. Hepatoma. (A) Arterial phase of a selective celiac arteriogram demonstrates marked displacement of the intrahepatic arterial branches involving primarily the right and middle lobes. (B) During the capillary phase, an intense tumor stain is seen associated with many abnormal tumor vessels. (C) During the late capillary phase, abnormal "laking" is seen within the tumors with persistence of contrast material within abnormally dilated veins (*arrows*).

Primary Malignant Tumors

Hepatomas

Primary carcinoma of the liver, or hepatoma, is almost always seen arteriographically as a vascular tumor.[38–40] The hepatic artery feeding the tumor is usually wider than normal, and the intrahepatic branches are gener-

ally displaced. During the arterial phase of a selective hepatic arteriogram the abnormal neovasculature, unlike that of hemangiomas, exhibits a chaotic and disorganized pattern. During the capillary phase of the examination, there is generally an intense tumor blush (Figs. 57-19 through 57-21). Marked arteriovenous shunting is a common finding in hepatomas (Figs. 57-

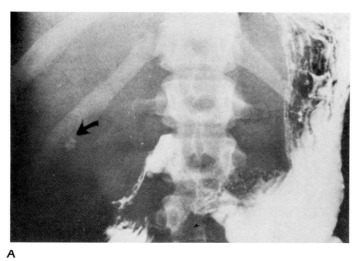

A

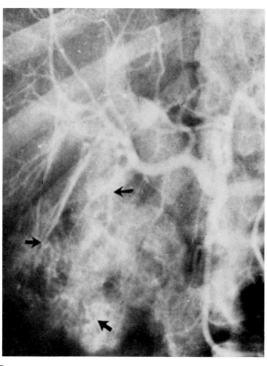

B

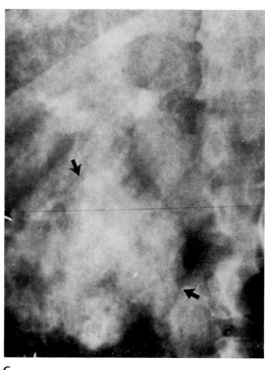

C

Figure 57-20. Calcification within a hepatoma. (A) An upper gastrointestinal study in a 22-year-old man demonstrates a large right upper quadrant mass displacing the first and second portions of the duodenum. Calcification is noted within the mass (*arrow*). Calcification within hepatomas is seen more often in children and young adults. (B) Selective hepatic arteriography demonstrates tumor vessels arising from the right hepatic artery (*arrows*) supplying this large, vascular tumor. (C) During the capillary phase of the study, an intense tumor blush is seen (*arrows*). The patient underwent successful resection of this lesion, which necessitated removal of the entire right lobe of the liver.

22 and 57-23), and on occasion the shunting into the portal venous system may be so great as actually to delineate tumor thrombi within the portal vein (Fig. 57-24).[41] Primary hepatic neoplasms derive almost all of their blood supply from the hepatic arteries. The portal venous system, which usually contributes approximately 75 percent of the blood supply to the normal liver, does not form the neovasculature of tumor masses.[42] As a result, splenoportography or arterial portography gives only indirect evidence of a mass, which is seen as a filling defect in an otherwise homogeneous portal hepatogram. Approximately 75 percent of patients with hepatomas have preexisting alcoholic or postnecrotic cirrhosis. The very distorted arterial pattern of advanced liver disease sometimes makes it difficult to detect a superposed carcinoma. A modification of the technique of hepatic arteriography for patients with suspected tumors has been the intrahepatic arterial administration of a vasoconstricting drug before the injection of contrast material (Fig. 57-25). This is based on the principle that tumor vessels, unlike normal vessels, do not react to vasoactive drugs.

1447

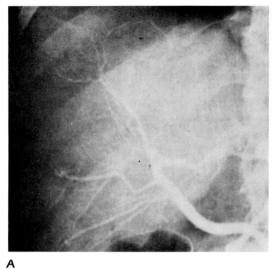

A

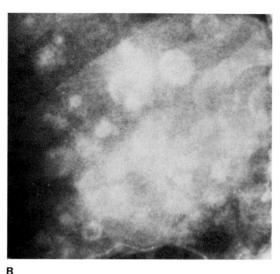

B

Figure 57-21. Multicentric hepatoma. (A) Selective hepatic arteriography fails to demonstrate tumor vessels or arteriovenous shunting. (B) During the capillary phase of the study, multiple tumor stains of various sizes can be identified. The arteriographic pictures resemble those of hepatic metastases. At surgery this was found to be a diffuse hepatoma. (Courtesy of Sidney Wallace, M.D.)

Figure 57-22. Hepatoma involving the left lobe of the liver. Selective injection into a common left hepatic–left gastric artery in a patient with cirrhosis and portal hypertension demonstrates marked arteriovenous shunting as a result of a hepatoma in the left lobe of the liver. The shunting into the portal venous system demonstrates hepatofugal flow.

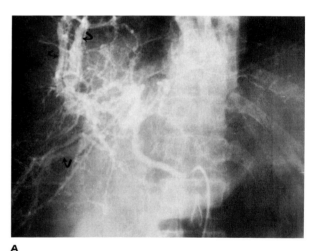

A

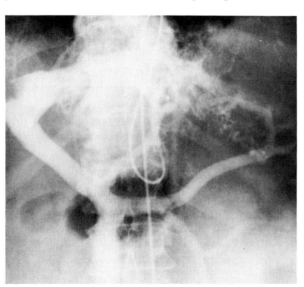

B

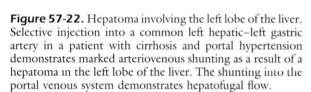

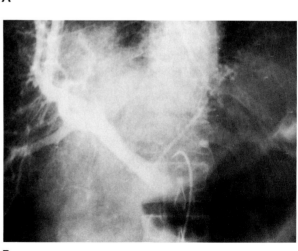

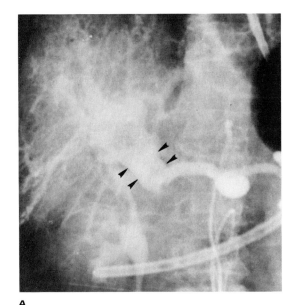

A

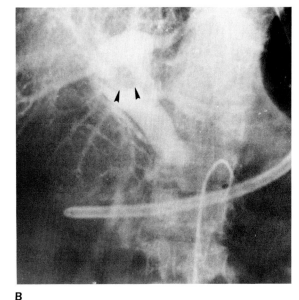

B

Figure 57-24. Hepatoma exhibiting marked arteriovenous shunting and a tumor thrombus in the portal vein. The patient presented with bleeding in the esophageal varices. (A) Selective celiac arteriography shows abundant tumor vascularity within the right lobe of the liver associated with arteriovenous shunting and opacification of the portal vein (*arrowheads*). (B) During the hepatographic phase of the injection a large filling defect can be seen within the main portal vein; this proved to be a tumor thrombus (*arrowheads*). (C) During the late phase of a selective inferior pancreaticoduodenal artery injection once again retrograde opacification of the portal vein can be seen due to arteriovenous shunting within the tumor. The tumor thrombus (*arrowheads*) is again identified extending upward into the liver.

C

◄ **Figure 57-23.** Hepatoma with marked hepatic arterial–portal venous shunting. (A) Selective hepatic arteriogram in a patient with cirrhosis and portal hypertension demonstrates hepatic arterial–portal venous shunting (*arrows*) secondary to a hepatoma. (B) During the hepatographic phase of the examination there is complete filling of the portal venous radicals with hepatofugal flow and filling of the coronary vein.

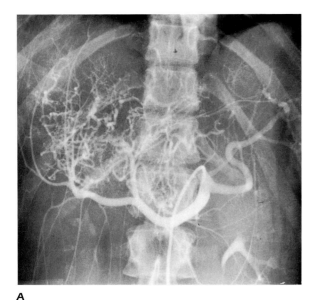

A

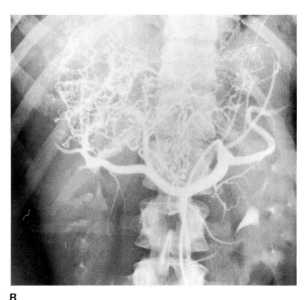

B

Figure 57-25. Hepatoma seen best after the injection of 1 unit of vasopressin. (A) Selective hepatic arteriography in a patient with cirrhosis of the liver and a superimposed hepatoma. Abnormal tumor vessels are seen within the liver as outlined by an irregular mass. (B) After injection of 1 unit of vasopressin into the hepatic artery there is vasoconstriction of the normal branches without any significant change of the tumor vessel diameter in the mass itself. Because of the vasoconstriction of the normal vessels more of the contrast is shunted to the mass, making it more clearly visible.

Small doses of epinephrine (5–10 µg) or vasopressin (1 pressor unit) injected into the hepatic artery immediately before injection of contrast material are often useful for the demonstration of tumor vessels.[43]

Because of the trend in surgery to attempt hepatectomies in this disease, it is important for the arteriographer to assess the operability of these tumors and to determine the plane of the tumor in relation to the plane of division of the liver, the so-called lobar fissure. It is also important to delineate clearly which branches of the hepatic artery supply the tumor. Since as many as 35 percent of hepatomas have macroscopic invasion of the portal vein, percutaneous splenoportography is of value in determining the extent of portal venous invasion and hence the feasibility of surgical resection.

Primary Bile Duct Carcinoma

Primary tumors of the biliary system are less vascular than hepatomas and do not exhibit the arteriovenous shunting that is so often seen in hepatomas.[44,45] The arterial branches going to the primary tumor of the common duct or gallbladder show displacement, margin irregularity, and on occasion complete obstruction (Fig. 57-26). During the capillary phase of the study, a tumor stain can frequently be seen, but it tends not to be as dense as that seen in hepatomas.

The angiographic findings in hepatomas and cholangiomas correlate well with their histologic appearance. Hepatomas have extremely rich capillary stroma, whereas cholangiomas are hard tumors with a predominance of connective tissue overgrowth and few capillaries. Since cholangiocarcinomas can spread through the biliary ducts, large and extensive tumors may be present without angiographic evidence of a large mass.

Angiosarcoma

Whelan et al.[46] have described the angiographic and radionuclide-uptake characteristics of hepatic angiosarcoma found following vinyl chloride exposure. The few cases described had a normal appearance of the hepatic artery associated with very small, fine tumor vessels around the periphery of the tumor. Contrast material persisting within the tumor extended very late into the venous phase of the examination. Areas of the tumor appeared hypovascular. The latter finding was probably a result of the central necrosis that frequently accompanies angiosarcomas.

Malignant Disease Metastatic to the Liver

Hepatic metastases, like primary tumors of the liver, are almost exclusively supplied by the hepatic artery. The metastatic lesion usually exhibits the same angio-

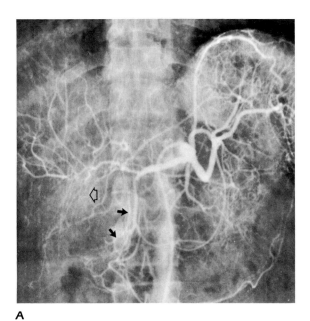

A

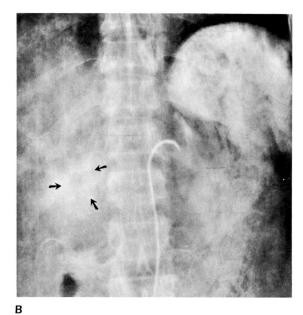

B

Figure 57-26. Carcinoma of the common duct. (A) The arterial phase of the selective celiac arteriogram demonstrates spreading of the common duct branches of the gastroduodenal artery (*solid black arrows*). Small, indistinct, irregular vessels are seen extending from the right hepatic artery (*open*

arrow). (B) During the capillary phase of the study, a tumor stain can be identified in the area of the abnormal vasculature (*arrows*) that is irregular and extends into the liver parenchyma. This was an inoperable carcinoma of the common duct infiltrating deeply within the liver.

graphic characteristics as the primary tumor. If the primary tumor is very vascular, as is renal cell carcinoma, carcinoid tumor (Fig. 57-27), or leiomyoma (Fig. 57-28) of the gastrointestinal tract, the metastatic deposits in the liver are also vascular. Poorly vascularized tumors, like adenocarcinoma of the gastrointestinal tract, when metastatic to the liver, may appear as either avascular masses or tumors exhibiting very small tumor vessels that stain sparsely during the capillary phase (Fig. 57-29). The latter changes are generally seen only when most of the hepatic parenchyma has been replaced by metastatic disease. The diagnosis of small scattered metastatic deposits within the liver is usually difficult to establish during arteriography. Rarely, as in carcinoma of the pancreas, the metastatic lesion to the liver is more vascular than the primary tumor.

Hepatic Trauma

Although only 15 to 20 percent of abdominal injuries damage the liver, more than 50 percent of deaths from abdominal trauma are caused by hepatic rupture.[47] The

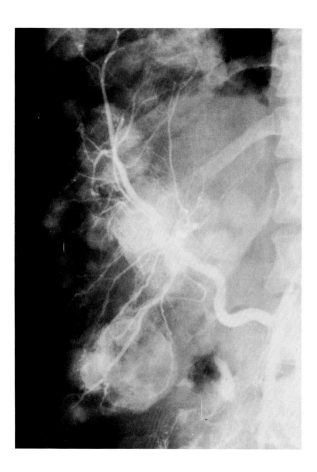

Figure 57-27. Ileal carcinoid tumor metastatic to the liver. Hepatic arteriography demonstrates multiple vascular metastases to the liver from a carcinoid tumor of the small bowel.

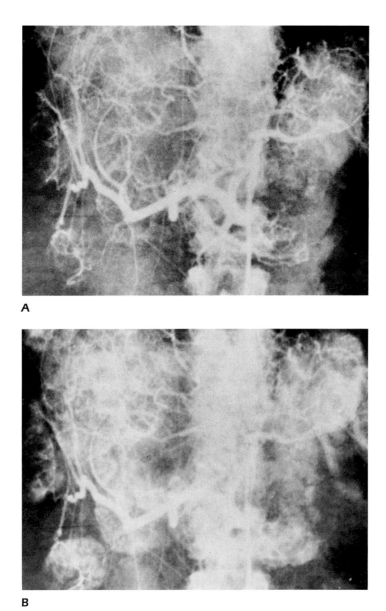

A

B

Figure 57-28. Leiomyosarcoma metastatic to the liver. (A) Selective hepatic arteriography demonstrates marked enlargement of the liver associated with displacement of intrahepatic arterial branches. Numerous irregular large tumor vessels can be identified. (B) During the late arterial phase of the examination, tumor stains of various sizes are seen. This patient had a primary leiomyosarcoma in the small intestine.

mortality is even higher in blunt hepatic trauma than in perforating injury and may go as high as 70 percent. Because of this high mortality, emergency surgery is frequently indicated and often lifesaving in patients with hepatic rupture. Since it may well be impossible to evaluate the extent of the injury at surgery—in fact, sometimes it is not even possible to identify the lesion within the liver—emergency hepatic arteriography should be performed if at all feasible.[48] The indications for angiography are as follows:

1. To document the presence of liver damage and to evaluate and localize its extent
2. To follow the natural course of an angiographically diagnosed lesion if surgery is not performed
3. To evaluate for complications of trauma, whether they be aneurysms, subcapsular hematomas, or hemobilia, following either conservative or surgical management
4. To control hepatic bleeding by the use of transcatheter embolization techniques (Fig. 57-30)

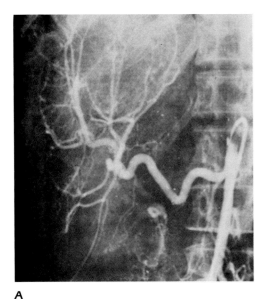 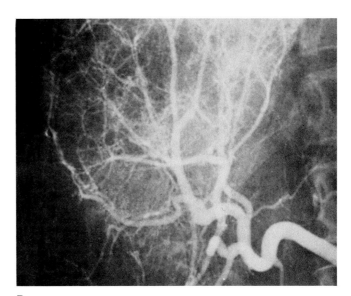

A   **B**

Figure 57-29. Adenocarcinoma of the colon metastatic to the liver. (A) The hepatic artery arises from the superior mesenteric artery. Selective superior mesenteric arteriography demonstrates displaced intrahepatic branches associated with a mottled appearance of the finer intrahepatic radicles. (B) Direct serial magnification arteriography demonstrates small tumor vessels as well as displacement of the intrahepatic branches to much greater advantage. Vessels of approximately 100 μ in diameter can be visualized with direct radiographic magnification using a fractional focal-spot x-ray tube.

Figure 57-30. Bleeding false aneurysm of the hepatic artery treated by transcatheter arterial embolization. (A) Selective hepatic arteriogram demonstrates a large false aneurysm of the right hepatic artery. (B) Persistent contrast material in the false aneurysm can be seen 29 seconds after the start of the injection. (C) Repeat hepatic arteriogram after the injection of Gelfoam plugs fails to demonstrate any evidence of continued arterial extravasation. This child's hepatic bleeding was caused by blunt abdominal trauma sustained during a bicycle accident. The transcatheter embolization successfully controlled the bleeding.

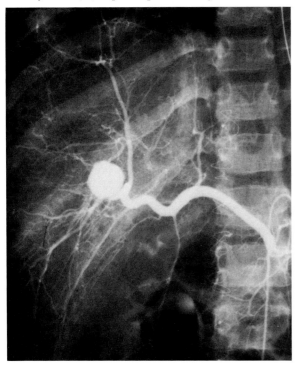

A   **B**

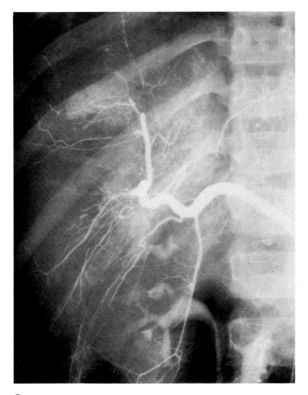

C

Figure 57-30 (continued).

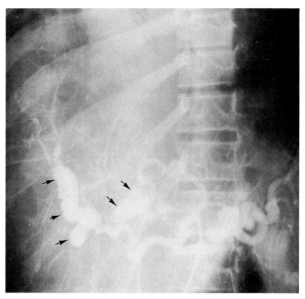

Figure 57-31. Traumatic false aneurysms of the right and middle hepatic arteries (*arrows*) in a patient who had sustained abdominal trauma several weeks earlier.

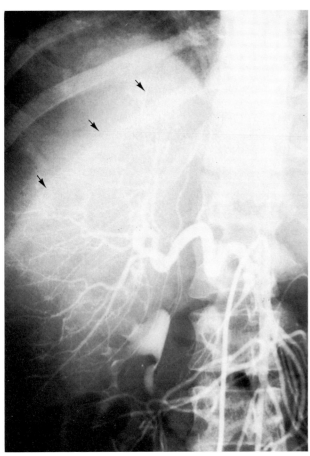

A

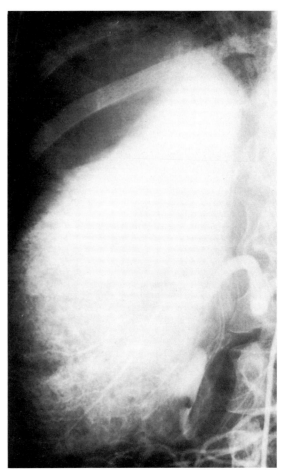

B

Any of the following angiographic findings may be seen in hepatic trauma:

1. Liver contusion
   a. Elongation and straightening of arterial branches
   b. Delay in hepatic blood flow to specific segments of the liver
   c. Small areas of contrast accumulation in affected areas
2. Liver laceration
   a. Hepatic arterial occlusion
   b. Contrast extravasation
   c. Pseudoaneurysm formation (Fig. 57-31)
   d. Arterioportal fistula
   e. Arteriobiliary fistula
3. Subcapsular or intrahepatic hematoma (Fig. 57-32)
   a. Arterial displacement
   b. Liver displacement
   c. Contrast extravasation

Small ruptures that are either subcapsular or central in location need no intervention if they are clinically silent. Boijsen et al.[49] reported that 11 of 25 patients with unequivocal angiographic signs of liver damage were not operated on and did well. Because of the high association of renal and splenic injuries following either blunt or penetrating abdominal trauma, hepatic arteriography is often combined with splenic and renal arteriography.

References

1. Bierman HR, Byron RL Jr, Kelly KH, Grady A. Studies on the blood supply of tumors in man: vascular patterns of the liver by hepatic arteriography in vivo. J Natl Cancer Inst 1951;12:107.
2. Seldinger SL. Catheter replacement of needle in percutaneous arteriography: a new technique. Acta Radiol 1953;39:368.
3. Ödman P. Percutaneous selective angiography of the celiac artery. Acta Radiol Suppl (Stockh) 1958;159:1.
4. Small WC, Chezmar JL, Bernardino ME. CT angiography and CT arterial portography in evaluation of hepatic adenomas. J Comput Assist Tomogr 1994;18(2):266–268.
5. Shamsi K, Deckers F, De Schepper A. Is it a haemangioma? Rofo Fortschr Geb Rontgenstr Neuen Bildgeb Verfahr 1993;159(1):22–27.
6. Finn JP, Clarke MP, Goldmann A. MR angiography of the liver. Semin Ultrasound CT MR 1992;13(5):367–376.
7. Aspestrand F, Kolmannskog F. CT and angiography in chronic liver disease. Acta Radiol 1992;33(3):251–254.
8. Michels NA. Blood supply and anatomy of the upper abdominal organs. Philadelphia: Lippincott, 1955.
9. Healey JE, Schroy PC. Anatomy of the biliary ducts within the human liver: analysis of the prevailing pattern of branchings and the major variations of the biliary ducts. Arch Surg 1953;66:599.
10. Nebesar RA, Kornblith PL, Pollard JJ, Michels NA. Anatomic considerations. In: Nebesar RA, et al, eds. Celiac and superior mesenteric arteries: a correlation of angiograms and dissections. Boston: Little, Brown, 1969.
11. Wagner D, Baum S. Preliminary arteriography in hepatic artery infusions for cancer. Surg Gynecol Obstet 1965;120:817.
12. Baum S, Roy R, Finkelstein AK, Blakemore WS. Clinical application of selective celiac and superior mesenteric arteriography. Radiology 1965;84:279.
13. Evans JA. Specialized roentgen diagnostic technics in the investigation of abdominal disease (Annual Oration in Memory of Clarence Elton Hufford). Radiology 1964;82:579.
14. Boijsen E, Ekman C-A, Lundh G. Selective splanchnic angiography. Adv Surg 1968;3:13.
15. Simmons JT, Baum S, Sheehan BA, Ring EJ, Athanasoulis CA, Waltman AC, Coggins PC. The effect of vasopressin on hepatic arterial blood flow. Radiology 1977;124:637.
16. Reuter SR, Redman HC. Gastrointestinal angiography. 2nd ed. Philadelphia: Saunders, 1977.
17. Rosenberg RF, Sprayregen S. The hepatic artery in cirrhosis: an angiographic pathophysiologic correlation. Angiology 1974;25:499.
18. Viamonte M Jr, Warren WD, Fomon JJ, Martinez LO. Angiographic investigations in portal hypertension. Surg Gynecol Obstet 1970;130:37.
19. Viamonte M Jr, Viamonte M. Liver circulation. Crit Rev Clin Radiol 1974;27:214.
20. Rabinowitz JG, Kinkabwala M, Ulreich S. Macroregenerating nodule in the cirrhotic liver. AJR 1974;121:401.
21. McNulty JG. Angiographic manifestations of hydatid disease of the liver: a report of two cases. AJR 1968;102:380.
22. Rizk GK, Tayyarah KA, Ghandur-Mnaymneh L. The angiographic changes in hydatid cysts of the liver and spleen. Radiology 1971;99:303.
23. Lomba Viana R. Selective arteriography in the diagnosis and evaluation of amebic abscess of the liver. Am J Dig Dis 1975;20:632.
24. Abrams RM, Beranbaum ER, Santos JS, Lipson J. Angiographic features of cavernous hemangioma of liver. Radiology 1969;92:308.
25. Alfidi RJ, Rastogi H, Buonocore E, Brown CH. Hepatic arteriography. Radiology 1968;90:1136.
26. Pantoga E. Angiography in liver hemangioma. AJR 1968;104:874.
27. Curry JL, Johnson WG, Feinberg DH, Updegrove JH. Thorium induced hepatic hemangioendothelioma: roentgenangiographic findings in two additional cases with clinical "informed consent" problems. AJR 1975;125:671.
28. McLoughlin MJ, Colapinto RF, Gilday DL, Hobbs BB, Korobkin MT, McDonald P, Phillips MJ. Focal nodular hyperplasia of the liver: angiography and radioisotope scanning. Radiology 1973;107:257.
29. Phillips MJ, Langer B, Stone R, Fisher M, Ritchie S. Benign liver cell tumors: classification and ultrastructural pathology. Cancer 1973;32:463.

◄ **Figure 57-32.** Traumatic subcapsular hepatic hematoma. (A) Arterial phase of a selective arteriogram demonstrates abrupt termination of the intrahepatic branches (*arrows*) before they reach the lateral body wall. (B) Capillary phase of the study shows the characteristic beaking due to compressed parenchyma and a radiolucent defect between the blush of the liver and the rib cage. The angiographic appearance of a subcapsular hepatic hematoma is identical to that of a subcapsular hematoma of the spleen.

30. Tate RC, Chacko MV, Singh S. Parenchymal hamartoma of the liver in infants and children. Am J Surg 1972;123:346.
31. Aronsen KF, Ericcson B, Lunderquist A, Malmborg O, Norden JG. A case of operated focal nodular cirrhosis of the liver. Scand J Gastroenterol 1968;3:58.
32. Galloway SJ, Casarella WJ, Lattes R, Seaman WB. Minimal deviation hepatoma: a new entity. AJR 1975;125:184.
33. Knowles DM, Wolff M. Focal nodular hyperplasia of the liver: a clinicopathologic study and review of the literature. Hum Pathol 1976;7:533.
34. Casarella WJ, Knowles DM, Wolff M, Johnson PM. Focal nodular hyperplasia and liver cell adenoma: radiologic and pathologic differentiation. AJR 1978;131:393.
35. Sorensen TI, Baden H. Benign hepatocellular tumors. Scand J Gastroenterol 1975;10:113.
36. Baum JK, Holtz F, Bookstein JJ, Klein EW. Possible association between benign hepatomas and oral contraceptives. Lancet 1973;2:926.
37. McLoughlin MJ, Phillips MJ. Angiographic findings in multiple bile duct hamartomas of the liver. Radiology 1975;116:41.
38. Boijsen E, Abrams HL. Roentgenologic diagnosis of primary carcinoma of the liver. Acta Radiol 1965;3:257.
39. Reuter SR, Redman HC, Siders DB. The spectrum of angiographic findings in hepatoma. Radiology 1970;94:89.
40. Neiman HL, Goldstein HM, Silverman PJ, Bookstein JJ. Angiographic features of peripancreatic malignant lymphoma. Radiology 1975;115:589.
41. Okuda K, et al. Demonstration of growing casts of hepatocellular carcinoma in the portal vein by celiac angiography: the thread and streaks sign. Radiology 1975;117:303.
42. Breedis C, Young G. The blood supply of neoplasms in the liver. Am J Pathol 1954;30:969.
43. Kahn PC, Frates WJ, Paul RE Jr. The epinephrine effect in angiography of gastrointestinal tract tumors. Radiology 1967;88:686.
44. Abrams RM, Meng CH, Firooznia H, Beranbaum ER, Epstein HY. Angiographic demonstration of carcinoma of the gallbladder. Radiology 1970;94:277.
45. Reuter SR, Redman HC, Bookstein JJ. Angiography in carcinoma of the biliary tract. Br J Radiol 1971;44:636.
46. Whelan JG Jr, Creech JL, Tamburro CH. Angiographic and radionuclide characteristics of hepatic angiosarcoma found in vinyl chloride workers. Radiology 1976;118:549.
47. Boijsen E, Judkins MP, Simay A. Angiographic diagnosis of hepatic rupture. Radiology 1966;86:66.
48. Aakhus T, Enge L. Angiography in rupture of the liver. Acta Radiol 1971;11:353.
49. Boijsen E, Kaude J, Tylén U. Angiography in hepatic rupture. Acta Radiol 1971;11:363.

58

Splenic Arteriography

HERBERT L. ABRAMS
MICHAEL F. MEYEROVITZ

The spleen is considered a vital element in the reticuloendothelial system. At one time, its removal was thought to cause no significant consequences. It is now clear, however, that asplenic patients may be subject to overwhelming sepsis and that the decreased immunologic competence that follows splenectomy cannot be ignored.[1,2] In portal hypertension the spleen may become huge and unwieldy; it is frequently involved in lymphoma; and in congenital hemolytic anemia it plays a central role in the disease process. The diagnosis of splenic lesions relies almost exclusively on noninvasive modalities, such as computed tomography (CT), ultrasound, and magnetic resonance imaging (MRI)[3,4]; angiography is rarely performed for assessment of the spleen itself, but it is useful for demonstrating pathology of the splenic artery and vein. In addition, transcatheter embolization techniques can be applied to the splenic circulation in selected patients.

Some years ago, one of the authors (HLA) participated in a study of the variations in the anatomy of the splenic artery, the frequency of visualization of its important branches, the variable sites of origin of the splenic artery branches, and the intrasplenic circulatory patterns recorded by serialographic filming.[5] It was hoped that an understanding of normal variations as visualized angiographically would provide a precise background for judging significant alterations in the splenic arterial patterns and their relationship to gastric, pancreatic, and splenic disease. This chapter is based on that analysis, as well as on the authors' accumulated experience and a review of the literature.

Anatomy of the Splenic Artery

The classic anatomic description of the splenic artery has been given by Michels on the basis of 100 human dissections.[6,7] Michels's descriptions have generally been confirmed and amplified in vivo in our clinical studies. The basic anatomic observations must first be summarized.

Origin

The splenic artery typically originates from the celiac artery via a hepatolienogastric trunk. This situation was found in 82 percent of the dissections. In the most common form, the left gastric artery is given off first and the splenic and hepatic arteries then form a common trunk. In about 25 percent of cases the left gastric, splenic, and hepatic arteries arise from the same point to form a tripod celiac configuration. Less often the dorsal pancreatic or middle colic artery arises from the same point to form a tetrapod configuration; this phenomenon occurred in 5 percent of the dissections. Occasionally the splenic artery arises from the aorta or the superior mesenteric artery, and, rarely, a double splenic artery is formed when a smaller branch to a superior pole of the spleen originates from the celiac axis.

Distribution

The arterial blood supply to the spleen is so varied that no two vascularization patterns were exactly alike in 100 dissections.[6,7] There are, however, two basic types of splenic arterial patterns.

1. A distributed type of spleen has a wide hilus, notches in the anterior and posterior borders, a thumblike lobe at the inferior pole, and a tubercle at the superior pole. This distributed configuration occurred in approximately 70 percent of dissections. The splenic trunk is relatively short, with terminal branching at any point from the celiac axis to the hilus of the spleen. The branches are usually numerous and small in caliber and enter 75 percent of the medial surface of the spleen.

2. A compact type of spleen has smooth, even borders with a narrow hilus, giving rise to a magistral configuration (found in approximately 30 percent of dissections). The splenic trunk is long; terminal division occurs near the hilus; and the terminal branches are few and large and enter 25 to 33 percent of the spleen's medial surface.

Measurements of the splenic artery have revealed an average length of 13 cm (with a range of 8–32 cm) and an average width of 7.5 mm (with a range of 5–12 mm).

Segmentation

The splenic artery can be divided into the following four main segments:

1. Suprapancreatic. This is the first 1 to 3 cm of the vessel.
2. Pancreatic. This portion of the vessel usually is found on the dorsal surface of the pancreas. It is the most tortuous of the segments, lies adjacent to the pancreas, and supplies the small pancreatic branches that enter the organ at frequent intervals.
3. Prepancreatic. This segment runs obliquely along the anterior surface of the tail of the pancreas. Terminal branching usually occurs in this segment and gives rise to a distributed pattern. In 80 percent of dissections the main trunk was divided into a superior terminal artery and an inferior terminal artery. In some cases an additional medial terminal artery was also present.
4. Prehilar. This segment is found between the tail of the pancreas and the spleen. If branching into a terminal division occurs at this point, the arterial pattern is magistral.

Tortuosity

One of the most pronounced characteristics of the splenic artery is its tortuosity, which is manifested in curves, loops, and spirals, primarily along the splenic trunk and secondarily in the terminal branches. Michels[7] feels that the tortuous appearance is correlated with age: it becomes progressively more marked in individuals over 50 years of age.

Branches of the Splenic Artery

Figure 58-1 depicts the major branches of the splenic artery.

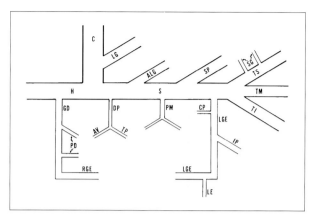

Figure 58-1. Schematic diagram of the major splenic arterial branches and their usual sites of origin. *C,* celiac trunk; *LG,* left gastric; *H,* hepatic; *S,* splenic; *GD,* gastroduodenal; *PD,* pancreaticoduodenal; *RGE,* right gastroepiploic; *DP,* dorsal pancreatic; *TP,* transverse pancreatic; *AV,* anastomotic vessels; *ALG,* accessory left gastric; *PM,* arteria pancreatica magna; *SP,* superior polar; *LGE,* left gastroepiploic; *CP,* caudal pancreatic; *IP,* inferior polar; *LE,* left epiploic; *SG,* short gastric; *TS,* superior terminal; *TM,* medial terminal; *TI,* inferior terminal.

Pancreatic Branches

Dorsal Pancreatic Branch (Superior Pancreatic Branch of Testut)

This vessel was described by Michels[7] as the "most varied of celiac-mesenteric vessels in its origin, branching and distribution." It measured 1 to 4 mm in width and originated from the splenic artery in 40 percent of dissections. Occasionally it arises from the celiac, hepatic, or superior mesenteric arteries. It supplies the dorsal and ventral surfaces of the pancreas in the region of the neck. Two right branches may originate from the dorsal pancreatic branch, one anastomosing with the superior pancreaticoduodenal artery and the other directly supplying the uncinate process. A left branch, the transverse pancreatic, runs along the inferior surface of the organ to its tail for an anastomosis with the arteria pancreatica magna and the caudal pancreatic vessels (Fig. 58-2).

A fourth branch may descend below the inferior pancreatic border to communicate with the superior mesenteric artery and thus constitute an important collateral pathway between the celiac and the superior mesenteric arteries (the artery of Bühler) (Fig. 58-3). In some instances, this descending branch is actually the middle colic artery or the accessory middle colic artery (the artery of Riolan), arising from the celiac artery. At times this vessel in its downward course gives rise to a pancreatic branch that functions as the dorsal pancreatic artery (Fig. 58-4).

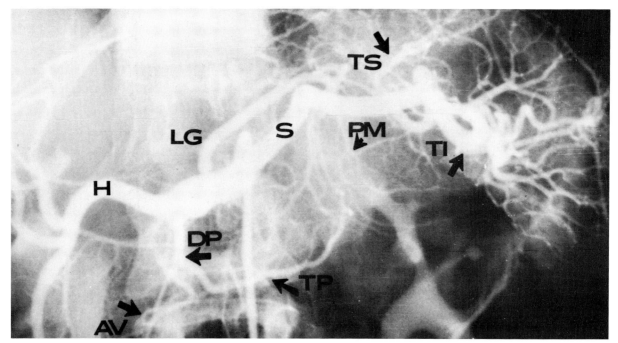

Figure 58-2. Normal splenic arterial anatomy. This 40-year-old woman was investigated for abdominal pain. *H,* hepatic artery; *LG,* left gastric artery; *S,* splenic trunk. Superior terminal (*TS*) and inferior terminal (*TI*) vessels supply numerous branches to the splenic parenchyma. The dorsal pancreatic branch (*DP*) is well visualized originating from the proximal splenic and dividing into the transverse pancreatic (*TP*) and anastomotic vessels (*AV*), which supply the head of the pancreas and anastomose with the pancreaticoduodenals. The arteria pancreatica magna (*PM*) originates from the second segment of the splenic trunk.

Figure 58-3. Normal splenic arterial anatomy in a 42-year-old man with abdominal pain. The left gastric artery (*LG*) is the first branch of the celiac trunk. Note the tortuous splenic trunk (*S*). A small dorsal pancreatic (*DP*) branch originates from the second segment. In addition, an inferior polar branch (*P*) is visualized originating from the distal second segment. The spleen is moderately enlarged. A direct communication between the hepatic artery (*H*) and the superior mesenteric artery represents the artery of Bühler (*B*). Numerous small, irregular tumor vessels (*arrows*) are identified. In addition, there is bowing of the gastroduodenal artery around a mass in the head of the pancreas and slight narrowing of this vessel in its descending limb (*upper left arrow*). Laparotomy revealed a carcinoma of the pancreatic head.

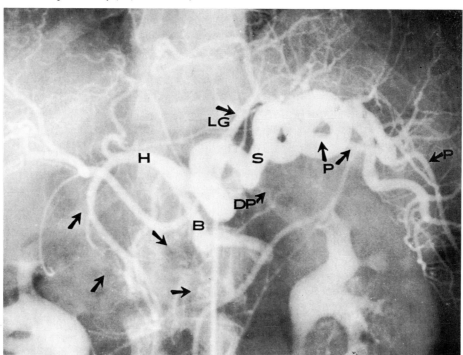

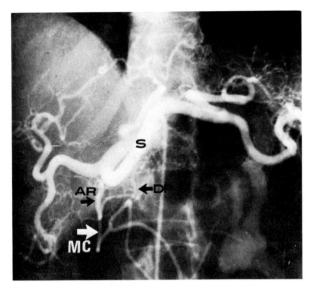

Figure 58-4. Variations in normal splenic arterial anatomy. This 3-year-old girl was studied for hypoglycemic attacks. An unusual normal variant was found. The middle colic artery (*MC*) originates from the junction of the celiac and splenic trunk (*S*) and gives off a dorsal pancreatic branch (*DP*). This configuration forms the artery of Riolan (*AR*).

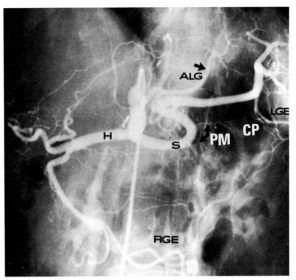

Figure 58-5. Variations in normal splenic arterial anatomy in a 51-year-old woman with abdominal pain. *H,* hepatic artery; *ALG,* accessory left gastric artery; *S,* splenic artery. Several small pancreatic branches (*PM*) take the place of a single arteria pancreatica magna trunk. The left gastroepiploic artery (*LGE*) originates from the third segment of the splenic trunk. A small caudal pancreatic branch (*CP*) supplies the tail of the pancreas. A small plaque can be visualized at the origin of the gastroduodenal artery. The greater curvature of the stomach appears to be supplied mainly from the right gastroepiploic artery (*RGE*).

Arteria Pancreatica Magna

This vessel is the largest branch to the pancreas. It measures 2 to 4 mm in width, arises often from the distal third of the splenic artery, and supplies the tail of the pancreas with most of its blood. The vessel frequently courses obliquely to the left after entering the pancreas. It then subdivides into right branches, which anastomose with the transverse pancreatic artery, and left branches, which anastomose with the caudal pancreatic artery (see Fig. 58-2).

Caudal Pancreatic Branch

This vessel originates from the distal splenic trunk or from the left gastroepiploic artery. It is usually short and may often be double. It supplies the tail of the pancreas or a small accessory spleen when present in the pancreaticolienal ligament. It anastomoses with the transverse pancreatic branch and the arteria pancreatica magna.

In addition, numerous small and inconsistent pancreatic branches from the splenic trunk supply the body of the organ (Fig. 58-5).

Splenic Terminal Branches

The splenic artery divides into two primary terminal branches (superior and inferior) in 86 to 93 percent of individuals, the remaining 7 to 14 percent having three primary terminal branches (superior, middle, and inferior) (Fig. 58-6); each of these primary terminal branches subdivides into two to six secondary branches.[8,9]

There is a good deal of variation in the pattern of terminal splenic branches.[10] The length of these primary terminal branches averages 4 cm but may vary from 1 to 12 cm. In the magistral configuration, the vessels originate 1 to 2 cm from the hilus, but in the distributed configuration they originate 2 to 12 cm from the hilus. The superior terminal branch is often much larger; it is the main direct blood supply to the spleen. Divisional patterns of the inferior terminal branch are more complicated, and frequently the left gastroepiploic and inferior pole arteries take origin from the inferior terminal branch.

Short Gastric Branches

These are very slender vessels, 2 to 10 in number, which supply the cardia and the fundus of the stomach. The most frequent origin of these vessels is the splenic terminals.

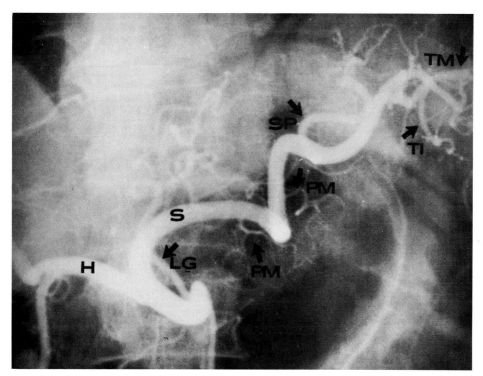

Figure 58-6. Variations in normal splenic arterial anatomy in a 79-year-old man with abdominal pain. The splenic trunk (*S*) is not unusually tortuous for a patient of this age. Two separate branches (*PM*) arise from the second portion and take the place of a single arteria pancreatica magna. A superior polar branch (*SP*) originates from the third portion and supplies the upper splenic pole. Medial terminal (*TM*) and inferior terminal (*TI*) branches supply the remainder of the spleen. *H*, hepatic artery; *LG*, left gastric.

Left Gastroepiploic Branch

In 72 percent of dissections this vessel arose from the splenic trunk 1 to 4 cm proximal to the primary terminal division; at other times it originated from an inferior terminal branch or one of its radicles. It descends along the right side of the greater curvature of the stomach in an anterior layer of the greater omentum, anastomosing with the right gastroepiploic branch to form the arcus arteriosus ventriculi inferior of Hyrtl. This vessel may supply an appreciable amount of blood to the spleen via inferior polar branches.

An important branch of the left gastroepiploic branch is the left epiploic. This vessel usually originates from the left gastroepiploic branch near the spleen and descends in the posterior layer of the greater omentum below the transverse colon to form the left limb of the arcus epiploicus magnus of Barkow, the right limb of which is formed by the right epiploic branch from the right gastroepiploic or the transverse pancreatic branch. This arch supplies the transverse colon by multiple ascending rami (Fig. 58-7).

Polar Arteries

A superior polar vessel was found in 65 percent of dissections, with the most common origin (75 percent of cases) from the splenic trunk proximal to its primary division. It may also originate from other portions of the splenic trunk or from the superior terminal artery (20 percent of cases). The length varies from 2 to 12 cm and the width from 1 to 5 mm. Rarely, this artery arises directly from the celiac artery to provide a double splenic artery (0.4 percent of cases). Frequently the vessel is tortuous and gives off numerous small branches to adjacent viscera.

The inferior polar branch was found in 82 percent of dissections, with the most frequent origin from the left gastroepiploic artery. At times it originates from the splenic trunk (see Fig. 58-3) or the inferior terminal artery, and on occasion it is multiple in origin. The length varies from 3 to 8 cm, with a slightly smaller width than that of the superior polar artery. This vessel is also usually tortuous, and it divides into two to four smaller branches.

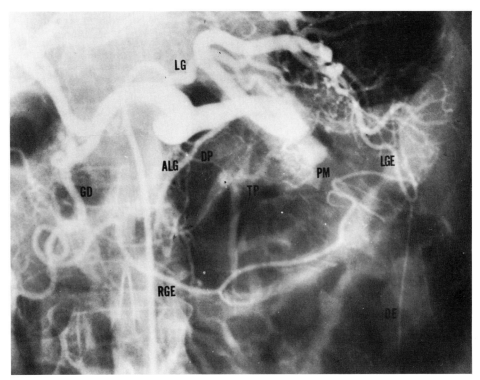

Figure 58-7. Normal splenic arterial anatomy. This 55-year-old woman was investigated because of abdominal pain. Her normal celiac arteriogram demonstrates a left descending epiploic branch (*DE*) originating from the left gastroepiploic artery (*LGE*). An anastomosis with the right gastro-epiploic artery (*RGE*) is also identified. *GD*, gastroduodenal artery; *ALG*, accessory left gastric artery; *DP*, dorsal pancreatic; *TP*, transverse pancreatic; *PM*, pancreatica magna; *LG*, left gastric.

Angiographic Analysis of Normal Vessels

Configuration of the Celiac Artery and Its Branches

The splenic artery arose from the distal end of the celiac axis in all 38 cases (Table 58-1). The origin of the left gastric artery was proximal to that of the splenic artery in 47 percent of cases. The left gastric artery was not visualized in 10 percent, but this does not imply any pathologic significance. In 37 percent of cases a common origin of the splenic, hepatic, and left gastric arteries was found (the tripod of Haller). This figure is somewhat greater than Michels's 25 percent. In only one case in this series did the hepatic artery arise independent of the celiac axis (from the superior mesenteric artery).

Origin and Incidence of Visualized Branches

Branches from the suprapancreatic segment were noted in 18 cases (Table 58-2). The dorsal pancreatic artery arose from this segment 16 times. Three additional dorsal pancreatic arteries were found: all originated from the second, or pancreatic portion, of the splenic artery. The common termination of the dorsal pancreatic artery—the transverse pancreatic artery—was occasionally visualized. In no case did the dorsal pancreatic artery originate from the hepatic artery or from an aberrant right hepatic artery. A surgically im-

Table 58-1. Configuration of the Celiac Artery and Its Branches (Analysis of 38 Cases)

Configuration	Number of Patients	Percent of Cases
Gastrohepatolienal with proximal origin of left gastric	18	47
Tripod (gastrohepatolienal with simultaneous origins)	14	37
Hepatolienal with nonvisualized left gastric	4	10
Lienogastric with superior mesenteric origin of hepatic	1	3
Undetermined	1	3
Total	38	100

Table 58-2. Origin and Incidence of Visualized Branches

Source	Number and Percent
From suprapancreatic segment	
Dorsal pancreatic	16 (42%)
Other: 1 left gastric; 1 inferior phrenic	
From pancreatic segment	
Pancreatic magna	21 (55%)
Short gastric	10 (26%)
Accessory left gastric	13 (34%)
Other: 2 left gastroepiploic; 3 superior polar; 3 dorsal pancreatic; 1 terminalis inferior; 1 inferior polar; 1 middle polar; 1 left gastroepiploic from accessory left gastric	
From prepancreatic segment	
Terminalis superior	30 (79%)
Terminalis inferior	29 (76%)
Caudal pancreatic	5 (13%)
Left gastroepiploic	7 (18%)
Terminalis media	6 (16%)
Other: 4 short gastric; 5 left epiploic; 3 superior polar; 1 accessory left gastric; 1 inferior polar	
Branches from the prehilar segment	
Terminalis superior	7 (18%)
Superior polar	1 (3%)
Terminalis inferior	7 (18%)
Inferior polar	1 (3%)
From inferior polar branch	
Caudal pancreatic	1 (3%)
Left gastroepiploic	1 (3%)
Left epiploic	2 (6%)
Magistral configuration	7 (18%)
Distributed configuration	31 (82%)

portant variation, origin of the dorsal pancreatic artery from the middle colic or accessory middle colic branch of the superior mesenteric artery, was not identified in this series. Additional branches of the first segment were one left gastric artery and one inferior phrenic artery.

The arteria pancreatica magna was the most common branch of the pancreatic segment (occurring in 21, or 55 percent, of the cases). An accessory left gastric artery was the next most common branch (13, or 34 percent, of the cases). Short gastric arteries were found in 26 percent of the cases, and one case showed numerous small branches constituting a substitute circulation for the arteria pancreatica magna (see Fig. 58-5). An unusual and previously undescribed branch was a "middle polar" branch, a long branch arising from the midportion of the main splenic trunk and resembling a proper superior polar artery, except that it ter-

minated in the middle part of the spleen. This might more correctly be considered an early origin of the medial terminal artery.

The most frequent branches originating from the prepancreatic, or third, segment were the superior terminal artery (79 percent of the cases) and inferior terminal artery (79 percent of the cases). These arteries, superior and inferior, each took origin from the prehilar segment in an additional 18 percent of the cases, establishing them as the most constant branches (see Fig. 58-2).

The left epiploic branch originated from the third segment or from a branch of the third segment in five cases and from the inferior polar in two additional cases (see Fig. 58-7). The origin from the left epiploic branch was given by Michels as the left gastroepiploic branch. It is unusual that three of the seven left epiploic branches visualized had other origins. That branch's directly descending course in the omentum aided in its recognition. The arch of Barkow, by which the branch anastomoses with the right epiploic artery in the inferior omentum, was not seen: it was probably too far caudal to be recorded.

The left gastroepiploic artery was filled in two cases from the pancreatic segment, in seven cases from the prepancreatic segment, and in one case from the inferior polar branch of the prehilar segment. It gave rise to the left epiploic artery in four cases.

The caudal pancreatic is a recurrent branch to the pancreas from the lower spleen. Consistently found in dissections, it was identified with certainty only once (see Fig. 58-5).

The pattern of blood vessels to the spleen was magistral in 18 percent of cases, as compared to the usual figures of about 30 percent noted in the angiographic studies of Ödman[11] and the dissections of Michels.[6] The remaining 82 percent were distributive in type.

Vessel Diameters

An analysis of the diameter of the vessels is given in Table 58-3. The diameter of the celiac axis averages 10.9 mm. Although this figure is slightly larger than Ödman's radiographic measurement of 8 to 11 mm, it agrees with Michels's postmortem measurement of 10 to 12 mm. The range in our series was wide (8–21 mm). The diameter of the origin of the splenic artery averaged 8.2 mm and ranged from 6 to 14 mm. Ödman's value was 4 to 9 mm, and Michels's postmortem dissections indicated 7 to 8 mm as the usual size. The average size of the splenic artery at its midportion was 7.3 mm, and at the hilus, 6.5 mm. In both segments, significant variation in size was observed.

Table 58-3. Vessel Diameters

Vessel	Diameter in Millimeters		
	Average	Maximum	Minimum
Celiac origin	10.9	21	8
Splenic origin	8.2	14	6
Splenic midportion	7.3	11	5
Splenic hilus	6.5	10	3

Length and Configuration of the Splenic Artery and Its Segments

The initial course of the first, or suprapancreatic, segment was analyzed (Table 58-4). Five configurations were observed: (1) upward clockwise, (2) downward clockwise, (3) horizontal, (4) upward counterclockwise, and (5) downward counterclockwise. Pancreatic masses were found in each category, and no particular disease process correlated with any specific configuration. On the other hand, narrowing and displacement of the celiac axis and its branches were observed in the presence of carcinoma of the pancreas.

The average age of the patients with the most tortuous vessels (four or more loops) was identical to the average age of the entire series (50 years). Michels's conclusion that tortuosity increased with age but was not necessarily associated with atherosclerosis was supported by this study. Patients with the straightest vessels (one loop) were on the average 10 years younger than the average age of the entire group. The pancreatic segment was consistently the most tortuous of the four segments of the artery.

The total length of the splenic artery averaged 17.3 cm and varied from 8.5 to 33 cm. Measurement of each of the four segments indicated that the pancreatic segment, with an average measurement of 10.4 cm, was by far the longest. The suprapancreatic and the prepancreatic segments were roughly equivalent in length (see Table 58-4).

Table 58-4. Length of the Splenic Artery and Its Segments

Artery	Length in Centimeters		
	Average	Maximum	Minimum
Total	17.3	33	8.5
Segment			
Suprapancreatic	2.5	7.0	1.0
Pancreatic	10.4	22.5	5.0
Prepancreatic	2.5	6.0	0.4
Prehilar	1.5	4.5	0.3

Table 58-5. Circulation Time[a]

Flow	Average			
	All	Cirrhosis	Maximum	Minimum
Anteroposterior view				
Beginning	8.3	8.0	18	4
Maximum	15.4	14.8	30	5
Difference[b]	7.1			
Oblique view				
Beginning	8.5	6.8	27	3
Maximum	15.4	14.3	36	7
Difference[b]	6.9			

[a]In seconds.
[b]Time from earliest visualization to maximum density.

Circulation Time

There was wide variation in the transit time of contrast agent from the splenic artery to its first appearance in the splenic vein (Table 58-5). The average circulation time was 8.3 seconds, and the range was 3 to 36 seconds. When patients with cirrhosis of the liver were compared with patients without cirrhosis, no significant difference in the circulation time was observed. The average times obtained were essentially the same in both projections, but considerable discrepancies were noted when the time was measured in both projections in a few individual cases. No correlation with recognized disease processes could be established. The wide variation observed indicated that any effort to study the splenic venous circulation using intraarterial injection should take into account the late phases of the study if maximal density is to be obtained.

Although it is generally held that the intrasplenic circulation is of an "open" type, with whole blood passing through pores in the splenic sinuses, arteriovenous shunting has been shown to play an important role in blood circulation, at least in patients with various splenic disorders.[12]

Angiographic Analysis of the Abnormal Splenic Artery: The Pancreas

The value of angiography in the diagnosis and surgical management of pancreatic carcinoma has been analyzed by several investigators.[13-23] The reader is referred to Chapter 55, Pancreatic Angiography, for a detailed discussion of pancreatic disease. We will deal here only briefly with certain arterial changes that must be recognized in the presence of pancreatic mass lesions.

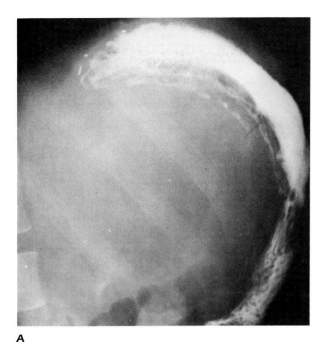

A

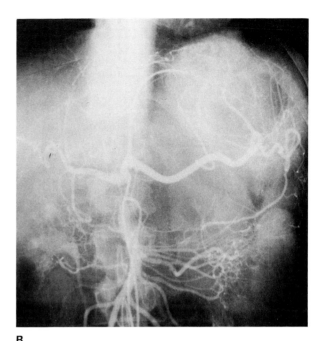

B

Figure 58-8. Pseudocyst of the pancreas. This 45-year-old man with chronic pancreatitis and ulcer disease had a recent onset of epigastric pain with a palpable left upper quadrant mass. Prior subtotal gastrectomy and gastroenterostomy, together with vagotomy, had been performed. (A) Upper gastrointestinal series, lateral projection. A large retrogastric mass is visible, displacing the stomach and anastomosed jejunum anteriorly. (B) Simultaneous celiac and superior mesenteric arteriogram. There is marked stretching and displacement of the left gastric and intrapancreatic branches of the splenic trunk. The splenic artery is straighter than normal, and the large mass is avascular. The diagnosis of pancreatic pseudocyst was made. Laparotomy revealed a large cyst of the pancreatic body and tail containing 500 ml of thick fluid.

Vascular Displacement

The normal range of variation in the course of the common hepatic, splenic, gastroduodenal, and pancreatic arcades is so wide that at times it is extremely difficult to recognize the slight degree of displacement that frequently accompanies an intrapancreatic neoplasm. A slight but definitive curvature of the gastroduodenal artery or straightening and bowing of the pancreaticoduodenal, dorsa pancreatic, or transverse pancreatic arteries frequently may be observed. A carcinoma in the body or the tail of the pancreas may elevate the entire celiac axis or the splenic artery. Vascular displacement indicates only enlargement of the pancreas and is certainly not specific for carcinoma. In cysts and pseudocysts, the displacement may be profound and may indicate the size of the lesion (Fig. 58-8).

Irregular Arterial Stenosis

This is a relatively common finding. It may involve the larger vessels about the pancreatic head and even the smaller intrapancreatic vessels, such as the dorsal or transverse pancreatic arteries. It is the most frequent sign of pancreatic carcinoma.[17] The normal contour of the affected vessel is lost by involvement of the vessel wall (sometimes simulating atherosclerosis). On occasion, the vessel may be completely occluded. It is generally agreed that such vascular encasement most often indicates a malignant tumor and, if present, will help make the differentiation from benign tumor, cyst, or pancreatitis (Figs. 58-9 and 58-10). Arterial narrowing due to tumor is sometimes associated with a smooth, tapered, elongated area of stenosis (Fig. 58-11). On the other hand, the intimal lesions of atherosclerosis will usually produce an irregularity of the internal lumen of the vessel that is limited to a short segment. Pancreatic carcinoma may, however, simulate arteriosclerosis in striking fashion (see Fig. 58-10).

It must be emphasized that vascular encasement is not always caused by neoplastic invasion of the vessel wall but instead sometimes represents a desmoplastic or fibrotic reaction to the adjacent tumor. Furthermore, it may be found in the presence of pancreatitis and therefore cannot be construed as pathognomonic of carcinoma.

Other findings, such as tumor vessels, tumor stain, and venous abnormalities, are discussed elsewhere in these volumes. Similarly, the changes in benign tumors

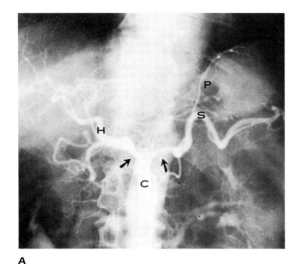

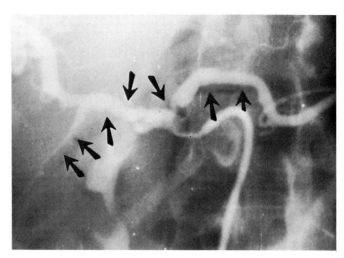

A   **B**

Figure 58-9. Carcinoma of the pancreas. (A) A 50-year-old man with abdominal pain. Visualization of the celiac axis (*C*) shows marked narrowing of the hepatic artery (*H*) and splenic artery (*S*) origins (*arrows*). At laparotomy, a large carcinoma of the pancreatic head encircled these vessels and caused external compression. An inferior phrenic branch (*P*)

originates from the splenic trunk. (B) A 52-year-old woman. There is marked narrowing of the splenic and hepatic vessels, including the gastroduodenal artery (*arrows*), simulating atherosclerotic disease. At laparotomy, carcinoma of the pancreatic head with compression of the celiac axis was discovered.

Figure 58-10. Splenic artery encasement in carcinoma of the pancreas. (A) Upper gastrointestinal series in an 80-year-old man showing a normal stomach and duodenum. (B) Arteriogram, same patient as in (A). From the origin of the splenic artery to about 5 cm along its course, the vessel wall

is strikingly irregular, with alternating areas of filling defects and eccentric narrowing. The appearance is quite similar to arteriosclerotic plaques. The patient proved at surgery to have carcinoma of the pancreas.

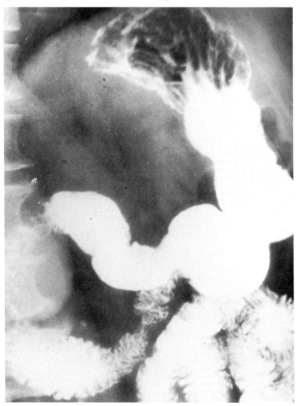

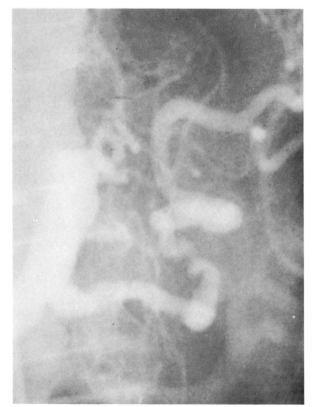

A   **B**

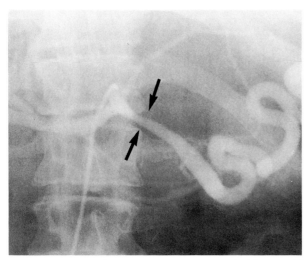

Figure 58-11. Splenic artery encasement. A 45-year-old woman with retroperitoneal lymphosarcoma. Note the smooth narrowing of the splenic artery beginning about 1 cm beyond its origin from the celiac artery (*arrows*).

Table 58-6. Causes of Splenomegaly

Inflammation
  "Acute splenic tumor" (acute infections)
  Chronic infections (e.g., tuberculosis, malaria)
  Miscellaneous inflammations (e.g., sarcoidosis, lupus erythematosus)
Cysts and tumors
  True cysts (e.g., congenital echinococcus)
  False cysts (posttraumatic)
  Benign tumors
  Malignant tumors
    Primary tumors (e.g., leukemia, lymphoma)
    Metastatic tumors
Infiltrative diseases
  Gaucher disease, Niemann-Pick disease
  Amyloidosis, hemosiderosis
Hyperplastic disorders
  Hemolytic anemias
  Myelofibrosis
  Polycythemia vera
  Thrombocytopenia purpura
  Other anemias (e.g., pernicious anemia)
Splenic vein hypertension
  Cirrhosis of the liver
  Portal or splenic vein thrombosis

and inflammation of the pancreas are reviewed in other chapters. Because the splenic artery and its branches are the source of a significant element of the pancreatic vascular supply, they are obviously affected by many of the lesions that involve the pancreas.

Angiographic Analysis of Abnormal Splenic Vessels: The Spleen

Splenomegaly

There are many causes of splenomegaly (Table 58-6; Figs. 58-12 and 58-13), and it is beyond the scope of this chapter to deal in detail with each one. Inflammation, such as in acute infections, chronic tuberculous or malarial infections, sarcoidosis, and autoimmune diseases (e.g., lupus erythematosus) are common causes of splenomegaly. Cysts are rare causes of splenomegaly, whereas tumors, such as lymphoma or leukemia, are more frequently associated with splenic enlargement. The infiltrative disorders, including Gaucher disease and amyloidosis, are relatively rare. The hyperplastic disorders are frequently associated with splenomegaly, including all the hemolytic anemias, except sickle cell disease, which in its most chronic form is generally associated with a small, infarcted spleen. Finally, splenic vein hypertension, such as that found in cirrhosis of the liver or in portal or splenic vein thrombosis, may be associated with splenic enlargement and hypersplenism.

Figure 58-12. Splenomegaly in Hodgkin disease. This 37-year-old man had peripheral adenopathy and splenomegaly due to Hodgkin disease. A celiac arteriogram demonstrates an enlarged spleen with stretching and distortion of the intrasplenic branches. Small dorsal pancreatic (*DP*) and large right gastroepiploic (*RGE*) branches are visualized. *S*, splenic artery.

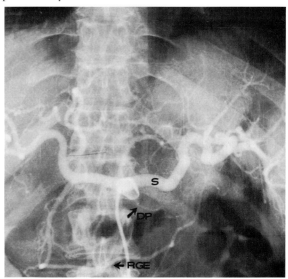

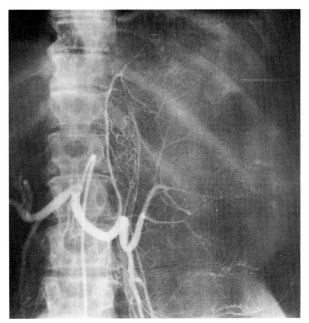

Figure 58-13. Splenomegaly in leukemia. A 56-year-old woman with hepatosplenomegaly. Arteriography demonstrates a huge spleen with compression of the splenic trunk and stretching of the peripheral splenic branches. A marrow biopsy confirmed the clinical diagnosis of myelogenous leukemia.

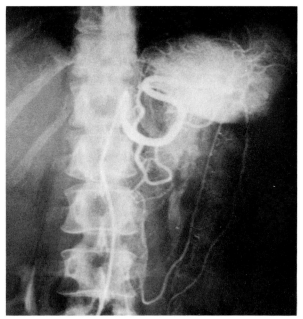

Figure 58-14. Transverse position of the spleen. The spleen lies in the left upper quadrant beneath the diaphragm in horizontal position, rather than in its usual vertical or oblique orientation. This represents a normal variation and has no pathologic significance.

The angiographic appearance of splenomegaly reflects to some degree the underlying cause of the disease. In all forms of splenomegaly, the most common appearance is of stretching and separation of the vessels, with a splenogram or capillary phase that is uniformly diminished in intensity. In the neoplastic or infiltrative disorders, there may be more or less uniform separation of the vessels, but, in addition, irregularity and encasement of arteries are visible at times. Inflammatory disorders, including arteritis, as well as cirrhosis of the liver, may be associated with aneurysmal change in the intrasplenic arteries, as well as with attenuation and wide separation of the vessels.

Congenital Anomalies

Anomalies of Position

Variants of Normal Spleen. In anomalies that are variants of the normal spleen, the spleen may be located transversely immediately below the diaphragm (Fig. 58-14), a finding of no pathologic significance. Similarly, the spleen may assume any level of obliquity (see Figs. 58-2, 58-3, and 58-6), or it may approach a vertical orientation. Radionuclide scanning with ^{99m}Tc sulfur colloid, ultrasonography, CT, and MRI can reliably establish the position of the spleen and assist in the diagnosis of such entities as situs inversus.[3,24–27]

Wandering Spleen. The spleen may be located aberrantly in the left flank (Fig. 58-15) of the midabdomen or the left lower quadrant or pelvis (Fig. 58-16).[28] Such instances of wandering spleen are rare, and they constitute a diagnostic challenge. The discovery of a mass in the midabdomen or near the lower pole of the left kidney on plain films, together with evidence of the splenic hump's absence on excretory urography and medial or anterior displacement of the spleen on barium examination, should prompt ultrasonography, radioisotope scanning, CT, or MRI. Angiography is not required for the diagnosis.

Patients with wandering spleen may be symptomatic or asymptomatic. Diagnosis is important in symptomatic cases because symptoms derive from torsion, which carries possible complications of infarction, gangrene, and abscess; the mortality is 50 percent in such cases.[29] In a case reported by Sorgen and Robbins,[30] bleeding fundal varices were associated with a wandering spleen in a 14-year-old girl. It was theorized that the varices developed as a result of splenic vein occlusion caused by torsion with consequent retrograde filling of short gastric and left gastroepiploic veins.

Wandering spleen has been reported in 0 to 0.4 percent of splenectomies.[31,32] Various causes have been suggested, including congenital anomalies of the lienogastric and lienorenal ligaments. In the case illus-

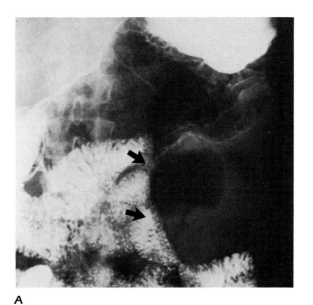

A

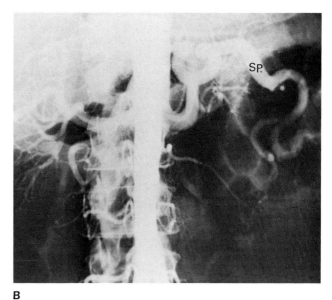

B

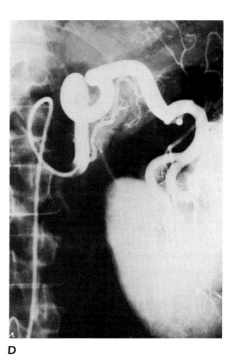

C   **D**

Figure 58-15. "Wandering," or ectopic, spleen. (A) Upper gastrointestinal series. The stomach fills the left upper quadrant in the area where the spleen normally is located. In addition, a mass is visible displacing small bowel loops (*arrows*) in the left midabdomen. (B) Aortogram. The coiled splenic artery (*SP.*), instead of being directed laterally and cephalad, extends in a caudal direction. (C) Splenographic phase. The spleen is visible in the left midabdomen (*arrows*), in precisely the area where the mass was noted on the upper gastrointestinal series. (D) Selective splenic arteriogram. The position of the spleen, well out of the left upper quadrant, is now clearly delineated. (Courtesy of David Levin, M.D.)

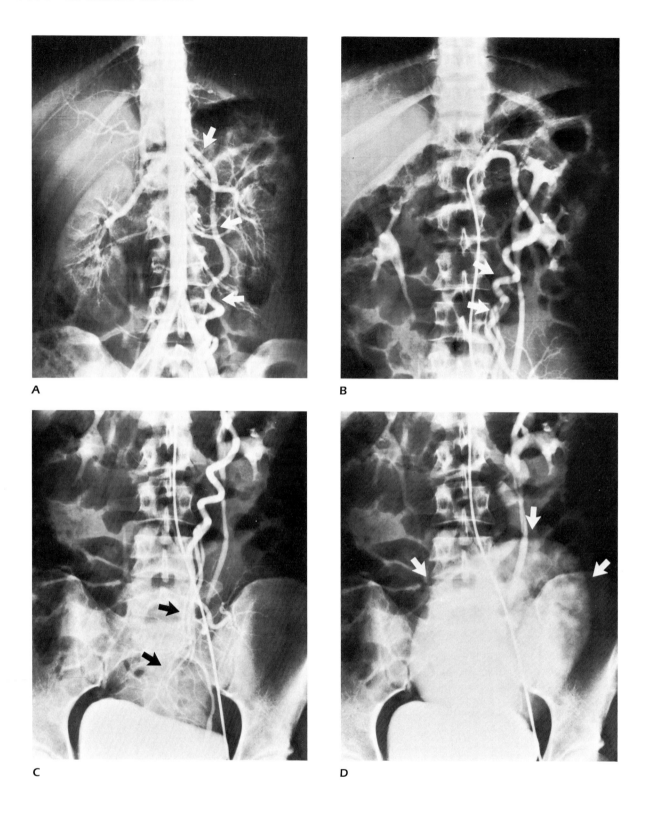

A

B

C

D

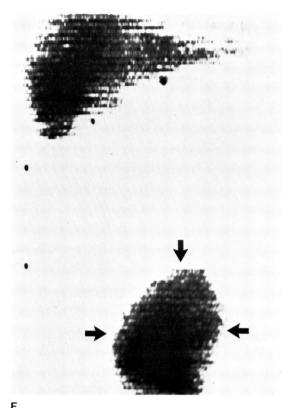

E

Figure 58-16. "Wandering," or ectopic, spleen. A mass was palpable in the pelvis. (A) Aortogram. A long, tortuous vessel extends toward the pelvis (*arrows*). (B) Selective arteriogram. The catheter tip is located in the mouth of this vessel (*arrows*), which is a branch of the celiac axis. (C) Selective splenic arteriogram, view of lower abdomen and pelvis. The tortuous vessel visualized on the prior two films arborizes extensively (*arrows*) in the pelvis. (D) Selective arteriogram, capillary phase. A large homogeneously dense mass (*arrows*) is visible in the pelvis above the contrast-filled bladder. The diagnosis of a wandering spleen was made because the vessel selectively catheterized was thought to be the splenic artery. (E) Radionuclide scan. The liver is visualized in its normal position in the right upper quadrant. No spleen is seen in the left upper quadrant. Instead, the wandering spleen in the pelvis is well visualized (*arrows*). (Courtesy of Melvin Clouse, M.D.)

trated in Figure 58-15, a left flank mass was palpated, and the absence of the normal spleen shadow on upper gastrointestinal series led to a tentative diagnosis of wandering spleen. The patient whose films are shown in Figure 58-16 had a palpable pelvic mass and lower abdominal pain. Angiography and radionuclide studies finally established the diagnosis.

Anomalies of Number

Accessory Splenic Tissue. Accessory spleens may be present in as many as 16 percent of people[31] and may be more common in people with hematologic disorders.[33] The classic accessory spleen is single and is located in the hilus of the spleen or adjacent to the tail of the pancreas. As a consequence, at the time of splenic surgery, accessory spleens may be readily recognized. Angiographically, these spleens are seen as small nodules with an arterial and a capillary phase similar to that of splenic tissue, which may be separate from and/or immediately adjacent to the hilus of the spleen or may be embedded in the pancreas. Computed tomography has also been able to identify accessory spleens, particularly during contrast enhancement. Radionuclide scanning with ^{99m}Tc sulphur coiled will identify the accessory splenic tissue.

The classic accessory spleen must be differentiated from "splenosis." Although approximately 20 percent of patients who have had splenectomy for hematologic indications have Howell-Jolly bodies or have "pitted" red cells, suggesting persistence of splenic activity, over 50 percent of children who have had splenectomy for splenic trauma have demonstrated persistent splenic activity. The fact that such patients develop splenosis may explain the relatively low incidence of sepsis in patients who have had splenectomy for traumatic indications.[34]

Although the presence of more than one spleen normally is of no significance, the accessory splenic tissue can occasionally present a diagnostic or therapeutic challenge. In one case reported by Fitzer,[35] a splenic hematoma could not be ruled out on radionuclide scans because of the presence of an accessory spleen, and arteriographic studies were necessary to arrive at a definitive diagnosis. Infarction of an accessory spleen, simulating acute appendicitis, has been reported,[36] and accessory spleens may cause recurrence of hematologic disorders after surgical removal of the primary spleen.[37] In addition, an accessory spleen can be a source of problems in treatment planning in Hodgkin disease.[38]

Asplenia. Although asplenia may appear as an isolated anomaly,[39] it most often occurs as part of the asplenia, or Ivemark, syndrome, in conjunction with complex, characteristic cardiovascular malformations and other anomalies.[40] The minimal incidence has been estimated as 1 in 40,000 live births.[41] The conjunction of anomalies in the asplenia syndrome has led some embryologists to postulate that it results from a teratogenic insult to the embryo between the 31st and 36th day of gestation.[42] It has also been suggested that the asplenia syndrome may represent an autosomal recessive trait.[43] Neither of these mechanisms can explain all cases of asplenia, however. In a case reported by Wilkinson et al.,[44] one monozygotic twin suffered from the asplenia syndrome and the other twin was normal; genetic factors could not have played a part in this instance, nor is it likely that a teratogen could have affected one twin and not the other.

The diagnosis of asplenia is suggested by a complex of cardiac and extracardiac anomalies, including some anomalies that represent a bilateral right-sidedness[45]: mesocardia or dextrocardia, bilateral superior vena cava, a single ventricle or two ventricles with a ventricular septal defect, a large atrial septal defect, transposition of the great vessels, total anomalous pulmonary venous return, bilateral trilobed lungs with bilateral eparterial bronchi, a symmetric liver, a midline gallbladder, and malrotation of the gastrointestinal tract. Cyanosis and heart failure are often evident soon after birth. Chest films usually reveal mesocardia or dextrocardia, decreased pulmonary vasculature, and a central symmetric liver.[46,47]

Although there have been reports of prolonged survival after surgery to repair complex cardiac anomalies in asplenic infants,[48,49] most such infants die soon after birth. In a series reported by Majeski and Upshur, the life span of 14 live-born asplenic infants averaged 38 days.[40] The first-year mortality of such infants was estimated in 1972 as being greater than 95 percent.[50]

In patients with isolated asplenia, the diagnosis may be more obscure. These patients have a high incidence of sepsis because of the absence of splenic tissue and the altered immunologic response early in life.[51] Honigman and Lanzkowsky[39] suggest that all infants and children with septicemia, especially of a pneumococcal or *Hemophilus influenzae* type, be assessed for the presence of Howell-Jolly bodies. Although isolated asplenia has been diagnosed in people as old as 69,[52] it can also predispose to early, sudden death.[43]

Polysplenia. Polysplenia syndrome is also a complex congenital disorder in which multiple discrete spleens are coupled with cardiac and extracardiac abnormalities. With polysplenia there is a tendency toward bilateral left-sidedness, with bilateral bilobed lungs and hyparterial bronchi. Interruption of the inferior vena cava with azygos or hemiazygos continuation is common. The liver is generally located centrally, and there is frequently malrotation of the bowel.

Although the cardiac disease is usually more benign in patients with polysplenia than in those with asplenia (because of the infrequent occurrence of transposition of the great arteries and total anomalous pulmonary venous return), the cardiac anomalies may lead to pulmonary vascular disease if they are not promptly corrected.

Radionuclide spleen scans will generally show abnormal results, but they usually do not suggest the diagnosis of polysplenia with any precision.[53] The diagnosis may be made on ultrasound, CT, or MRI. Arteriography can also demonstrate the diagnosis (Fig. 58-17).

Figure 58-17. Polysplenia. This young patient had congenital heart disease associated with an absent hepatic portion of the inferior vena cava. (A) Aortogram. The splenic artery extends into the right upper quadrant instead of the left upper quadrant. (B) Capillary phase. Two separate splenic shadows (*arrows*) are visible in the right upper quadrant. There is no evidence of a spleen located on the left upper quadrant.

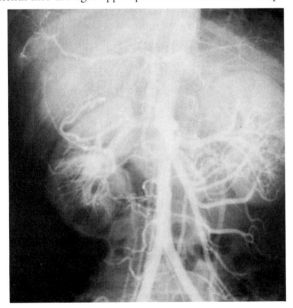

A

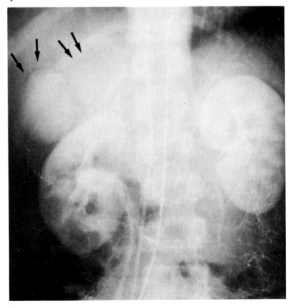

B

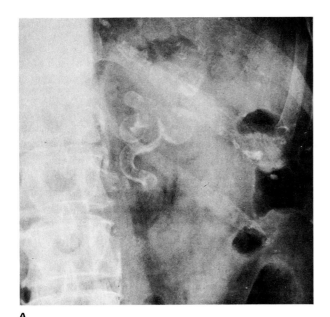

A

Figure 58-18. Arteriosclerosis of the splenic artery. (A) Calcified splenic artery. The splenic artery is grossly calcified throughout its course. Arteriosclerosis is manifested by both the tortuosity and the extensive calcium deposits in the wall. Note also the calcification of the abdominal aorta. See also Figure 58-9, in which carcinoma of the pancreas has invaded the wall of the splenic artery and resembles arteriosclerosis. (B) Calcified splenic artery (*arrowheads*). The tortuous vessel inserts at the lesser curvature of the stomach. (C) Arteriogram, same patient as in (B). Note the great elongation but relative absence of intimal filling defects.

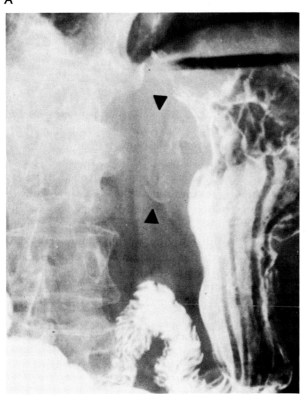

B

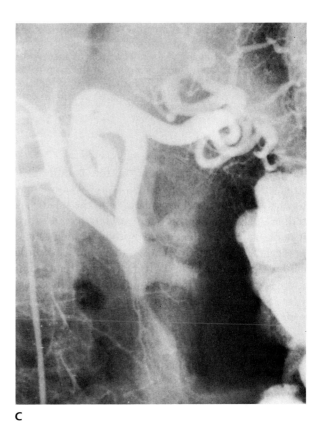

C

Primary Abnormalities of the Splenic Vascular Bed

Arteriosclerosis

The splenic artery is commonly affected by arteriosclerosis, and visible calcification of the highly tortuous vessels may be observed as an incidental finding on conventional films of the abdomen (Fig. 58-18). The involvement is largely medial rather than intimal, so that adequate lumen size is preserved in some of the most heavily calcified arteries. The splenic artery is particularly prone to elongation and tortuosity, which generally increase with age. Because the splenic artery is closely related to the stomach, tortuosity can pro-

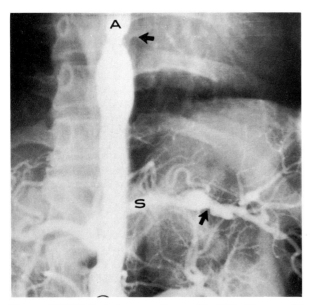

Figure 58-19. Splenic artery in arteritis. This 23-year-old hypertensive woman had a systolic bruit in the back. Aortography demonstrates marked irregularity in the lumen of the aorta (*A*), with a thickened wall (*arrow*). The splenic artery (*S*) is also irregular in appearance, with areas of aneurysmal dilatation (*arrow*) both along the course of the main trunk and in the peripheral branches. These changes were considered characteristic of an arteritis, a diagnosis consistent with the laboratory and biopsy data.

duce an extrinsic impression on the barium-filled stomach that may simulate a neoplasm.[54] Plaques may form and produce wall irregularities on the splenic arteriogram. Severe stenosis is unusual but occurs. When it does, it need produce no symptoms as long as it is gradual. Splenic arteriosclerosis, therefore, is of little clinical significance by itself. Its major importance clinically is determined by the extent to which it predisposes to aneurysm formation or, occasionally, to complete thrombosis.

Dysplasia of the Splenic Artery

The corrugated or string-of-beads pattern frequently described in the renal vessels may be visualized in the splenic trunk on rare occasions, as noted by Palubinskas and Ripley.[55] Splenic artery fibroplasia has been reported as an incidental finding in a 9-year-old boy.[56] When the lesion is localized, it may be impossible to differentiate from atherosclerosis.

Arteritis

Although primary arteritis of the splenic artery is rare, the artery may be involved in arteritis affecting the aorta (e.g., giant-cell arteritis) (Fig. 58-19) or other visceral branches. The inflammatory process involves the vessel wall to varying degrees, with destruction of media, areas of fibrosis and cicatrix, and at times aneurysm formation (see Fig. 58-19).

Splenic Artery Aneurysm

Splenic artery aneurysm is the most common intraabdominal aneurysm aside from those of the abdominal aorta and the iliac arteries. Splenic artery aneurysms may be multiple[57] and may occur in association with other visceral artery aneurysms.[58] They are observed most often in the third and sixth decades of life, and they are two to three times more common in the female. Half the women of childbearing age in whom they are discovered are pregnant at the time of discovery. Congenital splenic artery aneurysms rupture more commonly than any other visceral artery aneurysm in women, especially those under 45 years of age; rarely, they are responsible for hemorrhage in men.[59] Splenic artery aneurysms may be largely congenital in women and atherosclerotic in men.

The diagnosis may be made on the plain film by demonstration of a ringlike calcific shadow in the region of the splenic artery (Fig. 58-20; see also Fig. 58-23C). It is important to visualize this shadow in two projections because a tortuous splenic artery may simulate the ring of a splenic aneurysm.[60] Rupture of a splenic aneurysm may be well demonstrated by celiac arteriography. In a case described by Baum et al., diagnosis led to prompt surgical intervention that was almost certainly lifesaving.[61] Today, a ruptured splenic artery aneurysm is most rapidly controlled by transcatheter embolization using either Gianturco coils or detachable balloons. Embolization may also be the treatment of choice for intact splenic artery aneurysms[62–65] proximal to the splenic hilum. To completely obliterate the aneurysm, coils or detachable balloons should be placed either within the aneurysm or proximal and distal to it. Blood flow to the spleen is then maintained via gastric and pancreatic collaterals to the distal splenic artery.

Splenic artery aneurysms have been reported as incidental findings in 0.78 percent of all selective celiac axis angiographic examinations and in 0.1 percent of all autopsy studies.[66] Pollak et al., noting the benign course of most splenic artery aneurysms, suggest that resection of small, asymptomatic aneurysms in older patients is unnecessary.[59] In women who are pregnant or of childbearing age, resection or embolization is necessary because of the danger of rupture during pregnancy.[67] Laparoscopic ligation of a splenic artery aneurysm has also been reported.[68]

Figure 58-19 shows an unusual aneurysm in association with arteritis. Figure 58-20 demonstrates a calcified splenic artery aneurysm in a 68-year-old pa-

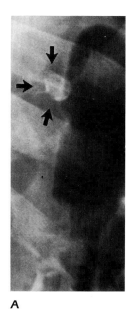
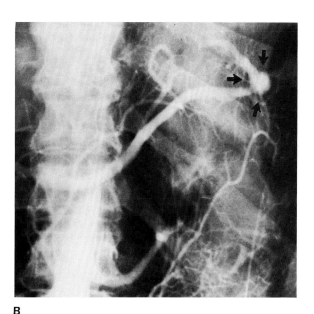

A　　　　　　**B**

Figure 58-20. Calcified splenic artery aneurysm. This 68-year-old woman had septicemia incidental to a renal abscess. (A) Film of the abdomen during an intravenous pyelogram shows a circumscribed area of calcification (*arrows*) in the left upper quadrant. (B) Abdominal aortogram to evaluate the renal arteries demonstrates filling of the calcified aneurysm (*arrows*) of the distal splenic artery.

tient with septicemia. The aneurysms shown in Figures 58-21 and 58-22 are large enough to warrant concern about rupture. Multiple aneurysms in a patient with celiac artery occlusion are seen in Figure 58-23. Figure 58-24 demonstrates numerous aneurysmal dilatations of the peripheral intrasplenic branches without early filling of veins in a patient with hypersplenism, and Figure 58-25 shows similar findings in a patient with cirrhosis.

Splenic Arteriovenous Fistula

Rarely, splenic arteriovenous fistulas are said to cause cardiac failure because the portal venous bed is much smaller than the systemic circulation and the return to the heart is delayed by the vascular resistance of the liver.[69] The fistulas may be congenital or acquired. The acquired lesions may be traumatic in origin, but they are also thought to result from rupture of splenic artery aneurysms. A bruit is usually heard in the left upper quadrant.[70] The spleen is commonly enlarged, and portal hypertension may be present.[71] Duplex Doppler sonography may aid in the diagnosis.[72]

Figure 58-26 shows an arteriovenous fistula in a lower part of the spleen in a 57-year-old woman. Acker et al.[73] described a traumatic fistula between the proximal splenic artery and the splenic vein through which a catheter was placed, which resulted in a transaortic portogram. Percutaneous occlusion of a large splenic arteriovenous fistula exacerbating portal hypertension

Figure 58-21. Splenic artery aneurysm. A large sacular aneurysm is visible (*arrows*) arising at the junction of the middle and distal thirds of the splenic artery. The caudal border of the aneurysm is irregular, suggesting the presence of thrombus within it.

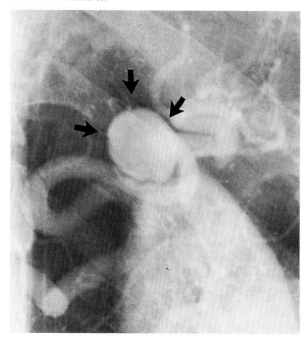

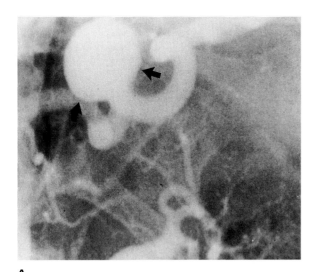

A

Figure 58-22. Splenic artery aneurysm. A large, smooth-walled sac (*arrows*) arises from the splenic artery at the junction of the proximal and middle thirds. The remainder of the artery is smooth-walled, strongly suggesting the congenital origin of this aneurysm.

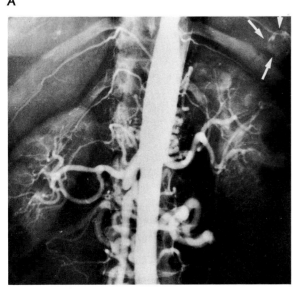

A

Figure 58-23. Multiple splenic artery aneurysms, associated with celiac artery occlusion. (A) Abdominal aortogram. The renal, superior mesenteric, and multiple lumbar arteries are visualized. No splenic artery is opacified following aortic injection. Note the ring-shaped calcification (*arrows*) in the left upper quadrant in the region of the spleen. (B) Aortogram, 3 seconds. Filling of the gastroduodenal artery has occurred from the common pancreaticoduodenal arteries arising from the superior mesenteric artery. There is retrograde flow into the common hepatic artery, with filling as well of the splenic artery, visualizing multiple aneurysms (*arrows*). (C) Lateral projection, abdominal aortogram. The calcified splenic artery is visible ventral to the aorta. In addition, there is complete occlusion of the celiac artery (*arrow*).

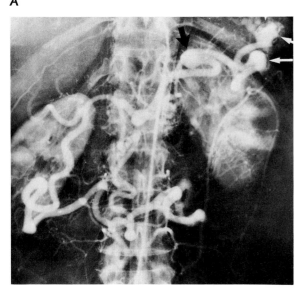

B

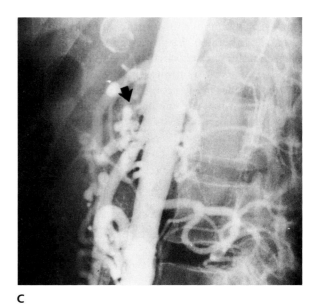

C

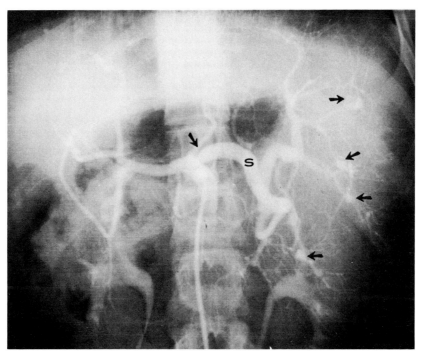

Figure 58-24. Intrasplenic arterial aneurysms. This 16-year-old girl had splenomegaly, leukopenia, thrombocytopenia, and a coagulation defect. The celiac arteriogram shows marked splenomegaly with slight stenosis (*single arrow at left*) at the origin of the splenic artery (*S*). There are numerous aneurysmal dilatations (*arrows*) of the peripheral intrasplenic branches. Early-draining veins were not identified, but multiple arteriovenous fistulas could not be completely ruled out.

was performed in a patient bleeding from esophageal varices after both mesocaval shunting and transthoracic esophageal and gastric devascularization with splenectomy (the Sugiura procedure); transhepatic obliteration of the varices was carried out at the same time.[74] Although a transcatheter approach was chosen in this case because of the patient's poor clinical status, the procedure may also be advantageously applied to other, less critically ill, patients.[75,76]

Splenic Infarction

Infarction of the spleen is relatively common in association with sickle cell anemia or emboli from the left atrium in mitral stenosis. Radionuclide studies and CT

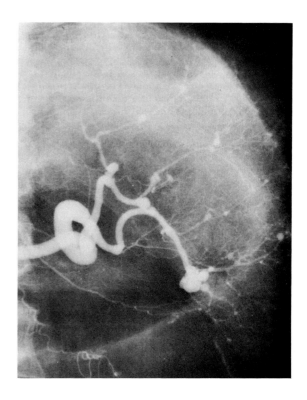

Figure 58-25. Intrasplenic branch artery aneurysms in cirrhosis of the liver. This 45-year-old chronic alcoholic had cirrhosis of the liver with chronic liver failure. He had had multiple bleeding episodes because of esophageal varices. Selective splenic arteriogram demonstrates multiple intrasplenic arterial aneurysms with profound narrowing of the intrasplenic arterial branches. The appearance resembles that in periarteritis but represents one of the findings sometimes associated with cirrhosis of the liver and portal hypertension.

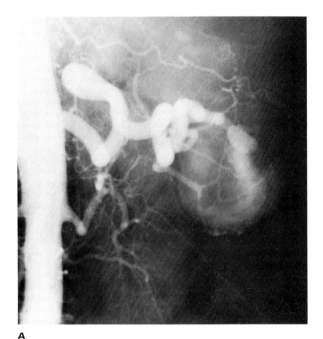

A

Figure 58-26. Splenic arteriovenous fistula in a 57-year-old woman complaining of weight loss, diarrhea, malaise, and an enlarging abdomen. Physical examination showed ascites without evidence of a mass and severe edema of both lower extremities. Angiography showed a large arteriovenous fis-

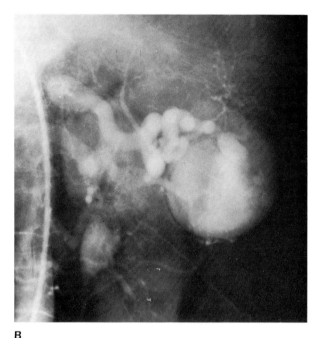

B

tula. (A) Early phase. A tortuous splenic artery fills a large blood sac in the spleen. (B) Late phase. The sac retains contrast, and its true size is now clearly defined. (Courtesy of Arthur Pryde, M.D.)

are useful screening methods (Fig. 58-27). Arteriographic studies demonstrate abrupt occlusion of intrasplenic branches associated with a localized ischemic zone, which is usually triangular (Fig. 58-28).[77]

Figure 58-27. Splenic infarction. CT scan demonstrates two wedge-shaped areas of diminished absorption in the spleen (*arrows*). These represent areas of splenic infarction in a patient with multiple embolic episodes.

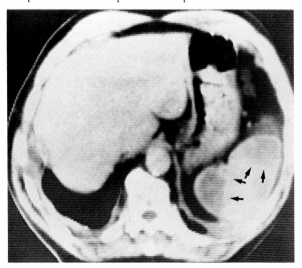

Splenic Artery Thrombosis

Splenic artery thrombosis is relatively rare. Arteriography reveals obstruction with filling of intrasplenic vessels through collateral channels (Figs. 58-29 and 58-30).

Changes After Surgery

After splenorenal arterial shunts, the proximal intrapancreatic branches of the splenic artery may undergo remarkable enlargement and provide a collateral supply to the distal portion of the previously divided splenic trunk (Fig. 58-31). Although immediate postoperative studies have shown little diversion of blood flow from the liver in patients with distal splenorenal venous (Warren) shunts,[78] 2-year follow-up studies have demonstrated reversal of portal venous flow from the liver to the low-pressure shunt.[79] In patients who had a Warren shunt performed that involved ligation of the left gastric and gastroepiploic veins, other collateral vessels formed postoperatively, whereas in patients who had a modified shunt without ligation of these branches, the left gastric and gastroepiploic veins enlarged and served as collateral vessels.[79]

Portal Hypertension

The splenic artery may enlarge in the presence of cirrhosis and portal hypertension. Intrasplenic branch aneurysms may also develop (see Fig. 58-28).

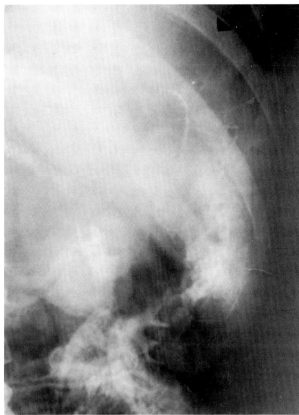

A

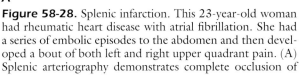

B

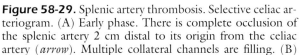

Figure 58-28. Splenic infarction. This 23-year-old woman had rheumatic heart disease with atrial fibrillation. She had a series of embolic episodes to the abdomen and then developed a bout of both left and right upper quadrant pain. (A) Splenic arteriography demonstrates complete occlusion of

the superior splenic arterial branch. No evidence of filling of the small vessels is observed in this area (*arrowhead*). (B) In the capillary phase, a large radiolucent area representing the zone of ischemia is apparent (*arrowhead*).

Figure 58-29. Splenic artery thrombosis. Selective celiac arteriogram. (A) Early phase. There is complete occlusion of the splenic artery 2 cm distal to its origin from the celiac artery (*arrow*). Multiple collateral channels are filling. (B)

Later phase at 1.5 seconds. The distal splenic artery (*arrows*) is densely opacified via collateral vessels and arborizes normally into the terminal branches in the spleen.

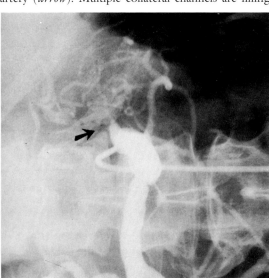

A

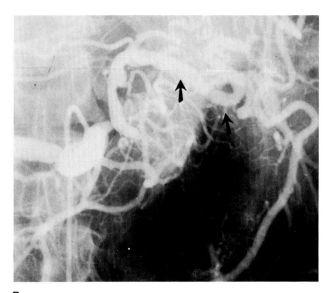

B

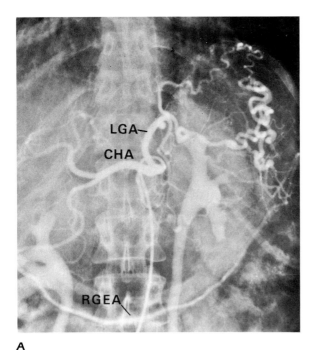

A

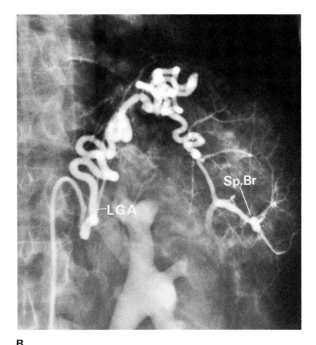

B

Figure 58-30. Splenic artery thrombosis. (A) Selective celiac arteriogram. There is complete occlusion of the splenic artery just beyond its origin. Collateral filling to the spleen via the left gastric artery (*LGA*) and the right gastroepiploic artery (*RGEA*) is apparent. *CHA*, common hepatic artery.

(B) Selective left gastric arteriogram, left posterior oblique projection. The left gastric artery is profoundly tortuous in its course and communicates with branches to the spleen, filling the rather thin intrasplenic arterial branches (*Sp. Br.*).

Splenic Vein Occlusion

Pancreatic and retroperitoneal disease may cause splenic vein occlusion with a consequent increase in intrasplenic and peripheral splenic vein pressures and venous flow to gastric varices through the splenoportal collateral vessels (the short gastric, coronary, and gastroepiploic veins).[80–83] Gastric varices may give rise to massive acute or recurrent hemorrhaging,[84] which can be forestalled by splenectomy.

Abdominal pain, weight loss, or iron-deficiency anemia is commonly associated with splenic vein occlusion.[82] Radiographic investigation may reveal a normal-size spleen[81,82] or splenomegaly. The presence of gastric varices in the absence of esophageal varices is evidence of splenic vein occlusion, whereas the coexistence of varices of both venous systems suggests portal hypertension.[80] In a study of 19 patients with angiographically demonstrated splenic vein occlusion, gastric varices were evident on barium examination in 74 percent as "broad, serpentine, redundant filling defects or clusters of polypoid defects, simulating thickened rugal folds."[80] Definitive diagnosis requires angiographic studies, although MRI may play an important role in diagnosis.

Cysts

Splenic cysts are rare lesions; fewer than 700 cases have been reported in the literature.[85] Although large splenic cysts have been found in neonates,[86] cysts in children are rare. Most cysts occur in people under 40 years of age,[87] and there is a female predominance.[88] Of six cases reported by Doolas et al.,[85] three were found in association with pregnancy.

Symptoms, including dyspnea, coughing, respiratory infections, nausea, vomiting, and urinary frequency, frequently arise as a result of visceral compression.[87] Twenty-five percent of splenic cysts rupture, and 45 percent are demonstrated as splenomegaly.[87] Although splenic cysts are usually diagnosed before surgery only when calcified, a high index of suspicion should be maintained because of the danger of cyst rupture. Excretory urography may demonstrate a splenic cyst as a suprarenal mass,[89] and, although nonspecific, the liver-spleen scan shows defects in 60 to 70 percent of cases of splenic cyst (Fig. 58-32).[90] Although ultrasonography plays a critical role in the evaluation of splenic cysts,[91] CT may also be of value if ultrasonography fails to adequately determine the location and characteristics of the cyst (Fig. 58-33).[92] As-

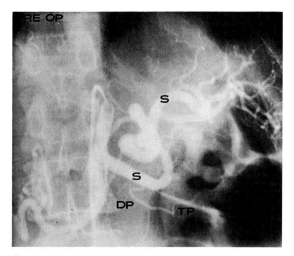

A

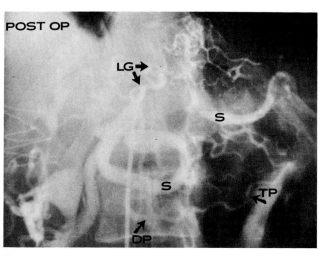

B

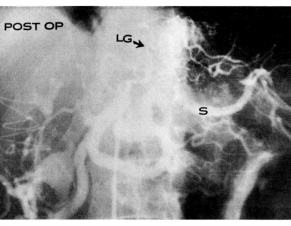

C

Figure 58-31. Postoperative changes in the splenic artery. This 46-year-old hypertensive man had severe left renal artery stenosis demonstrated by renal angiography. A splenorenal shunt was constructed at surgery. (A) Preoperative study. A normal, somewhat tortuous main splenic trunk (*S*) with dorsal pancreatic (*DP*) and transverse pancreatic (*TP*) branches is opacified. (B) Postoperative study 8 days after surgery. The splenic trunk (*S*) has been divided. The distal portion fills from the dorsal pancreatic (*DP*) and transverse pancreatic (*TP*) anastomosis, which has enlarged in the interval. *LG*, left gastric artery. (C) Later phase in the serialographic study. Additional collateral supply to the spleen via tortuous channels originating from the left gastric artery (*LG*) is evident.

piration of cyst fluid for diagnostic or therapeutic reasons may be safely performed using a 22-gauge needle in patients with normal coagulation parameters and nonhilar lesions.[93] However, this should be avoided if hydatid cyst is suspected because of the danger of leakage of cyst contents and anaphylaxis. Angiography (Fig. 58-34) has been superceded by ultrasound, CT, and MRI in the diagnosis of splenic cysts[94] but has in the past been valuable at times in excluding the diagnosis of abscess or neoplasm.[92,95]

Splenic cysts are divided into two large groups: (1) the true cysts, of either parasitic or nonparasitic origin, which have an epithelial lining; and (2) the false cysts, which frequently arise secondary to trauma and which lack an epithelial lining. The most common cause of splenic cysts is echinococcus infection; in such cysts peripheral calcification may be present in the cyst wall. In countries in which echinococcus disease is not endemic, false cysts have been reported to constitute 80 percent of splenic cysts.[92]

Characteristically, cysts cause compression and displacement of surrounding normal parenchyma. They are avascular,[96,97] and they may demonstrate large capsular vessels coursing over them. There is rarely any

Figure 58-32. Splenic cyst. Radionuclide scan demonstrates multiple round negative defects in the spleen, representing subcapsular cysts.

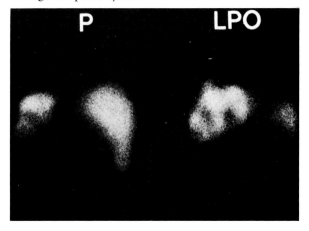

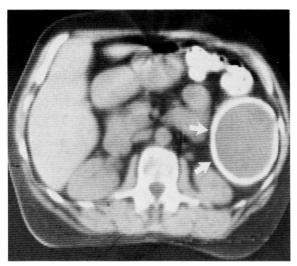

Figure 58-33. Calcified splenic cyst. CT scan shows a large cyst of the spleen (*arrows*) with a calcific wall. Although the appearance is compatible with an echinococcus cyst, this represented a congenital cyst of the kidney.

problem with the distinction from neoplasm because the intrasplenic vessels are smoothly compressed and displaced by the avascular cyst (Fig. 58-35).[96] Frequently there may be only a densely opacified shell of parenchyma during the capillary phase as a reflection of the high degree of replacement by the cyst.[98] The edge is usually sharp and smooth.

Neoplasms

Benign Tumors

The most common of primary benign tumors, although still rare, is the hemangioma. Histologically, hemangiomas consist of endothelially lined vascular channels of varying diameter and may be solid or cystic on gross pathology.[99] Solid hemangiomas are hyperechoic on ultrasound and hypo- or isodense on CT, where they enhance with contrast; the cystic hemangiomas have complex echo patterns with multiple cystic areas on ultrasound, and CT demonstrates a multicystic enhancing mass.[99]

On the few reported angiograms, hemangiomas are more often hypovascular than hypervascular, although both patterns may be seen.[99]

Other benign tumors of the spleen are of many varieties: fibromas, osteomas, chondromas, lymphangiomas, and hamartomas. Most of these tumors are round or oval and displace surrounding arterial branches significantly. Arteriography of the adjacent parenchyma may also be observed. A relative lack of vascularity in the parenchymal phase is generally apparent. The hamartomas, by contrast, may be richly vascular tumors with large, plexoid vessels that may simulate those of malignant neoplasms (Fig. 58-36). The vessels may be tortuous, with aneurysmal dilatations and multiple vascular lakes[95]: they ramify irregularly and may communicate directly with veins.[100] They resemble the

Figure 58-34. Cyst of the spleen. This 45-year-old man had left upper quadrant pain and a palpable mass. (A) Celiac arteriogram demonstrates a huge mass lesion, with distortion and compression of the peripheral splenic vessels. (B) A later phase of the same study shows a large, avascular area of mass compressing the remainder of the splenic parenchyma, which is filled with contrast medium. At laparotomy, the preoperative diagnosis of splenic cyst was confirmed.

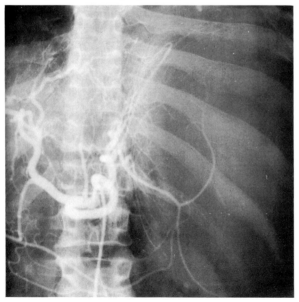

A

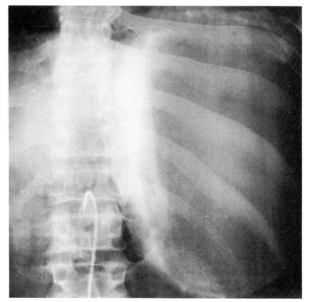

B

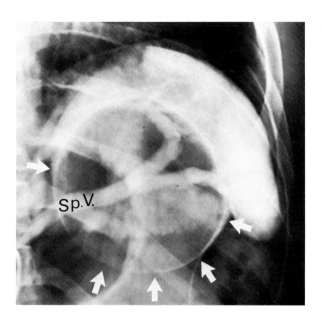

◄ **Figure 58-35.** Splenic cyst. Splenographic phase of a selective celiac arteriogram. A large lucent area is visible (*arrows*) in the hilus of the spleen, slightly compressing the visualized splenic vein (*Sp. V.*). Notice the thin rim of compressed splenic tissue around the congenital cyst.

neovasculature of malignant tumors of the kidney and other viscera.

Malignant Tumors

Malignant splenic neoplasms are characteristically those that involve the lymph nodes and the bone marrow (lymphosarcoma, Hodgkin disease, reticulum cell sarcoma, and the leukemias). The subject has been reviewed by Das Gupta et al.,[101] Rösch,[102] and Kishikawa et al.[54] In addition, hemangiosarcomas and fibrosarcomas may also be observed. All of these neoplasms,

Figure 58-36. Hamartoma of the spleen. (A) Arteriogram. This 4-year-old boy had an abdominal mass and the nephrotic syndrome. A retrograde abdominal aortogram showed splaying of the branches (*arrows*) of the splenic artery (*SPA*) around a tumor occupying approximately 50 percent of the splenic substance. In the early arterial phase, numerous large, tortuous vessels were visualized within the tumor mass. Vascular lakes and early venous filling were demonstrated on later serial films. The left renal artery (*LRA*) was also displaced superiorly and medially with

stretching of the lower pole branches. A diagnosis of congenital angiomatous malformation (hemangioma) or hemangiosarcoma was suggested. (B) Gross pathologic specimen. At laparotomy, the spleen weighed 300 g and contained a well-delimited 7-cm mass (*arrows*). On microscopic section, the appearance was considered characteristic of a hamartoma. The splenic mass was causing compression and stretching of the left renal vein. After splenectomy, proteinuria and hypoproteinemia disappeared.

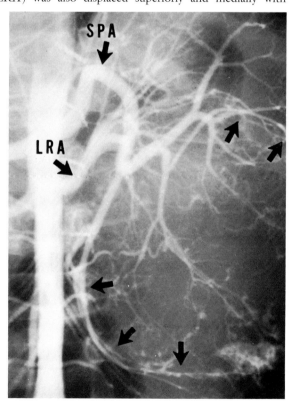

A

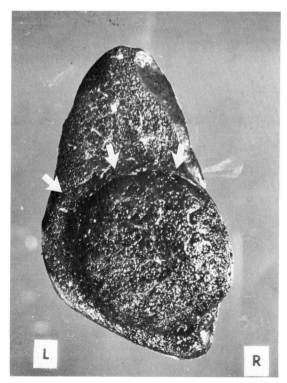

B

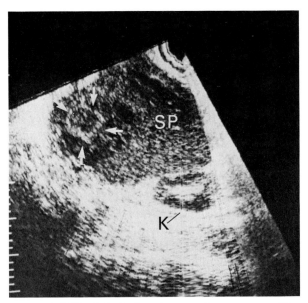

Figure 58-37. Splenic lymphoma, ultrasonogram. The spleen (*SP*) is grossly enlarged. A discrete echogenic tumor mass is visible within the splenic shadow (*arrows*). The kidney (*K*) is well visualized.

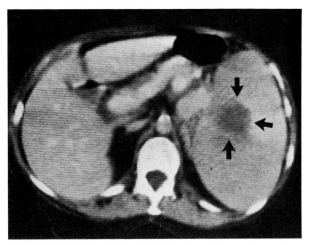

Figure 58-38. Hodgkin disease of the spleen, CT scan. The spleen is grossly enlarged, showing diffuse involvement by Hodgkin disease. In addition, there is an area of low atenuation (*arrows*) representing a localized implant of Hodgkin tissue.

with the exception of the hemangiosarcomas and the fibrosarcomas, cause a diffuse increase in the size of the spleen; the neoplastic tissue is distributed generally rather than localized.

Arteriography has not been commonly employed in the study of malignant neoplasms of the spleen because nonlymphomatous malignancies are unusual and because patients with metastases of epithelial neoplasms to the spleen generally have disseminated metastases. In 1954, Edsman[103] described the first case of malignant tumor of the spleen studied by angiography. The histology was that of a malignant splenic endothelioma.

As in malignant tumors elsewhere, the vessels may be irregularly narrowed, amputated, and displaced. By far the most common finding is displacement: stretching and distortion of the vessels by diffuse tumor infiltration. The appearance demonstrated in Figure 58-12, splenomegaly with Hodgkin disease, is typical. There is more or less stretching and distortion of the major branches of the splenic artery, with distinct separation of the distal small branches and frequently rather sriking narrowing as well.

In a study of the angiographic findings in splenic neoplasms, Kishikawa et al.[95] noted similar angiographic appearances in five cases of reticulum cell sarcoma and one case of Hodgkin disease. In these cases, the lesions were visualized as "multiple, poorly defined round defects in the splenic parenchymograms." Arte-

rial encasement was shown in all cases, and fine tumor vessels and venous obstruction were evident in, respectively, three and two of the cases of reticulum cell sarcomas. Splayed intrasplenic branches, vascular lakes in the late arterial-to-venous phase, and no obvious tumor vessels or stains were found in two cases of hemangiosarcoma.[54]

Vascular changes may also occur in the leukemias. In Figure 58-13, the stretching of the intrasplenic branches is obvious, and the capsular circulation is somewhat richer than is normally seen. The opacification of the spleen is relatively less than normal because of the replacement of a significant volume of tissue by the leukemic infiltrates.

Both CT and ultrasonography yield valuable information in splenic lymphoma (Figs. 58-37 and 58-38). As has been demonstrated in a case reported by Cunningham,[104] ultrasonography cannot reliably distinguish lymphoma from abscess; however, when angiography shows typical neovascularity and irregular, encased vessels, as in the reticulum cell sarcoma illustrated in Figure 58-39, an unequivocal diagnosis of malignancy can be made. CT has proved helpful in detecting moderate-size splenic metastases (Fig. 58-40), as has angiography (Fig. 58-41). On angiography metastases may displace vessels but more commonly are demonstrated as round, lucent areas in the capillary phase. The concept that the spleen is immune to metastases from epithelial neoplasms and that such metastases are rare has not been borne out by autopsy studies.[105]

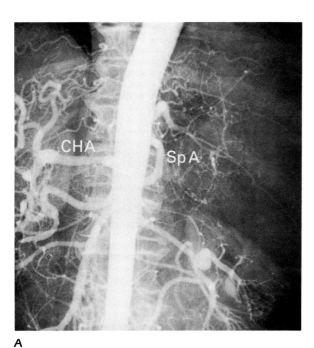

A

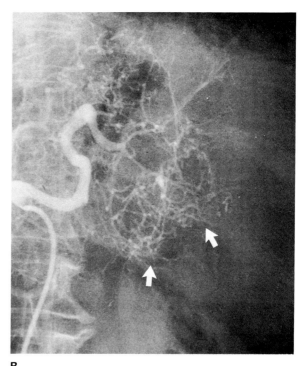

B

Figure 58-39. Reticulum cell sarcoma of the spleen and retroperitoneum. (A) Abdominal aortogram. The splenic artery (*SpA*) is visualized arising from the celiac axis and extending into the left upper quadrant. It then becomes obscured by a meshwork of malignant vessels extending into the spleen. Incidentally noted are extension of the tumor to involve the common hepatic artery (*CHA*) with encasement and an an- eurysm of the left renal artery. (B) Selective splenic arteriogram, magnification view, shows encasement of the splenic artery, reflected in the areas of narrowing and irregularity. The tumor has completely surrounded the vessel, which gives rise to a large cluster of tumor vessels (*arrows*) extending into the spleen.

Trauma

The spleen is ruptured more often than any other intraabdominal organ in nonpenetrating abdominal injuries, and it is also frequently injured in penetrating trauma. In a review of 335 consecutively studied patients undergoing splenectomy for trauma,[106] 57 percent of the patients had three or more associated injuries. Although no patient with only a splenic injury died, the mortality was greater than 30 percent among patients with more than three associated injuries. In penetrating tumor the chest is the most common site of associated injury; in blunt trauma, the skeletal system is the most common site (Table 58-7).[107] In both blunt and penetrating splenic trauma, shock and pulmonary complications are the most common causes of death (Table 58-8). It is likely that blunt trauma leads to splenic fractures in the areas between the intrasplenic arteries because the arteries serve as the major structural supports of the parenchyma[1]; if this is true, it would mean that the injuries themselves follow a natural segmental distribution.

Although diagnostic paracentesis may establish the

Figure 58-40. Metastasis to the spleen, CT scan. The splenic shadow (*Sp*) is well visualized, with a round nodule (*arrows*) representing metastasis from an ovarian carcinoma. The negative filling defects in the spleen (*barred arrows*) also represent metastatic disease.

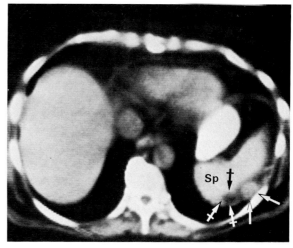

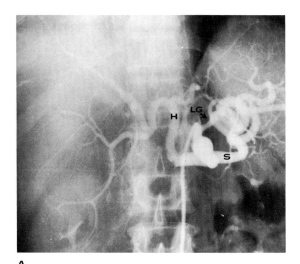

A

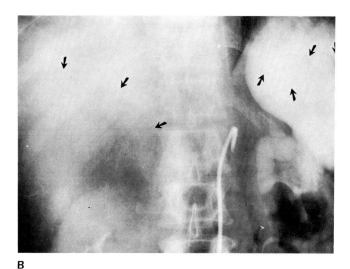

B

Figure 58-41. Metastases to the spleen and liver. This 50-year-old man had a diagnosis of malignant melanoma established on skin biopsy several years prior to the present study. He was admitted to the hospital complaining of malaise, anorexia, and abdominal pain. On physical examination, hepatosplenomegaly was found to be present, and the patient was subsequently found to have widespread metastatic disease.

(A) Celiac arteriogram demonstrates enlargement of the liver and spleen. Hepatic branches (*H*) are stretched peripherally. The splenic trunk (*S*) is tortuous and compressed by the enlarged spleen. *LG,* left gastric artery. (B) Later phase of same study reveals filling defects (*arrows*) in the opacified parenchyma of both the liver and the spleen due to metastatic deposits.

presence of blood in the peritoneal cavity and permit a presumptive diagnosis of splenic rupture,[106] imaging methods are frequently applied both for making the primary diagnosis and for defining the associated injuries. Indications of splenic trauma include depression of the splenic flexure of the colon, elevation of the diaphragm, obliteration of the splenic shadow, and prominent gastric rugae. Rib fractures, pleural fluid at the base of the left lung, and free peritoneal fluid may also be observed. However, these signs are not always present.

The prime diagnostic modalities for the diagnosis of splenic traumatic injury are CT and ultrasound, and these have displaced radioisotope studies and angiography for this purpose. In a series of 50 patients, CT has been shown to have a sensitivity of 96 percent for detecting splenic injury.[108] CT also enables one to evaluate the other intraabdominal viscera for associated injuries. Radioisotope studies lack specificity and cannot demonstrate very small subcapsular hematomas. Angiography, although assuming less importance as a diagnostic modality for the diagnosis of splenic rupture or laceration, may nevertheless be important for localizing the exact site of hemorrhage and offers an alternative method for arresting this bleeding by transcatheter embolization.

A positive angiographic diagnosis can best be made when extravasation is visualized. "Mottling," or apparent areas of subcapsular ischemia or fluid collection, is a less reliable sign,[109] although Scatliff has pointed out that mottling is frequently present and probably represents stasis of contrast material and blood in the

Table 58-7. Associated Injuries with Splenic Trauma

Blunt Injuries (150 patients)		Penetrating Injuries (186 patients)	
Orthopedic	79	Chest	104
Chest	64	Stomach	71
Central nervous system	48	Liver	52
Liver	31	Colon	46
Genitourinary	28	Genitourinary	36
Pancreas	19	Pancreas	32
Diaphragm (ruptured)	11	Extremity	26
Intestine	15	Small bowel	20

From Naylor R, Coln D, Shires GT. Morbidity and mortality from injuries to the spleen. J Trauma 1974;14:773–778. Used with permission.

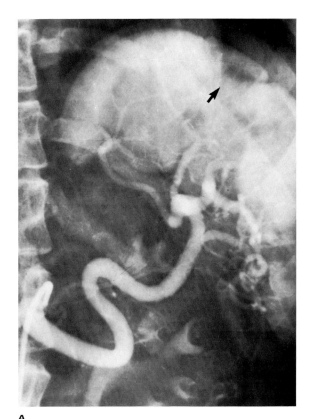

A

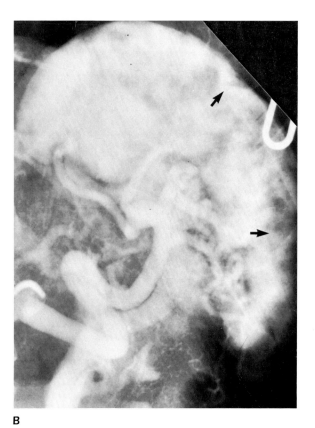

B

Figure 58-42. "Notching" of the spleen. This patient was in an automobile accident and was suspected of having splenic rupture. A splenic arteriogram was performed. (A) Early phase. There appears to be a defect in the contour of the spleen (*arrow*) located just below the diaphragm, and originally interpreted as possibly representing splenic hema-

toma consequent to trauma. (B) Splenographic phase. The spleen is densely but nonuniformly opacified, and a number of areas of lucency are visible at the edge of the spleen (*arrows*). Splenectomy was performed on this patient, and no evidence of splenic trauma was visible. Instead, congenital notching of the spleen was found.

marginal sinuses of the traumatized spleen.[110] Splenic "notching," or lobulation, may be incorrectly considered as evidence of splenic rupture (Fig. 58-42).[109] Extravasation is usually unmistakable (Fig. 58-43), but at times may be best demonstrated by intraarterial ad-

Table 58-8. Breakdown of Causes of Death Following Splenic Trauma

	Number of Deaths		Total Number of Deaths
Cause of Death	Blunt Trauma	Penetrating Trauma	
Shock	16	5	21
Pulmonary disorder	13	3	16
Central nervous system disorder	5	1	6
Sepsis	1	3	4
Unknown	1	1	2
Total	36	13	49

From Naylor R, Coln D, Shires GT. Morbidity and mortality from injuries to the spleen. J Trauma 1974;14:773–778. Used with permission.

ministration of epinephrine or vasopressin. Increasing the resistance at the precapillary arteriolar level may enhance contrast leakage (Fig. 58-44). The site of bleeding may be demonstrated by the leakage of contrast medium into the splenic pulp (Fig. 58-45).[14,111] Characteristic findings also include (1) a large, avascular area with spreading of the intrasplenic branches (see Figs. 58-45 and 58-47); (2) irregularities in the opacified spleen in the region of the hematoma (Fig. 58-46); (3) loss of the continuous splenic contour (see Fig. 58-43); (4) simultaneous visualization of the splenic artery and vein (see Fig. 58-45); (5) extravasation of contrast material in the spleen (see Figs. 58-43 through 58-45); (6) a clear break ("fracture") in the splenic contour (Fig. 58-47); and (7) an increased distance between the spleen and the left flank (see Figs. 58-43 through 58-46).[11] The spleen may be displaced medially and the kidney inferiorly.[112] In subacute or chronic trauma, intrasplenic "channels" may be visualized (see Fig. 58-47).

Arteriography can also be used to assess the degree of splenic injury (Fig. 58-48),[112-114] although this is

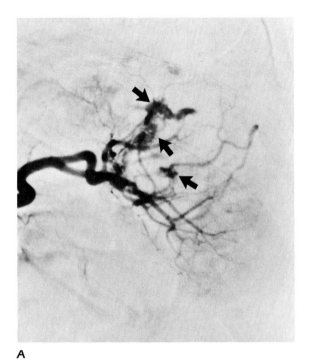

A

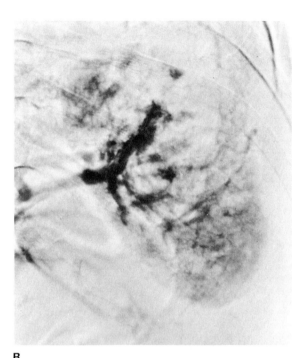

B

Figure 58-43. Splenic trauma. Selective splenic arteriography. (A) Early phase. Subtraction demonstrates unequivocal extravasation (*arrows*) of contrast agent outside the vascular bed into the splenic tissue. (B) Later phase. The contrast agent puddles within the splenic tissue, indicating the presence of gross splenic trauma. Notice that the lateral wall of the spleen is separated from the lateral abdominal wall by a subcapsular collection of blood.

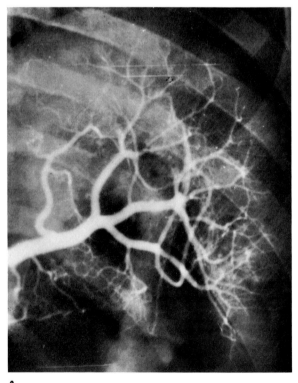

A

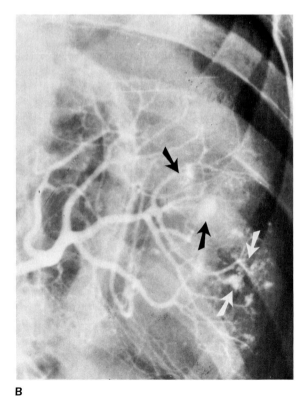

B

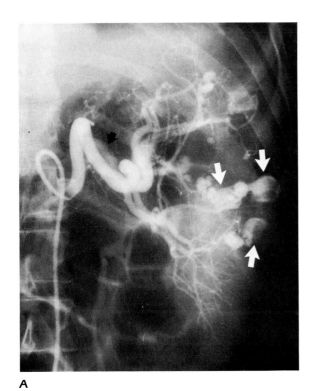

A

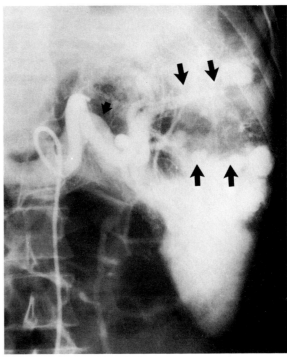

B

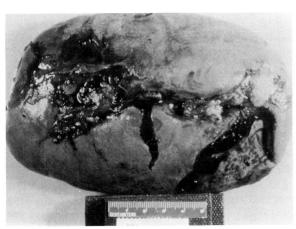

C

Figure 58-45. Splenic trauma. (A) Selective splenic arteriogram, early phase. Gross extravasation is visible within the splenic tissue (*white arrows*), as are profound separation of vessels and early filling of the splenic vein (*black arrow*). (B) Selective splenic arteriogram, splenographic phase. In addition to the gross extravasation, there is a large area of nonfilling (*large arrows*), representing intrasplenic hemorrhage. The splenic vein is densely visualized (*small arrow*). (C) Specimen of ruptured spleen. Multiple rents are visible in the surface of the spleen, with gross intrasplenic hemorrhage also demonstrated.

◄ **Figure 58-44.** Splenic trauma. (A) Selective splenic arteriogram. Although there is some spreading of the intrasplenic vessels, there is no definite evidence of extravasation or local collections of blood within the spleen. (B) Selective splenic arteriogram 15 seconds after the administration of 6 g of epinephrine. With the increase in the intrasplenic arterial resistance there is clear evidence of multiple areas of extravasation (*arrows*) throughout the spleen. The epinephrine, by raising the vascular resistance at the precapillary level, has helped establish an unequivocal diagnosis of splenic trauma. (Courtesy of Stanley Baum, M.D.)

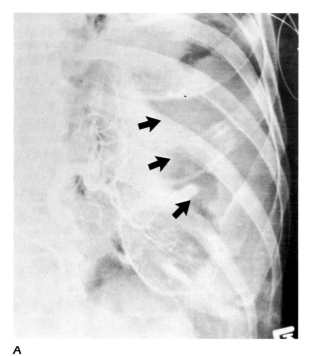

A

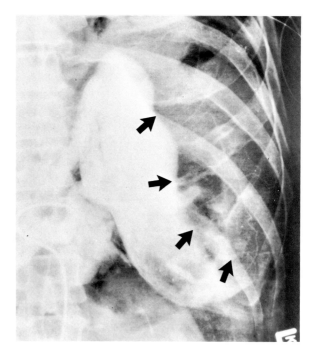

B

Figure 58-46. Splenic rupture with subcapsular hematoma. Selective splenic arteriogram. (A) Arterial phase. The splenic arterial branches are clumped together at the medial aspect of the kidney, and a large area of nonfilling is visible (*arrows*). (B) Splenographic phase. The splenic tissue is grossly compressed and very densely opacified. A large subcapsular hematoma is well visualized (*arrows*). It separates the opacified splenic tissue from the lateral abdominal wall to striking degree.

Figure 58-47. Splenic trauma. This patient was in an automobile accident and had multiple fractures. Although there was a suspicion of splenic trauma, arteriographic studies were delayed until 3 weeks after the accident. (A) Selective splenic arteriogram shows profound separation of intrasplenic arterial branches, with clumping and compression of splenic parenchyma. (B) Capillary phase shows striking evidence of splenic trauma. A large laceration of the spleen is visible, with intrasplenic hemorrhage (*arrows*). The splenic edge is separated from the lateral abdominal wall because of a subcapsular collection of blood. Intrasplenic tracts of contrast agent representing channels in an otherwise hemorrhagic area are clearly visible (*barred arrows*).

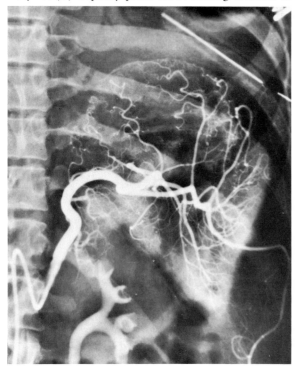

A

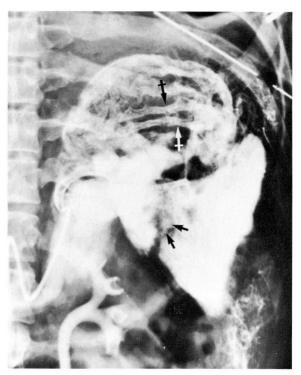

B

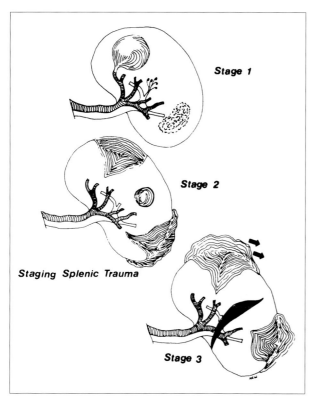

Figure 58-48. Diagrammatic representation of splenic trauma. (Courtesy of Mark Wholey, M.D.) *Stage 1,* intrasplenic hemorrhage; *stage 2,* subcapsular and extracapsular hemorrhage; *stage 3,* splenic fraction with extracapsular bleeding.

more accurately and less invasively accomplished by CT.

In view of the important role the spleen plays in immunocompetence (particularly with respect to prevention of infection due to encapsulated organisms), in recent years increased emphasis has been placed on splenic preservation. This is particularly true in children: a nonoperative approach is standard practice in isolated blunt splenic injuries whenever feasible, and when surgical intervention is necessary, splenorrhaphy is preferred over splenectomy.[115-117] Although controversial, a similar approach is being employed by some in adults.[118-122] The decision on whether to operate is based more on clinical grounds than on imaging studies,[121,123,124] and if surgery is required, splenorrhaphy is again preferred.[119,125,126] Sclafani et al. reported on the use of arteriography and transcatheter embolization in the management of 36 hemodynamically stable patients with splenic injury.[127] Their algorithm suggests emergency arteriography in hemodynamically stable patients with CT-diagnosed splenic injury and without associated abdominal trauma that would require laparotomy. If the arteriogram demonstrates extravasation

of contrast medium within or extending beyond the spleen, they embolize the splenic artery proximally with coils, their rationale being that hemostasis in the spleen will result while allowing continued splenic perfusion through the collateral circulation to the distal splenic artery. With this approach they report a splenic salvage rate of 97 percent, and exploratory laparotomy was avoided in 94 percent of patients.[127]

In recent years, occult rupture of the spleen has been recognized as a diagnostic challenge. Although splenic injury results in immediate rupture in 85 percent of patients and in delayed rupture (some days or weeks later) in 14 percent of patients, in 1 percent of patients the splenic rupture may take place without immediate symptoms and become clinically evident months or years after the trauma in a confusing welter of symptoms. In such cases of occult rupture, the hemorrhage is contained by an intact capsule or adhesions to adjacent organs.[128] Again, ultrasound or CT is the modality of choice for the diagnosis. Angiography is rarely performed, but the characteristic angiographic pattern comprises a peripheral avascular splenic area, tortuosity of the splenic artery with hilar vessel compression, and a smooth filling defect between the diaphragm and the spleen.[128]

Trauma is not necessarily implicated in all cases of splenic rupture[128]; in five cases collected by McMahon,[129] infectious mononucleosis was the underlying cause in two patients, Hodgkin disease in one, and amyloidosis in one, and in one patient no cause was ever determined. Preoperative diagnosis is important. In a case reported by Moskovitz[130] in which the diagnosis was not established preoperatively, extensive resection was carried out because the organized hematoma resembled infiltrating neoplasm.

Abscess

Splenic abscess is a rare but serious lesion that before the widespread availability of CT and ultrasound was frequently difficult to diagnose. Angiography is no longer performed for the diagnosis of splenic abscess, but two angiographic patterns have been described: (1) an avascular mass with tortuous peripheral arteries as well as collateral veins if the splenic vein is narrowed or obstructed[131] and (2) splenomegaly with an irregular mass lacking a vascular rim in association with normal veins and stretched arteries without encasement.[132] In some cases, the angiographic findings may be nonspecific or misleading, suggesting, for example, the presence of a subcapsular hematoma. Miller et al.,[133] noting that a mycotic aneurysm has been associated with a splenic abscess in a number of cases, have suggested that abnormal splenic arteriographic findings in the presence of a mycotic aneurysm should be interpreted as evidence of a splenic abscess. Today the diagnosis of splenic abscess is made by CT or ultrasound and can be confirmed by diagnostic fluid aspiration with a 20- or 22-gauge needle under guidance using these modalities.[93] If pus is obtained on aspiration, percutaneous catheter drainage can be undertaken with an expectant success rate of 76 percent, which is somewhat lower than the expected success rate of percutaneous abscess drainage in other locations (possibly because of multiloculation).[93]

Interventional Techniques

Interventional techniques with regard to the spleen relate to splenic embolization, fine-needle aspiration cytology, and fluid aspiration or drainage. Fluid aspiration and drainage have been discussed in text preceding on cysts and abscesses.

Fine-needle aspiration for cytologic examination of intrasplenic lesions can be accomplished safely using ultrasound or CT guidance. In a series of 42 patients in whom this technique was used under ultrasound guidance, the sensitivity was 69 percent and the specificity was 100 percent in differentiating between benign and malignant conditions.[134] No complications were encountered. The authors conclude that, although this is a safe technique with high specificity, it has relatively low sensitivity.[134]

Transcatheter splenic embolization techniques can be categorized into three groups: (1) splenic artery occlusion, (2) distal splenic artery branch occlusion, and (3) partial splenic ablation.

Splenic Artery Occlusion

Splenic artery occlusion refers to occlusion of the main trunk of the splenic artery, either with coils or detachable balloons, proximal to the hilum of the spleen. We prefer the use of coils rather than detachable balloons because of the considerable expense of the latter. Occasionally it may be possible to maneuver a detachable balloon to the intended site when it is not possible to reach that site with a catheter for coil placement. The size of coil deployed depends on the size of the splenic artery, but in most circumstances 8-mm coils are used. Placement of several coils is usually required to achieve thrombosis. The indications for splenic artery occlusion are (1) splenic artery aneurysm or splenic artery rupture,[62–65] (2) splenic trauma,[127] and (3) presplenectomy for massive splenomegaly.[135–137] After occlusion of the splenic artery in its proximal or mid region, the spleen is kept alive by collateral flow entering the distal splenic artery via the pancreatic branches (arteria pancreatica magna and caudal pancreatic branch), left gastroepiploic artery, and short gastric branches, depending on the exact site of the occlusion. Splenic artery embolization is probably the procedure of choice for focal splenic artery aneurysm or splenic artery rupture. Its use in trauma has been discussed in the section on trauma. Massive splenomegaly (10 times usual weight) may lead to technical difficulties during splenectomy and can result in massive hemorrhage. Preoperative splenic artery embolization may facilitate surgery.[135,136]

Selective Distal Splenic Artery Branch Occlusion

This refers to selective embolization of an intrasplenic branch with Gelfoam pledgets, coils, or detachable balloons. The indications are (1) traumatic rupture of a particular branch, (2) intrasplenic artery branch aneurysm, and (3) branch arteriovenous fistula. Because Gelfoam will resorb within approximately 3 weeks and result in recanalization, it should not be used for embolizing aneurysms or arteriovenous fistulas. To reach distal splenic branches it is often necessary to use a coaxial catheter such as the Tracker 18 catheter (Target Therapeutics) or the Cragg Fx (Meditech). The former will follow placement of 0.018-inch coils, and the latter will allow placement of 0.025-inch coils.

Partial Splenic Ablation

This refers to partial obliteration of the peripheral intrasplenic vascular bed by injection of particulate matter through the angiographic catheter selectively placed in the splenic artery. The indications are (1) hypersplenism,[138–142] (2) massive splenomegaly causing discomfort (e.g., beta-thalassemia major, myelofibrosis),[140,142] and (3) gastric and esophageal varices due to splenic vein thrombosis in patients who are not candidates for splenectomy.[142] The technique has been described in detail by Spigos and associates.[139,142,143] Their patients are pretreated with polyvalent pneumococcal vaccine at least 10 days before the procedure. In addition they receive prophylactic antibiotics (gentamycin and penicillin or a cephalosporin) in the periprocedural period. The spleen is embolized with 2-mm Gelfoam pledgets suspended in an antibiotic solution of gentamycin plus penicillin or a cephalosporin. Sixty to 70 percent of the splenic parenchyma is ablated. The majority of their patients who were embolized were renal transplantation candidates, but, with the widespread use of cyclosporine (which does suppress the bone marrow significantly), partial splenic ablation is now uncommonly used in this group of patients. Earlier reports of splenic ablation indicated high complication rates, with splenic abscess, rupture, septicemia, and pneumonia.[144-146] However, with the technique described by Jonasson and Spigos et al., the complication rate is acceptably low (13 percent): pleural effusion (7 percent), pancreatitis (1.5 percent), splenic abscess (1.5 percent), pancreatic pseudocyst (1.5 percent), and splenic hematoma (1 percent).[142] Patients commonly have pain postprocedurally and develop a fever, leukocytosis, and elevated serum amylase levels, but these all resolve. To avoid the complication of pancreatitis, it is important to place the catheter distally in the splenic artery beyond the pancreatic branches so as to prevent Gelfoam pledgets from entering the pancreatic arterial bed.[139,147] A video-dilution technique has been described to monitor the reduction in splenic blood flow during the embolization procedure and may be useful in determining when to stop injecting Gelfoam pledgets.[148]

Diagnostic Decision Pathway

Radiologic methods play an important role in establishing the presence or absence of splenic disease, as well as in defining its character when present. Splenomegaly may be well depicted by plain abdominal films, the upper gastrointestinal series, the barium enema, and the intravenous urogram. In trauma, multiple associated injuries may be detected. The conventional examinations, however, shed little light on the nature of the splenic abnormality that is present, and they may show entirely normal findings in many types of splenic disease.

Radionuclide scintigraphy and angiography were once commonly used methods for evaluating splenic lesions. The former, however, is insensitive for the detection of intrasplenic lesions and is uncommonly used in primary splenic pathology, except for the detection of accessory spleens. Angiography, because of its invasive nature, is reserved for the evaluation of the splenic artery and vein, and for splenic trauma if embolization is considered. The primary diagnostic modalities for evaluation of the spleen are CT and ultrasound. Both are noninvasive and provide excellent definition of intrasplenic lesions. In addition, other intraabdominal organs can be examined at the same time. MRI has not been proven to be more valuable than CT for intrasplenic pathology, although it is very useful for demonstrating patency of the splenic vein and the presence of collateral venous channels. In the future, it may be useful for tissue characterization of intrasplenic lesions.

References

1. Dixon JA, Miller F, McCloskey D, et al. Anatomy and techniques in segmental splenectomy. Surg Gynecol Obstet 1980; 150:516–520.
2. Morgenstern L, Shapiro SJ. Techniques of splenic conservation. Arch Surg 1979;114:449–454.
3. Taylor AJ, Dodds WJ, Erickson SJ, et al. CT of acquired abnormalities of the spleen. AJR 1991;157:1213–1219.
4. Rolfes RJ, Ros PR. The spleen: an integrated imaging approach. Crit Rev Diagn Imaging 1990;30:41–83.
5. Kupic EA, Marshall WH, Abrams HL. Splenic arterial patterns: angiographic analysis and review. Invest Radiol 1967; 2:70–98.
6. Michels NA. The variational anatomy of the spleen and splenic artery. Am J Anat 1942;70:21.
7. Michels NA. Blood supply and anatomy of the upper abdominal organs. Philadelphia: Lippincott, 1955.
8. Katritsis E, Parashos A, Papadopoulos N. Arterial segmentation of the human spleen by post-mortem angiograms. Angiology 1982;11:720–727.
9. Garcia-Parrero JA, Lemes A. Arterial segmentation and subsegmentation in the human spleen. Acta Anat (Basel) 1988; 131:276–283.
10. Mikhail Y, Kamel R, Nawar NN, et al. Observations on the mode of termination and parenchymal distribution of the splenic artery with evidence of splenic lobulation and segmentation. J Anat 1979;128:253–258.
11. Ödman P. Percutaneous selective angiography of the coeliac artery. Acta Radiol Suppl (Stockh) 1958;159:1.
12. Barnhart MI, Baechler CA, Lusher JM, et al. Arteriovenous shunts in the human spleen. Am J Hematol 1976;1:105–114.
13. Baum S, Kuroda K, Roy RH. Value of special angiographic techniques in the management of patients with abdominal neoplasms. Radiol Clin North Am 1965;3:583–599.
14. Baum S, Roy R, Finkelstein AK, et al. Clinical application of selective celiac and superior mesenteric arteriography. Radiology 1965;84:279.
15. Evans J. Techniques in the detection and diagnosis of malignant lesions of the liver, spleen and pancreas. Radiol Clin North Am 1965;3:567.
16. Lunderquist A. Angiography in carcinoma of the pancreas. Acta Radiol Suppl (Stockh) 1965;235:1.
17. Ranniger K, Saldino RM. Arteriographic diagnosis of pancreatic lesions. Radiology 1966;86:470–474.
18. Rösch J, Bret J. Arteriography of the pancreas. AJR 1965;94: 182.
19. Jafri SZ, Aisen AM, Glazer GM, et al. Comparison of CT angiography in assessing resectability of pancreatic carcinoma. AJR 1984;142:525–529.
20. Appleton GV, Bathurst NC, Virjee J. The value of angiography in the surgical management of pancreatic disease. Ann R Coll Surg Engl 1989;71:92–96.
21. Dooley WC, Cameron JL, Pitt HA. Is preoperative angiography useful in patients with periampullary tumors? Ann Surg 1990;211:649–654.
22. Warshaw AL, Gu ZY, Wittenberg J. Preoperative staging and assessment of resectability of pancreatic cancer. Arch Surg 1990;125:230–233.
23. Paul RE Jr, Miller HH, Kahn PC, et al. Pancreatic angiography, with application of subselective angiography of the celiac or superior mesenteric artery to the diagnosis of carcinoma of the pancreas. N Engl J Med 1965;272:283.
24. Chandramouly BS, Kihm RH, Flesh LH. Dextrocardia with

total situs inversus: radionuclide imaging and ultrasonography of liver and spleen. NY State J Med 1980;80:655–677.

25. Dodds WJ, Taylor AJ, Erickson SJ, et al. Radiologic imaging of splenic anomalies. AJR 1990;155:805–810.

26. Hernanz-Schulman M, Abrosino MM, Genieser NB. Pictorial essay: current evaluation of the patient with abnormal viscero-atrial situs. AJR 1990;154:797–802.

27. Allen KB, Gay BB Jr, Skandalakis JE. Wandering spleen: anatomic and radiologic considerations. South Med J 1992;85: 976–984.

28. Gordon DH, Burrell MI, Levin DC, et al. Wandering spleen—the radiological and clinical spectrum. Radiology 1977;125:39–46.

29. Abell I. Wandering spleen with torsion of the pedicle. Ann Surg 1933;98:722.

30. Sorgen RA, Robbins DI. Bleeding gastric varices secondary to wandering spleen. Gastrointest Radiol 1980;5:25–27.

31. Eraklis AJ, Filler RM. Splenectomy in childhood: a review of 1413 cases. J Pediatr Surg 1972;7:382–388.

32. Pugh HL. Collective review, splenectomy with special reference to historical background; indications and rationale, and comparison of reported mortality. Intern Abstr Surg 1946; 83:209.

33. Olsen WR, Beaudoin ED. Increased incidence of accessory spleens in hematologic disease. Arch Surg 1969;98:762–763.

34. Pearson HA, Johnston D, Smith KA, et al. The born-again spleen: return of splenic function after splenectomy for trauma. N Engl J Med 1978;298:1389–1392.

35. Fitzer PM. Accessory spleen simulating splenic hematoma. Va Med 1977;104:782–783.

36. Onuigbo WIB, Ojukwu JO, Eze WC. Infarction of accessory spleen. J Pediatr Surg 1978;13:129–130.

37. Bart JB, Appel MF. Recurrent hemolytic anemia secondary to accessory spleens. South Med J 1978;71:608–609.

38. Jacobson JM, Reynolds RD. Accessory spleen in Hodgkin's disease. JAMA 1978;240:2081.

39. Honigman R, Lanzkowsky P. Isolated congenital asplenia: an occult case of overwhelming sepsis. Am J Dis Child 1979;133: 552–553.

40. Majeski JA, Upshur JK. Asplenia syndrome: a study of congenital anomalies in 16 cases. JAMA 1978;240:1508–1510.

41. Rose V, Izukawa T, Moes C. Syndrome of asplenia and polysplenia: a review of cardiac and non-cardiac malformations in 60 cases with special reference to diagnosis and prognosis. Br Heart J 1975;37:840–852.

42. Okayasu I, Mori W, Kajita A. A study on so-called splenic agenesis syndrome—pathological examination of 27 autopsy cases. Acta Pathol Jpn 1974;24:495–513.

43. Katcher AL. Familial asplenia, other malformations, and sudden death. Pediatrics 1980;65:633–635.

44. Wilkinson JL, Holt PA, Dickinson DF, et al. Asplenia syndrome in one of mono-zygotic twins. Eur J Cardiol 1979;10: 301–304.

45. Majeski JA. Asplenia associated with a congenital diaphragmatic defect and neurologic anomalies. South Med J 1978; 71:1448.

46. Lucas RV Jr, Neufeld HN, Lester RG, Edwards JE. The symmetrical liver as a roentgen sign of asplenia. Circulation 1962; 25:973.

47. Roguin N, Auslaender L, Zeiter M, Katzir J, Sujov P, Riss E. Asplenia syndrome: report of two cases. Isr J Med Sci 1979; 15:451.

48. Albert HM, Fowler RL, Glass BA, et al. Cardiac anomalies and splenic agenesis. Am Surg 1968;34:94–98.

49. Ando F, Shirotani H, Kawai J, et al. Successful total repair of complicated cardiac anomalies with asplenia syndrome. J Thorac Cardiovasc Surg 1976;72:33–38.

50. Van Mierop LHS, Gessner I, Schiebler G. Asplenia and polysplenia syndromes. Birth Defects 1972;8:5.

51. Waldman JD, Rosenthal A, Smith AL, et al. Sepsis and congenital asplenia. J Pediatr 1977;90:555–559.

52. Kishikawa T, Numaguchi Y, Tokunaga M, et al. Hemangiosarcoma of the spleen with liver metastases: angiographic manifestations. Radiology 1977;123:31–35.

53. Roguin N, Pelled B, Amikam S, Auslaender L, Riss E. Polysplenia syndrome: a study of five new cases. Isr J Med Sci 1978;14:948.

54. Childress MH, Cho KJ, Newlin N, et al. Arterial impression on the stomach. AJR 1979;132:769–772.

55. Palubinskas AJ, Ripley HR. Fibromuscular hyperplasia in extrarenal arteries. Radiology 1964;82:451.

56. Garti IJ, Meiraz D. Fibromuscular dysplasia of the splenic artery in a child; case report. Vasa 1979;8:83–84.

57. Bücherl ES, Rucker G. Das Aneurysma der Arteria Coeliaca und ihre Äste. Chirurg 1964;35:354.

58. Boontje AH. Multiple aneurysms of the visceral branches of the abdominal aorta. Vasa 1979;8:42–50.

59. Pollak EW, Michas CA. Massive spontaneous hemoperitoneum due to rupture of visceral branches of the abdominal aorta. Am Surg 1979;45:621–630.

60. Otto WJ. Calcification in the left upper quadrant, or "All that glisters. . . ." JAMA 1965;193:1406.

61. Baum S, Greenstein RH, Nusbaum M, et al. Diagnosis of ruptured, noncalcified splenic artery aneurysm by selective celiac arteriography. Arch Surg 1965;91:1026–1028.

62. Tihansky DP, Lluncar E. Transcatheter embolization of multiple mycotic splenic artery aneurysms: a case report. Angiology 1986;37:530–534.

63. Reidy JF, Rowe PH, Ellis FG. Splenic artery aneurysm embolization—the preferred technique to surgery. Clin Radiol 1990;41:281–282.

64. Tarazov PG, Polysalov VN, Ryzhkov VK. Transcatheter treatment of splenic artery aneurysms (SAA): report of two cases. J Cardiovasc Surg (Torino) 1991;32:129–131.

65. Baker KS, Tisnado J, Cho SR, et al. Splanchnic artery aneurysms and pseudoaneurysm: transcatheter embolization. Radiology 1987;163:135–139.

66. Reuter SR, Fry WJ, Bookstein JJ. Mesenteric artery branch aneurysms. Arch Surg 1968;97:497–499.

67. Schug J, Bankin RP. Rupture of the splenic artery aneurysm in pregnancy. Obstet Gynecol 1965;25:717.

68. Hashizume M, Ohta M, Ueno K. Laparoscopic ligation of splenic artery aneurysm. Surgery 1993;113:352–354.

69. Stone HH, Jordan WD, Aker JJ, et al. Portal arteriovenous fistulas, review and case report. Am J Surg 1965;109:191.

70. Shah VV, Mehtalia SD, Shah KD, Hansoti RC. Splenia arteriovenous fistula. Angiology 1967;18:23.

71. Murray MJ, Thol AJ, Greenspan R. Splenic arteriovenous fistulas as a cause of portal hypertension. Am J Med 1960;29: 849.

72. Cantarero JM, Llorente JG, Hidalgo EG. Splenic arteriovenous fistula: diagnosis by duplex Doppler sonography. AJR 1989;153:1313–1314.

73. Acker JJ, Galambos JT, Weens HS. Selective celiac angiography. Am J Med 1964;37:417.

74. Keller FS, Rösch J, Dotter CT. Bleeding from esophageal varices exacerbated by splenic arterial-venous fistula: complete transcatheter obliterative therapy. Cardiovasc Intervent Radiol 1980;3:97–102.

75. Reuter SR. Embolization of gastrointestinal hemorrhage. AJR 1979;133:557–558.

76. Gartside R, Gamelli RE. Splenic arteriovenous fistula. J Trauma 1987;27:671–673.

77. Rösch J. Roentgenology of the spleen and pancreas. Springfield, IL: Thomas, 1967.

78. Reichle FA, Owen OE. Hemodynamic patterns in human hepatic cirrhosis: a prospective randomized study of the hemodynamic sequelae of distal splenorenal (Warren) and mesocaval shunts. Ann Surg 1979;190:523–524.

79. Widrich WC, Robbins AH, Johnson WC, et al. Long-term follow-up of distal splenorenal shunts: evaluation by arteriography, shuntography, transhepatic portal venography, and cinefluorography. Radiology 1980;134:341–345.

80. Cho KJ, Martel W. Recognition of splenic vein occlusion. AJR 1978;131:439–443.

81. Itzchak Y, Glickman MG. Splenic vein thrombosis in patients with a normal size spleen. Invest Radiol 1977;12:158–163.

82. Muhletaler C, Gerlock AJ Jr, Goncharenko V, et al. Gastric varices secondary to splenic vein occlusion: radiographic diagnosis and clinical significance. Radiology 1979;132:593–598.

83. Bernades P, Baetz A, Levy P, et al. Splenic and portal venous obstruction in chronic pancreatitis: a prospective longitudinal study of a medical-surgical series of 266 patients. Dig Dis Sci 1992;37:340–346.

84. Khan AH, O'Reilly CJ, Avakian VA, et al. Splenic vein thrombosis: an unusual case of gastric bleeding. Angiology 1977;28:725–727.

85. Doolas A, Nolte M, McDonald OG, et al. Splenic cysts. J Surg Oncol 1978;10:369–387.

86. Griscom NT, Hargreaves HK, Schwartz MZ, et al. Huge splenic cyst in a newborn: comparison with 10 cases in later childhood and adolescence. AJR 1977;129:889–891.

87. Qureshi MA, Hafner CD. Clinical manifestations of splenic cysts: a study of 75 cases. Am Surg 1965;31:605.

88. Fowler RH. Nonparasitic benign cystic tumors of the spleen. Internat Abstr Surg 1953;96:209–227.

89. Breslin JA, Turner BI, Rhamy RK, et al. Splenic cysts in the differential diagnosis of suprarenal masses. J Urol 1978;119:559–560.

90. Eisenstat TE, Morris DM, Mason GR. Cysts of the spleen: report of a case and review of the literature. Am J Surg 1977;134:635–637.

91. Propper RA, Weinstein BJ, Skolnick ML. Ultrasonography of hemorrhagic splenic cysts. J Clin Ultrasound 1979;7:18–20.

92. Faer MJ, Lynch RD, Lichtenstein JE, et al. Traumatic splenic cyst: radiologic-pathologic conference from the Armed Forces Institute of Pathology. Radiology 1980;134:371–376.

93. Quinn SF, vanSonnenberg E, Casola G. Interventional radiology in the spleen. Radiology 1986;161:289–291.

94. Dachman AH, Ros PR, Murari PJ. Nonparasitic splenic cysts: a report of 52 cases with radiologic-pathologic correlation. AJR 1986;147:537–542.

95. Kishikawa T, Numaguchi Y, Watanabe K, et al. Angiographic diagnosis of benign and malignant splenic tumors. AJR 1978;130:339–344.

96. Poller S, Wholey MH. Splenic cysts: confirmation by selective visceral angiography. AJR 1966;96:418–420.

97. Rösch J. Roentgenologic possibilities in spleen diagnosis. AJR 1965;94:453.

98. King MC, Glick BW, Freed A. The diagnosis of splenic cysts. Surg Gynecol Obstet 1968;127:509–612.

99. Ross PR, Moser RP Jr, Dachman AH, et al. Hemangioma of the spleen: radiologic-pathologic correlation in ten cases. Radiology 1987;162:73–77.

100. Wexler L, Abrams HL. Hamartoma of the spleen: angiographic observations. AJR 1964;92:1150.

101. Das Gupta T, Coombes B, Brasfield RD. Primary malignant neoplasms of the spleen. Surg Gynecol Obstet 1965;120:947.

102. Rösch J. Tumors of the spleen: the value of selective arteriography. Clin Radiol 1966;17:183–190.

103. Edsman G. Malignant tumor of the spleen diagnosed by lienal arteriography. Acta Radiol 1954;42:461.

104. Cunningham JJ. Ultrasonic findings in isolated lymphoma of the spleen simulating splenic abscess. J Clin Ultrasound 1978;6:412–414.

105. Abrams HL. The incidence of splenic metastasis of carcinoma. Calif Med 1952;76:281.

106. Fry DE, Garrison RN, Williams HC. Patterns of morbidity and mortality in splenic trauma. Am Surg 1980;46:28–32.

107. Naylor R, Coln D, Shires GT. Morbidity and mortality from injuries to the spleen. J Trauma 1974;14:773–778.

108. Jeffrey RB, Laing FC, Federie MP, et al. Computed tomography of splenic trauma. Radiology 1981;141:729–732.

109. Lepasoon J, Olin T. Angiographic diagnosis of splenic lesions following blunt abdominal trauma. Acta Radiol 1971;11:257–273.

110. Scatliff JH, Fisher ON, Guilford WB, et al. The "starry night" splenic angiogram: contrast material opacification of the malpighian body marginal sinus circulation in spleen trauma. AJR 1975;125:91–98.

111. Haertel M, Ryder D. Radiologic investigation of splenic trauma. Cardiovasc Radiol 1979;2:27–33.

112. Love L, Greenfield GB, Braun TW, et al. Arteriography of splenic trauma. Radiology 1968;91:96–102.

113. Berk RN, Wholey MH. The application of splenic arteriography in the diagnosis of rupture of the spleen. AJR 1968;104:662.

114. Redman HC, Reuter SR, Bookstein JJ. Angiography in abdominal trauma. Ann Surg 1969;169:57–66.

115. Schiffman MA. Nonoperative management of blunt abdominal trauma in pediatrics. Emerg Med Clin North Am 1989;7:519–535.

116. Lally KP, Rosario V, Majour GH. Evolution in the management of splenic injury in children. Surg Gynecol Obstet 1990;170:245–248.

117. Ein SH, Shandling B, Simpson JS. Nonoperative management of traumatized spleen in children: how and why. J Pediatr Surg 1978;13:117–119.

118. Hebler RF, Ward RE, Miller PW, et al. The management of splenic injury. J Trauma 1982;22:492–495.

119. Lucas CE. Splenic trauma: choice of management. Ann Surg 1991;213:98–112.

120. Longo WE, Baker CC, McMillen MA. Nonoperative management of adult blunt splenic trauma: criteria for successful outcome. Ann Surg 1989;210:626–629.

121. Elmore JR, Clark DE, Isler RJ. Selective nonoperative management of blunt splenic trauma in adults. Arch Surg 1989;124:581–585.

122. Kidd WT, Lui RC, Khoo R, et al. The management of blunt splenic trauma. J Trauma 1987;27:977–979.

123. Umlas SL, Cronan JJ. Splenic trauma: can CT grading systems enable prediction of successful nonsurgical treatment? Radiology 1991;178:481–487.

124. Brick SH, Taylor GA, Potter BM. Hepatic and splenic injury in children: role of CT in the decision for laparotomy. Radiology 1987;165:643–646.

125. Kreis DJ Jr, Montero N, Saltz M, et al. The role of splenorrhaphy in splenic trauma. Am Surg 1987;53:307–309.

126. Rappaport W, McIntyre KE Jr, Carmona R. The management of splenic trauma in the adult patient with blunt multiple injuries. Surg Gynecol Obstet 1990;170:204–208.

127. Sclafani SJ, Weisberg A, Scalea TM, et al. Blunt splenic injuries: nonsurgical treatment with CT, arteriography, and transcatheter arterial embolization of the splenic artery. Radiology 1991;181:189–196.

128. Budd DC, Fouty WJ Jr, Johnson RB, et al. Occult rupture of the spleen: a dilemma in diagnosis. JAMA 1976;236:2884–2885.

129. McMahon MJ, Lintott JD, Mair WSJ, et al. Occult rupture of the spleen. Br J Surg 1977;64:641–643.

130. Moskovitz M. Occult splenic rupture: presentation as a gastric pseudotumor. Conn Med 1978;42:498–499.

131. Reuter SR, Redman HC. Gastrointestinal angiography. Philadelphia: Saunders, 1972:202.

132. Jacobs RP, Shanser JD, Lawson DL, et al. Angiography of splenic abscesses. AJR 1974;122:419–424.

133. Miller FJ, Rothermel FJ, O'Neil MJ, et al. Clinical and roentgenographic findings in splenic abscess. Arch Surg 1976;111:1156–1159.

134. Siniluoto T, Paivansalo M, Tikkakoski T, et al. Ultrasound-guided aspiration cytology of the spleen. Acta Radiol 1992;33:137–139.

135. Fujitani RM, Johs SM, Cobb SR, et al. Preoperative splenic artery occlusion as an adjunct for high risk splenectomy. Am Surg 1988;54:602–608.

136. Hiatt JR, Gomes AS, Machleeder HI. Massive splenomegaly:

superior results with a combined endovascular and operative approach. Arch Surg 1990;125:1363–1367.

137. Levy JM, Wasserman P, Pitha N. Presplenectomy transcatheter occlusion of the splenic artery. Arch Surg 1979;114:198–199.

138. Kumpe DA, Rumack CM, Pretorius DH. Partial splenic embolization in children with hypersplenism. Radiology 1985;155:357–362.

139. Spigos DG, Jonasson O, Mozes M, et al. Partial splenic embolization in the treatment of hypersplenism. AJR 1979;132:777–782.

140. Pringle KC, Spigos DG, Tan WS, et al. Partial splenic embolization in the management of thalassemia major. J Pediatr Surg 1982;17:884–891.

141. Brandt CT, Rothbarth LJ, Kumpe D. Splenic embolization in children: long-term efficacy. J Pediatr Surg 1989;24:642–644.

142. Jonasson O, Spigos DG, Mozes MF. Partial splenic embolization: experience in 136 patients. World J Surg 1985;9:461–467.

143. Mozes MF, Spigos DG, Pollak R: Partial splenic embolization, an alternative to splenectomy—results of a prospective, randomized study. Surgery 1984;96:694–702.

144. Goldstein HM, Wallace S, Anderson JH, et al. Transcatheter occlusion of abdominal tumors. Radiology 1976;120:539–545.

145. Castaneda-Zuniga WR, Hammerschmidt DE, Sanchez R, et al. Nonsurgical splenectomy. AJR 1977;129:805–811.

146. Wholey MH, Chamorro HA, Rao G. Splenic infarction and spontaneous rupture of the spleen after therapeutic embolization. Cardiovasc Radiol 1978;1:249–253.

147. Mazer M, Smith CW, Martin V. Distal splenic artery embolization with a flow-directed balloon catheter. Radiology 1985;154:245.

148. Link DP, Seibert JA, Gould J, et al. On-line monitoring of sequential blood flow reduction during splenic embolization. Acta Radiol 1989;30:101–103.

59

Splenoportography and Portal Hypertension

GEOFFREY A. GARDINER, JR.
INGEMAR BERGSTRAND

Splenoportography

Indications

Opacification of the portal system by means of percutaneous injection of contrast material into the splenic pulp was first reported in humans by Boulvin et al.[1] in 1951 and Leger et al.[2] in 1955. This followed extensive studies in animals by Abeatici and Campi and others.[3,4] The term *splenoportography* was introduced in 1952 by Sotgiu.[5] Historically, splenoportography has been a commonly used method for studying the portal system, especially in Europe and Latin America. Experience with large series of procedures have been reported by several authors.[6–10] However, within the past decade, indirect (arterial) portography (the venous phase of contrast injections in the splenic or superior mesenteric arteries) and direct transhepatic portography have become the preferred techniques for invasively evaluating the portal vein and its branches. This is partly related to the hemorrhagic complications associated with splenoportography but also because of the diagnostic limitations of this technique. The inability of splenoportography to determine the status of the portal vein in cases with hepatofugal portal blood flow or when large collaterals originate from the splenic vein represents an important shortcoming of this technique. In addition, the development of noninvasive techniques such as Doppler ultrasound and magnetic resonance angiography have reduced the need for invasive contrast studies of the portal system in general.

However, in certain clinical situations splenoportography remains a valuable technique that can provide useful information not easily obtainable by other methods. Although its role in evaluating the portal system is limited, improvements in technique introduced over the past few years have made this a safer procedure, and technically it is simpler and easier to perform than other invasive techniques. Important changes in technique have involved the use of smaller and more flexible needles,[11,12] the use of digital subtraction imaging, which allows reduced injection rates and volumes,[10,13] and the use of Gelfoam to plug the needle track.[14,15]

One of the advantages of splenoportography compared to other invasive methods used for contrast portography is related to its ease of performance. Because splenoportography is technically less demanding, it is also less time-consuming and therefore reduces radiation exposure to the patient and staff. Burcharth et al. found that the time required for splenoportography averaged half the time required for transhepatic portography in a series of patients submitted to both procedures.[16] Compared to transhepatic portography, splenoportography produces better visualization of the portal system and collaterals when the portal vein is thrombosed. In contrast to arterial portography, portal vein pressure can be accurately assessed by measuring the splenic pulp pressure,[17,18] and splenoportography usually produces better opacification of the splenic and portal veins.

The disadvantages of splenoportography include its inability to visualize the mesenteric vein, which may be the source of large and important collaterals. In addition, nonvisualization of the portal vein or portions of the splenic veins may be difficult to interpret because it is not always possible to differentiate thrombosis from inflow of unopacified blood (Figs. 59-1 and 59-2). In a large series of patients, Burchell found that the portal vein was not visualized in 6.5 percent of procedures, and in those with severe portal hypertension who were operative candidates, this number increased to 17.8 percent.[10] In this series, 84 percent of nonvisualized portal veins were patent at autopsy or surgery. Burcharth reported an 18 percent incidence of a false-positive diagnosis of portal or splenic vein thrombosis at splenoportography using transhepatic portography to study the same patients.[18] Therefore, failure to visualize portions of the portal venous system by splenoportography is not absolute evidence of thrombosis unless intraluminal thrombus is outlined or periportal collaterals (cavernous transformation) are visualized.

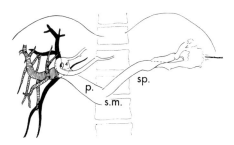

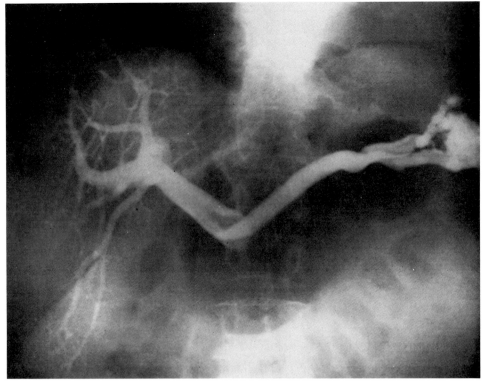

Figure 59-1. Normal splenoportogram. Exposure made 4 seconds after beginning of injection. Contrast medium has filled the entire right intrahepatic ramification but only part of the left. Note the filling defect in the portal vein caused by mesenteric blood. *p.,* portal vein; *s.m.,* superior mesenteric vein; *sp.,* splenic vein; *4,* left principal portal venous ramus. (Dorsocaudal branches are in *solid black* and ventrocaudal branches are *striated* in the diagrams of this chapter.)

Although splenoportography has definite limitations, it may be used to evaluate the splenic vein in cases of unexplained splenomegaly, investigate upper gastrointestinal bleeding of obscure origin, opacify the portal system for CT portography,[11] determine the status of the splenic vein in pancreatic disease, perform postoperative evaluation of portocaval shunts, and evaluate extrahepatic portal hypertension.

Contraindications include uncorrectable alterations of the blood-clotting mechanism, uncooperative patients who are not able to limit respiration when requested, patients with a history of severe contrast allergies, and patients with known tumors of the spleen. Ascites, a nonpalpable spleen, and overweight patients

are not considered contraindications, although they make the procedure more difficult.

Technique

Patient preparation is similar to that for most invasive procedures, including restrictions on oral intake and preprocedure sedation if needed. Some have recommended a bowel preparation before the study, but this is not commonly used. A CT scan or ultrasound may be helpful in localizing the spleen if splenomegaly is not present. Traditionally a scout film and fluoroscopy are used. The procedure is performed with the patient in the supine position, although improved filling of the portal vein, especially the left portal vein, may be pro-

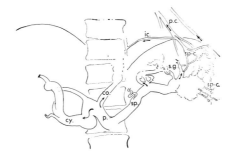

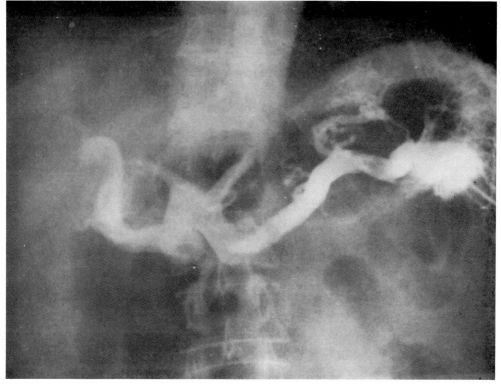

Figure 59-2. Portal thrombosis (verified at autopsy). Filling of splenic vein and hepatodistal part of portal vein from which contrast medium flows to the liver via dilated cystic veins. *sp.*, splenic vein; *p.*, portal vein; *cy.*, cystic vein; *co.*, coronary vein; *s.g.*, short gastric veins; *sp-c.*, collateral veins connecting spleen and hepatodistal part of splenic vein to systemic veins in the lateral abdominal wall; *p.c.*, pericardial veins; *ic.*, intercostal veins.

vided by placing the patient in the prone position because contrast tends to layer in the dependent portion of the portal system.[19,20] After the patient is appropriately prepared and draped and the skin is locally anesthetized, a 20- to 23-gauge, 10- to 15-cm-long needle is inserted. Generally the needle is inserted through the 8th, 9th, or 10th intercostal space, in the mid to posterior axillary line. The needle is angled cranially, usually 15 to 20 degrees. The goal is to place the needle tip centrally in the spleen near the hilum. Respiration is stopped during needle placement, and the patient is asked not to breathe deeply while the needle is in place. Sheathed needles are available and are considered by some to be less traumatic during respiratory

excursions. They are also useful if Gelfoam embolization of the needle track is planned. Once the needle is properly positioned, a slow drip of blood should occur through the needle hub. Occasionally a brisk injection of 1 to 2 ml of saline will facilitate this occurrence. A small test injection of contrast will confirm proper positioning of the needle with puddling of contrast at the needle tip followed by opacification of the splenic vein. Subcapsular injections of contrast generally do not produce good opacification of the splenic or portal veins, and are also painful. With optimal needle position, most patients feel nothing or only minimal discomfort during injections. Severe discomfort suggests malposition of the needle or extravasation of contrast.

Using digital subtraction angiography, 40- to 60-ml injections of dilute contrast (30 percent) are made at injection rates of 4 to 6 ml per second. Injection rates and volumes vary according to the patient, but usually 8- to 10-second injections are recommended. Successful splenoportograms using contrast injection by hand have been reported.[9] Although this may be facilitated by digital subtraction angiography, the small needles currently recommended make this more difficult. Filming up to 30 seconds after contrast injection is begun has been recommended to ensure visualization of collateral pathways. Judging the appropriate duration of filming is much easier using digital angiography because images can be viewed as they are acquired.

After the needle has been removed, the patient is placed at bedrest with careful monitoring of vital signs for a minimum of 8 to 12 hours. Having the patient lie on his or her left side for 4 hours after the procedure may help tamponade the puncture site.

Failure to successfully place a needle in the spleen or to opacify the portal system on contrast injection occurs in about 4 to 5 percent of procedures[7,10,14,21] but has been reported in as many as 16 percent[9] of procedures. Although failure rates of transhepatic or arterial portography are difficult to compare, there is probably little significant difference. Causes of failure include large patients or patients with small or difficult-to-localize spleens, complications such as extrasplenic injections or extravasation of contrast from the spleen, and, rarely, poor venous opacification despite adequate needle placement.

Complications

Complications related to splenoportography have been reported in approximately 6 percent of procedures.[7,8] The most feared complication is hemorrhage. This may occur as intraperitoneal bleeding or perisplenic or subcapsular hematoma. The prevalence of bleeding complications requiring transfusion is reportedly 2 to 3 percent.[7,8,16,18] Clinically it may present as persistent pain, but often a falling hemoglobin and hematocrit are the only findings. In the large majority of cases, transfusion is the only treatment necessary, although there are reported cases of patients requiring laparotomy or splenectomy. Uncorrected coagulation defects significantly increase the risk of this complication.

Other complications are only rarely associated with clinically significant consequences.[7,8] These include puncture of adjacent organs, which may involve the colon, liver, or kidney. Thoracic complications may occur because the pleural space is often traversed by the needle. In the midaxillary line the pleura is found as low as the 10th rib.[22] Complications such as pneumothorax and pleuritis have been reported,[8] but usually no treatment is required. Pyrogenic reactions may also occur.[7] If they are persistent, antibiotic therapy should be instituted.

Intrasplenic arterial aneurysms have been reported in one-third of patients with portal hypertension following splenoportography,[23] but their clinical significance and long-term course are unknown. These may be related in part to the presence of long-standing portal hypertension because splenic artery aneurysms have been documented in almost 20 percent of patients with cirrhosis and portal hypertension.[24]

Normal Hemodynamics

During the injection, contrast medium flows continuously into those veins draining the punctured part of the spleen. After successful puncture only a very small portion of the contrast injected persists in the splenic parenchyma and disappears within half an hour. The velocity and direction of flow recorded are measures of the actual hemodynamic conditions. Judging from clinical experience as well as from experiments on dogs, intrasplenic injection by the technique described does not disturb portal hemodynamics.[25] Thus, in normal subjects the contrast medium never fills the vessels emptying into the splenoportal pathway, such as the coronary vein and the mesenteric veins. On the contrary, on its way to the liver the contrast medium is diluted more and more by blood from these veins (Figs. 59-1 and 59-3 through 59-6).

The velocity of portal flow is sometimes changed, even in an early stage of portal obstruction. Normally the contrast medium reaches the porta hepatis 1 to 2 seconds after its passage through the splenic vein radicles (see Fig. 59-4A and B). This means a relatively high venous velocity (10–20 cm/second), which, like the relatively high oxygen tension of splenic venous blood, may be explained by the low resistance of the capillary splenic bed to arterial flow. Within 3 to 5 seconds after the beginning of the injection, the intrahepatic vessels of the right portion of the liver are optimally filled (see Fig. 59-1). The branches to the left portion fill somewhat later, and the filling obtained there is often less dense (see Fig. 59-4C). After another 3 to 5 seconds (3 to 5 seconds after the *end* of the injection), the contrast medium has left the intrahepatic portal branches and fills the hepatic sinusoids. The liver is then opacified diffusely (see Fig. 59-4D). At the end of the hepatographic phase, the hepatic veins are faintly visible (about 20–30 seconds after the beginning of the injection). Opacification of the liver disappears completely about 30 to 40 seconds after the beginning of the injection. The velocity of flow may be influenced to some extent by straining during the injection of contrast medium.

The width of the splenic and portal veins is often influenced by conditions such as portal stasis and increased intraabdominal pressure (for example, in patients with ascites). In normal studies we conducted, the width of the splenic vein, as measured in the films proximal to the liver, did not exceed 15 mm. The diameter of the portal vein, as measured distal to the liver, was 15 to 22 mm.

Normal Anatomy

The technique described demonstrates the vessels in frontal projection only. Because of incomplete intermixture between contrast-free blood from the mesenteric veins and opacified blood from the splenic vein, the portal vein and its ventrally situated intrahepatic branches are often less well opacified than the dorsal branches. This discrepancy, however, facilitates orientation in the ventrodorsal direction, as do differences in geometric enlargement and blur.

Figure 59-3. Vessels normally demonstrated by splenoportography; portal and splenic tributaries and systemic veins capable of forming important collateral pathways. *Arrows* indicate normal direction of flow. The names of the vessels are abbreviated as follows:

sp. = splenic vein
p. = portal vein
i.m. = inferior mesenteric vein
s.m. = superior mesenteric vein
co. = coronary vein
s.g. = short gastric veins
g.e. = gastroepiploic vein

cy. = cystic vein
pu. = parumbilical vein
sp. r. = connections between the splenic vein and the left renal vein
sp. c. = collateral veins connecting the spleen and hepatodistal part of the splenic vein to systemic veins in the lateral abdominal wall
I.V.C. = inferior vena cava
haz. = hemiazygos vein
e. = esophageal veins
d. = diaphragmatic veins
p.c. = pericardial veins
r. = left renal vein

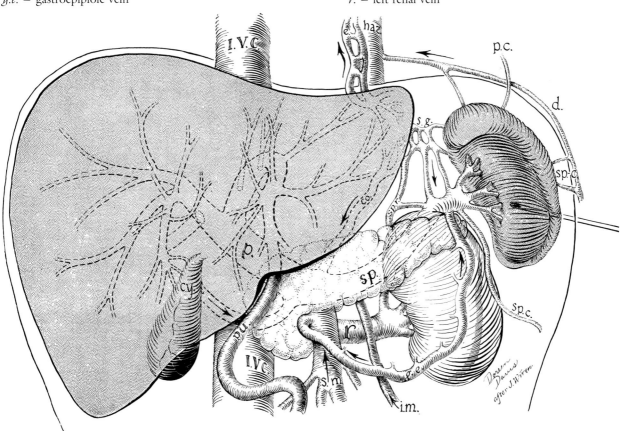

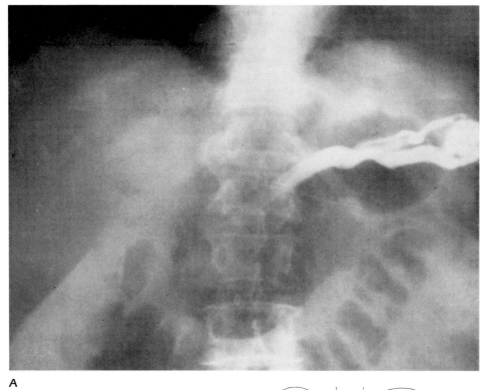

A

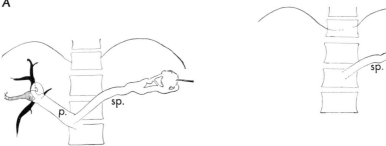

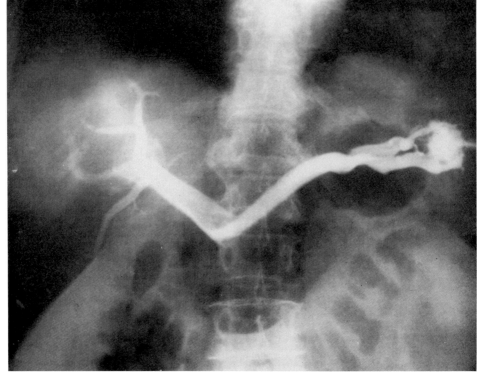

B

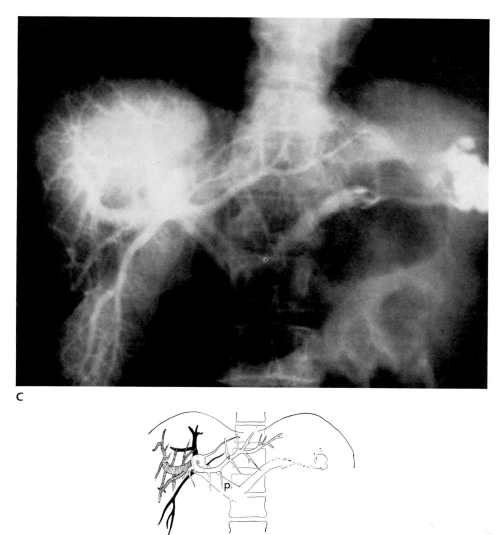

C

Figure 59-4. Normal splenoportogram. (A) Exposure made 1 second after beginning of injection. Contrast medium has filled the splenic vein (*sp.*). (B) Two seconds. Contrast medium has filled the splenic and portal veins and has entered the intrahepatic branches. *p.*, portal vein; *sp.*, splenic vein. (C) Six seconds. Contrast medium begins to fill the liver pa-renchyma. The entire left intrahepatic ramification is filled. *p.*, portal vein; *9*, ventrolateral portal venous ramus. (D) Eight seconds (4 seconds after the end of injection). Contrast medium has left the intrahepatic portal branches and is accumulated evenly in the liver parenchyma. Note the contrast defect corresponding to the fossa venae cavae.

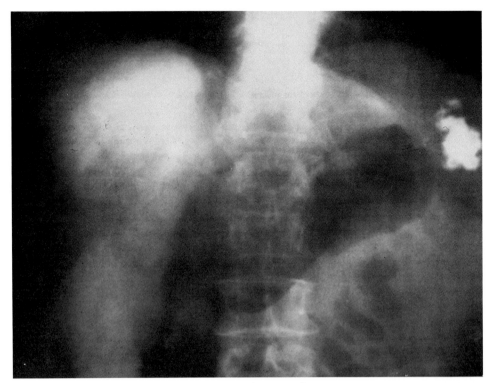

D **Figure 59-4** (continued).

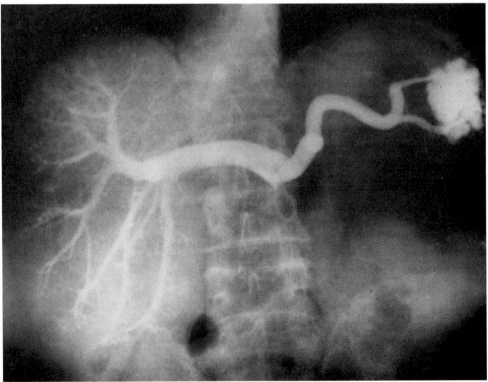

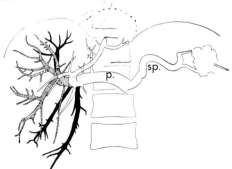

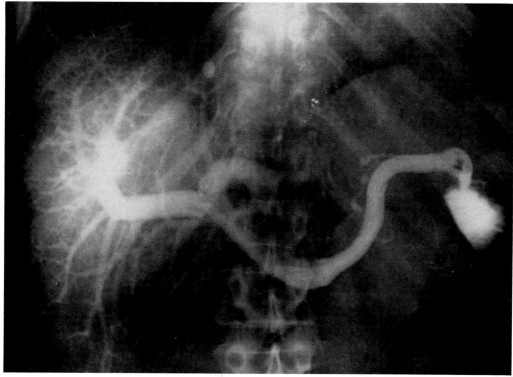

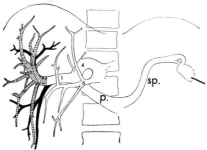

Figure 59-6. Normal splenoportogram. Note the good filling of the ventral vpr but no filling of the dorsolateral and ventrolateral vpr. Careful palpation of the left part of the liver at laparotomy and 1-year follow-up revealed no signs of tumor. *sp.,* splenic vein; *p.,* portal vein; *1,* right principal vpr; *4,* left principal vpr; *6,* ventral vpr.

Extrahepatic Vascular Anatomy

The normal variations of the splenic and portal veins, as well as of their tributaries, have been studied in living subjects and cadavers.[26] Knowledge of these variations is a prerequisite for detecting the presence of any space-occupying lesion in the vicinity of these vessels.

The splenic vein is formed by convergence of the short splenic radicles. The course of the splenic vein varies; sometimes it is straight, sometimes tortuous (see Figs. 59-1 and 59-3 through 59-6). It regularly meets the termination of the mesenteric vein and forms a caudally convex curve. The diameter of the splenic vein increases only slightly during its course toward the portal vein.

The portal vein is formed by the convergence of the splenic vein and the superior mesenteric vein. The blood from the latter causes a filling defect in the splenoportogram that should not be confused with mural thrombosis. This point, which marks the hepatodistal and widest end of the portal vein, is projected over the spine at the level of the first to second lumbar

◄ **Figure 59-5.** Normal splenoportogram showing a slight cranially convex curve of the portal vein. Note the straight vessel projected along the right margin of the spine and running to the liver, presumably a dorsal portal venous ramus (vpr). *sp.,* splenic vein; *p.,* portal vein; *7,* dorsal vpr.

vertebrae. The portal vein, 6 to 8 cm in length, usually pursues a straight dextrocranial course to form an angle of 40 to 90 degrees with the vertebral spine. Sometimes the vein is slightly curved, with the convexity cranial and to the left (see Fig. 59-5).

Intrahepatic Vascular Anatomy

A brief outline of the basic features of human liver anatomy will facilitate the description of the intrahepatic vascular anatomy.

The intrahepatic vascular tree is divided into two main parts. The plane of division passes to the right of the left sagittal fissure and the insertion of the falciform ligament and passes through the bed of the gallbladder to the inferior vena cava. The portal ramification of the right main part is divided into two main segments, one situated dorsocaudally and the other ventrocranially. These segments are then subdivided in different ways by different anatomists.[27-29] The left main part consists of two portions divided by a fissure corresponding to the insertion of the falciform ligament and the left sagittal fissure. The lateral portion is that part generally called the left liver lobe, and the central portion consists mainly of the ventrally situated quadrate lobe and the dorsally situated caudate lobe. The main branches of the hepatic veins run in the fissures formed between the different portal parts and segments.

The intrahepatic vascular nomenclature used here is based on an anatomic investigation by Hjortsjö.[29] It has been somewhat simplified[30] to suit roentgen diagnostic requirements. Figure 59-7 illustrates the nomenclature used and shows some usual types of intrahepatic portal vascular arrangement.

The extent to which different parts of the liver are opacified during the hepatographic phase depends on the amount of contrast medium actually passing through the sinusoids in the various parts of the liver and on the varying thickness of the liver. The left part of the liver is thin and located ventrally, so that it receives a relatively small amount of contrast medium. It is therefore only slightly opacified compared with the right part (see Figs. 59-4D and 59-15D). In the right part the ordinarily deep fossa for the gallbladder and the fossa venae cavae will often appear as well-defined defects.

Portal Hemodynamics in Vascular Obstruction

Venous stasis is roentgenographically manifested by a low velocity of flow, dilatation of the veins, and a filling of collateral vessels. Of these signs, filling of collaterals is the most important and reliable. In our own investigation of patients with venous stasis verified in other ways—for example, by pressure measurements—all showed filling of collaterals.[31] In another study, however, a few exceptions to this rule were found.[32] The direction of collateral flow is always such as to bypass the occluded part of the vascular pathway. This can be demonstrated by the way contrast medium fills and leaves the collaterals.

The velocity of flow is usually, although not always, abnormally low, and the vascular diameters are often abnormally large in vascular stasis with portal hypertension. In patients with ascites, however, the dilatation is usually slight at most.

The extent and capacity of the collateral circulation as judged by the number of the collaterals, vascular size, and velocity of flow are difficult to estimate. The large variations observed are apparently due mainly to differences in the duration and severity of the obstruction and to individual differences in the readiness with which a collateral circulation can be formed. Even in patients with a well-developed collateral circulation, its inability to drain the congested vascular bed adequately is apparent from a low velocity of flow and pathologically high pressures.

Intrahepatic Obstruction

In cirrhosis of the liver the portal intrahepatic ramifications are often involved to such a degree as to cause venous stasis and portal hypertension. Even widespread intrahepatic metastases cause only comparatively slight signs of vascular obstruction, probably because of the rapid and fatal course of the obstructing disease.

When the vascular obstruction is intrahepatic, the collateral vessels will drain the congested vascular area toward the low-pressure systemic veins and not to the liver. This is called a *hepatofugal* (away from the liver) collateral circulation. On the other hand, when the obstruction is extrahepatic, the collateral circulation will usually develop toward the portal system behind the obstruction and toward the liver where, in both locations, the portal pressure is normal. This is called a *hepatopetal* (toward the liver) collateral circulation.[33]

In intrahepatic obstruction the most common of the collateral connections demonstrable establish communication with the superior caval system via the coronary vein and short gastric veins on the one hand and the esophageal venous plexus on the other (Fig. 59-8; see Figs. 59-19, 59-20A, 59-21A, and 59-22A). Some cases, however, despite large esophageal varices, show no cranially directed collaterals. The absence can almost always be ascribed to imperfect contrast filling.[34] Demonstrable communications with the inferior caval system via the inferior mesenteric vein and hem-

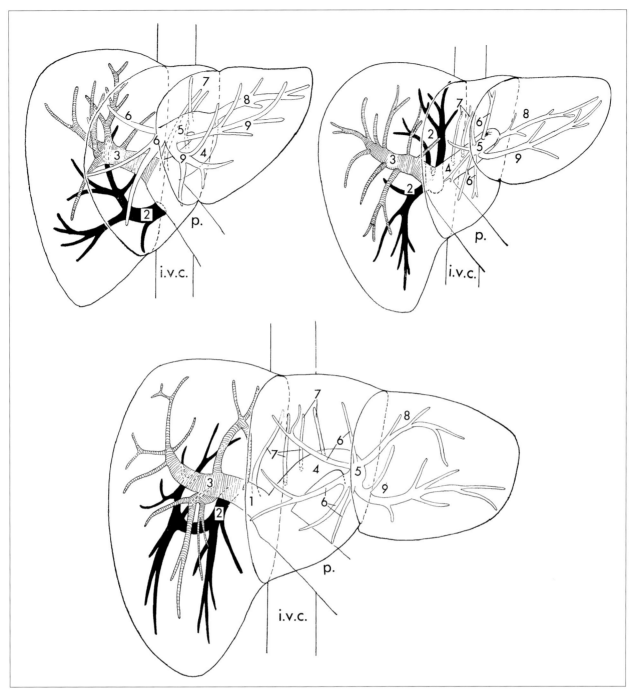

Figure 59-7. Schematic drawings showing normal intrahepatic portal vascular arrangement. The contours of the liver are roughly depicted with the two main fissures drawn in anatomic position. The drawings also show the intrahepatic portal nomenclature used by the author.

(A) The dorsocaudal vpr is an arcuate vessel that leaves the portal vein before the origin of the left principal vpr. Thus the right principal vpr is missing. The ventroflexed vpr is visible cranial to the left principal vpr. (B) Three dorsocaudal vpr's leave the portal vein at the same level as the left principal vpr. The ventroflexed vpr is projected over the left principal vpr. (C) The ventroflexed vpr projects to the left of the left principal vpr.

  p. = portal vein
i.v.c. = inferior vena cava
  1 = right principal portal venous ramus (vpr) ⎫ right main part
  2 = dorsocaudal vpr (*black*)   ⎬ of the liver
  3 = ventrocranial vpr (*striated*)   ⎭
  4 = left principal vpr
  5 = ventroflexed vpr
  6 = ventral vpr ⎫ central portion
  7 = dorsal vpr ⎭
  8 = dorsolateral vpr ⎫ lateral portion
  9 = ventrolateral vpr ⎭

left main part of the liver

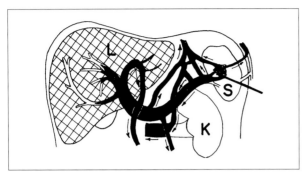

Figure 59-8. Diagram of a splenoportogram indicating intrahepatic obstruction. The main types of hepatofugal collateral vessels are delineated. *K*, kidney; *L*, liver; *S*, spleen. (From Bergstrand I. The localization of portal obstruction by splenoportography. AJR 1961;85:1111. Used with permission.)

orrhoidal vein plexus or via retroperitoneal connections with the left renal vein are less common (see Figs. 59-19 and 59-20A). In advanced intrahepatic obstruction, a collateral communication may be demonstrated between the portal venous ramus ventroflexus and the caval system via recanalized remnants of the umbilical vein and veins in the abdominal wall (see Fig. 59-22). Such a picture is suggestive of the Cruveilhier-Baumgarten syndrome.[35] Even in cases of advanced obstruction, filling may be obtained of at most a few centimeters of the superior mesenteric vein (see Fig. 59-20A). The contrast medium slowly returns by the same route, indicating the impossibility of significant collateral flow through that channel.

With complete intrahepatic obstruction the portal blood is entirely diverted to the caval system by the routes mentioned earlier without any filling of the occluded intrahepatic vessels. In the patent extrahepatic part of the pathway, blood flow is sometimes reversed toward the collaterals draining the splenic vein. Because contrast medium cannot fill a vessel against the blood flow, this patent part of the pathway is not demonstrated in the films and may falsely indicate extrahepatic obstruction (Figs. 59-9A and B). Arterial portography with injection of contrast medium via the superior mesenteric artery may reveal the true intrahepatic site of obstruction and other collaterals. This splenoportographic picture was found in 6 of 91 patients with verified intrahepatic portal obstruction.[33]

Extrahepatic Obstruction

Extrahepatic obstruction is usually caused by thrombosis, malformations, or both, which are long-standing conditions with well-developed signs of stasis. But extrahepatic obstruction may also be caused by other diseases, such as malignant tumors or pancreatic cysts, producing relatively slight signs of stasis. In partial vascular obstruction its exact site and extent are visible in the roentgenogram. In complete obstruction blood flow is sometimes reversed, so that its site may be deduced only from the type of the collateral circulation.

In most patients with complete obstruction of the portal vein, the correct diagnosis is made by demonstration of a hepatopetal circulation (Fig. 59-10) via paraportal tortuous collaterals (Figs. 59-2 and 59-11). In some of these patients, however, only a hepatofugal collateral circulation is demonstrated (Fig. 59-12).

In complete obstruction of the splenic vein or of the splenic and portal veins, the correct diagnosis is made by the demonstration of a hepatopetal collateral circulation and an absent filling of the obstructed part of the portal system (Figs. 59-13 through 59-15). Many times, however, the splenoportogram is not informative or is misleading in those patients in whom only hepatofugal collateral vessels are filled (Fig. 59-16). Connections with the inferior vena cava via retroperitoneal veins and emptying into the left renal vein are not uncommon (Fig. 59-17).

In intrahepatic combined with extrahepatic obstruction (such as cirrhosis with complicating portal thrombosis), all collaterals run to the caval system (Fig. 59-18).

Text continues on page 1512

Figure 59-9. Cirrhosis of the liver (verified at laparotomy). (A) Splenoportogram shows filling of tortuous collateral veins draining the splenic vein. There is no filling of the portal vein. Only small, cranially directed collaterals are visible despite the presence of large esophageal varices. *sp.*, splenic vein; *sp-r.*, connections between splenic vein and left renal vein. (B) Eight seconds later. Contrast medium has reached the left renal vein and enters the inferior vena cava. *r.*, left renal vein; *i.v.c.*, inferior vena cava; *sp-r.*, connections between splenic vein and left renal vein. (C) Portography during laparotomy. (Contrast medium was injected in the superior mesenteric vein via catheter.) Filling of a patent portal vein and a large coronary vein running to the esophageal veins. Contrast medium has also reached the splenorenal connection demonstrated in the splenoportogram. *sp.*, splenic vein; *sp-r.*, connections between splenic vein and left renal vein; *p.*, portal vein; *co.*, coronary vein; *s.m.*, superior mesenteric vein.

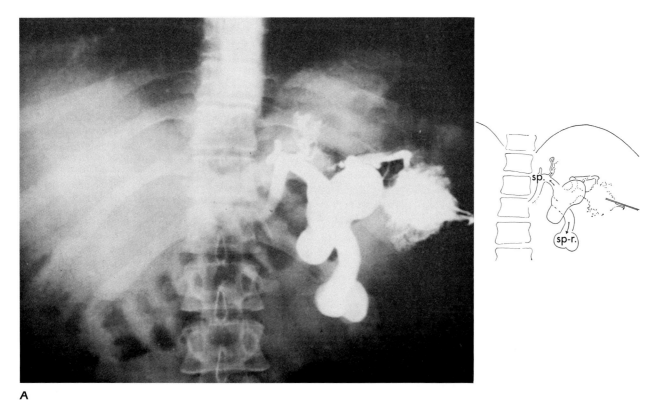

A

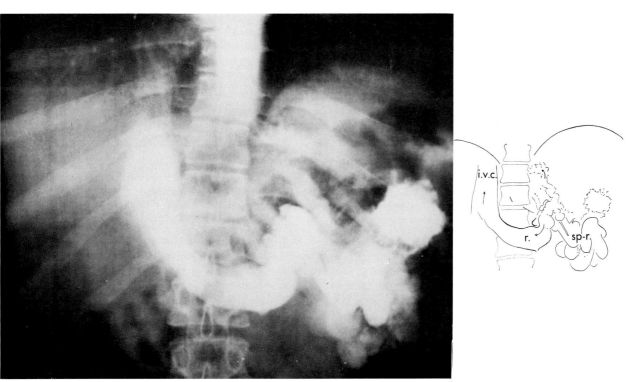

B

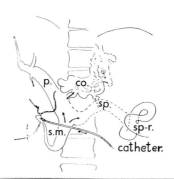

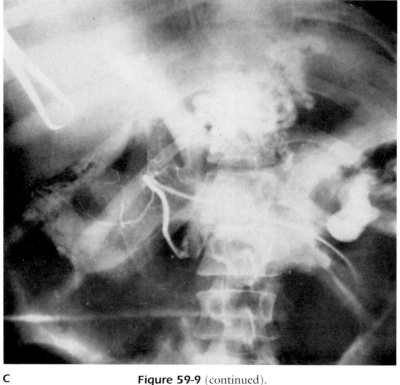

C   **Figure 59-9** (continued).

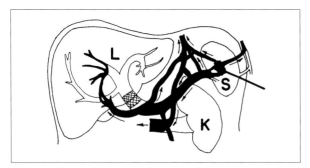

Figure 59-10. Diagram of a splenoportogram indicating extrahepatic portal vein obstruction. *K*, kidney; *L*, liver; *S*, spleen. (From Bergstrand I. The localization of portal obstruction by splenoportography. AJR 1961;85:1111. Used with permission.)

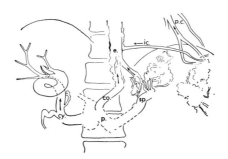

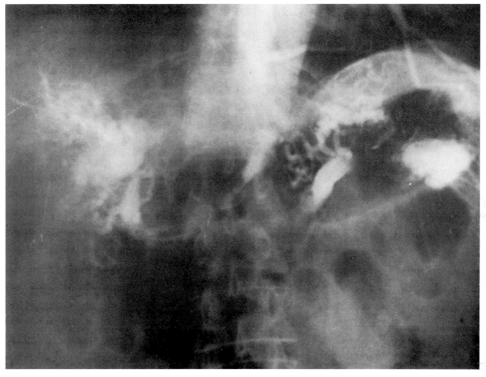

Figure 59-11. Collateral circulation to the superior vena cava via the coronary vein, short gastric veins, intercostal veins, and pericardial veins. *sp.,* splenic vein; *p.,* portal vein; *cy.,* cystic vein; *co.,* coronary vein; *p.c.,* pericardial veins; *ic.,* intercostal veins; *e.,* esophageal veins.

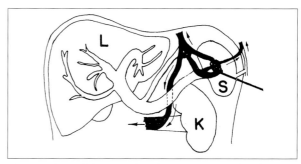

Figure 59-12. Diagram of a splenoportogram that does not indicate the site of obstruction (extrahepatic, intrahepatic, or both). *K,* kidney; *L,* liver; *S,* spleen. (From Bergstrand I. The localization of portal obstruction by splenoportography. AJR 1961;85:1111. Used with permission.)

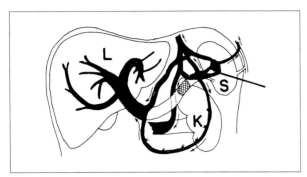

Figure 59-13. Diagram of a splenoportogram indicating extrahepatic splenic vein obstruction. *K,* kidney; *L,* liver; *S,* spleen. (From Bergstrand I. The localization of portal obstruction by splenoportography. AJR 1961;85:1111. Used with permission.)

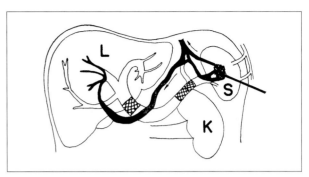

Figure 59-14. Diagram of a splenoportogram indicating extrahepatic obstruction (splenic, portal, or both). *K,* kidney; *L,* liver; *S,* spleen. (From Bergstrand I. The localization of portal obstruction by splenoportography. AJR 1961;85: 1111. Used with permission.)

A surgically established shunt between the portal vein and the inferior vena cava is directly demonstrable in splenoportography. In adequately functioning shunts, no filling of collaterals is obtained (see Fig. 59-21B). If the portacaval shunt is inefficient because of thrombosis or obstruction of flow in the inferior vena cava, collaterals are filled. The obstructing lesion is usually directly demonstrable.

Intrahepatic Anatomic Changes

Diseases affecting the size of the liver can be diagnosed only to a limited degree by splenoportography. The normally wide variation in the size of the liver in the frontal plane, however, diminishes this possibility. In certain conditions with liver cell injury causing hepatic failure, neither the size of the liver nor its vascular tree is affected. On the other hand, liver function tests may be normal in patients with severe vascular changes as seen by roentgenography.

There are two main groups of common diseases in which the actual intrahepatic vascular changes may be demonstrable by splenoportography: cirrhosis of the liver and intrahepatic malignant tumors.

Cirrhosis of the Liver

The circulatory disturbances in advanced human cirrhosis have been described by McIndoe[36] on the basis of corrosion preparations and perfusion experiments. He stressed the noticeable diminution in the hepatic vascular bed and the irregularity of the main branches. He also described the formation of direct intrahepatic connections between the portal and hepatic veins, which impaired the nutrition of the liver cells that were then dependent entirely on the arterial supply. Vascular intrahepatic obstruction may also be caused by compression of the smaller vessels by regenerating nodules or else by secondary thrombosis.

In the author's pathoanatomically verified material[37] derived from cirrhosis mainly combined with portal hypertension, two-thirds of the patients showed changes consisting of narrow branches (Fig. 59-19) or abruptly ending or irregularly tapering portal vessels whose course markedly deviated from the main direction (Fig. 59-20A). In several cases thrombi were directly visible or suggested by occlusion of branches (Fig. 59-21A). The left principal portal venous ramus and ventroflexed portal venous ramus were often wider than vessels of corresponding importance in the right main part and projected more dextrocranially than

Text continues on page 1521

Figure 59-15. Thrombosis of splenic vein (verified at laparotomy). (A) Exposure made 2 seconds after beginning of injection shows filling of collaterals from hilus of the spleen. *s.g.,* short gastric veins; *sp-c.,* collateral veins connecting spleen and hepatodistal part of splenic vein to systemic veins in the lateral abdominal wall. (B) Five seconds. Collaterals empty into the hepatoproximal part of the splenic vein. *sp.,* splenic vein; *p.,* portal vein; *s.g.,* short gastric veins; *g.e.,* gastroepiploic vein; *sp-c.,* collateral veins connecting spleen and hepatodistal part of splenic vein to systemic veins in the lateral abdominal wall. (C) Nine seconds. Filling of the portal vein and of intrahepatic portal branches. Note filling of the gastroepiploic vein emptying into the superior mesenteric vein. *p.,* portal vein; *g.e.,* gastroepiploic vein; *s.m.,* superior mesenteric vein; *6,* ventral vpr. (D) Twelve seconds. Hepatogram showing intense and even contrast accumulation in normal liver parenchyma. Note fossa for the gallbladder. ▶

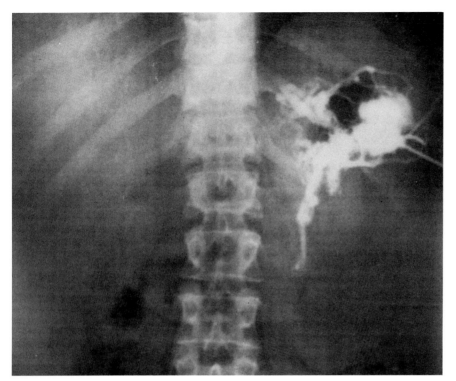

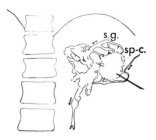

A

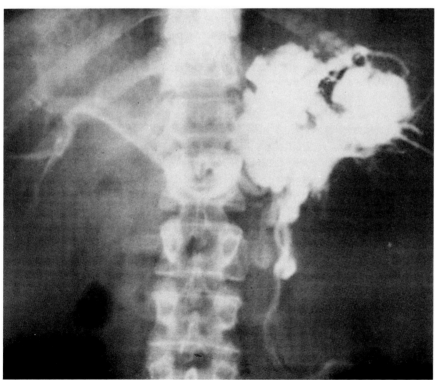

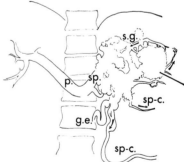

B

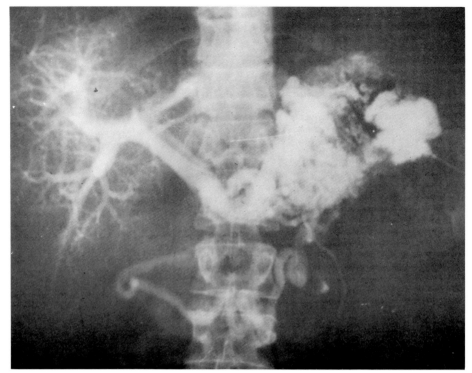

C

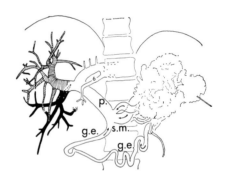

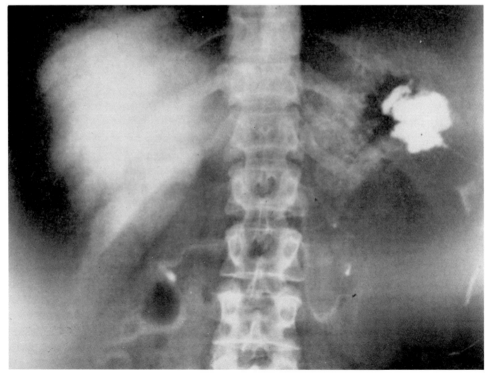

D

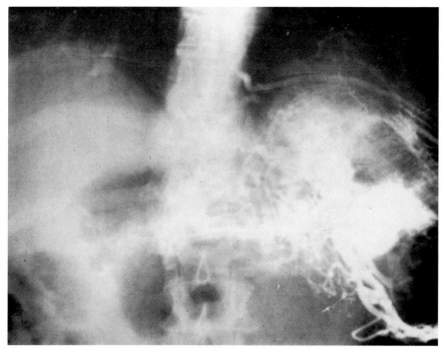

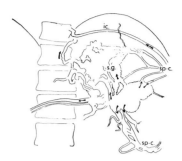

Figure 59-16. Thrombosis of splenic vein (verified at laparotomy). There is filling of numerous collaterals to the superior vena cava, such as the short gastric veins and connections to intercostal veins. There is no filling of the splenic vein. *s.g.*, short gastric veins; *sp-c.*, collateral veins connecting spleen and hepatodistal part of splenic vein to systemic veins in the lateral abdominal wall; *ic.*, intercostal veins.

Figure 59-17. Thrombosis of splenic vein (verified at laparotomy). Contrast medium empties via dilated, tortuous retroperitoneal connections from the hilus of the spleen into the left renal vein and inferior vena cava. There is no filling of splenic and portal veins. *sp-r.*, connections between splenic vein and left renal vein; *r.*, left renal vein; *i.v.c.*, inferior vena cava.

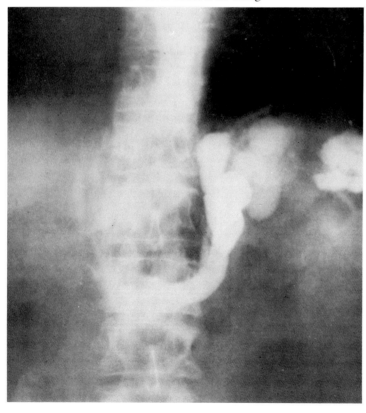

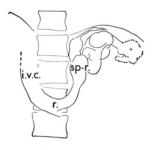

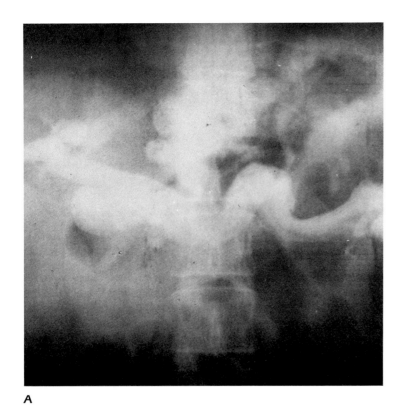

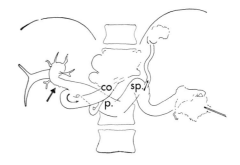

A

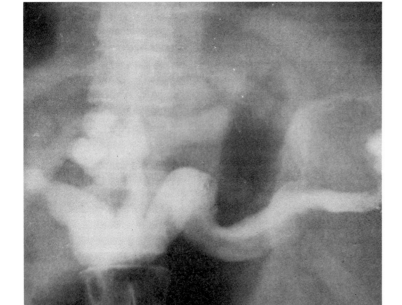

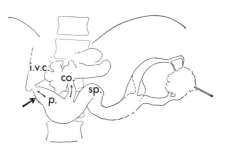

B

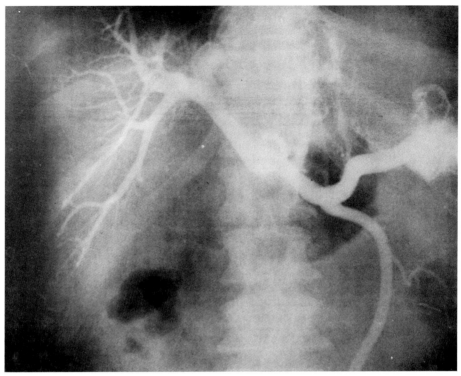

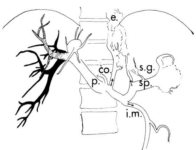

Figure 59-19. Cirrhosis of the liver. Splenoportogram shows narrow intrahepatic portal branches spread less than normally. Filling of collaterals toward superior vena cava (coronary vein, short gastric veins) and toward inferior vena cava (inferior mesenteric vein) indicates marked venous stasis. *sp.*, splenic vein; *p.*, portal vein; *co.*, coronary vein; *s.g.*, short gastric veins; *i.m.*, inferior mesenteric vein; *e.*, esophageal veins.

◀ **Figure 59-18.** Liver cirrhosis and mural portal thrombosis (verified at laparotomy). (A) Splenoportogram before portacaval shunt shows mural thrombosis in the portal vein (*arrow*) and a thick, tortuous coronary vein emptying in a cranial direction. *sp.*, splenic vein; *p.*, portal vein; *co.*, coronary vein. (B) Splenoportogram after portacaval shunt shows the shunt partly obstructed by thrombosis (*arrow*), resulting in persistent filling of the coronary vein. *sp.*, splenic vein; *p.*, portal vein; *co.*, coronary vein; *i.v.c.*, inferior vena cava.

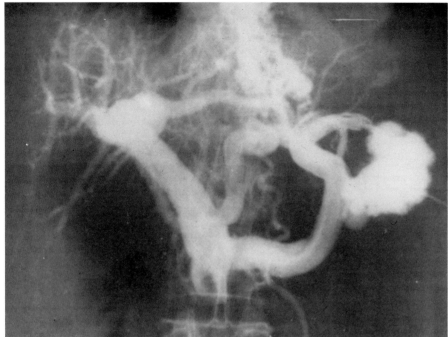

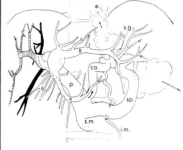

A

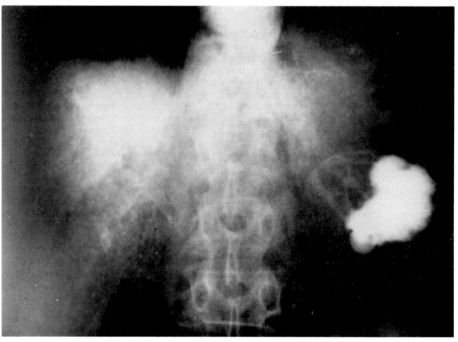

B

Figure 59-20. Cirrhosis of the liver. (A) Splenoportogram showing narrow and irregular intrahepatic portal branches. The left main part of the liver is abnormally large. There is filling of collateral vessels (coronary vein, short gastric veins, inferior mesenteric vein), indicating marked venous stasis.

(B) Hepatogram of mottled appearance. *sp.,* splenic vein; *p.,* portal vein; *co.,* coronary vein; *s.g.,* short gastric veins; *i.m.,* inferior mesenteric vein; *s.m.,* superior mesenteric vein; *e.,* esophageal veins; *6,* ventral vpr; *8,* dorsolateral vpr; *9,* ventrolateral vpr.

Figure 59-21. Cirrhosis of the liver. (A) Splenoportogram shows filling of only a few intrahepatic branches and no filling of the left principal vpr. Collateral circulation via the coronary vein and esophageal veins shows portal congestion. *sp.,* splenic vein; *p.,* portal vein; *co.,* coronary vein; *i.m.,* inferior

mesenteric vein; *e.,* esophageal veins; *1,* right principal vpr. ▶ (B) Splenoportogram after portacaval shunt shows no filling of collaterals. The contrast medium empties into the inferior vena cava. *sp.,* splenic vein; *p.,* portal vein; *i.v.c.,* inferior vena cava.

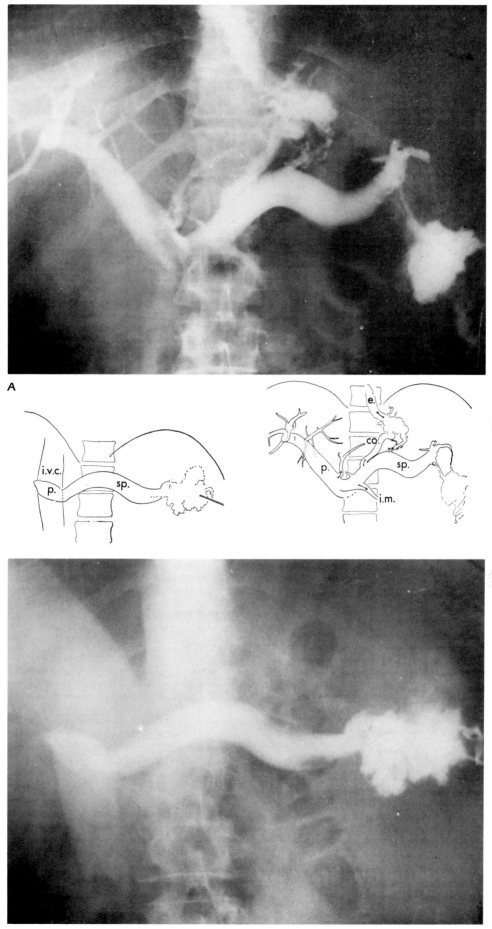

A

B

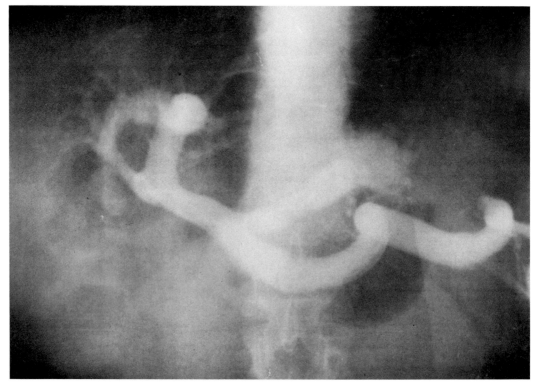

A

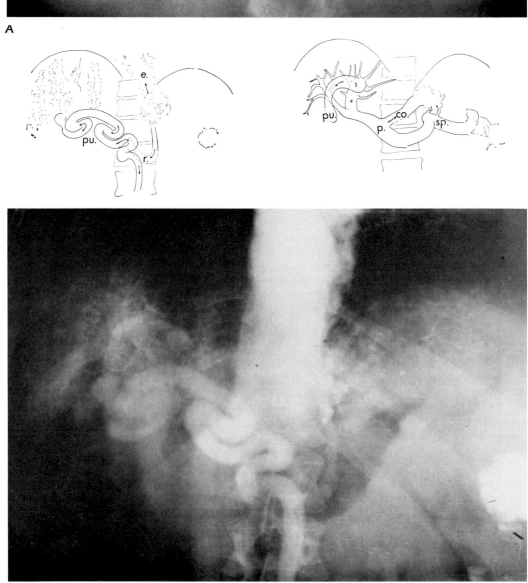

B

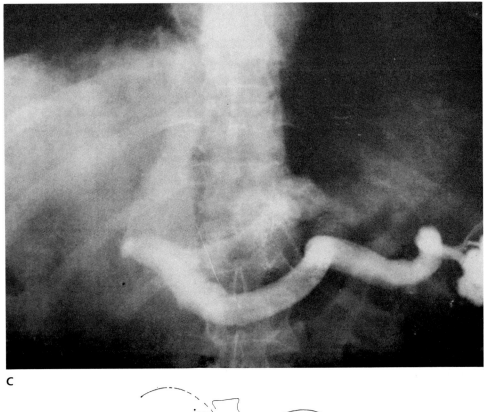

C

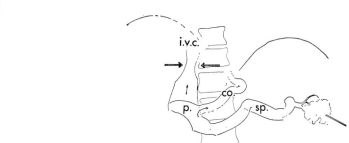

Figure 59-22. Cirrhosis of the liver. (A) Splenoportogram shows markedly changed intrahepatic ramification with few, narrow, and irregularly tapering vessels. Filling of a large coronary vein extending from the portal vein and a dilated parumbilical vein from ventroflexed vpr indicate portal stasis. *sp.*, splenic vein; *p.*, portal vien; *co.*, coronary vein; *pu.*, parumbilical vein; *4*, left principal vpr; *5*, ventroflexed vpr. (B) Six seconds later. Filling of the tortuous parumbilical vein is obtained. Contrast medium in the coronary vein plexus is emptying cranially into the esophageal veins and caudally via a retroperitoneal connection to the left renal vein. Note the mottled hepatographic appearance. *pu.*, parumbilical vein; *e.*, esophageal veins; *r.*, left renal vein. (C) Splenoportogram after portacaval shunt still shows filling of the coronary vein despite a broad portacaval communication. This may be explained by the narrowing of the inferior vena cava on its passage behind the liver, probably caused by cirrhotic nodules (*arrows*). The incapacity of the inferior vena cava was also evidenced by a relatively small decrease in portal pressure after establishment of the portacaval shunt (from 37 to 30 mmH$_2$O) and by edema of the legs postoperatively. *sp.*, splenic vein; *p.*, portal vein; *co.*, coronary vein; *i.v.c.*, inferior vena cava.

usual (Fig. 59-22A). The dilatation can often be attributed to a demonstrable collateral circulation from the ventroflexed portal venous ramus to the caval system via the parumbilical vein (see Fig. 59-22B). About one-third of the patients with cirrhosis show no definite vascular changes intrahepatically.

Hepatographic changes in cirrhosis must be judged with caution. In many instances the appearance of the liver is mottled (see Fig. 59-20B). This should be regarded as a definite sign of cirrhosis. Less distinct differences in contrast density are, however, also ob-

served in normal subjects. The hepatographic density is often poor in cirrhosis. It is most commonly explained by an extrahepatic collateral circulation so that the liver receives an abnormally small quantity of contrast medium. In several cases, however, a poor hepatographic density and an abnormally early appearance of hepatic veins are observed in patients with at most a small collateral circulation.[31,37] These signs are probably the roentgenographic manifestation of the intrahepatic shunts from portal to hepatic veins, bypassing the sinusoids in cirrhosis.[36,38,39]

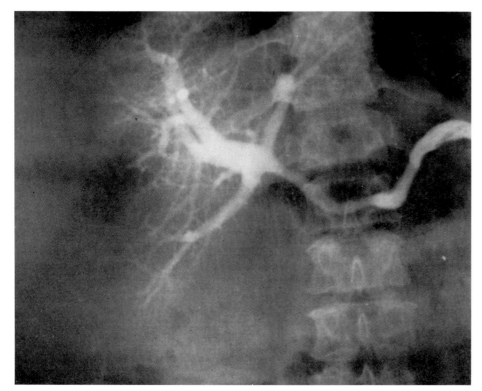
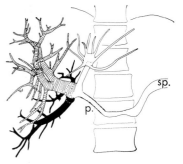

A

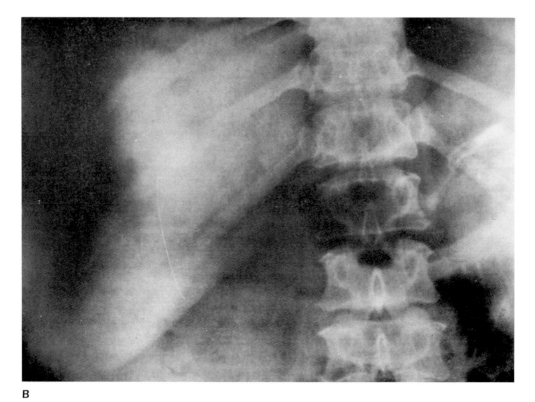

B

Figure 59-23. Tumor metastases. (A) Splenoportogram shows marked constriction of the portal vein. *sp.,* splenic vein; *p.,* portal vein. (B) Hepatogram shows one large filling defect corresponding to the lateral part of the ventrocranial segment.

Figure 59-24. Liver metastases. (A) Splenoportogram shows marked enlargement of the liver and displacement of the portal vein and intrahepatic branches. *sp.,* splenic vein; *p.,* portal vein; *1,* right principal vpr; *8,* dorsolateral vpr; *9,* ventrolateral vpr. (B) Hepatogram shows several filling defects corresponding approximately to displacement of the intrahepatic portal branches. ▶

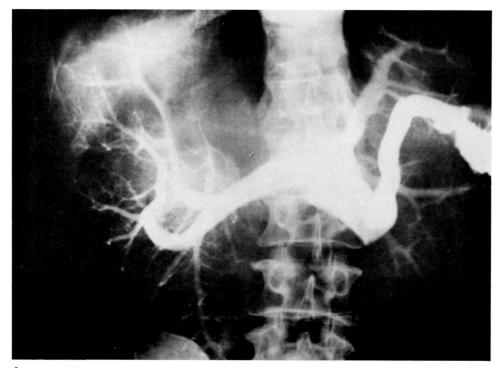

A

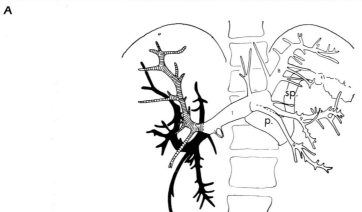

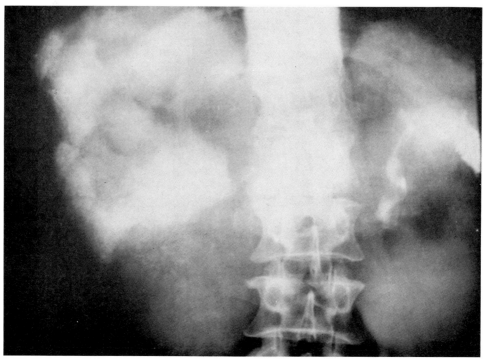

B

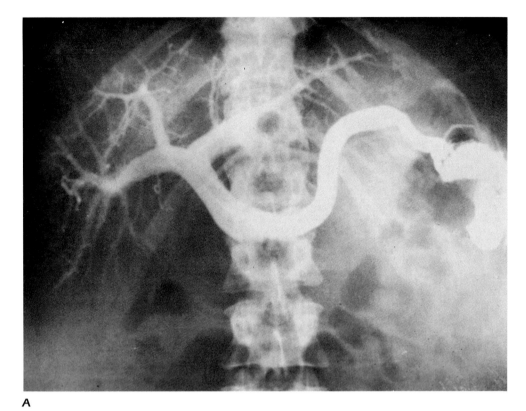

A

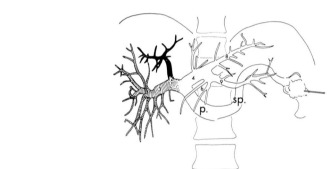

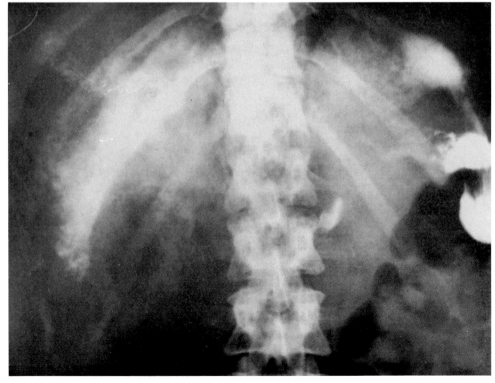

B

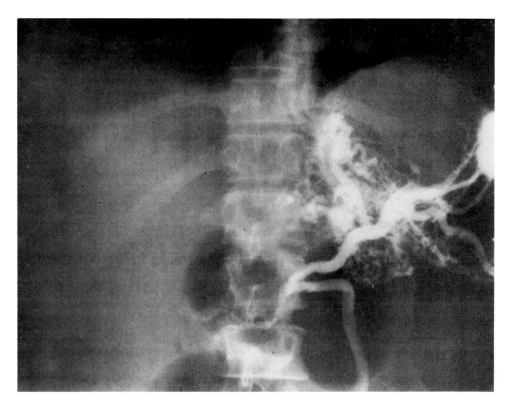

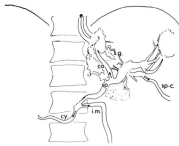

Figure 59-26. Portal occlusion caused by tumor metastases. Splenoportogram shows filling of collaterals (coronary vein, mesenteric vein, cystic vein). *sp.*, splenic vein; *s.g.*, short gastric veins; *co.*, coronary vein; *i.m.*, inferior mesenteric vein; *cy.*, cystic vein; *sp-c.*, collateral veins connecting spleen and hepatodistal part of splenic vein to systemic veins in the lateral abdominal wall; *e.*, esophageal veins.

Intrahepatic Malignant Tumors

Liver metastases as well as primary intrahepatic malignant growths affect the intrahepatic venous ramification mainly by their tendency to invade and occlude veins rapidly. Because the supply to these tumors is almost entirely arterial,[40] a contrast filling of tumor vessels in splenoportography is hardly to be expected.

The earliest change demonstrable by splenoportography usually consists of one or more clearly outlined, more or less irregular defects in the hepatogram (Figs. 59-23 through 59-25). This is a manifestation of invasion and occlusion of vessels too small to cause gross vascular changes. Sometimes tumor thrombi are seen in the vessels before obstruction is complete. A deficient filling of the left principal portal venous ramus

◄ **Figure 59-25.** Liver metastases. (A) Splenoportogram shows occlusion of smaller intrahepatic branches. There is no dislocation. *sp.*, splenic vein; *p.*, portal vein; *2*, dorsocaudal vpr (*black*); *3*, ventrocranial vpr (*striated*); *4*, left principal vpr; *6*, ventral vpr; *8*, dorsolateral vpr; *9*, ventrolateral vpr. (B) Hepatogram shows several major filling defects and numerous smaller ones.

or its branches should be interpreted with caution since this is also common in normal subjects (see Fig. 59-6). Sometimes a direct connection between portal and hepatic veins is demonstrable at the site of the tumor. Dislocation of vessels and signs of hepatomegaly are comparatively late signs (see Fig. 59-24A). In the absence of the above-mentioned signs of tumor invasion, any expansive process is probably not malignant. If the metastases are small and are evenly distributed, they do not appreciably change the roentgenogram.

Extrahepatic Anatomic Changes

The normally large variation in the course of the splenic vein makes it difficult to detect any dislocation.

Dislocation of or pressure on the portal vein, on the other hand, may be readily demonstrated because of the regularly straight or slightly curved normal course of this vessel. Such a change may, for example, be produced by tumor masses in the porta hepatis (Fig. 59-26; see also Fig. 59-23A) or in adjacent parts of the liver parenchyma.

References

1. Boulvin R, Chevalier M, Gallus P, et al. La Portographie par voie splénique transpariétale. Acta Chir Belg 1951;50:534.
2. Leger L, Albot G, Arvay N. La Phlébographie portale dans l'exploration des affections hépato-spléniques. Presse Med 1955;142:954.
3. Abeatici S, Campi L. Sur les possibilities de l'angiographie hépatique—la visualisation du système portal. Acta Radiol 1951;36:383.
4. Bahnson HT, Sloan RD, Blalock A. Splenic-portal venography. Johns Hopkins Bull 1953;92:331.
5. Sotgiu G, Cacciari C, Frassineti A. Splenoportographie. Press Med 1952;60:1295.
6. Bergstrand I. Splenoportography. In: Abrams HL, ed. Abrams angiography: vascular and interventional radiology. 3rd ed. Boston: Little, Brown, 1983:1573–1604.
7. Panke WF, Bradley EG, Moreno AH, et al. Technique, hazards and usefulness of percutaneous splenic portography. JAMA 1959;169:1032.
8. Foster JH, Conkle DM, Crane JM, et al. Splenoportography: an assessment of its value and risk. Ann Surg 1974;179:773–781.
9. Figley MM. Splenoportography: some advantages and disadvantages. Am J Roentgenol 1958;80:313–323.
10. Burchell AR, Moreno AH, Panke WF, et al. Some limitations of splenoportography: incidence, hemodynamics and surgical implications of the nonvisualized portal vein. Ann Surg 1965;162:981–995.
11. Sawada S, Nakamura K, Tanigawa N, et al. Technical note. Computed tomographic percutaneous transsplenic portography. Acta Radiol 1993;34:529–531.
12. Braun SD, Newman GE, Dunnick NR. Digital splenoportography. AJR 1985;144:1003.
13. Farid N, Balkanci F, Gruan S. A digital splenoportography: more sensitive method of detecting spontaneous splenorenal shunt. Angiology 1991;20:154–759.
14. Brazzini A, Hunter DW, Darcy MD, et al. Safe splenoportography. Radiology 1987;162:607–609.
15. Probst P, Rysavy JA, Amplatz K. Improved safety of splenoportography by plugging of the needle tract. AJR 1978;131:445–449.
16. Burcharth F, Neilbo N, Andersen B. Percutaneous transhepatic portography: II. Comparison with splenoportography in portal hypertension. AJR 1979;132:183–185.
17. Atkinson M, Sherlock S. Intrasplenic pressure as index of portal venous pressure. Lancet 1954;1:1325–1327.
18. Burcharth F, Aagaard J, Sorensen TIA, et al. Comparison of splenoportography and transhepatic portography in the diagnosis of portal vein thrombosis. J Hepatol 1986;2:351–357.
19. Baron MG, Bernard SW. Splenoportography. JAMA 1968;206:629–634.
20. Moskowitz H, Chait A, Margulies M, et al. Prone splenoportography. Radiology 1968;90:1132–1142.
21. Zamir O, Mogle P, Lernau O, et al. Splenoportography: a reappraisal. Am J Gastroenterol 1984;79:283.
22. Neff CC, Mueller PR, Ferrucci JT Jr, et al. Serious complications following transgression of the pleural space in drainage procedures. Radiology 1984;152:335–341.
23. Boijsen E, Efsing HO. Intrasplenic arterial aneurysms following splenoportal phlebography. Acta Radiol 1967;6:487–496.
24. Boijsen E, Efsing HO. Aneurysm of the splenic artery. Acta Radiol 1969;8:29–41.
25. Bergstrand I, Ekman C-A. Lieno-portal venography in the study of portal circulation in the dog. Acta Radiol 1957;47:257.
26. Doehner GA, Ruzicka FF, Hoffman G, Rousselot LM. The portal venous system: its roentgen anatomy. Radiology 1955;64:675.
27. Couinaud C. Étude de la veine porte intrahépatique. Presse Med 1953;61:1434.
28. Healey JE. Clinical anatomic aspects of radical hepatic surgery. J Int Coll Surg 1954;22:542.
29. Hjortsjö C-H. Die Anatomie der intrahepatischen Gallengänge beim Menschen, mittels Röntgen- und Injektions-technik studiert. Lunds Univ Årsskr N F 1948;44:3.
30. Bergstrand I. Roentgen anatomy of the intrahepatic portal ramification: a study on autopsy material. Kgl Fysiograf Sällskap Lund Förh 1957;27:85.
31. Bergstrand I, Ekman C-A. Portal circulation in portal hypertension. Acta Radiol 1957;47:1.
32. Turner MD, Sherlock S, Steiner RE. Splenic venography and intrasplenic pressure measurement in the clinical investigation of the portal system. Am J Med 1957;23:846.
33. Bergstrand I. The localization of portal obstruction by splenoportography. AJR 1961;85:1111.
34. Bergstrand I. Die portale Kollateralzirkulation und Ösophagusvarizen. In: Transactions of the Ninth International Congress of Radiology. Stuttgart: Thieme, 1960.
35. Armstrong EL, Adams WL Jr, Tragerman LJ, Townsend EW. The Cruveilhier-Baumgarten syndrome; review of the literature and report of two additional cases. Ann Intern Med 1942;16:113.
36. McIndoe AH. Vascular lesions of portal cirrhosis. Arch Pathol 1928;5:23.
37. Bergstrand I. Liver morphology in percutaneous lienoportal venography. Kgl Fysiograf Sällskap Lund Förh 1957;27:105.
38. Daniel PM, Prichard ML, Reynell PC. The portal circulation in experimental cirrhosis of the liver. J Pathol 1952;64:53.
39. Popper H, Elias H, Petty DE. Vascular pattern of the cirrhotic liver. Am J Clin Pathol 1952;22:717.
40. Breedis C, Young G. The blood supply of neoplasms in the liver. Am J Pathol 1954;30:969.

60

Arterial Portography

KLAUS M. BRON
RICHARD A. BAUM

*E*valuation of the portal venous system is essential for the management of patients with portal hypertension and its complications. Portal venography, although primarily useful for the investigation of portal hypertension, is also at times helpful in the assessment of pancreatic and other retroperitoneal masses. The relative inaccessibility of the portal venous system has prompted the search for a variety of techniques, both intraoperative and nonsurgical, to explore this circulation. The objective of these procedures is to determine the anatomic patency of the splenomesoportal axis and the hemodynamic alterations caused by the development of extrahepatic portosystemic collateral channels (a response to portal hypertension).

The earliest technique for portal vein visualization in humans was devised by Blakemore and Lord[1] in 1945 (at the suggestion of Whipple[2]) and consisted of the direct injection of contrast material into the portal vein or one of its mesenteric tributaries at laparotomy. Further reports in the early 1950s[3–5] attested to the value of operative portal angiography at laparotomy, but it quickly became apparent that this method was cumbersome, time-consuming, and less than satisfactory. More important, it did not aid in the preoperative diagnosis of the patient and thus was of no use in planning the surgical approach.

During the 1950s, the nonoperative technique of percutaneous splenoportography was developed after Abeatici and Campi[6] in 1951 demonstrated this method in dogs. To Leger[7] goes the credit for the first successful percutaneous splenoportogram in humans. Thereafter, this method became firmly entrenched as the preoperative diagnostic technique for investigating patients with portal hypertension. Numerous reviews have appraised the indications, hazards, and results of its use in large series of patients.[8–13]

Arterial portography, an alternative nonoperative technique, developed gradually after the observation in 1953 by Rigler et al.[14] that the portal venous system was occasionally visualized after injection of contrast material into the abdominal aorta. The technique was largely neglected because aortic injection resulted in low contrast concentration in the splenoportal axis, resulting in poor visualization of the portal vein. In 1958 Ödman[15] refined the technique by selective catheterization of the celiac axis and obtained excellent splenic and portal vein visualization. Two further modifications of the arterial technique were suggested with the intent of improving visualization of the portal circulation: simultaneous selective contrast injection of the celiac and superior mesenteric arteries[16] and selective splenic artery injection.[17] Selective arteriography, principally of the splenic and superior mesenteric arteries, is the technique presently used to visualize the portal circulation and has replaced all prior techniques.

Current noninvasive imaging procedures such as ultrasonography with Doppler flow, computed tomography (CT), and magnetic resonance imaging (MRI) are used to evaluate the anatomic status of the portal circulation. Often they suffice, but when questions of portal circulation patency or partial thrombosis remain, definitive anatomic evaluation is required by arteriography. At present, only selective arteriography of the celiac-splenic, common hepatic, and superior mesenteric arteries provides definitive preoperative evaluation of the portal venous circulation when noninvasive imaging is inconclusive. In the future, promising noninvasive techniques such as spiral computed tomography and magnetic resonance arteriography may obviate invasive arteriography.

Principles of Arterial Portography

The rationale inherent in arterial portography is that contrast material injected selectively into the celiac-splenic or superior mesenteric arteries will remain sufficiently concentrated to demonstrate the venous portion of the circulation. This requires an adequate amount of contrast and a rate of injection sufficient to form a contrast bolus that overcomes the diluting effect of the nonopacified blood.

The method is physiologically sound because it takes advantage of the normal, patent circulatory pathways between the splanchnic arteries and the portal venous system. When the normal routes are altered by disease, creating venous obstruction and portosystemic collateral vessels, the angiogram will reflect and demonstrate these abnormalities. The technique of arterial portography uses the specific anatomy of the portal vein. This vessel, which is formed by the confluence of the splenic and superior mesenteric veins, receives blood from both the splenic and mesenteric circulations. Thus the portal vein may be visualized after selective injection of either the celiac-splenic or the superior mesenteric arteries or both.

Selective arterial injection of the celiac-splenic artery axis is a more remote form of percutaneous splenoportography because in both instances the splenoportal axis is visualized. However, after arterial injection, additional information may be derived by the demonstration of the hepatic arterial circulation and splenic size. In the patient with a previous splenectomy, neither selective celiac arteriography nor percutaneous splenoportography will effectively demonstrate the splenoportal axis. However, selective injection of the superior mesenteric artery demonstrates the portal vein via blood returning to the liver in the superior mesenteric vein. This is an advantage because the absence of a spleen does not preclude portal vein visualization by this technique. Therefore, the status of the portal circulation may still be investigated in patients who have had a simple splenectomy or splenectomy in combination with an operative portosystemic shunt.

In a small group of patients with severe portal hypertension and a patent portal vein, the vein may not be visualized after selective celiac, splenic, or superior mesenteric arteriography. It should be recalled that the portal venous circulation is anatomically devoid of any venous valves. Blood flow in the portal circulation is determined by the pressure gradient between the liver sinusoids and the splanchnic veins. If this gradient is altered by pathology in the liver such as cirrhosis, the normal flow pattern may be changed.

The nonvisualization of a patent portal vein results from reversal or hepatofugal blood flow in the portal vein. Thus, instead of the normal forward or hepatopetal flow, the portal vein functions as an outflow tract for the liver in an effort to decompress the portal hypertension. This type of nonvisualization of a patent portal vein, or "pseudoocclusion," must be distinguished from true thrombotic occlusion.

When patency of the extrahepatic portal vein is questionable because of reversal of flow or an anatomic thrombosis, there are three diagnostic procedures that can resolve the question: (1) hepatic vein wedge injection; (2) selective common or proper hepatic artery injection; or (3) percutaneous transhepatic portal vein injection. One or more of these procedures may be necessary to provide a definitive answer.

Technique

Patient Preparation

All patients, adults and children, should be thoroughly familiarized with the procedure to allay unnecessary anxiety. All solid food is proscribed after the evening meal on the evening prior to the examination until conclusion of the study. Clear liquids are encouraged and not restricted. Cleansing enemas may be ordered for constipated patients if barium has been administered within 48 hours prior to the scheduled portogram. A surgical preparation of both groin areas is performed; occasionally the left axilla is prepared if both femoral artery pulses are absent. The femoral artery is the site of choice from which to selectively catheterize the various splanchnic arterial branches, but these vessels may also be catheterized from the left axillary artery.[18]

Analgesia and sedation are administered intravenously prior to the procedure. In adults this consists of Versed (midazolam hydrochloride) and fentanyl citrate in amounts appropriate to the patient's age and weight. For children general anesthesia is usually used.

Because patients with portal hypertension or retroperitoneal masses are frequently anemic from acute or chronic blood loss, the examination is postponed until the hemoglobin and hematocrit levels are in the range of 7 to 8 g and 25 to 30 percent, respectively. This consideration, however, is waived in the critically ill, emergency patient, who may be examined in a state of clinical shock with blood replacement flowing in an effort to determine the bleeding source. Coagulopathies and bleeding tendencies are frequent in patients with cirrhosis and portal hypertension. The platelet count should be corrected to 50,000, if necessary, by the infusion of platelets, and the prothrombin time should not exceed 15; otherwise fresh-frozen plasma is required to correct the deficit.

The patient's renal function, namely, the blood urea nitrogen and creatinine levels, should be obtained. This is important in determining the type of radiopaque contrast material to inject, since ionic contrast may exacerbate poor renal function. In addition, it may be useful to administer mannitol to mitigate the deleterious effects of radiopaque contrast in patients with compromised renal function.

Catheters and Catheterization

The percutaneous Seldinger technique[19] is used to puncture and catheterize the femoral artery. In adults a 5 French (5F) Cobra 2 or a 5F Simmons I catheter is used to selectively catheterize the celiac axis or its branches and also the superior mesenteric artery. These catheters are available in varying lengths (65 or 80 cm) from various well-known commercial manufacturers. In children the technique of introducing the catheter is slightly modified,[20] and a Formocath RPX 045 (Becton, Dickinson and Co.) catheter (40 cm long and similarly precurved) is used. Under fluoroscopic control the catheter is selectively manipulated into the specific splanchnic artery. The celiac-splenic and the superior mesenteric arteries are selectively catheterized and injected in most patients. When prior splenectomy has been performed, only the superior mesenteric artery is catheterized, since injection of the celiac axis will yield no information concerning the portal vein or portosystemic collaterals.

Assessment of extrahepatic portal vein patency in instances of either hepatofugal flow or anatomic thrombosis may require a variant of the usual technique. One of the following three procedures may be performed: (1) the hepatic artery may be selectively catheterized; (2) a hepatic vein wedge injection may be performed; or (3) a portal vein branch may be catheterized transhepatically. The common or proper hepatic artery can usually be subselectively catheterized after the celiac axis is catheterized. A hepatic vein wedge injection is performed by selectively catheterizing the right hepatic vein, either from a femoral or internal jugular vein approach. A 5F Cobra 2 catheter is used and the tip is advanced into a peripheral wedge position. The wedge position is identified when a small amount of hepatic parenchymal staining is observed fluoroscopically after a hand injection of 4 to 7 ml of contrast and when no blood can be aspirated. The third diagnostic procedure to visualize the portal vein is percutaneous transhepatic portal vein catheterization. This requires transhepatic puncture of a portal vein branch with a 22- or 18-gauge needle and then replacing the needle with a 4F catheter. With any of the three procedures described, the extrahepatic portal vein, if patent, fills with contrast in a retrograde direction rather than in the normal forward or hepatopetal flow pattern.

The choice of contrast material is influenced by the status of the patient's renal function and the history of a previous allergic contrast reaction. If the renal function is compromised or the allergic history is positive, then low-osmolar contrast is injected. Low-osmolar contrast is also used in children less than 6 years of age and adults above the age of 65.

At the conclusion of the examination, the catheter is withdrawn and manual pressure is exerted at the arterial puncture site to prevent bleeding and hematoma formation. In most patients, pressure need be maintained no longer than for 10 to 15 minutes after catheter withdrawal. Once bleeding has stopped, a pressure dressing is applied to the puncture site and the patient is returned to bed. The vital signs are monitored regularly, and the puncture site must be examined for evidence of bleeding during the 5 hours of bedrest prescribed after the examination.

Contrast and Filming

In adults, the contrast is injected selectively into the splenic or superior mesenteric arteries at a rate of 6 to 8 ml per second in amounts ranging from 50 to 70 ml. The larger quantities are used in patients with splenomegaly or proven varices. In children, contrast is injected at a rate of 6 ml per second for a total of 25 to 30 ml per injection.

Position and Film Program

A scout film is obtained prior to any sequential filming to check exposure factors and position. The top of the film should include at least 2 to 3 inches of the distal esophagus to visualize any esophageal varices.

A series of films in the anteroposterior position of a selective injection into the splenic and superior mesenteric arteries is routinely obtained. Another series of the superior mesenteric artery may be exposed in the right posterior oblique position. The latter study permits better visualization of the junction of the superior mesenteric and portal veins because the vessels in this position are displaced from the vertebral bodies. The oblique projection of the superior mesenteric artery is often recorded by digital subtraction angiography, and then less radiopaque contrast is required to obtain adequate vessel visualization.

Sequential films are obtained by means of a rapid serial film changer and programmed to expose films through the arterial, capillary, and venous phases. Films are usually exposed for a period of 40 seconds after the onset of contrast injection, with filming at the rate of 1 film per 2 seconds for a total of 20 films.

The film programming may have to be prolonged in extremely slow portal circulation. Unfortunately, this variation is unpredictable, but it occurs more frequently in association with marked splenomegaly and is due to severe portal hypertension.

Pharmacoangiography in the Portal System

The degree of contrast visualization of the portal venous circulation and gastroesophageal varices following selective splenic or superior mesenteric arteriography is not always adequate to delineate the anatomic detail of these structures. This deficiency is particularly distressing in patients with previous splenectomy and/or a proximal splenorenal shunt, which prevents the use of selective splenic arteriography to assess the portal venous anatomy. The use of various pharmacologic vasodilator agents has been advocated to enhance mesenteric and portal vein visualization. In 1966 Boijsen and Redman[21] reported on the effects of infusing bradykinin into the celiac and superior mesenteric arteries prior to angiography to enhance portal vein visualization.

Subsequently, infusions of tolazoline,[22] isoproterenol and phentolamine,[23] glucagon,[24] epinephrine,[25] papaverine,[26] and prostaglandin E_1[27] prior to arteriography have been reported to improve contrast visualization of the portal venous system. Since 1972 the author (Bron) has infused papaverine hydrochloride before selective superior mesenteric arteriography to improve the contrast visualization of the superior mesenteric and portal veins, as well as of gastroesophageal varices. This has proved to be extremely effective and safe in doses ranging from 0.6 to 1.1 mg per kilogram. My experience with this drug includes nearly 2500 patients with portal hypertension, pancreatic carcinoma, hepatic tumors, gastrointestinal bleeding, and retroperitoneal tumors.

The papaverine is prepared in a solution of nonheparinized normal saline in a concentration of 1.8 mg/ml. The papaverine solution is infused with an automatic pump or by hand at the rate of 20 ml per minute for 2 minutes. Occasionally a very mild transient drop in systemic blood pressure has been observed with this dose. The papaverine causes a 40 percent increase in the superior mesenteric artery blood flow, but this effect is very transient. Because the vasodilatory effect of papaverine in the mesenteric circulation is so transient, the solution is infused immediately prior to the contrast injection. If a repeat papaverine infusion is re-

quired, it can be safely done about 15 minutes after the first administration.

Complications

The complications of arterial portography are those caused by the technique of percutaneous catheterization and those produced by an allergic reaction to the contrast material. Among the minor hazards of the procedure are the formation of hematomas at the puncture site, intramural contrast deposition, inadvertent transmural passage of a guidewire, and arterial spasm. These are not generally associated with an increased morbidity, and their frequency is inversely proportional to the experience and skill of the angiographer.

One might anticipate that postcatheterization hematomas would be a more serious problem in portal hypertension patients with increased bleeding tendencies due to thrombocytopenia. In 52 percent of the author's (Bron's) patients with portal hypertension and thrombocytopenia with platelet counts of less than 100,000 and in 32 percent with thrombocytopenia with counts of less than 60,000, no significant increase in the rate or degree of hematoma formation was discerned.

A more serious complication is postcatheterization thrombosis at the puncture site, which occurs more often in elderly individuals with predisposing severe atherosclerosis. Because the majority of patients with portal hypertension usually do not fall into this category, this complication is infrequent. Generally, the complication rate from the technique of percutaneous catheterization ranges from 1 to 3 percent.[28-30]

Contraindications

A documented anaphylactic reaction to contrast material constitutes the single serious relative contraindication to any type of elective contrast study. The hazard of an allergic reaction, however, must be weighed against the danger of insufficient information concerning the portal circulation if a therapeutic operative procedure is being contemplated. If anatomic delineation by angiography is necessary, then the procedure can be performed under general anesthesia. In patients who have previously experienced urticaria, itching, faintness, and transient hypotension from a contrast injection, premedication with steroids, an antihistamine, and an alpha blocker are usually sufficient precautions.

Indications

The aim of arterial portography is to establish the anatomy and the possible etiology of the condition and to indicate a potential course of surgical management in patients with portal hypertension or retroperitoneal tumors. This is possible because the technique permits visualization of the component vessels of the portal circulation—the splenic, superior mesenteric, and portal veins—and the pathologic portosystemic collaterals.

One report[31] of the arterial technique for portal hypertension established specific indications (Table 60-1). They have withstood the test of subsequent experience.[32–36] The arterial approach should be the method of choice in examining patients with portal hypertension, especially children with this disorder.

Table 60-1. Indications for Arterial Portography

Portal hypertension
  Preoperative evaluation
    Differentiate intrahepatic and extrahepatic portal obstruction
    Demonstrate gastric and/or esophageal varices
    Evaluate technical failure of splenoportography
    Determine cause of nonvisualization of portal circulation by splenoportography
    Consider the relative contraindications for splenoportography (i.e., ascites, thrombocytopenia, and small spleen)
  Postoperative evaluation
    Demonstrate the function of shunts in nonsplenectomized patients
    Evaluate portal circulation after splenectomy
Extrahepatic tumors
  Pancreatic
    Carcinoma
    Pseudocyst

Normal Arterial Portograms

In an arterial portogram the common venous pathways visualized are the extra- and intrahepatic portal veins. Only occasionally are the hepatic veins demonstrated. When the splenic artery is injected (splenic portography), there is additional visualization of its arterial branches, the splenic parenchyma, and the splenic vein. Similarly, injection of the superior mesenteric artery (mesenteric portography) demonstrates the arterial branches, the mesenteric wall phase, and the superior mesenteric vein. Injection of the celiac axis (celiac portography) demonstrates the same regional blood flow pattern as a selective splenic artery injection, but in addition the hepatic and left gastric artery circulations are also displayed.

In the venous phase of the celiac and splenic portograms (Fig. 60-1), the tributaries and then the main splenic and portal veins are visualized. The normal flow is toward the liver, or hepatopetal. The splenic portion of splenic vein crossing the vertebrae may be indistinct, but note the caliber and straight course of the remainder of both vessels.

Figure 60-1. Celiac portogram. A normal venous phase after injection of the celiac artery (*C*). *Arrows* indicate the direction of blood flow from the spleen (*Sp*) into the splenic vein (*S*) and then into the extrahepatic portal vein (*PV*). The

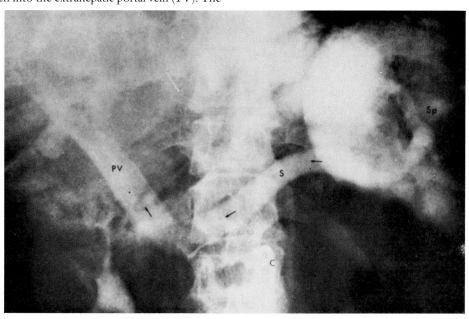

and portal veins are usually noted almost simultaneously, so that separate splenic and portal vein transit times cannot be established. The contrast density usually increases to a maximum in these vessels and then gradually fades. The splenic vein normally follows a slight undulating course. The portion of the splenic vein that overlies the vertebral body may be less dense. The degree of intrahepatic portal vein filling is variable. The main right and left lobe intrahepatic branches are noted at their origins, but the peripheral vessels are less perceptible. The right intrahepatic branch may be better filled with contrast than the left because in the supine position the right branch is more dependent. This position enhances the gravitational effect upon the contrast material. The hepatic veins draining the liver lobules into the systemic venous circulation are usually not visualized, except in children. The coronary vein (left gastric), which drains the lesser curvature and cardia of the stomach, is normally infrequently visualized. It may enter the splenic or portal vein. Another seldom noted vessel is the right gastroepiploic vein, which drains the greater curvature of the stomach. The pancreatic veins are never clearly visualized as distinct vessels. The inferior mesenteric vein, a tributary of the splenic vein, is not normally visualized.

Injection of contrast into the superior mesenteric artery (mesenteric portography) demonstrates a different group of regional vessels before the contrast reaches the portal vein. In the arterial phase the vessels to the duodenum and pancreas (the inferior pancreatic arcade arteries) are filled, and these in turn may demonstrate the gastroduodenal artery. The entire small bowel, except for the duodenum, is supplied by jejunal and ileal branches that arise primarily along the left side of the main superior mesenteric artery. The colon, from the cecum to the splenic flexure area, receives its blood supply from vessels that arise from the right side of the superior mesenteric artery. In the capillary phase the contrast is distributed in the wall of the various loops of bowel and when visualized on end may be mistaken for tumor staining.

As the contrast proceeds into the venous phase of the mesenteric portogram (Fig. 60-2), the different mesenteric tributaries draining the various portions of the small bowel and colon are visualized. These branches are named for the parts of the gut that they drain, and although a general pattern exists, there is marked variability in the individual patient. These regional veins coalesce into the main superior mesenteric vein, which joins with the splenic vein to form the portal vein.

There is usually no difference in the frequency of visualization of the intrahepatic branches of the portal

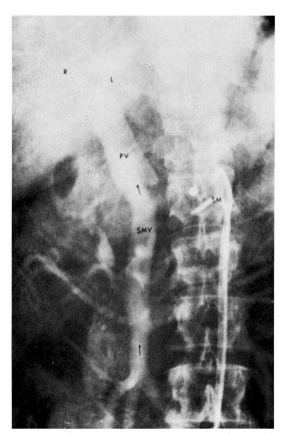

Figure 60-2. Superior mesenteric portogram. A normal venous phase after injection of the corresponding artery (*SM*). *Arrows* indicate the hepatopetal blood flow from the venous tributaries into the superior mesenteric vein (*SMV*), then into the extrahepatic portal vein (*PV*), and finally into the right (*R*) and left (*L*) intrahepatic branches.

and hepatic veins after either celiac-splenic or superior mesenteric artery injection. The portal vein may demonstrate a streaming effect caused by mixing of the two separate blood flows from the splenic and superior mesenteric veins when only one of these regional flows is opacified. This may render visible only a portion of the total diameter of the portal vein.

Abnormal Portograms

Intrahepatic Portal Obstruction and Collaterals

The most frequent cause of portal hypertension is intrahepatic obstruction, secondary to cirrhosis of the portal, biliary, or postnecrotic type. The pathologic changes cause distortion of the hepatic parenchyma with intermingling of necrotic, fibrotic, and regenerating areas of liver tissue. This progressive process even-

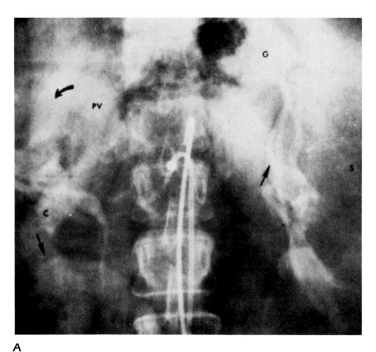

A

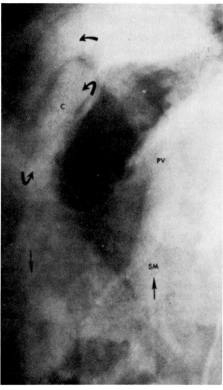

B

Figure 60-3. Collateral drainage. (A) Celiac portogram demonstrates two types of collaterals: gastric varices (*G*) and a dilated, tortuous umbilical vein (*C*). The gastric varices are supplied by vessels directly from the lower pole of the spleen (*arrows*). The splenic vein has emptied, and only the portal vein (*PV*) and the collateral vessel (*C*) remain visualized. The direction of blood flow is indicated by the *arrows. S,* spleen.

(B) The superior mesenteric portogram also shows the umbilical vein collateral (*C*), and its extent is better appreciated in the oblique view. This collateral vessel originates from the left branch of the portal vein (*PV*). *Arrows* indicate the direction of blood flow from the superior mesenteric vein (*SM*) toward the umbilicus.

tually results in impaired circulation of blood through the liver with consequent portal hypertension. The normal direction of portal blood flow is toward the liver (hepatopetal), but as the intrahepatic circulation becomes progressively impaired, portosystemic collateral vessels develop and blood flows away from the liver (hepatofugal).

The function of collaterals in the portal circulation is to decompress the hepatic circulation and divert splanchnic blood flow from the portal to the systemic circulation. The most frequent pathways eventually terminate in the superior vena cava via the esophageal, gastric, and azygos veins. Also important, though less frequent, are the pathways entering the inferior vena cava via the renal, iliac, and hemorrhoidal veins.

The major types of collateral channels are the esophagogastric, splenorenal, retroperitoneal, and umbilical varieties. These are formed by vessels that are normally present but that are unused in the absence of elevated portal pressure, rather than from the

growth of new vessels. The vessels that constitute the collateral circulation generally become dilated and markedly tortuous, and the blood flow through them is sluggish. Esophagogastric varices occur most frequently. More than one type of collateral circulation is often present (Fig. 60-3), and there seems to be no correlation between the degree of portal hypertension and the type of collateral developed. The esophagogastric varices (Fig. 60-4) are formed by either the coronary or short gastric veins or both. It is not unusual for either the esophageal or the gastric varices to appear more prominent than the other because both may not be developed to the same degree. The umbilical vein collateral arises from the left portal vein branch, since during embryologic development this anatomic connection existed. Occasionally an intestinal varix (Fig. 60-5) occurs because of the development of mesenteric collaterals.

The esophagogastric, splenorenal, and retroperitoneal collaterals are frequently best demonstrated by a

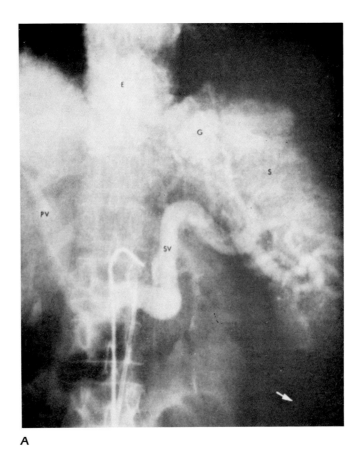

A

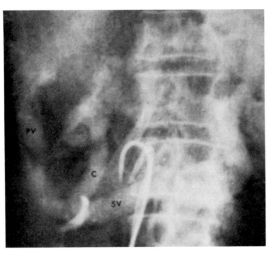

B

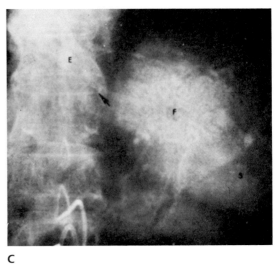

C

Figure 60-4. Esophagogastric varices. (A) A celiac porto-gram in the anteroposterior position demonstrates gastric (*G*) and esophageal (*E*) varices, supplied by the short gastric vessels from the spleen (*S*). The splenic vein (*SV*) is tortuous and dilated, reflecting the portal hypertension. The portal vein (*PV*) is patent. A dilated retroperitoneal vein (*arrow*) that functions as a collateral is visible at the caudal margin of the spleen. (B) A celiac portogram in the right posterior oblique position demonstrates a dilated coronary vein (*C*) that feeds esophageal varices. This vessel and the varices were not evident in the anteroposterior view. The splenic (*SV*) and portal (*PV*) veins are dilated. (C) Esophageal varices (*E*) are supplied by a vessel (*arrow*) directly from the cardia (*F*) of the stomach; this latter structure overlies the medial portion of the spleen (*S*).

celiac or splenic artery injection because these abnormal vessels are formed by branches of the splenic vein. However, when the coronary vein arises from the portal vein, the esophagogastric varices may be better seen after a superior mesenteric artery injection. The umbilical vein collateral may be equally well demonstrated after a celiac-splenic or superior mesenteric artery injection because the abnormal venous connection arises from the left intrahepatic branch of the portal vein.

These collaterals represent a natural mechanism that attempts to reduce the portal pressure by diverting the portal circulation away from the abnormal liver. That the attempt is eventually unsuccessful is attested to by the development of hematemesis, melena, and ascites, the clinical complications of portal hypertension.

Extrahepatic Portal Obstruction

The portal circulation may be obstructed by partial or complete occlusion of the extrahepatic portion of the portal and/or splenic veins. Obstruction of the hepatic veins is a less frequent cause, and rarely is the superior mesenteric vein directly included in the obstructive process. Unlike intrahepatic obstruction, which is secondary to hepatic tissue destruction, extrahepatic obstruction is the result of intrinsic vascular pathology in the form of thrombosis caused by infection, congenital malformation, tumor compression, cirrhosis, and postsurgical complications.

The portal vein is more often affected than the splenic vein. Neonatal umbilical vein infection and congenital malformation are responsible for the high incidence of portal vein obstruction and are the leading causes of portal hypertension in children. In adults there is associated portal vein obstruction in about 10 percent of patients with portal cirrhosis of the liver. Extrahepatic portal obstruction is considerably less frequent than intrahepatic obstruction as the cause of portal hypertension. A biopsy of the liver in extrahepatic portal obstruction, unless associated with hepatic cirrhosis, will usually reveal normal liver histology.

Recanalization may follow portal vein thrombosis and may cause a smaller than normal caliber, an irregular contour, or replacement by multiple channels (Fig. 60-6). There may also be evidence of calcification reflecting the previous thrombosis (see Fig. 60-13A).

The collateral vessels reflect the site of venous occlusion. When the splenic vein is occluded but the portal vein remains patent, collaterals will attempt to bypass the occlusion in order to reconstitute the portal vein (Fig. 60-7). If both the portal and splenic veins are occluded (Fig. 60-8), drainage from the spleen may be via esophagogastric, retroperitoneal, or spleno-

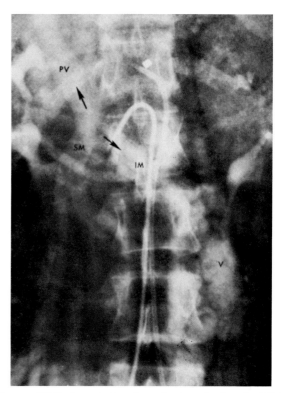

Figure 60-5. Intestinal varices. An intestinal varix (*V*) is present in the course of the inferior mesenteric vein (*IM*). This is a localized area of venous dilatation and tortuosity. The mesenteric portogram reveals that the blood flow from the superior mesenteric vein (*SM*) continues to be hepatopetal (*arrow*) in the portal vein (*PV*) but is hepatofugal (*arrow*) in the inferior mesenteric vein (*IM*).

renal collateral vessels. If the recanalized portal vein cannot accommodate the portal circulation, portal hypertension ensues with consequent collateral vessels and varices.

Prior Splenectomy

In the patient with a prior splenectomy it is important to evaluate the status of the portal circulation. These patients have usually had one or more surgical procedures in an attempt to alleviate the complications of portal hypertension. Splenectomy alone is a form of therapy for portal hypertension with hypersplenism, but more often a splenorenal shunt is performed or attempted in conjunction with splenectomy. Recurrence of hematemesis, melena, or ascites generally signals failure of the previous therapy, and before any further surgical intervention is done the existing portal circulation must be carefully evaluated (Fig. 60-9).

When the spleen is absent, the splenoportal axis has been interrupted. Any attempt to visualize the portal

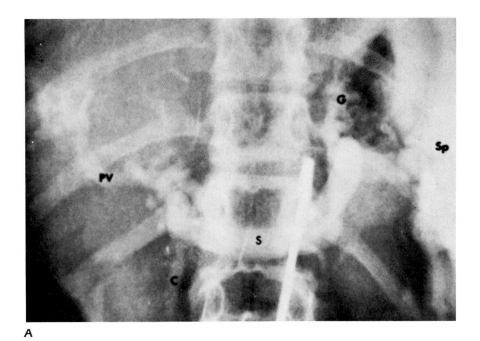

A

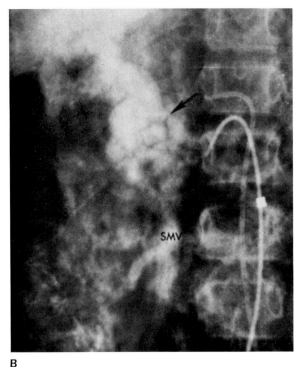

B

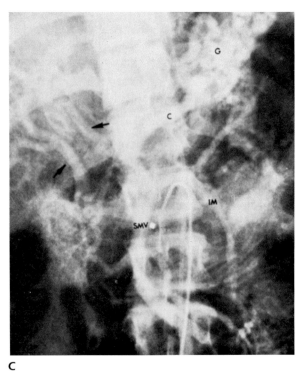

C

Figure 60-6. Extrahepatic portal obstruction. The vein displays a variety of changes reflecting the antecedent pathology. (A) The portal vein (*PV*) is reduced in caliber, and its junction with the splenic vein (*S*) is abnormal. A collateral vessel (*C*) and gastric varices (*G*) are present. The spleen (*Sp*) was enlarged. (B) The portal vein has been deformed into a tortuous tangle of vessels (*arrow*) at its origin from the superior mesenteric vein (*SMV*). (C) A previous splenectomy in this patient precluded any nonoperative evaluation of the status of the portal vessel other than superior mesenteric portography. The portal vein (*arrows*) consists of multiple channels that fill from the superior mesenteric vein (*SMV*). A dilated coronary vein (*C*) demonstrates gastric varices (*G*). The direction of blood flow in the inferior mesenteric vein (*IM*) is retrograde from the superior mesenteric vein.

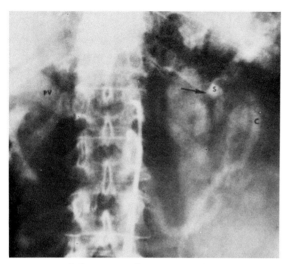

Figure 60-7. Splenic vein obstruction. The splenic vein (*S*) is occluded proximally (*arrow*). Dilated, tortuous collateral vessels (*C*) originate from the spleen and bypass the splenic vein obstruction to reconstitute the patent portal vein (*PV*).

Figure 60-8. Splenic and portal vein obstruction. The splenic and portal veins are occluded, with resultant splenomegaly (*Sp*) and venous drainage into esophageal varices (*E*) via the short gastric veins (*arrowhead*). The spleen is also decompressed by retroperitoneal collaterals (*C*). The metallic clips are from a partial gastrectomy and vagotomy that confirmed the venous occlusion.

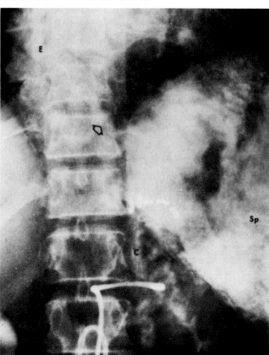

vein from the celiac-splenic circulation is therefore unsuccessful, and percutaneous splenoportography is impossible. In this situation the value of arterial portography via the superior mesenteric artery has been pointed out by Boijsen et al.[16] It is a safe and effective nonoperative technique for demonstrating the anatomy of the portal vein, any varices, and the patency of a splenorenal shunt that may be present after a prior splenectomy (see Fig. 60-6C).

Surgical Shunts

Therapy aimed at relieving portal hypertension and its complications—gastrointestinal bleeding, encephalopathy, and ascites—is based on reducing the portal pressure by the creation of portosystemic shunts. These surgically formed shunts may be of the portacaval, splenorenal, or mesocaval variety. The surgical shunts generally reduce portal pressure when the natural shunts (varices) become inadequate to lower the pressure. Unfortunately, shunt surgery is likely to afford relief only from acute life-threatening symptoms; it generally does not provide a permanent cure. Recurrent symptoms subsequent to surgery raise the question of shunt patency or shunt size adequacy to handle the portal circulation.

Figure 60-9. Postsplenectomy status. The patient presented with recurrent hematemesis after failure of a previous portacaval shunt and a subsequent unsuccessful splenorenal shunt that resulted in splenectomy. A superior mesenteric portogram demonstrates the status of the portal venous system. The superior mesenteric (*SM*) and portal (*PV*) veins are patent, and no evidence of a functioning portacaval shunt is observed. Gastric varices (*G*) are supplied by the coronary vein (*arrow*).

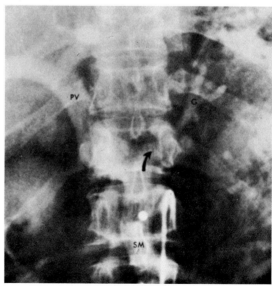

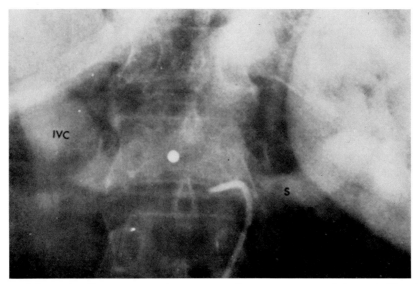

Figure 60-10. Portacaval shunt. A celiac portogram demonstrates the patent portacaval shunt. A dilated splenic vein (*S*) and the end-to-side anastomosis between the portal vein and inferior vena cava (*IVC*) are noted.

A variety of shunt procedures are available to effect a portosystemic shunt; all use various veins of the portal circulation. The portal and splenic veins are the principal vessels used to create surgical portosystemic

Figure 60-11. Splenorenal shunt. A superior mesenteric portogram is required to demonstrate patency of a splenorenal shunt. The arrows indicate the direction of blood flow from the superior mesenteric vein (*SMV*), which then continues into both the portal vein (*PV*) and splenorenal shunt (*S–R*). Dilution of the contrast by nonopacified renal vein blood causes poor visualization of the inferior vena cava. (Courtesy of Sam E. Morris, M.D.)

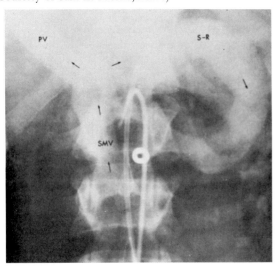

shunts. The end-to-side portacaval shunt is the preferred type of anastomosis when anatomically and technically feasible. There are two types of splenorenal shunts, a proximal or central and a distal or peripheral splenic vein anastomosis. In the proximal type the spleen is also resected, and thus this type of shunt is preferred when hypersplenism is present. A mesocaval shunt is created by anastomosing the superior mesenteric vein to the inferior vena cava with an interposed graft in an "H-type" shunt. This type of shunt is usually reserved for when a portacaval or splenorenal shunt fails.

When the spleen is intact, portacaval shunts may be demonstrated by either celiac-splenic (Fig. 60-10) or superior mesenteric arteriography (see Fig. 60-12A). After splenectomy the proximal splenorenal shunt and mesocaval shunts are demonstrated only by the mesenteric artery route (Fig. 60-11).

The demonstration of shunt patency can be rendered difficult by the rapid return of nonopacified lower extremity blood in the inferior vena cava. To prevent this problem, one may attempt to reduce the rate of return by applying vein-occluding tourniquets to both thighs. This reduces the contrast dilution in the inferior vena cava and improves the visualization of shunt patency (Fig. 60-12). The injection of tolazoline, a vasodilator, into the superior mesenteric artery just prior to angiography has been reported to accomplish the same result in the demonstration of portacaval shunts.[22]

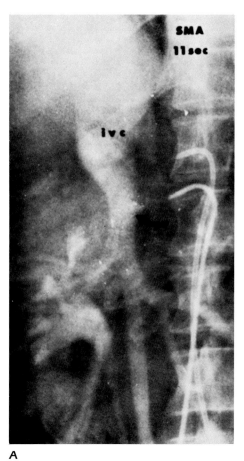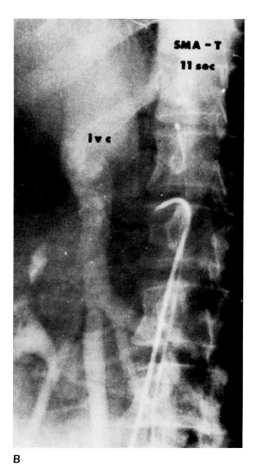

A   **B**

Figure 60-12. Portacaval shunt. (A) Patency of the portacaval shunt is demonstrated by the superior mesenteric portogram with filling of the inferior vena cava (*Ivc*) from the portal vein (*pv*). (B) Visualization of a patent portacaval shunt may be enhanced by reducing the dilution effect of nonopacified blood returning in the inferior vena cava. Tying tourniquets around both thighs accomplishes this by decreasing the venous return from the extremities. *SMA*, control superior mesenteric arteriogram; *SMA–T*, arteriogram with tourniquets around thighs. (From Bron KM, Fisher B. Arterial portography: indications and technique. Surgery 1967;61: 137. Used with permission.)

Patent but Nonvisualized Splenoportal Axis

When the splenic and portal veins are not visualized by percutaneous splenoportography but the portosystemic collaterals are, it is generally assumed that the splenoportal axis is anatomically occluded. Shortly after the introduction of percutaneous splenoportography, however, it became apparent that, in a definite percentage of patients in whom splenic or portal vein occlusion had been suspected on the basis of nonvisualization by this technique, these vessels were anatomically patent at surgery or autopsy.[37,38] The frequency of nonvisualization of the splenoportal axis by percutaneous splenoportography in the face of anatomic patency has been estimated at 17 percent[39] of such studies in patients who might benefit from a portacaval shunt. This serious limitation of percutaneous splenoportography must be recognized and not be lightly dismissed, because the decision of whether to perform a portacaval shunt or splenorenal shunt is based on the demonstration of a patent splenic or portal vein.

Several explanations have been advanced to account for this hemodynamic abnormality in portal hypertension. Ekman states that there is reversal of blood flow in the portal vein so that this vessel serves as a hepatic outflow tract instead of fulfilling its normal function as an inflow tract.[40] Other investigators[41] claim that the bulk of the splenic blood flow is diverted into the portosystemic collaterals; thus an insufficient quantity flows into the splenoportal axis to demonstrate these vessels. Burchell et al.,[39] by measuring portal vein blood flows at surgery with an electromagnetic flow-

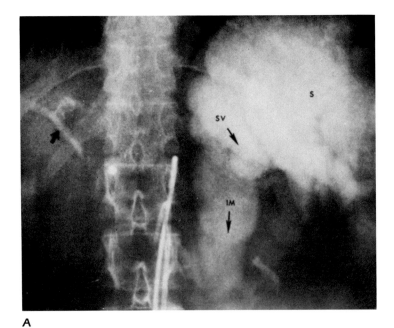

A

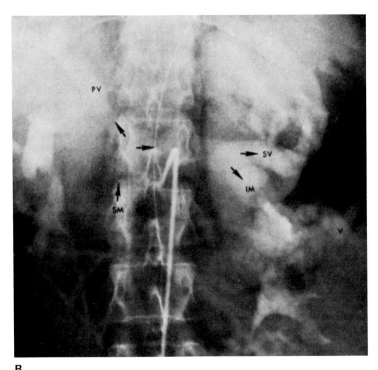

B

Figure 60-13. Splenic and/or portal vein thrombosis was suspected because a previous percutaneous splenoportogram had failed to demonstrate these vessels; calcification of the portal vein (*thick arrow*, A) was noted. (A) The celiac portogram demonstrates splenomegaly (*S*) and a dilated, tortuous splenic vein (*SV*) that empties into the inferior mesenteric vein (*IM*). *Thin arrows* indicate direction of blood flow. This study tends to confirm the conclusions of the percutaneous splenoportogram. (B) The superior mesenteric portogram, however, revealed that the splenic (*SV*) and portal (*PV*) veins were patent. The returning blood in the superior mesenteric vein (*SM*) flows antegrade in the portal vein but retrograde in the splenic and inferior mesenteric (*IM*) veins (*arrows*). Note the intestinal varix (*V*).

meter, were unable to demonstrate any reversal in blood flow, but found extremely low portal vein blood flows in patients with portal hypertension. Their observations tend to support the conclusion that the splenic and mesenteric venous blood flows were diverted through collaterals and thus caused nonvisualization of the splenic and portal veins.

In this situation of apparent splenoportal axis occlusion, arterial portography[42] can be very helpful in demonstrating that the vessels are patent. Because the superior mesenteric vein blood flow still maintains its hepatopetal direction despite elevation of portal pressure, arterial portography can demonstrate patency of these vessels in patients with portal hypertension and altered hemodynamics. In other words, the superior mesenteric vein, unlike the splenic and inferior mesenteric veins, does not generally function as a collateral channel to relieve portal hypertension. Thus, when the superior mesenteric artery is injected, the contrast returns in the vein and is distributed into the patent portal vessels and varices. Injection of contrast into the celiac axis or splenic artery in this situation will yield the same result as percutaneous splenoportography and will lead to a false conclusion of probable splenoportal vessel occlusion. This is also called *pseudoocclusion* of the portal vein. The celiac-splenic artery injection (Fig. 60-13A) will demonstrate the marked portosystemic collaterals that accompany the hemodynamic alterations in the portal circulation. But injection of the superior mesenteric artery (Fig. 60-13B) will reveal the true nature of the alteration and will dispel any doubt concerning patency of the splenic and portal veins.

CT During Arterial Portography

Increased 5-year survival rates have been described in patients who undergo resection of hepatic tumors. This has been found with both metastatic colorectal as well as primary hepatocellular carcinoma.[43–47] This aggressive surgical approach has placed increased demands on the radiologist to identify small intrahepatic lesions. The size, segmental location, and neoplastic extent of disease are very important to the surgeon contemplating partial liver resection. The efficacies of various imaging modalities to identify lesions less than 2 cm in size have been the subject of extensive review.[48–53] Despite recent advances in MRI, ultrasound, and nuclear medicine, CT remains the gold standard for diagnosing and staging intrahepatic disease.[54]

Soon after the introduction of CT, it was found that increased liver-to-lesion definition could be obtained with the administration of iodinated contrast material.

Table 60-2. Hepatic CT Contrast Enhancement Techniques

Intraarterial
  CT during arterial portography (CTAP); superior mesenteric arterial infusion with dynamic scanning with or without delayed images
  Hepatic arterial infusion with dynamic scanning
  Celiac axis infusion with dynamic scanning
  Splenic arterial infusion with dynamic scanning
  Delayed scanning after hepatic arterial infusion with iodinated oil
Intravenous
  Single intravenous bolus with routine scanning
  Dynamic scanning during intravenous infusion
  Delayed scanning after intravenous infusion

Although there is little debate that contrast material is an aid in evaluating primary and metastatic hepatic disease, there is no consensus on how best to administer it. Many CT imaging techniques have been introduced over the years that claim to have increased sensitivity for visualizing small intrahepatic lesions (Table 60-2). CT arterial portography (CTAP), first described over a decade ago, has emerged as the most sensitive imaging technique for the preoperative evaluation of patients with primary or metastatic liver disease.[55–66]

Principles of CT Arterial Portography

Normal hepatocytes derive 80 percent of their blood supply from the portal vein. Hepatic neoplasms, however, are supplied by the hepatic artery. The neovascularity demonstrated within hepatic tumors during selective hepatic arterial angiography is a result of this arterial supply.

During CT arterial portography, contrast material is infused directly into the superior mesenteric artery via an intraarterial catheter. The contrast circulates through the intestinal capillary bed and drains through the portal vein. This results in portal venous enhancement of the liver. CT images of the liver are obtained during the portal phase of the bolus (Fig. 60-14). Normal hepatocytes will demonstrate contrast enhancement, whereas neoplasms will remain unenhanced. Primary and metastatic disease, therefore, will appear as hypodense areas in a contrast-enhanced liver (Fig. 60-15).

In addition to visualizing intrahepatic masses, CT portography can be used to define hemodynamics and anatomic relationships of portal venous flow. Evidence of portosystemic shunting, cavernous transformation, and portal vein thrombosis all can be easily recognized on CT portography. This information has been used

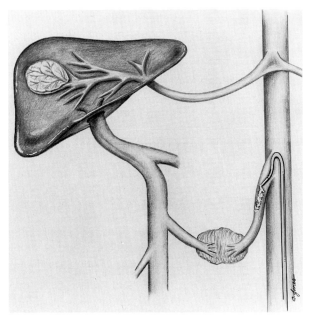

Figure 60-14. During CT arterial portography, contrast material is infused directly into the superior mesenteric artery via an intraarterial catheter. This contrast circulates through the intestinal capillary bed and drains via the portal vein, resulting in portal venous enhancement of the liver. It is during this phase of the examination that CT images of the liver are obtained.

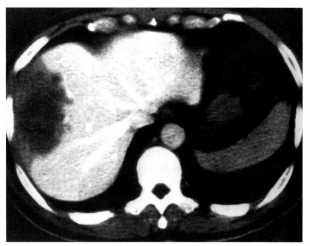

Figure 60-15. Metastatic adenocarcinoma demonstrated by CT portography. A large hypodense area involving both the anterior segment of the right hepatic lobe and the medial segment of the left hepatic lobe represents metastatic disease in this patient with a history of colon carcinoma.

by some to determine which patients are candidates for portosystemic shunt placement and which type of shunt would be most beneficial.[66–68]

Technique

Although CT portography is an exquisitely sensitive method for demonstrating small intrahepatic neoplasms, it can be a technically demanding examination. A recent report cites a technical failure rate of 26 percent.[69] There is currently no well-established imaging protocol for CT portography. Variations in technique are based on institutional preferences as well as differences in angiographic equipment and CT scanners. This explains the wide range of reported injection rates, delay times, and amount of contrast administered.

Typically, the superior mesenteric artery is selectively catheterized via a retrograde common femoral arterial approach. A limited superior mesenteric artery arteriogram is performed to define the patient's vascular anatomy. This is best accomplished using digital technique, since this decreases the amount of contrast used in this phase of the examination. Catheter place-

ment is critical in obtaining a diagnostic CT portogram. The tip of the catheter must be distal to the pancreaticoduodenal arcade but proximal to the jejunal and ileal branches to achieve optimal enhancement without artifacts.

A 5 to 6 French Simmons catheter is well suited for CT portography. Cobra catheters also are frequently used. Both have primary curves that allow for easy selective catheterization of the superior mesenteric artery. Their secondary and tertiary curves provide stability when positioned in the superior mesenteric artery. This is of great importance when transporting the patient to and from the CT scanner with the catheter in place.

Once the patient is on the CT table, a dose of tolazoline hydrochloride (10–20 mg) can be administered via the intraarterial catheter to increase superior mesenteric arterial flow and thereby portal venous return. The catheter is then connected to a power injector, and 30 percent iodinated contrast material is infused at a rate of 1.5 to 3.0 ml per second for a total volume of approximately 100 to 150 ml. An alternate approach would be the injection of 60 percent contrast at a rate of 0.5 to 1.0 ml per second for a total volume of approximately 75 to 100 ml. After a delay time of 9 to 30 seconds after the injection, dynamic scanning is begun with 10-mm-thick contiguous slices. The amount of delay depends on the type of contrast, the injection rate, and the patient's mesenteric flow rate as seen on the preliminary arteriogram.

Pitfalls of Interpretation

The primary advantage of CT portography over other imaging techniques is its high sensitivity for identifying and localizing small intrahepatic lesions (Fig. 60-16). However, several recent reports discuss high false-positive rates associated with CT portography. A wide range of hepatic perfusion abnormalities may cause hypodense intrahepatic lesions, which can mimic malignant hepatic disease.[70–77] Decreased portal perfusion, either focal or diffuse, may be related to failures of technique, venous obstruction, or anomalous hepatic arterial supply.

Failures of Technique

Catheter malposition, inadequate injection rates, and improper delay times all will cause segmental attenuation differences that may result in false-positive examinations. Recognizing the anatomic distribution of lesions can be essential in determining whether an apparent abnormality represents a true finding or simply a pseudolesion due to faulty technique. For example, streaky enhancement involving dependent hepatic segments is most likely related to catheter malposition. When the catheter is positioned too distally in an isolated jejunal or ileal branch, laminar portal flow occurs, leading to layering of contrast and an inhomogeneous enhancement pattern (Fig. 60-17). A catheter that is positioned proximal to the pancreaticoduodenal arcade can result in hepatic arterial enhancement via this collateral pathway (Fig. 60-18).

Injection rates that are too slow will fail to produce sufficient contrast between normal and abnormal hepatic tissue to delineate lesions. This is of particular importance when trying to identify and stage small intrahepatic lesions.

Improperly short delay times result in the acquisition of images prior to filling of hepatic veins with contrast material. This is recognized as hypodense linear defects in a hepatic venous distribution. Prolonged delay times result in recirculation of contrast causing mixed hepatic arterial and portal venous enhancement.

Portal Venous Obstruction

Obstruction of portal venous return can occur either extrinsically by tumor mass effect or intrinsically by thrombosis. Portal obstruction results in a characteristic linear variation in contrast enhancement termed the *straight-line sign*. The hypodensity typically originates centrally and extends to the periphery and is related to partial portal venous obstruction (Fig. 60-19). This finding has been reported in 36 percent of patients undergoing CT portography in a recent series.[78] It is an important lesion to recognize preoperatively, since the area of peripheral hypodensity does not represent tumor but is a result of central portal venous obstruction.[79,80]

Anomalous Hepatic Arterial Supply

Ten to 15 percent of the normal population have a right hepatic artery that originates from the proximal

Figure 60-16. Small intrahepatic focus of metastatic adenocarcinoma. A small area of decreased attenuation is identified within the lateral segment of the left hepatic lobe during CTAP (*arrows*).

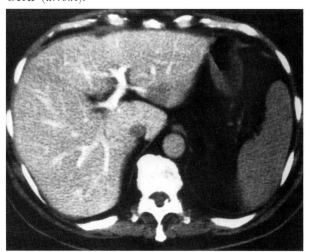

Figure 60-17. Inhomogeneous enhancement pattern due to catheter malposition. The catheter was inadvertently positioned in an isolated jejunal branch of the superior mesenteric artery, resulting in patchy enhancement of the liver.

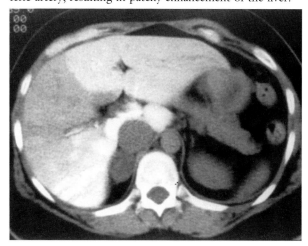

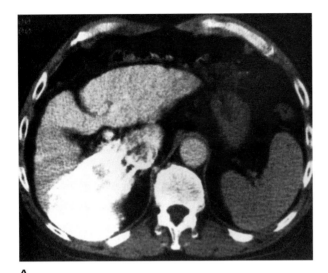

A

Figure 60-18. Hepatic arterial enhancement due to catheter malposition in the inferior pancreaticoduodenal artery (IPD). (A) Dense enhancement of the posterior segment of the right hepatic lobe resulted from IPD arterial injection.

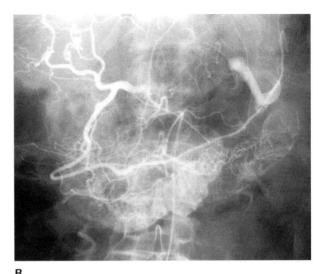

B

(B) Catheter malpositioned in the IPD branch of the superior mesenteric artery causing retrograde filling of the hepatic artery.

superior mesenteric artery, rather than from the proper hepatic artery. If CT portography is performed with the catheter positioned proximal to the "replaced right hepatic artery," an arterial enhancement pattern will occur in the right lobe of the liver. A portal venous enhancement pattern will predominate in the remainder of the liver, and the net result will be a confusing, nondiagnostic examination (Fig. 60-20). It is the responsibility of the angiographer to identify a replaced right hepatic artery prior to CT portography and to

properly position the tip of the infusion catheter distal to its origin.

Left Hepatic Lobe Pseudolesion

A characteristic area of decreased attenuation in the medial segment of the left hepatic lobe has been reported. This is located immediately anterior to the porta hepatis and does not correspond to an area of

Figure 60-19. "Straight-line sign" due to large hepatocellular carcinoma. CTAP reveals a large central hypodense mass causing partial portal venous obstruction. This results in a well-delineated area of decreased attenuation of the right hepatic lobe laterally (*arrows*).

Figure 60-20. Enhancement pattern caused by injection into a replaced right hepatic artery. Inadvertent injection into a replaced right hepatic artery caused arterial enhancement of the right hepatic lobe. Therefore, there is arterial ring enhancement of a metastatic adenocarcinoma within the posterior segment of the right hepatic lobe (*arrow*). The left hepatic lobe remains unenhanced.

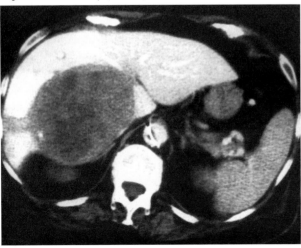

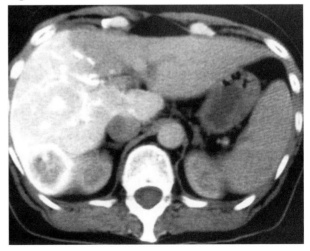

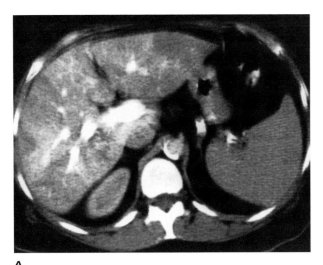

A

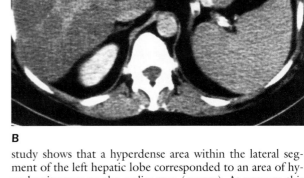

B

Figure 60-21. Value of delayed scanning in a nondiagnostic CTAP examination. (A) Technical difficulties resulted in this image, which had patchy enhancement throughout all lobes and several hypodense areas, which were of uncertain significance. (B) An image obtained 5 hours after the initial study shows that a hyperdense area within the lateral segment of the left hepatic lobe corresponded to an area of hypodensity seen on the earlier scan (*arrows*). At surgery, this was found to be the only area of metastatic disease in this patient with colorectal carcinoma.

disease on other imaging modalities or intraoperatively. A recent series identified this hypoperfused area in 14 percent of CT portograms.[81] A possible explanation for this pseudolesion is a normal variation in the portal venous flow to the medial segment of the left hepatic lobe. Another theory is that this area represents focal periligamentous fat. Whatever the etiology, it is important that this pseudolesion not be confused with neoplastic disease.

CT Portography in Cirrhosis

CT portography is of limited value in patients with cirrhotic liver disease. Regenerating nodules can appear as hypodense areas, which cannot be reliably distinguished from malignancy. In addition, patients with advanced disease will have decreased uptake of contrast due to poor hepatocyte function. For these reasons, CT portography has not been proven to have any benefit over other modalities in diagnosing hepatocellular carcinoma in these high-risk patients.[82]

Delayed Scanning

When conventional CTAP produces images that are equivocal or nondiagnostic, the examination may sometimes be salvaged by obtaining delayed images 4 to 6 hours after the initial study. Contrast will enter the systemic circulation after its initial first pass through the portal vein. The entire liver, including diseased segments, will become enhanced due to this mixed portosystemic delivery of contrast. Contrast will be eliminated from the normal hepatocytes in several

hours via the reticuloendothelial system. Neoplasms have a defective reticuloendothelial system and are unable to excrete contrast in the usual manner. Therefore, an area of malignant disease will appear bright on delayed imaging when compared with the normal liver parenchyma (Fig. 60-21).

In a related technique, iodinated oil is infused selectively into the hepatic artery, and delayed CT imaging is performed 1 to 4 weeks later. Kupffer cells in normal liver parenchyma will remove the oil-based contrast over time, whereas areas of disease will have defective excretion and will remain enhanced for several weeks. This technique is reported to have sensitivities comparable to CTAP and is performed frequently in Japan, where there is a high incidence of hepatic neoplasms.[51]

New Techniques

CT portography using three-dimensional reconstruction recently has been reported.[83,84] In a limited series, three-dimensional imaging demonstrated increased accuracy in determining the segmental location of hepatic neoplasms when compared with conventional two-dimensional methods. This is due to the better definition of anatomic landmarks and lesion extension that can be seen in three dimensions. This technique may gain further importance as surgeons become increasingly aggressive in treating hepatic cancers for cure.

A preliminary study using magnetic resonance portography demonstrates increased liver-to-lesion definition when compared with conventional MRI techniques.[85] This is performed using the same principles as CTAP. A low dose of gadopentetate dimeglumine is infused into the superior mesenteric artery during breath-holding gradient-echo or rapid acquisition spin-echo imaging. With the anticipated introduction of organ-specific MRI contrast agents and advanced MRI pulse sequencing, the future role of this invasive MRI technique is unclear.

Conclusion

The imaging options available to diagnose and stage patients with liver disease are extensive. MRI, conventional CT, nuclear medicine, angiography, conventional and intraoperative ultrasound, and CT during arterial portography all play pivotal roles in hepatic imaging. An important distinction must be made between screening patients for hepatic disease and staging patients with known malignancies. CTAP is the most sensitive technique for the preoperative identification of small intrahepatic lesions. However, because of its invasive technique and increased cost, CTAP is reserved for staging patients with known hepatic tumors and for planning operative procedures. Although it is a technically demanding procedure to perform and interpret, CTAP provides preoperative anatomic information not available from any other imaging modality.

Acknowledgments

Portions of this chapter (pages 1541–1546), including Table 60-2 and Figures 60-15 to 60-21, were reprinted with permission from Baum RA. CT during arterial portography: a review. Applied Radiology 1992 (March): 43–48.

References

1. Blakemore AH, Lord JW Jr. Technique of using vitallium tubes in establishing portacaval shunts for portal hypertension. Ann Surg 1945;122:476.
2. Whipple AO. The problem of portal hypertension in relation to the hepatosplenopathies. Ann Surg 1945;128:449.
3. Child CG III, O'Sullivan WD, Payne MA, McClure RD Jr. Portal venography: preliminary report. Radiology 1951;57:691.
4. Moore GE, Bridenbaugh RB. Portal venography. Surgery 1950;28:827.
5. Rousselot LM, Ruzicka FF Jr, Doehmer GA. Portal venography via portal and percutaneous splenic routes: anatomical and clinical studies. Surgery 1953;34:557.
6. Abeatici S, Campi L. Sur les possibilités de l'angiographie hépatique—la visualisation du système portal (recherches expérimentales). Acta Radiol 1951;36:383.
7. Leger L. Phlébographie portale par injection splénique intraparenchymateuse. Mem Acad Chir (Paris) 1951;77:712.
8. Bergstrand I, Ekman C-A. Percutaneous lieno-portal venography. Acta Radiol 1957;47:269.
9. Bookstein JJ, Whitehouse WM. Splenoportography. Radiol Clin North Am 1964;2:447.
10. Figley MM. Splenoportography: some advantages and disadvantages. AJR 1958;80:313.
11. Kogutt MS, Jander HP. Splenoportography—a valuable diagnostic technic revisited. South Med J 1977;70:1210.
12. Panke WF, Bradley EG, Moreno AH, Ruzicka FF Jr, Rousselot LM. Technique, hazards and usefulness of percutaneous splenic portography. JAMA 1959;169:1032.
13. Weitzman JJ, Stanley P. Splenoportography in the pediatric age group. J Pediatr Surg 1978;13:707.
14. Rigler LG, Olfelt PC, Krumbach RW. Roentgen hepatography by injection of a contrast medium into the aorta. Radiology 1953;60:363.
15. Ödman P. Percutaneous selective angiography of the coeliac artery. Acta Radiol (Stockh) 1958;Suppl 159.
16. Boijsen E, Ekman C-A, Olin T. Coeliac and superior mesenteric angiography in portal hypertension. Acta Chir Scand 1963;126:315.
17. Pollard JJ, Nebesar RA. Catheterization of the splenic artery for portal venography. N Engl J Med 1964;271:234.
18. Bron KM. Selective visceral and total abdominal arteriography via the left axillary artery in the older age group. AJR 1966;97:432.
19. Seldinger SI. Catheter replacement of needle in percutaneous arteriography: new technique. Acta Radiol 1953;39:368.
20. Bron KM, Riley RR, Girdany BR. Pediatric arteriography in abdominal and extremity lesions: clinical experience, indications and technic. Radiology 1969;92:1241.
21. Boijsen E, Redman HC. Effect of bradykinin on celiac and superior mesenteric angiography. Invest Radiol 1966;1:422.
22. Redman HC, Reuter SR, Miller WJ. Improvement of superior mesenteric and portal vein visualization with tolazoline. Invest Radiol 1969;4:24.
23. Cioffi CM, Ruzicka FF Jr, Carillo FJ, Gould HR. Enhanced visualization of the portal system using phentolamine and isoproterenol in combination. Radiology 1973;108:43.
24. Danford RO, Davidson AJ. The use of glucagon as a vasodilator in visceral angiography. Radiology 1969;93:173.
25. Boijsen E, Redman HC. Effect of epinephrine on celiac and superior mesenteric angiography. Invest Radiol 1967;2:184.
26. Widrich WC, Nordahl DL, Robbins AH. Contrast enhancement of the mesenteric and portal veins using intra-arterial papaverine. AJR 1974;121:374.
27. Jonsson K, Wallace S, Jacobson ED, Anderson JH, Zornoza J, Granmayeh M. The use of prostaglandin E₁ for enhanced visualization of the splanchnic circulation. Radiology 1977;125:373.
28. Folin J. Complications of percutaneous femoral catheterization for renal angiography. Radiologe 1968;8:190.
29. Halpern M. Percutaneous transfemoral arteriography. AJR 1964;92:918.
30. Lang EK. A survey of the complications of percutaneous retrograde arteriography. Radiology 1963;81:257.
31. Bron KM, Fisher B. Arterial portography: indications and technique. Surgery 1967;61:137.
32. Herlinger H. Arterioportography. Clin Radiol 1978;29:255.
33. Kuroyangi Y, Takagi H, Imanaga H. Significance of selective arteriographic patterns in the celiac axis and superior mesenteric artery in portal hypertension. Am J Surg 1976;132:664.
34. Levine E. Preoperative angiographic assessment of portal venous hypertension. S Afr Med J 1977;52:103.
35. Nebesar RA, Pollard JJ. Portal venography by selective arterial catheterization. AJR 1966;97:477.
36. Ruzicka FF Jr, Rossi P. Arterial portography: patterns of venous flow. Radiology 1969;92:777.
37. Leger L. L'inversion du courant portal—les fausses images

d'obstacle à la circulation sur le tronc porte. Presse Med 1956; 64:1189.

38. Moreno AH, Burchell AR, Reddy RV, Steen JA, Panke WF, Nealon TF. Spontaneous reversal of portal blood flow. Ann Surg 1975;181:346.
39. Burchell AR, Moreno AH, Panke WF, Rousselot LM. Some limitations of splenic portography. Ann Surg 1965;162:981.
40. Ekman C-A. Portal hypertension, diagnosis and surgical treatment. Acta Chir Scand 1957;Suppl 222.
41. Atkinson M, Barnett E, Sherlock S, Steiner RE. The clinical investigation of the portal circulation with special reference to portal venography. OJ Med 1955;24:77.
42. Bron KM, Jackson FC, Haller J, Perez-Stable E, Eisen HB, Poller S. The value of selective arteriography in demonstrating portal and splenic vein patency following nonvisualization by splenoportography. Radiology 1965;85:448.
43. Morrow CE, Grage TB, Sutherland DER, et al. Hepatic resection from secondary neoplasms. Surgery 1982;92:610–614.
44. Adson MA. Hepatic neoplasms in perspective. AJR 1983;140: 695–700.
45. Adson MA, Van Heerden JA, Adson MH, et al. Resection of hepatic metastases from colorectal cancer. Arch Surg 1984;119: 647–651.
46. Hughes KS, Rosenstein RB, Songhorabod S, et al. Resection of the liver for colorectal carcinoma metastases: a multi-institutional study of indications for resection. Surgery 1988;103: 278–288.
47. Takayasu K, Moriyama N, Muramatsu Y, et al. The diagnosis of small hepatocellular carcinomas: efficacy of various imaging procedures in 100 patients. AJR 1990;155:49–54.
48. Nelson RC, Chezmar JL, Sugarbaker PH, et al. Hepatic tumors: comparison of CT during arterial portography, delayed CT, and MR imaging for preoperative evaluation. Radiology 1989;172:27–34.
49. Miller DL, Simmons JT, Chang R, et al. Hepatic metastasis detection: comparison of three CT contrast-enhancement methods. Radiology 1987;165:785–790.
50. Heiken JP, Weyman PJ, Lee JKT, et al. Detection of focal hepatic masses: prospective evaluation with CT, delayed CT, CT during arterial portography, and MR imaging. Radiology 1989; 171:47–51.
51. Merine D, Takayasu K, Wakao F. Detection of hepatocellular carcinoma: comparison of CT during arterial portography with CT after intraarterial injection of iodized oil. Radiology 1990; 175:707–710.
52. Onik GM, Zemel R, Weaver MD, et al. Comparison of CT portography with intraoperative hepatic US. Presented at the 77th Scientific Assembly and Annual Meeting of the Radiological Society of North America, December 1991, Chicago, Illinois.
53. Garbagnati F, Spreafico C, Marchiano A, et al. Staging of hepatocellular carcinoma by ultrasonography, computed tomography, and angiography: the role of CT combined with arterial portography. Gastrointest Radiol 1991;16:225–228.
54. Ferrucci JT. Liver tumor imaging. Cancer 1991;67:1189–1195.
55. Hisa N, Hiramatsu K, Narimatsu Y, et al. Detection of hepatic neoplasms by computed tomography in portal hepatogram phase. Jpn J Clin Radiol 1980;25:529–534.
56. Matsui O, Kadoya M, Suzuki M, et al. Work in progress: dynamic sequential computed tomography during arterial portography in the detection of hepatic neoplasms. Radiology 1983;146:721–727.
57. Yamaguchi A, Ishida T, Nishimura G, et al. Detection by CT during arterial portography of colorectal cancer metastases to liver. Dis Colon Rectum 1991;34:37–40.
58. Lundstedt C, Götberg, Lunderquist A, et al. Computed tomographic angiography of the liver via the coeliac axis. Acta Radiol 1986;27:285.
59. Freeny PC, Marks WM: Computed tomographic arteriography of the liver. Radiology 1983;148:193–197.
60. Nakao N, Miura K, Takayasu Y, et al. CT angiography in hepa-

tocellular carcinoma. J Comput Assist Tomogr 1983;7:780–787.
61. Prando A, Wallace S, Bernardino ME, et al. Computed tomographic arteriography of the liver. Radiology 1979;130:697–701.
62. Matsui O, Takashima T, Kadoya M, et al. Dynamic computed tomography during arterial portography: the most sensitive examination for small hepatocellular carcinomas. J Comput Assist Tomogr 1985;9:19–24.
63. Matsui O, Takashima T, Kadoya M, et al. Liver metastases from colorectal cancers: detection with CT during arterial portography. Radiology 1987;163:65–69.
64. Nelson RC, Chezmar JL, Sugarbaker PH, et al. Preoperative localization of focal liver lesions to specific liver segments: utility of CT during arterial portography. Radiology 1990;176: 89–94.
65. Oliver JH, Baron RL, Dodd GD III, et al. Efficacy of CT portography in the evaluation of cirrhotic patients for hepatocellular carcinoma. Presented at the 77th Scientific Assembly and Annual Meeting of the Radiological Society of North America, December 1991, Chicago, Illinois.
66. Soyer PA, Vavasseur D, Breittmayer F Sr, et al. Influence of CT portography on surgical decision-making in liver metastases from colorectal cancer. Presented at the 77th Scientific Assembly and Annual Meeting of the Radiological Society of North America, December 1991, Chicago, Illinois.
67. Reinig JW, Sanchez FW, Vujic I. Hemodynamics of portal blood flow shown by CT portography. Radiology 1985;154: 473–476.
68. Itai Y, Furui S, Ohtomo K. Dynamic CT features of arterioportal shunts in hepatocellular carcinoma. AJR 1986;146:723–727.
69. Paulson EK, Baker ME, Meyers W, et al. CT arterial portography: causes of technical failures and enhancement variability. Presented at the 77th Scientific Assembly and Annual Meeting of the Radiological Society of North America, December 1991, Chicago, Illinois.
69a. Van Beers B, Pringot J, Trigaux JP, et al. Hepatic heterogeneity on CT in Budd-Chiari syndrome: correlation with regional disturbances in portal flow. Gastrointest Radiol 1988;13:61–66.
70. Fernandez MP, Bernardino ME. Pseudolesions versus neoplasm on CT arterial portography: aids in diagnosis. Presented at the 77th Scientific Assembly and Annual Meeting of the Radiological Society of North America, December 1991, Chicago, Illinois.
71. Peterson MS, Baron RL, Zajko AB, et al. Imaging-pathologic correlation of hepatic parenchymal perfusion defects detected with CT arterial portography. Presented at the 77th Scientific Assembly and Annual Meeting of the Radiological Society of North America, December 1991, Chicago, Illinois.
72. Freeny PC, Marks WM. Hepatic perfusion abnormalities during CT angiography: detection and interpretation. Radiology 1986;159:685–691.
73. Itai Y, Moss AA, Goldberg HI. Transient hepatic attenuation difference of lobar or segmental distribution detected by dynamic computed tomography. Radiology 1982;144:835–839.
74. Itai Y, Hachiya J, Makita K, et al. Transient hepatic attenuation differences on dynamic computed tomography. J Comput Assist Tomogr 1987;11:461–465.
75. Thompson GH, Nelson RC, Chezmar JL, et al. CT during arterial portography: gamut of perfusion abnormalities (exhibit). Presented at the 77th Scientific Assembly and Annual Meeting of the Radiological Society of North America, December 1991, Chicago, Illinois.
76. Van Beers B, Pringot J, Gigot J-F, et al. Nontumorous attenuation differences on computed tomographic portography. Gastrointest Radiol 1990;15:107–111.
77. Savader BBI, Fishman EK, Savader SJ: Hepatic cavernous hemangioma: potential pitfall of CT angiographic portography. Presented at the 77th Scientific Assembly and Annual Meeting of the Radiological Society of North America, December 1991, Chicago, Illinois.

78. Tyrrel RT, Kaufman SL, Bernardino ME. Straight line sign: appearance and significance during CT portography. Radiology 1989;173:635–637.

79. Matsui O, Takashima T, Kadoya M, et al. Segmental staining on hepatic arteriography as a sign of intrahepatic portal vein obstruction. Radiology 1984;152:601–606.

80. Itai Y, Ohtomo K, Kokubo T, et al. Segmental intensity differences in the liver on MR images: a sign of intrahepatic portal flow stoppage. Radiology 1988;167:17–19.

81. Fernandez MP, Bernardino ME. Hepatic pseudolesion: appearance of focal low attenuation in the medial segment of the left lobe at CT arterial portography. Radiology 1991;181:809–812.

82. Matsui O, Kadoya M, Kameyama T, et al. Benign and malignant nodules in cirrhotic livers: distinction based on blood supply. Radiology 1991;178:493–497.

83. Soyer P, Roche A, Gad M, et al. Preoperative segmental localization of hepatic metastases: utility of three-dimensional CT during arterial portography. Radiology 1991;180:653–658.

84. Soyer PA, Breittmayer F Sr, Gad MM Sr, et al. Three-dimensional CT imaging of hepatic metastases (exhibit). Presented at the 77th Scientific Assembly and Annual Meeting of the Radiological Society of North America, December 1991, Chicago, Illinois.

85. Pavone P, Siuliani S, Cardone G, et al. Intraarterial portography with gadopentetate dimeglumine: improved liver-to-lesion contrast in MR imaging. Radiology 1991;179:693–697.

61

Superior Mesenteric Angiography

ERIK BOIJSEN

Superior mesenteric angiography is performed less often today than it was when the previous edition of *Angiography*[1] became available. During the 1980s, noninvasive methods, including ultrasonography (US), computed tomography (CT), radionuclide imaging (RNI), and magnetic resonance imaging (MRI), have replaced most abdominal angiographic diagnostic procedures, particularly of abdominal parenchymatous organs. The gastrointestinal tube is not examined to the same extent by noninvasive methods (except with RNI) because endoscopy and barium studies in most cases give adequate information. One reason for the diminished use of superior mesenteric angiography is that RNI has become a primary method for diagnosing gastrointestinal hemorrhage and inflammatory bowel lesions. Another reason is that the information from color Doppler imaging, duplex Doppler, and magnetic resonance angiography (MRA) continuously improves, reducing the need for the more invasive angiographic techniques.

Despite these changes, the spatial resolution and the total vascular display are still better with conventional superior mesenteric angiography than with any other method. For this reason, there will always be a place for superior mesenteric angiography in the diagnosis of bowel disease. The technique will be different, mainly with digital subtraction, than it was a decade ago. The most important indications are to confirm the exact site of hemorrhage and its cause so that one can preoperatively map the vascular morphology and treat bowel lesions with various interventional methods. An intense clinical research program was initiated by Stanley Baum and his collaborators.[2-4] This chapter is intended to show the central role superior mesenteric angiography has taken in the diagnosis of intestinal disease. Its role in gastrointestinal hemorrhage is described in Chapter 25 of *Abrams' Angiography: Interventional Radiology*.

Anatomy

Anatomic and topographic studies of the blood supply of the small and large bowel through dissection, corrosion, and arteriography of autopsy specimens have extensively demonstrated the normal variations of the superior mesenteric artery.[5-14] However, the anatomic studies cannot replace a well-documented analysis of a series of normal superior mesenteric angiograms, especially when correlations are made to dissection studies.[15,16]

Arteries

The extensive work of Michels et al.[14,15] provides detailed information on the anatomy of the superior mesenteric artery. The following description is based mainly on their work.

The superior mesenteric artery originates from the anterior aspect of the aorta at the level of the 12th thoracic to the 2nd lumbar vertebral bodies.[7] It arises 1 to 20 mm below the origin of the celiac artery. Rarely, the superior mesenteric artery arises from the celiac artery as a celiomesenteric trunk. The first part of the superior mesenteric artery is immediately posterior to the body of the pancreas and can be surrounded by this organ when the uncinate process extends medially. The relationship of the superior mesenteric artery to surrounding structures is well observed on CT, particularly when the artery is enhanced after intravenous contrast medium injection.[17] Without contrast enhancement the artery was observed in 89 percent of cases,[18] whereas with enhancement the superior mesenteric artery was shown in 98 percent.[19] At US the superior mesenteric artery was observed in 91 percent of cases.[18]

The width of the main stem varies from 6 to 16

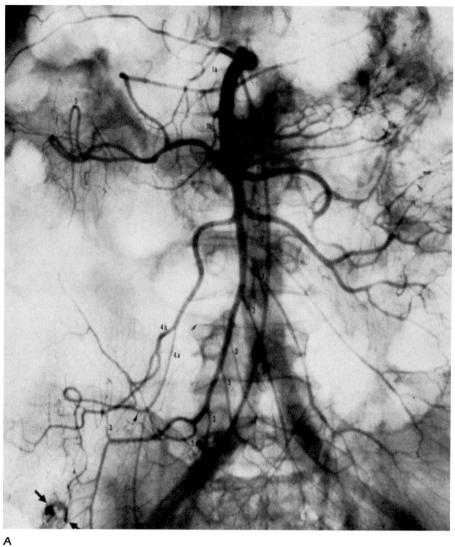

A

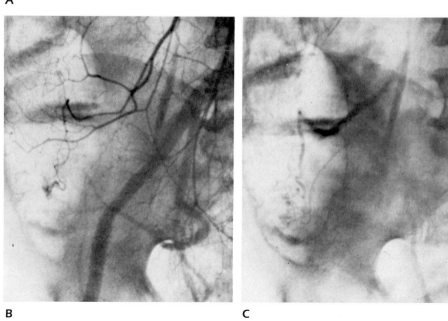

B   C

mm[14] or from 8.0 to 15.5 mm.[7] At angiography the width of the artery has been observed to be 8 to 10 mm,[20] 5 to 13 mm,[21] and 6.7 to 12.3 mm (mean 9.5).[22] The slightly lower figures found at angiography may depend on the fact that the measurements were made in the anteroposterior projection. In this view the first part of the superior mesenteric artery is not observed because the vessel runs more or less parallel to the central ray. Hearn[23] found in a small series of angiographic studies that the artery normally coursed in a 45- to 60-degree angle to the aorta. The author has often observed a 90-degree angle. The course of the first part of the superior mesenteric artery depends mainly on the amount of adipose tissue in the abdomen.

Certain anatomic landmarks are seen at superior mesenteric angiography, and they should always be defined (Fig. 61-1). These are the inferior pancreaticoduodenal artery, the jejunal arteries, the ileal arteries, and the ileocolic artery. Less often found but usually present are the right and the middle colic arteries. Finally, the hepatic, pancreatic, and gastric arteries may occasionally arise from the superior mesenteric artery.

With color Doppler imaging and MRA the origin and flow through the first part of the superior mesenteric artery and its relation to the aorta can be well demonstrated.

Inferior Pancreaticoduodenal Artery

This vessel arises either from the main stem or from the first jejunal artery. It may arise as a single artery or as one anterior and one posterior branch with separate origins. When arising from the first jejunal artery, it passes behind the superior mesenteric artery; when directly from the superior mesenteric artery, it passes from the right side directly to the duodenum and pancreas. An intercommunicating arterial arcade between the inferior pancreaticoduodenal artery and the first jejunal artery, according to Michels et al.,[14] is present in approximately 60 percent of individuals. This arcade, which supplies the fourth part of the duodenum, represents an important anastomotic arcade in occlusive disease.

Jejunal and Ileal Arteries

These vessels vary in number and size. Because there is no distinct anatomic border between the jejunum and the ileum, there is no way to decide where the jejunal arteries end and the ileal arteries begin. As a general rule, it is simplest to regard those arteries that arise from the superior mesenteric artery before the origin of the ileocolic artery as jejunal arteries, and those distal to this origin as ileal arteries. The jejunal arteries number between 2 and 7, and the ileal arteries between 7 and 17, not including those supplying the terminal ileum. The latter is supplied by 3 to 15 branches originating from the ileal branch of the ileocolic artery. This ileal branch anastomoses directly with the distal part of the superior mesenteric artery, forming a distal arcade (see Fig. 61-1).

The presence of intraarterial arcades is characteristic of the mesenteric circulation. The number of arcades varies at different levels from one to five; the largest number is observed in the midportion of the small bowel, the smallest in the terminal ileum. The long vasa recta of the small bowel arise from the last arcades, which are close to the mesenteric border. These vasa recta pass to the anterior and posterior surface of the bowel wall, but in humans they usually do not communicate at the antimesenteric border because they penetrate the bowel wall and enter the submucosal layer earlier. The short vasa recta arising from the last arcade directly or branching from the long vasa enter the submucosa of the intestinal wall at its mesenteric border. A rich interarterial anastomotic network among the vasa recta is present in the small bowel wall, but the connections in the large bowel are poor.[8] Angiographically the vasa recta of the jejunum appear wider and more tortuous than those of the ileum (see Fig. 61-1). Usually the width of the ileal arteries decreases distally, and the smallest vessels are observed in the terminal ileum.

Because of the large number of intercommunicating arcades in the mesenteric circulation, there is, as in the large bowel, an arterial channel running parallel to the mesenteric border. The vasa recta take their origin from this channel. It has the same importance in

---

◄ **Figure 61-1.** Angiomatous lesion of the cecum in a 55-year-old man with melena and anemia for 3 months. Gastrointestinal studies were normal. (A) At superior mesenteric arteriography a 10 × 10 mm area of the cecum showed an abnormal blood supply with wide, tortuous arteries and early shunting to the veins (*lower arrows*). Anatomic landmarks: The posterior inferior pancreaticoduodenal artery (*1a*) arises from the aberrant branch of the right hepatic artery. The anterior inferior pancreaticoduodenal artery (*1b*) arises from the first jejunal artery (*2*). Four jejunal (*2*) and eight ileal arteries (*3*) are observed. The ileocolic artery divides into ileal (*4a*) and colic (*4b*) branches. A short arcade (*upper arrow*) is present between the two arteries. The right colic artery (*5*) arises from the middle colic artery (*6*). (B and C) After injection of 5 μg of norepinephrine, a repeat angiogram demonstrates a general decrease in the width of all arteries, but the dysplastic lesion is not affected by the drug and is therefore better observed.

maintaining the viability of the small intestine as the marginal artery of Drummond has for the large intestine. The two channels communicate via the arcades in the terminal ileum and thus form an uninterrupted pathway from the duodenum to the rectum. Because these channels can be demonstrated with angiography and represent important collateral pathways in vascular disease or after surgery, they should be identified at superior mesenteric angiography. Because there are few communications between the vasa recta of the large bowel, preservation of the marginal artery is essential in colonic resection.[13]

Ileocolic Artery

This is the only constant artery from the right side of the superior mesenteric artery. It supplies the terminal ileum, the appendix, the cecum, and the proximal part of the ascending colon. Distal extension of supply may occur when the right colic artery is absent or originates from the ileocolic artery.

The ileocolic artery divides into one colic and one ileal artery. Usually there is an ileocolic arcade between them. The ileal artery communicates directly with the superior mesenteric artery. The terminal ileum has a precarious blood supply because the arcade at the mesenteric border, the recurrent ileal artery, is missing in 61 percent of individuals, and in 16 percent there is a 3- to 5-cm segment of distal ileum without vasa recta.[14] At arteriography of autopsy specimens this area is hard to fill adequately.[12] At superior mesenteric angiography the vasa recta of the terminal ileum are difficult or impossible to define, and the accumulation of contrast medium in the wall is often insignificant. With magnification techniques, however, more information is obtained about these small vessels.[24]

Right Colic Artery

This vessel has a variable origin from the superior mesenteric, middle colic, or ileocolic artery. It supplies the ascending colon and hepatic flexure.

Middle Colic Artery

This vessel supplies the transverse colon. It usually arises from the first part of the superior mesenteric artery at the level of the first jejunal artery but may originate more distally or from the celiac artery. An accessory middle colic artery is rarely present, and then is named the middle mesenteric artery.[25] The left branch of the middle colic artery is in direct communication with the left colic artery from the inferior mesenteric artery. This channel is the most important collateral in the mesenteric circulation. It proceeds in a proximal direction as the right branch of the middle colic artery, the right colic artery, and the ileocolic artery. A second collateral pathway is the marginal artery of Drummond, which represents the arcades along the mesenteric border of the colon. This marginal artery is usually not complete because the vasa recta of the transverse colon often arise directly from the middle colic artery. Riolan's artery is a third anastomosis between the superior and inferior mesenteric arteries. It is a short, direct connection running retroperitoneally from the root of the superior mesenteric artery or one of its primary branches to the inferior mesenteric artery or one of its branches.[10]

The common hepatic or, more often, the right hepatic artery may originate from the superior mesenteric artery. According to Michels et al.,[14] this occurs in 16 percent of individuals, which finding is in agreement with angiographic observations.[21,26-28] Not uncommonly seen are the dorsal pancreatic, transverse pancreatic, and gastroduodenal arteries with their origin from the first part of the superior mesenteric artery.

Collateral Arteries

"A knowledge of collateral circulation is of fundamental importance in surgical interference with the intestinal blood supply."[14] The same is true for the proper understanding of the angiographic study. More than 50 collateral pathways are listed by Michels et al. in the small and large bowels, and for complete information the reader is referred to their work.[14] In addition to those arcades in the mesenteric circulation mentioned previously, the pancreatic and pancreaticoduodenal arteries serve as collaterals in stenosis or occlusion of the main stem of the superior mesenteric artery (Figs. 61-2 and 61-3). The collateral arteries from the inferior mesenteric artery are also important in this type of lesion. Further connections are the epiploic arteries, at least in more distal occlusion of the superior mesenteric artery. Retroperitoneal parietal arteries, including renal capsular arteries, inferior phrenic arteries, and arteries supplying the adipose tissue of the mesentery, are also collateral vessels that may take part in the bowel supply in vascular occlusion (see Fig. 61-2).[12,29,30]

The dilatation of the collateral arteries may be extreme, and aneurysm formation may occur. Extirpation of an aneurysm of the widened pancreaticoduodenal artery in a patient with complete stenosis of the celiac artery can lead to a disaster with hepatic, gastroduodenal, and pancreatic necrosis.

Veins

The superior mesenteric vein follows the course of the superior mesenteric artery. The veins following the vasa recta are usually duplicated. At superior mesen-

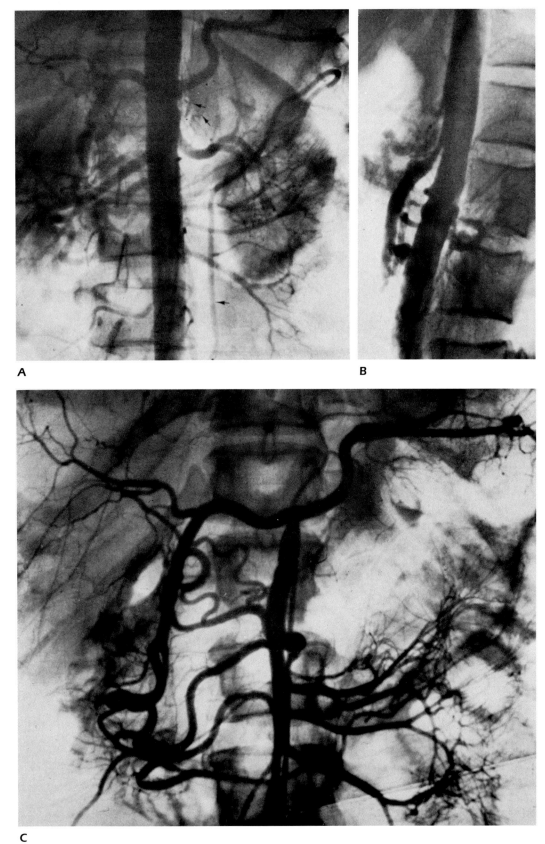

A

B

C

Figure 61-2. Occlusion of celiac axis and marked concentric stenosis of the superior mesenteric artery in a 31-year-old woman with postprandial pain and malabsorption. (A and B) At lumbar aortography the arterial constrictions are observed, as well as collateral circulation from the inferior mesenteric artery (*lower arrow*, A). Retroperitoneal collaterals are present to the left of the aorta (*upper arrows*, A). (C) At superior mesenteric angiography the complete celiac arterial system is contrast-filled via wide pancreaticoduodenal arcades. The stenosis is not observed in this view.

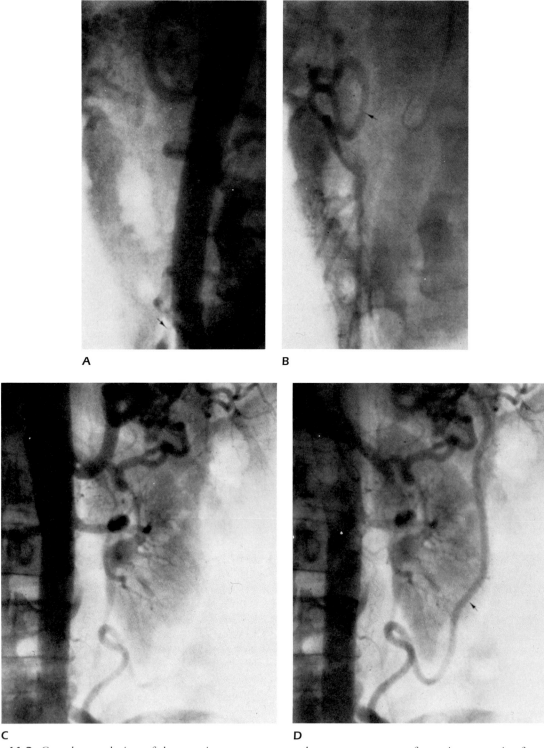

A

B

C

D

Figure 61-3. Complete occlusion of the superior mesenteric artery and of the common hepatic artery at its origin from the celiac artery and marked stenosis of the celiac and inferior mesenteric arteries in a 58-year-old man who had no gastrointestinal symptoms. Aortography in lateral (A and B) and left posterior oblique (C to E) projections was performed after percutaneous puncture of the left axillary artery to demonstrate patency of a previous operation for occlusion at the aortic bifurcation. Wide pancreatic arterial collaterals from the splenic artery supply the hepatic artery. The wide left and middle colic arteries (*arrows,* B, D, and E) supply the superior mesenteric artery from the stenotic inferior mesenteric artery (*arrow,* A).

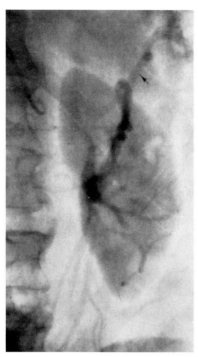

E   **Figure 61-3** (continued).

teric angiography the mesenteric veins are seldom well demonstrated unless a lesion is present or special techniques are used to delineate them.

Both anatomy and flow are best demonstrated by duplex and color Doppler or MRA. On transverse sections at US and CT, the superior mesenteric vein is usually observed to the right and anterior to the superior mesenteric artery. This important landmark is changed in malrotation.[17,31,32] This malalignment has been observed in MRA.[33]

Physiologic Considerations

Superior mesenteric blood flow is two to three times greater than blood flow to one renal artery.[34] The total capacity of the splanchnic circulation, of which the superior mesenteric artery conveys the main part, is as great as the entire blood volume.[35] The regulation of the mesenteric circulation is complex. Although humoral, neurogenic, and cardiovascular factors play the dominant roles, autoregulation and arteriovenous shunting are also important components of this control process that must be recognized in order to understand the variations in splanchnic blood flow in normal and pathologic situations.[35–37]

In vascular shock the size of the vascular bed is markedly reduced.[38–40] Vasoactive substances administered by intravenous or intraarterial injection cause a complex response in the superior mesenteric vascular bed that depends on autoregulatory escape and on the tone of the intestinal wall.[35,41] The effects of such substances have in part been confirmed by intraarterial injections in combination with superior mesenteric angiography.[42–52] Bowel distention and increased intraluminal pressure have a profound influence on intestinal blood flow[53,54]; at angiography a decreased flow and arteriovenous shunting are observed.[24]

Superior mesenteric artery blood flow can be examined with a variety of methods in vivo. The first techniques using a spill-over flowmeter[55] or dye dilution[51] are now replaced by duplex Doppler and pulsed Doppler.[56] For the blood flow in the superior mesenteric and portal veins, Doppler US and MRI are used most often.[57]

Technique and Complications

Originally, selective angiography was performed with antegrade technique after cutdown of the brachial artery.[58,59] The retrograde technique with percutaneous puncture of the femoral artery, as recommended by Ödman,[60] has replaced the antegrade method. Only in selected cases, when the femoral technique has failed because of advanced atherosclerosis, is the antegrade method used; percutaneous puncture of the axillary artery is then employed,[61–63] (see Fig. 61-3).[61–63] A thin-walled red Ödman-Ledin catheter (inner diameter 1.4 mm; outer diameter 2.2 mm) was previously used irrespective of the percutaneous route taken.[64] During the past decade, because of the improved resolution in the image-intensifier–television system, the catheters and guidewires used for superior mesenteric angiography are smaller (4–5 French), and coaxial catheters (3 French) are used at superselective catheterization of branches of the superior mesenteric artery with steerable guidewires (0.41 mm) and with open-end guidewires.[65–68] With these small instruments the catheterization may be performed from the brachial artery.

The optimal type and amount of contrast media have been extensively considered because serious complications in terms of bowel necrosis have been observed both clinically and experimentally.[69–73] Initially, out of concern for possible bowel injury, small amounts of dilute contrast media were commonly used, although the information provided was incomplete. Because no complications were observed, larger doses and more concentrated contrast media were used. A reevaluation of previous complications suggested that they were largely caused by the technique employed and the effects of the earlier, more toxic contrast agents. The experimentally produced bowel necroses seemed to be the result of temporary vascular occlusion, which permitted prolonged contact of the toxic contrast medium with the intima. A repeat experimental study could not reproduce the toxic effects when the superior mesenteric artery was not occluded by the catheter, even when larger contrast doses were used.[74] Temporary occlusion of the superior mesenteric artery with a balloon catheter during contrast medium injection did not damage the bowel.[75] However, electron microscopic analysis has shown mitochondrial changes caused by contrast media injected into the superior mesenteric artery of the rabbit, suggesting damage to the intracellular enzyme production.[76] The significant elevation of SGOT and alkaline phosphatase observed in dogs after contrast injection suggests possible liver damage in these animals.[77]

The clinical use of 40 to 50 ml of a 76 percent solution of methylglucamine salts of metrizoate, diatrizoate, or iothalamate has not caused any complications, even when the dose is repeated. During the past decade the high-osmolar ionic contrast media have been almost completely replaced by the low-osmolar ionic media (ioxaglate) or nonionic media (iopamidol, iohexol). They are used with about the same concentration of iodine (300 mg I/ml), but they cause less pain.[78] Whatever contrast medium is used, it should be delivered at a rate of 7 to 10 ml per second. The transit of the contrast medium to the veins is followed by a series of exposures in the anteroposterior projection for at least 20 seconds. For complete evaluation of the superior mesenteric artery, a short series with approximately 15 ml of contrast medium in the lateral view is necessary. Before the full dose of contrast medium is delivered, a test injection with 10 ml should be performed under fluoroscopic control to avoid subintimal injection. Despite this precaution, subintimal deposition of contrast medium may occur, but in the author's experience it has not had any severe sequelae. After translumbar aortography, however, several serious accidents with bowel necrosis or paralytic ileus have been reported.[79-81]

When there is simultaneous injection into the celiac and superior mesenteric arteries, the flow of the contrast medium is commonly observed to be slower through the superior mesenteric artery than through the splenic or hepatic arteries.[82] The reason is not clear, and the variance is contradictory to the physiologic findings of superior mesenteric flow. The contrast medium may cause an initial vasoconstriction in the superior mesenteric arterioles, which may also explain the usually poor opacification of the superior mesenteric vein. Or it may be that the deformed red blood cells have greater difficulty in passing through the mesenteric vascular bed as compared with that of the splenic or hepatic. The prolonged contact of the hypertonic contrast medium with the capillaries results in an increase in intravascular fluid with consequent dilution of the medium. The response to selective injection will within 20 seconds be vasodilation with increased mesenteric flow lasting for 15 minutes.[83] Thus, when a larger amount of contrast medium is used and the injection period is markedly extended, the vasodilating effect is dominant. The contrast medium is less diluted and the venous information is consequently enhanced.[84,85] The poor visualization of the superior mesenteric vein is also observed with the nonionic contrast media. The reason is probably the effect on red blood cell crenation rather than the tonicity of the contrast medium.

There is no objection to single doses of larger amounts of contrast medium than were just recommended, but a complete angiographic study usually includes repeated injections into the superior mesenteric artery and also into the celiac axis. The total dose of contrast medium may then be too high. There is no defined upper limit to the total amounts of contrast medium that can be given to a patient over a period of 1 hour. The author's present policy is not to exceed a single dose of 1 ml per kilogram of body weight and to keep the total amount given to less than 3 ml per kilogram of body weight.

During the 1980s 100-mm photofluorography and digital subtraction angiography (DSA) have slowly replaced the conventional full-sized film-screen radiography in abdominal angiography. Eventually DSA will be the main type of filming because with this technique examination time decreases considerably.[86-90] The digital technique also means increased contrast resolution, so that contrast media can be injected in a smaller amount and at a lower concentration; consequently, smaller catheters are used. However, the method has some drawbacks, the most important being reduced spatial resolution, limited field of view, and misregistration artifacts due to respiratory and bowel movements.[86,87,89,90] Improvements in the digital technique have limited these drawbacks and will therefore rarely give any problems.

Other techniques for superior mesenteric angiography include the noninvasive imaging methods. Visualization of the superior mesenteric vessels with duplex Doppler and/or color Doppler,[91,92] CT,[17-19] and MRI[93,94] is now well established and will further reduce the indications for conventional superior mesenteric angiography.

Pharmacoangiography

Pharmacoangiography is now a well-established method and should be used in the mesenteric circulation whenever increased information about the mesenteric vein is required.

Vasodilation has been employed to improve the visualization of, for example, angiodysplastic lesions of the bowel.[95] Various vasodilating drugs have been used. The best and most consistent results are obtained with bradykinin and tolazoline,[42,46,74] but prostaglandin E_1 and F_2-alpha, isoproterenol, secretin, glucagon, cholecystokinin, and extended epinephrine infusion have been used with good results.[48–50,85,96–102] Injection of 20 to 30 ml of normal saline containing 5 ml of 2 percent Xylocaine immediately before the injection of contrast medium is said to cause good opacification of the superior mesenteric vein.[103]

Improved venous opacification may also be achieved when superior mesenteric angiography is performed during digestion.[104] The most reliable technique, not yet fully tested in humans, is to inject contrast medium after balloon occlusion of the superior mesenteric artery with release of the occlusion at the end of the contrast medium injection.[75,105] Higher venous concentrations of contrast have also been achieved experimentally by balloon occlusion of the celiac axis and contrast injection into the superior mesenteric artery.[106]

Injection of 5 to 10 μg of bradykinin into the superior mesenteric artery within 30 seconds before angiography has been, in the author's experience with more than 1000 patients, a reliable and safe method for demonstrating the superior mesenteric and portal veins. Although the bradykinin produces such an increased flow that arterial detail is lost, it usually causes a marked accumulation of contrast medium in the bowel wall, giving an "intestinogram," which can aid in demonstrating local abnormalities of the gut.

Because bradykinin is not widely available, tolazoline is sometimes substituted. Tolazoline enhances the venous opacification to approximately the same extent as bradykinin. The author's technique for obtaining maximum information about the venous system is to inject 25 mg tolazoline followed by 70 to 80 ml of the contrast medium, beginning at a slow rate of 2 to 3 ml per second and then increasing slowly to a rate of 10 ml per second. With this technique, advantage is taken of the dilating effect of both tolazoline and the contrast medium (Fig. 61-4). Tolazoline, however, may also be difficult to obtain, but prostaglandins may be available for use in this technique.

To enhance arterial detail and to differentiate an in-flammatory lesion from a tumor, *vasoconstrictive substances* may be helpful[43,45,52,107–112] (Fig. 61-5). Although no consistent advantage of this method has been demonstrated, it appears that the vessels of an active inflammatory lesion are more susceptible to constriction than are normal or tumor vessels.

Other methods of superior mesenteric angiography have also been used, including operative mesenteric angiography.[113–115] Because of the complicated procedures required during operation and the lack of serial films, the information afforded is less than that of conventional superior mesenteric angiography, despite the better arterial detail of operative angiography.

Routine superior mesenteric angiography does not always necessitate administration of drugs before contrast medium injection. On the contrary, in a routine study a small amount of contrast medium (20–30 ml) injected at a rate of 8 to 10 ml per second without any previous injection of drugs will often give the required information. A series of films covering about 20 seconds should be taken with a film speed of two frames per second for 5 seconds, one frame per second for 5 seconds, and one frame every other second for 10 seconds.

The arteriogram contains morphologic as well as functional information about the splanchnic vasculature; therefore, the emptying time of the arteries as well as the appearance time of the veins should be recorded. There is a sequential arterial emptying of contrast medium from the proximal jejunal to the distal ileal and colic arteries.[42,43,116,117] The appearance times for the veins are approximately in the same sequence. The contrast medium of the jejunal, ileal, and colic arteries disappears within 2 seconds after the end of injection, and the veins of the small bowel usually appear within 8 to 10 seconds after the start of the injection. Abnormalities in the sequence of filling and emptying of mesenteric arteries and veins can be a guide to the diagnosis of a variety of bowel disorders.[107,116–119]

Mesenteric Vascular Insufficiency

Stenosis or occlusion of the main stem or branches of the superior mesenteric artery produces symptoms of various types and severity. The results of surgical correction have been improving, in large part because angiography is being employed with greater frequency. The main clinical problem is to know when the patient has a vascular insufficiency and, if it is acute, to suspect a lesion early enough for adequate diagnosis and treatment. Angiography is the only method by which a

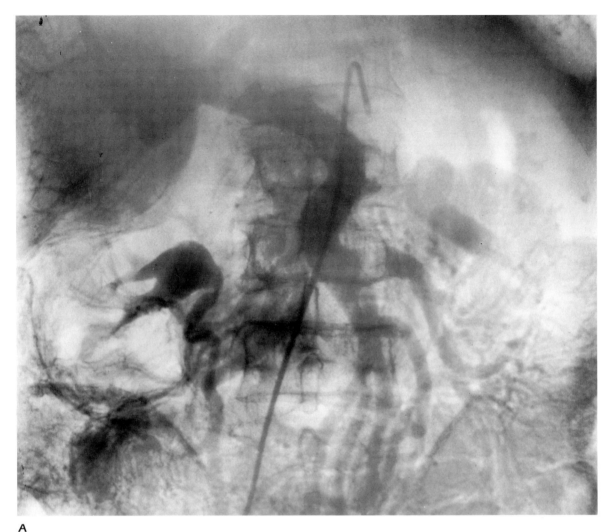

A

Figure 61-4. Venous phase of superior mesenteric angiogram after 25 mg tolazoline and 60 ml contrast medium were injected into the artery. (A) Normal venogram. (B) Portal hypertension with dilatation and reversal of flow in inferior mesenteric vein (*arrows*) in a patient with cholangiocarcinoma infiltrating the portal vein in the hilus of the liver.

reliable diagnosis can be made and is therefore an important part in the understanding of the morphologic and functional events that occur.

Acute Occlusion

Acute obstruction of the superior mesenteric artery or its branches causes symptoms that are difficult to interpret clinically. Diagnosis is therefore likely to be delayed, with serious consequences.[120] An important support for an early diagnosis of acute mesenteric ischemia is CT, which has an 85 percent sensitivity for bowel infarction.[121,122] On MRI information may be obtained of the aorta and the first part of the mesenteric arteries.[123]

Bowel ischemia may be due to acute arterial occlu-

sion (thrombosis or embolization), venous obstruction, and "nonocclusive ischemia." The clinical symptomatology is basically the same for all three causes and depends mainly on the duration of the ischemia. Because the therapeutic approach is contingent on whether an occlusion is present, the specific cause should be defined as precisely as possible. Even if plain films and CT may suggest a vascular catastrophe, angiography is the only method that provides information of importance for therapeutic activity. Although the patients are usually in poor general condition, angiography does not cause any additional risks to the patient or any essential delay in the therapy.[124–127]

Mortality is extremely high in this disease. Abnormalities are observed in the mucosa within minutes of the occlusion, followed by extensive necrosis with sub-

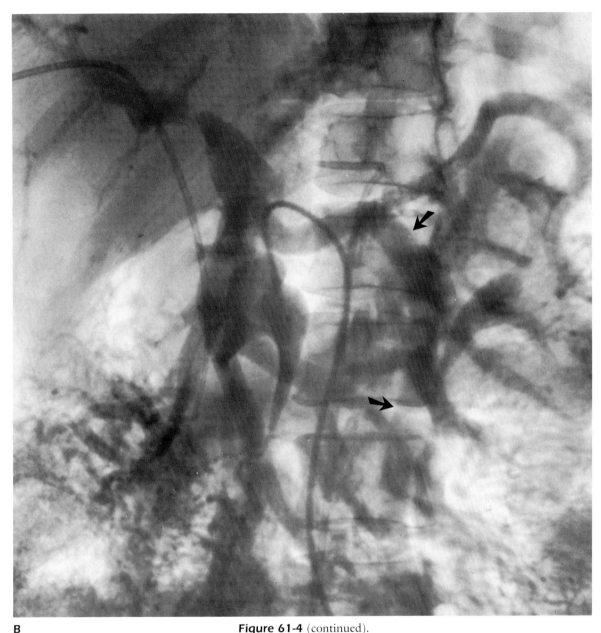

B   **Figure 61-4** (continued).

mucosal edema and hemorrhage. In the literature the maximum time delay between onset of occlusion and operation for successful result varies. Although it appears that irreversible damage to the bowel may occur within 12 hours of the occlusion,[128] good results have been obtained in patients who had angiography and operation within 24 hours of the occlusion.[129] In the world literature there are few cases of successful removal of emboli or thrombi; in 1974 there were 49 out of 69 patients surviving this type of operation.[130] An aggressive clinical approach will, however, reveal

more operable cases, consequently yielding a better outcome.[129,131,132] In the acute stage both CT and Doppler imaging will give indications for angiography, at which time also intraarterial infusion of streptokinase may be attempted before surgery is contemplated.[133,134]

The *angiographic examination* should start with a lumbar aortogram in lateral and frontal projections to define the degree of aortic atherosclerosis and occlusions of the main stems and first branches of the splanchnic arteries. If the main stem of the superior

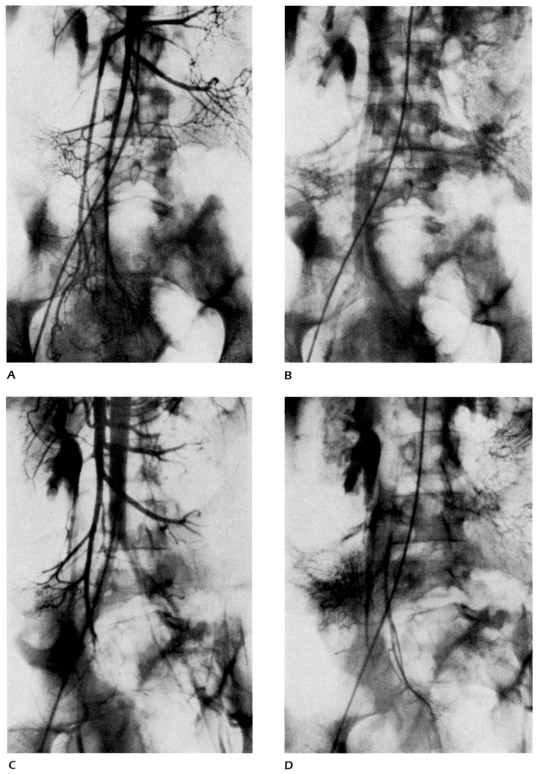

A

B

C

D

Figure 61-5. Granulomatous enterocolitis of terminal ileum and cecum in a 17-year-old boy. (A and B) At conventional superior mesenteric angiography, irregular, stenosed arteries are present within the field of supply of the ileocolic and distal superior mesenteric arteries. There is marked hypervascularization with early transit of contrast medium to the veins, especially in the terminal ileum but also in the remaining part of the small bowel. (C and D) After injection of 1 IU of vasopressin into the superior mesenteric artery, angiography reveals marked constriction of all peripheral branches, but it is most pronounced in the region of the terminal ileum.

mesenteric artery is patent, a superior mesenteric angiogram should be performed in frontal projection (Fig. 61-6).

The incidence of various causes of bowel ischemia varies in different series. The incidence of nonocclusive mesenteric infarction is recognized in 50 to 75 percent of patients with acute bowel ischemia, whereas venous thrombosis is rarely seen.[125,135-137]

Acute arterial occlusion is caused by either an embolus or a thrombus (see Fig. 61-6). The site of the occlusion observed at angiography may give some information about the cause, but in most cases angiography alone will not achieve a firm diagnosis.[126] As a rule, moderate to severe aortic atherosclerosis is associated with thrombotic occlusion, whereas minimal atherosclerosis strongly suggests embolic disease. Thrombosis is usually situated at the origin of the superior mesenteric artery, but branch thrombosis is frequently encountered in autopsy series.[138]

Occlusion of multiple splanchnic and renal arteries speaks in favor of embolic disease. Embolic occlusion of the superior mesenteric artery is angiographically observed at the level of the middle colic artery or within the first 10 cm of the main stem,[124,126,127] but single or multiple emboli can occur in branches of the superior mesenteric artery. Arteries proximal and distal to an embolic occlusion show marked constriction, and collateral flow may not be present.[124,126,127,139] Consequently, there is increased resistance to flow with delayed arterial visualization and decreased vascularity.[119] Apparently spasm does not occur immediately after embolization; in iatrogenic embolization it was never observed when angiography was performed soon after occlusion.[140]

When present, the angiographic characteristics of the collateral circulation are the same as in chronic obliterative disease of the splanchnic arteries.[30,141-146] If adequate collateral circulation is established in an acute occlusion, operation appears to be unnecessary.

Extensive experimental and clinical research has shown that the degree and extent of bowel damage depend largely on the duration of the occlusion and its site and extent.[129,140,147-152] An acute occlusion proximal to the origin of the middle colic artery may not cause any necrosis, and the result of surgery is also good in cases of ischemia.[129] The incidence of emboli is probably higher than reported, because large emboli may pass unnoticed and without symptoms in iatrogenic embolism[140] and in therapeutic embolism in patients with intestinal hemorrhage.[153-155] This is particularly the case for the small bowel when segmental arteries are occluded, and intentional occlusions of the large bowel arteries have caused necrosis.[155] Occlusion of arteries close to the bowel wall may thus not cause

alarming symptoms but may nevertheless result in serious complications such as perforation, ulceration, stenosis, or hemorrhage, depending on the extent of the vascular compromise (Fig. 61-7).[116,149,156-158] Stenosis of the bowel may later cause malabsorption or small bowel obstruction.[119,150,159,160] It is essential to realize that a patient with "intestinal angina" may be subject to acute occlusion of the superior mesenteric artery, be it by thrombosis or embolism.[161] About 50 percent of patients who have an acute infarction secondary to a thrombus had had previous symptoms of abdominal angina.[162,163] The poor correlation between the incidence of stenosis of splanchnic arteries and intestinal angina is well known, but any patient with abdominal symptoms and arteriographic evidence of significant arterial obstruction should be considered a candidate for percutaneous angioplasty,[164,165] urokinase in the superior mesenteric artery,[166] or reconstructive surgery to prevent a later catastrophe.[125,163]

In patients with atrial fibrillation or myocardial infarction, the emboli usually originate from the heart. It has been suggested that the primary heart disease may favor a complicating spasm in the mesenteric circulation, thus decreasing the bowel perfusion, with a consequently greater risk of bowel necrosis.[129,140] Paradoxical embolism to the superior mesenteric artery from venous thrombosis has also been observed.[129] Cholesterol embolism is another, perhaps too often overlooked, cause of occlusion of the mesenteric artery.[167,168]

Thrombosis of the superior mesenteric artery is most often secondary to the atheromatosis, but increased activity in vasopressin therapy has caused thrombosis of both arteries and veins in the mesenteric circulation.[169-171]

In addition to embolus and thrombosis secondary to atherosclerosis, a wide variety of other disorders may cause acute occlusion of small mesenteric arteries. Mesenteric angiography can provide information about abnormalities due to lupus erythematosus, polyarteritis nodosa, rheumatoid disease, and other types of vasculitis.[158,172-175] Intimal arterial hyperplasia and thrombus formation in small mesenteric arteries may also cause infarction.[176] Bowel ischemia due to operation,[158] catheterization,[140] and trauma[177,178] are other causes of vascular occlusions that can be defined by angiography.

It should be realized that occlusion of branches of the superior mesenteric artery can occur without causing any symptoms at all (Fig. 61-8).[179]

Occlusion of the superior mesenteric vein may be secondary to hematologic or intraabdominal disease or to vasopressin infusion. In primary occlusion no obvious cause is found. The angiographic findings are constric-

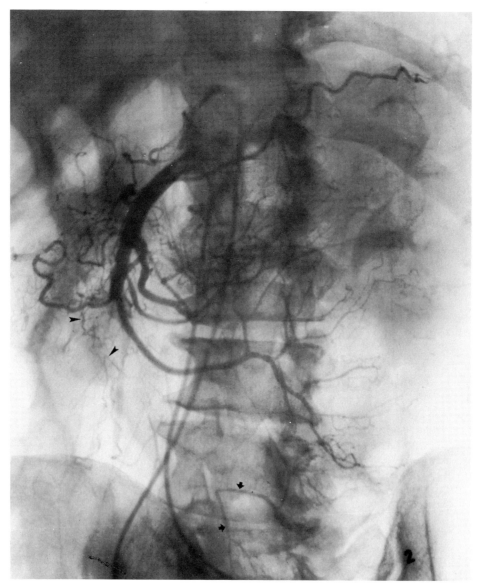

A

Figure 61-6. Short thrombosis of the superior mesenteric artery at the level of the third jejunal artery in a 77-year-old man with progressive abdominal pain during the previous week. Marked atheromatosis was observed at lumbar aortography, but the first part of the superior mesenteric artery was patent. (A) At superior mesenteric angiography, collateral circulation to the distal jejunal and ileal arteries is shown to be incomplete and insufficient via arcades (*arrows*) or vessels in the mesentery (*arrowheads*). (B) At inferior mesenteric angiography, the right colon and distal small bowel are found to be supplied via the left colic–middle colic–right colic artery. At operation 50 cm of jejunum had to be removed because of partial necrosis in the wall.

tion of superior mesenteric artery branches, delayed emptying, and absence of the venous phase.[114,180–182] Preoperative phlebography will demonstrate the extension of a thrombus,[183] whereas the venous phase of superior mesenteric angiography, if anything, will show a venous collateral circulation.[184] The diagnosis of superior mesenteric vein thrombus with angiography is notoriously difficult, and therefore the number of preoperatively diagnosed cases are rarely reported with angiography. The number has increased remarkably since the introduction of US and CT.[185–188] MRA will also prove to be of value in superior mesenteric vein thrombosis.[188–190] Direct visualization of a thrombus may be obtained after percutaneous transhepatic introduction of a catheter into the superior mesenteric vein. Urokinase through the catheter may then cause

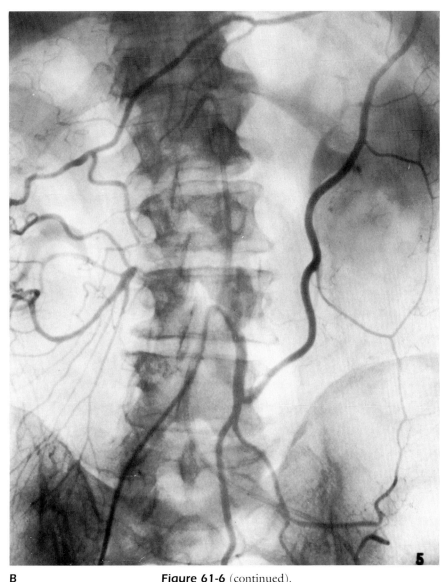

B **Figure 61-6** (continued).

thrombolysis and restoration of flow.[191] Vascular compromise—particularly venous, but also arterial—is noted in bowel intussusception, strangulated bowel obstruction, intestinal volvulus, and midgut malrotation. Clinical and experimental angiographic work has demonstrated the abnormal circulation.[117,192–196] Clinical as well as angiographic symptomatology may mimic occlusive or nonocclusive ischemia, leading to a wrong preoperative diagnosis. However, typical findings with an abnormal course of mesenteric vessels should direct the radiologist's attention to the lesions.[194,196–198] Displacement of the superior mesenteric vein in relation to the superior mesenteric artery will be observed on CT.[31]

Nonocclusive mesenteric ischemia usually occurs in patients with low-flow syndromes due to myocardial insufficiency, hypotension, and low cardiac output.[40,199–203] It is probably the most common cause of bowel necrosis today. Damage to the bowel occurs despite patency of the major intestinal arteries and veins. The pathologic lesions are similar to those found in dogs dying of shock.[38,204] Enteritis gravis is another entity probably caused by shock and spasm in the peripheral branches of the superior mesenteric artery.[205,206] A severe pancreatitis may display features like those of nonocclusive ischemia.[126,207] A persistent vasoconstriction is regarded as being responsible for bowel necrosis,[131,208] but a shunt mechanism in the bowel wall has

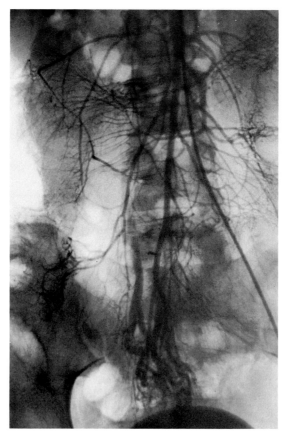

A

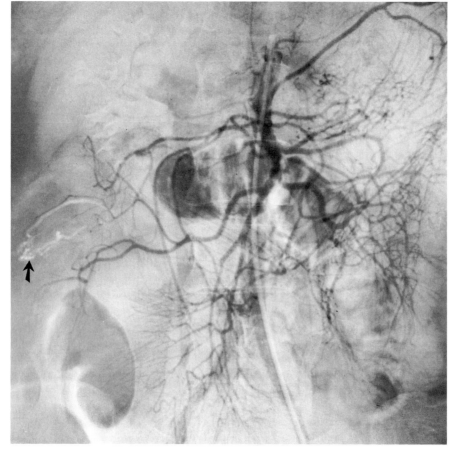

B

1564

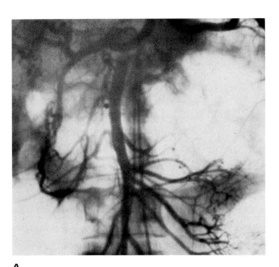

A

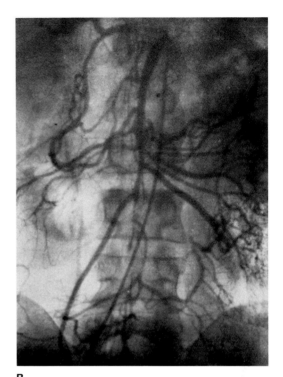

B

Figure 61-8. Thrombosis of the superior mesenteric artery in a man who at the age of 25, after an upper respiratory infection and recurrent fever, had arthritis in multiple joints. Weight loss and an elevated sedimentation rate indicated the need for celiac and superior mesenteric angiography. (A) Except for some irregular pancreatic arteries and moderately widened pancreaticoduodenal arcades, nothing abnormal was observed. After a period of improvement, hypertension and multiple pulmonary lesions appeared. With medical treatment the pulmonary lesions disappeared. At the age of 29 the patient was in good health, but he was continuously treated for hypertension. (B) Repeat superior mesenteric angiography was performed. The main stem was reduced in width and was occluded distal to the origin of the ileocolic artery. The ileum was supplied from peripheral arterial collaterals via jejunal and ileocolic arteries. Similar changes were present in the renal arteries. The patient had no symptoms from the gastrointestinal tract.

also been claimed as the cause of nonocclusive ischemia.[209] Digitalis has a definite constrictive effect on the mesenteric circulation.[210] Because it is a common prescription, it may produce bowel necrosis, especially when given in too high a dose.[211]

The angiographic findings vary. Usually, a generalized narrowing of the superior mesenteric tree is present with smooth tapering of jejunal and ileal branches. These arteries may also show a pattern of repetitive narrowings, producing a beaded appearance (Fig. 61-9).[1,124,126,127,131,132,202,203,211–213] Such findings are, however, not present in all cases.[126]

Early operation should not be performed because there is no vascular occlusion to correct and the degree and extent of bowel lesion are difficult to determine at an early stage.[214] Because the prognosis is extremely poor, many suggestions have been made for improving the circulation by intraarterial injection of vasodilating drugs.[131,132,135,202,212,213,215] The most successful therapy reported so far was achieved by the infusion of 30 to 60 mg of papaverine per hour for 16 to 24 hours.[131,132]

Ischemic colitis is a specific vascular disorder of the large bowel, usually present within the supply of the inferior mesenteric artery but often observed in the splenic flexure and sometimes more proximally.[216–218] Plain film and barium enema examination provide

◄ **Figure 61-7.** (A) Superior mesenteric angiography in a 24-year-old woman with repeated episodes of intestinal hemorrhage. An angiomatous lesion is present in the distal small bowel with early venous filling. At operation and histopathologic examination, an ischemic stricture with ulceration and thrombosed arteries in the wall of the bowel was found but no malformation. There were no further hemorrhages from the bowel, but reevaluation was made 4 years later because of hypertension. (B) At renal angiography an aneurysm was found on the renal artery, and repeated mesenteric angiography showed a dysplastic lesion in the right colon (subtraction film, *arrow*).

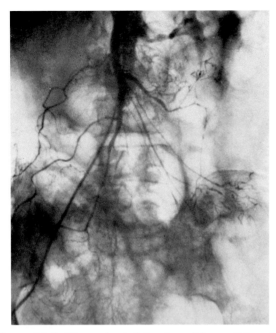

Figure 61-9. Hemorrhagic infarction of the small bowel in a 77-year-old woman who had had severe abdominal pain for the previous 24 hours. Superior mesenteric angiography showed that the main stem was patent but reduced in width. Marked constriction of all arteries to the small bowel is noted as well as signs of increased peripheral resistance. Multiple small branches and arcades are occluded, and there is insufficient collateral supply. Ileocolic and right colic arteries are less constricted, whereas blood supply of the transverse colon is missing. The angiographic findings were almost the same after injection of 10 μg of bradykinin into the superior mesenteric artery with only slight improvement of blood flow. At autopsy no occlusion was observed. Hemorrhagic necrosis was present in the small bowel and transverse colon. An old myocardial infarction was also found.

important information on its site and extent.[216,219,220] Angiography is of less importance because it does not provide a therapeutic implication.[218] The pathoanatomic abnormalities are mucosal necrosis and submucosal edema and hemorrhage.[221] Compared with other types of ischemic disease, ischemic colitis has a relatively good outcome, with recovery in about two-thirds of the cases without acute resection. The lesion may heal completely or cause a fibrous narrowing that later requires resection. The etiology may be an arterial occlusion brought about by atherosclerosis, vasculitis, aortic surgery, or catheterization for angiography.[216,222-225] Often, however, no vascular occlusion is observed, but instead increased blood flow with dilated arteries and early venous filling (Fig. 61-10).[107,218,225-227] This type of ischemic colitis should not be confused with the very serious forms of colitis that occur in nonocclusive ischemia, which usually include

the small bowel as well as the right part of the large bowel.

Chronic Obstruction

Congenital lesions such as prenatal occlusion of the superior mesenteric artery[228] are not observed at angiography because collateral supply to the duodenum and proximal jejunum is absent; the child will therefore not survive. Abdominal coarctation with marked stenosis or occlusion of the large trunks arising from the proximal lumbar aorta is a congenital lesion diagnosed by lumbar aortography.[22,229] The celiac and mesenteric lesions are usually accidental findings, the main symptom being hypertension. A well-developed collateral circulation to the abdominal viscera eliminates bowel ischemia and the typical symptoms following it.

Chronic obstruction of the superior mesenteric artery is ordinarily of arteriosclerotic origin and is most often located in the first 1 to 2 cm of the artery.[230-232] The stenosis is best observed at angiography in the lateral projection (see Fig. 61-2). Contrast medium should therefore be injected in the lumbar aorta at the origin of the superior mesenteric artery.[157,158,233-236]

Autopsy studies of arteriosclerotic changes in the mesenteric circulation have shown that they are less pronounced and less common than in the coronary arteries or the aorta.[138,230] Various opinions are on record concerning the frequency of arteriosclerotic narrowing of the celiac and superior mesenteric arteries. Derrick et al.[231] found approximately the same frequency in both vessels in a consecutive series of patients (44 percent and 37 percent, respectively). In patients above 50 years of age, on the other hand, Goertler[237] found moderate and severe stenosis in more than 25 percent in the superior mesenteric artery and in only 6 percent in the celiac axis.

These findings are at variance with angiographic studies, in which celiac stenoses are much more frequently seen than stenoses of the superior mesenteric artery. Thus, in a series of 713 patients Bron and Redman[235] found celiac stenoses in 12.3 percent and stenoses of the superior mesenteric artery in only 3.4 percent. This report may be explained by the observations of Dunbar et al.[238] and Rob[158] that the celiac stenosis is usually not arteriosclerotic but rather is caused by a compression of the crura of the diaphragm or of the celiac ganglion. On the other hand, the high frequency of superior mesenteric stenosis found at autopsy cannot be verified by angiography, perhaps because small plaques at the orifice are not angiographically demonstrable. Although the most common angiographic finding due to atherosclerosis is a concentric constric-

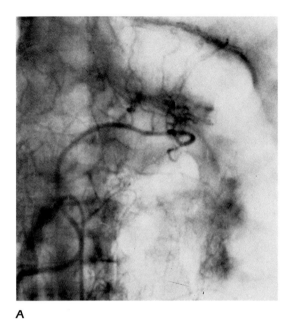

A

B

Figure 61-10. Reversible infarction of the splenic flexure of the colon in a 64-year-old man with acute rectal bleeding and abdominal pain. Two years previously he had had a myocardial infarction. At barium study typical findings of bowel infarction of the splenic flexure were observed. (A and B) At superior mesenteric angiography 10 days after onset of symptoms, no vascular occlusion is present but there is marked hypervascularization of the diseased area. Later examination with barium enema showed a complete regression.

tion at or near the origin (see Fig. 61-2), the earliest morphologic appearance is an eccentric, degenerative lesion.[237] Duplex Doppler sonography and MRA will give information about the direction of flow in diastole and also anatomic information about the abnormalities in the celiac and superior mesenteric arteries.[92,94,239,240]

Arteriosclerotic stenosis or occlusion in the branches of the superior mesenteric artery has been considered rare by some observers.[158,230] Reiner et al.,[12,138] using arteriography of autopsy specimens, frequently found peripheral arteriosclerotic disease of the mesenteric circulation but mentioned that dissection studies alone did not give adequate information.

A stenosis or occlusion of the main stem of the superior mesenteric artery is not an uncommon finding at autopsy in patients who have had no symptoms related to the gastrointestinal tract.[138,241] In fact, occlusion of two or three main stems does not necessarily cause symptoms of ischemic bowel disease.[235,242] Stenosis of the superior mesenteric artery alone may, on the other hand, cause abdominal symptoms—most commonly postprandial pain and malabsorption with fatty stools and weight loss. Some authors believe that at least two main stems must be occluded for these symptoms to be produced.[179,233,243] The first reports on malabsorption in connection with vascular disease showed, however, occlusion of only the superior mesenteric artery.[177,244] This finding has been verified by others.[157,158,245] Partial ligation of the superior mesenteric artery produced intestinal malabsorption in dogs with partial villous atrophy.[246] Improvement of mucosal changes and symptoms of malabsorption after 3 weeks agrees with the clinical observations by Connolly et al.[247] that these symptoms depend on the potentialities of the collateral supply. The varying ability of each individual to develop a collateral circulation may be the most important factor in determining whether the syndrome of abdominal angina will appear.[248]

Obstruction of peripheral branches of the superior mesenteric artery may also cause intestinal ischemia with malabsorption.[158,160,249] Reiner,[179] on the other hand, found peripheral occlusion due to local arteriosclerosis and thrombosis that were often silent during life. Joske et al.[250] reported two patients who developed malabsorption after temporary occlusion of the superior mesenteric artery. Aortography in one of the patients revealed a widely patent superior mesenteric artery, but peripheral branches could not be observed in detail. The importance of using aortography to demonstrate the stenosis in abdominal angina or malabsorption has been stressed by all authors, but selective angiography is required to evaluate the malabsorption syndrome fully, especially when the main stem of the superior mesenteric artery is patent.

Experimental experience suggests that malabsorption may appear also when the superior mesenteric artery is patent, that is, when a relative insufficiency is present or there is mesenteric steal due to stenosis of the celiac and inferior mesenteric arteries.[246] Mesenteric steal causing relative ischemia of the villi may likewise be due to aortoiliac steal,[251] to stenosis of the celiac and inferior mesenteric arteries, or to arteriovenous shunting in the mesenteric circulation.

Celiac and superior mesenteric angiography was performed in patients with signs of malabsorption.[252] In these patients, all of whom had steatorrhea, there were different types of alterations in the mesenteric circulation that could cause relative anoxia of the villi. In one group shunting of blood was due to Crohn disease (see Fig. 61-5), ileocecal carcinoma, colitis, or arteriovenous fistula (Fig. 61-11). Because of the shunting, a form of mesenteric steal was present with relative anoxia to the otherwise normal bowel. In another group of patients with gluten-induced steatorrhea, the superior mesenteric artery was wider than normal but there was no evidence of shunting because the veins were not observed early and were poorly opacified (Fig. 61-12). An explanation for the dilated artery may be the special anatomic and physiologic arrangements in the bowel wall.[36,39,62] Gluten-induced steatorrhea is probably a form of allergy.[253] It is postulated that because of this allergic reaction vasospasm occurs in the villi and blood is short-circuited to the veins. Anoxia and villous atrophy, which are characteristic for sprue, result. The contrast medium may be pooled in the mesenteric blood reservoir and therefore diluted so that early filling of veins cannot be observed during angiography. General increased width of the superior mesenteric artery and marked general venous shunting have been reported in a few cases of nontropical sprue[254] and in patients with *Strongyloides stercoralis* enteritis.[255] Patients with reticulum cell sarcoma of the bowel, a disease related to idiopathic sprue, may also have a wide superior mesenteric artery.[256]

Another common finding in the ischemic syndrome is occult blood in the feces.[257–259] Angiography of the superior mesenteric artery should therefore be performed in every patient with unexplained bleeding from the gastrointestinal tract. Boijsen and Reuter[18] found a high percentage of vascular stenosis in patients with this symptom, which later was verified by others.[260–262] Because collateral circulation is often observed at angiography, this observation in patients with hemorrhage to the gastrointestinal tract is difficult to evaluate.

Although narrowing of the superior mesenteric artery is ordinarily atherosclerotic in origin, other causes are known. The most common are tumor encasement,

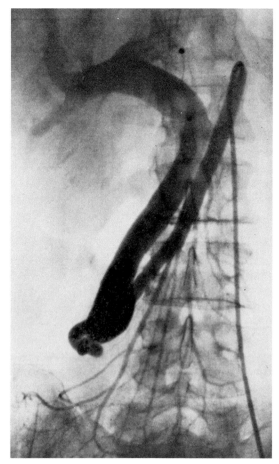

Figure 61-11. Arteriovenous fistula between the superior mesenteric artery and vein in a 61-year-old woman with gluten-induced steatorrhea who had a normal gastrointestinal barium study. The fistula was secondary to a previous bowel resection for intussusception due to a lipoma of the ileum with gangrene.

usually due to pancreatic carcinoma, and stenosis secondary to chronic pancreatitis. Splanchnic angiography is the best preoperative method for diagnosis of these lesions (Fig. 61-13). Although aortography may demonstrate the local constriction, for detailed analysis selective angiography is necessary. The malabsorption syndrome often seen in pancreatic disease may be related not only to a reduction of pancreatic exocrine function but also to a stenosis of the superior mesenteric artery.

Distal stenoses of the superior mesenteric artery or its branches are common in carcinoma infiltrating the mesentery. The stenosis is different from that caused by arteriosclerosis because the vessels are irregularly infiltrated by the tumor.[107] Fibromuscular hyperplasia,[248,263,264] pseudoxanthoma elasticum,[265] thromboangiitis obliterans,[266] and other types of arteritis[267] (see

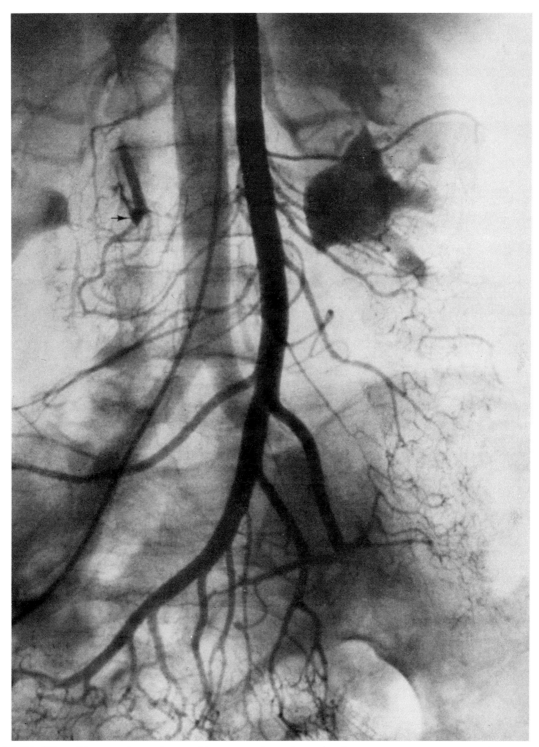

Figure 61-12. Idiopathic sprue in a 63-year-old woman. At angiography the superior mesenteric and the ileal arteries are seen to be unusually wide, whereas the jejunal arteries are small. No shunting is observed, but there is an aneurysm of the gastroduodenal artery (*arrow*).

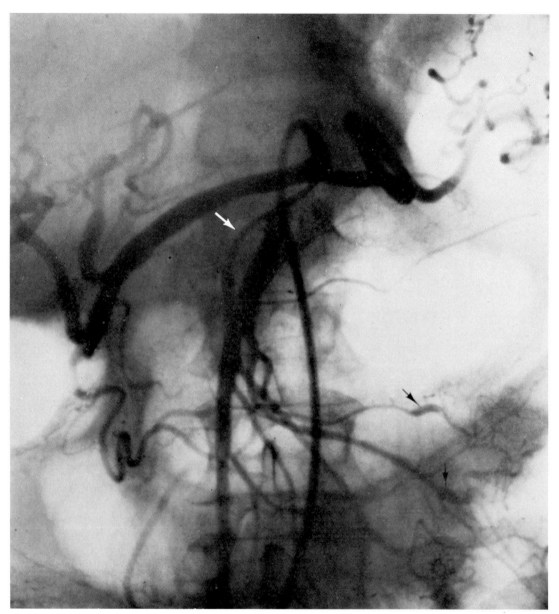

Figure 61-13. Chronic pancreatitis in a 66-year-old woman with abdominal pain. At celiac angiography the superior mesenteric artery is filled in a retrograde direction from a dilated dorsal pancreatic artery, also called the anastomosis of Bühler (*upper arrow*). Irregular arterial walls are present within the splenic, common hepatic, dorsal pancreatic, superior mesenteric, and first jejunal arteries. Peripheral aneurysms are visible in the jejunal arteries (*lower arrows*).

Fig. 61-8) cause narrowing or occlusion of the main stem or branches of the superior mesenteric artery, sometimes with abdominal angina. More peripheral arteries are stenosed or occluded in systemic amyloidosis,[228] polyarteritis nodosa,[268] necrotizing angiitis due to drug abuse,[269] carcinoid tumors,[270,271] and peritoneal carcinomatosis.[107] In granulomatous enterocolitis, irregular stenosis of the vasa recta may be observed at angiography,[84,107,272–274] an observation that is not verified by microangiography.[275,276]

With the development of modern therapeutic dilatation technique in diagnostic radiology, it appears that some of the central stenoses of the superior mesenteric artery can be treated percutaneously.[164,165,251]

Aneurysms

Aneurysms of the superior mesenteric artery or its branches are seldom observed at autopsy or operation.

In a review of the literature Rob[158] found that approximately 20 percent of aneurysms in the splanchnic viscera were located in the superior mesenteric artery. The aneurysms reported were mycotic and located in the main stem. Previous experience gave the impression that most aneurysms of the main stem were syphilitic or necrotic,[277,278] but with the increasing use of angiography, these lesions seem to be arteriosclerotic. Furthermore, with today's indications for mesenteric angiography, particularly performed in patients with gastrointestinal hemorrhage, few aneurysms are reported.[262,279–281] One reason is that most aneurysms are silent; another is that angiography of the superior mesenteric artery is not performed as often as it should be in patients with disease entities complicated with aneurysms, that is, polyarteritis nodosa,[174,268] necrotizing angiitis,[48] and pancreatitis (see Fig. 61-13). Aneurysms of the branches of the superior mesenteric artery, when large enough, can also be detected by US,[282] but in pancreatitis they may be difficult to differentiate from pseudocysts. Destruction of the arterial wall by pancreatic enzymes or by neoplasms may cause large pseudoaneurysms of the mesentery or pancreas, or the aneurysms may rupture into the peritoneal cavity. The small arteriosclerotic aneurysms of the superior mesenteric artery and its branches rarely cause any symptoms, but rupture may occur without previous symptoms (Fig. 61-14). They may also cause thrombotic occlusion of branches of the superior mesenteric artery, which may or may not elicit abdominal symptoms.

The aneurysms of polyarteritis nodosa have a varying appearance at angiography. They are usually small (1–5 mm) and situated in peripheral branches close to the mesenteric border, but secondary or tertiary branches may also be engaged, with extensive, irregular destruction of the arterial wall and thrombotic occlusion of branches[268] (Fig. 61-15).

Arteriovenous Communications

Angiomatous Lesions

A large variety of benign vascular lesions with abnormal arteriovenous connections may be recognized at selective superior mesenteric angiography: angioma, hemangioma, hamartoma, angiodysplasia, phlebectasia, and telangiectasia. Some of them (e.g., angiodysplasia and phlebectasia) are thus benign vascular tumors that have a different histologic appearance in which widened mucosal or submucosal veins are the most characteristic finding. These lesions are often called *vascular malformations. Angiomatous lesions*

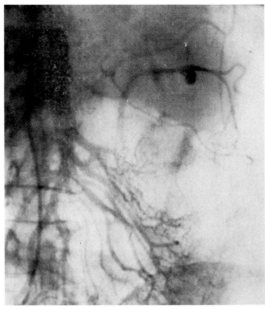

Figure 61-14. Aneurysm of the left branch of the middle colic artery in a 56-year-old man with hypertension and sudden bleeding into the abdominal cavity. At superior mesenteric angiography a 7 × 7 mm aneurysm is visible surrounded by a hematoma displacing the marginal artery. Collateral circulation was demonstrated in the area at angiography. The aneurysm could therefore be extirpated without compromising the bowel circulation.

would be a better name because some of the lesions are hereditary (hereditary hemorrhagic telangiectasia), others are congenital (blue rubber bleb nevus, Klippel-Trenaunay syndrome), and still others are acquired (old age, congestive heart failure, aortic stenosis). The latter are usually called *angiodysplasia*. A distinction between these lesions based on angiography alone is usually not possible.

The angiomatous lesions have other characteristics in common. They usually cause gastrointestinal hemorrhage and they are difficult or impossible to find at exploratory laparotomy. Since the first description in 1960 by Margulis et al.,[283] based on operative angiography, a large number of reports have shown that selective splanchnic angiography, particularly superior mesenteric angiography, is a useful method to demonstrate these lesions.[2,16,116,118,262,284–291]

The characteristic and most frequent angiographic observation of the *angiodysplastic lesion* is that of a small (less than 1 cm) vascular lesion of the cecum or ascending colon. It is fed by a slightly enlarged vasa recta, and early filling of a widened draining vein is seen (see Fig. 61-1).[289–291] Delayed emptying of the early-filled draining vein is also noted.[290,291] This has been believed to be an indication of venous stasis, presumably induced by increased luminal bowel pressure,

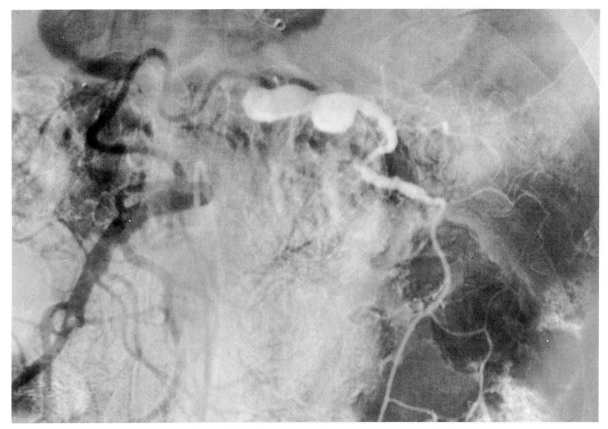

Figure 61-15. Aneurysm formation in the middle colic artery in a 56-year-old man, previously operated on for a lumbar aortic aneurysm. The complicated operation involved the left renal artery, and reoperation was necessary because of insufficiency in graft anastomosis. Four months later, he rebled to the gastrointestinal tract, and a long irregular aneurysm of the type found in polyarteritis nodosa was observed in the middle colic artery at superior mesenteric angiography. The aneurysm was resected. It was probably the result of the complicated operation.

and a cause of the phlebectasia observed.[292] Another hypothesis is that the lesion is secondary to mucosal ischemia,[289] because most lesions occur in elderly patients and shunting has been found in cases in which arteries in the region were thrombosed (see Fig. 61-7).[116] This hypothesis is also in line with the observation that some of the lesions occur in patients with aortic stenosis[293] or in patients with cardiac, vascular, or pulmonary insufficiency.[294]

The diagnosis of the angiodysplastic lesions is thus made by angiography of the superior mesenteric artery. In many patients repeated gastrointestinal barium studies and colonoscopy have failed to demonstrate the lesions.[289,291] On the other hand, it is known that angiography may be falsely negative and that colonoscopy may reveal the lesion.[295] Magnification angiography or pharmacoangiography may improve the diagnostic accuracy (see Fig. 61-1).[291,295] With increasing experience the angiodysplastic lesions have also been observed at angiography in the small bowel and in the left colon and rectosigmoid area, and new lesions are seen to appear after resection of the primary lesion (see Fig. 61-7).[289,291] Of particular interest is the fact that angiodysplastic lesions also occur in the upper gastrointestinal tract, as has been observed at endoscopy in patients with aortic stenoses.[296] Certainly, some of the unexplained recurrent gastrointestinal hemorrhages with negative angiography could be referred to these lesions. Perhaps the local hypervascularization of the stomach or duodenum sometimes observed in otherwise unexplained hemorrhage[118] could be accounted for by similar lesions.

The angiomatous lesions discovered at angiography in patients with *hereditary hemorrhagic telangiectasia* occur in all abdominal organs, including the gastrointestinal tract.[285,291] At superior mesenteric angiography multiple punctate lesions may be observed but usually only single lesions are noted, looking much like angiodysplasia of the colon. Often the vascular tufts are too small to be observed. Angiography may then show a localized early filling of the vein, or the angiogram may appear normal.

A *diffuse angiomatous lesion* of the small bowel in infants is a particular entity that appears angiographically as a general shunting from the widened superior mesenteric artery.[291]

In *Klippel-Trenaunay syndrome*,[288,291] *blue rubber bleb nevus*,[297] and other congenital angiomatous lesions of the small or large bowel, the angiographic findings are not similar to those of angiodysplasia. Usually there is no arteriovenous shunting, and the feeding arteries are not dilated.

In localized lesions such as angiodysplasia of the large bowel, resection has been the method of choice. During the past few years, however, embolization[298] or electrocoagulation via the endoscope[294,296] has been successful.

Acute and chronic hemorrhage to the gastrointestinal tract is one of the main indications for superior mesenteric angiography. The most common causes of hemorrhage within the field of supply of the superior mesenteric artery have been mentioned in the previous sections of this chapter, but varices and tumors should also be included. The approach to diagnosing bleeding sources in the small bowel and colon depends on a number of factors, among which the general condition of the patient and the degree of hemorrhage are the most important. It is important to realize that the RN tracers (^{99m}Tc red blood cells or ^{99m}Tc sulfur colloid)[299,300] give better information about the bleeding point than angiography. Some controversy exists regarding which type of tracer should be preferred,[301] but both have a relatively high sensitivity. In addition, intraarterially injected RN tracers (dynamic radionuclide angiography)[302] and conventional pharmacoangiography aggravating or reactivating bleeding[303,304] will improve information. However, the main purpose of angiography is not only to confirm the exact site and reason for the hemorrhage, but also to institute treatment by vasopressin infusion or embolization.[305,306]

Arteriovenous Fistulas

Whereas the angiomatous lesion rarely grows to be a shunt of hemodynamic import, the arteriovenous fistula may very well shunt significant amounts of blood. This fistula represents a direct communication between the main stem or branches and their respective veins and is of traumatic origin. The main stem fistulas are secondary to direct violence,[307,308] whereas those of the peripheral branches are secondary to previous complicated operations.[309–311] Congenital arteriovenous fistula of the mesentery has also been described.[312] Because of a markedly increased flow, the superior mesenteric artery becomes wider and a shunt can be observed even at lumbar aortography.[307,308,310] The exact site of the fistula may be difficult to define by aortography,[307] but selective angiography readily delineates the exact position of the lesion (see Fig. 61-11).[311]

Although malabsorption has been reported in patients with arteriovenous fistula,[309,310] it is not a constant finding. One patient with the disorder had a gluten-induced steatorrhea, which disappeared after ligation of the fistula. Biopsy showed that the villi were normal, but the enzymes in the villi were reduced. Thus decreased peripheral resistance due to the fistula can reduce perfusion pressure in the bowel wall, resulting in reduction of the enzymes.[252]

Portal Hypertension

The redistribution of flow in portal hypertension before operation was previously documented by arterioportal angiography and by various direct percutaneous portographic techniques. After shunt operation, direct venographic demonstration of shunt patency was made via the femoral vein. Today duplex Doppler and color Doppler imaging are used to show the dynamics of the portal circulation as well as the postoperative shunt patency.[91,92,313] MRA will show not only the patency of the superior mesenteric vein but also the increased mesenteric circulation, the entire collateral system, the portosystemic connections, and, postoperatively, patency of the shunts.[314–318]

Tumor and Inflammatory Disease

Inflammatory and neoplastic disease of the intestine has been studied by microangiography, and differences in the vascular pattern of the lesions have been observed.[275,276,319,320] Although it does not achieve the same detailed vascular anatomy as microangiography, conventional selective angiography adds more information about the pathophysiologic changes within these lesions (Fig. 61-16). Changes in the vascular patterns are seen during selective angiography in most neoplastic[248,270,284,321–327] and inflammatory lesions within the bowel.[84,107,272–274,328–330] The differential diagnosis of a specific neoplastic or inflammatory origin, however, may be difficult. From the present collected experience it seems that certain angiographic findings are characteristic, but at times it is impossible to make a definite diagnosis.

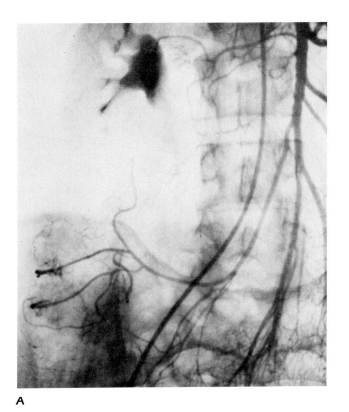

A

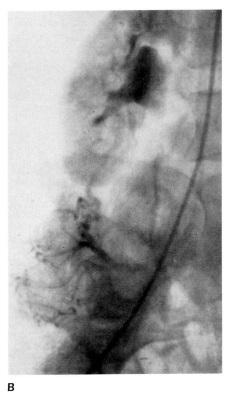

B

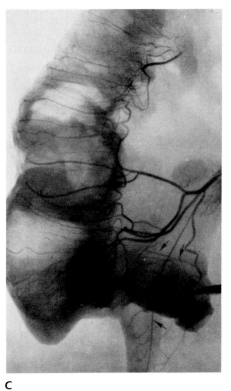

C

Figure 61-16. Carcinoma of the cecum in a 52-year-old woman. (A and B) At superior mesenteric angiography tumor vessels and early venous filling are observed in a 5 × 5 cm area of the cecum. (C) Arteriography of the operative specimen demonstrates that the slight arterial changes can hardly be seen with this method and that the pathophysiologic changes due to the tumor are far better observed with serial angiography. Note in the specimen the recurrent ileal artery supplying the terminal ileum (*upper arrows*) and the artery supplying the appendix (*lower arrow*).

Inflammation

The two main types of inflammatory disease, regional enterocolitis and ulcerative colitis, have distinct angiographic patterns when they are fully developed. The pathologic and microangiographic changes explain the angiographic findings. In Crohn disease degenerative vascular changes are observed, with granulomatous reaction and diffuse fibrosis of all layers of the bowel as well as the mesentery.[276] Inflammatory vascular changes are relatively few in the early stages of the disease, when there is a nonspecific inflammatory reaction. Conversely, in ulcerative colitis the inflammatory vascular reaction dominates, and degenerative vascular changes are nonexistent. Thus, at angiography in advanced stages of Crohn disease with stenosis, the long vasa recta and the arteries near the mesenteric border appear irregularly stenosed or occluded, and collateral circulation with tortuous arteries in the gut wall is found.[84,107,272,276] These observations are not in agreement with other reports.[330] Microangiography and histoangiography have definitely shown that there is no occlusion of the vasa recta even in advanced stages of Crohn disease.[275,276] Since they are crowded, tortuous, and reduced in width, they will not be seen on routine angiograms. Other findings in Crohn disease are wide-angle branching between the long vasa recta[329] and small vascular tufts in the bowel wall and mesentery.[331] The arterial changes in idiopathic ulcerative colitis[328,329] are wide vasa recta and signs of hypervascularization. In cases of "zoning"[329,330] (i.e., hypervascular areas present in the submucosa and serosa), the diagnosis of Crohn disease can be made. Otherwise it is rarely possible to make a distinction between the two disease entities. Hypervascularization with shunting to densely opacified veins is observed in both types when activity is present (Fig. 61-17; see Fig. 61-5). This phenomenon may also be noted where there is delayed transit of contrast medium through the arteries of the diseased bowel.[116] Absence of early venous filling is frequently observed in the advanced stage of Crohn disease.

To summarize, the interesting and somewhat controversial angiographic changes observed in inflammatory bowel disease are usually not specific.[276,330] The extension of disease can be defined quite well as a rule,

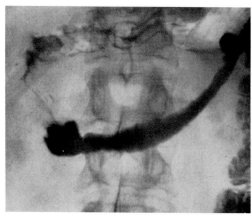

A

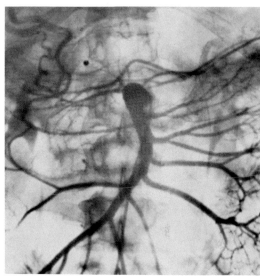

B

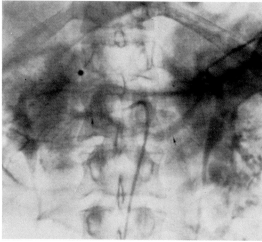

C

Figure 61-17. Regional enteritis of the duodenum in a 31-year-old man. (A) Typical changes observed at upper gastrointestinal barium study. (B and C) At superior mesenteric angiography slightly irregular changes are observed in the peripheral branches of the pancreaticoduodenal arteries and gastroduodenal artery. Hypervascularization with early shunting to the veins is visible (*arrows*).

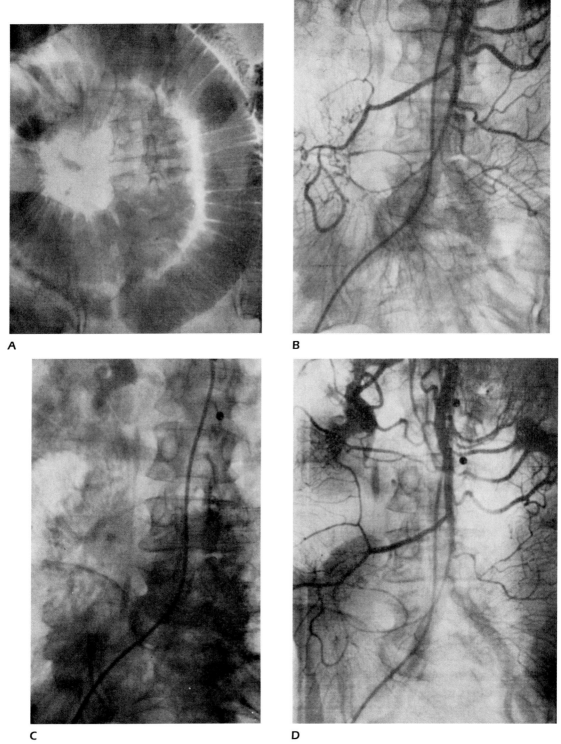

A

B

C

D

Figure 61-18. Carcinoid of ileum in a 64-year-old woman with malabsorption and a palpable mass to the right in the abdomen. (A) Small bowel study demonstrates dilated ileal loops surrounding a tumor. (B and C) At superior mesenteric angiography the terminal part of the artery as well as peripheral branches and arcades are found to be irregularly infiltrated. The mesentery is infiltrated with consequent typi-cal radiation of the vasa recta toward the tumor. Collateral supply is present from the infiltrated ileocolic artery. Ileal and ileocolic veins are occluded by tumor (C). (D) At phar-macoangiography using 0.5 IU of vasopressin, the irregular arterial infiltrations of larger branches are somewhat better observed but fewer tumor vessels are seen.

but the rather complicated procedure and the radiation risks of the method have made the indications for angiography obsolete in young patients. There is a certain risk of malignant change in the bowel of these patients. However, it occurs late in the disease, and then other diagnostic methods will usually give the diagnosis.

Tumors

Tumors of the small bowel are rare and often overlooked or misinterpreted at barium examination. Superior mesenteric angiography plays an important role in diagnosis, in preoperative evaluation of local extent, and in locating the exact site of the tumor in the small bowel wall.[326,327]

The most common primary tumor of the small bowel is the *carcinoid,* usually present in the ileum. Because of a marked desmoplastic reaction of the mesentery, the tumor has a typical angiographic pattern when it extends outside the bowel wall (Fig. 61-18).[112,270,271,332,333] Ileal mesenteric arteries and veins are stenosed or occluded. Often the ileocolic artery is narrowed in its entire length. Because of a mesenteric retraction the distal arcades and the vasa recta are arranged in a stellate pattern. Tumor vessels have been observed, but they are probably collateral channels opened up because of occlusion of arterial arcades. Tumor stain is usually not discerned but may occur.[112,332,337] Pharmacoangiography may enhance the

information.[52,112] Although in small tumors without the desmoplastic change of the mesentery, the primary lesion will not be seen,[271,332,333] local metastases in the mesentery as well as hepatic metastases will nevertheless be shown.[332] The angiographic findings are thus, as a rule, typical, but similar findings in mesenteric fibrosis have been noted.[334] It appears, however, that vascular displacement and distortion are more typical for this lesion than is incasement.[335-337]

Carcinoid tumors of the large bowel within the superior mesenteric territory are rarely examined by angiography despite the fact that the most frequent site is in the appendix. Only two cases are reported,[332] with the same findings as in small bowel tumors.

Leiomyoma or neurinoma of the small bowel has a characteristic appearance.[107,284,286,322,326,338-340] The tumor has well-circumscribed margins. Prominent feeding arteries and draining veins are observed, and many irregular tumor vessels give rise to a dense stain (Fig. 61-19). Malignancy can rarely be ruled out, but if the tumor is small (3–4 cm) it is probably benign. Angiography appears to be extremely reliable and is not infrequently used in the diagnosis of chronic, otherwise unexplained, melena. Only one case of angiography of a leiomyoma of the large bowel has been reported.[326]

The *hamartoma* in patients with Peutz-Jeghers disease is a vascular tumor, but at angiography it is usually noted as a hypovascular mass with lack of venous drainage.[341-343]

Adenocarcinoma of the small bowel is a rare lesion,

Figure 61-19. Leiomyoma of the jejunum in a 67-year-old man with repeated bleeding from the bowel. Previous operation for diverticula of the colon did not stop the bleeding. Repeated small bowel studies were reported negative. (A and

B) At superior mesenteric angiography a 3.5 × 2.5 cm richly vascularized tumor was found to be supplied by the first jejunal artery.

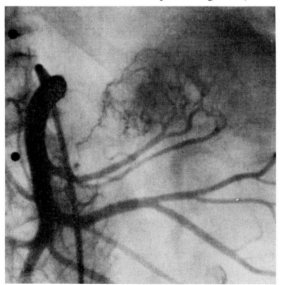

A

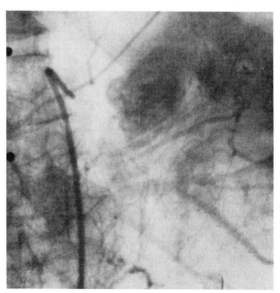

B

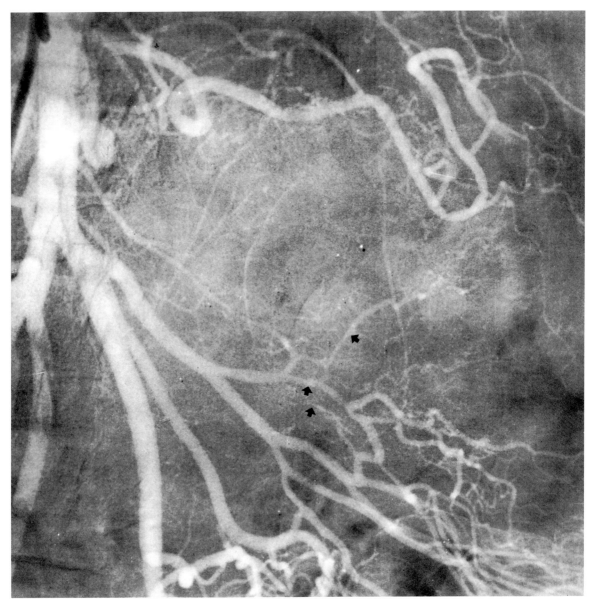

Figure 61-20. Adenocarcinoma of the jejunum with marked infiltration of jejunal arteries (*arrows*). Few tumor vessels are observed, but there is a slight accumulation in the tumor. (2.5× magnification, subtraction film)

and angiography is therefore seldom reported.[344] The large bowel adenocarcinoma has been frequently observed at superior mesenteric angiography.[107,109,260,262] The angiographic appearance varies with the type of growth. Thus the infiltrating, scirrhous tumor is avascular or hypovascular and infiltrates the vasa recta with no tumor stain and no early venous filling. This is most often seen in the small bowel adenocarcinoma (Fig. 61-20). Tumors of the large bowel supplied from the superior mesenteric artery are, on the other hand, usually hypervascular and show tumor stain as well as dense and early venous drainage (see Fig. 61-16). In-

filtration of arteries of the mesentery signifies extension of tumor outside the bowel wall.

Villous tumor of the ascending colon may have a slightly different appearance from that of carcinoma.[345]

Lymphoma, lymphosarcoma, and *reticular cell sarcoma* of the bowel are rarely examined by mesenteric angiography. Findings in the few cases reported are noncharacteristic.[107,256,262,336,346] Vascular displacement and incasement are reported as well as early shunting, but occasionally no abnormality is observed despite the extensive involvement of the mesentery.[256]

Cystic lesions of the mesentery cause vascular displacement, and sometimes accumulation of contrast medium in the wall may be noted.[336,347]

Miscellaneous Conditions

Besides primary vascular lesions, tumors, and inflammatory disease, angiography may reveal the presence of *internal herniation, intussusception, volvulus, malrotation,* or *adhesions.* These are of particular importance to define when there is a vascular compromise[117,192–198,260,344,348–350] that may cause acute bowel ischemia, symptoms of gastrointestinal hemorrhage, or abdominal pain.

Meckel diverticulum may also be revealed by angiography, particularly in acute bleeding when extravasation or accumulation of contrast medium in the ectopic gastric mucosa is observed.[260,262,351–353]

Radiation enteritis is another lesion of the bowel that appears angiographically as irregular stenosis or occlusion of superior mesenteric artery branches including the vasa recta. The latter are often tortuous and crowded.[354,355] The bowel wall appears hypovascular, and the veins are often stenosed.

Ileal varicosities may be seen at angiography in patients with portal hypertension. In the venous phase of the superior mesenteric angiogram large venous varicosities are observed in the bowel wall.[336,356,357] Aneurysm of the superior mesenteric vein may also occur in portal hypertension but can also be congenital or acquired secondary to pancreatitis. This aneurysm has been observed at US and CT and confirmed by superior mesenteric angiography.[358,359]

Superior mesenteric angiography is thus a useful method for detecting a variety of gastrointestinal lesions. It should be taken advantage of particularly in situations in which other approaches, including CT, MRI, and US, have failed.

References

1. Boijsen E. Superior mesenteric angiography. In: Abrams HL, ed. Angiography: vascular and interventional radiology. 3rd ed. Boston: Little, Brown, 1983.
2. Nusbaum M, Baum S. Radiographic demonstration of unknown sites of gastrointestinal bleeding. Surg Forum 1963; 14:374.
3. Baum S, Nusbaum M, Clearfield HR, Kuroda K, Tumen HJ. Angiography in the diagnosis of gastrointestinal bleeding. Arch Intern Med 1967;119:16.
4. Baum S, Nusbaum M. The control of gastrointestinal hemorrhage by selective mesenteric arterial infusion of vasopressin. Radiology 1971;98:497–505.
5. Drummond H. Some points relating to the surgical anatomy of the arterial supply of the large intestine. Proc R Soc Med 1913;7:185.
6. Steward JA, Rankin FW. Blood supply of the large intestine: its surgical considerations. Arch Surg 1933;26:843.
7. Cauldwell EW, Anson BJ. The visceral branches of the abdominal aorta: topographical relationships. Am J Anat 1943; 73:27.
8. Ross AJ. Vascular patterns of small and large intestine compared. Br J Surg 1952;39:330.
9. Basmajian JV. The marginal anastomoses of the arteries to the large intestine. Surg Gynecol Obstet 1954;99:614.
10. Basmajian JV. The main arteries of the large intestine. Surg Gynecol Obstet 1955;101:585.
11. Mayo CW. Blood supply of the colon: surgical considerations. Surg Clin North Am 1955;35:1117.
12. Reiner L, Rodriguez FL, Platt R, Schlesinger MJ. Injection studies on mesenteric arterial circulation: I. Technique and observations on collaterals. Surgery 1959;45:820.
13. Griffiths JD. Extramural and intramural blood supply of colon. Br Med J 1961;1:323.
14. Michels NA, Siddarth P, Kornblith PL, Parke WW. The variant blood supply to the small and large intestines: its import in regional resections. J Int Coll Surg 1963;39:127.
15. Nebesar RA, Kornblith PL, Pollard JJ, Michels NA. Celiac and superior mesenteric arteries: a correlation of angiograms and dissections. Boston: Little, Brown, 1969.
16. Baer JW, Ryan S. Analysis of cecal vasculature in the search for vascular malformations. AJR 1976;126:394–405.
17. Zerin JM, DiPietro MA. Mesenteric vascular anatomy at CT: normal and abnormal appearances. Radiology 1991;179: 739–742.
18. Kolmannskog F, Swenson T, Vatne MH, Larsen S. Computed tomography and ultrasound of the normal pancreas. Acta Radiol 1982;23:443–451.
19. Carrington BM, Martin DF. Position of the superior mesenteric artery on computed tomography and its relationship to retroperitoneal disease. Br J Radiol 1987;60:997–999.
20. Olivero S. Angiografia selettiva dell'arteria mesenterica superiore. Minerva Cardioangiol 1960;8:55–66.
21. Voorthuisen AE van. Ervaringern met selectieve arteriografie van de arteria coeliaca en de arteria mesenterica superior. Leiden: Staflen's Wetenschappelijke Uitgeversmaatschappij N.V., 1967.
22. Boijsen E, Larini GP. Aortic hypoplasia combined with coarctation of the thoracic and lumbar aorta. J Can Assoc Radiol 1966;17:81.
23. Hearn JB. Duodenal ileus with special reference to superior mesenteric artery compression. Radiology 1966;86:305–310.
24. Baum S. Magnification arteriography in intestinal vascular disease. In: Boley SJ, Schwartz SS, Williams LF Jr, eds. Vascular disorders of the intestine. New York: Appleton-Century-Crofts, 1971.
25. Lawdahl RB, Keller FS. The middle mesenteric artery. Radiology 1987;165:371–372.
26. Lunderquist A. Angiography in carcinoma of the pancreas. Acta Radiol Suppl (Stockh) 1965;235:1.
27. Lunderquist A. Arterial segmental supply of the liver: an angiographic study. Acta Radiol Suppl (Stockh) 1967;272:1.
28. Suzuki T, Imamura M, Kawabe K, Honjo J. Selective demonstration of the variant hepatic artery. Surg Gynecol Obstet 1972;135:209–215.
29. Turner W. On the existence of a system of anastomosing arteries between and connecting the visceral and parietal branches of the abdominal aorta. Br Foreign Med Chir Rev 1963;32:222.
30. Sacks RP, Sheft DJ, Freeman JH. The demonstration of the mesenteric collateral circulation in young patients. AJR 1968; 102:401.
31. Nichols DM, Li DK. Superior mesenteric vein rotation: a CT sign of midgut malrotation. AJR 1983;141:707–708.
32. Gaines PA, Saunders AJS, Drake D. Midgut malrotation diagnosed by ultrasound. Clin Radiol 1987;38:51–53.
33. Shatzkes D, Gordon DH, Haller JO, Kantor A, De Silva R. Malrotation of the bowel: malalignment of the superior mes-

enteric artery-vein complex by CT and MR. J Comput Assist Tomogr 1990;14:93.

34. Texter EC. Small intestinal blood flow. Am J Dig Dis 1963; 8:587.

35. Jacobson ED. Physiologic aspects of the intestinal circulation. In: Boley SJ, Schwartz SS, Williams LF Jr, eds. Vascular disorders of the intestine. New York: Appleton-Century-Crofts, 1971.

36. Sweifach BW. Functional behavior of the microcirculation. Springfield, IL: Charles C Thomas, 1961.

37. Johnson PC. Autoregulation in the intestine and mesentery. In: Boley SJ, Schwartz SS, Williams LF Jr, eds. Vascular disorders of the intestine. New York: Appleton-Century-Crofts, 1971.

38. Lillehei RC. The intestinal factor in irreversible hemorrhagic shock. Surgery 1957;42:1043.

39. Gilbert RP. Mechanisms of the hemodynamic effects of endotoxin. Physiol Rev 1960;40:245.

40. Corday E, Irving DW, Gold H, Bernstein H, Skelton RBT. Mesenteric vascular insufficiency. Am J Med 1962;33:365.

41. Green HD, Kepchar JH. Control of peripheral resistance in major systemic vascular beds. Physiol Rev 1959;39:617.

42. Boijsen E, Redman HC. Effect of bradykinin on celiac and superior mesenteric angiography. Invest Radiol 1966;1:422–430.

43. Boijsen E, Redman HC. Effect of epinephrine on celiac and superior mesenteric angiography. Invest Radiol 1967;2:184–199.

44. Nusbaum M, Baum S, Kuroda K, Blakemore WS. Control of portal hypertension by selective mesenteric arterial drug infusion. Arch Surg 1968;97:1005.

45. Steckel RJ, Ross G, Grollman JH Jr. A potent drug combination for producing constriction of the superior mesenteric artery and its branches. Radiology 1968;91:579–581.

46. Redman HC, Reuter SR, Miller WJ. Improvement of superior mesenteric and portal vein visualization with tolazoline. Invest Radiol 1969;4:24–27.

47. Rösch J, Dotter CT, Rose RW. Selective arterial infusions of vasoconstrictors in acute gastrointestinal bleeding. Radiology 1971;99:27–36.

48. Cioffi CM, Ruzicka FF Jr, Carillo FJ, Gould HR. Enhanced visualization of portal venous system using phentolamine and isoproterenol in combination. Radiology 1973;108:43–49.

49. Widrich WC, Nordahl DL, Robbins AH. Contrast enhancement of the mesenteric and portal veins using intraarterial papaverine. AJR 1974;121:374–379.

50. Redman HC. Mesenteric arterial and venous blood flow changes following selective arterial injection of vasodilators. Invest Radiol 1974;9:193–198.

51. Norryd C, Dencker H, Lunderquist A, Olin T. Superior mesenteric blood flow in man following injection of bradykinin and vasopressin into the superior mesenteric artery. Acta Chir Scand 1975;141:119–128.

52. Boijsen E, Göthlin J. Effect of vasopressin on celiac and superior mesenteric angiography. Acta Radiol 1980;21:523–533.

53. Noer RJ, Derr JW, Johnston CG. The circulation of the small intestine: an evaluation of its revascularizing potential. Ann Surg 1949;130:608.

54. Boley SJ, et al. Pathophysiologic effects of bowel distension on intestinal blood flow. Am J Surg 1969;117:228.

55. Olin T, Redman H. Spillover flowmeter. Acta Radiol 1966; 4:217–222.

56. Sato S, Ohnishi K, Sugita S, Okuda K. Splenic artery and superior mesenteric artery blood flow: nonsurgical Doppler US measurement in healthy subjects and patients with chronic liver disease. Radiology 1987;164:347–352.

57. Tamada T, et al. Portal blood flow: measurement with MR imaging. Radiology 1989;173:639–644.

58. Bierman HR, Miller ER, Bryon RL Jr, Dod KS, Kelly KH, Black DH. Intra-arterial catheterization of viscera in man. AJR 1951;66:555.

59. Morino F, Tarquini A, Olivero S. Artériographie abdominale

60. Ödman P. Percutaneous selective angiography of the superior mesenteric artery. Acta Radiol 1959;51:25–32.

61. Hanafee W. Axillary artery approach to carotid, vertebral, abdominal aorta, and coronary angiography. Radiology 1963; 81:559.

62. Roy P. Percutaneous catheterization via the axillary artery: a new approach to some technical roadblocks in selective arteriography. AJR 1965;94:1.

63. Boijsen E. Selective visceral angiography using a percutaneous axillary technique. Br J Radiol 1966;39:414–421.

64. Boijsen E, Bron KM. Visceral arteriography. Ann Rev Med 1964;15:273–286.

65. Sos TA, Cohn DJ, Srur M, Wengrover SI, Saddekni S. A new open-ended guidewire/catheter. Radiology 1985;154:817–818.

66. Meyerovitz MF, Levin DC, Boxt LM. Superselective catheterization of small-caliber arteries with a new high-visibility steerable guide wire. AJR 1985;144:785–786.

67. Chuang VP. Superselective hepatic tumor embolization with Tracker-18. J Intervent Radiol 1988;3:69.

68. Okazaki M, et al. Emergent embolization for control of massive hemorrhage from a splanchnic artery with a new coaxial system. Acta Radiol 1992;33:57–62.

69. McAfee JG. A survey of complications of abdominal aortography. Radiology 1957;68:825–838.

70. Grayson T, Margulis AR, Heinbecker P, Saltzstein SL. Effects of intra-arterial injection of Miokon, Hypaque, and Renografin in the small intestine of the dog. Radiology 1961;77: 776.

71. Saltzstein SL. The effects of intra-arterial injection of contrast media on canine intestine. AJR 1963;89:730.

72. Cooley RN, Schreiber MH, Brown RW. Effects of transaortic catheter injection of Renografin, Urokon, Hypaque and Miokon into the superior mesenteric arteries of dogs. Angiology 1964;15:107.

73. Sewell RA. Small bowel injury by angiographic contrast media. Surgery 1968;64:459.

74. Redman HC, Berg NO, Boijsen E. Absence of toxicity of contrast media in the superior mesenteric artery: a pathologic study in rabbits. Invest Radiol 1967;2:123–125.

75. Phillips DA, Adams DF, Beckmann CF, Abrams HL. Balloon-occlusion superior mesenteric arteriography for improved visualization of the mesenteric and portal venous anatomy of dogs. Invest Radiol 1980;15:129–133.

76. Moss AA, Margulis AR, Lee JC, Youker JE. The effect of intra-arterial contrast media on the small intestine of rabbit: an electron microscopic study. Radiology 1973;108:279–284.

77. Bonakdarpour A, Shea FJ, Esterhai JL, Siplet H. Serum enzyme changes following selective superior mesenteric arteriography in dogs. Radiology 1972;104:427–428.

78. Skjennald A, Heldaas J, Höiseth A. Comparison of iohexol and meglumine-Na-Ca metrizoate in visceral angiography. Acta Radiol Suppl (Stockh) 1983;366:158–165.

79. Wagner FB Jr, Price AH. Fatality after abdominal arteriography: prevention by new modification of technique. Surgery 1950;27:621.

80. Melick WF, Byrne JE, Boler TD. The experimental and clinical investigation of various media used in translumbar aortography. J Urol 1952;67:1019.

81. Grainger K, Aber C. Dissection of the superior mesenteric artery during aortography with recovery—report of a case. Br J Radiol 1961;34:265–268.

82. Boijsen E. Selective visceral angiography with Isopaque B. Acta Radiol Suppl (Stockh) 1967;270:121–131.

83. Siegelman SS, Warren A, Veith FJ, Boley SJ. The physiologic response to superior mesenteric angiography. Radiology 1970;96:101–105.

84. Lunderquist A, Lunderquist A, Knutsson H. Angiography in Crohn's disease of the small bowel and colon. AJR 1967;101: 338.

sélective par le cathétérisme de l'artère humérale. Presse Med 1956;64:1944.

85. Steckel RJ, Rösch J, Ross G, Grollman JH Jr. New developments in pharmacoangiography (and arterial pharmacotherapy) of the gastrointestinal tract. Invest Radiol 1971;6:199–211.

86. Crummy AB, Stieghorst MF, Turski PA, et al. Digital subtraction angiography: current status and use of intraarterial injection. Radiology 1982;145:303–307.

87. Foley WD, Stewart ET, Milbrath JR, SanDretto M, Milde M. Digital subtraction angiography of the portal venous system. AJR 1983;140:497–499.

88. Chang R, Kaufman SL, Kadir S, Mitchell SE, White RI Jr. Digital subtraction angiography in interventional radiology. AJR 1984;142:363–366.

89. Katzen BT. Peripheral, abdominal, and interventional applications of DSA. Radiol Clin North Am 1985;23:227–241.

90. Rees CR, Palmaz JC, Alvarado R, Tyrrel R, Ciaravino V, Register T. DSA in acute gastrointestinal hemorrhage: clinical and in vitro studies. Radiology 1988;169:499–503.

91. Needleman L, Rifkin MD. Vascular ultrasonography: abdominal applications. Radiol Clin North Am 1986;24:461–484.

92. Scoutt LM, Zawin ML, Taylor KJW. Doppler US: Part II. Clinical applications. Radiology 1990;174:309–319.

93. Edelman RR, Zhao B, Liu C, et al. MR angiography and dynamic flow evaluation of the portal venous system. AJR 1989; 153:755–760.

94. Vock P, Terrier F, Wegmüller H, Mahler F, Gertsch PH, Souza P, Dumoulin CL. Magnetic resonance angiography of abdominal vessels: early experience using the three-dimensional phase-contrast technique. Br J Radiol 1991;64:10–16.

95. Sniderman KW, Baxi RK, Saddekni S, Sos TA. Use of tolazoline enhanced superior mesenteric arteriography to improve opacification of a cecal vascular ectasia: a case report. Gastrointest Radiol 1979;4:339–341.

96. Danford RO, Davidson AJ. The use of glucagon as a vasodilator in visceral angiography. Radiology 1969;93:173–175.

97. Kahn PC, O'Halloran JF Jr, Paul RE Jr. Improved portography by delayed postepinephrine celiac and mesenteric arteriography. Radiology 1969;92:86–89.

98. Udén R. Effect of secretin in celiac and superior mesenteric angiography. Acta Radiol 1969;8:497–513.

99. Udén R. Cholecystokinin-pancreozymin in celiac and superior mesenteric angiography. Acta Radiol 1972;12:363–374.

100. Cho KJ, Chuang VP, Reuter SR. Prostaglandin E$_1$ as a pharmacoangiographic agent for arterial portography. Radiology 1975;116:207–209.

101. Davis LJ, Anderson JH, Wallace S, Gianturco C, Jacobson ED. The use of prostaglandin E$_1$ to enhance the angiographic visualization of the splanchnic circulation. Radiology 1975; 114:281–286.

102. Dencker H, Göthlin J, Hedner P, Lunderquist A, Norryd C, Tylén U. Superior mesenteric angiography and blood flow following intra-arterial injection of Prostaglandin F$_2\alpha$. AJR 1975;125:111–118.

103. Hernandez C, Morin G, Ecarlat B. L'émbol pulsé en artériographie sélective digestive. Presse Med 1965;73:2889.

104. Lunderquist A, Lunderquist A, Nommesen N. Angiographic changes during digestion. AJR 1969;107:191–197.

105. Weber J, Novak D. Occlusion arteriography: diagnostic and therapeutic applicability of balloon catheters. Cardiovasc Intervent Radiol 1980;3:81–96.

106. Jensen R, Olin T. Balloon catheters in angiography: an experimental investigation in rabbits. Acta Radiol 1972;12:721–736.

107. Boijsen E, Reuter SR. Mesenteric angiography in the evaluation of inflammatory and neoplastic disease of the intestine. Radiology 1966;87:1028–1036.

108. Kahn PC, Frates WJ, Paul RE Jr. The epinephrine effect in angiography of gastrointestinal tract tumors. Radiology 1967; 88:686–690.

109. Miller WJ, Reuter SR, Redman HC. Epinephrine effect in angiography of colonic carcinoma: an inconsistent aid in diagnosis. Invest Radiol 1969;4:246–251.

110. Kaplan JH, Bookstein JJ. Abdominal visceral pharmacoangiography with angiotensin. Radiology 1972;103:79–83.

111. Ekelund L, Lunderquist A. Pharmacoangiography with angiotensin. Radiology 1974;110:533–540.

112. Goldstein HM, Miller M. Angiographic evaluation of carcinoid tumors of the small intestine: the value of epinephrine. Radiology 1975;115:23–28.

113. Schobinger R, Blackman G, Kan Lin R. Operative intestinal arteriography. Acta Radiol 1957;48:330–336.

114. Margulis AR, Heinbecker P. Mesenteric arteriography. AJR 1961;86:103.

115. McAlister WH, Margulis AR, Heinbecker P, Spjut H. Arteriography and microangiography of gastric and colonic lesions. Radiology 1962;79:769.

116. Boijsen E, Härtel M. Kontrastmittelpassagezeiten im Versorgungsgebiet der Arteria mesenterica superior. ROEFO 1972;118:491–498.

117. Scott WW Jr, Harrington DP, Siegelman SS. Functional abnormalities of mesenteric blood flow: a guide to organic disease of the bowel. Gastrointest Radiol 1977;1:367–374.

118. Boijsen E, Reuter SR. Angiography in diagnosis of chronic unexplained melena. Radiology 1967;89:413–419.

119. Bonakdarpour A. Angiography of mesenteric arterial occlusion. Invest Radiol 1970;5:316–328.

120. Mavor GE, Chrystal KMR. Problems in mesenteric infarction. J Cardiovasc Surg (Torino) 1962;3:250.

121. Federle MP, Chun G, Jeffrey RB, Rayor R. Computed tomographic findings in bowel infarction. AJR 1984;142:91–95.

122. Shaff MI, Tarr RW, Partain CL, James AE. Computed tomography and magnetic resonance imaging of the acute abdomen. Surg Clin North Am 1988;68:233–254.

123. Fishman MC, Naidich JB, Stein HL. Vascular magnetic resonance imaging. Radiol Clin North Am 1986;24:485–501.

124. Aakhus T, Brabrand G. Angiography in acute superior mesenteric arterial insufficiency. Acta Radiol 1967;6:1–12.

125. Williams LF Jr. Vascular insufficiency of the intestines. Gastroenterology 1971;61:757.

126. Wittenberg J, Athanasoulis CA, Shapiro JH, Williams LF Jr. A radiological approach to the patient with acute extensive bowel ischemia. Radiology 1973;106:13–24.

127. Aakhus T, Evensen A. Angiography in acute mesenteric arterial insufficiency. Acta Radiol 1978;19:945–954.

128. Boley SJ, Sprayregen S, Veith FJ, Siegelman SS. An aggressive roentgenologic and surgical approach to acute mesenteric ischemia. In: Nyhus LM, ed. Surgery annual. New York: Appleton-Century-Crofts, 1973. Vol. 5, pp. 355–378.

129. Kaufman SL, Harrington DP, Siegelman SS. Superior mesenteric artery embolization: an angiographic emergency. Radiology 1977;124:625–630.

130. Bergan JJ, Dean RH, Conn J, Yao JST. Revascularisation in treatment of mesenteric infarction. Ann Surg 1975;182:430.

131. Siegelman SS, Sprayregen S, Boley SJ. Angiographic diagnosis of mesenteric arterial vasoconstriction. Radiology 1974;12: 533–542.

132. Siegelman SS. An aggressive approach to acute small bowel ischemia. In: Margulis AR, Gooding CH, eds. Diagnostic radiology. San Francisco: University of California Printing Department, 1977:85–97.

133. Flickinger EG, Johnsrude IS, Ogbrun NL, Weaver MD, Pories WJ. Local streptokinase infusion for superior mesenteric artery thromboembolism. AJR 1983;140:771–772.

134. Pillari G, Doscher W, Fierstein J, Ross W, Loh G, Berkowitz BJ. Low-dose streptokinase in the treatment of celiac and superior mesenteric artery occlusion. Arch Surg 1983;118: 1340–1344.

135. Ottinger LW, Austen WG. A study of 136 patients with mesenteric infarction. Surg Gynecol Obstet 1967;124:251.

136. Britt LG, Cheek RC. Non-occlusive mesenteric vascular disease: clinical and experimental observations. Ann Surg 1969; 169:704.

137. Pierce GE, Brockenbrough EC. The spectrum of mesenteric infarction. Am J Surg 1970;119:233.

138. Reiner L, Rodriguez FL, Jimenez FA, Platt R. Injection studies on mesenteric arterial circulation: III. Occlusions without intestinal infarction. Arch Pathol 1962;73:461.

139. Pollard JJ, Nebesar RA. Abdominal angiography. N Engl J Med 1968;279:1148.

140. Lande A, Meyers MA. Iatrogenic embolization of the superior mesenteric artery: arteriographic observations and clinical implications. AJR 1976;126:822–828.

141. Muller, RF, Figley MM. The arteries of the abdomen, pelvis, and thigh: I. Normal roentgenographic anatomy. II. Collateral circulation in obstructive arterial disease. AJR 1957;77:296.

142. Brolin I, Paulin S. Abdominal communications between splanchnic vessels. Acta Radiol 1964;2:460–472.

143. Diemel H, Rau G, Schmitz-Dräger H-G. Die Riolansche Kollaterale: Ihre diagnostische Bedeutung für die Angiographie bei Verschlusskrankheiten der Mesenterialarterien. ROEFO 1964;101:253–264.

144. Baum S, Stein GN, Baue A. Extrinsic pressure defects on the duodenal loop in mesenteric occlusive disease. Radiology 1965;85:866–874.

145. Bron KM. Thrombotic occlusion of the abdominal aorta: associated visceral artery lesions and collateral circulation. AJR 1966;96:887.

146. Bücheler E, Düx A, Rohr H. Mesenteric-steal-syndrom. ROEFO 1967;106:313.

147. Kameron GR, Khanna SD. Regeneration of the intestinal villi after extensive mucosal infarction. J Pathol 1959;77:505.

148. Reiner L, Platt R, Rodriguez FL, Jimenez FA. Injection studies on the mesenteric arterial circulation: II. Intestinal infarction. Gastroenterology 1960;39:747.

149. Reeves JD, Wang CC. The stages of mesenteric artery disease. South Med J 1961;54:541.

150. Boley SJ, Krieger H, Schultz L, Robinson K, Siew FP, Allen AC, Schwartz S. Experimental aspects of peripheral vascular occlusion of the intestine. Surg Gynecol Obstet 1965;121:789–794.

151. Bosniak MA, Farmelant MH, Bakos C, Hasiotis CA, Williams LF Jr. Experimental in vivo photographic magnification angiography of the canine kidney and bowel. Invest Radiol 1968;3:120.

152. Noonan CD, Rambo ON, Margulis AR. Effect of timed occlusions at various levels of mesenteric arteries and veins: correlative study of arteriographic and histologic patterns of rat gut. Radiology 1968;90:99–106.

153. Katzen BT, Rossi P, Passariello R, Simonetti G. Transcatheter therapeutic arterial embolization. Radiology 1976;120:523–531.

154. Bookstein JJ, Naderi MJ, Walter JF. Transcatheter embolization for lower gastrointestinal bleeding. Radiology 1978;127:345–349.

155. Walker WJ, Goldin AR, Shaff MI, Allibone GW. Per catheter control of a haemorrhage from the superior and inferior mesenteric arteries. Clin Radiol 1980;31:71–80.

156. Teicher I, Arlen M, Muehlbauer M, Allen AC. The clinical-pathological spectrum of primary ulcers of the small intestine. Surg Gynecol Obstet 1963;116:196.

157. Varay A, Orcel L, Périer E, Blondon J, Durand F, Roland J. La malabsorption d'origine vasculaire: contribution à l'étude des artériopathies ostiales mésentériques supérieures et des ulcères primitifs du grêle. Arch Fr Mal App Dig 1964;53:937–958.

158. Rob C. Surgical diseases of the celiac and mesenteric arteries. Arch Surg 1966;93:21.

159. Rosenman LD, Gropper AN. Small intestine stenosis caused by infarction: an unusual sequel of mesenteric artery embolism. Ann Surg 1955;141:254.

160. Hawkins CF. Jejunal stenosis following mesenteric artery occlusion. Lancet 1957;2:121–122.

161. Perdue GD Jr, Smith RB. Intestinal ischemia due to mesenteric arterial disease. Am Surg 1970;36:152.

162. Bergan JJ. Recognition and treatment of intestinal ischemia. Surg Clin North Am 1967;47:109.

163. Buchardt Hansen HJ, Christoffersen JK. Occlusive mesenteric infarction. Acta Chir Scand Suppl 1976;472:102.

164. Roberts L Jr, Wertman DA Jr, Mills SR, Moore AV Jr, Heaston DK. Transluminal angioplasty of the superior mesenteric artery: an alternative to surgical revascularization. AJR 1983;141:1039–1042.

165. Odurny A, Sniderman KW, Colapinto RF. Intestinal angina: percutaneous transluminal angioplasty of the celiac and superior mesenteric arteries. Radiology 1988;167:59–62.

166. Köhler M, et al. Erfolgreiche Behandlung einer Thrombose der Arteria mesenterica superior durch lokale, hochdosierte Urokinasetherapie. Klin Wochenschr 1985;63:722–727.

167. Perdue GD Jr, Smith RB. Atheromatous microemboli. Ann Surg 1969;169:954.

168. Schwartz S, Waters L. Cholesterol embolization. Radiology 1973;106:37–41.

169. Renert WA, Button KF, Fuld SL, Casarella WJ. Mesenteric venous thrombosis and small-bowel infarction following infusion of vasopressin into the superior mesenteric artery. Radiology 1972;102:299–302.

170. Berardi RS. Vascular complications of superior mesenteric artery infusion with Pitressin in treatment of bleeding oesophageal varices. Am J Surg 1974;127:757.

171. Roberts C, Maddison FE. Partial mesenteric arterial occlusion with subsequent ischemic bowel damage due to pitressin infusion. AJR 1976;126:829–831.

172. Rabinovitch J, Rabinovitch S. Infarction of the small intestine sequent to polyarteritis nodosa of the mesenteric vessels. Am J Surg 1954;88:896.

173. Adler RH, Norcross BM, Lockie LM. Arteritis and infarction of the intestine in rheumatoid arthritis. JAMA 1962;180:922.

174. Chudacek Z. Angiographic diagnosis of polyarteritis nodosa of the liver, kidney, and mesentery. Br J Radiol 1967;40:864–865.

175. Philips JC, Howland WJ. Mesenteric arteritis in systemic lupus erythematosus. JAMA 1968;206:1569.

176. Aboumrad MH, Fine G, Horn RC Jr. Intimal hyperplasia of small mesenteric arteries. Arch Pathol 1963;75:196.

177. May AG, Lipchik EO, Deweese JA. Repair of injured visceral arteries. Ann Surg 1965;162:869.

178. Ledgerwood A, Lucas CE. Survival following proximal superior mesenteric artery occlusion from trauma. J Trauma 1974;14:622.

179. Reiner L. Mesenteric arterial insufficiency and abdominal angina. Arch Intern Med 1964;114:765.

180. Goldstone J, More WS, Hall AP. Chronic occlusion of the superior and inferior mesenteric veins. Ann Surg 1970;36:235.

181. Matthews AE, White RR. Primary mesenteric venous occlusive disease. Am J Surg 1971;122:579.

182. Rankin RS, Hussey JL. Idiopathic inferior mesenteric venous thrombosis demonstrated by angiography. Gastrointest Radiol 1976;1:275–276.

183. Bergentz SE, Ericsson B, Hedner U, Leandoer L, Nilsson JM. Thrombosis in the superior mesenteric and portal veins: report of a case treated with thrombectomy. Surgery 1974;76:286–290.

184. Tey PH, Sprayregen S, Ahmed A, Chan KF. Mesenteric vein thrombosis: angiography in two cases. AJR 1981;136:809–811.

185. Merritt CRB. Ultrasonographic demonstration of portal vein thrombosis. Radiology 1979;133:425–427.

186. Kidambi H, Herbert R, Kidambi AV. Ultrasonic demonstration of superior mesenteric and splenoportal venous thrombosis. J Ultrasound 1986;14:199.

187. Vogelzang RL, Gore RM, Anschuetz SL, Blei AT. Thrombosis of the splanchnic veins: CT diagnosis. AJR 1988;150:93.

188. Haddad MC, Clark DC, Sharif HS, Al Shahed M, Aideyan O, Sammak BM. MR, CT, and ultrasonography of splanchnic venous thrombosis. Gastrointest Radiol 1992;17:34.

189. Hricak H, Amparo E, Fisher MR, Crooks L, Higgins CB. Abdominal venous system: assessment using MR. Radiology 1985;156:415–422.

190. Arrivé L, et al. Diagnosis of abdominal venous thrombosis by means of spin-echo and gradient-echo MR imaging: analysis with receiver operating characteristic curves. Radiology 1991; 181:661–668.

191. Yankes JR, Uglietta JP, Grant J, Braun SD. Percutaneous transhepatic recanalization and thrombolysis of the superior mesenteric vein. AJR 1988;151:289–291.

192. Aakhus T. Angiography in experimental strangulating obstruction of the small intestine in dogs. Acta Radiol 1967;6: 337–347.

193. McPhedran NT, Holliday R, Colapinto RF. Angiographic diagnosis of strangulated bowel obstruction. Can J Surg 1970; 13:90.

194. Buranasiri SI, Baum S, Nusbaum M, Tumen H. The angiographic diagnosis of midgut malrotation with volvulus in adults. Radiology 1973;109:555–556.

195. Chang T, Huang T. Arteriographic diagnosis of intussusception: three case reports. AJR 1973;117:317.

196. Kadir S, Athanasoulis CA, Greenfield AJ. Intestinal volvulus: angiographic findings. Radiology 1978;128:595–599.

197. Cohen AM, Patel S. Arteriographic findings in congenital transmesenteric internal hernia. AJR 1979;133:541–543.

198. Seo KW, Bookstein JJ, Brown HS. Angiography of intussusception of the small bowel. Radiology 1979;132:603–604.

199. Ende N. Infarction of the bowel in cardiac failure. N Engl J Med 1958;258:879.

200. Hoffman FG, Zimmerman SL, Cardwell ES Jr. Massive intestinal infarction without vascular occlusion associated with aortic insufficiency. N Engl J Med 1960;263:436.

201. Gooding RA, Couch RD. Mesenteric ischemia without vascular occlusion. Arch Surg 1962;85:186.

202. Boley SJ, Siegelman SS. Experimental and clinical non-occlusive mesenteric ischemia: pathogenesis, diagnosis, and management. In: Hilal S, ed. Symposium on small vessel angiography. St. Louis: Mosby, 1973.

203. Barth K, Strecker EP, Schmidt-Hieber M, Brobmann GF, Schmidt HA. Klinische und experimentelle Beiträge zum Krankheitsbild der non-occlusive mesenteric Ischemia. Radiologe 1974;14:431–434.

204. Laufman H, Nora PF, Mittelpunkt AI. Mesenteric blood vessels: advances in surgery and physiology. Arch Surg 1964;88: 1021.

205. Penner A, Bernheim AI. Acute postoperative enterocolitis: a study on the pathologic nature of shock. Arch Pathol 1939; 27:966.

206. Wilson R, Qualheim RE. A form of acute hemorrhagic enterocolitis afflicting chronically ill individuals: a description of twenty cases. Gastroenterology 1954;27:431.

207. Boijsen E, Tylén U. Angiography in diagnosis in the exocrine pancreas. Clin Gastroenterol 1972;1:85.

208. Williams LF Jr, Anastasia LF, Hasiotis CA, Bosniak MA, Byrne JJ. Experimental nonocclusive mesenteric ischemia. Arch Surg 1968;96:987.

209. Waltman AC, Jang GC, Athanasoulis CA, Ring EJ, Baum S. Emergency gastrointestinal angiography. Geriatrics 1974;29: 48.

210. Strecker E-P, Schmidt-Hieber M, Barth K, Brobmann GF, Birg W, Schmidt HA. Strophantineffekt auf die Mesenterialarterien (zur Pathogenese der non-occlusive-disease). Vasa 1975;4:391–396.

211. Voegeli E, Binswanger R. Angiographie bei akuten Dunndarmischämien. Schweiz Med Wochenschr 1975;105:1258.

212. MacGregor AMC, Abney HT, Morris L. Pharmacodynamic response in nonocclusive mesenteric ischemia. Am Surg 1974; 40:381–384.

213. Athanasoulis CA, Wittenberg J, Bernstein R, Williams LF. Vasodilatory drugs in the management of nonocclusive bowel ischemia. Gastroenterology 1975;69:146–150.

214. Williams LF Jr, Kim J-P. Nonocclusive mesenteric ischemia. In: Boley SJ, Schwartz SS, Williams LF Jr, eds. Vascular disorders of the intestine. New York: Appleton-Century-Crofts, 1971.

215. Ulano HB, Treat E, Shanbour LL, Jacobson ED. Selective dilatation of the constricted superior mesenteric artery. Gastroenterology 1972;62:39.

216. Boley SJ, Schwartz S, Lash J, Sternhill V. Reversible vascular occlusion of the colon. Surg Gynecol Obstet 1963;116:53–60.

217. Boley SJ, Schwartz SS. Colonic ischemia: reversible ischemic lesions. In: Boley SJ, Schwartz SS, Williams LF Jr, eds. Vascular disorders of the intestine. New York: Appleton-Century-Crofts, 1971.

218. Wittenberg J, Athanasoulis CA, Williams LF Jr, Paredes S, O'Sullivan P, Brown B. Ischemic colitis: radiology and pathophysiology. AJR 1975;123:287–300.

219. Wang CC, Reeves JD. Mesenteric vascular disease. AJR 1960; 83:895.

220. Shippey SH Jr, Acker JJ. Segmental infarction of the colon demonstrated by selective inferior mesenteric angiography. Am J Surg 1965;109:671.

221. Morson BC. Pathology of ischemic colitis. Clin Gastroenterol 1972;1:765.

222. Dunbar JD. Reversible cecal infarction. Am J Surg 1966;112: 447.

223. Farman J. Vascular lesions of the colon. Br J Radiol 1966;39: 575–582.

224. Andersen PE. Ischemic colitis caused by angiography. Clin Radiol 1969;20:414–417.

225. Reuter SR, Kanter JE, Redman HC. Angiography in reversible colonic ischemia. Radiology 1970;97:371–373.

226. DeDombal FT, Fletcher DM, Harris RS. Early diagnosis of ischemic colitis. Gut 1969;10:131.

227. Herlinger H. Angiography of visceral arteries. Clin Gastroenterol 1972;1:547.

228. Schroeder FM, Miller FJ, Nelson JA, Rankin RS. Gastrointestinal angiographic findings in systemic amyloidosis. AJR 1978;131:143–146.

229. Janson R, Beltz L. Abdominelle Aortakoarktation, kombiniert mit Abgangsstenosen des Truncus coeliacus, der Arteria mesenterica superior und der Arteria renalis beidseits. ROEFO 1973;118:690–696.

230. Carucci JJ. Mesenteric vascular occlusion. Am J Surg 1953; 85:47.

231. Derrick JR, Pollard HS, Moore RM. The pattern of arteriosclerotic narrowing of the celiac and superior mesenteric arteries. Ann Surg 1959;149:684.

232. Leymarios J. Contribution à l'étude de la pathologie de l'artère mésentérique supérieure: l'ischémie intestinale non nécrosante. Thèse Médicine, Paris, 1960.

233. Morris GC Jr, DeBakey ME. Abdominal angina—diagnosis and surgical treatment. JAMA 1961;176:89.

234. Fontaine R, Kieny R, Japy C, Warter P. Etude angiographique des oblitérations de l'artère mésentérique supérieure. J Radiol Electrol Med Nucl 1966;47:1.

235. Bron KM, Redman HC. Splanchnic artery stenosis and occlusion: incidence; arteriographic and clinical manifestations. Radiology 1969;92:323–328.

236. Fontaine R, Kim M, Kiney R. Le traitement chirurgical des oblitérations des artères mésentériques: aspect clinique, artériographique et indications chirurgicales. Lyon Chir 1962;58: 641.

237. Goertler K. Das Gefässystem in Bauchraum aus der Sicht des Pathologen. In: Bertelheimer H, Heisig N, eds. Aktuelle Gastroenterologie. Stuttgart: Thieme, 1968.

238. Dunbar JD, Molnar W, Beman FF, Marable SA. Compression of the celiac trunk and abdominal angina: preliminary report of 15 cases. AJR 1965;95:731.

239. Nicholls SC, Kohler TR, Martin RL, Strandness BE. Use of hemodynamic parameters in the diagnosis of mesenteric insufficiency. J Vasc Surg 1986;3:507.

240. Lewin JS, Laub G, Hausmann R. Three-dimensional time-of-flight MR angiography: applications in the abdomen and thorax. Radiology 1991;179:261–264.

241. Johnsson CC, Baggenstoss AH. Mesenteric vascular occlu-

sion: II. Study of 60 cases of occlusion of arteries and of 12 cases of occlusion of both arteries and veins. Mayo Clin Proc 1949;24:649.

242. Koikkalainen K, Köhler R. Stenosis and occlusion in the celiac and mesenteric arteries. Ann Chir Gynaecol 1971;60:9–24.

243. Fry WJ, Kraft RO. Visceral angina. Surg Gynecol Obstet 1963;117:417.

244. Mavor GE, Michie W. Chronic midgut ischaemia. Br Med J 1958;2:534.

245. Busson A, Natali J, Charleux H, Davezac J-F. Syndrome douloureux hyperalgique péri-ombilical par sténose de l'origine du tronc de l'artère mésentérique supérieure, traité par pontage entre l'aorte et la mésentérique supérieure. Arch Fr Mal App Dig 1964;53:1089.

246. Passi RB, Lansing AM. Experimental intestinal malabsorption produced by vascular insufficiency. Can J Surg 1964;7:332.

247. Connolly JE, Abrams HL, Kieraldo JH. Observations on the diagnosis and treatment of obliterative disease of the visceral branches of the abdominal aorta. Arch Surg 1965;90:596.

248. Reuter SR, Redman HC. Gastrointestinal angiography. Philadelphia: Saunders, 1977.

249. Carron DB, Douglas AP. Steatorrhoea in vascular insufficiency of the small intestine. Q J Med 1965;34:331.

250. Joske RA, Shamma'a MH, Drummey GD. Intestinal malabsorption following temporary occlusion of the superior mesenteric artery. Am J Med 1958;25:449–455.

251. Furrer J, Grüntzig A, Kugelmeier J, Goebel N. Treatment of abdominal angina with percutaneous dilatation of an arteria mesenterica superior stenosis: preliminary communication. Cardiovasc Intervent Radiol 1980;3:43–44.

252. Boijsen E, Tylén U. Angiographic findings in malabsorption. Unpublished results, 1969.

253. Taylor KB, Truelove SC. Immunological reactions in gastrointestinal disease: a review. Gut 1962;3:277.

254. Cynn W-S, Herasme VM, Levin BL, Gureghian PA, Schreiber MN. Mesenteric angiography of non-tropical sprue. AJR 1975;125:442–446.

255. Louisy CL, Barton CJ. The radiological diagnosis of *Strongyloides stercoralis* enteritis. Radiology 1971;98:535–541.

256. Lunderquist A, Lunderquist A, H:son Holmdahl K, Clemens F. Selective superior mesenteric arteriography in reticulum cell sarcoma of the small bowel. Radiology 1971;98:113–115.

257. Mandell HN. Abdominal angina: report of a case and review of the literature. N Engl J Med 1957;257:1035.

258. Keeley FX, Misanik LF, Wirts CW. Abdominal angina syndrome. Gastroenterology 1959;37:480.

259. Morris GC Jr, Crawford ES, Cooley DA, DeBakey ME. Revascularization of the celiac and superior mesenteric arteries. Arch Surg 1962;84:95.

260. Klein HJ, Alfidi RJ, Meaney TF, Poirier VC. Angiography in the diagnosis of chronic gastrointestinal bleeding. Radiology 1971;98:83–91.

261. Williams LF Jr. Chronic intestinal ischemia. In: Boley SJ, Schwartz SS, Williams LF Jr, eds. Vascular disorders of the intestine. New York: Appleton-Century-Crofts, 1971.

262. Sheedy PF II, Fulton RE, Atwell DT. Angiographic evaluation of patients with chronic gastrointestinal bleeding. AJR 1975;123:338–347.

263. Wylie EJ, Binkley FM, Palubinskas AJ. Extrarenal fibromuscular hyperplasia. Am J Surg 1966;112:149.

264. Ripley HR, Levin SM. Abdominal angina associated with fibromuscular hyperplasia of the celiac and superior mesenteric arteries. Angiology 1966;17:297.

265. Bardsley JL, Koehler PR. Pseudoxanthoma elasticum: angiographic manifestations in abdominal vessels. Radiology 1969; 93:559–562.

266. Rosenberger A, Munk J, Schramek A, Arieh JB. The angiographic appearance of thromboangiitis obliterans (Buerger's disease) in the abdominal visceral vessels. Br J Radiol 1973; 46:337–343.

267. Gotsman MS, Beck W, Schrire V. Selective angiography in

arteritis of the aorta and its major branches. Radiology 1967; 88:232–248.

268. D'Izarn JJ, Boulet CP, Convard JP, Bonnin A, Ledoux-Lebard G. L'artériographie dans la périartérite noueuse: a propos de 15 cas. J Radiol Electrol 1976;57:505–509.

269. Citron BP, et al. Necrotizing angiitis associated with drug abuse. N Engl J Med 1970;283:1003.

270. Reuter SR, Boijsen E. Angiographic findings in two ileal carcinoid tumors. Radiology 1966;87:836–840.

271. Boijsen E, Kaude J, Tylén U. Radiologic diagnosis of ileal carcinoid tumors. Acta Radiol 1974;15:65–82.

272. Brahme F. Mesenteric angiography in regional enterocolitis. Radiology 1966;87:1037–1042.

273. Miller MH, Lunderquist A, Tylén U. Angiographic spectrum in Crohn's disease of the small intestine and colon. Surg Gynecol Obstet 1975;141:907–914.

274. Katzen BT, Sprayregen S, Chisolm A, Rossi P. Angiographic manifestations of regional enteritis. Gastrointest Radiol 1976; 1:271–274.

275. Brahme F, Lindström C. A comparative radiographic and pathological study on intestinal vaso-architecture in Crohn's disease and in ulcerative colitis. Gut 1970;11:928–940.

276. Kalima TV, Peltokallio P, Myllärniemi H. Vascular pattern in ileal Crohn's disease. Ann Clin Res 1975;7:23–31.

277. McClelland RN, Duke JH. Successful resection of an idiopathic aneurysm of the superior mesenteric artery. Ann Surg 1966;164:167.

278. Weidner W, Fox P, Brooks JW, Vinik M. The roentgenographic diagnosis of aneurysms of the superior mesenteric artery. AJR 1970;109:138.

279. Reuter SR, Fry WJ, Bookstein JJ. Mesenteric artery branch aneurysms. Arch Surg 1968;97:497.

280. Boijsen E, Göthlin J, Hallböök T, Sandblom P. Preoperative angiographic diagnosis of bleeding aneurysms of abdominal visceral arteries. Radiology 1969;93:781–791.

281. Stanley JC, Thompson NW, Fry WJ. Splanchnic artery aneurysms. Arch Surg 1970;101:689–696.

282. Kovac A, Zali MR, Geshner J. False aneurysm of the superior mesenteric artery—a complication of pancreatitis. Br J Radiol 1979;52:836–838.

283. Margulis AR, Heinbecker P, Bernard HR. Operative mesenteric arteriography in the search for the site of bleeding in unexplained gastrointestinal hemorrhage: a preliminary report. Surgery 1960;48:534.

284. Kanter IE, Schwartz AJ, Fleming RJ. Localization of bleeding point in chronic and acute gastrointestinal hemorrhage by means of selective visceral arteriography. AJR 1968;103:386.

285. Halpern M, Turner AF, Citron BP. Hereditary hemorrhagic telangiectasia: an angiographic study of abdominal visceral angiodysplasia associated with gastrointestinal hemorrhage. Radiology 1968;90:1143–1149.

286. Wenz W, Roth F-J, Brückner U. Die Angiographie bei der akuten Gastrointestinalblutung: Experimentelle Voraussetzung und klinische Ergebnisse. ROEFO 1969;110:616–629.

287. Alfidi RD, Esselstyn CD, Tarar R, Klein HJ, Hermann RE, Weakley FL, Turnbull RB Jr. Recognition and angiosurgical detection of arteriovenous malformations of the bowel. Ann Surg 1971;174:573.

288. Ghahremani GG, Kangarloo H, Volberg F, Meyers MA. Diffuse cavernous hemangioma of the colon in the Klippel-Trenaunay syndrome. Radiology 1976;118:673–678.

289. Baum S, Athanasoulis CA, Waltman AC, Galdabini J, Schapiro RH, Warshaw AL, Ottinger LW. Angiodysplasia of the right colon: a cause of gastrointestinal bleeding. AJR 1977; 129:789–794.

290. Boley SJ, Sprayregen S, Sammartano RJ, Adams A, Kleinhaus S. The pathophysiologic basis for the angiographic signs of vascular ectasias of the colon. Radiology 1977;125:615–621.

291. Nyman U, Boijsen E, Lindström C, Rosengren J-E. Angiography in angiomatous lesions of the gastrointestinal tract. Acta Radiol 1980;21:21–31.

292. Boley SJ, Sammartano R, Adams A, Dibiase A, Kleinhaus S,

Sprayregen S. On the nature and etiology of vascular ectasias of the colon: degenerative lesions of aging. Gastroenterology 1977;72:650–660.

293. Galloway SJ, Casarella WJ, Shimkin PM. Vascular malformations of the right colon as a cause of bleeding in patients with aortic stenosis. Radiology 1974;113:11–15.

294. Rogers BH. A newly recognized syndrome: (1) lower intestinal blood loss of obscure cause, (2) hemangiomas of the right large bowel and (3) cardiac vascular or pulmonary insufficiency. Gastrointest Endosc 1979;25:47.

295. Hagihara PF, Chuang VP, Griffen WO. Arteriovenous malformation of the colon. Am J Surg 1977;133:681–687.

296. Weaver GA, Alpern HD, Davis JS, Ramsey WH, Reichelderfer M. Gastrointestinal angiodysplasia associated with aortic valve disease: part of a spectrum of angiodysplasia of the gut. Gastroenterology 1979;77:1.

297. Baker AL, Kahn PC, Binder SC, Patterson JF. Gastrointestinal bleeding due to blue rubber bleb nevus syndrome: a case diagnosed by angiography. Gastroenterology 1971;61:530.

298. Sniderman KW, Franklin J Jr, Sos TA. Successful transcatheter Gelfoam embolization of a bleeding cecal vascular ectasia. AJR 1978;131:157–159.

299. Alavi A. Scintigraphic demonstration of acute gastrointestinal bleeding. Gastrointest Radiol 1980;5:205–208.

300. McKusick KA, Froelich J, Callahan RJ, Winzelberg GG, Strauss HW. ^{99m}Tc red blood cells for detection of gastrointestinal bleeding: experience with 80 patients. AJR 1981;137:1113–1118.

301. Bunker SR, et al. Scintigraphy of gastrointestinal hemorrhage: superiority of ^{99m}Tc red blood cells over ^{99m}Tc sulfur colloid. AJR 1984;143:543–548.

302. Berger RB, Zeman RK, Gottschalk A. The technetium-99m-sulfur colloid angiogram in suspected gastrointestinal bleeding. Radiology 1983;147:555–558.

303. Rösch J, Keller FS, Wawrukiewicz AS, Krippaehne WW, Dotter CT. Pharmacoangiography in the diagnosis of recurrent massive lower gastrointestinal bleeding. Radiology 1982;145:615–619.

304. Glickerman DJ, Kowdley KV, Rösch J. Urokinase in gastrointestinal tract bleeding. Radiology 1988;168:375–376.

305. Gomes AS, Lois JF, McCoy RD. Angiographic treatment of gastrointestinal hemorrhage: comparison of vasopressin infusion and embolization. AJR 1986;146:1031–1037.

306. Encarnacion CE, Kadir S, Beam CA, Payne CS. Gastrointestinal bleeding: treatment with gastrointestinal arterial embolization. Radiology 1992;183:505–508.

307. Sumner RG, Kistler PC, Barry WF Jr, McIntosh HD. Recognition and surgical repair of superior mesenteric arteriovenous fistula. Circulation 1963;27:943.

308. Taylor RMR, Douglas AP, Hacking P, Walker FC. Traumatic fistula between a main branch of the superior mesenteric artery and vein. Am J Med 1965;38:641.

309. Mowitz D, Finne B. Postoperative arteriovenous aneurysm in mesentery after small bowel resection. JAMA 1960;173:42.

310. Munnell ER, Mota CR, Thompson WB. Iatrogenic arteriovenous fistula: report of a case involving the superior mesenteric vessels. Am Surg 1960;26:738.

311. Steinberg I, Tillotson PM, Halpern M. Roentgenography of systemic (congenital and traumatic) arteriovenous fistulas. AJR 1963;89:343.

312. Anderson RD, Liebeskind A, Lowman RM. Arteriovenous fistula of the mesentery. Am J Gastroenterol 1972;57:453–458.

313. Hederström E, Forsberg L, Ivancev K, Lundstedt C, Stridbeck H. Ultrasonography and Doppler duplex compared with angiography in follow-up of mesocaval shunt patency. Acta Radiol 1990;31:341–345.

314. Bernardino ME, Steinberg HV, Pearson TC, Gedgaudas-McClees RK, Torres WE, Henderson JM. Shunts for portal hypertension: MR and angiography for determination of patency. Radiology 1986;158:57–61.

315. Ohtomo K, Itai Y, Makita K, Yashiro N, Yoshikawa K, Ko-

kubo T, Iio M. Portosystemic collaterals on MR imaging. J Comput Assist Tomogr 1986;10:751–755.

316. Williams DM, Eckhauser FE, Aisen A, Knol JA, Strodel WE. Assessment of portosystemic shunt patency and function with magnetic resonance imaging. Surgery 1987;102:602–607.

317. Gehl H-B, Bohndorf K, Klose K-C, Günther RW. Two-dimensional MR angiography in the evaluation of abdominal veins with gradient refocused sequences. J Comput Assist Tomogr 1990;14:619.

318. Johnson CD, Ehman EL, Rakela J, Ilstrup DM. MR angiography in portal hypertension: detection of varices and imaging techniques. J Comput Assist Tomogr 1991;15:578–584.

319. Spjut HJ, Margulis AR, McAlister WH. Microangiographic study of gastrointestinal lesions. AJR 1964;92:1173.

320. Spjut HJ, Margulis AR. Microangiographic patterns of chronic ulcerative colitis. Dis Colon Rectum 1965;8:215.

321. Boijsen E, Olin T. Zöliakographie und Angiographie der Arteria mesenterica superior. In: Schinz HR, Glauner R, Rüttiman A, eds. Ergebenisse der medizinischen Strachlenforschung. Stuttgart 1964;112–142.

322. Debray C, Leymarios J, Hernandez C, Marche C, Hardouin J-P, Pironneau A. Tumeur bénigne de l'intestine grêle (léiomyome) diagnostiquée par artériographie mésentérique supérieure. Presse Med 1964;72:3005.

323. Nebesar RA, Pollard JJ, Edmunds LH Jr, McKhann CF. Indications for selective celiac and superior mesenteric angiography: experience with 128 cases. AJR 1964;92:1100.

324. Baum S, Roy R, Finkelstein AK, Blakemore WS. Clinical application of selective celiac and superior mesenteric arteriography. Radiology 1965;84:279–295.

325. Koehler PR, Salmon RB. Angiographic localization of unknown acute gastrointestinal bleeding sites. Radiology 1967;89:244–249.

326. Kaude J, Silseth Ch, Tylén U. Angiography in myomas of the gastrointestinal tract. Acta Radiol 1972;12:691–704.

327. Ekberg O, Ekholm S. Radiography in primary tumors of the small bowel. Acta Radiol 1980;21:79–84.

328. Lunderquist A, Lunderquist A. Angiography in ulcerative colitis. AJR 1967;99:18.

329. Herlinger H. Angiography in Crohn's disease. Clin Gastroenterol 1972;1:383.

330. Brahme F, Hildell J. Angiography in Crohn's disease revisited. AJR 1976;126:941–951.

331. Dombrowski H, Korb G. Das Gefässbild bei Enteritis regionalis (Morbus Crohn) und sein diagnostische Bedeutung. Radiologe 1970;10:17–24.

332. Kinkhabwala M, Balthazar EJ. Carcinoid tumors of the alimentary tract: II. Angiographic diagnosis of small intestinal and colonic lesions. Gastrointest Radiol 1978;3:57–61.

333. Collatz Christensen S, Stage JG, Henriksen FW. Angiography in the diagnosis of carcinoid syndrome. Scand J Gastroenterol Suppl 1979;14:111–114.

334. Gold RE, Redman HC. Mesenteric fibrosis simulating the angiographic appearance of ileal carcinoid tumor. Radiology 1972;103:85–86.

335. Carillo FJ, Ruzicka FF Jr, Clemett AR. Value of angiography in the diagnosis of retractile mesenteritis. AJR 1972;115:396–398.

336. Diamond AB, Meng C-H, Goldin RR. Arteriography of unusual mass lesions of the mesentery. Radiology 1974;110:547–552.

337. Sacks B, Joffe N, Harris N. Isolated mesenteric dermoids (mesenteric fibromatosis). Clin Radiol 1978;29:95–100.

338. Debray C, et al. Tumeurs de l'intestine grêle diagnostiquées exclusivement par l'artériographie sélective de la mésentérique supérieure: a propos de 2 cas. Arch Fr Mal Appar Dig 1965;54:593.

339. Meyers MA, King MC. Leiomyosarcoma of the duodenum: angiographic findings and report of a case. Radiology 1968;91:788–790.

340. Ramer M, Mitty HA, Baron MG. Angiography in leiomyomatous neoplasms of the small bowel. AJR 1971;113:263–268.

341. Robert PE, Pradel E, Hernandez C, Chemali A. Utilisation et enseignement de l'artériographie sélective dans un syndrome de Peutz-Jeghers. Semin Hop Paris 1966;42:1975.

342. Gasquet C, Barbier J. L'artériographie séléctive mésentérique supérieure dans le syndrome de Peutz-Jeghers. Semin Hop Paris 1968;44:1953.

343. Fenlon JW, Schackelford GD. Peutz-Jeghers syndrome: case report with angiographic evaluation. Radiology 1972;103: 595–596.

344. Ekberg O, Ekholm S. Radiology in primary small bowel adenocarcinoma. Gastrointest Radiol 1980;5:49–53.

345. Riba PO, Lunderquist A. Angiographic findings in villous tumors of the colon. AJR 1973;117:287–291.

346. Albrechtsson U, Tylén U. Angiography in reticulum cell sarcoma. Acta Radiol 1977;18:210–216.

347. Gordon RB, Capetillo A, Principato DJ. Angiographic demonstration of a lymphatic cyst of the mesentery: a case report. AJR 1968;104:870.

348. Lunderquist A, Lunderquist A. Arteriographic appearance of intestinal adhesions. AJR 1968;103:354–358.

349. Meyers MA. Arteriographic diagnosis of internal (left para-duodenal) hernia. Radiology 1969;92:1035–1037.

350. Lande A, Schechter LS, Bole PV. Angiographic diagnosis of small intestinal intussusception. Radiology 1977;122:691–693.

351. Cornet A, et al. Diverticule de Meckel à form hémorrhagique: dépistage artériographique. Semin Hop Paris 1967;43:3441.

352. Bree RL, Reuter SR. Angiographic demonstration of a bleeding Meckel's diverticulum. Radiology 1973;108:287–288.

353. Friedmann G, Bützler HO, Wehrle J. Angiographische Befunde bei zwei rezidivierend blutenden Meckelschen Divertikeln (MD). ROEFO 1974;120:446–452.

354. Dencker H, H:Son Holmdahl K, Lunderquist A, Olivecrona H, Tylén U. Mesenteric angiography in patients with radiation injury of the bowel after pelvis irradiation. AJR 1972; 114:476–481.

355. Rogers LF, Goldstein HM. Roentgen manifestations of radiation injury to the gastrointestinal tract. Gastrointest Radiol 1977;2:281–291.

356. Gray RK, Grollman JH Jr. Acute lower gastrointestinal bleeding secondary to varices of the superior mesenteric venous system: angiographic demonstration. Radiology 1974;111:559–561.

357. Barth V, Kölmel B. Blutende Dunndarmvarizen bei portaler Hypertension als seltene Komplikation nach abdominellen Operationen. ROEFO 1980;132:219–221.

358. Schild H, Schweden F, Braun B, Lang H. Aneurysm of the superior mesenteric artery. Radiology 1982;145:641–642.

359. Mathias KD, Hoffmann J, Krabb HJ, Polonius MJ. Aneurysm of the superior mesenteric vein. Cardiovasc Intervent Radiol 1987;10:269–271.

62

Inferior Mesenteric Arteriography

HERBERT L. ABRAMS
MICHAEL F. MEYEROVITZ

Within recent years, mesenteric vascular disease has emerged as an important and difficult medical problem.[1-9] While the need for clinical recognition of abdominal angina has been emphasized, the capacity to define obstructive disease of the mesenteric arterial branches has simultaneously been enhanced.[10,11] The frequency of occlusive disease has become apparent,[3,12] and the inferior mesenteric artery has become recognized as a major collateral channel. Nonocclusive ischemic colitis has been clearly documented as a syndrome with multiple inciting factors.[4] Interest has also grown in the study of the tumor vascular bed and inflammatory disease of the colon. In 1962, Ström and Winberg demonstrated that selective mesenteric arteriography was technically feasible, and they devised a preshaped catheter for easy entrance into the vessel. They summarized their experience with carcinoma of the colon and diverticulitis.[13] Halpern indicated his enthusiasm for the method in a report of a limited series of cases.[14] Kahn and Abrams later discussed in detail the normal inferior mesenteric artery and the changes found in occlusive disease of the mesenteric vessels.[11] Wholey et al. noted the indications,[15] and Boijsen and Reuter attempted to distinguish inflammatory disease and neoplastic disease.[16] Brahme has studied the changes in regional enterocolitis.[17] Perhaps of greatest importance, the detection and treatment of left colic bleeding via the angiographic catheter has become a central aspect of the management of such disorders.[18-21]

This chapter summarizes the technique, normal anatomy, indications, and value of inferior mesenteric arteriography.

Technique

Percutaneous transfemoral catheter insertion from the left femoral artery is preferred when attempting to catheterize the inferior mesenteric artery, except when there is femoral artery occlusive disease. The transaxil-lary or transbrachial approach may then be employed. The inferior mesenteric circulation can be readily shown by intraaortic injection below the level of the renal arteries, although the distal inferior mesenteric branches may not be well demonstrated and bleeding sites cannot be reliably shown with nonselective arteriography. If this method is used when selective studies are not feasible, 35 ml of contrast medium should be injected over a 2-second period. If the orifice of the inferior mesenteric vessel is to be seen dependably, an intraaortic injection must be obtained, and by far the best projection is the lateral one. When vascular occlusive disease is suspected, it is often essential to place the catheter at the level of the celiac artery and to define the orifices of the celiac, superior mesenteric, and inferior mesenteric arteries simultaneously.

The preferable approach to selective arteriography is to employ a preshaped catheter so designed as to permit ready entry into the inferior mesenteric artery. The orifice is usually located on the left anterolateral wall of the aorta at the level of the third lumbar vertebra. The most commonly used catheter shapes are a Simmons 1, a cobra 1, or a simple C curve similar to that described by Ström and Winberg[13] (illustrated in Fig. 62-2). For filming, 15 ml of contrast medium is injected at a rate of 3 ml per second unless the artery is large and supplying collateral circulation, in which case the rate and volume can be increased. Our normal filming sequence for mesenteric arteriography is two films per second for 2 seconds, one film per second for 5 seconds, and then one film every other second for 20 seconds. This sequence will show the arterial, capillary, and venous phases to good advantage and will allow bleeding sites to be clearly distinguished. The images may be acquired either with cut film or digitally. If digital subtraction imaging is used, bowel motion will give rise to artifacts.[22] The field of interest must be carefully collimated to obtain maximal detail, and with cut film the kilovoltage should be kept appropriately low to obtain good contrast. Frequently it will be desirable to perform a second study with the patient in a left posterior oblique projection to refine to a greater degree the analysis of the vessels and their distribution.

After the initial examination, it may be desirable to use a vasodilating drug to visualize the small vascular bed and venous drainage more effectively.

Normal Anatomy

Although the anatomy of the inferior mesenteric artery in cadavers has been well described,[23–26] there have been few serious, systematic attempts to analyze the angiographic anatomy and its variations. Some years ago, therefore, Abrams and Kahn undertook a review of 142 consecutive angiographic studies of the abdominal aorta and its branches. Such a study seemed warranted not only because there was considerable interest in inferior mesenteric artery insufficiency but also because the potential application of chemotherapeutic agents to bowel tumors by direct perfusion depends on a precise knowledge of the anatomy of the vascular bed. Furthermore, there was reason to believe that angiographic studies in vivo might yield information not attainable from postmortem studies and not necessarily in accord with conventional anatomic data.[27] In all except 6 of the 142 cases, analysis of the inferior mesenteric circulation was feasible. The material that follows on normal anatomy is drawn from that review.[11]

The inferior mesenteric artery originates from the left anterior wall of the abdominal aorta at about the level of the third lumbar vertebra. After descending parallel to the aorta for 3 to 4 cm, it gives off an ascending branch. This branch may consist of the left colic artery alone or one or more sigmoid branches as well. In 60 percent of the cases studied, the left colic artery and one or more sigmoid branches arose jointly as a single major trunk; in about 40 percent of cases, the left colic artery arose as a separate and distinct vessel (Figs. 62-1 and 62-2). The descending branch is the continuation of the inferior mesenteric artery and gives off the sigmoid branches not originating from the left colic artery. As it courses over the common iliac vessels, it becomes the superior hemorrhoidal artery. Branches of the left colic and sigmoid arteries participate in the large anastomosing channel of the mesocolon known as the *marginal artery*. This vessel, probably first described by Von Haller in 1786[28] and subsequently reemphasized by Drummond in his classic paper in 1914,[29] is almost invariably visualized with good opacification of the inferior mesenteric artery. From it, as well as from the other arcades of the mesocolon, originate the vasa recta that supply the bowel wall. They are best demonstrated by selective arteriog-

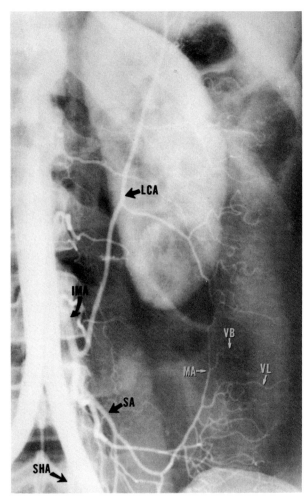

Figure 62-1. Normal inferior mesenteric arteriogram, aortic injection. The inferior mesenteric artery (*IMA*) gives off the left colic (*LCA*) and sigmoid branches (*SA*) and becomes the superior hemorrhoidal artery (*SHA*) after passing over the iliac vessels. The first branch of the left colic artery is the marginal artery (*MA*), which is continuous with the marginal branch of the sigmoid artery. The vasa brevia (*VB*) and vasa longa (*VL*) arise from the marginal artery and supply the wall of the colon.

raphy (see Fig. 62-2), but they may also be well seen after intraaortic injection.

The so-called marginal artery has been the source of much confusion in the literature. As Drummond described it, it represents a system of arcades to which the ileocolic, right colic, middle colic, left colic, and upper sigmoid arteries contribute. Although the colic arteries parallel the marginal artery at times, they also represent integral components of the marginal system. Thus, in injected specimens and in vivo, the colic arteries or their branches may give rise to the vasa recta of the colon directly and hence act as a marginal artery. In such instances it is impossible to define where the colic arteries and their branches end and the marginal

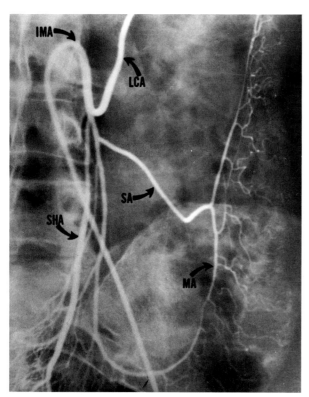

Figure 62-2. Normal inferior mesenteric arteriogram, selective injection. The left colic artery (*LCA*) originates as a single branch. Immediately thereafter, a sigmoid trunk arises, which subsequently divides into three sigmoid arteries (*SA*). The marginal artery (*MA*) follows the course of the sigmoid colon and the descending colon. The inferior mesenteric artery (*IMA*) continues into the pelvis as the superior hemorrhoidal artery (*SHA*).

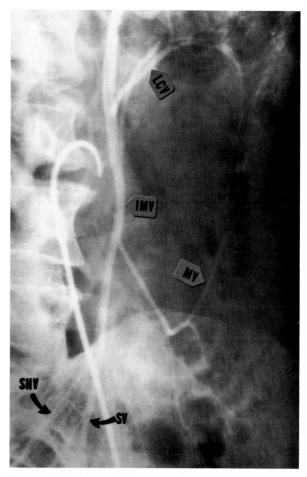

Figure 62-3. Normal inferior mesenteric venogram, selective injection. The venous phase demonstrates the superior hemorrhoidal vein (*SHV*), sigmoid veins (*SV*), left colic branches (*LCV*), and marginal vein (*MV*) draining into the inferior mesenteric vein (*IMV*). The inferior mesenteric vein empties into the splenic vein.

artery begins. The authors have therefore chosen to speak of the marginal artery as the total complex of arcades from which the nutrient vessels of the colon derive (particularly because the marginal artery connects the colon branches and merges imperceptibly with them). When the marginal system functions as a major collateral pathway in humans between the superior and inferior mesenteric arteries, we have designated the large major trunk as the *marginal artery,* although elements of the left colic and middle colic arteries clearly may independently play an important role.

The inferior mesenteric vein is a continuation of the superior hemorrhoidal vein; it receives the drainage from the left colon through the left colic and sigmoid veins (into which the marginal vein empties) (Fig. 62-3). It lies in the retroperitoneal space to the left of the spine and empties into the splenic vein after passing behind the pancreas.

The circulation time through the inferior mesenteric system has been studied both by cine and large-

film techniques. The time required for the development of threshold density in the inferior mesenteric vein after contrast injection into the inferior mesenteric artery is about 6 to 7 seconds in the normal individual.

Level of Origin of the Inferior Mesenteric Artery

The inferior mesenteric artery may arise at any level from the second to the fourth lumbar vertebra. In 66 percent of all cases, it arose at the level of the third lumbar vertebra, and in 87 percent, between the lower border of the second and the upper border of the fourth lumbar vertebra (Fig. 62-4). Thus in most instances its origin is sufficiently above the aortic bifurcation that thromboobliterative disease at the

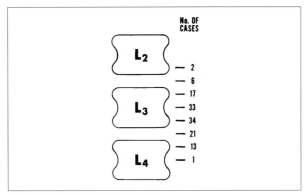

Figure 62-4. Level of aortic origin of the inferior mesenteric artery. The number of cases in which the artery arose at the level of the second, third, and fourth lumbar vertebrae (L2, L3, L4) is indicated.

bifurcation need not involve the inferior mesenteric circulation.

Segments of Colon Supplied by the Inferior Mesenteric Artery

In about 20 percent of the cases analyzed, the inferior mesenteric artery supplied the distal colon up to the middle or the lower descending colon. In 25 percent of cases, the area of supply reached but did not include the splenic flexure. In 44 percent of cases, the splenic flexure was included in the area of supply, and in an additional 10 percent the branches extended proximal to the splenic flexure. In only 3 percent of cases was the middle portion of the transverse colon supplied by the inferior mesenteric artery; the overwhelming bulk of cases demonstrated supply by the middle colic branch of the superior mesenteric artery.

Size of the Inferior Mesenteric Artery and Its Branches

There is great variability in the size of the inferior mesenteric artery in adults (1.2–5.5 mm in diameter) (Table 62-1). The same is true for the branches of the inferior mesenteric artery. The size bears no relationship to the degree of atheromatous disease of the aorta or of the inferior mesenteric artery. There is a rough correlation between the size of the left colic artery and the length of the colic segment supplied: the smaller diameters are found in patients in whom only the middle or the low descending colon is supplied by the left colic artery, whereas the larger diameters are found in those patients in whom the left colic branches are distributed to the splenic flexure and the transverse colon.

Table 62-1. Size of Inferior Mesenteric Artery Branches in Normal Subjects*

Mesenteric Branch	Number of Patients	Range (mm)	Mean (mm)
Inferior mesenteric artery	110	1.2–5.5	3.34
Ascending branch (LC & S)	57	1.2–4.0	2.60
Ascending branch (LC)	35	1.0–3.1	2.07
Ascending branch (overall)	97	1.0–4.0	2.39
Left colic	106	1.0–2.8	1.70
Descending branch (part S)	53	1.0–4.0	2.47
Descending branch (all S)	36	1.2–4.4	2.58
Descending branch (overall)	95	1.0–4.4	2.54
Superior hemorrhoidal	37	1.0–3.0	2.02

*Patients under the age of 16 and those with occlusion have been excluded.
LC = left colic artery; S = sigmoid artery.

Indications for Arteriography

Mesenteric Vascular Disease

In those cases in which intestinal ischemia is thought to be present, the demonstration of the mesenteric vessels by arteriography is the only definitive method other than surgery to define the site and degree of luminal compromise. In acute ischemia, arteriography may establish the presence or absence of occlusion of the inferior mesenteric artery and the extent of the collateral circulation. It may corroborate or rule out embolic occlusion.

Colic Bleeding of Undetermined Etiology

Mesenteric arteriography may demonstrate the site of bleeding or the presence of an angiomatous malformation in the bowel wall. Transcatheter therapy may then be undertaken.

Adequacy of Blood Supply of Bowel Segment to Be Transplanted for Esophageal Prosthesis

If there is significant atherosclerotic narrowing of the vessels supplying the bowel segment to be used, the chances of a successful operation are significantly reduced.

Primary Vascular Abnormalities

Intestinal Ischemia

The classic clinical picture of chronic intestinal ischemia includes postprandial pain, weight loss, and bowel dysfunction. A history of cramping upper abdominal pain that is worse after a large meal is helpful if present, but the symptoms may be relatively nondescript, and the character of the pain is not always specific. Even in cases displaying classic symptoms, the diagnosis has frequently been missed until acute vascular insufficiency supervened.[4] Because the mortality is far higher for emergency than for elective surgical procedures,[2] a high index of suspicion must be maintained for ischemic bowel disease, and symptoms suggestive of acute bowel ischemia should prompt immediate angiographic studies.

In the analysis of visceral ischemic syndromes, and of bowel infarction as well, emphasis traditionally has been on the superior mesenteric artery,[30,31] partly because it supplies such a large segment of the intestine. Nevertheless, it is clear that the inferior mesenteric artery is also a frequent site of atheromatous change and, at times, of occlusion. Perhaps a major factor in the persistent viability of the gut associated with significant disease of the inferior mesenteric artery is the richness of the collateral system.

The syndrome of mesenteric artery insufficiency of the colon or the rectum has been described with increasing frequency as a spontaneous occurrence[2,32,33] or as a result of aortic surgery[34-39] or translumbar aortography.[40-44] Characteristically, the patient complains of left lower quadrant pain, melena, and often diarrhea.[45] Sigmoidoscopy may be diagnostic (showing bluish-black areas of ischemia, most often at the rectosigmoid junction).[46] Because the surgical approach to mesenteric vascular disease is becoming more sophisticated,[30,32,47-52] the role of arteriography has been significantly amplified as a means of defining the site and the degree of major vessel narrowing. When arterial surgery is contemplated, an arteriographic map is essential. Once the presence of stenosis or occlusion of one of the mesenteric arteries has been established, the question still remains as to its relationship to the patient's symptoms. It is clear that significant degrees of stenosis and occlusion of the mesenteric arteries may be present without symptoms.[3,11,51,53,54] A major determinant of the sufficiency of the blood supply is the extent of the collateral circulation.

Collateral Circulation to Left Colon

The collateral circulation used after inferior mesenteric artery occlusion comprises primarily the marginal ar-

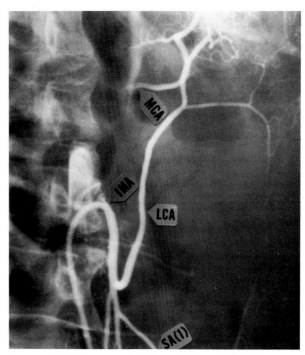

Figure 62-5. Retrograde filling of the middle colic artery from the inferior mesenteric artery. After selective injection into the inferior mesenteric artery (*IMA*), the left colic artery (*LCA*) and the marginal branches opacify, with retrograde flow into the middle colic artery (*MCA*). There is no evidence of mesenteric vascular disease. The inferior mesenteric artery trunk, after the origin of the left colic, divides into the sigmoidal artery (*SA*) and the superior hemorrhoidal artery.

tery, which, adjacent to the splenic flexure, communicates with the middle colic branch of the superior mesenteric artery.[55] In addition, a short retroperitoneal loop connecting the superior and inferior mesenteric arteries or their major branches may be an important collateral element. Below the termination of the marginal artery and the lower sigmoid colon, connections with the middle and inferior hemorrhoidal branches of the hypogastric artery and the middle sacral artery give rise to a rich collateral source in the rectum.

Among the 136 cases in which satisfactory inferior mesenteric arteriograms were obtained, there were 93 normal studies, 6 of which showed filling of potential collateral channels.[11] Such filling was best demonstrated by selective inferior mesenteric arteriography. After opacification of the inferior mesenteric and the left colic arteries, the middle colic artery filled from the marginal vessel, a continuation of the left colic artery (Fig. 62-5). Conversely, retrograde filling of an apparently normal left colic artery was seen on selective superior mesenteric arteriography (Fig. 62-6). In addition, connections between the inferior mesenteric artery and the celiac axis were sometimes visible in the

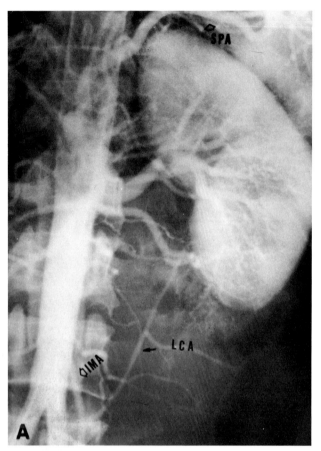
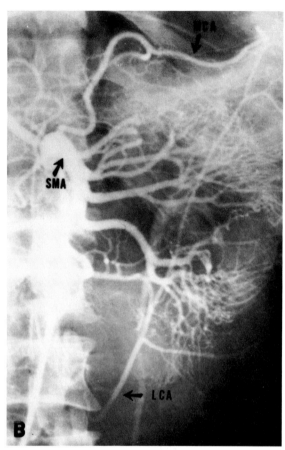

Figure 62-6. Retrograde filling of the left colic artery from the superior mesenteric artery. (A) Aortic injection. There is normal prograde filling of the inferior mesenteric (*IMA*) and left colic (*LCA*) arteries. Other branches of the aorta, such as the splenic artery (*SPA*) and the superior mesenteric and renal arteries, are also filled. (B) Selective superior mesenteric arteriogram. After injection into the superior mesenteric artery (*SMA*), the middle colic artery (*MCA*) opacifies in continuity with the marginal loop, from which the left colic branch (*LCA*) of the inferior mesenteric artery fills.

presence of otherwise normal mesenteric vessels (Fig. 62-7).

With occlusive disease of one or more of the major mesenteric arteries, the marginal loop may become strikingly prominent. In this way, the inferior mesenteric artery may supply the superior mesenteric channels (Fig. 62-8) or both the superior mesenteric and the celiac circulations (Fig. 62-9). By the same token, occlusive disease of the inferior mesenteric artery permits flow from the middle colic artery into the marginal artery and hence an adequate supply to the branches of the inferior mesenteric artery (Fig. 62-10). Under these circumstances, the enlargement of the marginal artery is not as great as it is when a patent inferior mesenteric artery functions as a major avenue of supply to the proximal large bowel.

The degree to which the mesenteric arteries may function as an effective collateral network either prograde or retrograde has been emphasized in several ar-

ticles.[10,11,56] The number of collateral vessels demonstrated by angiography was found by Hansen and Efsen to serve as a crude index of the significance of mesenteric vascular disease.[3] In their study, patients with symptomatic disease had, on the average, twice as many collateral vessels as did asymptomatic patients. The relationship was not consistent, however; just as some symptomless patients exhibited collateral vessels, so some patients with symptomatic disease had none identified. Presumably, the intestinal blood supply was maintained through collateral vessels that were not angiographically evident. The major cause of a developed collateral circulation is arteriosclerotic narrowing or occlusion, but congenital lesions, vasculitis, emboli, neoplastic disease, and inflammatory lesions may all alter regional flow to the bowel.[57] Even with acute occlusion of the superior mesenteric artery, the inferior mesenteric artery may function as a collateral channel.[58] Collateral flow from the inferior mesenteric and celiac arteries is of vital importance because the superior mesenteric artery receives no extramesenteric collateral flow.[3]

The inferior mesenteric artery also participates as a collateral channel in occlusive disease of the aorta and the iliac arteries. If the abdominal aorta is obstructed below the level of the superior mesenteric artery, the marginal loop may form one of the major pathways for blood to the lower aorta and the lower extremities (Fig. 62-11). When the obstruction in the aorta is below the origin of the inferior mesenteric artery, the superior hemorrhoidal anastomoses to the hypogastric artery become prominent and serve as important collateral vessels to the lower extremities (Fig. 62-12). The major supply to the rectum is through the middle and inferior hemorrhoidal arteries arising from the hypogastric artery. If the anastomoses between the superior and the middle hemorrhoidal arteries are inadequate, ischemia of the rectum may develop after distal aortic surgery or iliac artery ligation, even when the marginal artery supplies the remainder of the left colon.

Arteriosclerosis, Stenosis, and Occlusion

The angiographic findings in arteriosclerosis of the inferior mesenteric arteries may be summarized as follows: (1) eccentric plaques; (2) eccentric filling defects, probably incorporating both plaque and thrombus; (3) concentric narrowing; (4) occlusion; and (5) segmental stenosis. Dysplasia involving the mesenteric arteries is rare. In two cases of nonocclusive intestinal infarction, histologic examination of distal branches of the superior mesenteric artery revealed ultrastructural changes similar to those that have been experimentally produced in the renal arteries by hypertension.[59] It is likely that such lesions may also occur in the inferior mesenteric artery in some hypertensive individuals. Thrombotic occlusion of the abdominal aorta may be associated with inferior mesenteric artery occlusion.[60]

One of the major questions with regard to mesenteric artery insufficiency is the degree to which arterial lesions are found in asymptomatic patients as well as in symptomatic patients. A significant amount of information has been accumulated on this subject. In the series under discussion, total occlusion of the inferior mesenteric artery was present in 9 (6.6 percent) of 136 patients with satisfactory studies (see Fig. 62-10).[11] In an additional 23 patients (17 percent), stenosis or atheromatous change of a significant degree was visible in the inferior mesenteric artery (Fig. 62-13), but none of these patients had symptoms of intestinal ischemia. In association with arteriosclerosis of the inferior mes-

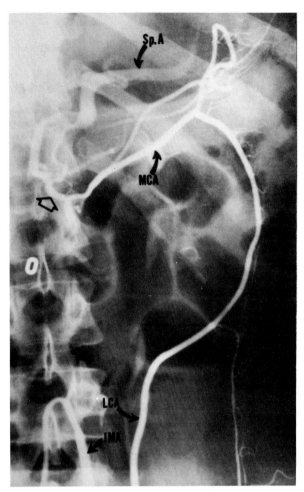

Figure 62-7. Retrograde filling of the splenic artery from the inferior mesenteric artery as shown by a selective inferior mesenteric arteriogram. After injection of the inferior mesenteric artery (*IMA*), good filling of the left colic artery (*LCA*) and the middle colic artery (*MCA*) is demonstrated. Through a retroperitoneal connection (*open arrow*), the splenic artery (*Sp. A*) is filled with contrast material and can be outlined throughout most of its course.

enteric artery, a characteristic plaque at the origin of this vessel was often seen. This plaque was usually best defined in the left posterior oblique projection (see Fig. 62-13B). Arteriosclerotic change in the inferior mesenteric artery was unusual in the absence of significant atheromata in the aortic wall at other levels. In a review of 2029 abdominal aortograms by Hansen and Efsen, 118 (5.6 percent) were found to show stenoses or occlusions in one or more of the three major visceral arteries.[3] Only 32 (27 percent) of the patients with arteriographically demonstrated abdominal vascular disease had symptoms of intestinal ischemia.

Text continues on page 1600

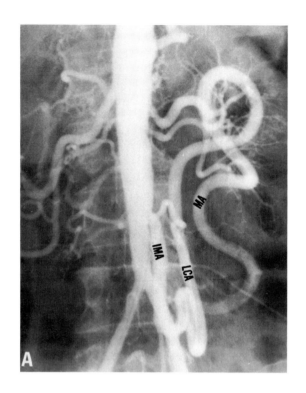

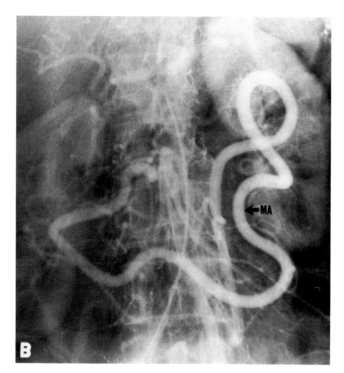

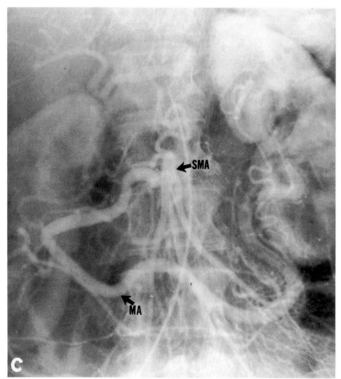

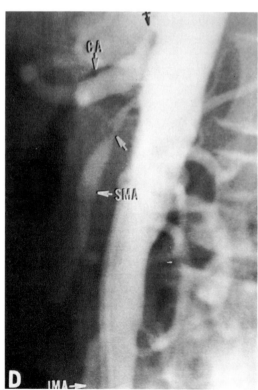

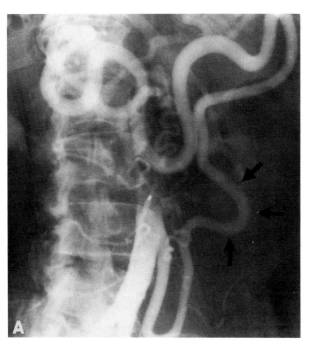 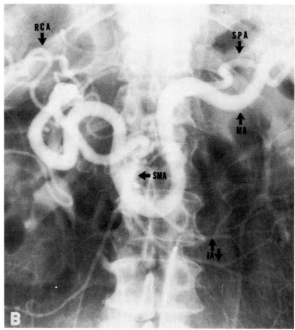

Figure 62-9. The intestinal collateral circulation in occlusive disease: stenosis of the celiac and superior mesenteric arteries. This 52-year-old woman had a 25-year history of hypertension and had noted the onset of intermittent claudication of both lower extremities a few months before admission. Femoral arteriography demonstrated arteriosclerotic disease with stenosis of the left external iliac and the left common femoral arteries and both hypogastric arteries. Aortography revealed the marginal artery as the source of blood to both the celiac and the superior mesenteric circulations. (A) Abdominal aortogram, right posterior oblique projection. The catheter has deliberately been placed below the renal arteries near the mouth of the inferior mesenteric artery. From the inferior mesenteric artery, a grossly dilated marginal artery (*arrows*) is visible. It pursues a circuitous course following the distribution of the left colic and the middle colic arteries. (B) Abdominal aortogram, anteroposterior projection, 2.5 seconds. The large marginal artery (*MA*) is seen to fill the branches both of the superior mesenteric artery (*SMA*) and the celiac artery. Filling of the splenic artery (*SPA*), the right colic artery (*RCA*), and the intestinal branches (*IA*) of the superior mesenteric artery is clearly demonstrated. A subsequent aortogram in the lateral projection demonstrated virtually complete occlusion of both the celiac and superior mesenteric arteries just distal to their origin.

◄ **Figure 62-8.** The intestinal collateral circulation in occlusive disease. Superior mesenteric artery stenosis. This 50-year-old woman had intermittent claudication of both lower extremities. Femoral arteriography demonstrated marked arteriosclerotic disease in both superficial femoral arteries. No symptoms referable to the abdomen were present. Aortography demonstrated a huge marginal artery as an important collateral system. (A) At 1 second after injection, moderate atheromatous changes are visible in the aortic wall. The inferior mesenteric artery (*IMA*) is dilated and may be seen in continuity with an enlarged left colic (*LCA*) and marginal artery (*MA*). In spite of the excellent filling of the abdominal aortic branches, the superior mesenteric artery is not visualized. (B) At 2.5 seconds, the marginal artery is in continuity with the middle colic artery and follows the transverse mesocolon to the right. (C) At 4.5 seconds, the marginal artery (*MA*) can now be seen to anastomose with the superior mesenteric artery (*SMA*), which fills quite densely only after a long interval. (D) Lateral projection at 1 second. Stenosis of both the celiac artery (*CA*) and the superior mesenteric artery is clearly defined. The flow through the celiac artery seems adequate in spite of stenosis (*upper barred arrow*). The flow distally in the superior mesenteric artery, however, is significantly diminished, and, as can be seen from (A), (B), and (C), most blood reaches the superior mesenteric circulation through the marginal artery. The proximal segment of the superior mesenteric artery is significantly narrowed (*arrow*). The inferior mesenteric artery (*IMA*) is not the site of stenosing lesions.

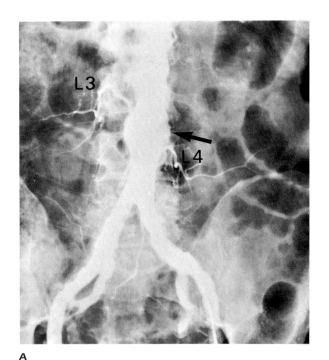

A

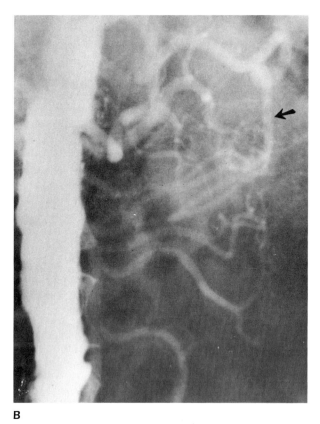

B

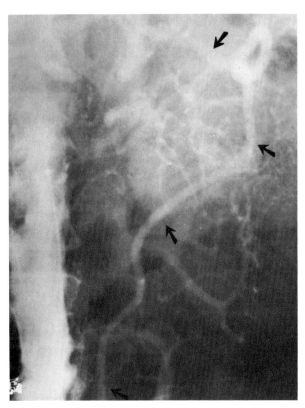

C

Figure 62-10. The collateral circulation in occlusive disease: inferior mesenteric artery occlusion. (A) Abdominal aortogram. There is extensive atheromatous disease of the abdominal aorta. The left third lumbar and the right fourth lumbar arteries are obstructed, together with the inferior mesenteric artery origin (*arrow*). (B and C) Collateral filling from the superior mesenteric artery. (B) At 1 second, gross atheromatous disease in the abdominal aorta, together with complete occlusion of the inferior mesenteric artery, is visible. A large marginal artery (*arrow*) may be seen filling during this phase of the study. (C) At 2 seconds, the left colic artery is now defined (*multiple arrows*), in continuity with the middle colic artery and the inferior mesenteric artery below. (D to G) Obstruction of the inferior mesenteric artery and the left common iliac artery.

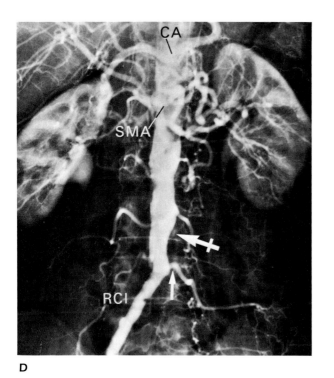

D

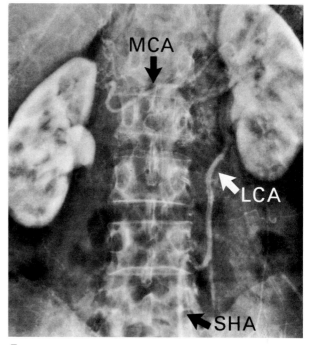

E

F

G

Figure 61-10 (continued). (D) The right common iliac (*RCI*) artery is opacified, but the left common iliac artery is not visualized because it was obstructed at its origin (*arrow*). A large plaque is seen on the left side of the aorta in the region of the origin of the inferior mesenteric artery, which is occluded (*barred arrow*). Filling of the superior mesenteric artery (*SMA*) and the celiac artery (*CA*) is well demonstrated. (E) At 3 seconds, the middle colic artery (*MCA*, *black arrow*) is opacified and may be seen extending to fill the left colic artery (*LCA*, *white arrow*). The left colic artery in turn is clearly in continuity with the superior hemor-

rhoidal artery below (*SHA, black arrow*). (F) The left colic (*LCA, white arrow*) and the inferior mesenteric (*IMA, black arrow*) arteries represent the channel whereby blood reaches the superior hemorrhoidal artery (*SHA, white arrow*) and the middle hemorrhoidal artery (*MHA*) below. (G) With opacification of the middle hemorrhoidal artery (*MHA*), the left obturator artery is the channel whereby the internal iliac and the common femoral arteries are filled and opacified. Thus, with complete obstruction of the common iliac artery, the circulation to the left limb is maintained largely via the inferior mesenteric and the superior hemorrhoidal arteries.

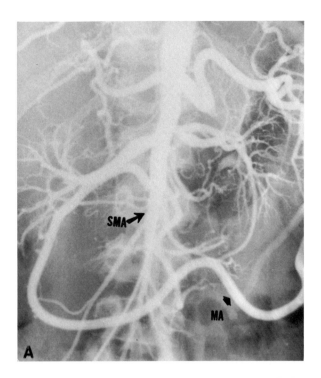

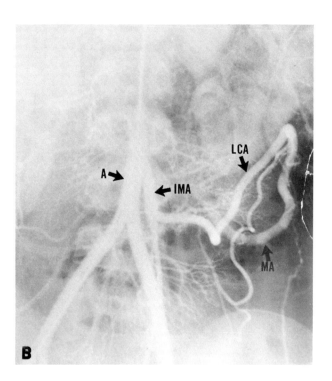

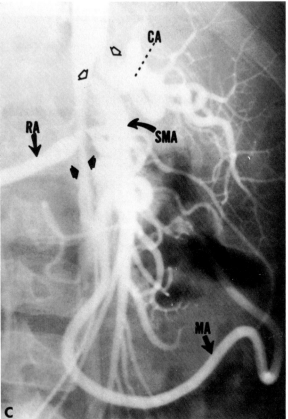

Figure 62-11. The intestinal collateral circulation in occlusive disease: stenosis of the upper abdominal aorta. This 6-year-old girl had a blood pressure of 180/110 mmHg in the upper extremities and diminished femoral pulses. (A) Abdominal aortogram, anteroposterior projection, 1 second. The superior mesenteric artery (*SMA*) is large and is in continuity with a dilated marginal loop (*MA*). Notice the prominence of the intercostal arteries above, adjacent to the ribs. (B) Abdominal aortogram, anteroposterior projection, 2.5 seconds. Contrast has moved from the marginal artery (*MA*) into the left colic and inferior mesenteric arteries and retrograde to fill the distal abdominal aorta and the common iliac arteries. *A,* aorta; *IMA,* inferior mesenteric artery; *LCA,* left colic artery. (C) Abdominal aortogram, left posterior oblique projection. The oblique projection shows that there is gross narrowing of the abdominal aorta (*solid arrows*), with stenosis as well of the origin of the celiac artery and the superior mesenteric arteries (*open arrows*). Both renal arteries (*RA*) are also narrowed at their origin. The dilated marginal artery in continuity with the superior mesenteric artery (*SMA*) is clearly seen in the oblique projection. In this case of abdominal coarctation, the origins of virtually all the great visceral vessels from the abdominal aorta were also involved. The marginal artery provided an avenue of distal aortic filling. *CA,* celiac artery.

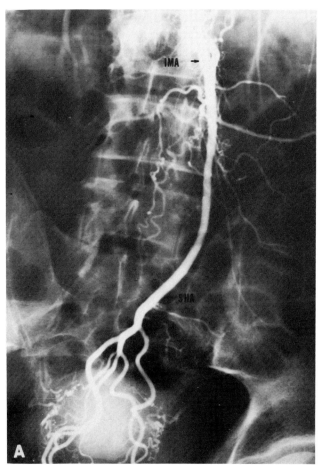

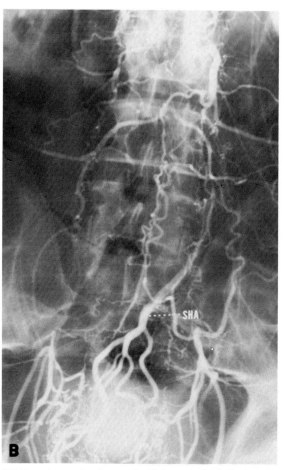

Figure 62-12. The intestinal collateral circulation in occlusive disease: occlusion of the distal abdominal aorta. This 40-year-old man had claudication of both legs and absent femoral pulses. Abdominal aortography was performed with percutaneous transaxillary catheterization of the distal aorta. (A) Intraaortic injection demonstrated complete occlusion of the distal aorta with a large inferior mesenteric artery (*IMA*) and superior hemorrhoidal artery (*SHA*). (B) At 2 seconds, the superior hemorrhoidal artery (*SHA*) and its branches are well delineated. There is retrograde filling of branches of the hypogastric arteries, and subsequent studies demonstrated that the inferior mesenteric artery was an important channel of blood flow to the lower extremities.

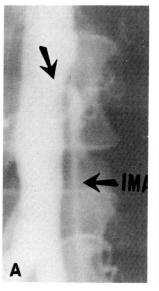

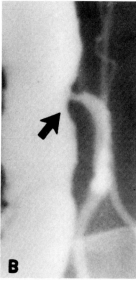

Figure 62-13. Stenosis of the inferior mesenteric artery. (A) Anteroposterior projection. A typical plaque is seen at the origin of the inferior mesenteric artery (*IMA, arrow*), with resulting stenosis of the vessel (*arrow*). (B) Left posterior oblique projection. In another case the plaque is again well defined (*arrow*). The stenosis of the origin of the inferior mesenteric artery is associated with slight poststenotic dilatation.

In contrast to the above patients without symptoms is a significant group in which mesenteric vascular disease is clearly associated with symptoms and in which the disease may be catastrophic if allowed to go unchecked. Some years ago Abrams and colleagues reported a group of such cases.[48] In one patient, celiac artery stenosis and superior mesenteric artery occlusion were associated with absence of the inferior mesenteric artery, which had been sacrificed during a previous aortic resection. The basis for this patient's symptoms was not recognized until an acute exacerbation of signs and symptoms led to exploration and the discovery of gangrene. Earlier recognition might have avoided this sequence. In another patient, the presence of profound stenosis of the superior mesenteric artery as a cause of the patient's symptoms was not recognized even at surgery. Subsequently the patient developed infarction of the bowel and died. A more satisfying course was exemplified by a third patient. This woman had the classic symptoms of pain, diarrhea, and weight loss. Careful study led to a precise diagnosis. Surgical correction of a stenosis of the aortograms by superior mesenteric artery was followed by cure.[48]

Nevertheless, the author's own data support the concept that inferior mesenteric artery insufficiency rarely accompanies chronic, sustained, luminal compromise. Among the 32 individuals who had either occlusion or gross atheromatous change in the inferior mesenteric artery, none had the clinical signs of vascular insufficiency of the colon or rectum. Although three patients in a surgical series reviewed by Hansen and Christoffersen had intestinal angina as a result of occlusion of the inferior mesenteric artery alone,[2] isolated inferior mesenteric artery disease was not associated with symptoms in any of the patients in Hansen and Efsen's angiographic series.[3] The relative rarity of symptomatic inferior mesenteric artery disease is explained by the rich collateral circulation available to the left colon. With slow diminution of the blood supply through the inferior mesenteric artery, the marginal artery may receive the bulk of its flow from the middle colic branch of the superior mesenteric artery and therefore continue to supply the small vessels of the colon with adequate oxygen and nutrients. Almost certainly, an acute insult, such as surgical trauma, acute thrombosis, or embolism, must be superimposed on an already compromised vascular bed to produce significant ischemia.

Several reports indicate that all three major arteries can be occluded without accompanying symptoms. In one patient described,[54] the celiac and mesenteric circulations were filled by large retroperitoneal collateral vessels arising from the aorta. Although it had been clear that splanchnic vessel stenosis or occlusion may be asymptomatic, it had been assumed that occlusion of two major vessels is usually accompanied by symptoms. Apparently, if time permits the development of an adequate collateral circulation, ischemia can be avoided.

The work of Hansen and Efsen also demonstrates that triple-vessel disease is not necessarily associated with symptoms of intestinal angina.[3] In 14 percent of their asymptomatic patients, all three vessels were diseased. Similarly, in a case reported by Hildebrand, an extensive collateral network from the internal iliac and the superior hemorrhoidal arteries supplied the visceral vessels retrogradely through their branches, preserving intestinal viability despite complete occlusion of the celiac artery, superior mesenteric artery, and inferior mesenteric artery. The patient, who also had marked aortoiliac stenosis that diminished the collateral flow, was symptomatic. In another reported case, the patient had occlusion of all three visceral arteries as well as of the right common iliac artery.[4] The entire gastrointestinal tract was supplied through a stenotic left iliac artery and through an artery of Drummond.

Bron and Redman have reported on 730 patients studied by aortography.[12] In 123 patients (17.3 percent), there was stenosis or occlusion of one or more vessels: the celiac artery was involved in 90 patients (12.5 percent), the superior mesenteric artery in 24 patients (3.4 percent), and the inferior mesenteric artery in 36 patients (5.5 percent). Of the last group, 25 patients showed stenosis, and 11 patients had occlusion. Hypertension or peripheral vascular disease was the major indication for aortography; abdominal pain was the indication in 18 percent of the patients. Among those with vessel obstruction, abdominal pain was present in 39 percent. The authors drew the inference that this pain was attributable to the vessel involvement, although no patients had typical abdominal angina.

In the 118 patients found by Hansen and Efsen to have occlusive disease of the visceral arteries, lesions were found in 210 vessels: 90 in the celiac axis, 65 in the superior mesenteric artery, and 55 in the inferior mesenteric artery.[3] Although stenoses were frequent in the celiac axis and the superior mesenteric artery, occlusions occurred four times as frequently as stenoses in the inferior mesenteric artery.

An interesting quantitative approach to abdominal angina was described by Dick et al.[53] They studied the splanchnic vessels by lateral lumbar aortography and attempted to estimate the sum of the cross-sectional areas of the celiac, superior mesenteric, and inferior mesenteric arteries. A significant difference was found in the cross-sectional areas of the group with ischemic gut disease as compared to a control group (27 patients with no evidence of arterial disease, 56 hypertensive patients, and 12 patients with known arteriosclerosis but without evidence of intestinal ischemia). A normal cross-sectional area was established, and, in cases of intestinal ischemia, the cross-sectional area of the main arterial trunks was less than two-thirds of this normal level.

The patterns of involvement of the inferior mesenteric artery by arteriosclerosis must be kept in mind in the surgical management of the elderly patient.[61] The marginal artery may be a vital source of collateral supply in such a patient; it cannot be sacrificed without careful consideration.[62] Conversely, the inferior mesenteric artery may be a major source of blood to the viscera or even the lower extremities,[63,64] and the availability of other collateral channels should be ensured before it is ligated. It is possible to compromise the collateral circulation of the left lower extremity by left colectomy when the inferior mesenteric artery is a major source of blood supply to this area. At least one case is on record in which gangrene followed such a procedure.[65] In addition, in those instances in which stenosis of the celiac and superior mesenteric arteries is accompanied by a large mesenteric collateral system, surgery on the common iliac or femoral arteries may permit blood to be shunted away from the mesenteric circulation and into the periphery and thus create the so-called aortoiliac syndrome. In patients with complete occlusion of the infrarenal aorta and flow to the lower extremities through a central anastomotic artery connecting with the superior mesenteric artery, walking after meals may elicit symptoms of intestinal angina.[36]

In six of the patients studied, a local dilatation of the abdominal aorta was visible directly opposite the origin of the inferior mesenteric artery (Fig. 62-14).[11] This had the appearance of a small saccular aneurysm. In the presence of a large fusiform aneurysm, the inferior mesenteric artery origin was frequently within the wall of the aneurysm. Nevertheless, in six of seven patients with large aneurysms, the inferior mesenteric artery filled directly from the aorta and was therefore not occluded (Fig. 62-15).

Figure 62-14. Early aneurysm formation near the origin of the inferior mesenteric artery. A localized dilatation opposite the origin of the inferior mesenteric artery was visible in six cases. (A) The *upper arrow* points to the local bulge; the inferior mesenteric artery (*IMA*) is patent. (B) Similar local dilatation (*upper arrow*) is another subject. Notice that beyond the origin of the inferior mesenteric artery (*IMA*) there is a large plaque.

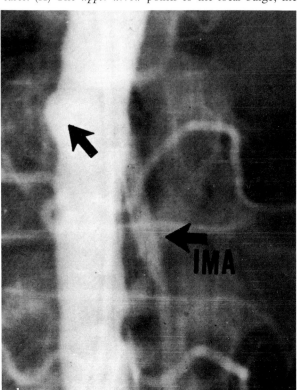

A

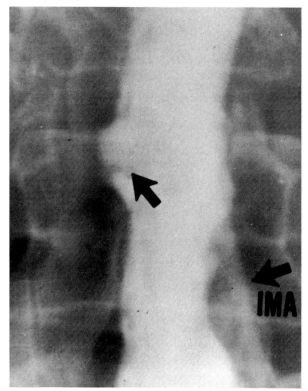

B

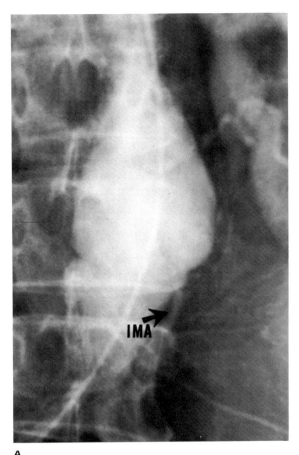

A

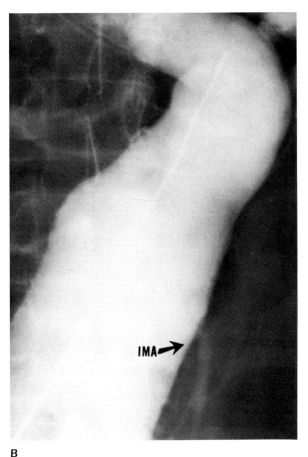

B

Figure 62-15. The inferior mesenteric artery in the presence of abdominal aortic aneurysm. (A) The inferior mesenteric artery (*IMA*) arises directly from the aneurysm and is clearly patent. (B) With a long, fusiform aneurysm of the abdominal aorta, the inferior mesenteric artery (*IMA*) arises from the midportion of the aneurysm. Contrast filling directly from the aorta indicates that it is patent.

Acute Vascular Occlusion

The incidence of acute embolic occlusion of the inferior mesenteric artery is much lower than occlusion of the superior mesenteric artery. Not only is the latter a much larger vessel, but it also runs parallel to the aorta and is ideally located for collecting emboli. Acute occlusion of the inferior mesenteric artery is well tolerated if the occlusion is limited to its proximal portion and if collateral vessels to the superior mesenteric artery are functional.[49]

Acute occlusion may occur, however, as a consequence of arterial thrombosis. When it does, infarction of variable segments of the left colon may develop, with subsequent gangrene and death unless successful surgical intervention is possible. In some patients, occlusion may follow surgery; in others, it may be associated with atheromatous plaques, blood dyscrasias, saccular aortic aneurysm, and sepsis.[33] Clinically, the course of such patients is characterized by the onset of sudden, severe, lower abdominal pain, tenderness, rigidity, and bloody rectal discharge. The mortality is high,[2,4] and an aggressive surgical approach is called for when the diagnosis is recognized. Arteriography is the only means of defining the precise lesion and the degree of collateral development.

Acute ischemia has been noted, particularly after resection of abdominal aortic aneurysms.[34,38,65] It has been treated by reattachment of the inferior mesenteric artery with a button of the aorta.[49] Although ligation of the inferior mesenteric artery alone need not be catastrophic if the marginal system is intact, ligation of the hypogastric arteries may be disastrous if the channels between the superior and the inferior hemorrhoidal arteries are not well established. Even temporary clamping of the hypogastric arteries after sacrifice of the inferior mesenteric artery for aortic aneurysm surgery may produce severe ischemia in about 10 percent of cases.[39] Asymptomatic patients with two- or three-vessel obstruction can develop gangrene after periods of hypotension, as may occur during intraab-dominal surgery.[49]

In the presence of acute embolic obstruction of the superior mesenteric artery, the inferior mesenteric artery may maintain a blood supply to the intestine via the marginal artery, but the blood supply is unlikely to be adequate in most cases.[58]

Boley and colleagues have pointed out that the course of the ischemic episode cannot be predicted from the initial clinical or radiographic findings.[66,67] The patient should be observed carefully, the bowel placed at rest, and antibiotics and intravenous fluids administered. Steroids, which increase the chance of perforation, should not be given. The damage is considered irreversible if the patient's clinical state deteriorates or if symptoms persist for more than 2 weeks. In such cases, surgical treatment, involving resection of the involved intestinal segment with primary anastomosis of the remaining bowel, should be carried out. In Boley's series of 150 cases of colonic ischemia, 44.7 percent had reversible disease, 18.7 percent had persistent colitis, 12.7 percent had ischemic stricture, and 18.7 percent suffered gangrene or perforation. In 5.3 percent the follow-up was incomplete.[66]

Carcinoma of the Colon

The importance of lesions of the segment of the gut supplied by the inferior mesenteric artery is hardly reflected by the volume of literature on this vascular bed. Over 75 percent of all polyps and cancers of the colon occur in the distribution area of the inferior mesenteric artery. Although it is possible to identify these lesions by arteriographic technique,[13–16] less invasive and more sensitive and specific diagnostic techniques (i.e., double-contrast barium enema and endoscopy) make arteriography unnecessary. Computerized tomography (CT), magnetic resonance imaging (MRI), and endoluminal ultrasound can be used to assist in staging colorectal tumors and to detect postoperative recurrence.[68]

In all cases studied arteriographically by Boijsen and Reuter,[16] tumor vessels were observed. The tumors varied in vascularity and consequently in the number of abnormal vessels visualized. The vessels were tortuous in course, random in distribution, irregular in appearance, and abnormally tapered (Fig. 62-16). These findings are a requisite for the diagnosis of carcinoma. The contrast agent accumulates in the tumor, and many carcinomas also demonstrate premature venous filling.[13] Nevertheless, the density of the venous phase is significantly less than that seen in inflammatory disease.

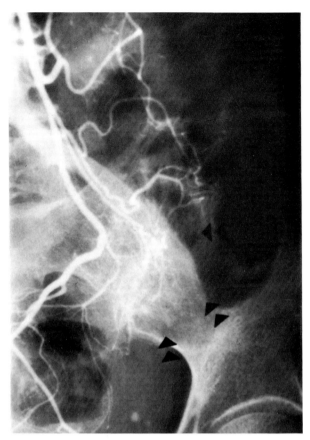

Figure 62-16. Carcinoma of the colon. This 65-year-old woman was admitted to the hospital because of rectal bleeding. Barium enema examination revealed a short, stenotic segment of sigmoid colon (*arrowheads*), and the differentiation between carcinoma and diverticulitis was not clear. Inferior mesenteric angiography demonstrated unequivocal tumor vessels in the neoplasm, displacement of large branches, and profuse staining of the neoplastic mass. (Courtesy of Stewart Reuter, M.D.)

Extension of the tumor through the bowel wall may be diagnosed by demonstrating irregularity of the arterial branches and marginal artery. Encasement of the marginal artery may occur, but this does not necessarily mean that the tumor is unresectable.[69] In addition, it is possible to demonstrate invasion of draining veins using pharmacoangiography.[70] However, angiographically demonstrated vascular involvement may not necessarily reflect tumor invasion but rather inflammatory changes, adhesions, and fibrosis around the tumor.[71] Depending on the size of the tumor, there may be varying degrees of large-vessel displacement.

The distinction of recurrent tumor from scar formation at the site of the previous anastomosis may be difficult.[12,15] Tumor vessels will usually be observed if there is a recurrence.[16]

Arteriography following intraarterial injection of

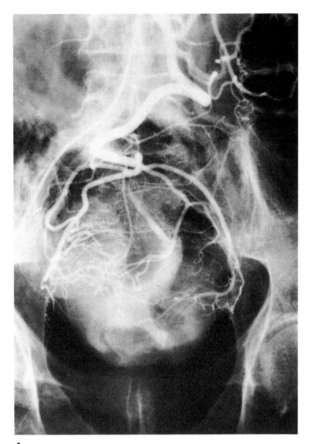

A

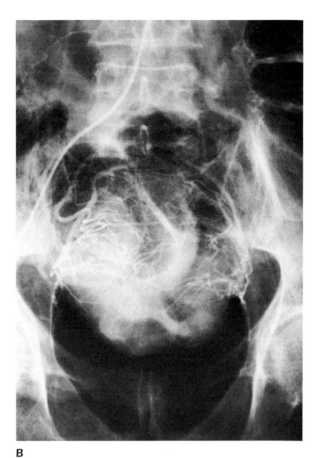

B

Figure 62-17. Villous adenoma of the colon. This 68-year-old man entered the hospital because of mucoid, watery diarrhea, persistent weakness, and occasional nausea and vomiting. Bowel movements varied from 10 to 50 a day, most of them watery. There was no history of rectal bleeding. Sigmoidoscopy revealed a lesion in the right lateral rectal wall about 15 to 18 cm from the mucocutaneous junction. Biopsy showed a villous adenoma. Angiography demonstrated a profusion of blood vessels to the tumor and gross displacement of the adjacent supplying vessels, indicating the size and extent of the tumor. There was contrast staining of the neoplastic mass. (A) Early phase. The hypervascularity of the tumor is clearly demonstrated, as are the tortuous vessels, their irregularity, and the displacement of adjacent large vascular trunks. (B) Later phase. There is persistent filling of many of the large branches and contrast accumulation in the tumor, somewhat difficult to define because of the opacified bladder. (Courtesy of Stewart Reuter, M.D.)

prostaglandin F_2 alpha in normal subjects demonstrates vasodilatation of colonic vessels, whereas in patients with neoplastic or inflammatory colonic disease, there is vasoconstriction at the affected sites in response to this drug.[72]

Figure 62-16 demonstrates the local vascular pattern in a 65-year-old woman in whom the clinical distinction between diverticulitis and carcinoma was not clear. Arteriography demonstrated unequivocal tumor vessels and a profound tumor stain.

Figure 62-17 shows the angiograms of a 68-year-old man admitted to the hospital because of mucoid, watery diarrhea, persistent weakness, and occasional nausea and vomiting. Angiography demonstrated a profusion of blood vessels—some of them tortuous and abnormal in their course. The extent of the tumor and the displacement of the adjacent vessels were clearly indicated. Biopsy showed a villous adenoma.

Figure 62-18 is an angiographic study of a 76-year-old man in whom polyps were noted in the descending colon on barium enema study. Selective inferior mesenteric angiography demonstrated abnormal vessels to the polyps. At surgery this area was resected, and the polyps were found to be adenocarcinomatous.

It is clear, then, that inferior mesenteric arteriography may present unequivocal evidence of malignancy in certain instances in which the differential diagnosis from diverticulitis is difficult. The relative lack of an extensive vascular supply in diverticulitis is also helpful in the differentiation. However, clinical signs and symptoms combined with current diagnostic techniques such as barium enema examinations, CT, MRI,

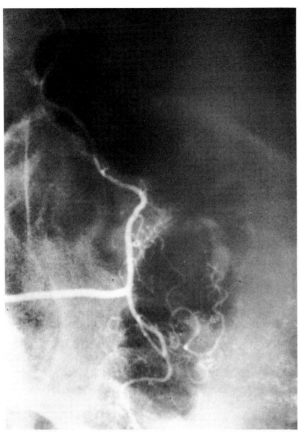

Figure 62-18. Malignant polyps of the colon. This 76-year-old man had polyps in the descending colon. Angiography demonstrated tortuous, abnormal vessels subserving these polyps. At resection the polyps were found to be adenocarcinomatous. (Courtesy of Stewart Reuter, M.D.)

ultrasound, and colonoscopy with biopsy enable the correct diagnosis to be made in the vast majority of cases without resorting to arteriography.

Inflammatory Disease of the Colon

Schobinger, on the basis of operative intestinal arteriography in diverticulitis, pointed out that mild degrees of inflammation had a vascular pattern similar to that of the surrounding normal bowel.[73] With acute inflammation, local hyperemia was visible but not the altered characteristics of the vascular bed seen with malignancy. No pooling of contrast agent was observed, nor were there arteriovenous shunts. Ström and Winberg also noted the absence of early venous filling in diverticulitis.[13]

Boijsen and Reuter demonstrated that in regional enterocolitis the arteries and veins filled more rapidly than those in the surrounding normal bowel, increased

vascularity was present, and there was slight dilatation of the supplying arteries and some dilatation and tortuosity of the veins draining the diseased segments.[16] During the capillary phase, thickened bowel could be seen in the presence of active disease. In ulcerative colitis there was also increased vascularity of the involved segment, but the vasa recta were smooth and regular (Figs. 62-19 through 62-21). In contrast to those in the normal bowel, there was relatively little tapering in the width of these vessels. In diverticulitis there was only a slight increase in the vascularity of the diseased segment, and irregularity and distortion of the vasa recta were apparent.

Brahme, in describing the findings in regional enterocolitis, distinguished between (1) the changes in the ileum, in which the arteries of the bowel wall were reduced in number and the capillary phase was fainter than normal, and (2) inflammation in the colon, in which hypovascularization was not evident.[17] He pointed out that hypervascularization was also not seen (in contrast to the appearance in ulcerative colitis). The major changes were in the number of vessels and in the distorted course of those remaining. Relatively little accumulation of contrast medium in the intestinal wall was observed. In the colon the vasa longa and the vasa brevia were tortuous and irregular in caliber (Fig. 62-22). Venous return appeared within a normal time.

Lunderquist and Lunderquist have reported detailed studies of angiography in ulcerative colitis.[74] In symptomatic cases, the inferior mesenteric artery and the vasa recta were widened. The vasa recta failed to taper toward the periphery, as they do in the normal colon. In some instances they terminated abruptly. A moderate increase in the thickness of the bowel wall was noted during the capillary phase. The veins were dilated, and their course was irregular. The large veins were abnormally wide and the contrast filling was unusually dense. These changes have been thought to be related to increased blood flow to the colon in ulcerative colitis.[75] In two symptom-free patients with ulcerative colitis, the angiographic studies were not dissimilar from the normal. The authors pointed out that the absence of tapering of the vasa recta might be useful in distinguishing ulcerative from granulomatous colitis, in which the peripheral arteries in the intestinal wall are abnormally narrow and tortuous and have an irregular lumen. Erikson et al. found that the angiographic appearances in ulcerative colitis and Crohn disease were similar, although there was more shunting, venous filling, and hypervascularity in ulcerative colitis on inferior mesenteric angiography.[76] Tsuchiya et al. studied 25 patients with ulcerative colitis and found that the angiographic changes were correlated with the

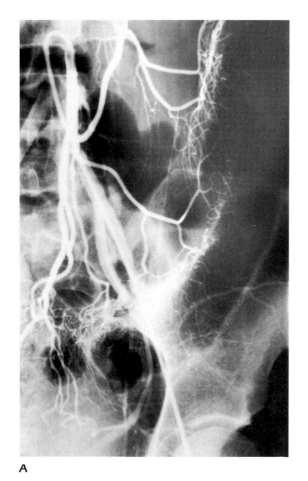

A

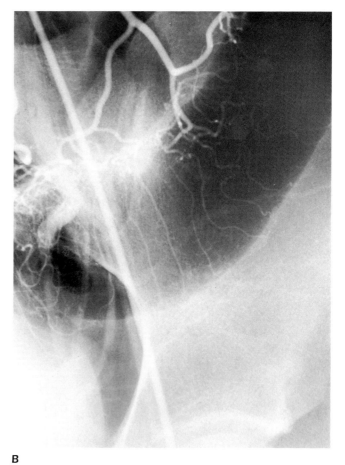

B

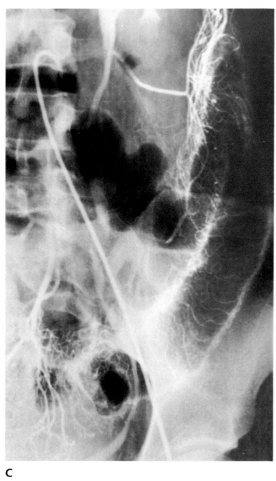

C

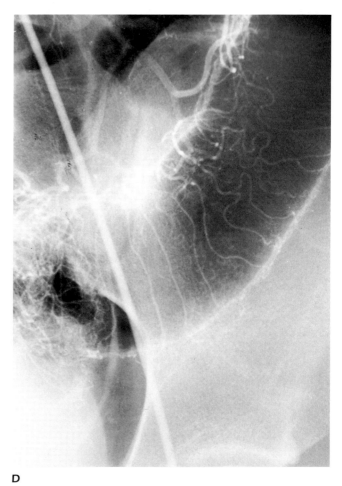

D

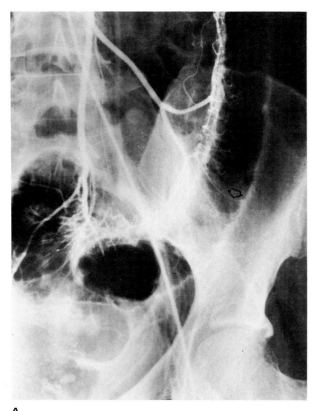

A

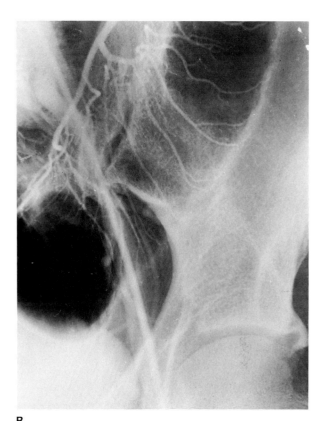

B

Figure 62-20. Ulcerative colitis. (A) Selective inferior mesenteric arteriogram. Augmented vascularity is apparent, and the capillary phase is increased. Loss of normal tapering is apparent (*arrowhead*). (B) Magnified view. Later films showed an early, intense venous phase. (Courtesy of Stanley Baum, M.D.)

severity and activity of the disease, rather than with the duration or extent of involvement.[75]

In summary, ulcerative colitis is distinguished by the findings of inflammation: dilated vessels, increased blood flow, augmented capillary phase, and large draining veins. In the chronic phase, the appearance may be normal. Granulomatous colitis reflects the involvement of the entire wall, with tortuous vessels, narrowing and sometimes stretching of smaller branches, and irregularity of the vessel wall. The arteriogram may at times show a longer segment of involvement than does the barium enema examination.

Intraarterial infusion therapy of prednisone via the superior and inferior mesenteric arteries has been described with a 57 percent effective response rate in patients with ulcerative colitis refractory to conventional medical therapy.[77]

Ischemic colitis, an unusual vascular disease that may cause occult bleeding and that may represent a phase of segmental ulcerative colitis, may also be distinguished angiographically.[78]

Cytomegalovirus colitis may occur in patients with acquired immunodeficiency syndrome and may cause lower gastrointestinal bleeding. Arteriography in this instance has been reported to demonstrate hypervascularity of the affected colonic segments.[79]

◄ **Figure 62-19.** Ulcerative colitis. This 24-year-old woman had long-standing ulcerative colitis. (A) Selective inferior mesenteric arteriogram. There is good visualization of the major vessels to the left colon and the sigmoid. (B) Magnified view of (A). (C) Later phase. (D) Magnified view of (C).

The vasa recta are prominent and exhibit a nontapered appearance indicative of increased vascularity. The wall is slightly thickened, and the capillary phase is more intense than normal. The findings are nonspecific and less striking than in the acute phase. (Courtesy of Stanley Baum, M.D.)

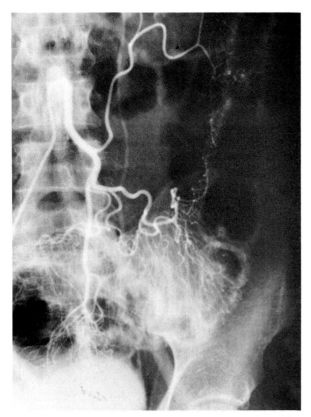

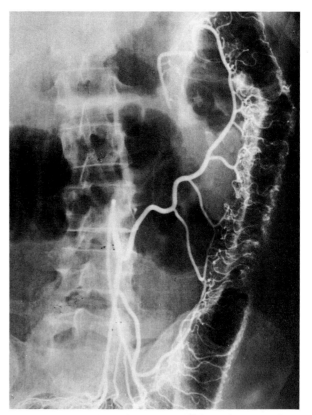

Figure 62-21. Ulcerative colitis in a 53-year-old man, selective inferior mesenteric arteriogram. There is a marked increase in vascularity, particularly to the sigmoid colon. The capillary blush is intense and the wall slightly thick. The vessels are relatively straight and do not taper normally. A small inflammatory polyp is visible in the descending colon. (Courtesy of Stanley Baum, M.D.)

Figure 62-22. Granulomatous colitis, selective inferior mesenteric arteriography. The inflammatory changes are not as marked as they are in ulcerative colitis. There is marked tortuosity of the vasa recta, with some loss of the normal smooth appearance of the walls. The vessels are somewhat stretched to the affected area of the bowel. The smaller mesenteric vessels may be narrowed in regional enteritis, and as the disease becomes chronic, irregularity and beading may be seen in some of the narrowed vessels. Note the marked thickening of the wall in the involved area and compare the tortuous vessels with those in the adjacent normal colon. (Courtesy of Stanley Baum, M.D.)

Bleeding in the Left Colon

The subject of gastrointestinal bleeding is treated in Chapter 25 of *Abrams' Angiography: Interventional Radiology,* to which the reader is referred for a detailed discussion. Bleeding in the left colon is associated most commonly with diverticular disease and angiodysplasia.[21] Other causes include neoplasms, ulcerative colitis, Crohn disease, radiation proctitis, ischemic colitis, colonic varices, and infectious or inflammatory ulceration.[80] In idiopathic bleeding, associated factors include immunosuppression, chemotherapy, and anticoagulation for various disorders.[80]

Diverticular Bleeding

This is the most common cause of bleeding in the large bowel, occurring generally in individuals over the age of 60. Although diverticula are more common in the left colon, bleeding from diverticula occurs three times more often in the right colon than in the left colon.[21]

The cause of diverticular bleeding is thought to be erosion of a peridiverticular arteriole by fecal material within the diverticulum. Contrast extravasation is the only certain means of defining the precise site; when seen in the left colon in the absence of angiodysplasia or neoplasm, the cause is most likely diverticular. Vasopressin infusion may control diverticular bleeding,[20,81] but it is not always successful (Fig. 62-23),[81,82] presumably because of age and arteriosclerotic changes in the vessels.

Angiodysplasia

Angiodysplasia is a vascular malformation of the bowel wall in which dilated vascular channels—arterial, capil-

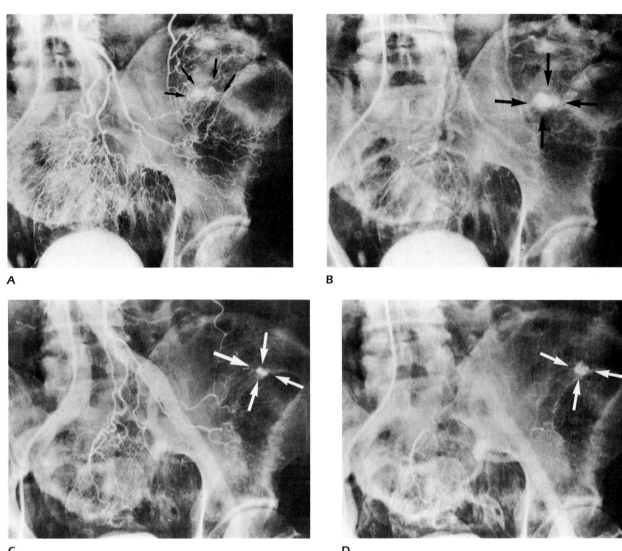

A

B

C

D

Figure 62-23. Left colic bleeding and diverticulosis. This 60-year-old man had massive bleeding into his lower gastrointestinal tract, and he required transfusion to maintain his blood volume. Superior mesenteric arteriography failed to disclose a bleeding site. Inferior mesenteric arteriography was then performed. (A) Inferior mesenteric arteriogram, 1 second. A discrete area of accumulation of contrast material in the lower descending colon is clearly visible (*arrows*). (B) At 3 seconds, during the venous phase, the accumulation of contrast material has become somewhat more dense (*arrows*). (C) Arteriogram following the administration of

0.2 U of vasopressin per minute for 45 minutes directly into the inferior mesenteric artery. Note the diminished caliber of the branch arteries. In spite of the response of the arteries to vasopressin infusion, evidence of bleeding is still visible in the descending colon (*arrows*). (D) Arteriogram during the venous phase. There is dense extravasation (*arrows*) in the descending colon, clearly less than on the initial examination but without cessation of bleeding. The patient was taken to surgery. Resection of the descending colon in the area of the bleeding demonstrated multiple diverticula, one of which had eroded at its base and destroyed the arterial wall.

lary, or venous—are present. These may be either gross or microscopic. Many terms, including *vascular ectasia, dysplasia,* or *malformation, telangiectasia,* and *arteriovenous fistula or malformation,* have been applied to these unique lesions, which are frequently a cause of chronic or recurrent gastrointestinal bleeding.[19] Most lesions have been found in the right side of the colon,[83–85] but in some series left colic vascular

malformations have represented an important group (Fig. 62-24), emphasizing the need for inferior mesenteric arteriography.[19,86]

The most important angiographic features of angiodysplasia are an early-filling vein; a slowly emptying, tortuous intramural vein; a dilated feeding artery or arteries; a local wall stain; a vascular tuft; and prolonged venous opacification.[83]

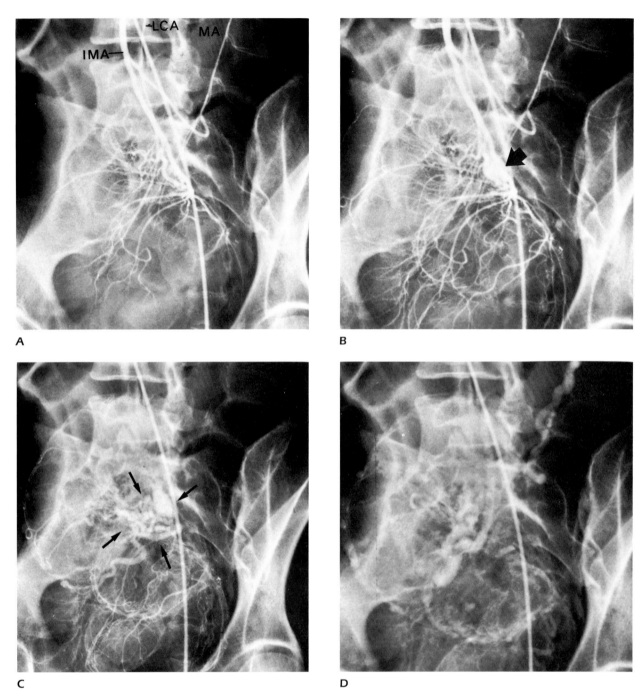

A

B

C

D

Figure 62-24. Angiodysplasia of the left colon. The patient had a history of recurrent bleeding. Superior mesenteric arteriography demonstrated no abnormalities. Inferior mesenteric arteriography was therefore performed. (A) Arteriogram, 0.5 second. No definite abnormalities are visible. (B) At 1 second, an area of contrast material accumulation (*arrow*) within a vascular wall is well demonstrated. (C) At 2 seconds, multiple tortuous vessels are opacified, with premature venous drainage at the site of the angiodysplastic lesion (*arrows*). (D) At 5 seconds, draining veins are now visu- alized, some of which are rather large and tortuous. These are particularly prominent in the region of the angiodysplasia. Thus this lesion demonstrates many of the classic features of colon angiodysplasia. Dilated feeding arteries are visible, together with an intense local wall stain, an early-filling vein, dilated intramural veins, prolonged venous opacification, and a large vascular tuft. Identification of this lesion permitted a direct surgical approach to controlling chronic gastrointestinal bleeding in this patient.

In chronic gastrointestinal bleeding with normal barium enema studies, angiodysplasia is a potentially correctable cause of bleeding if it can be correctly diagnosed. It is essential, in such patients, that the inferior mesenteric artery as well as the superior mesenteric and celiac arteries be investigated angiographically.

Ischemic Colitis

Although there is good evidence that ischemic colitis may cause occult or massive bleeding,[21] it must be considered an unusual cause of severe gastrointestinal hemorrhage. Occlusive mesenteric vascular disease has been thoroughly investigated, but nonocclusive mesenteric vascular insufficiency is not as well understood.[4] Particularly in the presence of central shock and low cardiac output, shunting of blood away from the mucosa may be associated with mucosal necrosis and, ultimately, erosion of vessels to the intestinal wall, with resultant bleeding into the bowel.

One type of ischemic colitis is illustrated in Figure 62-25. The woman whose case is illustrated had acute leukemia and was under treatment with cytotoxic drugs when she began to pass bright red blood per rectum. She was hospitalized, and the bleeding increased 2 days after admission. Superior mesenteric arteriography was normal, but the inferior mesenteric arteriogram (see Fig. 62-25) demonstrated the bleeding site in the sigmoid colon. Vasopressin infusion was initiated, and the bleeding was controlled. The infusion was tapered over 4 days; with the removal of the catheter, however, bleeding began anew, and the patient was taken to surgery. A segment of the sigmoid colon was resected. It demonstrated vasculitis and thrombosis of multiple small vessels, with ischemic sigmoiditis and ulcer formation (see Fig. 62-25C). Thus thrombosis of the small arteries was associated with mucosal ischemia and necrosis, ulcer formation, and ultimately with bleeding from a small and eroded artery.

Among the causes of nonocclusive ischemic colitis, the use of digitalis, certain vasopressors that constrict the splenic bed, antihypertensive medication, congestive heart failure, and low blood volume have been identified. Other factors may be related to small-vessel disease, with inflammation of small arteries producing mucosal damage, as in diabetes, lupus erythematosus, rheumatoid arthritis, polyarteritis nodosa, and radiation colitis. In these disorders, angiography frequently will not yield distinctive or diagnostic features. Barium enema studies may show the classic thumb printing, ulcerations, and strictures at the end stage, but the precise source of bleeding is frequently not well defined by angiography.[87,88]

Angiographic Detection Rates in Colonic Bleeding

In a study of 30 patients with massive gastrointestinal bleeding, Giacchino et al. were able to localize a site of bleeding in 23 patients (77 percent). Angiography was successful in 11 patients, barium enema study in 5 patients, and proctoscopy in 7 patients.[80] Best et al. analyzed angiographically 60 patients' studies for chronic gastrointestinal bleeding and noted a detection rate of 38 percent.[19] As is pointed out by Baum in Chapter 25 of *Abrams' Angiography: Interventional Radiology,* for successful visualization of a bleeding site the patient must be actively bleeding at a rate of at least 0.5 ml per minute.

Because radionuclide scans are more sensitive than arteriography in determining the presence of active lower gastrointestinal bleeding,[89,90] the scan should precede the arteriogram, the latter only being performed if the scan is positive. The purpose of the arteriogram is to define exactly the bleeding location and to provide the option of transcatheter therapy. Selection injection of ^{99}Tc colloid into the mesenteric arteries has been described in patients in whom conventional arteriography is negative.[91]

It is important when performing an inferior mesenteric arteriogram to include the entire region supplied by this vessel, including the low rectum and anal verge, because endoscopy can miss these low bleeding sites.[92]

Barium enema studies should be avoided before arteriography, not only because of their low yield in acute lower gastrointestinal bleeding, but also because the presence of barium in the bowel will make arteriography difficult if not impossible to interpret.

In chronic lower gastrointestinal bleeding, arteriography should be reserved for those patients in whom all other investigations prove negative. In such a patient the purpose of the arteriogram is to define a structural vascular abnormality because in this situation active bleeding at the time of the arteriogram is unusual, and therefore extravasation of contrast medium into the bowel lumen is usually evident. In patients with chronic gastrointestinal bleeding of obscure origin, arteriography will reveal a source in approximately 45 percent, with arteriovenous malformations accounting for about half of these[93,94]; the majority of the lesions are found in the jejunum, ileum, cecum, and ascending colon[94] and are therefore discovered on superior mesenteric arteriography. If there is a history of recurrent massive lower gastrointestinal bleeding and the arteriogram is negative, angiography can be performed following a fibrinolytic agent such as urokinase in an attempt to demonstrate the resultant precipitated hemorrhage[95]; this approach obviously carries some risk.

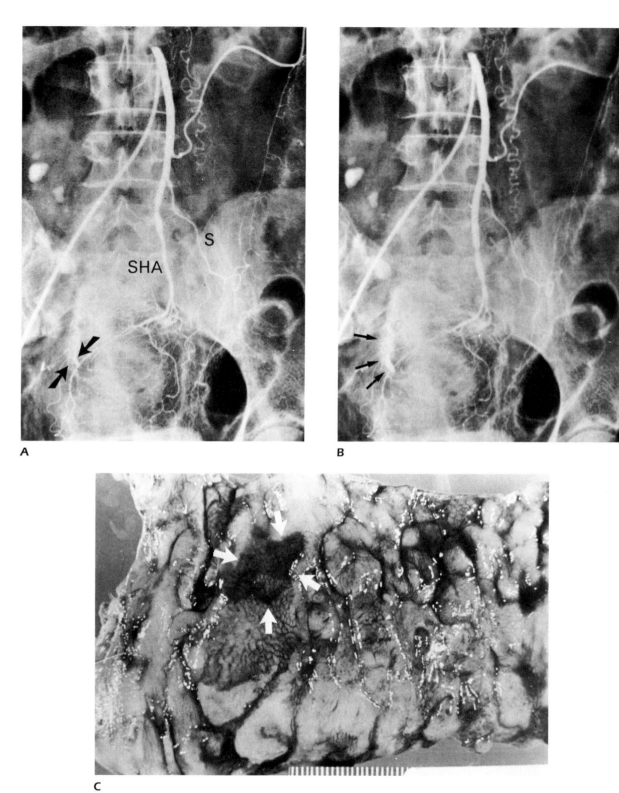

Figure 62-25. Ischemic colitis. This 60-year-old woman with acute leukemia was placed on cytotoxic agents for her blood dyscrasia. She began to pass bright red blood per rectum, so she was hospitalized. Two days later, there was a sudden increase in bleeding, and arteriography was performed. The superior mesenteric arteriogram was normal. The inferior mesenteric arteriogram demonstrated a bleeding site and was followed by vasopressin infusion for 4 days, with cessation of bleeding. At the time of catheter removal, however, the bleeding was reinitiated, and the patient was taken to surgery. Sigmoid resection was performed, and the involved segment demonstrated multiple thrombosed small vessels, with ischemic sigmoiditis and ulcer formation. (A) Inferior mesenteric arteriogram, 1 second. The inferior mesenteric artery and its left colic, sigmoid (*S*), and superior hemorrhoidal (*SHA*) arterial branches are well demonstrated. A branch of the superior hemorrhoidal artery to the sigmoid colon demonstrates a discrete area of intraluminal

Acknowledgments

Many of the illustrations in this chapter were reproduced with permission from Kahn P, Abrams HL. Inferior mesenteric arterial patterns: an angiographic study. Radiology 1964;82:429.

References

1. Bernstein WC, Bernstein EF. Ischemic ulcerative colitis following inferior mesenteric arterial ligation. Dis Colon Rectum 1963;6:54.
2. Hansen HJB, Christoffersen JK. Occlusive mesenteric infarction: a retrospective study of 83 cases. Acta Chir Scand Suppl 1976;472:103–108.
3. Hansen HJB, Efsen F. Occlusive disease of the mesenteric arteries: a clinical and radiological study. Dan Med Bull 1977; 24:117.
4. Hildebrand HD, Zierler RE. Mesenteric vascular disease. Am J Surg 1980;139:188–192.
5. Miller WH, Maloriello JJ, Stein DB Jr. Mesenteric vascular occlusion in infancy and childhood: review of literature and report of an additional case. J Pediatr 1961;59:567.
6. Morris GC Jr, DeBakey ME, Bernhard V. Abdominal angina. Surg Clin North Am 1966;46:919–930.
7. Ratner IA, Swenson O. Mesenteric vascular occlusion in infancy and childhood. N Engl J Med 1960;263:1122.
8. Schwartz S, Boley SJ, Robinson K, et al. Roentgenologic features of vascular disorders of intestines. Radiol Clin North Am 1964;2:71.
9. Wang CC, Reeves JD. Mesenteric vascular disease. AJR 1960; 83:895.
10. Brolin I, Paulin S. Abnormal communications between splanchnic vessels. Acta Radiol 1964;2:460.
11. Kahn P, Abrams HL. Inferior mesenteric arterial patterns: an angiographic study. Radiology 1964;82:429.
12. Bron KM, Redman HC. Splanchnic artery stenosis and occlusion: incidence; arteriographic and clinical manifestations. Radiology 1969;92:323–328.
13. Ström BG, Winberg T. Percutaneous selective arteriography of the inferior mesenteric artery. Acta Radiol 1962;57:401.
14. Halpern N. Selective inferior mesenteric arteriography. Vasc Dis 1964;1:294.
15. Wholey MH, Bron KM, Haller JB. Selective angiography of the colon. Surg Clin North Am 1965;45:1283–1291.
16. Boijsen E, Reuter SR. Mesenteric arteriography in the evaluation of inflammatory and neoplastic disease of the intestine. Radiology 1966;87:1028.
17. Brahme F. Mesenteric angiography in regional enterocolitis. Radiology 1966;87:1037–1042.
18. Baum S, Rösch J, Dotter CT, et al. Selective mesenteric arterial infusions in the management of massive diverticular hemorrhage. N Engl J Med 1973;288:1269.
19. Best EB, Teaford AK, Rader FH Jr. Angiography in chronic/recurrent gastrointestinal bleeding: a nine year study. Surg Clin North Am 1979;59:811–829.
20. Shaff MI, Becker H. Diagnosis and control of diverticular bleeding by arteriography and vasopressin infusion. S Afr Med J 1979;56:72–74.
21. Casarella WJ, Kanter IE, Seaman WB. Right-sided colonic diverticula as a cause of acute rectal hemorrhage. N Engl J Med 1972;286:450.
22. Rees CR, Palmaz JC, Alvarado R, et al. DSA in acute gastrointestinal hemorrhage; clinical and in vitro studies. Radiology 1988;69:499–503.
23. Goligher JC. The blood supply to the sigmoid colon and rectum. Br J Surg 1949;37:157.
24. Griffiths JD. Surgical anatomy of the blood supply of the distal colon. Ann R Coll Surg Engl 1956;19:214.
25. Steward JA, Rankin FW. Blood supply of the intestine: its surgical considerations. Arch Surg 1933;26:843.
26. Sunderiand S. Blood supply of the distal colon. Aust N Z J Surg 1942;11:253.
27. Boijsen E. Angiographic studies of the anatomy of single and multiple renal arteries. Acta Radiol Suppl (Stockh) 1966;183:1028.
28. Von Haller A. Cited by Steward JA, Rankin FW. Blood supply of the intestine: its surgical considerations. Arch Surg 1933;26:843.
29. Drummond H. The arterial supply of the rectum and pelvic colon. Br J Surg 1914;1:677.
30. Stoney RJ, Wylie EJ. Recognition and surgical management of visceral ischemic syndromes. Ann Surg 1966;164:714–722.
31. Trotter LBC. Embolism and thrombosis of the mesenteric vessels. London: Cambridge University Press, 1913.
32. Bergan JJ, Dean RH, Conn J Jr, et al. Revascularization in treatment of mesenteric infarction. Ann Surg 1975;182:430–438.
33. Carter R, Vannix R, Hinshaw DB, et al. Acute inferior mesenteric vascular occlusion, a surgical syndrome. Am J Surg 1959; 98:271.
34. Bernatz PE. Necrosis of the colon following resection for abdominal aortic aneurysm. Arch Surg 1960;81:373.
35. Cole FH Jr, Richardson RL. Mesenteric thrombosis after penetrating cardiac trauma. South Med J 1976;69:1517–1518.
36. Connolly JE, Kwaan JHM. Prophylactic revascularization of the gut. Ann Surg 1979;190:514–522.
37. Ernst CB, Hagihara PF, Daugherty ME, et al. Inferior mesenteric artery stump pressure: a reliable index for safe IMA ligation during abdominal aortic aneurysmectomy. Ann Surg 1978;187:641–646.
38. Perdue GD, Lowry K. Arterial insufficiency to the colon following resection of abdominal aortic aneurysms. Surg Gynecol Obstet 1962;115:39.
39. Smith RF, Szllagyi DE. Ischemia of the colon as a complication in surgery of the abdominal aorta. Arch Surg 1960;80:806.
40. Baum V, Eufrate SA. Inferior mesenteric artery injury: a complication of translumbar aortography. NY State J Med 1962; 62:3931.
41. McAfee JC. A survey of complications of abdominal aortography. Radiology 1957;68:825.
42. McDowell RFC, Thompson ID. Inferior mesenteric artery occlusion following lumbar aortography. Br J Radiol 1959;32:344.
43. Padhi RK. Fatal infarction of the descending colon after lumbar aortography. Can Med Assoc J 1960;82:199.
44. Sumner DS. Successful revascularization of mesenteric infarction following aortography. Am Surg 1977;43:743–750.
45. Selby DK, Bergan JJ. Colonic infarction due to inferior mesenteric artery occlusion. Q Bull Northwest Univ Med Sch 1960; 34:244.
46. Carter R, Vannix R, Hinshaw DB, et al. Inferior mesenteric vascular occlusion: sigmoidoscopic diagnosis. Surgery 1959;46:845.

extravasation (*arrows*). (B) Inferior mesenteric arteriogram, 1.5 seconds. The contrast extravasation has increased (*arrows*). Note that in both (A) and (B) there are segments of irregular narrowing of the inferior mesenteric and superior hemorrhoidal branches, reflecting spasm in these branches.

(C) Specimen of resected sigmoid colon. The mucosa is grossly inflamed, and an area of ulceration is visible (*arrows*). Beneath the area of ulceration, multiple thrombosed arteries were found, producing an ischemic sigmoiditis.

47. Atwell RB. Superior mesenteric artery embolectomy. Surg Gynecol Obstet 1961;112:257.
48. Connolly JE, Abrams HL, Kieraido JH. Observations on obliterative disease of the visceral branches of the abdominal aorta. Arch Surg 1965;90:596.
49. Crawford ES, Morris GC Jr, Myhre HO, et al. Celiac axis, superior mesenteric artery, and inferior mesenteric artery occlusion: surgical considerations. Surgery 1977;82:856–866.
50. Danesh S. Abdominal angina and mesenteric insufficiency. Angiology 1979;30:281–283.
51. Eidemiller LR, Nelson JC, Porter JM. Surgical treatment of chronic visceral ischemia. Am J Surg 1979;138:264–268.
52. Webb WR, Hardy JD. Relief of abdominal angina by vascular graft. Ann Intern Med 1962;57:289.
53. Dick AP, Graff R, Gregg DM, et al. An arteriographic study of mesenteric arterial disease: I. Large vessel changes. Gut 1967;8:206–220.
54. Matz EM, Kahn PC. Occlusion of the celiac, superior mesenteric and inferior mesenteric arteries: angiographic demonstration in an asymptomatic patient. Vasc Dis 1968;5:130–136.
55. Basmajian JV. The marginal anastomoses of the arteries to the large intestines. Surg Gynecol Obstet 1954;99:614.
56. Moskowitz M, Zimmerman H, Felson B. Meandering mesenteric artery of colon. AJR 1964;92:1088.
57. Sacks RP, Shaft DJ, Freeman JH. The demonstration of the mesenteric collateral circulation in young patients. AJR 1968;102:401–406.
58. Aakhus T. The value of angiography in superior mesenteric artery embolism. Br J Radiol 1966;39:928–932.
59. McGregor DH, Pierce GE, Thomas JH, et al. Obstructive lesions of distal mesenteric arteries: a light and electron microscopic study. Arch Pathol Lab Med 1980;104:79–83.
60. Bron KM. Thrombotic occlusion of the abdominal aorta: associated visceral artery lesions and collateral circulation. AJR 1966;96:887.
61. Demos NJ, Bahuth JJ, Urnes PD. Comparative study of arteriosclerosis in the inferior and superior mesenteric arteries: with a case report of gangrene of the colon. Ann Surg 1962;155:599.
62. Harrison AW, Croal AE. Left colon ischemia following occlusion or ligation of the inferior mesenteric artery. Can J Surg 1962;5:293.
63. Edwards EA, LeMay M. Occlusion patterns and collaterals in arteriosclerosis of the lower aorta and iliac arteries. Surgery 1955;38:950.
64. Lindstrom BL. The value of the collateral circulation from the inferior mesenteric artery in obliteration of the lower abdominal aorta. Acta Chir Scand 1950;100:367.
65. Schobinger R. Personal communication, 1964.
66. Boley SJ, Brandt LJ, Veith FJ. Ischemic disorders of the intestines. Curr Probl Surg 1978;15:1–85.
67. Boley SJ, Schwartz S, Krieger H, et al. Further observations on reversible vascular occlusion of the colon. Am J Gastroenterol 1965;44:260–268.
68. Thoeni RF. Colorectal cancer: cross-sectional imaging for staging of primary tumor and detection of local recurrence. AJR 1991;156:909–915.
69. Karlsson S, Jonsson K, Rosengren JE, et al. Angiography in colonic carcinoma. Dis Colon Rectum 1984;27:648–650.
70. Iijima T. Pharmacoangiographic diagnosis of venous invasion of carcinoma of the colon with reference to liver metastases. Dis Colon Rectum 1988;31:718–722.
71. Iijima T. Angiographic diagnosis of the degree of serosal invasion of carcinoma of the colon. Dis Colon Rectum 1988;31:46–49.
72. Yuasa Y, Kohda E, Ido K, Kodera K, et al. Vasoconstrictive effects of prostaglandin F_2 alpha angiography on colonic lesions. Radiology 1984;151:305–309.
73. Schobinger R. Operative intestinal arteriography in the diagnosis of diverticulitis of the colon. Acta Radiol 1959;5:28.
74. Lunderquist A, Lunderquist A. Angiography and ulcerative colitis. AJR 1967;99:18.
75. Tsuchiya M, Miura S, Asakura H, et al. Angiographic evaluation of vascular changes in ulcerative colitis. Angiology 1980;31:147–153.
76. Erikson U, Fagerberg S, Krause U, et al. Angiographic studies in Crohn's disease and ulcerative colitis. AJR 1970;110:385–392.
77. Momoshima S, Kohda E, Hiramatsu K, et al. Intraarterial prednisolone infusion therapy in ulcerative colitis. AJR 1985;145:1057–1060.
78. Todd GJ, Forde KA. Lower gastrointestinal bleeding with negative or inconclusive radiographic studies: the role of colonoscopy. Am J Surg 1979;138:627–628.
79. Sharma VS, Valji K, Bookstein JJ. Gastrointestinal hemorrhage in AIDS: arteriographic diagnosis and transcatheter treatment. Radiology 1992;185:447–451.
80. Giacchino JL, Geis WP, Pickleman JR, et al. Changing perspectives in massive lower intestinal hemorrhage. Surgery 1979;86:368.
81. Walker WJ, Goldin AR, Shaff MI, et al. Per catheter control of haemorrhage from the superior and inferior mesenteric arteries. Clin Radiol 1980;31:71–80.
82. Browder W, Cerise EJ, Litwin MS. Impact of emergency angiography in massive lower gastrointestinal bleeding. Ann Surg 1986;204:530–536.
83. Boley SJ, Sprayregen S, Sammartano RJ, et al. The pathophysiologic basis for the angiographic signs of vascular ectasias of the colon. Radiology 1977;125:615–621.
84. Baum S, Athanasoulis CA, Waltman AC, et al. Angiodysplasia of the right colon: a cause of gastrointestinal bleeding. AJR 1977;129:789.
85. Moore JD, Thompson NW, Appleman HD, et al. Arteriovenous malformation of the gastrointestinal tract. Arch Surg 1976;111:381–389.
86. Emanuel RB, Weisner MM, Shenoy SS, et al. Arteriovenous malformations as a cause of gastrointestinal bleeding: the importance of triple-vessel angiographic studies in diagnosis and prevention of rebleeding. J Clin Gastroenterol 1985;7:237–246.
87. Bartram CI. Obliteration of thumbprinting with double-contrast enemas in acute ischemic colitis. Gastrointest Radiol 1979;4:85–88.
88. Gore RM, Calenoff L, Rogers LF. Roentgenographic manifestations of ischemic colitis. JAMA 1979;241:1171–1173.
89. McKusick KA, Froelich J, Callahan RJ, et al. ^{99m}Tc red blood cells for detection of gastrointestinal bleeding: experience with 80 patients. AJR 1981;137:1113–1118.
90. Alavi A, Ring EJ. Localization of gastrointestinal bleeding superiority of ^{99m}Tc-sulfur colloid compared with angiography. AJR 1981;137:741–748.
91. St. George JK, Pollak JS. Acute gastrointestinal hemorrhage detected by selective scintigraphic angiography. J Nucl Med 1991;32:1601–1604.
92. Jaques PF, Fitch DD. Anal verge and low rectal bleeding: a diagnostic problem. J Clin Gastroenterol 1986;8:38–42.
93. Sheedy PF, Fulton RE, Atwell DT. Angiographic evaluation of patients with chronic gastrointestinal bleeding. AJR 1975;123:338–347.
94. Rollins ES, Picus D, Hicks ME, et al. Angiography is useful in detecting the source of chronic gastrointestinal bleeding of obscure origin. AJR 1991;156:385–388.
95. Rösch J, Keller FS, Wawrukiewicz AS, et al. Pharmacoangiography in the diagnosis of recurrent massive lower gastrointestinal bleeding. Radiology 1982;145:615–619.

63

Mesenteric Ischemia

SCOTT J. BOLEY
LAWRENCE J. BRANDT

As our population has achieved a longer life span the greater number of elderly patients has been accompanied by an increasing frequency in the diagnosis of ischemic disorders of the intestines. In part this is due to a real increase in their incidence; importantly, it is the result of the belated recognition of the many clinical manifestations that have as their common etiology interference with intestinal blood flow.

Although chronic intestinal ischemia was the subject of many articles in the 1960s, it has become evident that relatively few patients suffer from this problem. Far more common are episodes of acute mesenteric ischemia with either immediate or delayed effects of the circulatory insult. Angiography plays a major role in both the diagnosis and the management of mesenteric ischemia, especially in its acute forms.[1]

Pathophysiologic Changes Accompanying Intestinal Ischemia

Reduction in blood flow to the intestine may be a reflection of generalized poor perfusion, as in shock or with a failing heart, or it may result from either local morphologic or functional changes. Narrowings of the major mesenteric vessels, focal atheromatous emboli, vasculitis as part of a systemic disease, and mesenteric vasoconstriction can all lead to inadequate circulation. However, whatever the cause, intestinal ischemia has the same end results—a spectrum ranging from completely reversible functional alterations to total hemorrhagic necrosis of portions of the bowel or all of it.

The intestines are protected from ischemia to a great extent by their abundant collateral circulation, which has been discussed in detail in Chapter 61, Superior Mesenteric Angiography.

Communications between the celiac and the superior and inferior mesenteric beds are numerous, and a general rule that has proved valid is that in gradual occlusion at least two of these vessels must be compromised to produce symptomatic intestinal ischemia.

Moreover, occlusion of two of the three vessels occurs frequently without evidence of ischemia, and total occlusion of all three vessels in asymptomatic patients has been observed.

Collateral pathways around occlusions of smaller arterial branches in the mesentery are provided by the primary, secondary, and tertiary arcades in the small bowel and the marginal arterial complex of Drummond in the colon. Within the bowel wall, there is a network of communicating submucosal vessels that can maintain the viability of short segments of the intestine where the extramural arterial supply has been lost.

When a major vessel is occluded, collateral pathways open immediately in response to the fall in arterial pressure distal to the obstruction. Increased blood flow through this collateral circulation continues as long as the pressure in the vascular bed distal to the obstruction remains below the systemic pressure. If vasoconstriction develops in the distal bed, the arterial pressure there rises and causes diminution of collateral flow. If normal blood flow is reestablished, the flow through collateral channels ceases.

In the resting state, the splanchnic circulation receives 28 percent of the cardiac output. This may increase modestly after eating or may decrease during exercise, but major changes are usually related to increased sympathetic activity. Vasomotor control of the mesenteric circulation is mediated primarily through the sympathetic nervous system. Although beta-adrenergic receptors are present in the splanchnic vascular bed, alpha-adrenergic receptors predominate, and increased sympathetic activity produces vasoconstriction, which increases resistance and decreases blood flow. Folkow et al.[2] have shown that vasoconstriction induced by sympathetic nervous stimulation can virtually stop blood flow for brief intervals. Although vasoconstriction occurs in both the arterioles and venules, the increase in precapillary resistance is relatively greater than the increase in postcapillary resistance, and thus hydrostatic pressure within the capillary bed falls during prolonged vasoconstriction. This decrease in capillary pressure usually results in loss of plasma volume into the mesenteric bed.

In vascular disorders of the intestines, there is a frequently changing interrelationship between blood flow, the mesenteric vessels, and intestinal cellular viability. Mesenteric vasoconstriction may be present and cause a reduction in blood flow but not produce a fall to inadequate levels (ischemia). Similarly the lumen of a short segment of the superior mesenteric artery (SMA) may be reduced by 80 percent with no diminution in blood flow. Moreover, intestinal ischemia can be present without intestinal necrosis, and intestinal necrosis may be present with normal blood flow if blood flow is determined after a transient episode of ischemia has been relieved.

Intestinal ischemia may result from a reduction in blood flow, from redistribution of blood flow, or from a combination of both. With hypotension, there is decreased splanchnic blood flow due to vasoconstriction and also arteriovenous shunting within the bowel wall.[3] A similar situation occurs with intestinal distention.[4] In both the small and the large bowels, after an intraluminal pressure of 30 mmHg is reached, further stepwise increases in pressure result in parallel decreases in intestinal blood flow. However, 20 to 35 percent of control blood flow remains even at a pressure of 210 mmHg. Bowel injected with silicone rubber during distention and cleared to permit visualization of blood vessels reveals almost complete shunting away from the mucosa and muscularis propria, with filling of only the submucosal and serosal arteries. Thus the remaining blood flow is redistributed away from the oxygen-consuming components of the intestine. This redistribution is reflected in a decreasing arteriovenous oxygen difference that parallels this fall in blood flow. The highly oxygenated blood flowing through the serosal arteries and veins results in a normal pink external appearance of the bowel, even when the total blood flow is only 20 percent of control. This phenomenon explains the frequent clinical observation of bowel that appears normal externally but in which there is pronounced hemorrhagic infarction of the mucosa.

The effects of intermittent distention on both a distended segment of small bowel and the rest of the small intestine are profound.[5] Intermittent increases in intraluminal pressure significantly reduce blood flow not only to the distended segment but also to the entire small bowel, and this diminution in flow persists for hours after relief of the distention.

Episodes of mesenteric ischemia may have delayed or protracted effects. Clinically, these effects are demonstrated by the occurrence of nonocclusive intestinal ischemia hours to days after the cardiovascular problem has been alleviated and by the well-documented progression of bowel infarction after an arterial occlusion has been corrected. In extensive animal experiments, *persistent mesenteric vasoconstriction* has been shown to be one explanation for these phenomena.[6–8]

These investigations showed that when the SMA blood flow is decreased 50 percent with a hydraulic occluder, the mesenteric arterial pressure in the peripheral bed immediately falls proportionately, and blood flow through the sources of collateral blood supply (i.e., the celiac and the inferior mesenteric arteries) rises. However, a decreased SMA flow of several hours' duration results in mesenteric vasoconstriction, the pressure in the mesenteric bed rises to the level of the systemic arterial pressure, and blood flow through the arteries supplying collateral flow returns to normal. Initially, the mesenteric vasoconstriction is reversible with release of the SMA occlusion, but after it has been present for several hours the vasoconstriction persists even after the occlusion is removed. Thus a low SMA flow initially produces mesenteric vascular responses that tend to maintain adequate intestinal blood flow, but if the diminished flow is prolonged, active vasoconstriction develops and may persist even after the primary cause of mesenteric ischemia is corrected.

Further studies showed that this persistent mesenteric vasoconstriction can be reversed by the selective injection of papaverine, a vasodilator, into the SMA. Such papaverine injections, therefore, could interrupt the vicious cycle that might result in persistent mesenteric ischemia following a transient fall in cardiac output or other temporary local or systemic causes of decreased mesenteric blood flow. This active and often persistent vasoconstriction can be identified angiographically and is the basis for the diagnosis of nonocclusive mesenteric ischemia.[9–11]

Acute Mesenteric Ischemia

Emergency angiography is one of the cornerstones of the authors' approach to acute mesenteric ischemia (AMI).[12] Emboli, thromboses, and mesenteric vasoconstriction can be diagnosed and the adequacy of the splanchnic circulation evaluated. The angiographic catheter also provides a route for the intraarterial administration of vasodilators.

The angiographic technique used for diagnosing AMI is similar to that used for routine SMA arteriography, with the exception of the volume of contrast material employed. Because the initial angiographic examination and follow-up studies include multiple injections, and because most of the patients already

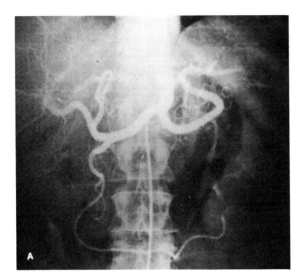

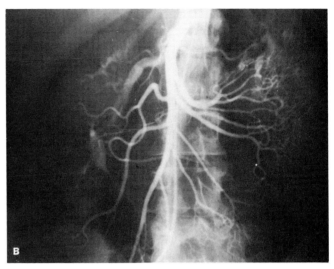

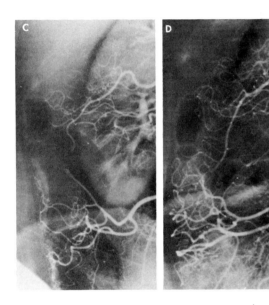

Figure 63-1. (A) Celiac angiogram from a 51-year-old woman with rheumatic heart disease, atrial fibrillation, and right lower quadrant pain of sudden onset. The embolus in the distal splenic artery was suspected on the flush aortogram. (B) Initial selective superior mesenteric arteriogram from the same patient, midarterial phase. The jejunal and ileal arcades are filled, but there is no filling of the arcades of the right colon. (C) Repeat angiogram after a bolus injection of papaverine shows a marked improvement in the circulation to the right colon. (D) Repeat angiogram after papaverine infusion for 20 hours shows excellent circulation with good visualization of the arcades and the intramural vessels. By this time, the abdominal pain had disappeared. (From Siegelman SS, Sprayregen S, Boley SJ. Angiographic diagnosis of mesenteric arterial vasoconstriction. Radiology 1974; 112:553. Used with permission.)

have reduced renal blood flow, one-half the usual volume of contrast material is used in all selective studies to reduce renal damage. An initial flush aortogram with biplane filming is obtained to evaluate the aorta and the origin of the major aortic branches. The aortogram is important because renal or splenic arterial emboli can also appear with abdominal pain of sudden onset. Such pain may reflect renal or splenic infarction or intestinal ischemia due to reflex mesenteric vasoconstriction (Fig. 63-1). Aortography is also used to evaluate the collateral circulation between the superior mesenteric, celiac, and inferior mesenteric arteries. Because mesenteric vasoconstriction may accompany hypotension, angiography is performed only in patients who are normotensive. A selective SMA angiogram is performed to identify emboli, thromboses, or mesenteric vasoconstriction and to assess the perfusion of the vascular bed distal to any obstruction. If an occlusion or a vasoconstriction is found, the angiogram is repeated after a single bolus of 25 mg of tolazoline is administered into the SMA catheter. This bolus of vasodilator permits better visualization of the peripheral circulation and indicates the potential effectiveness of a papaverine infusion. The response to tolazoline does not affect the decision to use a papaverine infusion in patients with nonocclusive mesenteric ischemia, but it may indicate the possibility of employing nonoperative therapy for patients with embolic obstructions. Initially, papaverine (60 mg) was used as the bolus, but tolazoline was substituted because of its more rapid effect. Tolazoline is not used for continuous infusions because it is neither as effective nor as safe as papaverine by this method of administration.

In three of the authors' patients with nonocclusive ischemia, the abdominal pain and marked peritoneal signs resulting from mesenteric vasoconstriction disappeared within 20 minutes after the tolazoline injection. The relief of pain and physical signs led to cancellation of scheduled laparotomies, and both patients survived without operation.

Nonocclusive Mesenteric Ischemia

From 1958, when Ende first described nonocclusive mesenteric ischemia (NOMI),[13] to the late 1970s, the proportion of mesenteric vascular accidents resulting from this entity rose from 12 percent[14] to over 50 percent in several series.[15,16] In the early 1980s, however, the authors and others found a marked decline in the incidence of nonocclusive mesenteric ischemia, probably because of the use of downstream unloading drugs in coronary and intensive care units. These drugs would prevent the splanchnic vasoconstriction believed to be responsible for this condition, which occurs in response to a decrease in cardiac output, hypovolemia, dehydration, vasopressor agents, or hypotension. This vasoconstriction may persist even after the initiating cause has been corrected. Predisposing conditions include myocardial infarction, congestive heart failure, aortic insufficiency, renal and he-

patic disease, and major abdominal or cardiac operations. In addition, a more immediate precipitating cause, such as pulmonary edema, cardiac arrhythmia, or shock, is usually present, although the intestinal ischemic episode may not become manifest until hours to days later.

Treatment of nonocclusive mesenteric ischemia has been ineffective in reducing its 90 percent mortality. The patients are generally elderly and extremely ill, and in the majority of cases the underlying cause of the inadequate blood flow is not amenable to surgical correction. Because many of the patients are in coronary or intensive care units, there has been an understandable reluctance in the past to subject such patients to aggressive invasive diagnostic studies and therapy. However, despite their critical condition, a significant number of these patients survive the major cardiac insult only to succumb to intestinal infarction.

Angiographically, nonocclusive mesenteric ischemia is diagnosed when the signs of mesenteric vasoconstriction are seen in a patient who has a clinical picture suggestive of intestinal ischemia but who is neither in shock nor receiving vasopressors. Reliable angiographic criteria for the diagnosis of mesenteric vasoconstriction include (1) narrowings at the origins

Figure 63-2. Angiographic appearance of mesenteric vasoconstriction. (A) Spasm at the origins of the major superior mesenteric artery (SMA) branches and multiple areas of intermittent spasm (*arrowheads*) and dilatation ("string of sausages"). (Courtesy of S. S. Siegelman, M.D.) (B) Typical appearance of marked constriction of the entire SMA and its major branches.

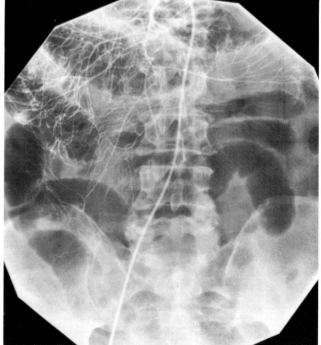

A   B

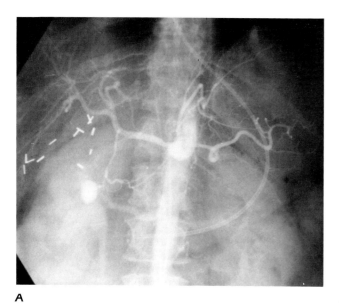

A

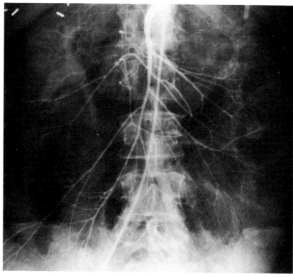

B

Figure 63-3. (A) Celiac angiogram from a patient with upper gastrointestinal tract bleeding and hypertension. Extravasation of contrast material from a branch of the gastroduodenal artery indicates the site of the duodenal bleeding.

(B) Superior mesenteric arteriogram from the same patient showing mesenteric vasoconstriction in response to the hypotension.

of multiple branches of the SMA, (2) irregularities in intestinal branches, (3) spasms of arcades, and (4) impaired filling of intramural vessels.[9–11] The angiographic findings may vary from localized spasm to a "pruned" appearance of the entire mesenteric tree (Fig. 63-2). Mesenteric vasoconstriction does occur with other conditions, such as hemorrhage (Fig. 63-3) and pancreatitis, but when it is present in patients without these disorders in whom intestinal ischemia is suspected, it is strong evidence of nonocclusive mesenteric ischemia. Thus, if angiography is performed sufficiently early in the course of their illnesses, patients with AMI of a nonocclusive origin, as well as patients with surgically correctable lesions, can be identified before bowel infarction occurs.

Superior Mesenteric Artery Embolus

Today, superior mesenteric artery emboli (SMAE) are responsible for 40 to 50 percent of episodes of acute mesenteric ischemia; they usually originate from a mural or an atrial thrombus.[17,18] In the past, such thrombi were most commonly associated with rheumatic valvular disease, but in a review of the authors' experience with 47 patients with SMAE, arteriosclerotic heart disease was the cause in all but one case.[17] Many patients have a previous history of peripheral arterial embolism, and 20 percent or more have synchronous emboli in other arteries.

In a normal angiographic study, the major branches of the SMA, the intestinal arcades, the intramural arteries, and the mesenteric veins are all visualized. Emboli typically appear as sharp, rounded defects, but the duration of symptoms can influence this angiographic appearance. When angiography is performed immediately after the onset of abdominal pain, the emboli are apt to be sharply defined (Figs. 63-4A, 63-5B), but if the study is delayed for several days, secondary thrombus may build up proximally and distally and obscure the typical configuration (Figs. 63-4B, 63-5A). The artery may be completely occluded (Fig. 63-4A and B), but more often the embolus only partially obstructs blood flow (Fig. 63-4C). Mild to marked vasoconstriction is often present in arteries both proximal and distal to the embolus.[9,10] The degree of vasoconstriction affects the retrograde filling of the SMA and its branches distal to the embolus, which, together with the adequacy of the perfusion of the intestinal mural branches, should be evaluated before and after the injection of the tolazoline bolus.

Arterial emboli tend to lodge at points of normal anatomic narrowings, usually just distal to the origin of a major branch. In the authors' series, the most frequent sites were just above the origin of the inferior pancreaticoduodenal artery, occluding all the main branches of the SMA, at or just above the origin of the middle colic artery, and just above or including the origin of the ileocolic artery. Approximately 10 per-

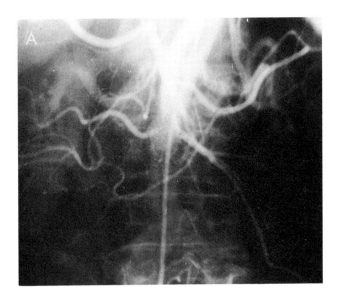
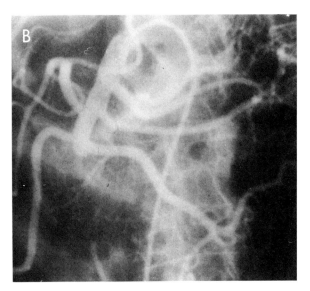
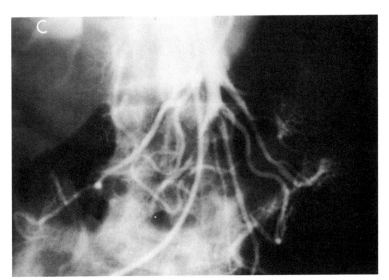

Figure 63-4. Angiographic appearance of superior mesenteric artery emboli. (A) Recent embolus lodged at the level of origin of the middle colic artery shows a well-defined round contour and a complete occlusion of the main artery. (B) Older embolus just below the origin of the right colic artery shows a complete obstruction, but the sharp contour seen in (A) is absent. (C) Recent embolus at the level of the ileocolic artery and extending into it. Well-defined round edges can be seen at the top and bottom of the embolus. The artery is only partially obstructed. (From Boley SJ, Brandt LJ, Veith FJ. Ischemic disorders of the intestines. Curr Probl Surg 1978;15:1. Used with permission.)

cent of patients had more peripheral emboli, and in two patients the emboli were multiple (Fig. 63-5C).

Acute Superior Mesenteric Artery Thrombosis

The incidence of acute superior mesenteric artery thrombosis (SMAT) varies in different reports. For example, Ottinger[16] and Jackson[14] found thromboses to be almost as common as emboli, whereas we found emboli to be three to four times more frequent. SMAT almost always is superimposed on severe atherosclerotic narrowing, most commonly in the region of the origin of the main artery. Because the acute episode represents the end stage of a chronic problem, it is not surprising that 30 to 50 percent of patients have had abdominal pain during the preceding weeks or months. Most patients have severe diffuse arterio-

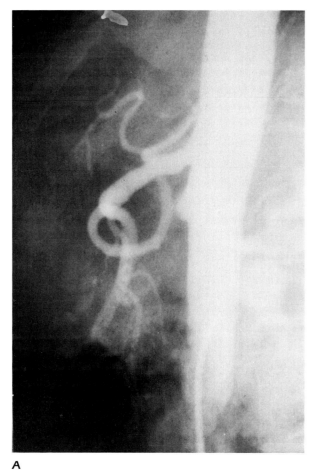

A

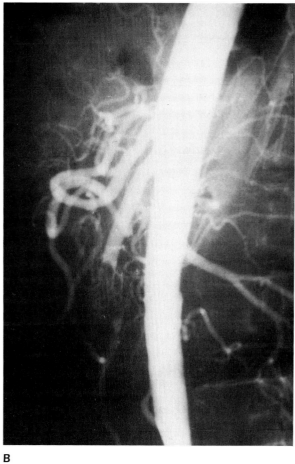

B

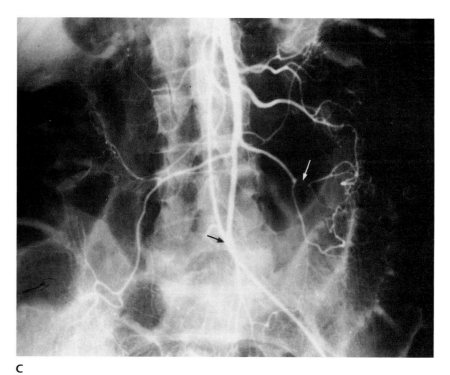

C

Figure 63-5. Angiographic appearance of superior mesenteric emboli. (A) Totally occluding embolus just distal to the origin of the SMA. (B) Embolus more distal in the main SMA with a well-defined round contour. (C) Multiple emboli to the ileocolic artery and the peripheral jejunal branch (*arrows*). (From Kieny R, Cinqualbre J. Les ischemies intestinales signes. Paris: Expansion Scientifique Française, 1979. Used with permission.)

sclerosis, and a prior history of coronary, cerebral, or peripheral arterial ischemia is frequent.

Identification of SMAT is usually made from the flush aortogram, which most often shows total occlusion of the SMA within 1 to 2 cm of its origin. Some filling of the artery distal to the obstruction is almost always present because of collateral circulation. Branches both proximal and distal to the occlusion may show local spasm or diffuse constriction. Angiographic differentiation between a thrombosis and an old embolus may be difficult; in such instances, the patients are treated initially as if they had emboli. A more difficult problem arises when a total occlusion of the SMA is demonstrated by angiography in a patient with abdominal pain but no abdominal findings. In such an instance it is important to differentiate between an acute and a long-standing occlusion, because the latter may be coincidental to an unrelated presenting illness. Prominent collateral vessels between the superior mesenteric and the celiac or inferior mesenteric circulations are characteristic of chronic SMA oc-

clusion. If large collaterals are present and there is good filling of the SMA on the late films during the angiogram, the occlusion can be considered to be chronic, and the abdominal pain is probably unrelated to mesenteric vascular disease (Fig. 63-6). In the absence of peritoneal signs, such patients are treated expectantly. The absence of collateral vessels or the presence of collaterals within inadequate filling of the SMA indicates an acute occlusion. In the latter instance, the middle colic artery probably has occluded, interrupting the collateral circulation to an already marginal system. Prompt intervention is indicated irrespective of the abdominal findings in these cases (Fig. 63-7).

Acute Mesenteric Venous Thrombosis

Acute mesenteric venous thrombosis is a distinct form of intestinal ischemia, which although cited as the most frequent cause of intestinal infarction 70 years ago,[19] is responsible for only a few cases today. Much

Figure 63-6. (A) Angiogram from a patient with a superior mesenteric artery occlusion. The prominent "meandering artery" shows that collateral channels have been present for some time and that the occlusion is not acute. (From Boley SJ, Brandt LJ, Veith FJ. Ischemic disorders of the intestines.

Curr Probl Surg 1978;15:1. Used with permission.) (B) Meandering artery is seen in another patient communicating with and supplying the SMA, establishing that there has not been an acute occlusion of the collateral blood supply to a chronically occluded SMA.

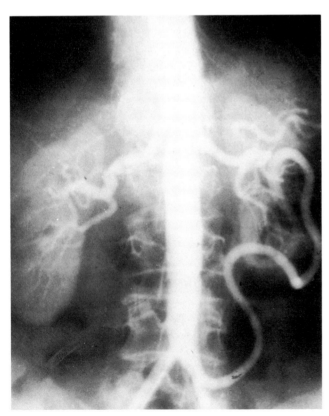

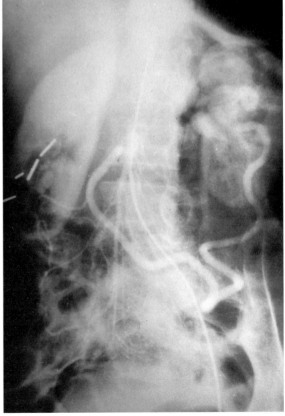

A

B

of this decline is due to the fact that in the past infarction in the absence of arterial occlusion was interpreted as being the result of venous thrombosis, whereas today nonocclusive mesenteric ischemia is usually recognized as the cause.

Although many conditions were associated with mesenteric venous thrombosis in older studies, as many as 55 percent of patients were thought to have no etiologic factor. However, in more recent reports, contributing disorders were identified in 81 percent.[20] This discrepancy can be explained by the fact that many of the cases in retrospective reviews occurred before new conditions such as deficiency of antithrombin III, protein S, or protein C had been described. It can be expected that with increasing knowledge the number of cases of primary mesenteric venous thrombosis in which no cause can be identified will decrease further. Hypercoagulable states are especially important,

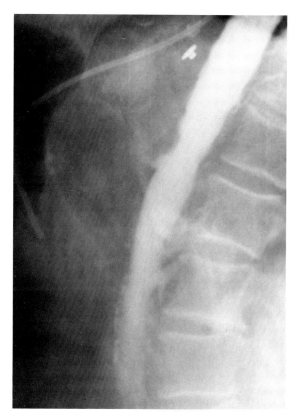

Figure 63-7. (A) Flush aortogram (lateral view) from another patient showing an occlusion of both celiac and superior mesenteric arteries. (B) Anteroposterior view shows no apparent prominent collateral vessels. (C) Late phase lateral view shows a small-caliber "meandering artery." The absence of large collateral vessels indicates an acute rather than a chronic occlusion.

A

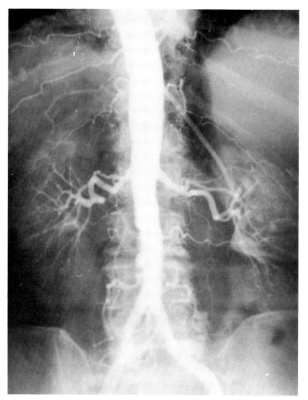

B

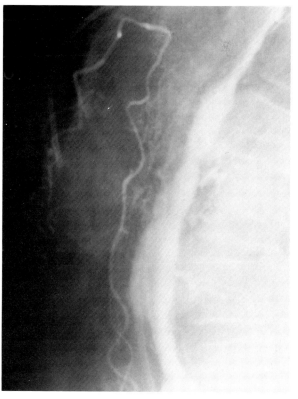

C

having been found in 14 of 16 patients in a 1989 report.[21]

Mesenteric venous occlusion produces a spectrum of clinical presentations, the most common of which is the acute onset of abdominal pain with progressive signs and symptoms of bowel infarction. Compared with other forms of acute mesenteric infarction, this acute form of mesenteric venous thrombosis occurs in younger patients, typically has a more indolent and nonspecific course, involves shorter segments of bowel, and has a lower mortality rate. In the past, most patients presented with this clinical picture of an acute abdomen, and the diagnosis was made only at laparotomy or postmortem. However, recent discoveries have altered our concepts of the disorder, and we now recognize that thrombosis of the superior mesenteric vein (SMV) can develop slowly with no symptoms, in a more subacute manner with pain but no intestinal infarction, or acutely with the classic presentation.[22] In the past, in 90 to 95 percent of patients the correct diagnosis was made only at laparotomy. In more recent series, the use of newer diagnostic modalities has enabled the diagnosis to be made without or before operation in most patients.[21] Imaging studies can definitively establish the diagnosis of mesenteric venous thrombosis before intestinal infarction occurs. Selective mesenteric arteriography can establish a definitive diagnosis before bowel infarction, can differentiate venous thrombosis from arterial forms of ischemia, and can provide access for the administration of intraarterial vasodilators if relief of the associated arterial vasoconstriction is deemed important in a specific patient.[23] The angiographic findings of mesenteric venous thrombosis have been determined experimentally and clinically[24-26] and include (1) demonstration of a thrombus in the SMV with partial or complete occlusion; (2) failure to visualize the SMV or portal vein; (3) slow or absent filling of the mesenteric veins; (4) arterial spasm; (5) failure of arterial arcades to empty; (6) reflux of contrast into the artery; and (7) a prolonged blush in the involved segment. In addition, the angiogram may show reconstitution of venous blood flow above the thrombus, which can be an important factor in selecting therapy.

Ultrasonography,[27-29] computed tomography (CT),[21,28,30] and magnetic resonance imaging (MRI) have all been used to demonstrate thrombi in the superior mesenteric and portal veins before bowel infarction. Gastrointestinal CT scanning[21] can establish a diagnosis in more than 90 percent of patients with mesenteric venous thrombosis by demonstrating the thrombus, venous collateral circulation, and abnormal segments of intestine. Some authors[30] believe that when a diagnosis of mesenteric venous thrombosis is made on CT, little is gained by a subsequent selective mesenteric angiogram. However, the better delineation of thrombosed veins and the access for potential administration of intraarterial vasodilators that this technique provides may make it of value in some patients.

Thus there is no firm information on the desirability of performing angiography and CT in the patient with acute mesenteric venous thrombosis. A small number of patients identified just by imaging techniques and without abdominal findings have been treated successfully without angiography or operation. MRI has been used to diagnose mesenteric venous thrombosis in a few patients, but its only apparent advantage is that it avoids the use of ionizing radiation.

Plan for Diagnosis and Therapy

All patients suspected of having AMI are promptly treated for associated cardiovascular problems and are sent for plain radiographic studies of the abdomen. Subsequent abdominal angiography is routinely performed unless some other intraabdominal condition is diagnosed on the plain film examination. On the basis of the angiographic findings and the presence or absence of signs of peritoneal irritation on physical examination, the individual patient is then treated according to the proposed plan of Figure 63-8.

Selection of Patients

AMI is most likely to develop in patients over 50 years of age with (1) valvular or arteriosclerotic heart disease; (2) long-standing congestive heart failure, especially with unsatisfactory control of digitalis therapy or prolonged use of diuretics; (3) cardiac arrhythmias of any cause; (4) hypovolemia or hypotension of any origin, such as burns, pancreatitis, or gastrointestinal or postoperative hemorrhage; or (5) recent myocardial infarctions.

Patients in any of these high-risk categories who have abdominal pain that started suddenly and has lasted more than 2 or 3 hours are started on the management protocol. Less absolute indications for an aggressive investigation are unexplained abdominal distention or gastrointestinal bleeding. These broad selection criteria are essential if early diagnosis and treatment are to be achieved, because the presence of more extensive and specific signs and symptoms usually signifies irreversible intestinal damage.

Even when the decision to operate has been made, an angiogram must be obtained to manage the patient properly at operation. Moreover, the relief of mesenteric vasoconstriction is an integral part of the therapy for emboli and thromboses, as well as for low-flow

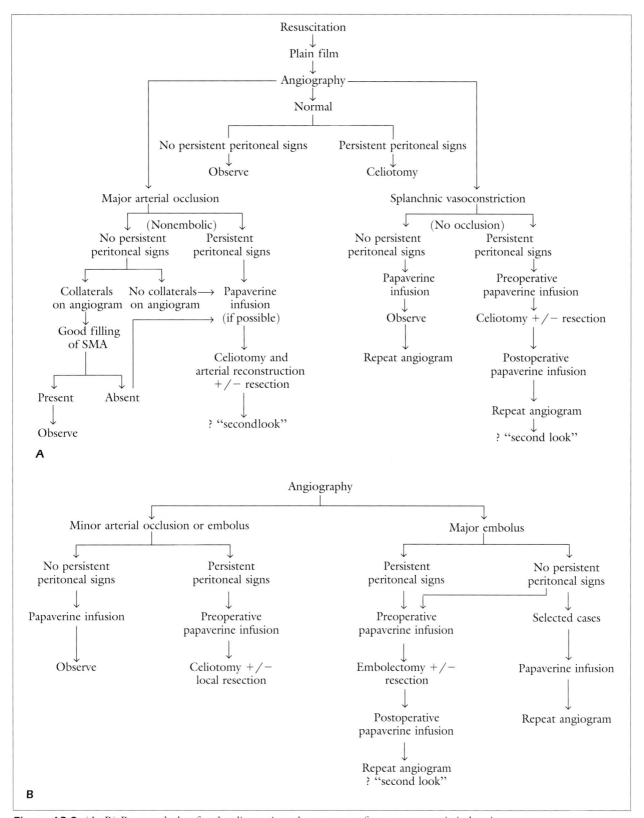

Figure 63-8. (A, B) Proposed plan for the diagnosis and treatment of acute mesenteric ischemia.

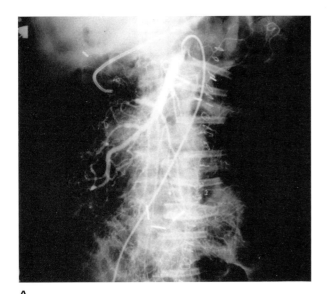

A

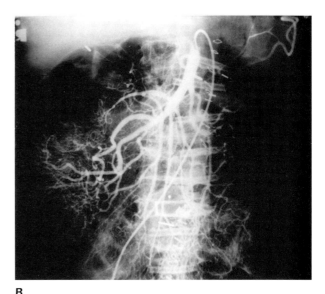

B

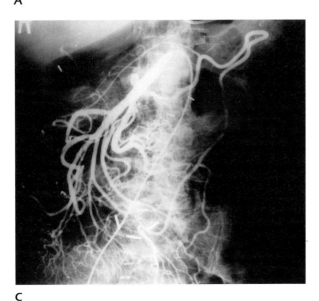

C

Figure 63-9. Patient with embolus in main SMA who was operated upon for acute diverticulitis. An embolectomy was performed and a superior mesenteric arteriogram was obtained postoperatively. (A) Immediate postoperative angiogram showing patent SMA but marked constriction of its branches. (B) Angiogram after 14 hours of SMA papaverine infusion showing much less, but still significant, vasoconstriction. (C) Angiogram after 50 hours of papaverine infusion showing complete relief of vasoconstriction. The patient had an uneventful recovery.

states, and can best be achieved by intraarterial infusion of papaverine through the angiography catheter (Fig. 63-9).

Initial Preparation and Resuscitation

The initial treatment is directed toward correcting the predisposing or precipitating causes of the mesenteric ischemia. Relief of acute congestive heart failure, correction of cardiac arrhythmias, and replacement of blood volume precede any diagnostic studies. In general, efforts at increasing intestinal blood flow will be futile if low cardiac output, hypotension, or hypovolemia persists. On rare occasions, the authors have combined dopamine administered intravenously into a peripheral vein with papaverine administered intraarterially into the SMA, and we have been able to im-

prove both systemic and mesenteric blood flow. Patients in shock should not undergo angiography because mesenteric vasoconstriction will always be evident, even without intestinal ischemia. Such patients should not receive papaverine intraarterially since it will increase the size of the vascular bed and aggravate the hypovolemia (Fig. 63-10). The management of congestive heart failure or shock that is complicated by mesenteric ischemia is especially difficult because the use of digitalis or vasopressors may further aggravate the diminished intestinal blood flow. Digitalis preparations all have a direct vasoconstrictor action on SMA smooth muscle, especially with the blood levels observed during rapid digitalization or with digitalis intoxication. The decision to discontinue digitalis is often a difficult one to make because the drug may be required to control rapid ventricular rates associated with atrial fibrillation or to manage severe congestive heart failure. Vasopressors are contraindicated in the treatment of shock if mesenteric ischemia is suspected.

When intestinal ischemia has progressed to the extent that systemic alterations associated with bowel infarction are present, appropriate correction of plasma volume deficits and fluid loss, gastrointestinal decom-

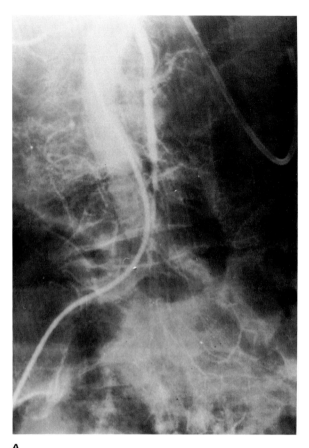

A

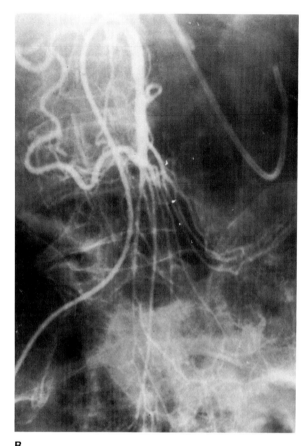

B

Figure 63-10. (A) Superior mesenteric arteriogram from a patient with moderate hypovolemic hypotension. Marked vasoconstriction is apparent. (B) Repeat angiogram after a bolus infusion of papaverine shows relief of the mesenteric vasoconstriction. In the absence of correction of the hypovo-lemia, the relief of the vasoconstriction was accompanied by a further fall in blood pressure. This sequence of events emphasizes the importance of adequate resuscitation before angiography is performed for suspected mesenteric ischemia.

pression, and parenteral antibiotics are included in the preparation prior to roentgenologic studies.

After the initial corrective and supportive measures have been completed, roentgenographic studies are undertaken irrespective of the abdominal physical findings or the surgeon's decision on whether to operate.

Plain Film Studies

The initial examination includes a chest roentgenogram and roentgenograms of the abdomen with the patient in the supine, erect, and both lateral decubitus positions. Signs of intestinal ischemia on plain film studies occur late and usually indicate bowel infarction. In series of cases in which a significant portion of the patients have had such signs, the mortality has been dismaying.[31-33]

A normal plain film of the abdomen does not exclude AMI, and, ideally, all patients should be studied before roentgenographic signs of ischemia develop. Thus *the primary purpose of these plain film studies is not to help in the diagnosis of AMI but to exclude other radiographically diagnosable causes of abdominal pain* (e.g., a perforated viscus or an intestinal obstruction). If no other acute abdominal condition is detected, angiography is performed.

Therapeutic Papaverine Infusion

When the therapeutic regimen includes the use of papaverine, the drug is infused through the angiography catheter, which is left in the SMA. To prevent dislodgment, the catheter is sutured to the skin at its point of entry in the thigh. The papaverine is administered at a constant rate of 30 to 60 mg per hour using an infusion pump. The drug is usually diluted in saline to a concentration of 1 mg per ml, but the concentration may vary according to the patient's fluid limitations or requirements. Continuous monitoring of systemic arterial pressure and cardiac rate and rhythm is indicated because these amounts of papaverine theoretically could have systemic effects. The authors have not observed such problems in either our experimental or clinical studies, probably because the drug is metabolized in the liver before it reaches the general circulation. Infusion at these rates has been used clinically for as long as 5 days without untoward systemic changes.

Heparin is not added to the infusion because it is not compatible with papaverine hydrochloride and we have not found it necessary to prevent thrombus formation within the SMA. No other medications or fluids should be administered through the arterial catheter, and the patient must be observed carefully for evidence of dislodgment of the catheter.

The duration of the papaverine infusion varies with both the purpose for its use and the response of the patient. In conjunction with the embolectomy or arterial reconstruction, the infusion is continued for 12 to 24 hours if a "second-look" operation is not planned. After 12 to 24 hours, the angiogram is repeated, and, unless some specific indication for more prolonged vasodilator therapy is demonstrated, the infusion is discontinued. When a second-look operation is to be performed, the papaverine is continued until the abdomen is reopened, but a repeat angiogram is obtained before operation. The need for an additional period of infusion is determined intraoperatively, depending on the state of the bowel and the results of the preoperative angiogram.

When papaverine infusion is used as the primary treatment for nonocclusive mesenteric ischemia, it is continued for approximately 24 hours. Then the infusion is changed to isotonic saline without papaverine, and, 30 minutes after the change, a repeat angiogram is performed. On the basis of the clinical course of the patient (i.e., abdominal distention, bowel functioning, abdominal findings, and evidence of blood in the stools) and the response of the vasoconstriction to therapy as indicated by the angiogram, the infusion is discontinued or maintained for another 24 hours; the patient's condition is then reevaluated (Figs. 63-11 and 63-12). Infusions have been continued for up to 5 days, but usually they can be stopped after 24 hours. When papaverine is used in conjunction with laparotomy for nonocclusive disease, a second-look operation is frequently necessary. In such cases, the infusion is continued as described previously for second-look operations following embolectomy. The papaverine infusion is discontinued when no signs of vasoconstriction are present on an angiogram that is obtained 30 minutes after the vasodilator infusion is temporarily replaced by saline alone. The SMA catheter is removed promptly when the intraarterial infusion is stopped.

Supportive Therapy

An essential aspect of the supportive therapy of patients with AMI is the maintenance of an adequate plasma volume. Just as massive losses of protein-rich fluids occur with early bowel infarction, so they may occur after revascularization of ischemic bowel. Hence is it important to correct continually for losses before undertaking treatment during papaverine infusions and following surgical relief of arterial occlusions. The use of low-molecular-weight dextran may serve a dual purpose because of its effect as a plasma expander and because of its potential value in decreasing sludging in the microcirculation.

The value of both systemic and locally administered antibiotics in improving the viability of compromised bowel is well accepted. For this reason, and because of the high incidence of positive blood cultures with AMI, systemic antibiotics are started as soon as the diagnosis is established.

Intestinal decompression by nasogastric suction, the use of furosemide and mannitol to maintain urinary output, and specific therapy for the cardiac problems all play a role in the management of most patients. Digitalis, as previously mentioned, must be used cautiously, and vasopressors should be avoided. Anticoagulant therapy during and immediately after operation is specifically avoided (except in venous thrombosis) because of the danger of intestinal hemorrhage. Early in the authors' experience we had two patients who bled massively as a result of heparin therapy after successful embolectomy. Anticoagulant therapy is begun after 48 hours when a revascularization operation has been performed. In mesenteric venous thrombosis, however, heparin therapy is started immediately.

Prognosis

Although mortalities of 70 to 90 percent were reported through 1980 using traditional methods of diagnosis and therapy, the aggressive approach described above can reduce these catastrophic figures.[24,34,35] Of the authors' first 50 patients managed by this approach, 35 (70 percent) proved to have AMI. Of these, 33 had angiographic signs of ischemia. The remaining 2 patients had normal angiograms. Of 65 patients from two institutions using this protocol, 36 (55 percent) survived, including 14 of 26 with NOMI, 14 of 23 with SMAE, 4 of 6 with SMAT, and 4 of 6 with superior mesenteric venous thrombosis. Most of the survivors lost no bowel or less than 3 feet of small intestine.

In a separate review of 47 patients with intestinal ischemia resulting from SMA emboli,[17] a survival rate

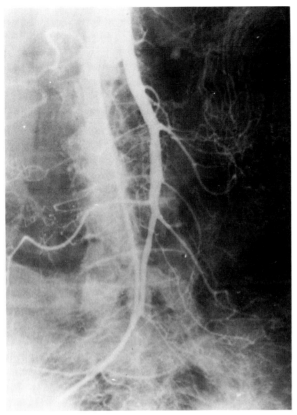
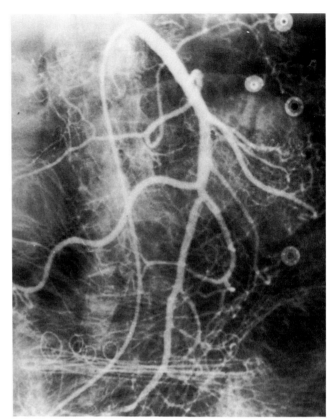

A

B

Figure 63-11. Patient with nonocclusive mesenteric ischemia managed with papaverine infusion for 3 days. (A) Initial angiogram showing a spasm of the main superior mesenteric artery, origins of branches, and intestinal arcades. (B) Angiogram after 36 hours of papaverine infusion. The study was obtained 30 minutes after papaverine was replaced with saline. At this time, the patient's abdominal symptoms and signs were gone. (From Boley SJ, Brandt LJ, Veith FJ. Ischemic disorders of the intestines. Curr Probl Surg 1978;15: 1. Used with permission.)

of 55 percent was achieved in patients managed according to our aggressive protocol, whereas only 20 percent of those patients treated by traditional methods survived. Intraarterial papaverine as the primary treatment was successful in 4 patients; 2 of these were not operated upon, and the other 2 had normal intestine at the time of delayed laparotomy. Of special interest in this study was the observation that of those patients with SMA emboli who were placed in the protocol within 12 hours of reporting their pain to their physician and who were managed strictly according to this protocol, two-thirds survived.

Using the aggressive approach outlined above, this catastrophic mortality has been substantially reduced. Overall, 50 percent or more of the patients presenting with AMI and treated according to the present algorithm survive, and approximately 70 to 90 percent lose less than a meter of intestine. Ninety percent of patients with AMI who had angiography but no signs of peritonitis have survived, demonstrating the potential value of early diagnosis. Ideally all patients with AMI should be studied at a time when the plain films of the abdomen are normal and before the development of an acute surgical abdomen. Other published reports that did not use vasodilator therapy have had significantly higher mortality rates. Therefore, a wider use of this aggressive protocol for the patients at risk for AMI may improve overall results of treatment for AMI.

The complications of the angiographic studies and prolonged infusions of vasodilator drugs have not been excessive. Of the first 50 patients, 3 developed transient acute tubular necrosis following angiography and treatment of their mesenteric ischemia. One patient developed arterial occlusions in both lower extremities during a papaverine infusion for an SMA embolus. These probably represented other emboli from the patient's primary source of embolization, but the SMA catheter could not be excluded as a factor. There were several instances of local hematomas at the arterial puncture site, but no other major problems were encountered with blood flow to the lower extremities.

Problems with prolonged papaverine infusions have

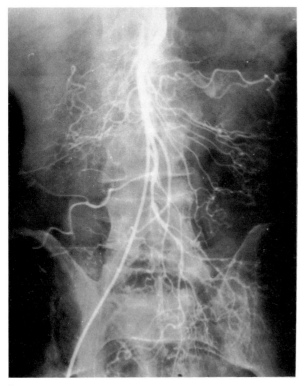

A

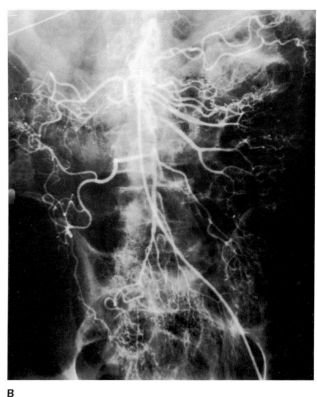

B

Figure 63-12. Patient with nonocclusive mesenteric ischemia following an episode of gastrointestinal hemorrhage and shock. (A) Initial superior mesenteric arteriogram showing diffuse vasoconstriction. (B) Repeat angiogram after papaverine infusion for 24 hours shows partial but not complete relief of the vasoconstriction. (C) Angiogram performed after 48 hours of papaverine infusion shows dilatation of all vessels. The patient was asymptomatic by that time. (Courtesy of Leon Schultz, M.D.)

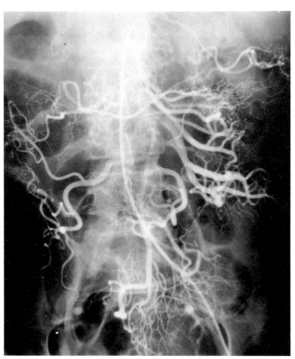

been minimal. Infusions for more than 5 days have been used without significant systemic effects. More than 90 percent of the drug is inactivated with each circulation through the liver, and so large doses can be given safely into the mesenteric circulation. Fibrin clots on the arterial catheter have been commonly observed but have not caused any difficulty. Three catheters clotted and had to be removed, but this complication can be avoided if a continuous infusion pump is used. Catheter dislodgment occurred several times and required replacement under fluoroscopy.

C

Chronic Intestinal Ischemia (Abdominal Angina, Intestinal Angina, Recurrent Mesenteric Ischemia)

The term *chronic intestinal ischemia* (CMI) includes a host of conditions in which there is insufficient blood flow to satisfy the demands of increased motility, secretion, and absorption that develop after meals. These disorders manifest themselves either by ischemic visceral pain or by abnormalities in gastrointestinal absorption or motility. Patients with CMI are actually experiencing recurrent acute episodes of insufficient blood flow during periods of maximum intestinal work load. Therefore, the pain is similar to that arising in the myocardium with angina pectoris or that in the calf muscles with intermittent claudication.

Angiography plays a less important role in the diagnosis of CMI than it does in the diagnosis of AMI, because the demonstration of narrowed or occluded visceral vessels is not proof of chronic intestinal ischemia. Angiographic evaluation includes flush aortography in frontal and lateral views and selective injections of the SMA, the celiac axis (CA), and, if possible, the inferior mesenteric artery (IMA). The degree of occlusive involvement of the three major arteries can be best assessed on the lateral projections, and the collateral circulation and pattern of flow are best seen on the frontal views. The presence of prominent collateral vessels indicates a significant stenosis of a major vessel, but it also denotes a chronic process.

Although partial or complete occlusions of the SMA, CA, and IMA have been identified frequently in autopsy and angiographic studies, there have been relatively few patients with documented chronic intestinal ischemia. Moreover, there are many patients with occlusion of two or even all three of these vessels who remain asymptomatic (Fig. 63-13). Hence, the clinical significance of the angiographic demonstration of occlusion of one or more of these vessels remains controversial. The dearth of objective means of determining the inadequacy of intestinal blood flow before the morphologic changes of ischemia occur is the major obstacle to identifying patients with CMI.

Dick et al.[36] attempted to establish objective guidelines for the presence of CMI by angiographic measurements of the total cross-sectional area of the SMA, CA, and IMA in control patients, in hypertensive and arteriopathic patients, and in patients with chronic intestinal ischemia. These authors found that all patients with intestinal ischemia had total cross-sectional areas reduced to below two-thirds of normal. However, patients without ischemia had similar reductions. The in-

exact nature of such measurements is obvious. Moreover, the length of the stenosis, which is also an important factor, was not considered. A major shortcoming of estimating intestinal blood flow from the patency of the individual major vessels is the equal importance and variability of the collateral blood supply. The significance of stenoses of the major arteries is reduced in the presence of prominent collateral anastomoses but is of great importance in their absence. Determining the presence or absence of these collateral circuits is an integral part of the angiographic evaluation of possible chronic intestinal ischemia. The absence of collateral vessels with occlusion of the SMA or CA is an ominous sign and suggests an acute rather than a chronic process.

A method of assessing the adequacy of splanchnic blood flow in which the angiographer plays a role is that described by Hansen et al.[37] *Splanchnic blood flow* is defined as the total blood flow through the three splanchnic arteries and extrasplanchnic collateral vessels, and it is determined by measuring hepatic blood flow with indocyanine-green, both in the fasting state and after a standard meal. Oxygen consumption in the splanchnic bed is also measured. This technique involves catheterization of the radial artery, an arm vein, and a hepatic vein. In their study of 15 patients with abdominal pain, there was a significant failure of patients with abdominal angina to increase their splanchnic blood flow after the test meal. After arterial reconstruction, the postprandial increase in flow was similar to that in the control group. The complexity and invasiveness of this procedure have limited its use.

CMI has been reported with aneurysms of the aorta, CA, and SMA, with congenital and traumatic arteriovenous fistulas involving the SMA and the hepatic arteries, with coarctation of the aorta, and with congenital anomalies of the splanchnic vessels. Such cases are rare, however, and atherosclerotic involvement of the mesenteric vessels is the usual cause of this form of intestinal ischemia.

Atherosclerosis commonly involves the splanchnic arteries in individuals over 45 years of age. Of 88 adult patients studied by Reiner, Jiminez, and Rodriguez, 77 percent had evidence of atherosclerosis of the splanchnic vessels.[38] Some degree of luminal stenosis was observed in 72 percent of those with atherosclerosis, and in 65 percent the SMA, CA, or IMA was involved. Narrowing of the major vessels was almost always due to a plaque at the aortic ostium or in the proximal 1 to 2 cm of the artery. Severe stenoses were uniformly associated with marked aortic atherosclerosis, and, as expected, patients with severe mesenteric involvement had a higher incidence of coronary artery disease and diabetes mellitus. There was little correla-

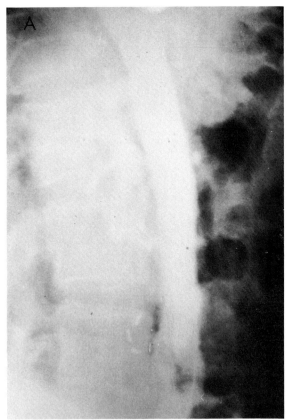

Figure 63-13. Angiogram from a patient with no abdominal symptoms. (A) Flush aortogram in lateral position shows an occlusion of the celiac axis, superior mesenteric artery (SMA), and inferior mesenteric artery. (B) Anteroposterior flush aortogram demonstrates filling from the middle hemorrhoidal arteries up to a large "meandering artery," with ultimate filling of the SMA and celiac axis through these collateral channels. (From Boley SJ, Brandt LJ, Veith FJ. Ischemic disorders of the intestines. Curr Probl Surg 1978;15: 1. Used with permission.)

tion between the degree of mesenteric atherosclerosis and the clinical course.

Diagnosis and Treatment

Because there has been no specific reliable diagnostic test for abdominal angina, the diagnosis has been based on clinical symptoms, arteriographic demonstration of splanchnic arterial occlusions, and exclusion of other gastrointestinal disease.

Conventional radiographic examinations of the gastrointestinal tract usually are unremarkable. Studies for malabsorption often show increased fecal fat and decreased D-xylose excretion. Although these tests identify absorption defects, none is specific for malabsorption caused by ischemia. Nonspecific abnormalities also have been detected in small bowel biopsies.

Balloon tonometers have been used indirectly to determine intestinal intramural pH (pH_1), which is a measure of the adequacy of oxygenation in relation to the tissue's metabolic demands. Intestinal angina probably results from a meal-induced increase in gastric blood flow that, with fixed splanchnic arterial inflow, is achieved by stealing from the blood flow to the intestines. The decrease in intestinal blood flow is reflected in a fall in intestinal pH_1; hence tonometric determination of small bowel pH_1 offers an ideal means of diagnosing intestinal ischemia after eating.

A new provocative test for CMI based on these concepts uses tonometers to determine intestinal intramural pH before and after a test meal.[39] The test also can be used after revascularization to determine the success of the operation.

The one essential clinical symptom of CMI is abdominal pain, which is usually postprandial, progressive, and associated with weight loss. Physical findings are limited and nonspecific. A systolic bruit is heard in the upper abdomen in approximately one-half the patients, but even when present its diagnostic significance must be questioned because similar bruits have

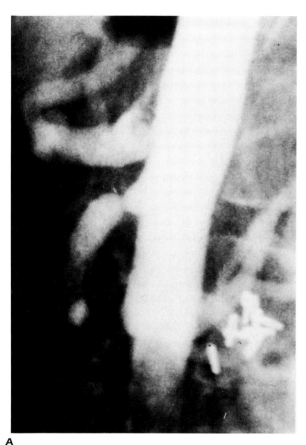

A

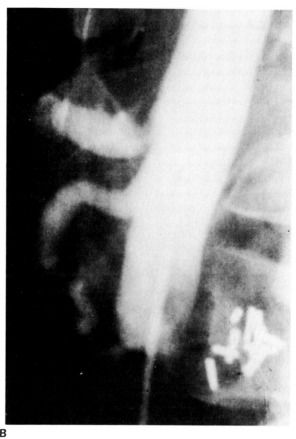

B

Figure 63-14. Transluminal angioplasty performed on a patient with symptoms of chronic intestinal ischemia. (A) Aortogram before dilatation shows stenosis and poststenotic dilatation of both celiac and superior mesenteric arteries.

(B) Aortogram performed after dilatation of the SMA shows correction of the SMA stenosis. The patient was relieved of her symptoms. (Courtesy of Christos Athanasoulis, M.D.)

been reported in 6.5 to 15.9 percent of healthy patients.[40]

In the past, the only treatment for CMI was some form of operative arterial reconstruction. Today, transluminal angioplasty may afford an alternative approach of lesser magnitude and risk.

Patients have been managed by transluminal dilatations, with good short-term responses (Fig. 63-14).[41–43] In the absence of a method for measuring intestinal blood flow, precise criteria to define the need for operative arterial reconstruction have been lacking. There is agreement that a patient who has classic abdominal angina and unexplained weight loss, whose diagnostic evaluation has excluded other gastrointestinal disease, and whose angiogram shows occlusive involvement of at least two of the three major arteries should be treated. The issue has been much less clear if only one major vessel has been involved or if the nature of the clinical presentation has been atypical. With the availability of transluminal angioplasty, dila-

tation of stenoses of the SMA and the CA at the time of the original angiography is possible, and thus the indications for treatment may be liberalized. Further experience and follow-up will reveal whether this method will be as helpful in the management of patients with CMI as it has been in those with angina pectoris and renovascular hypertension. Tests of blood flow described earlier or the provocative tonometric test may serve to identify patients who should have mesenteric angiography and who may benefit from revascularization procedures.

There is one special situation in which reconstruction or dilatation of obstructed splanchnic arteries is indicated in the absence of abdominal complaints. This indication arises in a patient who is undergoing an aortic operation for peripheral vascular disease and in whom aortography has demonstrated occlusive involvement of the SMA and/or the CA and the presence of a large "meandering artery." In such a patient, the latter artery is supplying most of the blood flow to the splanchnic circulation from the IMA. Because the IMA may be compromised during the aortic procedure, it is advisable to provide another source of blood flow as part of this operation. The occurrence of acute intestinal ischemia resulting from "aortoiliac steal syndromes" has also been described in this situation after successful restoration of blood flow to the legs, but when no reconstructive procedure has been performed on the visceral vessels. Although we question whether the acute intestinal ischemia in these reports[44] represents a true "steal," the occurrence of this complication indicates the need for prophylactic revascularization.

Total occlusions or long stenoses of the SMA not amenable to transluminal angioplasty require operative revascularization of the splanchnic bed. Endarterectomy, reimplantation, and bypass procedures have all been successfully employed. Many surgeons believe that, in the presence of CA and SMA occlusion, adequate management must include restoration of normal arterial pressures in both vessels and their branches.[45] The infrequency of fatal acute mesenteric infarction after a successful revascularization operation suggests that such procedures may prevent a major intestinal ischemic episode.

Results

Long-term follow-up information after operative revascularization is limited. In three reported series involving 70 patients, the combined operative mortality was 7 percent, and 70 percent of patients were relieved of their symptoms.[44,46,47] Late deaths occurred in 21 percent of patients and are a reflection of the generalized arteriosclerotic disease in these patients. In McCollum et al.'s series of 33 patients, 83 percent were alive 5 years after operation, and 62 percent were alive after 10 years.[44]

Properly selected patients with intestinal angina can be operated on successfully with a reasonable operative risk and a good long-term prognosis. Most will be relieved of their pain and malabsorption, although complete relief of the latter may take months.[1,48] Although it has not been shown definitively that revascularization will protect against a fatal acute mesenteric infarction, the infrequency of these catastrophes after a successful operation suggests that that may be so.

References

1. Kaleya RN, Sammartano RJ, Boley SJ. Aggressive approach to acute mesenteric ischemia. Surg Clin North Am 1992;72:157.
2. Folkow B, Lewis D, Lundgren O, Mellander S, Wallentin J. The effect of the sympathetic vasoconstrictor fibers on the distribution of the capillary blood flow in the intestine. Acta Physiol Scand 1964;61:458.
3. Chou CC, Yu LC, Yu LM. Effects of acute hemorrhage (H) and carotid artery occlusion (CAO) on compartmental microcirculation in the G-I tract. Presented at the First World Congress for Microcirculation, Toronto, Canada, 1975.
4. Boley SJ, et al. Pathophysiologic effect of bowel distention on intestinal blood flow. Am J Surg 1969;117:228.
5. Tunick PA, Treiber WF, Frank M, Veith FJ, Gliedman ML, Boley SJ. Pathophysiologic effects of bowel distention on intestinal blood flow: II. Curr Top Surg Res 1970;2:59.
6. Boley SJ, Regan JA, Tunick PA, Everhard ME, Winslow PR, Veith FJ. Persistent vasoconstriction—a major factor in nonocclusive mesenteric ischemia. Curr Top Surg Res 1971;3:425.
7. Boley SJ, Treiber W, Winslow PR, Gliedman ML, Veith FJ. Circulatory response to acute reduction of superior mesenteric arterial blood flow. Physiologist 1969;12:180.
8. Everhard ME, Regan JA, Veith FJ, Boley SJ. Mesenteric vasomotor response to reduced mesenteric blood flow. Physiologist 1970;13:191.
9. Aakhus T, Brabrand G. Angiography in acute superior mesenteric arterial insufficiency. Acta Radiol 1967;6:1.
10. Aakhus T, Evensen A. Angiography in acute mesenteric arterial insufficiency. Acta Radiol 1978;19:945.
11. Siegelman SS, Sprayregen S, Boley SJ. Angiographic diagnosis of mesenteric arterial vasoconstriction. Radiology 1974;112:553.
12. Boley SJ, Sprayregen S, Veith FJ, Siegelman S. An aggressive roentgenologic and surgical approach to acute mesenteric ischemia. In: Nyhus N, ed. Surgery annual. New York: Appleton-Century-Crofts, 1973.
13. Ende N. Infarction of the bowel in cardiac failure. N Engl J Med 1958;258:879.
14. Jackson BB. Occlusion of the superior mesenteric artery. In: American lectures in surgery. Springfield, IL: Charles C Thomas, 1963.
15. Boley SJ, Sprayregen S, Siegelman SS, Veith FJ. Initial results from an aggressive approach to acute mesenteric ischemia. Surgery 1977;82:848.
16. Ottinger LW, Austen WG. A study of 136 patients with mesenteric infarction. Surg Gynecol Obstet 1965;121:789.
17. Boley SJ, Feinstein RF, Sammartano RJ, Brandt LJ. New concepts in the management of emboli of the superior mesenteric artery. Surg Gynecol Obstet 1981;153:561.
18. Ottinger LW. The surgical management of acute occlusion of the superior mesenteric artery. Ann Surg 1978;188:721.
19. Cokkinis AJ. Mesenteric vascular occlusion. London: Baillière, Tindall and Cox, 1926.
20. Abdu RU, Zakhour BJ, Dallis DJ. Mesenteric venous thrombosis—1911 to 1984. Surgery 1987;101:383.
21. Harward TRS, Green D, Bergan JJ, et al. Mesenteric venous thrombosis. J Vasc Surg 1989;9:328.
22. Boley SJ, Kaleya RN, Brandt LJ. Mesenteric venous thrombosis. Surg Clin North Am 1992;72:183.
23. Lanthier P, Lepot M, Mahieu P. Mesenteric venous thrombosis presenting as a neurological problem. Acta Clin Belg 1984;29:92.
24. Clark RA, Gallant TE. Acute mesenteric ischemia: angiographic spectrum. AJR 1984;142:555.
25. Clavien PA, Durig M, Harder F. Venous mesenteric infarction: a particular entity. Br J Surg 1988;75:252.
26. Polk H. Experimental mesenteric venous occlusion. Ann Surg 1966;163:432.
27. Kidami H, Herbert R, Kidami AV. Ultrasonic demonstration of superior mesenteric and splenoportal venous thrombosis. J Clin Ultrasound 1986;14:199.
28. Matos C, Van Gansbeke D, Zalcman M, et al. Mesenteric venous thrombosis: early CT and ultrasound diagnosis and conservative management. Gastrointest Radiol 1986;11:322.
29. Verbanck JJ, Rutgeerts LJ, Haerens MH, et al. Partial splenoportal and superior mesenteric venous thrombosis: early sono-

graphic diagnosis and successful conservative management. Gastroenterology 1984;86:949.

30. Rosen A, Korobkin M, Silverman PM, et al. Mesenteric vein thrombosis: CT identification. AJR 1984;143:83.
31. Frimman-Dahl J. Roentgen examination in mesenteric thrombosis. AJR 1950;64:610.
32. Hessen I. Roentgen examination in cases of occlusion of the mesenteric vessels. Acta Radiol 1955;44:293.
33. Tomchik FS, Wittenberg J, Ottinger LW. The roentgenographic spectrum of bowel infarction. Radiology 1970;96:249.
34. Batellier J, Kieny R. Superior mesenteric artery embolism: 82 cases. Ann Vasc Surg 1990;4:112.
35. Levy PJ, Krausz MM, Manny J. Acute mesenteric ischemia: improved results: a retrospective analysis of 92 patients. Surgery 1990;107:373.
36. Dick AP, Graff R, Gregg DC, Peters N, Sarner M. An arteriographic study of mesenteric arterial disease. Gut 1967;8:206.
37. Hansen HJB, Engell HC, Ring-Larsen H, Raneck L. Splanchnic blood flow in patients with abdominal angina before and after arterial reconstruction. Ann Surg 1977;186:215.
38. Reiner L, Jiminez FA, Rodriguez FL. Atherosclerosis in the mesenteric circulation: observations and correlations with aortic and coronary atherosclerosis. Am Heart J 1963;66:200.
39. Boley SJ, Brandt LJ, Kosches D, Sales C. A new provocative test for the diagnosis of chronic mesenteric ischemia. Am J Gastroenterol 1991;86:888.
40. Edwards AJ, Hamilton JD, Nichol WD, Taylor GW, Dawson AM. Experience with coeliac axis compression syndrome: a phonoarteriographic study. Ann Intern Med 1973;79:211.
41. Athanasoulis C. Personal communication, 1980.
42. Furrer J, Grüntzig A, Kugelmeier J, Goebel N. Treatment of abdominal angina with percutaneous dilatation of an arteria mesenterica superior stenosis. Cardiovasc Intervent Radiol 1980;3:43.
43. Ring E. Personal communication, 1980.
44. McCollum CH, Graham JM, DeBakey ME. Chronic mesenteric arterial insufficiency: results of revascularization in 33 cases. South Med J 1976;69:1266.
45. Morris G, DeBakey M, Bernhard V. Abdominal angina. Surg Clin North Am 1966;46:919.
46. Hansen HJB. Abdominal angina. Acta Chir Scand 1976;142:319.
47. Reul GJ Jr, Wukasch DC, Sandiford FM, Chiarillo L, Hallman GL, Cooley DA. Surgical treatment of abdominal angina: review of 25 patients. Surgery 1974;75:682.
48. Dardik H, Seidenberg B, Parker JG, Hurwitt ES. Intestinal angina malabsorption treated with elective revascularization. JAMA 1965;194:1206.

64

Pelvic Angiography

ERICH K. LANG

Although the advent of new modalities such as magnetic resonance angiography, spiral computed tomographic angiography, and color Doppler ultrasound has affected the volume of patients referred for conventional diagnostic angiography, a concomitant massive increase in the number of interventional angiographic techniques in the pelvis has resulted in an overall further increase in diagnostic angiographic procedures.[1–7] In particular, the demand for superselective angiographic techniques, first to identify the precise location and vascular supply of neoplastic or traumatic lesions and then to limit therapeutic intervention to the vascular bed of the lesion while sparing adjacent normal tissues, has provided a large and new source of patients.[8–15] The now well-established technique of transluminal balloon dilatation of atherosclerotic lesions of pelvic vessels and more recently the placement of metallic stents to reconstitute the lumen have channeled a large number of patients toward these interventional procedures.[16–21] The availability of small balloon catheters capable of attacking arteriosclerotic lesions of the corporal and penile circulation, hitherto correctable only by microvascular surgical techniques, has further expanded the patient pool.[4,16] New techniques to attack venous leakage from the corpora cavernosa by transcatheter embolization have expanded not only interventional techniques but again have sharply increased the demand for detailed venographic assessment of the responsible vascular systems.[22,23] Reconstitution of flow in vessels occluded by blood clots by means of intraarterial and intraclot administration of agents such as urokinase is yet another example of a technique calling for intensified use of pelvic angiography.[24–26]

Magnetic Resonance Angiography

Two-dimensional time-of-flight magnetic resonance angiography (MRA) has been shown to have broad applicability in the diagnosis and follow-up of vascular disease and intervention involving pelvic and lower extremity vessels.[1,6,7,27–29] Although this approach using maximum intensity projection must yet overcome a number of bothersome artifacts such as phase ghosting, absent retrograde flow, slice and vessel misregistration, turbulence, and pseudostenosis, its overall place as a noninvasive screening technique, particularly in postoperative follow-up, appears to be established (Fig. 64-1).[6,7,30] The phase contrast method, another modality of MRA, uses additional magnetic field gradients to encode flow as shifts in the phase of NT, thus relying on base information rather than T1, the index for all time-of-flight techniques.[6,31] This method may further improve the detailed visualization of vessels.

Digital Angiography

Digital angiography is the arteriographic method of choice for all conditions except those mandating detailed assessment of exceedingly small vascular structures such as penile arteries, for which conventional enlargement arteriograms are preferred (Fig. 64-2A).[13,32–37]

Digital arteriograms of the pelvis and runoff angiograms are best performed under local anesthesia.[2] After the anesthetic agent has infiltrated the subcutaneous tissues and periarterial space, the artery is entered with a single entry puncture and a J-shaped guidewire is introduced. A small skin incision is made, subcutaneous tissues are dissected with a straight hemostat, and a tract to the arterial puncture site is dilated with a vessel dilator of appropriate size. The etiology of the underlying disease, the conditions of the vascular tree to be negotiated, and sometimes specific needs, such as the desire to extend the procedure to intervention, determine the approach (i.e., via the transaxillary or transfemoral route).[38–40] In patients who have sustained massive pelvic trauma causing hematomas that complicate the percutaneous approach to the femoral arteries or in those treated by pneumatic compression,

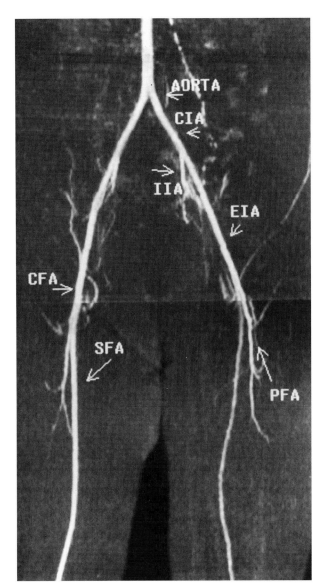

Figure 64-1. Two-dimensional time-of-flight magnetic resonance angiogram with maximum intensity projection (*MIP*) demonstrates excellent visualization of the distal aorta, common iliac artery (*CIA*), internal iliac artery (*IIA*), external iliac artery (*EIA*), common femoral artery (*CFA*), superficial femoral artery (*SFA*), and profunda femoral artery (*PFA*). Imaging parameters: TR/TE = 33/6.8 msec; flop angle = 60 degrees; FOV = 28 cm; matrix = 256 × 128; slice thickness = 2 mm; inferior saturation with spacing = 2 cm; GE signal, 1.5 Tesla System. (Courtesy of Drs. George Holland, M. Reblas, and E. Zerhouni.)

which makes the groin area inaccessible, an axillary approach is favored.[8,12,34,41–43] In patients in whom exchange for a different catheter and/or balloon catheters is anticipated, a vascular sheath of appropriate size is seated in the artery.

Engagement of the desired segmental arterial branch is made possible by a variety of precurved catheter tips, particularly by the use of a guidance system

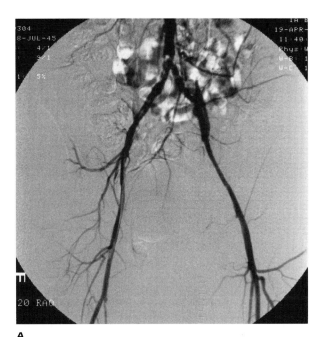

A

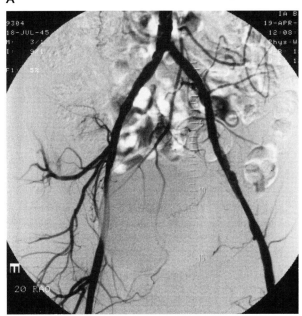

B

Figure 64-2. (A) Digital arteriogram demonstrates an eccentric plaque resulting in a 95 percent occlusion of the left common iliac artery. Additional atheromatous plaques are demonstrated in the region of the bifurcation involving both right and left common iliac arteries. (B) Control digital arteriogram after transluminal angioplasty demonstrates an excellent cosmetic effect of the intervention. Intraarterial pressure recordings and endovascular ultrasound velocity measurements confirmed the salutary result of the intervention.

and tip deflectors, which can alter the intrinsic curvature of the catheter tip and thus facilitate engagement of the desired vessel.

Coaxial catheter systems are favored for the superselective engagement of small vessels. A 3, 4, or 5 French catheter is advanced under fluoroscopic guidance into the desired major branch. A steerable coaxial catheter, such as the Tracker 18 system, is then positioned into the desired subsegmental vessel. The location of both the coaxial catheter and the Tracker catheter is ascertained by injecting a small bolus of dilute contrast medium recorded on digital angiograms. The diaphragms of the arterial sheath as well as the coaxial catheter prevent leakage of blood during the procedure; access ports allow flushing of both the sheath and the coaxial catheter, usually with a heparinized flush solution of 1000 ml of saline mixed with 3000 to 5000 units of heparin. This technique prevents clotting of blood in the sheath or around the catheter.

The amount of contrast medium needed for optimal opacification of the vascular system varies with the prevailing flow rate and the information sought by the study. In general, nonionic contrast media, diluted 1:1 with saline, are favored for digital angiography. The rate, speed, and amount of contrast medium injected vary greatly for different purposes and regions to be studied. Similarly, projections of roentgenographic recordings are governed by the information sought and vary for different pathologic conditions.

The pharmacologic manipulation of blood flow—the epinephrine arteriogram—has been found useful for the study and management of certain pathologic conditions.[44]

Arteriosclerotic Disease of Pelvic Arteries

The widespread use of aortofemoral bypass grafts, endarterectomy, transluminal angioplasty, and the placement of metallic stents to correct occlusion or compromise of major pelvic arteries has intensified the need for the detailed diagnostic categorization of such lesions, the assessment of the runoff vessels, and the documentation of the existence and magnitude of the collateral vascular supply.[21]

Although MRA and three-dimensional spiral CT angiography are the techniques of choice for screening and follow-up, the detailed assessment and categorization of these lesions are best done by digital angiography.[2,5,26,39] However, color Doppler studies and color flow duplex imaging offer additional physiologic information on the status of the vascular system.[2] The data provided by angiography—the categorization of the primary lesion and the status of the runoff vessels—determine the type of intervention (i.e., bypass graft,

endarterectomy, transluminal balloon dilatation, placement of metallic stents, or a combination thereof).[18,20,45] Although intravenous digital arteriography usually provides adequate anatomical detail of the lesion and of runoff vessels, arterial digital angiography is generally favored because it offers better detail of indeterminate segments, which are often in peripheral anatomic locations.[37] Moreover, the amount of contrast medium deployed can be kept to a minimum because the arterial catheter can be advanced to a more distal site for detailed assessment of a peripheral location. For mapping pelvic and runoff vessels, injecting 60 to 80 ml of nonionic contrast medium at a flow rate of 15 ml per second and recording on a step table is generally preferred. An injection of 20 to 30 ml of nonionic contrast medium at a flow rate of 15 ml suffices for the study of the pelvic vessels, which may be complemented by digital angiograms of both lower extremities (runoff study). This method may be favored in patients with marginal renal capacity because digital angiography allows one to use 1:1 dilute contrast medium, reducing the sum total contrast load to about 50 ml.[46] Obviously, the flow rate, speed of injection, and timing of roentgenographic recording are adjusted according to the magnitude of arteriosclerotic disease documented on the preliminary pelvic angiogram, taking into consideration demonstrated delay of runoff.

If complete occlusion of an iliac artery is suspected and recanalization by a one-stage procedure desired, venous digital arteriography is preferred since it does not pose the risk of an existing arterial puncture when using lytic therapy. In general, entry into the vascular system will be sought via the better side, and selective studies of the "bad side" carried out by advancing the catheter across the bifurcation into the contralateral common iliac artery.

Transluminal balloon dilatation or placement of metallic stents can be carried out in the contralateral common or external iliac artery. However, in general, it is better to perform these procedures via an ipsilateral retrograde approach even though this may mandate a second puncture of the artery (see Fig. 64-2B).[47]

To reestablish the lumen of a common or external iliac artery compromised by arteriosclerotic plaques, a guidewire is advanced across the lesion, usually in retrograde but sometimes in antegrade direction.[47] A J-shaped guidewire is favored for this purpose. If a J-shaped guidewire cannot negotiate the irregular and severely compromised lumen, a hydrophilic coated guidewire (glidewire) is recommended. Once the guidewire has been passed across the lesion, a 4 French catheter is advanced and an injection is carried out above the lesion to demonstrate the lesion in detail.

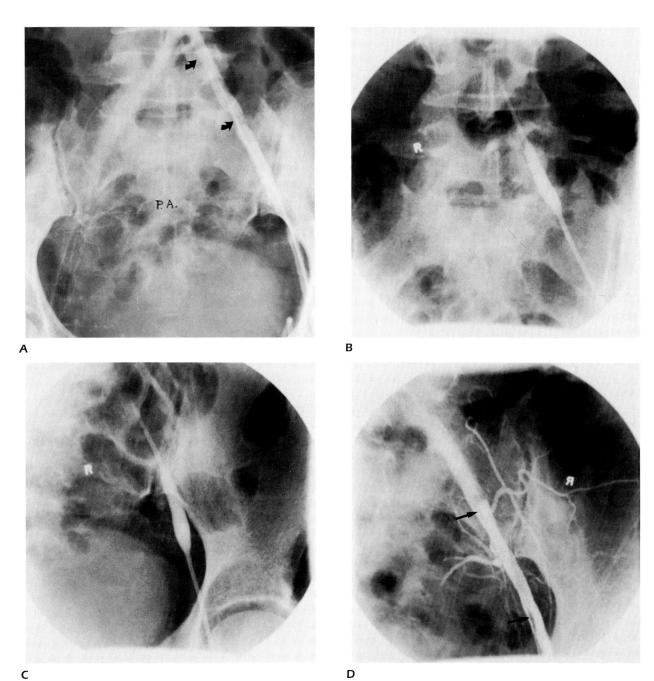

A

B

C

D

Figure 64-3. Extensive arteriosclerotic disease of the aortic bifurcation and common and external iliac arteries (*arrows,* A). (A to C) Transluminal dilatation is carried out with a high-pressure balloon at multiple levels. Initially the balloon shows a waistlike compression (C), indicating an as yet inadequate therapeutic result. (D) The postdilatation control arteriogram shows improvement of the lumen, although a small intimal flap has been created (*arrows*). Miniheparinization was instituted to prevent thrombosis and was maintained for several days. Thereafter the patient was put on 325 mg of aspirin.

Thereafter, a relatively stiff guidewire (Lunderquist, Amplatz) is once again passed through the catheter to a position above or distal to the lesion and a balloon of appropriate length and diameter is passed across the lesion. The balloon should extend beyond the lesion by 0.5 cm both in cephalad and caudal directions. The diameter of the balloon is chosen on the basis of measurements obtained from a normal segment of the artery above or below the lesion. Although overdilatation of the lesion has been advocated by some authorities, dilatation to the actual diameter of the artery is adequate and does not compromise VQSQ-

VQSQRQ.[17] The balloon is inflated with a pressure gauge using dilute contrast medium and retaining a pressure of 2 to 5 atm for 30 to 45 seconds. Salutary correction of the lesion is indicated by disappearance of any waist effect on the balloon and lack of reappearance of the waist when deflating the balloon. Heparinization, preferably via an intravenous route deploying 1000 units of heparin per hour for the next 24 hours, is favored as an immediate postoperative therapeutic measure. Thereafter, antiplatelet agglutination therapy by compounds such as aspirin is generally recommended (Fig. 64-3).

Placement of stents is advocated for eccentric plaques and plaques that do not yield to transluminal balloon dilatation.[48] If a stent of appropriate length is not available, multiple stents must be joined and overlapped to cover the lesion adequately. After the stent is placed, additional dilatation can be carried out by placing a high-pressure balloon inside the stent (Blue Max, Olbert) and further increasing the luminal diameter.[19] Care is advocated for both placement of stents and balloon dilatation so that existing collaterals are not interrupted.

The combination of lytic therapy and transluminal balloon dilatation in the management of completely occluded segments is discussed in the following section.

Intraarterial Fibrinolytic Therapy

Intraarterial fibrinolytic therapy of arterial occlusions has been advocated in the management of acute, subacute, and chronic femoropopliteal and some iliac artery occlusions, particularly those longer than 10 cm, as well as in the management of acute reocclusion and peripheral embolization during routine angioplasty.[25,49] The proximal end of the occlusion must be localized fluoroscopically and the catheter is advanced into the core of the organized clot to perfuse the thrombotic material with the fibrinolytic drug. Urokinase (UK) or a recombinant tissue type of plasminogen activator (RT-PA) is favored as a lytic agent. Both act directly on plasminogen to convert it into plasmin and are nonantigenic. For a single perfusion dose, 100,000 units per hour of UK or 2.5 mg per hour of RT-PA is advocated. This is carried to a maximal dose of 1.5 million units of UK or 20 mg of RT-PA. At this point, the treatment is terminated because systemic effects of the lytic drug might otherwise cause severe complications. To prevent acute rethrombosis, heparin or another aggregation inhibitor is administered.[25]

As lysis progresses, aspiration embolectomy can be undertaken to hasten recanalization. However, this carries an increased risk of embolizing thrombotic material to a more peripheral segment.

Low-dose thrombolytic therapy is mostly performed on thrombi in the femoropopliteal segment. Iliac occlusion is a less common indication because the success rate is slightly lower than for surgery. Nonetheless, a success rate in excess of 50 percent may be expected.[25]

Short-term ultrahigh streptokinase therapy combined with percutaneous transluminal angioplasty has been advocated to further increase the patency rate of treated iliac artery occlusions. Of patients thus treated, 62.3 percent responded favorably. Patients with occlusions less than 6 weeks old and less than 15 cm long showed an even more favorable response of 79.3 percent.[50] The method deploys an initial dose of 20,000 units per minute of streptokinase over 20 minutes followed by a maintenance dose of 1.5 million units of streptokinase per hour over 6 hours. A maximum of 26 hours of infusion may be carried out.[50]

Thrombolysis of an aortobifemoral arterial bypass graft addresses this same problem in a subset of patients (Fig. 64-4).[24,26]

Prelysis angiography must evaluate the proximal and distal vascular bed, giving particular attention to the status of distal runoff vessels.[26,50,51] Venous digital subtraction angiography has been advocated to avoid the need for an arterial puncture before the start of fibrinolytic therapy. Lytic treatment of an occluded bypass graft requires placing the catheter tip in the occluded segment. Whenever feasible, the catheter should be introduced via an antegrade approach into the occluded segment. At the onset of therapy, a bolus of fibrinolytic agent may be given to lace the thrombus and increase fibrinolysis. Coaxial techniques using a 5 French catheter at the proximal infusion site with a 2 or 3 French catheter or guidewire with delivery channel positioned into the mid or distal occluded segment are favored to simultaneously infuse the fibrolytic agent at different levels.[52] Sixty to 100,000 units of UK per hour are used as a low-dose infusion technique, and 4000 units per minute for 2 to 3 hours as a high-dose technique.[26] Although overall limb salvage is significantly improved (50 to 60 percent), there is a high rate of reocclusion, with a patency rate at 1 year of about 33 percent.[49] The initial restoration of blood flow through the occluded graft, however, tends to be in excess of 95 percent.[24] Balloon angioplasty should be performed to remove any distal anastomotic or poststenotic stenoses predisposing to rethrombosis.

Distal embolization is the major complication of local thrombolysis. Often continued thrombolytic therapy and heparinization will result in disappearance of ischemic symptoms attributable to distal embolization.

Fibrolytic therapy is also useful to hasten normaliza-

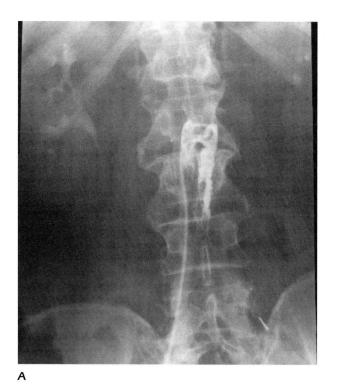

A

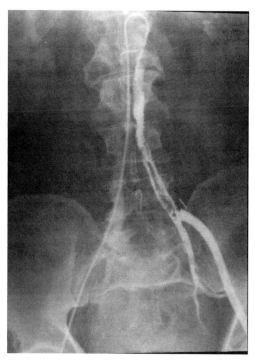

B

Figure 64-4. (A) Arteriogram demonstrates complete occlusion of the left limb of an aortofemoral bypass graft. (Courtesy of Prof. K. Mathias.) (B) The tip of the catheter has been advanced in an antegrade direction deep into the thrombus, and the clot has been laced with 250,000 units of urokinase. A follow-up arteriogram 6 hours after continuous infusion at a rate of 60,000 units per hour of urokinase shows incomplete restoration of the lumen. (C) After 48 hours of continued infusion of urokinase (60,000 units per hour) and heparin (1000 units per hour) as well as a transluminal dilatation to correct an obstructing plaque at the distal end of the thrombosis, there is now a nearly normal vascular lumen.

tion of perfusion in patients who have sustained torsion of the testes that has been corrected surgically within 4 hours after onset (Fig. 64-5).

Acute gastroduodenal ulcers, surgery within the previous 4 weeks, a history of stroke, hypertension, hemorrhagic diathesis, aneurysms, neoplasms, and arterial puncture within the previous 5 days are considered contraindications to such fibrinolytic therapy.[25]

Angiography in the Assessment of Male Impotence

Ten million American men are estimated to suffer from erectile dysfunction, the majority with an organic base for the dysfunction.[23,53] Abnormalities of the vascular system of the penis constitute the major cause for organic erectile dysfunction.[54,55] After endocrine and

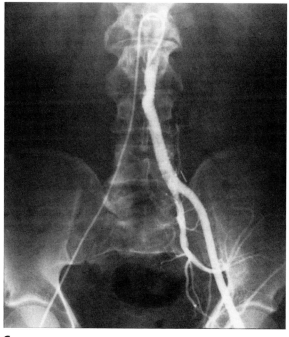

C

psychological causes are eliminated by endocrine screening and by the nocturnal penile tumescent test, the vascular system is studied by penile Doppler ultrasonography, dynamic infusion and pharmacocavernosometry and cavernosography, and selective arteriography.[32,56,57]

The erectile phenomenon of the penile vascular sys-

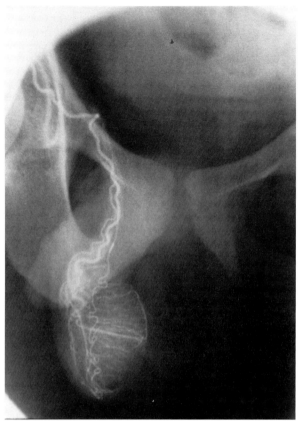

Figure 64-5. Selective follow-up arteriogram of the gonadal artery demonstrates a completely normal vascular pattern of the testis and the epididymis and its supply arteries. The study was obtained 6 hours after surgical correction of a torsion of the testis and selective thrombolytic therapy using 4000 units of urokinase per minute for 2 hours and 60,000 units of urokinase per hour with 1000 units of heparin per hour thereafter.

tem can be divided into three phases: (1) increased arterial flow via the cavernosal arteries; (2) sinusoidal relaxation and filling of corporal bodies; and (3) decrease in outflow and hence trapping of blood within the corpora, producing tumescence and rigidity.[35,55] The inability to increase the intracorporal pressure above the systolic blood pressure results in inadequate rigidity for vaginal penetration. A detailed study of the venous and arterial system of the penis and the corpora cavernosa is designed to pinpoint those lesions amenable to vascular surgical or interventional angiographic correction versus lesions that need to be treated by penile implants.[16,32,35,58]

On the basis of history, traumatic versus degenerative etiologies are suggested. Selective enlargement arteriography is usually reserved for patients who on dynamic infusion and pharmacocavernosography and cavernosometry demonstrate slowly rising or diminished corporal pressure in response to papaverine, ab-

sence of proximal corporal venous dysfunction, and a gradient of 35 mmHg between the cavernosal and brachial arteries' systolic occlusion pressures.[4]

Venous Anatomy

The deep dorsal penile vein, best visualized by injection into the glans penis, is located directly above the intercavernous septum within a sulcus formed by the corpora cavernosa. During Valsalva maneuver, the central portion of the deep dorsal vein may dilate to 4 to 5 mm.[22] The deep dorsal penile vein empties into the preprostatic plexus. These veins, in turn, form one or more vesical veins. At the junction between the deep dorsal penile vein and the preprostatic plexus, the deep dorsal vein is connected to several internal pudendal veins. The pudendal veins run parallel to the pudendal arteries. A characteristic oblique path across the obturator foramen identifies the obturator veins and differentiates them from the pudendal veins. The *deep system* refers to the deep dorsal penile vein, preprostatic (pudendal) plexus, and internal pudendal veins.[22] There are also communications between the internal pudendal vein and crural perforators.

A recent authoritative article states that there are no communications between the deep and superficial venous system of the penis.[22] The superficial dorsal vein lies above Buck fascia and drains the prepuce and skin into the external pudendal veins. The glans penis drains via the deep dorsal vein exclusively. The deep dorsal vein in the sulcus between the corpora cavernosa lies deep to Buck fascia and superficial to the tunica albuginea.[22] Small veins from the corpora cavernosa perforate and empty into the deep dorsal vein. At the root of the penis, the deep dorsal vein passes between suspensory ligaments and under the pubic symphysis. There it divides into right and left rami, forming the preprostatic plexus. The preprostatic plexus lies within the fascial sheet of the prostate and has communications to the vesical plexus as well as the rectal venous plexus. The lower part of the preprostatic plexus communicates to the internal pudendal veins. The corpora spongiosa are drained via bulbar veins that are also communicating with the internal pudendal vein.[22]

Opacification of the deep and superficial system observed after cavernosography proves conclusively that communications occur through the erectile bodies and small perforator veins.[22]

Arteriography

The internal pudendal artery has a variable origin, arising from the main hypogastric trunk, branches of the anterior division of the hypogastric trunk, or the infe-

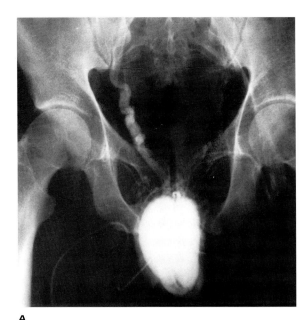

A

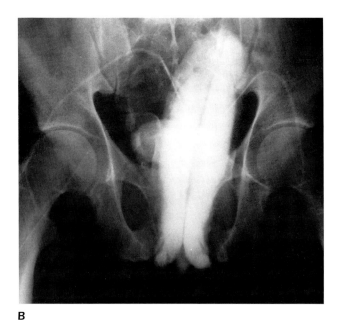

B

Figure 64-6. (A) Cavernosogram performed with an injection of 60 ml of a 50:50 mixture of contrast medium and saline after preperfusion of the corpora cavernosa with 120 ml of saline per minute for 1/2 minute. Note a large drainage vein apparently communicating to the crural perforators.

(B) After administration of 60 mg of papaverine into the corpora cavernosa, a repeat cavernosogram no longer shows abnormal venous drainage but rather demonstrates a prominent erection. Cavernosometry confirmed intracavernosal pressures in excess of arterial systolic pressures.

rior gluteal artery, or as an accessory internal pudendal artery.[4] The common penile artery arises from the distal internal pudendal artery, continuing as the proximal dorsal penile artery and cavernosal arteries.

Cavernosography and Cavernosometry

Dynamic infusion and pharmacocavernosometry and cavernosography are performed to demonstrate abnormal venous leakage or venous occlusive incompetence secondary to rupture of the tunica albuginea (Fig. 64-6).[57,59-62]

Cavernosography and cavernosometry are performed after intracorporal injection of 60 mg papaverine and after infusion of normal saline at a rate of 120 ml per minute for 1½ minutes. The infusion is carried out through 21-gauge needles placed into each corpus cavernosum. The needles are connected to a pressure transducer, which is connected to a digital pressure monitor. A baseline intracorporal pressure is recorded before the injection of papaverine; a second pressure is then recorded 90 seconds after commencing infusion of normal saline at the above-stated rate and intracorporal administration of papaverine. Continued pressure recordings are obtained 2, 3, 5, and 10 minutes after infusion, and the rate of decrease of intracorporal pressure is documented. Cavernosography is performed by injecting 60 ml of a 50:50 mixture of low-molecular-weight contrast medium and saline.[60]

Failure of normal corporal trapping and/or the presence of abnormal venous leaks are indicated by the following: failure to increase the intracorporal pressure over the systolic pressure after saline infusion and pharmacologic manipulation; a rapid decrease in intracorporal pressure, irrespective of the peak value, to baseline levels within 10 to 20 seconds after cessation of the saline infusion; demonstration of contrast medium in the dorsal penile, crural, or saphenous and iliac veins; and/or demonstration of abnormal drainage veins (see Fig. 64-6A).[23] Injection of papaverine into the corpora cavernosa results in smooth muscle relaxation and hence trapping of blood in the corpora cavernosa.[23,59] The venous drainage from the corpora cavernosa occurs via the deep dorsal vein or via the crural veins. The causes of venous leakage are as yet unknown. However, loss of elasticity due to ischemia of the tunica albuginea may be one cause for venous leakage. The incidence of venous leakage causing erectile impotence is estimated as 25 to 78 percent.[57] The disparity of dynamic balance between arterial inflow and venous leakage is assumed to be the cause of erectile impotence.[23,57] Traumatic rupture of the tunica albuginea will likewise result in venous occlusion incompetence because of failure of an adequate trapping mechanism.[35,60,61,63]

Arterial lesions are diagnosed on digital subtraction angiograms for the common and internal iliac arteries and on selective internal pudendal arteriograms for the more distal vessels.[37,54] The latter sequences are best

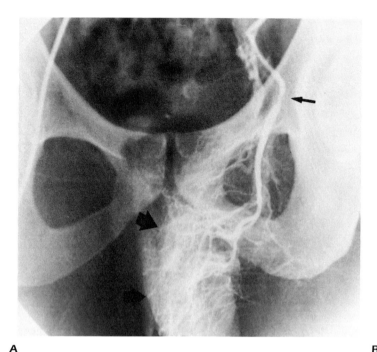

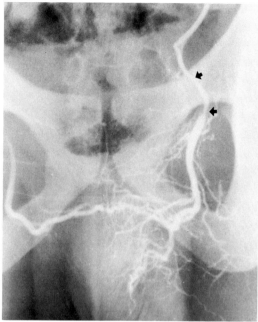

A

B

Figure 64-7. (A and B) Arteriogram obtained after intraarterial administration of 3 mg of Priscoline documents unabated concentric narrowing of the internal pudendal artery

(*arrows*). The pharmacoangiogram confirms the diagnosis of organic stricture and eliminates vascular spasm induced by passage of the guidewire as a possible cause.

Figure 64-8. Arteriogram showing an area of minor arteriosclerotic narrowing of the internal pudendal artery (*left arrow*). Lack of runoff into the deep cavernosal and corpus spongiosum branches indicates endarterial disease (*right arrow*).

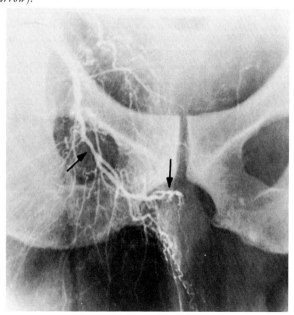

recorded on magnification angiograms (Fig. 64-7). Vasodilatation is ensured by intraarterial administration of papaverine (30 mg) and nitroglycerin (100–200 μg). In addition, intracavernosal injection of 60 mg papaverine hydrochloride is carried out in preparation for the arteriogram. The examination is undertaken to identify lesions that can be successfully treated by microsurgical bypass or angioplasty.[4,16] In contrast to earlier reports, the recent literature indicates that significant inflow arterial disease is rare.[4,36] This may be due in part to a bias by the selection profile; that is, arteriograms may have been performed only on patients who showed no other peripheral vascular disease or major risk factors for generalized arteriosclerosis. In this select group the most frequent occlusive site was in the cavernosal arteries (Fig. 64-8).[4] Conversely, the common penile artery, proximal penile vessels, and inflow arteries were largely free of hemodynamically significant disease.[4] Because of the frequency of asymmetric arterial disease, the supply to the penis from both sides needs to be assessed arteriographically.[36]

If lesions develop as a consequence of blunt perineal or pelvic trauma, involvement of the distal internal pudendal and common penile artery has been much more common than of the hypogastric or cavernous arteries.[64,65] Rupture of the puboprostatic ligament and/or rupture of the urogenital diaphragm can lead to damage of the arteries that lie within it. Therefore, isolated perineal trauma has been shown to cause solitary cavernous artery lesions without proximal arterial occlusive disease much more frequently than blunt pelvic trauma.[64] Relatively minor trauma can cause occlusions because the mechanism depends on endothelial damage and not necessarily on severance of the artery.[65]

In general, men who have sustained blunt pelvic trauma with resultant immediate impotence show a characteristic occlusive lesion involving the internal pudendal, common penile, cavernous, and dorsal penile arteries.[65] Conversely, men who have sustained perineal trauma with resulting delayed impotence tend to show a pattern of arterial occlusion involving the cavernous and dorsal penile arteries. However, even seemingly innocuous and minor trauma may be a risk factor for the later occurrence of "idiopathic" impotence.[64] The sometimes observed combination of arterial obstruction and venous leakage may in fact be due to ischemic changes of the tunica albuginea and hence loss of elasticity rather than the primary impact of trauma.[35,61,63] Venous leakage can be treated by surgical ligation or embolo- and sclerosing therapy delivered percutaneously into the deep dorsal penile vein. The latter method is favored because it produces obstruction of the deep dorsal vein as well as the prostatic plexus. Even the entry to crural perforators and the cranial portion of the preprostatic plexus may be occluded by this technique.

Although patients with extensive generalized atherosclerotic disease are considered ineligible for revascularization procedures, some beneficial results have been recorded from the combination of transluminal angioplasty for the proximal lesion of the common and internal iliac arteries and microvascular bypass techniques for the distal lesions.[16]

Arteriography in Pelvic Neoplasms

In the past, arteriography played an important role in the diagnosis and staging of pelvic neoplasms.[13,33,44,66–76] Today the diagnosis and staging of carcinoma of the bladder, carcinoma of the cervix, and endometrial and ovarian carcinoma are better achieved by CT, MRI, and ultrasound. Demonstration of tumor neovascularity on arteriograms has been useful for assessing local extension and for staging the primary tumor (Figs. 64-9 and 64-10).[33,69,72–76] Detail assessment of vascularity is also possible by spiral angio-CT, MRA, or MRI with gadolinium enhancement.[31,47,77] The differentiation of hypervascular benign neoplasms such as pheochromocytomas, hemangiopericytomas, hemangiomas, and arteriovenous malformations (AVMs) no longer relies on arteriography.[70,78–80]

However, arteriography remains most valuable for the assessment of hypervascular lesions for treatment, embolization, chemotherapeutic perfusion, and

Figure 64-9. Late phase film of an aortogram demonstrates tumor neovascularity and a dense stain in the left medial parametrium (*arrows*). This finding suggests extension of the carcinoma of the cervix to the medial parametrium, and hence a stage IIA lesion. (From Lang EK, Greer JL. The value of pelvic arteriography for the staging of carcinoma of the cervix. Radiology 1969;92:1027. Used with permission.)

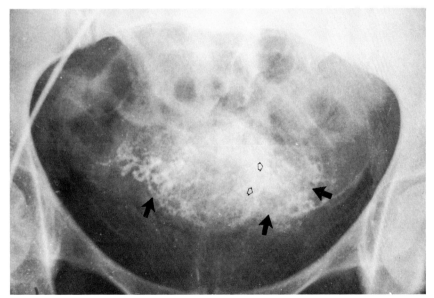

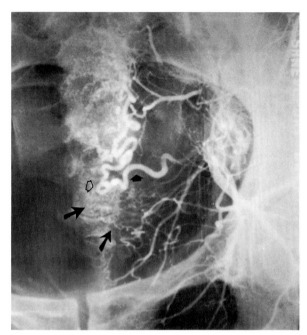

Figure 64-10. Selective arteriogram of the anterior division of the left hypogastric artery demonstrates tumor neovascularity (erratic caliber) in the normally avascular cervical segment of the uterus (*long arrows*). The parametrium (*short black arrow*) is free of tumor neovascularity. On the basis of the anteriograms, the neoplasm appears to be confined to the cervix and vaginal fornix.

skeletonization or resection.[81-88] Detail assessment of all vascular supply and drainage is particularly important when attacking pelvic AVMs.[15,89] Similarly, arteriography offers valuable information for superselective perfusion of trophoblastic neoplasms (Fig. 64-11).[38,68,90-92]

Pelvic Angiography in Obstetrics

Ultrasonography has largely replaced pelvic arteriography in the diagnosis of abnormal conditions of pregnancy. However, the latter technique is still favored for follow-up of chorioepithelioma and hydatidiform mole treated by chemotherapy.[11,33,38,66-68,82,90-92] Although titers of human gonadotropin are generally obtained for diagnosis and follow-up of treated hydatidiform mole and chorioepithelioma, arteriograms may sometimes identify residual trophoblastic elements while production of the hormone is still suppressed by chemotherapy.[11,91] The arteriographic diagnosis of hydatidiform mole is based on the demonstration of avascular spaces within the endometrial cavity. Arteriograms obtained 5 to 10 seconds after completion of contrast medium injection demonstrate filling of the intervillous spaces, which in patients with hydatidiform mole appear to be widely separated because of the large hydropic vesicles of the mole (Fig. 64-12). A discrepancy between enlarged spiral myometrial vessels and the relatively avascular uterine content is another arteriographic observation suggesting hydatidiform mole.[33,66,68,90,91] Perseverance of cavities within the uterine wall and arteriographic demonstration of persistent arteriovenous communications suggest incomplete evacuation of the mole or malignant degeneration.[66]

Chorioepithelioma and chorioadenoma destruens are characterized by an extensive pathologic vascularization of the myometrium. Hugely enlarged spiral myometrial arteries feed directly into vascular pools, which in turn communicate with prominent veins (see Fig. 64-11). The magnitude of the shunt across the arteriovenous fistulas is suggested by premature opacification of the ovarian veins.[91,92] Unlike in hydatidiform mole, the spiral arteries are enormously hypertrophied around areas of localized growth.[91] Extension into the parametrium is indicated by a massive neovascularity.

Diagnostic arteriography is often expanded to serve therapeutic purposes and to concentrate methotrexate into the tumor-bearing area.[11,84] Most recently, chemoembolization delivering an emulsate of the chemotherapeutic agent and Ethiodol superselectively into the tumor-bearing area has been advocated, with the purpose of retaining the chemotherapeutic agent for a prolonged period of time in the tumor and thus increasing its effect on the tumor (Fig. 64-13).[81,82,84]

The diagnosis of placenta previa is made by ultrasonography; however, diagnostic arteriography is useful for identifying the precise vascular supply of an anonymously located placenta (tubal pregnancy) (Fig. 64-14A).[67] Embolization of the placenta located in the fallopian tube or placental rests retained in the tube after evacuation can then be carried out by superselective techniques (see Fig. 64-14B).[10,12]

Pelvic Arteriography in Gynecology

CT, MRI, and ultrasonography have proven to be more sensitive than arteriography in the detection and categorization of gynecologic masses. Today, arteriography is reserved for identifying the bleeding sites in pelvic neoplasms and the vascular supply of pelvic neoplasms slated for selective chemotherapeutic perfusion and/or embolization. Advanced carcinoma of the cervix, in particular, benefits from arteriographic assessment because contiguous extensions of such tumors frequently tap into the circulation of adjacent organs such as the bladder, rectum, or vagina. Selective arte-

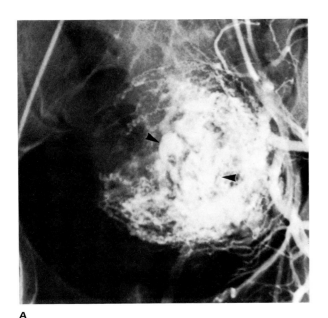

A

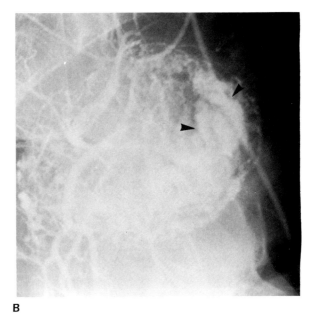

B

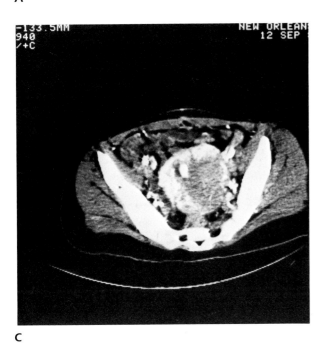

C

Figure 64-11. (A) A highly vascularized tumor (*arrowheads*) is demonstrated on an early phase selective arteriogram of the anterior division of the left hypogastric artery. (B) Cross-table lateral projection of the same arteriogram demonstrates intramural corkscrew arteries traversing the tumor (*arrowheads*). This appearance is characteristic of an intramural chorioepithelioma. (C) A dynamic computed tomogram demonstrates the densely opacified intramural elements of a choriocarcinoma destruens.

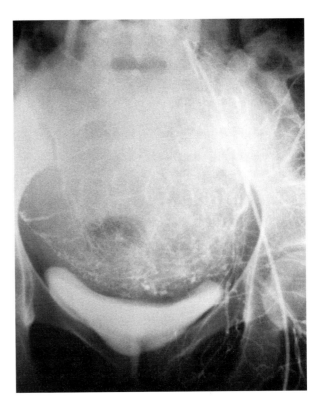

riographic studies will then demonstrate the contribution of vascular supply to the tumor from such vessels as the superior and inferior vesical artery, the internal pudendal artery, the obturator artery, branches of the inferior mesenteric artery, and sometimes branches

Figure 64-12. Selective left hypogastric arteriogram demonstrates abnormal vessels in a hugely enlarged uterine cavity separated by avascular spaces. The latter are caused by hydropic vesicles of a mole. The appearance is characteristic for a hydatidiform mole.

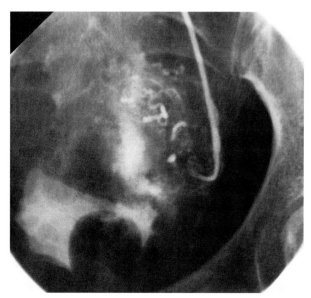

Figure 64-13. Opaque droplets in a tumor cavity indicate emulsate of doxorubicin and Ethiodol infused superselectively as chemoembolization therapy.

originating from the posterior division of the hypogastric group (Fig. 64-15).[11–13,33,42,44,76,82,84,86,87,93–96]

Detail angiographic assessment is also necessary to establish the prevalence of collateral supply and thereby to determine the degree of embolization that can be tolerated without risking necrosis of the af-

fected tissues (Fig. 64-16).[14,83,86,88,96–102] The presence and magnitude of documented collateral supply likewise influence the choice of embolic material (i.e., embolic material such as an autologous blood clot resulting in only a temporary occlusion versus material such as cyanoacrylate causing permanent occlusion).[102] Such detail studies also establish the level of collateral flow, whether through major vessels or precapillary arterioles, a fact that once again determines the choice of the embolic material and the level at which occlusion is set.

Arteriography in the Diagnosis of Pelvic Hemorrhage

Massive extraperitoneal hemorrhage is a common and not infrequently fatal complication of pelvic trauma.[8,9,34,39,40,43,48,81,103–105] In some studies, about 65 percent of patients who died as a result of pelvic fractures exsanguinated from related hemorrhage.[12,40] Postmortem injection studies have demonstrated multiple lacerations of small and medium-size arteries and veins.[41] Surgical ligation of the proximal internal iliac artery has only limited effect because of abundant collaterals.[41,98,99,106] However, the risk of incising the retroperitoneum is substantial because loss of this tissue barrier may release the tamponade, which is often the

Figure 64-14. (A) Superselective arteriogram demonstrates a highly vascularized tumor in the region of the left fallopian tube. Note the disparity in size of the vessel supplying the tumor and the normally much more prominent myometrial arteries. Elements of a retained placenta cause the vascularized tumor mass. (B) After superselective embolization,

an arteriogram of the left uterine artery no longer shows any tumor vascularity but rather a patent uterine artery and patent myometrial branches supplying the corpus of the uterus. The embolic therapy was carried out superselectively via a Tracker catheter using 6-cyanoacrylate diluted 1:1 with contrast medium.

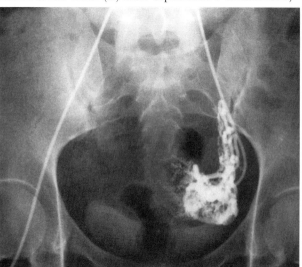

A

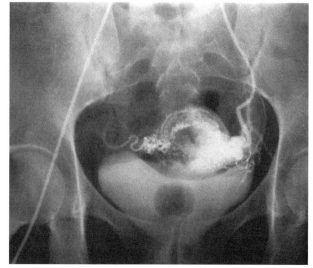

B

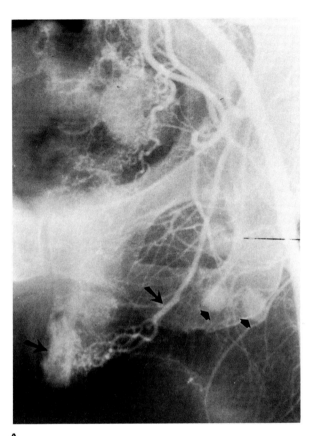

A

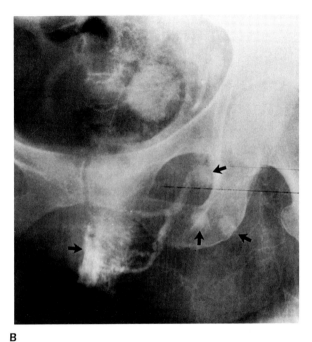

B

Figure 64-15. (A and B) Hypervascular tumor supplied from branches of the internal pudendal artery; other components of the tumor in the wall of bladder are supplied from the superior vesical artery. The delayed arteriogram demonstrates abnormal vessels and a staining tumor in the vaginal introitus and bladder wall (*long arrows*). Note the staining lymph nodes (*short arrows*).

only effective force of hemostasis for venous bleeding.[39,40,105-107]

In addition to external trauma, pelvic hemorrhage may be caused by advanced pelvic neoplasms and by iatrogenic injuries, such as those occurring during transurethral resection of the prostate, orthopedic surgery, childbirth, or even as a consequence of radiation therapy.[10,76,87,88,93,96,108-113]

Aortography and selective arteriography of pelvic vessels permit one to identify the bleeding sites and assess the magnitude of vascular injury and

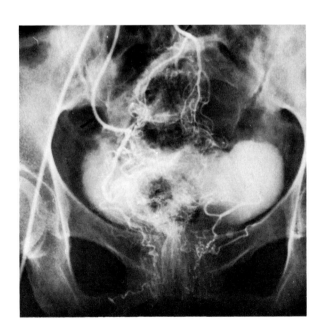

Figure 64-16. Selective injection of a main branch of the anterior division of the right hypogastric artery giving rise to the vesical arteries demonstrates opacification of the inferior mesenteric artery via collaterals from the hemorrhoidal group. This suggests obstruction of the proximal inferior mesenteric artery and dependence of the recto-sigmoid on collateral vascular supply via this pathway. (From Lang EK. Redefinition of goals and techniques of transcatheter embolization of pelvic vessels for control of intractable hemorrhage. Radiology 1981;140:331. Used with permission.)

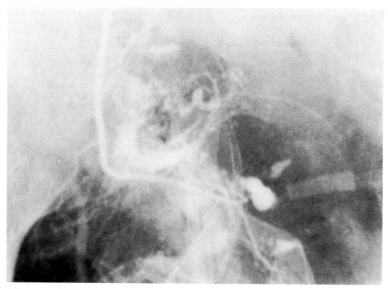

Figure 64-17. Selective injection of the right superior vesical artery demonstrates frank contrast medium extravasation, indicating severance of this vessel attendant upon pelvic trauma.

existing hematomas, and can be expanded to control hemorrhage by transcatheter embolization with autologous blood clot or a variety of inert embolic materials.[8–10,12,14,15,42,76,81,82,85–88,93–95,100,101,104,108,110,112–115]

Technique

Because of the frequent presence of large hematomas in the groin area or of orthopedic fixation devices or pneumatic compression suits, entry via the axillary artery is favored. A digital flush aortogram is recommended for the initial study. Superselective arteriograms are then obtained for detailed assessment of the vascular injury in preparation for transcatheter embolization (Figs. 64-17 and 64-18).

Intractable hemorrhage from advanced pelvic neoplasms mandates detailed study of the anterior divisions of both hypogastric arteries (Fig. 64-19). Conversely, hemorrhage attendant on hip replacement surgery calls for a study of the common iliac artery and the posterior division of the hypogastric artery because of the propensity for injury of the medial circumflex femoral artery (Figs. 64-20 and 64-21).[39]

Transcatheter Embolization for Uncontrollable Hemorrhage from Pelvic Organs

The aim of transcatheter embolization in the management of intractable bleeding from pelvic organs is to control hemorrhage and stabilize the patient without

Figure 64-18. Same patient as Figure 64-17. Following selective transcatheter embolization of the right superior vesical, internal pudendal, and several other smaller anterior division branches with Gelfoam particles, the control arteriogram confirms occlusion and cessation of extravasation of contrast medium, or active bleeding.

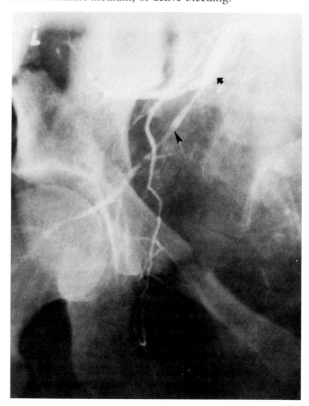

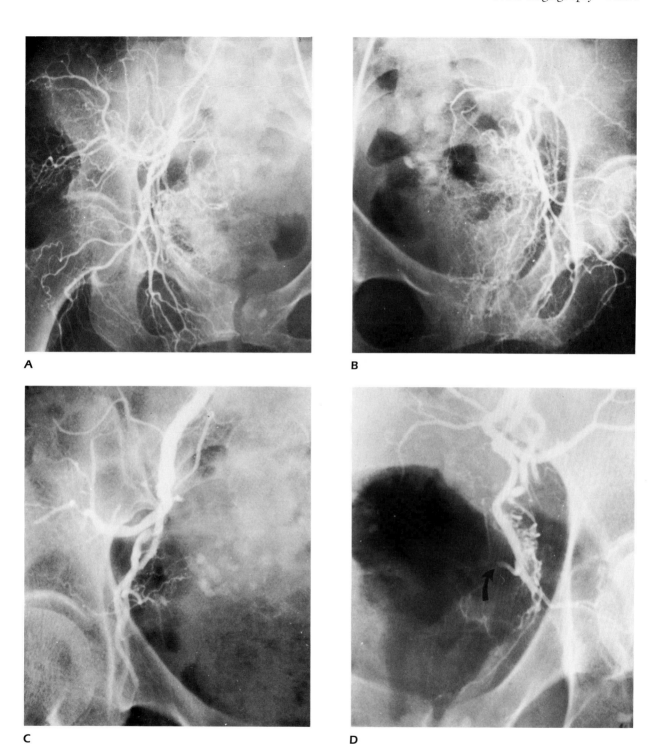

Figure 64-19. (A) Selective arteriogram of the anterior division of the right hypogastric artery demonstrates extensive tumor neovascularity involving the right half of the bladder. (From Lang EK, et al. Transcatheter embolization of hypogastric branch arteries in management of intractable bladder hemorrhage. J Urol 1979;121:30.) (B) A similar selective study on the left side demonstrates identical findings. (C) After transcatheter embolization of branches of the anterior division of the right hypogastric artery with Gelfoam particles, all tumor vessels appear to be occluded. Branches of the posterior division are patent. (D) A control arteriogram after selective embolization of most branches (*curved arrow*) of the left hypogastric artery shows only a few vessels that were left patent to minimize the risk of acute necrosis of the bladder.

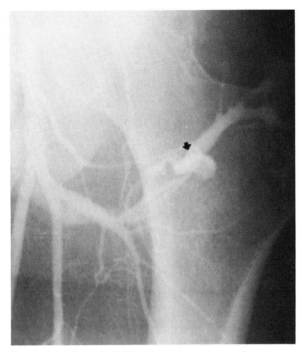

Figure 64-20. Actively bleeding traumatic pseudoaneurysm (*arrow*) of the left medial circumflex femoral artery caused by iatrogenic injury sustained during surgery on the joint capsule.

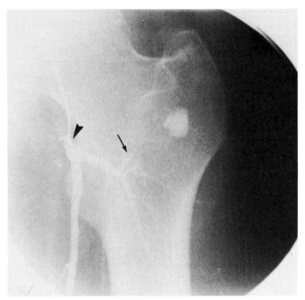

Figure 64-21. Same patient as Figure 64-20. The offensive branch of the medial circumflex femoral artery (*long arrow*) has been successfully embolized with autologous blood clot. Very origin of branch remains patent (*arrowhead*).

permanently disrupting vascular perfusion and risking irreversible tissue infarction. Disruption of blood flow therefore needs to be restricted to the smallest branch vessel so as to effectively curtail hemorrhage yet not compromise collateral perfusion. Embolization of vessels at the level of the capillary bed eliminates collateral flow via the precapillary plexus and can result in massive tissue necrosis.[83,97] To avoid this complication, transcatheter embolization is directed at vessels at the arteriolar level. The use of embolic material with the appropriate characteristics and size ensures lodging in vessels of the desired size and, if embolic material prone to dissolution is chosen, latter restoration of vascular continuity.[42]

Technique

Once the site of hemorrhage is defined, the catheter is advanced under fluoroscopic guidance, preferably using a digital road map, into the hypogastric artery and then into the offensive branch, usually of the anterior division. The size of the vessel to be embolized and the need for permanent or short-time occlusion determine the choice of material.[42,102]

Autologous blood clot has the advantage of nonantigenicity, ready availability, conformity to vessel size, and lysis within 8 to 24 hours. An admixture of Amicar

(epsilon-aminocaproic acid) extends the longevity of the clot, with lysis occurring within 72 to 96 hours. The relatively short longevity of occlusion makes this the embolic material of choice if restoration of vascular continuity is desired, such as in patients treated for intractable bleeding following orthopedic surgery, transurethral resection of the prostate, puerperal hemorrhage, or hemorrhage secondary to pelvic trauma (see Fig. 64-21).

Gelfoam and Ivalon (polyvinyl alcohol) are readily available substances suitable for semipermanent occlusion. If deployed in the form of 1-mm³ cubes, occlusion tends to occur at the level of the small arteries, ensuring collateral circulation via the precapillary plexus (see Figs. 64-18 and 64-19).[102] Gelfoam cubes have a propensity to fragment and therefore tend to embolize at a more distal site. The use of Gelfoam powder is contraindicated because this material tends to occlude the capillary bed and can cause massive tissue necrosis.

Isobutyl 6-cyanoacrylate monomer is useful if permanent occlusion is desired. Depending on the percentile mixture of contrast medium and monomer, the compound will set at different speeds. This feature can be used to set occlusion at different levels. In a mixture with contrast medium of 1:3, the compound released in a branch artery will drift to the level of the arterioles before setting. Conversely, if the mixture is diluted at a ratio of 1:1, setting will occur early and a mixture released at the same level will set at the level of major

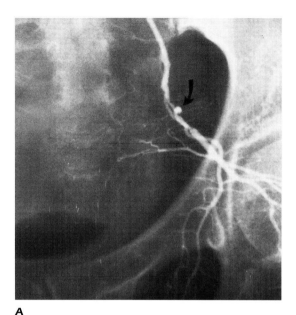

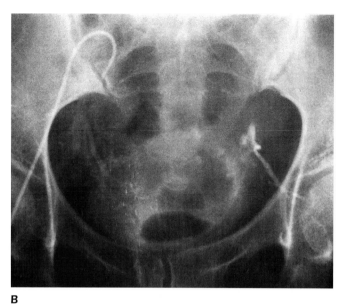

A   B

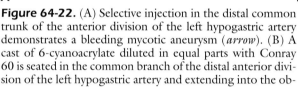

Figure 64-22. (A) Selective injection in the distal common trunk of the anterior division of the left hypogastric artery demonstrates a bleeding mycotic aneurysm (*arrow*). (B) A cast of 6-cyanoacrylate diluted in equal parts with Conray 60 is seated in the common branch of the distal anterior division of the left hypogastric artery and extending into the ob- turator and circumflex femoral arteries. The mycotic aneurysm is likewise occluded by the cast. A selective injection of the right hypogastric artery shows premature venous opacification and residual opacification of abnormal tumor vessels in the right half of the uterine fundus.

muscular arteries (Fig. 64-22). Thus branch arterial collaterals rather than those of the precapillary plexus will remain patent.

The potential danger of permanently fusing the catheter to the arterial wall mandates the use of a coaxial system. A 4 French catheter is usually advanced into the major branch; coaxially a Tracker 2 French catheter is advanced to a more distal position to release the embolisate. Through a separate channel the coaxial catheter can be flushed at all times with 5 percent glucose. The Tracker delivery catheter also must be flushed with 5 percent glucose immediately after the cyanoacrylate monomer is deployed.

For occlusion of larger vessels, coils or detachable balloons are favored. However, if a high-flow system exists distal to the site of occlusion, enforcement of the "barricade" with Gelfoam or Ivalon plugs is often necessary to establish an effective occlusion. Otherwise, massive flow through Gianturco coils has been observed attendant to the siphoning effect of a peripheral high-flow shunt.

If only temporary control of bleeding is desired to facilitate an immediate surgical intervention, a balloon catheter can be advanced to the appropriate position and large vessels can be temporarily occluded by inflating the balloon. Flushing of the peripheral bed and organs through the catheter with iced saline solution may reduce tissue damage and prolong the tolerated "ischemic time."

Embolization with autologous blood clot is the method of choice in the management of traumatic pelvic hemorrhage.[8,9] To channel the resulting fragments of blood clots selectively into medium-size arteries leading to the bleeding sites, pharmacologic manipulation of flow by intraarterial administration of epinephrine hydrochloride is advocated. This drug constricts normal arterioles but does not affect the vessels leading to a bleeding site. Thus a very selective flow pattern is created, limiting the volume of tissue embolized. The existence of collateral circulation via the precapillary plexus and particularly restoration of vascular continuity and flow shortly after lysis of the autologous clot are important factors toward prevention of tissue necrosis. The presence of hematomas compressing venous structures and possibly causing venous thrombosis is another complicating factor leading to tissue necrosis and hence emphasizes the need for moderation in intervention on the arterial side.

A specific relationship between fracture site and affected vessel often allows limited embolization of a branch artery, frequently the obturator artery (see Fig. 64-20).[39,104] If, however, the bleeding vessel cannot be identified, embolization should be limited to the anterior division of the hypogastric artery on the side of the fracture. Embolization of the posterior division of the hypogastric artery should be avoided because of intolerance of the gluteus muscle and ischial nerve to ischemia.[42] Hemorrhage occurring as a complication of orthopedic procedures can often be traced to bleeding from a specific branch artery, and embolization can be limited to the offensive branch (see Figs. 64-20 and 64-21).[42]

Hemorrhage attendant upon transurethral resection and refractory to conventional treatment can be managed by embolization of the anterior division of both hypogastric arteries, preferably, again, with autologous blood clot.[76,108,112]

Intractable puerperal hemorrhage is handled in an identical fashion, with limited embolization of branches of the anterior division of the hypogastric arteries and particularly of the uterine artery with autologous blood clot.[10,110]

Pelvic Arteriovenous Malformations

Pelvic AVMs can be divided on the basis of etiology into two large groups: (1) congenital pelvic AVMs and (2) traumatic AVMs. Traumatic AVMs in the pelvis occur as a consequence of penetrating trauma or of iatrogenic injury incurred during pelvic surgery. One or several usually large arteriovenous communications exist.

Congenital AVMs are caused by multitudinous embryonic connections between the arterial and lower resistance venous systems. The lesions are considered to be undifferentiated vascular structures resulting from arrested embryonic development at various stages. Hemangiomas form as a consequence of arrest at the primitive capillary stage of embryonic development, whereas microfistular and macrofistular AVMs are caused by arrest at the retiform stage.[89,109] The lesions may be isolated or may involve adjacent organs, specifically the uterus, bladder, or bowel (Fig. 64-23). These pelvic AVMs may be confined or may involve the buttocks and extend into the extremities or abdominal cavity (Fig. 64-24A and B). The massive shunting of blood to lower resistant veins produces massive venous and tissue engorgement. The resultant distended veins in the wall of the bladder, vagina, and rectum can cause hematuria, vaginal bleeding, or gastrointestinal hemorrhage. The turbulent blood flow through the arteriovenous channels produces bruit and thrill usually found during physical examination.

Figure 64-23. (A) Flush aortogram demonstrates a huge arteriovenous malformation involving the right bladder wall. (B) Late phase film demonstrates hugely dilated draining veins (*arrows*). (From Lang EK, et al. Transcatheter embolization of hypogastric branch artery in management of intractable bladder hemorrhage. J Urol 1979;121:30. Used with permission.)

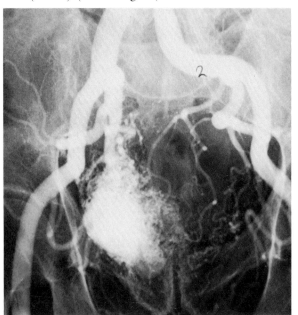

A

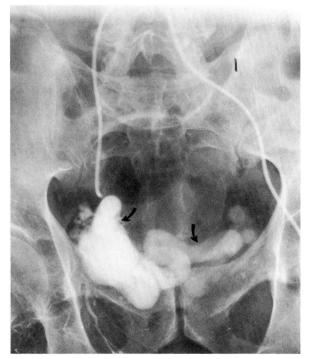

B

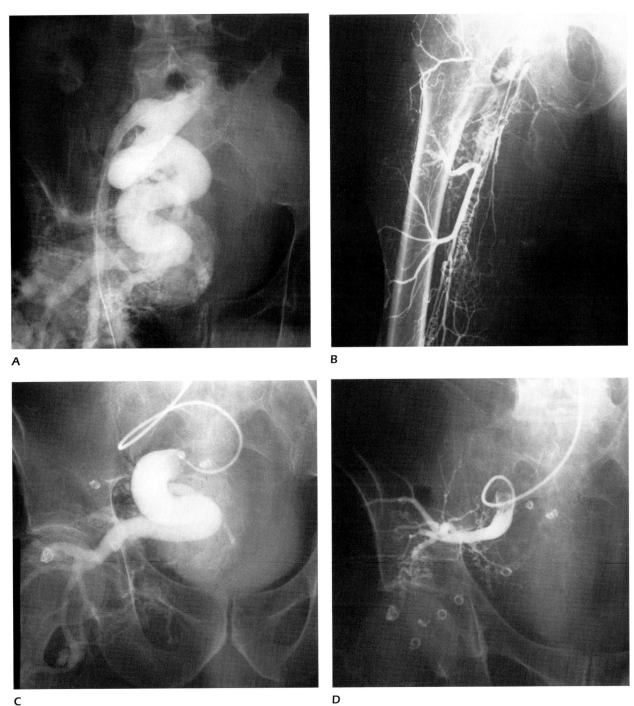

A

B

C

D

Figure 64-24. (A) Huge AVM in the right half of the true pelvis. (B) Extension of the AVM into the muscles of the right thigh. Note the dilated venous structures. (C and D) Selective percutaneous embolization of major feeders such as branches of the inferior and midgluteal artery is carried out with Gianturco coils reinforced with Gelfoam particles.

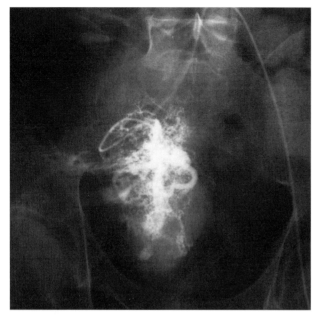

E

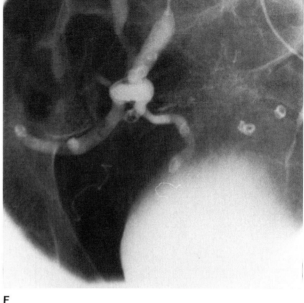

F

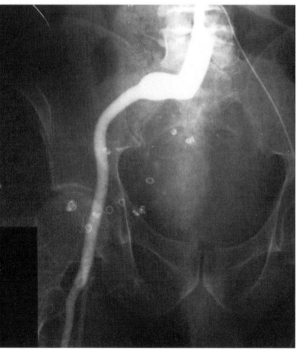

G

Figure 64-24 (continued). (E) The subsequent transcatheter embolization is directed against other components of the AVM in the presacral region. (F) At a subsequent session, selective catheterization with a coaxial system is used to occlude recanalized segments of feeder arteries with 6-cyanoacrylate (diluted at a ratio of 1:1 with Conray 60). (G) After nine selective transcatheter embolizations and seven surgical procedures resecting the venous elements of the embolized components as well as skeletonization of the arteries, complete eradication of the AVM is accomplished.

Pelvic examination, particularly in women, may reveal the presence of a soft, spongy mass.

Based on outcome of treatment as reported in the literature, these lesions are best subdivided into two groups: asymptomatic primary AVMs and symptomatic primary AVMs.

Currently recommended management protocols advocate conservative management of asymptomatic nonenlarging lesions.[89] However, the AVMs should be monitored with CT scans, MRI scans, or duplex color flow Doppler sonography.

Symptomatic or enlarging AVMs and lesions involving adjacent organs such as bladder or bowel mandate treatment. Isolated lesions not involving bladder or bowel and considered resectable are best treated by surgical excision, sometimes after preoperative embolization to reduce blood loss.[88] Lesions involving adjacent organs such as bowel and bladder or extremely diffuse lesions that are considered nonresectable are best treated by repeated transcatheter embolization (Figs. 64-25 and 64-26; see also Fig. 64-24C through E).[89,95] Repeated arterial transcatheter embolization followed by surgical skeletonization and resection of the venous structures may be the optimal method of eradicating large AVMs (see Figs. 64-24F and G). Surgical ligation of the internal iliac arteries has proven fruitless and should be avoided because it precludes subsequent transcatheter embolization of the AVM.[89]

Embolization must be directed at the level of arterioles and micro- and macrofistular communications.

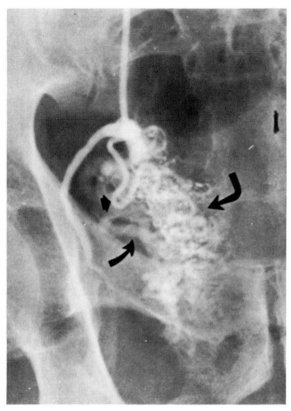

Figure 64-25. Selective arteriogram of feeder vessels originating from the anterior division of the right hypogastric artery shows a tumefactive AVM (*arrows*). (From Lang EK, et al. Transcatheter embolization of hypogastric branch artery in management of intractable bladder hemorrhage. J Urol 1979;121:30. Used with permission.)

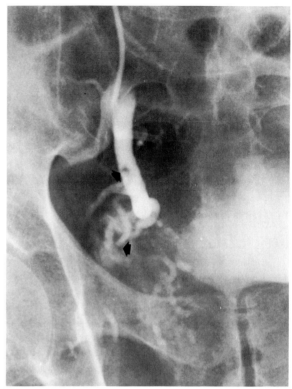

Figure 64-26. Same patient as Figure 64-25. After selective embolization of supply vessels to the AVM, there is cessation of flow into the AVM (*arrow*). However, reconstitution of flow from other branches mandated subsequent reembolization in 6 weekly intervals. (From Lang EK, et al. Transcatheter embolization of hypogastric branch artery in management of intractable bladder hemorrhage. J Urol 1979;121: 30. Used with permission.)

The 6-cyanoacrylate monomer is probably best suited to accomplish this task. However, because of the rapid flow existing through such AVMs, congealing of the compound must be set precisely so it does not wash through the AVM into the venous circulation. Technically this can be facilitated by using a coaxial system with a large balloon catheter placed into the feeding vessel and a coaxial Tracker catheter advanced further distally. After the balloon has been inflated, the flow is significantly reduced if not temporarily stopped. A mixture of 6-cyanoacrylate and contrast medium will then tend to flow slowly into the arterioles and micro- and macrofistular communications, where it sets. This causes optimal obliteration of the fistular communications (see Fig. 64-24F). It is often necessary to reposition the balloon catheter into multiple large feeding vessels and then to carry out embolization through the coaxial Tracker catheter at multiple different peripheral locations. Occlusion of a major vessel with a Gianturco metallic coil is contraindicated. These high-flow AVMs cannot be occluded by this measure. How-

ever, a combination of coils and Ivalon or Gelfoam cubes can be used to occlude such AVMs. Once again, reconstitution of flow via new collaterals will frequently occur within a period of 4 to 6 months, and repeated transcatheter embolizations may then be carried out to control the symptoms. However, surgical removal of the venous structures immediately following the transcatheter embolization of the arterial component of the AVM is the procedure of choice to eliminate recanalization of the AVM via new collaterals (see Fig. 64-24F).

A review of the literature suggests that with symptomatic AVMs recurrence may be anticipated in two-thirds of patients treated by only either surgery or transcatheter embolization.[89] A very limited experience with combined preoperative embolization and surgical excision of the venous component of the malformation suggests that the recurrence rate for this technique may be significantly lower.[89] Traumatic

AVMs, conversely, are usually manageable by transcatheter embolization.

Transcatheter Embolization for Intractable Hemorrhage from Neoplastic Disease

The clinical course of advanced pelvic neoplasms is often complicated by life-threatening hemorrhage.[113] The hemorrhage may originate from the organ giving rise to the neoplasm or from an organ involved by contiguous extension. Carcinoma of the cervix, for example, has a propensity for invading the vesicovaginal septum (Figs. 64-27 and 64-28). Massive bleeding may therefore occur from the primary site of the tumor, from vaginal metastases, and frequently from the bladder, the posterior wall of which has been permeated by neoplasm.[83,87,88,93,113] Contiguous extension of the tumor may also occur into the rectum and rectosigmoid with resulting hemorrhage. Hemorrhage is usually caused by extensive necrosis of the tumor, areas of sloughs, and bleeding from abnormal tumor vessels.

Advanced carcinoma of the bladder, carcinoma of the prostate, and bulky neoplasms of the recto-

Figure 64-27. Arteriogram demonstrating tumor neovascularity (*arrows*) in the left parametrium and involving the dome of the bladder and the right bladder wall. This establishes the diagnosis of recurrent and residual neoplasm rather than bleeding from radiation-induced fibrosis.

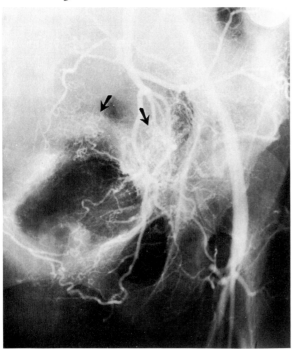

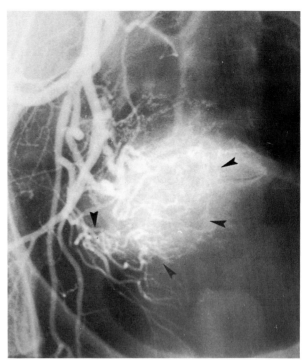

Figure 64-28. Tumor neovascularity in the parametrium (*arrowheads*), indicating the presence of a carcinoma of the cervix as a cause for bleeding. This patient had been subjected to a prior supracervical hysterectomy. (From Lang EK, et al. Arteriography, pelvic pneumography and lymphangiography augmenting assessments and staging of carcinoma of the cervix. South Med J 1970;63:1249. Used with permission.)

sigmoid may give rise to bleeding attendant upon a similar process (Fig. 64-29). Massive hemorrhage has also occurred in patients after radiation therapy for pelvic neoplasms.[111] In these patients the bleeding originates from telangiectatic vessels that have developed in pelvic organs as a consequence of the radiation (Fig. 64-30). Of course, such hemorrhage can be attributable to a combination of residual necrotic tumor elements and telangiectatic vessels.[111]

Transcatheter embolization is the procedure of choice for managing uncontrollable hemorrhage that has failed to respond to conservative treatment by "packing, silver nitrate irrigation or similar measures."[111] Depending on whether the specific bleeding site can be identified on the preliminary arteriograms, transcatheter embolization can be limited to a specific incriminated branch vessel or can involve all branches of the anterior division of both internal iliac arteries (Figs. 64-31 and 64-32). Overzealous use of embolization carries the risk of gangrene of the affected organ, which becomes deprived of its vascular supply.[83,97,102] Abundant collateral supply from the right to

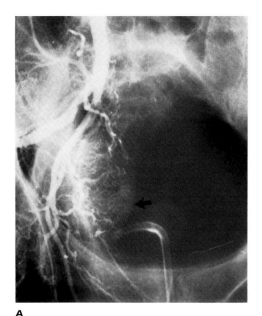
A

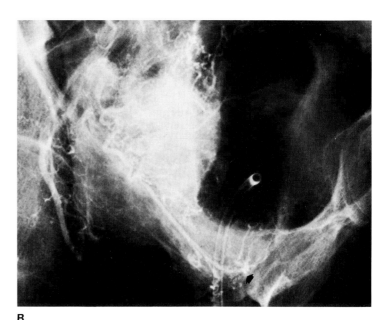
B

Figure 64-29. (A and B) Oblique projection of a selective right hypogastric arteriogram demonstrates massive tumor neovascularity involving the right lateral and posterolateral bladder wall and representing the probable source for bleeding. Note tumor extension into the base of the bladder (*arrow*).

the left internal iliac artery usually allows complete occlusion of all branches of one side without significantly compromising the vascular supply to such midline organs as the uterus or bladder.[97,98] The second important factor for maintaining collateral perfusion is the level of occlusion.[42,75,101] Occlusion at the level of the muscular branch arteries permits collateral flow via the precapillary plexus and hence maintains viability of the affected tissue. Moreover, pressure and flow will be adequately reduced to stop bleeding and allow clot

Figure 64-30. Telangiectatic vessels throughout the bladder (*arrows*) are felt to be responsible for intractable hemorrhage, a not uncommon complication of external radiation therapy of bladder neoplasms. (From Lang EK. Roentgeno graphic assessment of bladder tumors: a comparison of diagnostic accuracy of roentgenographic techniques. Cancer 1969;23:717. Used with permission.)

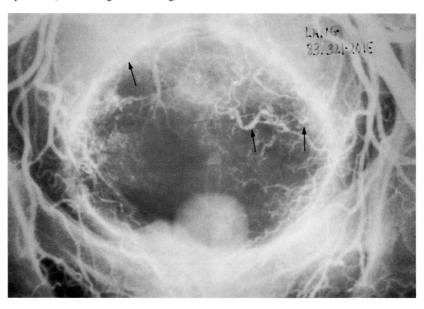

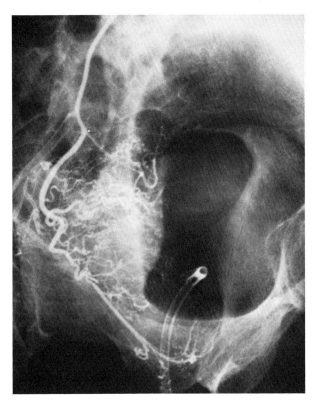

Figure 64-31. The superior vesical and internal pudendal arteries are identified as principal vascular supply to a tumor involving the right lateral bladder wall. Transcatheter embolization of these vessels should suffice to control bleeding.

formation at the bleeding site. The ultimate goal of transcatheter embolization in these patients is to control bleeding without compromising the vascular supply to a degree that risks avascular necrosis of the affected tissues (see Fig. 64-19).[42,75] Intractable hemorrhage from the bladder secondary to a massive primary neoplasm or neoplasms involving the bladder by contiguous extension is therefore best treated by transcatheter embolization of identifiable principal feeding arteries or of all branches of the anterior division of the internal iliac artery on the side harboring the predominant tumor mass but only partial embolization of some branches of the anterior division of the contralateral internal iliac artery, such as the superior vesical and internal pudendal arteries. Such conservative embolization will generally reduce the pressure and flow in the afflicted areas sufficiently to stop hemorrhage and form a clot without compromising viability.[12–14,42,75,81,87,88,93,94,96,97,100,101] In general, material prone to cause only temporary occlusion, such as Gelfoam, is favored.[75,101,102] Recanalization is known to occur after occlusion with the Gelfoam plugs in approximately 3 weeks, a feature that further reduces the risk

of late tissue necrosis. However, under certain circumstances, particularly if embolization of a specific incriminated branch vessel is desired, permanent occlusion with agents such as 6-cyanoacrylate may be the procedure of choice (see Fig. 64-22B).[81] Superselective catheterization of such incriminated vessels and deployment of 6-cyanoacrylate setting at the designated location will effectively eliminate flow through this vessel yet permit some collateral flow via the precapillary plexus as long as the occlusion has occurred at a proximal location in muscular arteries (see Fig. 64-22B). To reduce the incidence of rebleeding, some authors have advocated a more aggressive approach that involves embolizing both anterior divisions of the internal iliac arteries with a permanently occlusive agent.[101] This technique is said to be capable of achieving permanent control of bleeding in more than 70 percent of the patients (74 of 108 patients).[101]

Embolization should be carried out under fluoroscopic control with the catheter in the anterior division of the internal iliac artery or one of its branches. Fractionated and decreasing amounts of embolic material should be deployed to prevent regurgitation and inadvertent embolization of branches of the posterior division. Small test injections of contrast medium are used to evaluate the degree of completion of the embolization process. Once a to-and-fro motion of the contrast medium column is appreciated, the embolization process can be considered complete.

Intractable bleeding from the uterus, cervix, or vagina is handled in an identical fashion. If an offensive vessel can be identified, superselective embolization as outlined above with a permanent type of embolic material is advocated (see Fig. 64-22). If bleeding appears to be from a large diffuse tumor mass, embolization of both uterine arteries and in many instances complete embolization of the anterior division of one internal iliac artery and partial embolization of branches of the anterior division of the other internal iliac artery are indicated. In some instances the ovarian artery may be the major contributor to vascular supply and must be embolized to effectively control hemorrhage.[86]

In rare instances, transcatheter embolization with radioactive infarct particles may be the treatment of choice.[85] In these patients, treatment relies on the effect of radiation therapy by an interstitial implant that has been seeded via transcatheter arterial embolization. The method is particularly useful for managing bulky tumor extensions in the distal third of the vagina and/or labia that present with only moderate bleeding (Fig. 64-33). While awaiting the salutary effects of radiation therapy, the bleeding must be controllable by insertion of local packs.

Transcatheter embolization of tumors predomi-

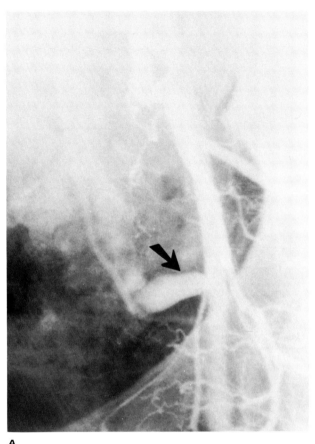

A

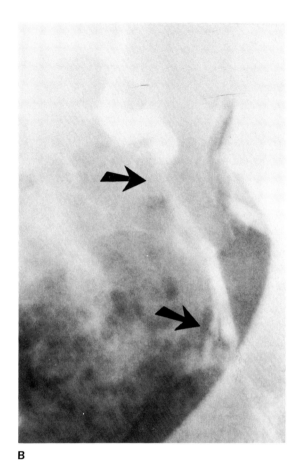

B

Figure 64-32. (A) Early phase arteriogram demonstrates contrast medium in a pseudoaneurysm (*arrow*) caused by tumor invasion of the wall of the artery. (B) Following transcatheter embolization with 2 × 2 × 2 mm Gelfoam particles, there is satisfactory occlusion of the incriminated branch of the anterior division of the left hypogastric artery (*arrows*). (From Lang EK. Redefinition of goals and techniques of transcatheter embolization of pelvic vessels for control of intractable hemorrhage. Radiology 1981;140:331. Used with permission.)

nately supplied by the inferior mesenteric artery and located in the rectum and sigmoid demands meticulous assessment of the total vascular supply. Reduction of pressure and flow to the tumor-bearing area is the desired result. However, care must be exercised to ensure viability of the tissues either via residual supply from branches of the inferior mesenteric group, left patent, or via collateral supply from the superior, middle, and inferior hemorrhoidal artery anastomoses and the internal iliac group (see Fig. 64-16).[42,75,98,116]

Transcatheter Embolization for High-Flow Priapism

In general, priapism results as a consequence of venous outflow obstruction. In rare instances, uncontrolled arterial inflow, often as a consequence of arterial trauma, may be responsible. Superselective transcathe-

ter embolization via a Tracker catheter advanced coaxially into the common penile artery with autologous blood clot has been successfully used to effect detumescence.[117]

Superselective Chemotherapy and Chemoembolization

Superselective chemotherapy has been advocated for advanced-stage pelvic neoplasms as both a definitive treatment and as a way to downstage the tumor and make possible later surgical resection.[38,118–131] In addition, selective chemotherapy using 5-fluorouracil delivered via both anterior divisions of the internal iliac arteries has been advocated to increase the sensitivity of neoplasms to radiation therapy.[124,130]

For definitive chemotherapy, the vessels supplying the bulk of the tumor are superselectively catheterized

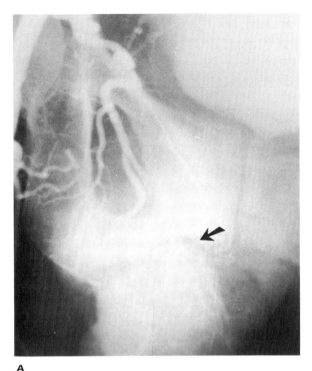

A

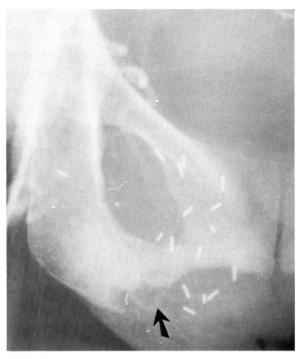

B

Figure 64-33. (A) An area of massive tumor neovascularity is supplied from the right internal pudendal and obturator arteries (*arrow*). (B) Transcatheter embolization with radon gold seeds creates an infarct implant designed to deliver a high dose to the tumor-bearing area. This resulted in marked regression in the size of the tumor and reepithelialization of denuded and excoriated areas in this octogenarian. This follow-up arteriogram obtained 3 months later shows the degree of regression of the tumor mass and reduced vascularity (*arrow*).

and receive 50 percent of the contemplated dose of the chemotherapeutic agent (Fig. 64-34). Then the catheter is withdrawn to a more proximal position in the anterior division of the internal iliac arteries, and the remainder of chemotherapeutic agent is delivered from this location to ensure distribution to tumor extensions supplied by other branches of the anterior division of the hypogastric artery. Perfusions may be carried out in daily increments for 5 to 6 days or as a single-dose infusion. In the former case, the catheter must be kept patent by perfusion with heparinized saline and its proper location must be confirmed daily before commencing infusion of the chemotherapeutic agent. Control arteriography or scintiscans after administration of some short-life radioactive microspheres are used for this purpose. Single-dose infusion therapy may, of course, be repeated after an appro-

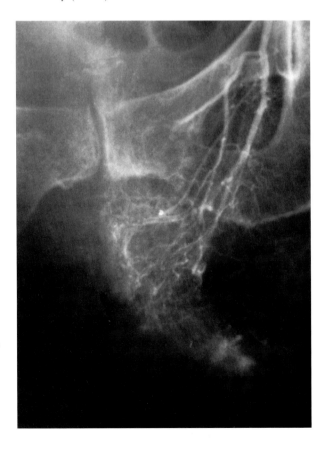

Figure 64-34. Superselective catheterization of the ▶ branches supplying a carcinoma of the vulva has been carried out to deliver 50 percent of the chemotherapeutic agent. The catheter will then be withdrawn to a location in the anterior division for delivery of the remaining 50 percent. This approach is designed to ensure coverage of tumor extensions by chemotherapy.

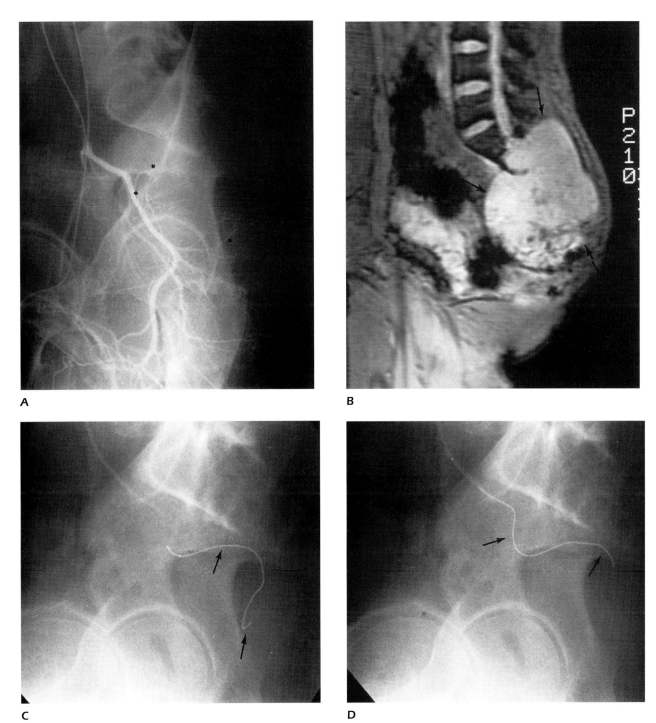

Figure 64-35. (A) Selective arteriogram of the posterior division of the right hypogastric artery demonstrates a relatively avascular chordoma extending anteriorly (*small arrows*). (B) A T1-weighted sagittal MRI scan demonstrates destruction of the sacrum as well as anterior, posterior, and superior (*arrow*) extension of this malignant chordoma. (C and D) Superselective catheterization of branches supplying the chordoma was carried out with a steerable Tracker 17 system (*arrows*) and subsequently followed by chemoembolization using a mixture of Ethiodol and doxorubicin or cisplatin or mitomycin C.

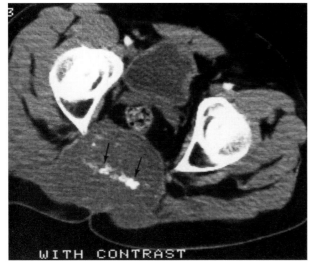

E

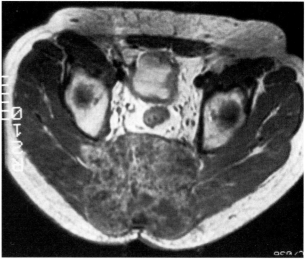

F

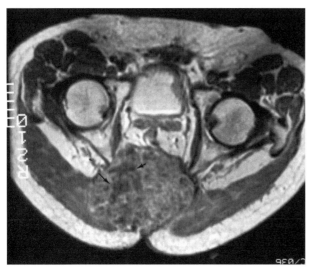

G

Figure 64-35 (continued). (E) Axial CT scan demonstrates opaque droplets (Ethiodol) in the large tumor (*arrows*). (F and G) T1-weighted axial MRI scans demonstrate areas of necrosis (*arrows*) in the tumor attendant to chemoembolization.

Figure 64-36. Transperineal injection of the prostatic venous plexus shows notable absence of filling of the right prostatic and pampiniform plexus (*arrows*). This was proven to be caused by carcinoma of the prostate extending through the capsule.

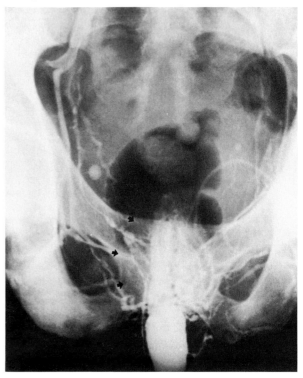

priate window of 4 to 6 weeks to reduce systemic ill effects.

Chemoembolization is another technique that extends the time of exposure of the embolized tissue to the chemotherapeutic agent.[127] An emulsion is prepared using Ethiodol and the desired chemotherapeutic agent and then delivered superselectively to the tumor-bearing area, usually using steerable Tracker catheters (Fig. 64-35A through D). The method has seen limited use with uterine neoplasms and more recently with malignant neurogenic and osseous tumors.[127] The ultimate location of the embolisate is most easily identified on computed tomograms showing the opaque Ethiodol droplets (see Fig. 64-35E). Computed tomograms and magnetic resonance images are best suited to assess the effectiveness of this therapy and to measure the regression of such tumors as malignant chordomas and other malignant neurogenic tumors (see Fig. 64-35E through G).

Pelvic Venography

Pelvic venography is useful for assessing pelvic vein thrombosis, a common source of pulmonary emboli, for determining traumatic injury of pelvic veins, and for staging pelvic neoplasms.[58,107]

Transfemoral catheterization of the external and common iliac veins followed by retrograde injection into the internal iliac veins usually gives adequate demonstration of the pelvic venous system to establish or exclude the diagnosis of pelvic vein thrombosis.

Detailed demonstration of uterine, parametrial, and internal pudendal veins is useful for staging neoplasms arising from the female organs. Transvaginal insertion of a needle into the myometrium and injection of contrast medium is the best technique for visualizing uterine parametrial veins and demonstrating direct invasion or encasement of these veins by tumor.

Cannulation of the dorsal vein of the penis or direct injection into the prostatic or pampiniform plexus offers optimal visualization of the perivesical and prostatic venous plexus and internal pudendal vein in the male.[58] Demonstration of filling defects within the veins may indicate early tumor extension and invasion through the prostatic capsule (Fig. 64-36).[132] Unfortunately, inflammatory disease can cause indistinguishable encasement and amputation of veins. Displacement of the internal pudendal vein may reflect the presence of a primary tumor mass or large metastatic nodes.

References

1. Borrello JA. MR angiography vs conventional x-ray angiography in the lower extremities: everyone wins. Radiology 1993; 187:615–617.
2. Cossman DA, Ellison JE, Wagner WH, et al. Comparison of contrast arteriography to arterial mapping with colorflow duplex imaging in the lower extremities. Vasc Surg 1989;10: 522–529.
3. Kalender WA, Seissler W, Klotz E, Vock P. Spiral volumetric CT with single breath holding technique, continuous transport and continuous scanner rotation. Radiology 1990;176: 181–183.
4. Rosen MP, Greenfield AJ, Walker TJ, Grant P, Guben JK, Dubrow J, Bettmann MA, Goldstein I. Arteriographic impotence: findings in 195 impotent men examined with selective internal pudendal angiography. Young investigators reward. Radiology 1990;174:1043–1048.
5. Rubin GD, Dake MD, Napel SA, McDonnell CH, Jeffrey RB. Three-dimensional spiral CT angiography of the abdomen: initial clinical experience. Radiology 1993;186:147–152.
6. Schiebler ML, Lisderud J, Holland J, Owen R, Baum R, Kressel HY. Magnetic resonance angiography of the pelvis and lower extremities: work in progress. Invest Radiol 1992; 27(Suppl):90–96.
7. Sivanathan UM, Rees MR, Ridgway J, Ward J, Bann K. Fast MR with turbo flash sequences in aortoiliac disease. Lancet 1992;338:1090–1091.
8. Ayella RJ, DuPriest RW Jr, Khaneja SC, Maekawa K, Sonderstrom CA, Rodriguez A, Cowley RA. Transcatheter embolization of autologous clot in the management of bleeding associated with fractures of the pelvis. Surg Gynecol Obstet 1978;147:849.
9. Barlow B, Rottenberg RW, Santulli TV. Angiographic diagnosis and treatment of bleeding by selective embolization following pelvic fracture in children. J Pediatr Surg 1975;10: 939.
10. Brown B, Heaston DK, Poulson AM, Gabert HA, Mineau DE, Miller FJ Jr. Uncontrollable postpartum bleeding: a new approach to hemostasis through angiographic arterial embolization. Obstet Gynecol 1968;54:642.
11. Cavanough D, Horadhouakul P, Comas MR. Regional chemotherapy—a comparison of pelvic perfusion and intra-arterial infusion in patients with advanced gynecologic cancer. Am J Obstet Gynecol 1975;123:435.
12. Hu G, Guo J, Huang Z, Zhou Y. Vascular embolization in cases of life-threatening bleeding in the true pelvis. Roentgenpraxis 1990;43(9):331–334.
13. Klein HM, Gunther RW. Angiography and angiotherapy in diseases of the pelvic organs. Roentgenblaetter 1990;43(8): 323–328.
14. Majewski VA, Luska G, Malasowsky B, Lelle R, Wagner HH. Results of percutaneous transluminal embolization in severe hemorrhage in the pelvis. Rofo 1987;147(6):591–598.
15. Van Poppel H, Claes H, Suy R, Wilms G, Oyen R, Baert L. Intraarterial embolization in combination with surgery in the management of congenital arteriovenous malformation. Urol Radiol 1988;10(2):89–91.
16. Goldstein I. Penile revascularization. Urol Clin North Am 1987;14:805–813.
17. Johnston KW. Iliac arteries: reanalysis of balloon angioplasty. Radiology 1993;186:207–212.
18. Kaufman SL, Barth KH, Kadir S, et al. Hemodynamic measurements in the evaluation and follow-up in transluminal angioplasty of the iliac and femoral arteries. Radiology 1982; 142:329–336.
19. Palmaz JC, Encarnacion CE, Garcia OJ, Schatz RA, et al. Aortic bifurcation stenosis: treatment with intravascular stents. J Vasc Intervent Radiol 1991;2:319–323.
20. Tegtmeyer CJ, Hartwell GD, Selby JB, Robertson R Jr, Kron IL, Tribble CG. Results and complications of angioplasty in aorto iliac disease. Circulation 1991;83(Suppl):153–160.
21. Wilson SE, Wolf GL, Cross AP. Percutaneous transluminal angioplasty vs operative intervention for peripheral arteriosclerosis. Vasc Surg 1989;9:1–9.
22. Bookstein JJ, Lurie AL. Selective penile venography: anatomical and hemodynamic observations. Urology 1988;140:55–59.
23. Rajfer J, Rosciszewski A, Mehringer M. Prevalence of corporal venous leakage in impotent man. Urology 1988;140:69–71.
24. Mathias K. Local thrombolysis for salvage of occluded bypass graft. Semin Thromb Hemostasis 1991;17(1):14–19.
25. Roth FJ, Rieser R, Scheffler A, Krings W. Intraarterial fibrinolytic therapy of chronic arterial occlusions. Semin Thromb Hemostasis 1991;17(1):39–46.
26. VanBreda A. Thrombolysis in arterial bypass grafts. Semin Thromb Hemostasis 1991;17(1):7–13.
27. Lewin JS, Laub G, Housemann R. Three dimension time of flight MR angiography: complications in the abdomen and thorax. Radiology 1991;179:261–264.
28. Siewert VB, Kaiser WA, Layer G, Traver F, Kania U, Hartlapp J. MR venography of deep leg and pelvic venous thrombosis: comparison of 2-D single image and 3-D MIP reconstruc-

tions with phlebography. Fortschr Roentgenstr Neuen Bildgeb Verfahr 1992;156(6):549–554.

29. Yucel EK, Dumoulin CL, Waltman AC. MR angiography of lower extremity: arterial disease, preliminary experience. J Magn Reson Imag 1992;2:303–309.

30. Price RR, Creasy JL, Lawrenz DH, Partain L. Magnetic resonance angiography techniques. Invest Radiol 1992;27(2):S27–S32.

31. Keller PJ, Drayer BP, Fram EK, Williams KD, Dumoulin CL, Souza SP. MR angiography with two-dimensional acquisition and three-dimensional display. Radiology 1989;173:527–532.

32. Bahren W, Gall H, Scherb W, Steif C, Thon W. Arterial anatomy and arteriographic diagnosis of arterial impotence. Cardiovasc Intervent Radiol 1988;11:195–210.

33. Borell U, Fernstrom I, Lindblom K, Westman A. The diagnostic value of arteriography of the iliac artery in gynaecology and obstetrics. Acta Radiol 1952;38:247.

34. Lang EK. The role of arteriography in trauma. Radiol Clin North Am 1976;14:353.

35. Lue TF, Tanagho EA. Physiology of erection and pharmacological management of impotence. J Urol 1987;137:829.

36. Schwartz AN, Friedenberg D, Harley JD. Nonselective angiography after intracorporal papaverine injection: alternative technique for evaluating penile arterial integrity. Radiology 1988;167:249–253.

37. Wilkins RA, Garvey CJ, Lewis JD. Peripheral vascular disease: prospective study of intraarterial digital subtraction angiography using a 9 inch intensifier. Radiology 1986;159:423.

38. Liukko P, Gronroos M, Satokari K, Pitkancy T. Pelvic angiography in the follow-up of chorioadenoma destruens. Ann Chir Gynecol 1978;67:147.

39. Roeren T, Hauenstein K, Dinkel E, et al. Intra-arterial digital subtraction angiography of renal transplants. Urol Radiol 1986;8:77.

40. Rothenberger DA, Fischer RP, Perry JF Jr. Major vascular injuries secondary to pelvic fractures: an unsolved clinical problem. Am J Surg 1978;136:660.

41. Flint LM Jr, Brown A, Richardson JD, Polk HC. Definitive control of bleeding from severe pelvic fractures. Ann Surg 1979;189:709.

42. Lang EK. Redefinition of goals and techniques of transcatheter embolization of pelvic vessels for control of intractable hemorrhage. Radiology 1981;140:331.

43. Margolies MN, Ring EJ, Waltman AC, Kerr WS Jr, Baum S. Arteriography in the management of hemorrhage from pelvic fractures. N Engl J Med 1972;287:317–321.

44. Lang EK. Angiography in the diagnosis and staging of pelvic neoplasms. Radiology 1980;134:353.

45. Udoff EJ, Barth KH, Harrington DP, Kaufman SL, White RI. Hemodynamic significance of iliac artery stenosis: pressure measurements during arteriography. Radiology 1979;132:289.

46. Smith TP, Cragg AH, Berbaum KS, Nakagawa N. Comparison of the efficacy of digital subtraction and film screen arteriography of the lower limb: prospective study in 50 patients. Am J Roentgenol 1992;152(2):431–436.

47. Kashdan BS, Trost DW, Jagust MB, Rackson ME, Sos TA. Retrograde approach for contralateral iliac and infrainguinal angioplasty: experience in 100 patients J Vasc Intervent Radiol 1992;3:515–521.

48. Raillat C, Rousseau H, Joffre F, et al. Treatment of iliac artery stenosis with the Wallstent endo prosthesis. AJR 1990;154:613.

49. Hess H, Mietschk A, Ingrisch H. Low dose thrombolysis for restitution of flow after arterial occlusion. Dtsch Med Wochenschr 1980;105:787–791.

50. Martin M, Fiebach O. Short term ultrahigh streptokinase treatment of chronic arterial occlusions in acute deep vein thromboses. Semin Thromb Hemostasis 1991;17(1):21–38.

51. Belkin M, Donaldson MC, Whittemore AD, Polak JF, Grassi CJ, Harrington DP, Mannick JA. Observations on the use of thrombolytic agents for thrombotic occlusion of infrainguinal vein grafts. J Vasc Surg 1990;11:289–296.

52. Bilbao JI, Aquerreta JD, Longo JM. Open ended guidewire as superselective catheter for intraarterial chemotherapy: experience in 190 procedures. Cardiovasc Intervent Radiol 1990;13:375.

53. Davis SS, et al. Evaluation of impotence in older men. West J Med 1985;142:499.

54. Ginestie J, Romieu A. Traitement des impuissance d'orgine vasculaire: la revascularisation des corp caverneau (English abstract). J Urol Nephrol (Paris) 1976;82:853.

55. Wagner G. Physiological, psychological and surgical diagnosis and treatment. In: Erection: physiology and endocrinology in impotence. Wagner G, Green R, eds. New York: Plenum, 1981:25–36.

56. King BF. Doppler sonography of erectile dysfunction. Lippincott's review. Radiology 1992;1(4):645.

57. Lue TF, Hricak H, Schmidt RA, Tanagho EA. Functional evaluations of penile veins by cavernosography in papaverine-induced erection. J Urol 1986;135:479.

58. Fitzpatrick TJ. Venography of the deep dorsal venous and valvular systems. J Urol 1974;111:518.

59. Buvat J, Buvat-Herbaut M, Dehaene JL, Lemaire A. Is intracavernous injection of papaverine a reliable screening test for vascular impotence? J Urology 1986;135:476–478.

60. Lewis RW. Cavernosography and cavernosometry. Lippincott's review. Radiology 1992;1(4):610.

61. Lurie AL, Bookstein JJ, Kessler WO. Angiography of post traumatic impotence. Cardiovasc Intervent Radiol 1988;11:232.

62. Virag R, Frydman D, Legman M, Virag H. Intracavernous injection of papaverin as a diagnostic and therapeutic method in erectile failure. Angiology 1984;35:79.

63. Lurie AL, Bookstein JJ, Kessler WO. Post traumatic impotence: angiographic evaluation. Radiology 1988;166(1):115–119.

64. Levine FJ, Greenfield AJ, Goldstein I. Arteriographically determined occlusive disease within the hypogastric-cavernous bed in impotent patients following blunt perineal and pelvic trauma. Urology 1990;144:1147–1153.

65. Sharlip ID. Penile arteriography and impotence after pelvic trauma. Urology 1981;126:477–481.

66. Borell U, Fernstrom I. Hydatidiform mole diagnosed by pelvic angiography. Acta Radiol 1961;56:113.

67. Borell U, Fernstrom I, Ohlson L. Diagnostic value of arteriography in cases of placenta previa. Am J Obstet Gynecol 1963;86:535.

68. Borell U, Fernstrom I, Westman A. The value of pelvic arteriography in the diagnosis of mole and chorionepithelioma. Acta Radiol 1955;44:378.

69. Braedel HU, Krauntzun K. Die Gefassdarstellung bosartiger Harnsblasengeschwulste unter besonderer Berucksichtigung ihrer ortlichen Ausbreitung. ROEFO 1964;100:209.

70. Christenson RR, Smith CW, Beuko H. Arteriographic manifestations of pheochromocytoma. AJR 1976;126:567.

71. Deklerk DP, Catalona WJ, Nime FA, Freeman C. Malignant pheochromocytoma of the bladder: late development of renal cell carcinoma. J Urol 1975;113:864.

72. Lang EK. Roentgenographic assessment of bladder tumors: a comparison of diagnostic accuracy of roentgenographic techniques. Cancer 1969;23:717.

73. Lang EK, Greer JL. The value of pelvic arteriography for the staging of carcinoma of the cervix. Radiology 1969;92:1027.

74. Lang EK. Intra-abdominal and retroperitoneal organ injuries diagnosed on dynamic computed tomograms obtained for assessment of renal trauma. J Trauma 1990;30(9):161.

75. Lang EK. Management of hemorrhaging pelvic neoplasms by transcatheter embolization. J Intervent Radiol 1989;4:113.

76. Pereiras RV Jr, Meier WL, Katz ER, Viamonte M Jr. Arteriographic embolization treatment for postprostatectomy hemorrhage. Urology 1977;9:705–709.

77. TNM classification of malignant tumors. 3rd ed. Geneva: Union Internationale Contre Cancer, 1978.

78. Hietala SO, Hazra T. Angiography in vesical and perivesical neoplastic and non-neoplastic lesions. Acta Radiol 1978;19:447.

79. Hietala SO, Texter JH Jr, Crane DB. Angiography in pheochromocytoma of the urinary bladder: report of a case. Acta Radiol 1977;18:313.

80. Klein TW, Kaplan TW. Klippel-Trenaunay syndrome associated with urinary tract hemangiomas. J Urol 1975;114:596.

81. Freeny PC, Bush WH Jr, Kidd R: Transcatheter occlusive therapy of genitourinary abnormalities using isobutyl 2-cyanoacrylate (bucrylate). AJR 1979;133:647–656.

82. Harima Y, Shiraishi T, Harima K, Tanaka Y. Long term results of transcatheter arterial embolization therapy in cases of recurrent and advanced pelvic cancer. Nippon Igaku Hoshasen Gakkai Zasshi 1991;51(3):935–941.

83. Hietala SO. Urinary bladder necrosis following selective embolization of the internal iliac artery. Acta Radiol 1978;19:316.

84. Lang EK. Therapeutic angiography in oncologic practice. In: Moossa AR, Robson MC, Schimpff SC, eds. Oncology. Baltimore: Williams & Wilkins, 1986:302.

85. Lang EK, Sullivan J. Management of primary and metastatic renal cell carcinoma by transcatheter embolization with iodine 125. Cancer 1988;62(2):279.

86. Marx MB, Picus D, Weyman PJ. Percutaneous embolization of the ovarian artery in the treatment of pelvic hemorrhage. AJR 1988;150:1337–1338.

87. Miller FJ Jr, Mortel R, Mann WJ, Jahshan AE. Selective arterial embolization for control of hemorrhage in pelvic malignancy: femoral and brachial catheter approach. AJR 1976;126:1028.

88. Schurhke TD, Barr JW. Intractable bladder hemorrhage: therapeutic angiographic embolization of the hypogastric arteries. J Urol 1976;116:523.

89. Calligaro KD, Sedlacek TB, Savarese RP, Carneval P, Delaurentis DA. Congenital pelvic arteriovenous malformations: long term follow-up in two cases and a review of the literature. J Vasc Surg 1992;16(1):100–108.

90. Cockshott WP, Evans KT, Hendrickse JP deV. Arteriography of trophoblastic tumors. Clin Radiol 1964;15:1.

91. Hendrickse JP deV, Cockshott WP, Evans KTE, Barton CJ. Pelvic arteriography in the diagnosis of malignant trophoblastic disease. N Engl J Med 1964;271:859.

92. Kolstad P, Liverud K. Pelvic arteriography in malignant trophoblastic neoplasia. Am J Obstet Gynecol 1969;105:175.

93. Goldstein HM, Meddin H, Ben-Menachem Y, Wallace S. Transcatheter arterial embolization in the management of bleeding in the cancer patient. Radiology 1975;115:603.

94. Grace DM, Pitt DF, Gold RE. Vascular embolization and occlusion by angiographic techniques as an aid or alternative to operation. Surg Gynecol Obstet 1976;143:469.

95. Lang EK, Deutsch JS, Goodman JR, Barnett TS, LaNasa J, Duplessis GH. Transcatheter embolization of hypogastric branch artery in management of intractable bladder hemorrhage. J Urol 179;121:30.

96. Smith DC, Wyatt JF. Embolization of hypogastric arteries in the control of massive vaginal hemorrhage. Obstet Gynecol 1977;49:317.

97. Braf ZF, Koontz WW Jr. Gangrene of bladder: complication of hypogastric artery embolization. Urology 1977;9:670.

98. Burchell RC. Physiology of internal iliac artery ligation. J Obstet Gynaecol Br Commonw 1968;75:642.

99. Fahmy K. Internal iliac artery ligation and its efficiency in controlling pelvic hemorrhage. Int Surg 1969;51:244.

100. Hald T, Mygind T. Control of life-threatening vesical hemorrhage by unilateral hypogastric artery muscle embolization. J Urol 1974;112:60.

101. Pisco J, Martins JM, Correia MG. Internal iliac artery embolization to control hemorrhage from pelvic neoplasms. Radiology 1989;172:337–339.

102. White RI Jr, Strandberg JV, Gross GS, Barth KH. Therapeutic embolization with long term occluding agents and their effects on embolized tissues. Radiology 1977;125:677.

103. Braunstein PW, Skudder PA, McCarroll JR, Musolino A, Wade PA. Concealed hemorrhage due to pelvic fracture. J Trauma 1964;4:832.

104. Ring EJ, Athanasoulis C, Waltman AC, Margolies MN, Baum S. Arteriographic management of hemorrhage following pelvic fracture. Radiology 1973;109:65.

105. Rothenberger DA, Fischer RP, Strate RG, Velasco R, Perry JF Jr. The mortality associated with pelvic fractures. Surgery 1978;84:356.

106. Ravitch MM. Hypogastric artery ligation in acute pelvic trauma. Surgery 1964;56:601.

107. Reynolds BM, Balano NA. Venography in pelvic fractures: a clinical evaluation. Ann Surg 1971;173:104.

108. Faysal M. Angiographic management of post-prostatectomy bleeding. J Urol 1979;122(1):129–131.

109. Fuleihan FM, Cordonier JJ. Hemangioma of the bladder: report of a case and review of the literature. J Urol 1969;102:581.

110. Heaston DK, Mineau DE, Brown BJ, Miller FJ Jr. Transcatheter arterial embolization for control of persistent massive puerperal hemorrhage after bilateral surgical hypogastric artery ligation. AJR 1979;133:152.

111. Kumar APM, Wrenn EL, Yayalakshmramma B, Quinn P, Cox C. Silver nitrate irrigation to control bladder hemorrhage in children receiving cancer therapy. J Urol 1976;116:85.

112. Mitchell ME, Waltman AC, Athanasoulis CA, et al. Control of massive prostatic bleeding with angiographic techniques. J Urol 1976;115:692.

113. Smith JC Jr, Kerr WS, Athanasoulis CA, Waltman AC, Ring EJ, Baum S. Angiographic management of bleeding secondary to genitourinary tract surgery. J Urol 1975;113:89.

114. Greenfield AJ, Athanasoulis CA, Waltman GAC, LeMoure ER. Transcatheter embolization: prevention of embolic reflux using balloon catheters. AJR 1978;131:651.

115. Schroder J, Terwey B, Buhr HJJ, Gerhardt P. Die Behandlung traumatischer Becken-blutungen durch Embolisation. Chirurg 1978;49:286.

116. Tajes RV. Ligation of the hypogastric arteries and its complications in resection of cancer of the rectum. Am J Gastroenterol 1956;26:612.

117. Walker TJ, Grant PW, Goldstein I, Crane R, Greenfield AJ. Highflow priapism: treatment with superselective transcatheter embolization. Radiology 1990;174:1053–1054.

118. Goldman JL, Bilbao MK, Rösch J, Dotter CT. Complications of indwelling chemotherapy catheters. Cancer 1975;36;1983.

119. Patt YZ, Peters RE, Chuang VP, Wallace S, Claghorn L, Mavligit G. Palliation of pelvic recurrence of colorectal cancer with intraarterial 5 fluorouracil and mitomycin. Cancer 1985;56:2175–2180.

120. Reichelt G, Gellhaar G, Eichenberg HU. Complicated situations with implantable catheter system for regional arterial infusion therapy of tumors in the pelvis (bladder carcinoma): radiologic and nuclear medicine assessment. Urologe A 1986;25(6):333–337.

121. Uyama T, Uxama T. Doxorubicin intraarterial chemotherapy combined with low dose radiation in bladder cancer. Gan To Kagaku Ryoho 1987;414(7):2293–2299.

122. Wallace S, Chuang VP, Samuels M, Johnson D. Hines catheter intraarterial infusion of chemotherapy in advanced bladder cancer. Cancer 1982;49:640.

123. Curry TS III. Real time ultrasound in the diagnosis of acute dissecting aneurysm of the abdominal aorta. AJR 1979;132:115.

124. Carlsson G, Hafstron L, Johnsson PE, Aask A, Kullum B, Lunderquist A. Unresectable and locally recurrent rectal cancer treated with radiotherapy or bilateral internal iliac artery infusion of 5 Fluorouracil. Cancer 1986;58:336–340.

125. Chatelain C. Adjuvant cytotoxic chemotherapy in association with radical surgery or radical radiation treatment

in presumably localized prostatic cancer. Acta Oncol 1991; 30:259.

126. Fiorentini G, Tienghi A, Emiliani E, Graziani G, Priori T, Turci D, Rosti G, Cruciani G, Marngolo M. Management of pelvic osteosarcoma: the sequence of neoadjuvant chemotherapy containing intraarterial cisplatin, local treatment and adjuvant chemotherapy. Reg Cancer Treat 1990;3:175–180.

127. Fiorentini G, Dazzi C, Tienghi A. Chemofiltration and chemoembolization: new techniques in advanced pelvic bone malignancies. Annals Oncol 1992;3(S2):S37–S38.

128. Jacobs SC, McLellan SL, Maher C, Lawson RK. Precystectomy intraarterial cis-diamminedichloroplatinum II with local bladder hyperthermia for bladder cancer. J Urol 1984;131: 473.

129. Jakse G, Frommhold H, Marberger H. Combined cisplatinum and radiation therapy in patients with stages PT3 and PT4 bladder cancer. Pilot study. J Urol 1983;129:502.

130. Muller H, Aigner KR. Palliation of recurrent rectal cancer with intraarterial mitomycin C and 5 fluorouracil via the jet port aortic bifurcation catheter. Reg Cancer Treat 1990;3: 147–151.

131. Nakamura K, Takashima S, Nakatsuka H, Onoyama W. Prostate cancer: arterial infusion chemotherapy and alteration of intrapelvic flow. Radiology 1992;185:885.

132. Stewart BJ, Eapen L, Hirte E, Futter NG, et al. Intraarterial cisplatinum for bladder cancer. J Urol 1987;138:302–305.

65

Retroperitoneal Arteriography in Adults

DAVID C. LEVIN

Retroperitoneal arteriography is sometimes performed to evaluate suspected retroperitoneal masses—principally malignant or benign tumors, abscesses and other inflammatory lesions, or hematomas. Retroperitoneal masses are rare. Armstrong and Cohn[1] reviewed 25,647 tumors recorded in the New Orleans Tumor Registry between 1948 and 1962. Only 41 of these tumors (0.16 percent) arose mainly in the retroperitoneal space. In this discussion and all referenced papers, masses arising in specific organs such as the kidneys, adrenals, duodenum, and pancreas are excluded. The term *retroperitoneal mass* is taken to include only those lesions arising in the amorphous retroperitoneal space in which these organs are contained.

Although retroperitoneal tumors are rare, they provide a distinct challenge from both diagnostic and therapeutic points of view. Because they do not arise in specific organs, symptoms do not occur until relatively late in their course, and the masses are usually rather large at the time of detection. The presenting clinical symptoms and signs can include weight loss, abdominal enlargement or fullness, a palpable mass, nausea, and back pain.

The retroperitoneal space contains a number of different types of tissues: fibrous tissue, muscle, areolar connective tissue, fat, lymph nodes, lymphatics, fascia, sympathetic nervous structures, blood vessels, mesothelial tissues, and remnants of the embryologic urogenital ridge. A wide histologic variety of primary retroperitoneal tumors therefore occur. These can be classified into five major types.

1. *Mesenchymal tumors.* Liposarcomas, leiomyosarcomas, fibrosarcomas, rhabdomyosarcomas, and spindle cell sarcomas are the most common. Undifferentiated sarcomas and carcinomas, chondrosarcomas, hemangiopericytomas, malignant fibrous histiocytomas, and mesotheliomas occur less commonly. The only benign mesenchymal tumor that appears with any frequency is lipoma.

2. *Lymphomas.* Between 5 and 10 percent of all lymphomas arise primarily within the abdomen, and approximately half of these occur in the retroperitoneal space.[2,3] This category does not include the more common cases of lymphoma (which are first detected elsewhere in the body and which occur secondarily in the retroperitoneal space) because these cases are generally not studied arteriographically.

3. *Metastatic tumors.*

4. *Neural tumors.* These can be benign or malignant and include neurofibroma, neurilemoma, extraadrenal neuroblastoma, and ganglioneuroma.

5. *Tumors of the urogenital ridge remnant.* On rare occasions, a tumor having the histologic appearance of a gonadal tumor develops in the retroperitoneal space when the gonads are normal. Such tumors are thought to arise in the embryonic urogenital ridge remnant.

The most prevalent benign, nonneoplastic causes of retroperitoneal masses are hematomas and inflammatory lesions such as abscesses. Cysts and retroperitoneal fibrosis also occur on rare occasions. Retroperitoneal hematomas may be signaled clinically by the sudden onset of back or flank pain, shock, and a falling hematocrit. They may result from trauma, be caused by rupture of a small metastatic tumor of the adrenal gland or other small retroperitoneal tumor, or occur entirely spontaneously. Retroperitoneal abscesses and other inflammatory masses often present clinically similar to retroperitoneal tumors, except that inflammatory masses are more likely to be accompanied by fever. In some cases of retroperitoneal inflammatory disease, symptoms may be largely or completely absent.

Approximately 80 to 85 percent of retroperitoneal masses are malignant.[1] Their prognosis is generally poor, in part because the lesions are usually rather far advanced before the patient seeks medical attention. Radical surgery is the treatment of choice, except in

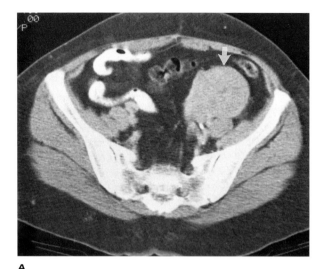

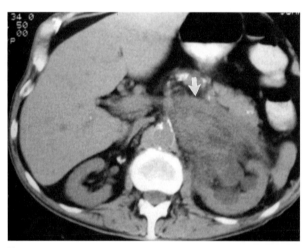

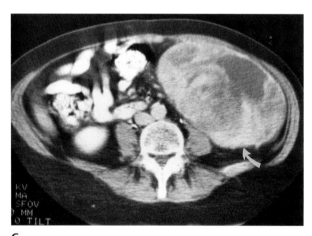

Figure 65-1. Three examples of retroperitoneal tumors demonstrated by CT scans. (A) Leiomyosarcoma of the left retroperitoneal space. (B) Spindle cell sarcoma of the left retroperitoneal space. (C) Liposarcoma of the left retroperitoneal space.

cases of lymphoma, which are best treated by radiation.

The emergence within the past 2 decades of noninvasive imaging modalities like computed tomography (CT), ultrasound, and more recently magnetic resonance imaging (MRI) has greatly altered the diagnostic approach to retroperitoneal lesions. Before the advent of CT and ultrasound, the retroperitoneal space was an exceedingly difficult area to visualize, and arteriography was frequently performed as a relatively early screening procedure in cases in which retroperitoneal lesions were suspected. At the present time, CT, ultrasound, and MRI can provide excellent visualization of retroperitoneal lesions, so that arteriography need no longer be used for screening purposes (Fig. 65-1). However, once CT or ultrasound has suggested the presence of a retroperitoneal mass, arteriography can still provide important information to help in surgical management. This is discussed in greater detail later in the chapter.

Angiographic Findings in Retroperitoneal Tumors

The arteriographic findings in retroperitoneal tumors have been described in considerable detail by the author and others.[4-10] Although often striking, they are nonspecific. These findings can generally be characterized in terms of degree of vascularity and displacement of arteries and/or the kidneys.

Displacement of arteries and/or the kidneys is seen in virtually all but very small retroperitoneal masses. This is not surprising because the abdominal aorta is a retroperitoneal structure and all its major branches pass through the retroperitoneal space for at least part of their course. The kidneys are the largest and most easily visible retroperitoneal organs angiographically, and their displacement also may be one of the first signs, and sometimes the only sign, of a retroperitoneal mass.

The vascularity exhibited by retroperitoneal tumors can be conveniently classified into three major types.

Type I tumors contain vessels that are large, coarse, highly irregular, and ragged and that fail to show progressive decrease in caliber as do normal vessels. Sinusoidal pooling of contrast and tumor staining may occur during the capillary phase. In the vast majority of cases exhibiting this type of vascularity, the lesion will prove to be a malignant tumor.[9] However, in rare instances benign neural tumors such as neurofibroma or neurilemoma will produce this same coarse hypervascularity.[4,6] Figure 65-2 shows a fibrosarcoma in a young woman. Extensive neovascularity is present

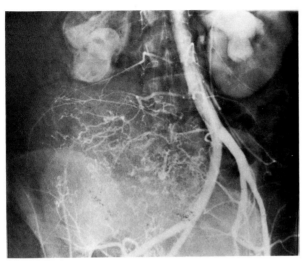

Figure 65-2. Right retroperitoneal fibrosarcoma. The tumor contains extensive coarse and irregular neovascularity, arising from several right lumbar arteries and both hypogastric arteries. (From Levin DC, Watson RC, Baltaxe HA. Arteriography of retroperitoneal masses. Radiology 1973;108: 543. Used with permission.)

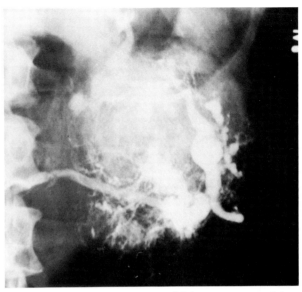

Figure 65-3. Left retroperitoneal leiomyosarcoma. Selective arteriography of a left lumbar artery demonstrates extensive and highly irregular neovascularity with multiple large vascular sinusoids, particularly along the lower and lateral aspects of the tumor. (Courtesy of Iraj Hooshmand, M.D.)

with supply from multiple lumbar arteries and the iliac arteries on both sides. Figure 65-3 shows a leiomyosarcoma in the left retroperitoneal space. Very large, irregular arteries and vascular sinusoids are present within the tumor. In the author's experience, among all retroperitoneal neoplasms, leiomyosarcomas and spindle cell sarcomas seem to contain the greatest degree of coarse neovascularity.

Type II tumors also display hypervascularity, but the vessels are of a finer, more reticular character and tend to be distributed in a more homogeneous manner. Diffuse staining is generally seen during the capillary phase, but contrast pooling or vascular sinusoids are usually not seen. As with type I lesions, most type II lesions prove to be malignant tumors. However, on rare occasions benign neural tumors and lipomas may demonstrate this vascular pattern.[8] Figure 65-4 shows a non-Hodgkins lymphoma arising primarily in the retroperitoneal space. Fine neovascularity and staining in the area of the tumor can be seen on selective left testicular and lumbar arteriograms. Figure 65-5 shows a leiomyosarcoma of the pelvic retroperitoneal space. The tumor was supplied by multiple arteries. Lymphomas are the most common lesions to exhibit type II hypervascularity.

Type III includes all retroperitoneal tumors that are hypovascular or avascular. Although absence of neovascularity is often considered a sign of a benign lesion, in the retroperitoneal space most hypovascular or avascular masses nevertheless prove to be malignant tumors. In the author's experience, slightly fewer than

half of all malignant retroperitoneal tumors are hypovascular or totally avascular. Figure 65-6 shows a large liposarcoma that is entirely avascular. Benign retroperitoneal tumors, such as neurofibroma and lipoma, can also have an avascular pattern.

It is apparent from the foregoing discussion that malignant retroperitoneal tumors can be characterized by a broad spectrum of vascularity, ranging from extremely hypervascular to totally avascular. In many instances, lesions of the same histologic type may exhibit widely varying degrees of vascularity in different patients. Any attempt at making a histologic diagnosis based on the vascular pattern of the tumor should therefore be avoided.

Angiographic Findings in Retroperitoneal Hematomas

Retroperitoneal hemorrhage may result from trauma or rupture of tumors (especially metastatic tumors of the adrenal gland) or may occur spontaneously. Angiography often fails to reveal the exact source of bleeding but demonstrates a mass effect with displacement and stretching of major vessels and/or the kidneys. As would be expected, the hematomas are entirely avascular.

Figure 65-7 shows a left retroperitoneal hematoma that was found at surgery to arise from rupture of a

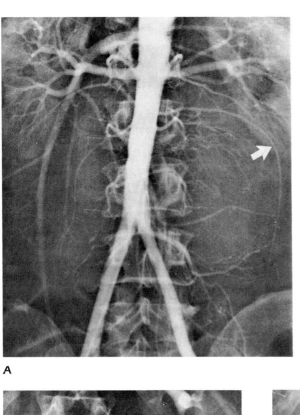

A

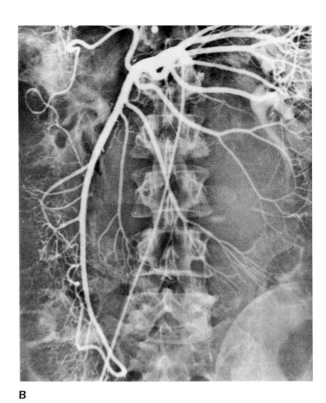

B

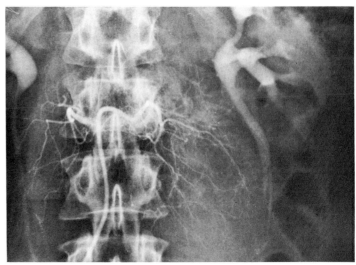

C   D

Figure 65-4. Retroperitoneal lymphosarcoma. (A) Initial abdominal aortogram demonstrates displacement of the superior mesenteric artery to the right and displacement of the left testicular artery (*arrow*) around a mass containing fine neovascularity. (B) Superior mesenteric arteriography shows that the artery is draped around the border of the retroperitoneal tumor but does not contribute any neovascularity to it. (C) Selective left testicular arteriogram again demonstrates displacement of the artery around the lateral border of the tumor. Some fine neovascularity arises from the proximal portion of the testicular artery as it passes medial to and slightly below the left kidney. (D) Selective left lumbar arteriogram demonstrates fine neovascularity arising from this lumbar branch as well. (A, C, D from Levin DC, Watson RC, Baltaxe HA. Arteriography of retroperitoneal masses. Radiology 1973;108:543. Used with permission.)

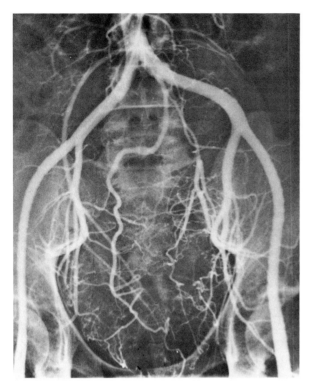

Figure 65-5. Leiomyosarcoma of the pelvic retroperitoneal space. Fine neovascularity is observed throughout the large mass, arising from both hypogastric arteries and the median sacral artery.

metastatic lesion of the left adrenal gland from a primary bronchogenic carcinoma. Figure 65-8 demonstrates an apparently spontaneous left retroperitoneal hemorrhage in a previously healthy 25-year-old woman. No specific cause or source of the hemorrhage was ever found at surgery.

Figure 65-6. Left retroperitoneal liposarcoma. (A) Initial ▶ abdominal aortogram shows downward displacement of the left renal artery and left kidney, upward displacement of the spleen, and displacement to the right of the lower abdominal aorta. No abnormal vascularity is seen. (B) Celiac axis arteriogram confirms the upward displacement of the spleen. No definite neovascularity is seen. (C) The venous phase of the celiac arteriogram confirms the absence of any tumor staining or pooling. (From Levin DC, Watson RC, Baltaxe HA. Arteriography of retroperitoneal masses. Radiology 1973; 108:543. Used with permission.)

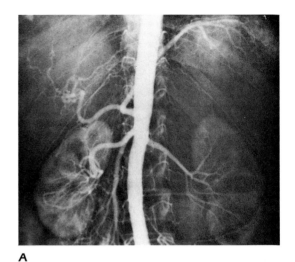

A

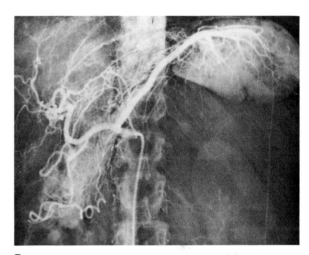

B

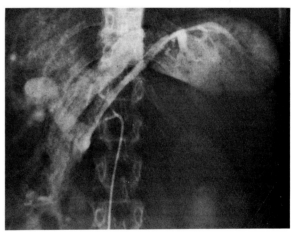

C

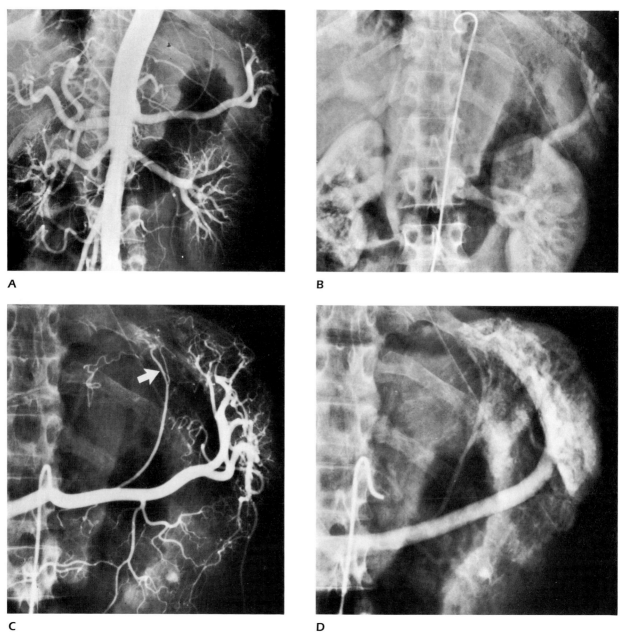

A

B

C

D

Figure 65-7. Left retroperitoneal hematoma resulting from rupture of the left adrenal gland. The patient had bronchogenic carcinoma, which metastasized to the left adrenal gland. (A and B) Abdominal aortogram, early and late phase films. No neovascularity is seen. The left renal artery is slightly straightened, and the left kidney is displaced downward slightly. (C and D) Selective splenic arteriogram, early and late phase films. A large avascular mass is present in the left upper quadrant retroperitoneal space. The splenic artery is stretched, particularly a small branch to the upper pole of the spleen (*arrow,* C). The spleen itself is draped over the lateral border of the mass. The late phase film shows that there is also displacement and stretching of the splenic vein.

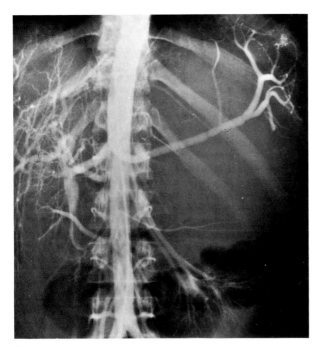

A

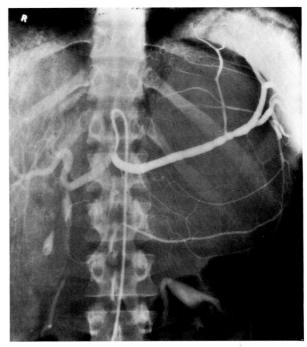

B

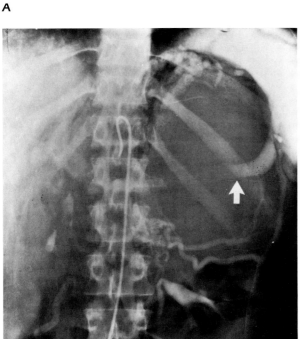

C

Figure 65-8. Spontaneous left retroperitoneal hemorrhage. (A) Initial abdominal aortogram demonstrates a large left upper quadrant avascular mass with marked downward displacement of the left renal arteries and left kidney. (B) Selective splenic arteriogram confirms the avascular nature of the mass. There is stretching of the splenic and pancreatic arteries. Several areas of narrowing are seen in the midportion of the splenic artery, but these were never explained. (C) The late phase of the splenic arteriogram demonstrates the avascular nature of the mass. The central portion of the splenic vein (*arrow*) is not opacified, and some collateral venous pathways are noted in the region of the gastric fundus and the upper pole of the left kidney. This finding suggests splenic vein obstruction, but at operation the splenic vein was noted to be patent. It was simply compressed by the large retroperitoneal hematoma.

Angiographic Findings in Retroperitoneal Inflammatory Disease

The angiographic findings in patients with retroperitoneal abscesses or other types of inflammatory disease are often somewhat more subtle than those in patients who have retroperitoneal tumors.[10] Displacement of vessels by the mass may be present, particularly if the lesion is a relatively large abscess under tension. On the other hand, if the inflammatory process is not encapsulated or confined, displacement of vessels and/or the kidneys may not occur.

The degree of vascularity is also variable. Retroperitoneal inflammatory lesions may be totally avascular or may show a mild degree of fine, somewhat irregular vascularity similar to the type II vascularity described above. If the abscess is vascularized, some staining may occur during the capillary phase, but this is unusual. The degree of vascularity is probably related partly to the proximity of the lesion to well-vascularized retroperitoneal organs such as the kidneys or pancreas. Thus perinephric or peripancreatic abscesses tend to be somewhat more vascular than psoas abscesses. The author has never seen an instance in which an inflammatory retroperitoneal mass contained extremely prominent, coarse type I vascularity. Figure 65-9 illustrates a staphylococcal perinephric abscess. Fine vascularity is seen medial to the kidney, but there was no staining.

Differential Diagnosis

The first sign that should alert the angiographer to the presence of a retroperitoneal mass is displacement of the retroperitoneal segments of major vessels (either arteries or veins) and/or the kidneys. This sign occurs in the vast majority of retroperitoneal mass lesions, although it may be absent in some cases of poorly confined retroperitoneal inflammatory processes.

If the mass, in addition to vascular and/or renal displacement, demonstrates coarse, ragged, highly irregular arteries (type I) with pooling or filling of sinusoids during the late phase, the diagnosis is most likely to be malignant tumor (there is a small possibility that such findings could be caused by a benign neural tumor). If the mass shows fine, somewhat more homogeneous vascularity (type II), the diagnosis is again ordinarily malignant tumor, but the cause could also be benign neural tumors, lipomas, or abscesses. If the mass is hypovascular or completely avascular, the dif-

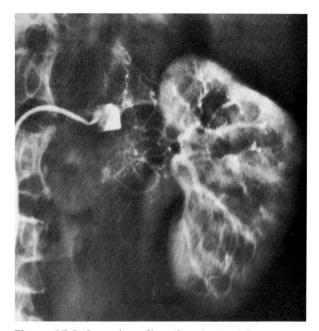

Figure 65-9. Late phase film of a selective left renal arteriogram in a patient with staphylococcal perinephric abscess. The density just lateral to the catheter tip is caused by overlying barium in the colon. Fine vascularity is seen medial to the upper pole of the left kidney. This case is an example of an inflammatory retroperitoneal lesion exhibiting type II neovascularity similar to that found in many malignant tumors. (Courtesy of Iraj Hooshmand, M.D.)

ferential diagnosis includes malignant tumors, benign neural tumors or lipomas, hematomas, and abscesses.

The actual cell type of a malignant retroperitoneal tumor cannot be predicted angiographically. As indicated earlier, the author has seen numerous examples of a given type of tumor exhibiting widely varying degrees of vascularity and ranging from totally avascular to extremely hypervascular.

Role of Angiography in Evaluation of Retroperitoneal Masses

Ultrasound, CT, and MRI have proved to be reliable in the detection of retroperitoneal masses.[11-20] Therefore, angiography is not necessary as a screening procedure in patients clinically suspected of having such lesions. Once a retroperitoneal mass is detected by ultrasound or CT, however, angiography may have a role to play before surgery.[7,11] Because the degree of vascularity of these masses is so highly variable, it is important that the surgeon know in advance whether excessive neovascularity is present. If it is, the surgeon must be aware of the source from which it arises. If there is significant arterial supply to the mass from renal, celiac, superior mesenteric, or inferior mesenteric arteries, these arteries may have to be sacrificed during the tumor resection, necessitating removal of devascularized organs such as the kidney or portions of bowel. Even if the mass is located posteriorly in the retroperitoneal space and is supplied only by lumbar arteries, it is important to know, before ligating them, whether any of these lumbar arteries supply portions of the spinal cord. In rare instances, avascular retroperitoneal masses may invade or encase major arteries or veins,[7] thereby necessitating resection of segments of those vessels at the time of resection of the tumor. In certain patients with highly vascular retroperitoneal masses, preoperative devascularization by transcatheter embolization might facilitate resection, although there has been little experience so far with the application of embolization in this area. Finally, Karp et al.[11] have pointed out that even with the current availability of sophisticated noninvasive imaging techniques, it may at times be impossible to differentiate intraperitoneal from retroperitoneal lesions if the mass is very large. In such instances the delineation of the source of blood supply by arteriography might indicate whether the mass arises primarily in the retroperitoneal space or is within the peritoneal cavity or one of the intraperitoneal organs.

For all the above reasons, surgeons experienced in treatment of retroperitoneal masses have found angiography to be valuable in preoperative planning of their approach and have advocated its routine use[16] in dealing with these difficult and dangerous lesions.

References

1. Armstrong JR, Cohn I Jr. Primary malignant retroperitoneal tumors. Am J Surg 1965;110:937.
2. Banfi A, Bonnadonna G, Carnevali G, Oldini C, Salvini E. Preferential sites of involvement and spread in malignant lymphoma. Eur J Cancer 1968;4:319.
3. Fuller LM. Results of large volume irradiation in management of Hodgkin's disease and malignant lymphoma originating in the abdomen. Radiology 1966;87:1058.
4. Bron KM, Sherman L. Arteriography in evaluating retroperitoneal mass lesions. NY State J Med 1967;67:1875.
5. Vinik MN Jr, Neal MP Jr, Freed TA. Retroperitoneal angiography. South Med J 1968;61:646.
6. Lowman RM, Grnja V, Peck DR, Osborn D, Love L. The angiographic patterns of the primary retroperitoneal tumors: the role of the lumbar arteries. Radiology 1972;104:259.
7. Levin DC, Watson RC, Baltaxe HA. Arteriography of retroperitoneal masses. Radiology 1973;108:543.
8. Damascelli B, Musumeci R, Botturi M, Petrillo R, Spagnoli I. Angiography of retroperitoneal tumors: a review. AJR 1975;124:565.
9. Levin DC, Gordon DH, Kinkhabwala M, Becker JA. Arteriography of retroperitoneal lymphoma. AJR 1976;126:368.
10. Lois JF, Levin DC, Hooshmand I. Angiography of non-neoplastic retroperitoneal masses. Cardiovasc Intervent Radiol 1982;5:312.
11. Karp W, Hafstrom LO, Jonsson PE. Retroperitoneal sarcoma: ultrasonographic and angiographic evaluation. Br J Radiol 1980;53:525.
12. Stephens DH, Sheedy PF II, Hattery RR, Williamson B Jr. Diagnosis and evaluation of retroperitoneal tumors by computed tomography. AJR 1977;129:395.
13. Carter BL, Wechsler RJ. Computed tomography of the retroperitoneum and abdominal wall. Semin Roentgenol 1978;13:201.
14. Bree RL, Green B. Gray scale sonographic appearance of intraabdominal mesenchymal sarcoma. Radiology 1978;128:193.
15. Korobkin M, Callen PW, Fisch AE. Computed tomography of the pelvis and retroperitoneum. Radiol Clin North Am 1979;17:301.
16. Duncan RE, Evans AT. Diagnosis of primary retroperitoneal tumors. J Urol 1977;117:19.
17. Lee JKT. Magnetic resonance imaging of the retroperitoneum. Urol Radiol 1988;10:48.
18. Demas BE, Hricak H. Magnetic resonance imaging in the evaluation of the retroperitoneum. Urol Radiol 1986;8:151.
19. Dodds WJ, Darweesh RMA, Lawson TL, Stewart ET, Foley WD, Kishk SMA, Hollworth M. The retroperitoneal space revisited. AJR 1986;147:1155.
20. Lane RH, Stephens DH, Reiman HM. Primary retroperitoneal neoplasms: CT findings in 90 cases with clinical and pathologic correlation. AJR 1989;152:83.

V

The Extremities and Lymphangiography

66

Arteriography of the Patient with Previous Aortoiliac Interventions

ANDREW B. CRUMMY
JOHN C. MCDERMOTT

The aging of our population and improvements in surgical, percutaneous, interventional, and anesthetic technique have increased the number of patients undergoing procedures for disease of the abdominal aorta and iliac vessels. In addition, sufficient years have passed so that many patients now have recurrent symptoms or have developed complications related to their previous interventions.[1–3] Therefore, the number of these patients who require arteriography is steadily increasing.

In patients with straightforward abdominal aortic and iliac artery disease, the problem can generally be assessed by a few pertinent questions and a simple physical examination. The diagnosis is seldom in doubt, and arteriography is done for staging. The arteriogram demonstrates (1) the exact site of obstruction, (2) whether the distal vessels are satisfactory for anastomosis, and (3) whether the outflow vessels will allow sufficient flow to maintain patency. In the patient who has had a previous intervention, detailed knowledge of its nature and the current clinical problem is essential for the performance of an adequate examination.[4]

Arteriographic Technique

The arteriographic technique for evaluation of the patient who has had previous therapy may differ significantly in several respects from the examination of the patient who has not had previous treatment. If either femoral artery is available for catheterization, this is the preferred route. As a practical matter, to avoid puncturing a graft if one is in place, at least one of the distal anastomoses will have to be to an iliac artery. Generally, then, the ipsilateral groin will not have an incision. Arteriography is performed in the usual manner,[1] with the positioning of the catheter varied according to the problem (Figs. 66-1 and 66-2).

When use of the femoral route is precluded, the authors' preference is for translumbar arteriography (Fig. 66-3). The puncture should be made in the aorta rather than the graft. Unless the patient has a graft that extends above the renal arteries, an unusual circumstance, one is generally in a satisfactory position if the entry is made at the L1-L2 level. It is also useful to check the vascular clips that are invariably present and to make the entrance cephalad to the most proximal clip. Fluoroscopic control during the placement of the needle greatly simplifies this maneuver.

The authors' technique of translumbar puncture is similar to that discussed in Chapter 43. An 18-gauge, 22-cm Teflon sheath needle with four very distal side holes is used. Injection rates as rapid as 20 ml per second can be readily accommodated by this catheter needle. Frequently, however, a slower injection rate is employed because obstruction is a major indication for these studies. The sleeve is flexible, so it can be passed either distally or proximally, depending on the particular problem. In the presence of an open aortic bifurcation graft and with the need to study runoff vessels (i.e., the vessels distal to the inguinal ligament), distal placement of the tip is preferred because this will prevent loss of contrast into the visceral vessels. On the other hand, in the presence of severe proximal obstruction or occlusion, one must fill the collateral vessels, which for the most part are the high lumbar, intercostal, and superior mesenteric arteries. Such filling is best achieved by passing the catheter tip cephalad so that the injection is made into the distal thoracic aorta (see Fig. 66-3).[5]

The direction of the catheter tip can usually be altered by manipulation with a 3-mm J guidewire.[6] On

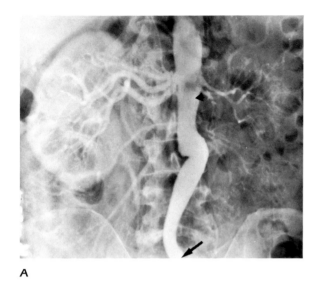

A

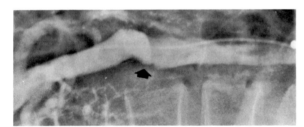

B

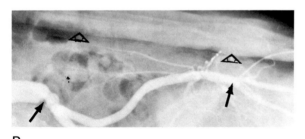

D

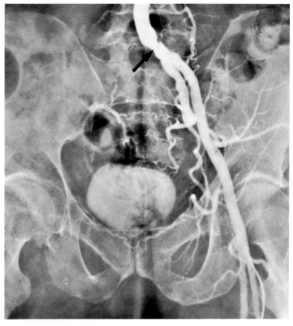

C

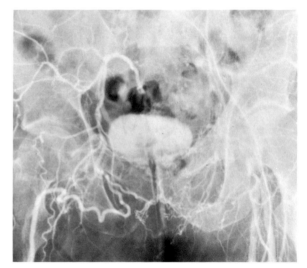

E

Figure 66-1. Patient with recurrence of claudication in the right lower extremity after placement of an aortobilateral common iliac graft. (A) Anteroposterior view of the graft, the right arm of which is obstructed. The *arrowhead* indicates an incidental left renal artery stenosis, and the *solid arrow* points to an irregularity of the left anastomosis. (B) Satisfactory appearance of the end-to-end aortic anastomosis (*arrow*). (C) Antegrade filling of the iliac system as well as opacification of cross-pelvic collaterals. The *arrow* identifies the anastomosis. (D) In lateral view, a large posterior plaque, not seen in the frontal view, is outlined at the anastomosis (*left arrow*). The *open arrowheads* indicate the interface between the bolus bags and the anterior aspect of the pelvis, and the *right arrow* points to the posterior origin of the profunda femoral artery, which is normal. (E) The right profunda femoral artery has now filled through collaterals and is the entire source of blood for that extremity.

occasion, a tip deflector, such as that marketed by Cook, is useful. If puncture of the aorta is made with a relatively acute angle between the needle and the distal aorta, proximal passage of the tip is usual. Entry with the needle almost perpendicular to the aorta facilitates distal passage.

The use of the axillary brachial artery system is a reasonable alternative; as a matter of fact, it is the pre-

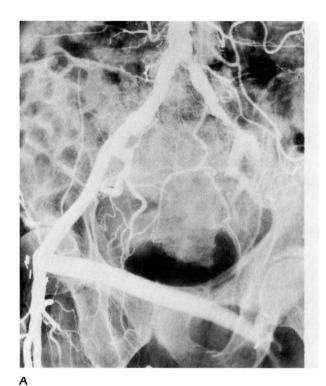

A

Figure 66-2. A femorofemoral graft was used to bypass the left iliac artery disease in an elderly patient who was not considered a candidate for an aortofemoral graft. Recurrent symptoms on the left prompted this examination. (A) The right common femoral artery has been entered below the graft. There is excellent filling of the distal aorta, pelvic vessels, collaterals, and graft. (B and C) Flow in the graft gradually opacifies the left femoral artery. The anastomoses are best seen in lateral projection.

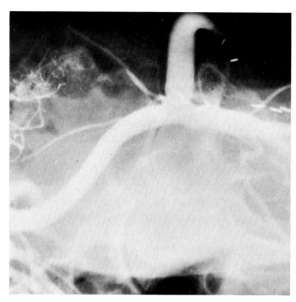

B

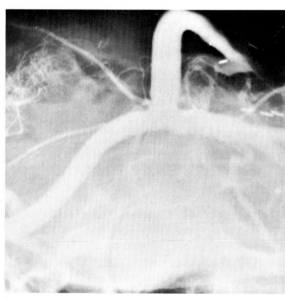

C

ferred approach of some angiographers for study of the abdominal aorta and pelvic vessels in lower extremity vascular disease. The authors find this is a technically more difficult puncture, and the passage around an elongated, ectatic aortic arch may be time-consuming. The upper extremity access is also the only approach that carries the risk of a cerebral vascular accident.

Only when a satisfactory alternative is not available do we puncture the aortobifemoral graft for access (Figs. 66-4 and 66-5). We are reluctant to puncture grafts because of two problems unique to prostheses.[7] Synthetic material or vein does not have the muscular wall of an artery and therefore lacks the ability to contract and close the puncture site. In addition, the neointima that lines the prostheses can be easily stripped away from the wall, possibly resulting in obstruction or embolization.

If catheterization of a graft is required (e.g., to study the lower extremity vessels in the presence of an axillofemoral bypass), the use of a needle without an obturator is recommended (see Fig. 66-5). This facili-

tates a single-wall puncture. The needle is passed slowly so that blood appears through the lumen before the posterior wall is punctured. There is generally a considerable amount of perigraft fibrosis, and the use of a Teflon dilator and a heavy duty wire (e.g., Rosen) is helpful in establishing a tract to the graft. The dilator has the additional advantage of being sharply tapered, minimizing the possibility of intimal stripping.

A Teflon-coated 3-mm J guidewire facilitates smooth passage and minimizes the possibility of guidewire disruption of the neointima. Generally, if no problem is encountered at the puncture site, pas-

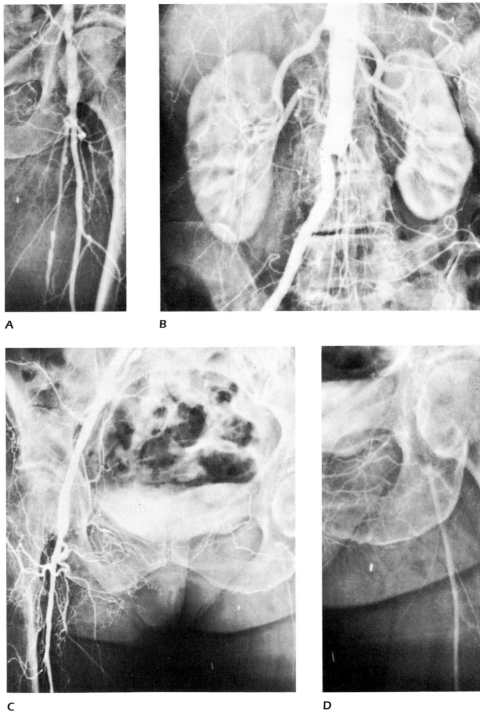

A

B

C

D

Figure 66-3. (A) Distal left iliofemoral system of a patient with bilateral lower extremity ischemia. There is significant obstruction in the common femoral artery just distal to the inguinal ligament and at its bifurcation. The patient had an aortofemoral graft placed. (B to D) Symptoms recurred on the left, and reexamination showed that the right limb of the graft was normal. The left limb was obstructed, but flow through anterior pelvic collaterals gradually filled the left profunda femoral system. Presumably progression of disease in the common femoral artery resulted in thrombosis of the vessel and the graft. The loss of runoff caused retrograde propagation of thrombus to the graft bifurcation.

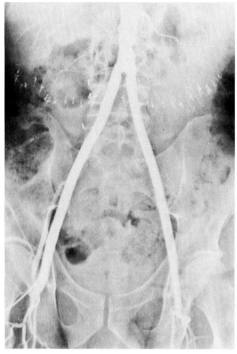
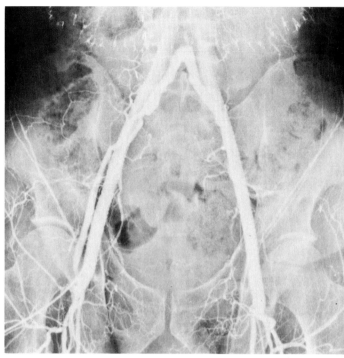

A   B

Figure 66-4. Arteriography of an aortofemoral graft performed through the right limb of the graft. (A) End-to-end aortic anastomosis and end-to-side femoral anastomoses. The graft is normal and provides excellent opacification of the femoral vessels. (B) Filling of the circumflex vessels and retrograde flow in the native external and common iliac systems.

Figure 66-5. Right axillofemorofemoral graft performed because of bilateral lower extremity ischemia. Recurrent left-sided symptoms resulted in reexamination. (A) A catheter is in place in the distal axillary limb. There is an intraluminal filling defect representing thrombus in the proximal portion of the femoral limb, and the thrombus extends proximally and distally in the axillary limb. The proximal right femoral vessels are filled. (B) Good opacification of the distal femoral limb and the left femoral system outlines a short segment of advanced disease just distal to the anastomosis. Note the retrograde filling of the common femoral and distal external iliac arteries as well as of the iliac circumflex vessel. Poor flow within the femoral limb of the graft was presumed to have resulted in thrombosis with retrograde propagation into the axillary portion.

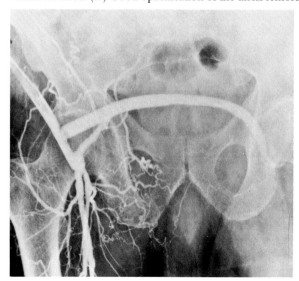
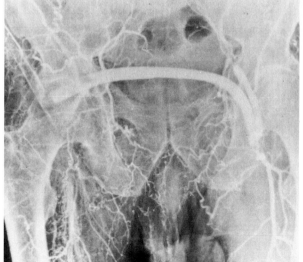

A   B

sage through the graft is problem-free. The smallest-diameter catheter that will deliver the required amount of contrast should be used. A 55-cm 5.3 French catheter allows for injection of 18 ml per second and is usually satisfactory. When the catheter is being moved, especially during removal, it is best to keep a guidewire within it to prevent catheter disruption as it passes through the synthetic material.

After removal of the catheter, particular care must be given to achieving hemostasis. It is important that pressure on the puncture site not bring about complete occlusion of the graft because this predisposes to thrombosis. Also, great care must be exercised to avoid a hematoma formation because an infected hematoma may necessitate removal of the prosthesis.

Digital subtraction angiography (DSA), developed by Mistretta and associates at the University of Wisconsin, is a technique for real-time digital processing of x-ray transmission data from image-intensified videofluoroscopy systems.[8-10] The signal from the iodine is logarithmically amplified and subtracted on-line by a small dedicated computer. Because amplification of the iodine signal is coupled with subtraction, satisfactory studies of the abdominal aorta and the pelvic vessels can be achieved by the intravenous injection of 40 ml of contrast agent (about 350 mg iodine/ml), delivered at the rate of 20 ml per second through a 5.2 French pigtail catheter preferably into the right

atrium. Exposures are made every 1.5 seconds as a bolus from the intravenous injection passes through the area. Motion interferes with subtraction, so the patient must remain still. Peristalsis can be suppressed if necessary by the intravenous administration of glucagon just before the study. Because the subtraction is done electronically, the images are available for immediate evaluation, and additional studies in other projections can be made as indicated. Moreover, the amount of subtraction can be varied so that some anatomic information can be left in the image to aid orientation.

With intravenous DSA (IVDSA), it is possible to detect aneurysms, false aneurysms (Fig. 66-6), stenoses, and occlusions (Fig. 66-7) and to determine the patency of grafts (Fig. 66-8). Such information is useful in the management of postintervention aortoiliac problems.

The IVDSA technique eliminates the risks associated with intraarterial catheterization. The major hazard is related to the intravascular administration of contrast agent, a risk common to both IVDSA and standard arteriography.

The authors are convinced that biplane filming is helpful in evaluating these complex problems (Figs. 66-9 through 66-11; see also Figs. 66-1 and 66-2). In areas such as the pelvis and proximal thigh, overlap of bilaterally symmetric arteries can be eliminated by angulating the tube for simultaneous biplane filming

Figure 66-6. An IVDSA arteriogram following injection of 60 ml of contrast agent at the rate of 14 ml per second. (A) The donor end of a femorofemoral graft is shown, with good delineation of the external iliac and common femoral arteries. (B) The distal end of the graft is shown to be patent. The endarterectomized segment of the left common femoral artery has become aneurysmal. The profunda vessel and its lateral femoral circumflex branch are well seen.

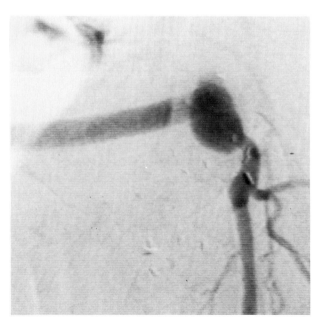

A

B

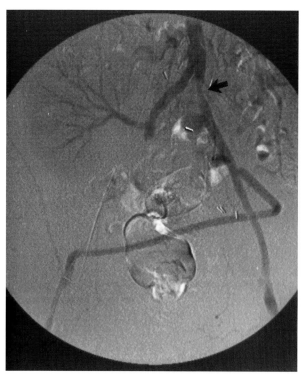

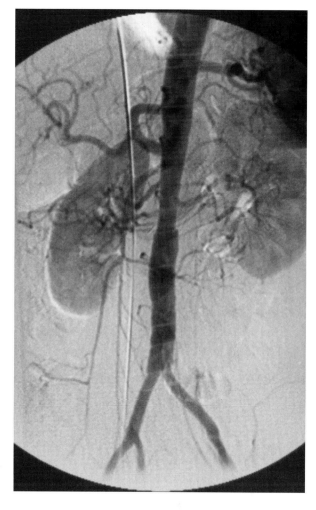

Figure 66-7. An IVDSA was performed to evaluate an ilio-femoral bypass graft. The right iliac system is obstructed distal to a transplant renal artery. The left common iliac artery has a moderate stenosis (*arrow*).

Figure 66-8. An IVDSA shows a well-functioning aortic ▶ tube graft that extends from the infrarenal portion of the aorta to the aortic bifurcation.

Figure 66-9. An elderly patient who had a previous axillo-bifemoral graft sought attention because of a groin mass, which he thought was an inguinal hernia. Anteroposterior (A) and lateral (B) projections show the aortobifemoral graft with a pseudoaneurysm arising at the origin of the femoral limb. Both projections were necessary to define accurately the relationships of the pseudoaneurysm. The *curved arrows* outline the endarterectomized portion of the common femoral and proximal profunda femoral arteries. The *straight arrows* point to the distal trunk of the profunda, which is severely involved with atherosclerosis. The *open arrowheads* identify the hypertrophied lateral femoral circumflex vessel, which is the main supply to the distal extremity. The *solid arrowheads* mark the pseudoaneurysm arising from the origin of the femoral limb. In (B), the *large arrow* points to the anastomosis of the graft to the left produnda artery. On the basis of this detailed pathoanatomic information, the surgeons were able to approach the graft in such a way that they could place one stitch to close the small leak that had occurred at the take-off of the femoral arm.

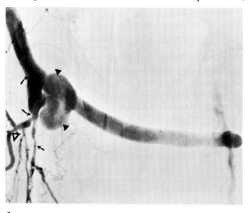

A

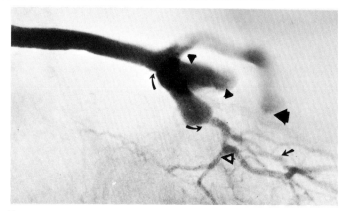

B

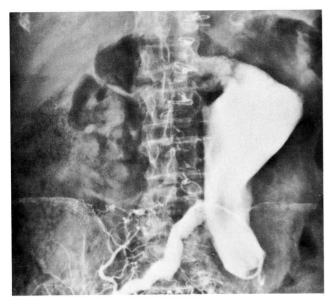

A

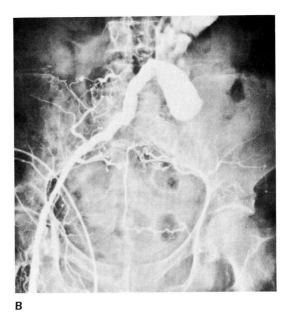

B

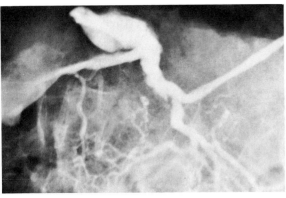

C

Figure 66-10. A patient who had had a well-functioning aorto–bilateral common iliac graft for a number of years noted pyrexia and malaise. At the time of admission, she was febrile and had an absent left femoral pulse; hematologic studies were compatible with an infection. The diagnosis of an infected graft was made, and arteriography was undertaken to delineate the anatomy. (A and B) Right transfemoral aortogram shows marked extravasation of contrast agent into a huge paravascular pseudoaneurysm. The pseudoaneurysm extended from L2 inferiorly along the left limb of the graft to the midportion of the sacroiliac joint. There is excellent filling of the vessels in the right hemipelvis that course to the left graft limb (B). (C) Lateral projection shows that the pseudoaneurysm extends into the posterior paraspinal area. No further attempts to delineate the anatomy were made. The diagnosis was an infected graft with a large pseudoaneurysm and obstruction of the left limb. At surgery, the aortic and left iliac anastomoses were disrupted, and the blood was contained by the large infected pseudoaneurysm. The graft was removed, and the patient was observed. Because her extremities did not show evidence of additional ischemia, an extraanatomic bypass was not required.

or by obtaining both oblique projections with separate runs. Angulation of the tube results in differences in the length of the beam path in tissue and causes unequal film exposure. This discrepancy can be overcome by using a water bolus on the anterior surface of the pelvis and thighs. Intravenous fluid bags are satisfactory for this purpose.[11]

Nonionic contrast agents are recommended because of the decrease in patient discomfort, especially when severe ischemia is present.

The choice of approach and filming sequence depends on the patient's problems. As a general rule, relatively large volumes of contrast introduced at moderate injection rates (about 40–50 ml at 15–20 ml/sec) are best used to fill vessels distal to obstructions as well as pseudoaneurysms that may have small communications with the vascular tree. Moderate to slow filming rates are adequate (one per second × 15 or one per second × 10, then one every second × 5). The contrast is usually injected into the lower thoracic aorta. Biplane films of the suprarenal aorta; a graft, if present, including the proximal and distal anastomoses; and the runoff vessels should be obtained. On occasion, particularly when the thrombosis is acute and collaterals are not fully developed, it may be difficult to fill the femoral vessels. The injection of 25 to 50 mg tolazoline or 60 mg papaverine just before contrast injection may increase collateral flow and aid opacification of the runoff vessels.[12] Despite acute ischemia, which may be severe, reactive hyperemia may induce additional vasodilatation and is the authors' preferred method.[11] A blood pressure cuff is placed around the thigh, inflated to above the systolic pressure for 7 minutes, and re-

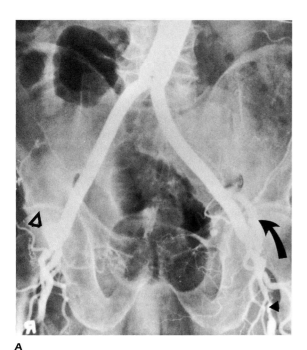

A

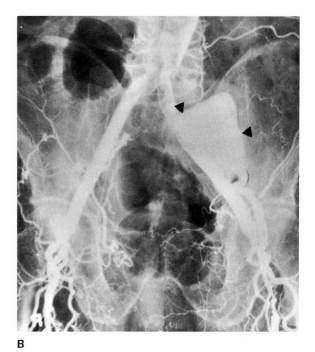

B

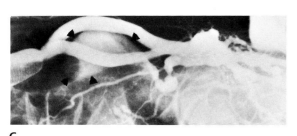

C

Figure 66-11. An 83-year-old patient had an aortobifemoral graft because of an abdominal aortic aneurysm 6 years previously. At that time, the right iliac artery was obstructed, and the left common iliac artery was aneurysmal. The iliac artery aneurysm was ligated proximally and distally and left in situ. The patient was seen at this time because of a palpable left pelvic mass. (A) Translumbar aortogram shows excellent filling of the aortobifemoral graft. The *solid arrowhead* points to distal profunda femoral artery obstruction. The *open arrowhead* shows a small pseudoaneurysm at the site of the anastomosis. The overall size of the pseudoaneurysm is best appreciated by combining both the anteroposterior (A and B) and lateral projections (C). The *straight arrow* (A) points to retrograde flow in the left common femoral and external iliac arteries. Frontal (B) and lateral (C) projections in a later phase show a large aneurysm of the left common iliac artery (*arrowheads*). Note that the left limb of the graft is displaced anteriorly by the aneurysm. (C) was taken with the patient prone so that the contrast is layered in the dependent portion of the graft. For ease of viewing, the film is displayed as if the patient were supine. It was presumed that the left iliac artery sutures had deteriorated and that the vessel had recanalized with increase in size of the aneurysm. The patient was explored by an extraperitoneal approach; the aneurysm was exposed and again ligated proximally and distally and evacuated. The patient did well.

leased just before the injection. During the vasoocclusive phase, patients may have some discomfort, but usually with reassurance they are willing to tolerate it.

Angiography suites are generally kept relatively cool for the comfort of the angiography team. In such circumstances, ischemic extremities may rapidly cool, with resultant vasoconstriction that will handicap the examination. This may be prevented by properly covering the extremities.

Postintervention Problems

Immediate Problems

Vascular problems immediately after aortoiliac interventions are generally related to technical failures that may result in thrombosis or hemorrhage. Graft thrombosis is usually secondary to an unsatisfactory anastomosis or poor distal outflow (runoff). Graft occlusion can also be due to obstruction secondary to dissection of intima that was inadequately reattached after endarterectomy, usually at or near the anastomotic site.[13] Acute graft thrombosis can usually be diagnosed on the basis of clinical information, occasionally supplemented by simple Doppler ultrasound studies; as a rule arteriography is omitted unless thrombolysis is indicated. Significant bleeding (i.e., an amount that would require reoperation) will be manifested clinically, and arteriography is not required.[4] However, if a patient is transferred from another institution because of graft failure in the immediate postoperative period, it is the authors' practice to perform an arteriogram to define exactly the pathoanatomic situation. Similarly, arteriography is performed in patients with postoperative bleeding if their clinical condition permits.

Acute failure of an aortoiliac angioplasty is usually due to thrombosis at the site secondary to an obstructing intimal flap. Because a catheter is generally in place, immediate assessment is usually possible with DSA. Treatment with thrombolytic agents and/or placement of an intravascular stent can salvage the procedure.

Late Postoperative Problems

At times it is difficult to know whether a problem is related to a therapeutic misadventure or to progression of the underlying disease. For example, thrombosis of a limb of a graft could be due to a poor anastomosis or to advancement of the atherosclerotic process. It also may be impossible to know whether a pseudoaneurysm is the cause of or the result of an infection. For the most part, the precipitating event is not important; rather, diagnosis of the problem with delineation of the extent of the process and the involved anatomy is paramount for potential repair.

Graft Thrombosis

Graft thrombosis, which is more prevalent in patients with occlusive than with aneurysmal disease, may occur either abruptly or insidiously after a satisfactory initial result.[1,14] Progression of the atherosclerotic process in the runoff vessels is the major cause (see Figs. 66-3 and 66-5). Poor surgical technique may also be a factor.[15] In the case of an angioplasty, progression of disease may occur at the site of angioplasty, in the vessel adjacent to the PTA site, or in the outflow vessels. In most circumstances, the profunda femoris artery provides sufficient flow for the graft or iliac arteries to remain patent.[16] Therefore, it is essential that the profunda vessel be adequately evaluated, including its orifice, which is a common site of occlusive disease. Because the profunda orifice is posterior in relation to the common femoral artery, a lateral or oblique view must be obtained (see Fig. 66-1D).

The profunda artery may have a main trunk obstruction as well as branch orifice stenosis distally (see Figs. 66-5 and 66-11).[17] Because these lesions may be accessible to an extended endarterectomy or angioplasty, the entire profunda should be studied. Biplane views of the distal profunda artery have not been found to consistently contribute useful information, and the authors therefore obtain them only on the rare occa-

sion when they appear to be necessary. If both limbs of an aortobifemoral graft are occluded, the thrombosis will extend proximally to the first branch vessels, usually a large pair of lumbar arteries or the renal arteries. Correction requires that technical problems be identified and rectified and any inadequacy of runoff corrected, or rethrombosis will occur. Removal of thrombus from the graft with a Fogarty catheter or thrombolytic therapy may be satisfactory. Otherwise, the graft will have to be replaced or a new bypass, such as an axillofemoral or a femorofemoral bypass, will have to be established.[14]

If one limb of the graft is open and thrombectomy fails, an iliofemoral or a femorofemoral bypass rather than replacement of the graft may be best. In these circumstances, it is mandatory to assess the status of the patent graft limb (see Fig. 66-1). If arteriography shows an obstruction of questionable hemodynamic significance, pressures should be measured before and after induced hyperemia to establish whether a gradient is present. If there is a pressure gradient at rest or a gradient of more than 15 mmHg after hyperemia, it is unlikely that the graft will accommodate flow to both extremities; in such cases, the gradient will have to be corrected or an alternative procedure will have to be done.

Progression of Disease

As previously discussed, progression of atherosclerotic disease may cause native vessel or graft thrombosis (see Figs. 66-3 and 66-5).[3,14,18] On the other hand, the profunda femoris artery may provide runoff adequate to maintain patency, but distal disease may cause claudication, rest pain, or tissue necrosis.[19] Arteriography is useful for confirming the status of the graft or native vessel and for visualizing the vessels of the extremity; it should be performed by injecting a large volume of contrast at the aortic or graft bifurcation and filming the extremity vessels.

After aortic–common iliac grafting, the internal and external iliac vessels fill in a normal antegrade manner (see Figs. 66-1 and 66-8). After an end-to-end aortic anastomosis and an end-to-side external iliac or femoral anastomosis, the iliac system fills by retrograde flow in the external and internal iliac arteries as well as through collaterals (see Figs. 66-4 and 66-10). With an end-to-end external iliac or femoral anastomosis, filling is largely retrograde through the profunda collaterals and antegrade through the lumbar collaterals. Because these vessels are perfused, the potential for aneurysm development persists (see Fig. 66-11). Aneurysms of these sites may be manifested in a variety of ways, including (1) by rupture, (2) as a mass, (3) through ureteral compression, and (4) by peripheral embolization.

Ultrasound may be helpful in delineating the nature, size, shape, and location of a mass as well as its acoustic characteristics. The relationship of the mass to vessels in the pelvis may, however, be difficult to define because of bowel gas. Computed tomography (CT) and magnetic resonance angiography (MRA) have the advantage of demonstrating clot in the aneurysm sac as well as contrast within the lumen of the aneurysm (Fig. 66-12). DSA can show the vessel as well as the aneurysm, whereas conventional arteriography affords better spatial resolution. It needs to be performed only if detailed resolution is required or peristalsis causes subtraction artifacts.

Pseudoaneurysms and Infected Grafts

It is difficult to consider pseudoaneurysms and infected grafts separately because they are so closely related. If blood extravasates slowly, a hematoma may form, providing some degree of tamponade. The outer layer of the hematoma may become fairly well organized and fibrotic, but the portion adjacent to the artery generally remains filled with liquid blood. Such a lesion is called a pseudoaneurysm because none of the layers of the vessel form part of the hematoma wall, and the hematoma communicates with the vascular lumen.

False aneurysms, when present in a patient with a graft, are usually seen in the region of an anastomosis (see Figs. 66-6 and 66-12).[20,21] They are the result of an insidious leak that remains occult until a mass is palpable or an associated complication such as an infection or massive bleed occurs. Infection may disrupt the suture line, resulting in bleeding; depending on the circumstances, including the rate of hemorrhage, a false aneurysm may form or exsanguination may occur.

Infection of a vascular prosthesis is a feared complication.[22] Szilagyi et al.[23] reported an incidence of 0.7 percent when the distal anastomoses were done through an abdominal incision, but the rate more than doubled to 1.6 percent when groin anastomoses were performed. Most infections are believed to be the result of contamination through the incision.[24] However, injury to the gastrointestinal tract and primary infection of an aneurysm at the time of surgery are also factors in graft infection.[25,26] Hematogenous seeding secondary to bacteremia, whatever the cause, likewise plays a role in late infection. Pressure necrosis of the gastrointestinal tract from pulsations of the relatively rigid prosthesis or a pseudoaneurysm may result in an aortoenteric fistula.

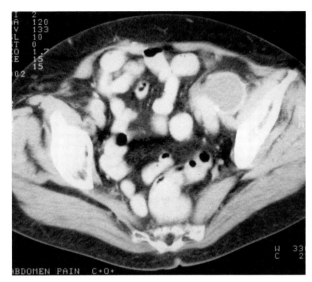

A

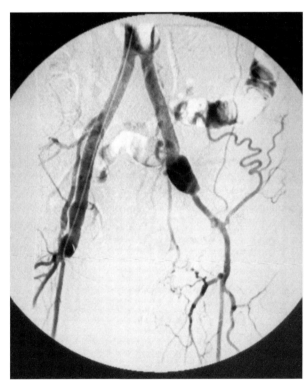

B

Figure 66-12. (A) CT scan through the pelvis of a patient with a previous aorto right femoral and left iliac graft. A pseudoaneurysm of the iliac anastomosis is seen on the left. The lumen of the pseudoaneurysm is partially filled with clot. (B) Arteriogram of the same patient, done through the graft, shows the pseudoaneurysm and its relationship to the anastomosis. Only part of the lumen is opacified because the major portion of the pseudoaneurysm contains clot. The true extent of the pseudoaneurysm is not as well appreciated as on the CT scan.

The clinical manifestations of an infected graft or a pseudoaneurysm are partly related to the virulence of the organisms, the response of the host, and the location. In the groin, the classic signs of infection are tenderness, erythema, and swelling, which may be seen early. If the skin breaks down, there may be extravasation of pus and some bleeding. The same process may occur in the abdomen, but early symptoms will be less likely and thus diagnosis will be more difficult.

Diagnosis

Any patient with a vascular graft and fever should be suspected of having an infected graft. A film of the involved area showing gas bubbles in the region of the graft is diagnostic. Ultrasound and CT scan may show fluid collections in the paraprosthetic region. However, it may be difficult to distinguish a pseudoaneurysm from an abscess unless there is associated gas.[27] In the presence of pyrexia, contamination must be presumed. An indium-labeled white blood cell scan demonstrating localization of the isotope in the paraprosthetic area is strongly suggestive of infection, especially if the location is near a suture line.[28,29]

If attention is drawn to an uninfected graft because of bleeding, palpable mass, or other sign, arteriography may provide valuable information. Malpositioned or unusual contour of the graft may suggest abnormality, and contrast may opacify an aneurysm or pseudoaneurysm (Figs. 66-12 and 66-13).[11] If surgery is

contemplated, knowledge of the vascular anatomy is helpful in planning possible removal of the graft and any corrective surgery (see Figs. 66-10 and 66-12).

With a firm clinical diagnosis of an infected graft, the primary role of arteriography is the definition of the vascular anatomy. Of particular importance is the state of the distal vessels, which determines the feasibility of the secondary repair. Demonstration of the presence and extent of a pseudoaneurysm is also helpful.[30] In a patient in whom the diagnosis is not clear, the demonstration of a pseudoaneurysm greatly enhances the possibility of an infected graft.

Aortoenteric Fistulas and Paraprosthetic Enteric Fistulas

Four years after aortic reconstructive surgery was initiated, the first aortoenteric fistula was reported.[22,31] The major clinical manifestations of this potentially catastrophic complication are gastrointestinal bleeding and sepsis. These symptoms in any patient who has had previous aortic surgery must raise the possibility of an aortoenteric fistula.[28,32]

The infrarenal aorta and the transverse part of the duodenum are juxtaposed, and it is necessary to interpose viable tissue between the duodenum and aortic suture line to prevent pressure necrosis of the bowel caused by pulsations of the relatively rigid prosthesis. Damage to the bowel wall compromises its integrity,

Figure 66-13. (A) Color Doppler examination of a pseudoaneurysm that resulted from a previous arterial puncture of the common femoral artery. The neck of the aneurysm and the main mass are well delineated. (B) After compression

of the neck of the pseudoaneurysm, thrombosis occurred, so that now there is no flow in the neck or in the pseudoaneurysm. (Courtesy of Fred T. Lee, Jr, M.D.)

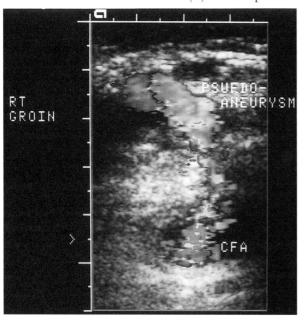

A

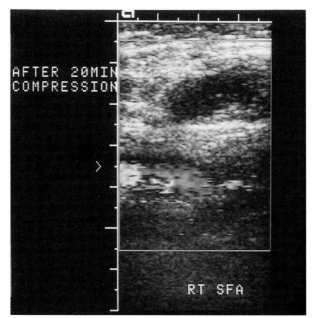

B

leading to contamination with enteric bacteria. In the presence of such an infection, disruption of the anastomosis will almost surely ensue. A frank, free communication of the vascular lumen and the bowel will result in rapid massive gastrointestinal bleeding, which may result in exsanguination. Fortunately, because the fistula is usually small and plugged with thrombus and other debris, bleeding is intermittent and generally not massive. There is little about the clinical circumstances to suggest a fistula except the history of prior aortic surgery and the combination of gastrointestinal bleeding and sepsis. Barium studies are of little use because the patients are likely to be in an age group in which many lesions with a potential for bleeding are found, necessitating that a lesion be proved responsible for the bleeding. An aortoenteric fistula can, of course, coexist with another source of bleeding. The presence of barium will handicap endoscopy, ultrasound, CT scanning, and arteriography.

Upper gastrointestinal endoscopy may identify many lesions and actually demonstrate the bleeding. On occasion, the gastrointestinal side of the fistula may be visualized. A major handicap to this approach is that manipulation of the duodenum may disrupt the precarious state of hemostasis existing in the fistula. Therefore, some recommend that endoscopy, if done, be carried out in the operating room with the patient prepared for surgery.

CT scanning may demonstrate air adjacent to the graft or a paraprosthetic fluid collection and may suggest the presence of a false aneurysm. Arteriography may demonstrate a false aneurysm or a paragraft extravasation of contrast agent, but, unless the patient is bleeding, it is unlikely to be identified. In a patient suspected of having graft complication who is briskly bleeding, the risks of surgery without angiographic information are probably less than the risk of exsanguination because of delay. A less common type of fistula, paraprosthetic enteric fistula, is caused by erosion of bowel remote from a suture line and is ordinarily without a false aneurysm.[33] A major predisposing factor is a graft that is too long, causing anterior bowing of the proximal portions of the iliac limbs with resultant pressure necrosis of the bowel. Under these circumstances, the manifestations of infection rather than bleeding are paramount.[11] The bleeding that occurs is the outcome of bowel necrosis and does not represent a communication with the vascular lumen through a disrupted suture line. Contamination of the area of necrosis with intestinal organisms is inevitable. [111]Indium or [99m]technetium hexamethylpropyleneamine oxime-labeled leukocytes may be helpful in localizing inflammation in the region of the prosthesis.[15,29]

The role of arteriography is preeminent in defining the vascular anatomy and the state of vessels that may be used for extraanatomic bypass.

Arteriovenous Fistulas

Arteriovenous (AV) fistulas are rare complications of aortoiliac surgery. They are generally recognized during surgery and immediately repaired, but they may also occur as a late complication, commonly manifested by (1) high-output cardiac failure, (2) distal ischemia, (3) a palpable mass, (4) bruit, and (5) thrill.[34,35]

Doppler ultrasound examination is the preferred method of delineating the presence of an AV fistula. Arteriography delineates the anatomy and determines the exact site of the fistula as well as the relationship of involved vessels and the presence of potential collaterals. Large-volume injections with multiple projections and very rapid filming (up to six per second) are essential aspects of the examination.

Pseudoaneurysms after Catheterization, Angioplasty, or Endarterectomy

Of particular interest are the pseudoaneurysms that occur after catheterization of a femoral vessel for diagnostic or therapeutic purposes. In the authors' experience, these are most often seen after cardiac catheterization. They can be suspected when a palpable mass and bruit are present after catheterization. The diagnosis can be readily confirmed by Doppler ultrasound examination. When the exact site of leak is identified, prolonged (20 minutes or more) extrinsic compression of the area with the ultrasound transducer may result in thrombosis of the pseudoaneurysm and closure of the defect (see Fig. 66-13).[36] If unsuccessful, surgery, frequently under local anesthesia, can easily close the puncture site. Meticulous attention to achieving hemostasis after the procedure is helpful in preventing this complication.

Aneurysms or pseudoaneurysms may be seen at angioplasty or endarterectomy sites (Fig. 66-14). Their manifestations and management are similar to those seen after graft surgery. Noninvasive methods are usually used for detection, and arteriography is performed to delineate the vascular anatomy.

Failure of Prosthetic Materials

Deterioration of prosthetic materials may be the source of clinical problems.[19] Aneurysmal dilatation of synthetic grafts or veins, which may lead to rupture or loss of integrity of the anastomoses due to deterioration of the suture material, is a well-recognized

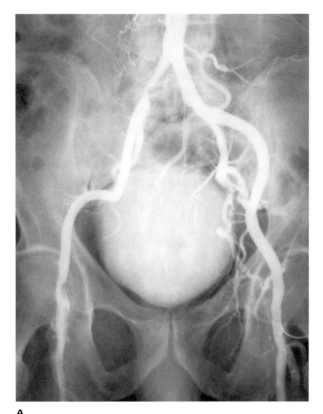

A

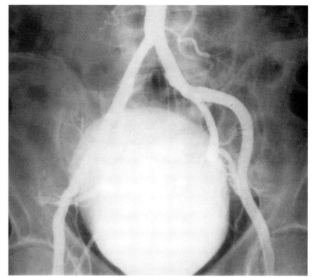

B

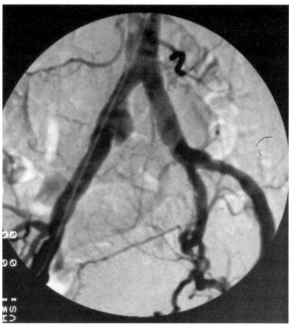

C

Figure 66-14. (A) Pelvic arteriogram showing an eccentric obstructive lesion of the right common iliac artery. (B) Post–percutaneous transluminal angioplasty (PTA) arteriogram shows an excellent result with a smooth lumen. (C) An arteriogram was repeated 16 months after the PTA because of recurrent symptoms. At the PTA site there is now an aneurysm that was clinically unsuspected.

Figure 66-15. This patient with a previously placed aortobifemoral graft was seen because of fever. CT-guided aspiration of the fluid contained within the aortic wall, which had been wrapped around the graft, was positive for *Staphylococcus aureus* on both Gram stain and culture.

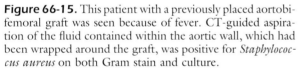

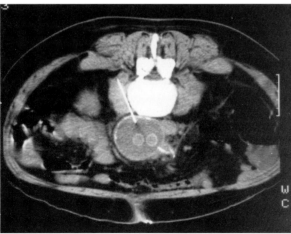

problem and is greatly reduced by the use of newer synthetics. Generally, the manifestations are those associated with true or false aneurysms of any cause, and the arteriographic approach is similar to that previously discussed.

Aspiration of Paraprosthetic Fluid

If a fluid collection is identified in a paraprosthetic position with ultrasound or CT guidance, it may be possible to aspirate some of it and subject the fluid to microbiological analysis (Fig. 66-15).[20,37] If an organism is recovered that is susceptible to antibiotic treatment, it may be possible to eradicate the infection without having to remove the prosthesis. However, removal of the graft is usually necessary and is done under appropriate antibiotic coverage.

Magnetic Resonance Imaging and Angiography

Magnetic resonance imaging (MRI) and angiography (MRA) are being extensively investigated. Catheter angiography with intravascular injection has not been replaced by MRA. However, MRA, which is undergoing rapid technical advances, may assume an important role in vascular evaluation in the near future.

In 1989, Auffermann and colleagues[38] reported encouraging work in the differentiation of perigraft infection from postoperative changes. This work was based on a small series, and confirmatory work has not been forthcoming.

References

1. Crawford ES, Manning LG, Kelley TF. "Redo" surgery after operations for aneurysm and occlusion of the abdominal aorta. Surgery 1977;81:41.
2. Naylor AR, Ah-See AK, Engeset J. Graft occlusion following aortofemoral bypass for peripheral ischaemia. Br J Surg 1989; 76(6):572–575.
3. van den Akker PH, van Schilfgaarde R, Brand R, van Bockel JH, Terpstra JL. Long term success of aortoiliac operation for atherosclerotic obstructive disease. Surgery 1992;174:485–496.
4. Thompson WM, Johnsrude IS, Jackson DC, Older TA, Wechsler AS. Late complications of abdominal aortic reconstructive surgery. Ann Surg 1977;183:326.
5. Vine HS, Sacks BA. Visualization of the distal arterial vessels in complete aortic occlusion. AJR 1980;134:847.
6. White RI Jr. Angiography of the abdominal aorta and its branches. In: White RI Jr, ed. Fundamentals of vascular radiology. Philadelphia: Lea & Febiger, 1976:53.
7. Eisenberg RL, Mani RL, McDonald EJ Jr. The complication rate of catheter angiography by direct puncture through aortofemoral bypass grafts. Am J Roentgenol 1976;126:814.
8. Crummy AB, et al. Computerized fluoroscopy: a digital subtraction technique for intravenous angiocardiography and arteriography. Am J Roentgenol 1980;135:1131.
9. Mistretta CM, Crummy AB. Digital fluoroscopy. In: Coulam CM, Erickson JJ, Rollo FD, James AE Jr, eds. The physical basis of medical imaging. New York: Appleton-Century-Crofts, 1981:107–122.
10. Strother CM, Sackett JF, Crummy AB, et al. Clinical applications of computerized fluoroscopy: the extracranial carotid artery. Radiology 1980;136:780.
11. Crummy AB, Rankin RS, Turnipseed WD, Berkoff HA. Biplane arteriography in ischemia of the lower extremity. Radiology 1978;126:111.
12. Crummy AB, Sherry JJ, Ahlstrand RA. A technique for peripheral arteriography using tolazoline. Australas Radiol 1973;17: 309.
13. Knudson JA, Downs AR. Reoperation following failure of aorto-iliofemoral arterial reconstruction. Can J Surg 1978;21: 316.
14. Downs AR. Management of aortofemoral graft limb occlusion. In: Bergan JJ, Yao JST, eds. Surgery of the aorta and its body branches. New York: Grune & Stratton, 1979:551.
15. Chung CJ, Hicklin A, Payan JM, Gordon L. Indium-111-labeled leukocyte scan in detection of synthetic vascular graft infection: the effect of antibiotic treatment. J Nucl Med 1991; 32:13–15.
16. Okike S, Bernatz PE. The role of the deep femoral artery in revascularization of the lower extremity. Mayo Clin Proc 1976; 51:209.
17. Hill DA, McGrath MA, Lord RSA, Tracy GD. The effect of superficial femoral artery occlusion on the outcome of aortofemoral bypass for intermittent claudication. Surgery 1980;87: 113.
18. Mani RL, Costin BS. Catheter angiography through aortofemoral grafts: prevention of catheter separation during withdrawal. Am J Roentgenol 1977;128:328–329.
19. Greenhalgh RM, Chir M. Dilation and stretching of knitted Dacron grafts associated with failure. In: Bergan JJ, Yao JST, eds. Surgery of the aorta and its body branches. New York: Grune & Stratton, 1979:621.
20. Harris KA, Kozak R, Carroll SE, Meads GE, Sweeney JP. Confirmation of infection of an aortic graft. J Cardiovasc Surg 1989;30(2):230–232.
21. Hollier LH, Batson RC, Cohn IJ Jr. Femoral anastomotic aneurysms. Ann Surg 1980;191:715.
22. Dubost C, Allary M, Oeconomos N. Resection of an aneurysm of the abdominal aorta: reestablishment of the continuity by a preserved human arterial graft with result after five months. Arch Surg 1952;64:405.
23. Szilagyi DE, Smith RF, Elliott JP, Vrandecic MP. Infection in arterial reconstruction with synthetic grafts. Ann Surg 1972; 176:321.
24. Veith FJ. Surgery of the infected aortic graft. In: Bergan JJ, Yao JST, eds. Surgery of the aorta and its body branches. New York: Grune & Stratton, 1979:521.
25. Jarrett F, Darling RC, Mundth ED, Austen WG. Experience with infected aneurysms of the abdominal aorta. Arch Surg 1975;110:1281.
26. Scher LA, Brener BJ, Goldenkranz RJ, Alpert J, Brief DK, Parsonnet V, Tiro AC. Infected aneurysms of the abdominal aorta. Arch Surg 1980;115:975.
27. Low RN, Wall SD, Jeffrey RB Jr, Sollitto RA, Reilly LM, Tierney LM Jr. Aortoenteric fistula and perigraft infection: evaluation with CT. Radiology 1990;175(1):157–162.
28. Bernard VM, Leinman LH. Aortoenteric fistulas. In: Bergan JJ, Yao JST, eds. Surgery of the aorta and its body branches. New York: Grune & Stratton, 1979:591.
29. Vorne M, Laitinen R, Lantto T, Jarvi K, Toivio I, Mokka R. Chronic prosthetic vascular graft infection visualized with technetium-99m-hexamethylpropyleneamine oxime-labeled leukocytes. J Nucl Med 1991;32:1425–1427.
30. Ehrenfeld WK, Wilbur BG, Olcott CN, Stoney RJ. Autogenous

tissue reconstruction in the management of infected prosthetic grafts. Surgery 1979;85:82.

31. Brock RC. Aortic homografting: a report of six successful cases. Guy's Hosp Rep 1953;102:204.

32. Calligaro KD, Bergen WS, Savarese RP, Westcott CJ, Azurin DJ, DeLaurentis DA. Primary aortoduodenal fistula due to septic aortitis. J Cardiovasc Surg 1992;33(2):192–198.

33. Thompson WM, Jackson DC, Johnsrude IS. Aortoenteric and paraprosthetic-enteric fistulas: radiologic findings. Am J Roentgenol 1976;127:235.

34. Igidbashian VN, Mitchell DG, Middleton WD, Schwartz RA, Goldberg BB. Iatrogenic femoral arteriovenous fistula: diagnosis with color Doppler imaging. Radiology 1989;170:749–752.

35. Littooy FN, Baker WH. Major arteriovenous fistulas of the aortic territory. In: Bergan JJ, Yao JST, eds. Surgery of the aorta and its body branches. New York: Grune & Stratton, 1979: 605.

36. Fellmeth BD, Roberts AC, Bookstein JJ, Freischlag JA, Forsythe JR, Buckner NK, Hye RJ. Postangiographic femoral artery injuries: nonsurgical repair with ultrasound guided compression. Radiology 1991;178:671–675.

37. Tobin KA. Aortobifemoral perigraft abscess: treatment by percutaneous catheter drainage. J Vasc Surg 1988;8:339–343.

38. Auffermann W, Olofsson PA, Rabahie GN, Tavares NJ, Stoney RJ, Higgins CB. Incorporation vs infection of retroperitoneal aortic grafts: MR imaging features. Radiology 1989;172(2): 359–362.

67

Femoral Arteriography

JOSEPH F. POLAK

Historical Background

Femoral arteriography remains the gold standard for depicting lower extremity arterial anatomy and the last step in the preoperative evaluation of patients with peripheral arterial disease. The focus of the examination has shifted somewhat since improvements in the techniques of revascularization, both by surgery[1] and by percutaneous transluminal angioplasty,[2,3] have created the need for a more careful delineation of the extent of arterial disease and better characterization of the distal runoff branches.

Noninvasive screening techniques now identify patients with clinically suspected peripheral vascular disease. Pressure measurements at rest and at exercise[4,5] as well as other noninvasive examinations such as Doppler waveform analysis and pressure volume recordings[6] have eliminated the need to obtain arteriograms in patients who have normal noninvasive studies. Because of its very high sensitivity in identifying patent distal target vessels in the leg and foot, peripheral vascular magnetic resonance angiography (MRA) is assuming an important role in the preoperative evaluation of patients undergoing distal bypass grafting.[7]

Technical Advances

Digital technology has been responsible for an interesting evolution in the way peripheral arteriography is performed. Efforts to eliminate the "invasive" entry of a catheter into an artery and therefore reduce complication rates led to the introduction of intravenous digital subtraction angiography. Although less invasive, this technique requires the injection of large amounts of iodinated contrast material. Because of this constraint and the fact that the concentration of agent finally reaching the leg arteries is low, the technical success rates and overall quality of the examinations are less than adequate. The realization that the "cut film" could be eliminated from the imaging chain, thereby decreasing costs without reducing accuracy,[8]

has led to the adoption of digital imaging as a critical component of modern arteriography. Rather than rely on subtraction techniques, the digital interface can now acquire and store images of diagnostic quality. This reduces the time taken for image processing and facilitates a wide variety of percutaneous interventions.[9]

Procedural Advances

The realization that digital subtraction techniques could be used to image after the injection of dilute amounts of iodinated contrast material parallels the development of smaller-caliber catheters. The outpatient procedures previously possible with the intravenous digital angiogram became more common with the smaller-caliber intraarterial catheters (4 or 5 French). Imaging time and catheter residence times are further reduced when the digital arteriogram is used.

Arterial access has also changed dramatically. The translumbar approach has been replaced by the common femoral artery access. Axillary and brachial approaches are common practice.[10–12] Percutaneous interventions—angioplasty and thrombolysis—in the femoral and infrapopliteal arteries also require newer approaches. Antegrade common femoral artery punctures have become routine, and so has the judicious use of tandem systems such as the arterial sheath and the coaxial small-caliber (3 French) catheters.

Arteriographic Anatomy

Normal Anatomy

The description of the normal arterial anatomy and collateral circulation of the pelvis and lower extremities is derived from several standard texts[13–15] and articles.[16,17]

The common femoral artery is the continuation of the external iliac artery distal to the inguinal ligament

1697

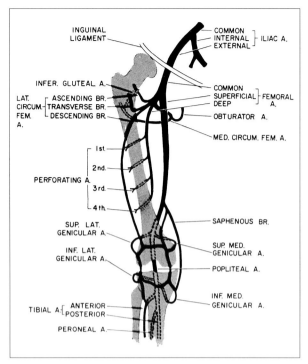

INGUINAL
LIGAMENT

COMMON
INTERNAL ⎤ ILIAC A.
EXTERNAL

INFER. GLUTEAL A.

COMMON
SUPERFICIAL ⎤ FEMORAL
DEEP   A.

LAT. ⎡ ASCENDING BR.
CIRCUM.┤ TRANSVERSE BR.
FEM. ⎣ DESCENDING BR.
A.

OBTURATOR A.

MED. CIRCUM. FEM. A.

1st.

2nd.

PERFORATING A.

3rd.

4th.

SUP. LAT.
GENICULAR A.

SAPHENOUS BR.

SUP. MED.
GENICULAR A.

INF. LAT.
GENICULAR A.

POPLITEAL A.

INF. MED.
GENICULAR A.

TIBIAL A.⎡ ANTERIOR
         ⎣ POSTERIOR

PERONEAL A.

Figure 67-1. Composite drawing of the normal anatomy of the femoral artery, its branches, the distal runoff arteries, and the potential collateral vessels.

(Fig. 67-1). The common femoral artery gives off a deep branch, the profunda femoris, medial to the neck of the femur. The continuation of the common femoral artery in the thigh is the superficial femoral artery, which runs medial and anterior to the femur. More traditional textbooks of anatomy do not favor the term *superficial femoral artery* but rather refer to the *femoral artery* when describing the main conduit artery between the common femoral and popliteal arteries.

The profunda femoris artery (see Fig. 67-1) is the most significant branch of the common femoral artery because it serves as the main blood supply to the thigh muscles. It is the prime collateral vessel to the leg when the superficial femoral artery is occluded. The profunda femoris and superficial femoral arteries are nearly equal in caliber at their origins. The profunda femoris divides rapidly into several branches: the medial circumflex femoral, lateral circumflex femoral, perforating, and muscular branches (see Fig. 67-1). The medial circumflex artery divides into several branches, one or more of which anastomose with the obturator and internal pudendal branches of the internal iliac artery.

The lateral circumflex femoral artery (see Fig. 67-1) divides into the ascending, transverse, and descending branches. These vessels anastomose with the superior and inferior gluteal branches of the internal iliac, the

deep iliac circumflex branch of the external iliac, and the first perforating arteries. The medial and lateral circumflex femoral branches constitute important collateral pathways when the common and external iliac or common femoral arteries are occluded. The lateral descending branch of the lateral circumflex artery supplies the more common donor site for myocutaneous flaps taken over the adductor muscle in the distal thigh.

The four perforating branches of the profunda femoris artery descend caudally along the posteromedial aspect of the femur and obliquely penetrate the adductor magnus muscle to reach the back of the thigh. The terminal branches of these perforating arteries anastomose freely with the small muscular branches of the superficial femoral artery (Fig. 67-2).

The superficial femoral artery functions primarily as a conduit to supply blood to the knee and calf areas. In the thigh it gives off some small muscular branches and the descending genicular or saphenous artery (see Fig. 67-1). The superficial femoral artery lies medial to the femur and in the lower third of the thigh runs posteriorly to pass through the adductor canal. As it passes through this tendinous hiatus in the adductor magnus muscle, the vessel becomes the popliteal artery.

The popliteal artery lies posterior in the intercondylar (popliteal) fossa (Fig. 67-3; see also Fig. 67-1) and continues across the knee joint to end in three terminal branches. The important anastomotic branches of the popliteal artery are the superior and inferior medial and lateral genicular vessels (see Figs. 67-3 and 67-4; see also Fig. 67-1). The genicular branches join with the descending branches of the lateral and circumflex arteries and the descending genicular branch of the superficial femoral artery to form collaterals around the knee when the popliteal artery is occluded. The sural branches supplying the lateral and medial heads of the gastrocnemius form another possible collateral pathway (see Fig. 67-3).

The distal runoff arteries, the anterior and posterior tibial and peroneal arteries, are the three terminal branches of the popliteal artery. These vessels supply blood to the several calf muscles. The anterior tibial artery runs anteriorly through the interosseous membrane between the tibia and the fibula (see Fig. 67-1). It is the only major artery in the anterior muscle compartment of the lower leg and continues into the foot as the dorsalis pedis artery. The posterior tibial artery is the direct continuation of the popliteal artery. It supplies the muscles of the posterior compartment and is the nutrient artery to the tibia; it continues into the foot along the medial malleolus. The peroneal artery is the third terminal branch of the popliteal artery

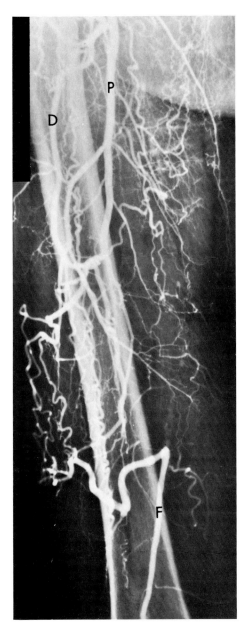

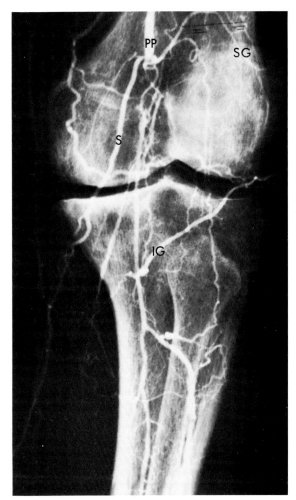

Figure 67-3. In response to a segmental occlusion of the popliteal artery (*PP*), several collateral branches have developed at the knee: the lateral superior genicular (*SG*), the lateral inferior genicular (*IG*), and the sural (*S*). Other, unnamed collateral branches are also present.

Figure 67-2. In the thigh, the profunda femoris artery (*P*) and its descending lateral circumflex branch (*D*) form the principal collateral circulation between the pelvis and the lower leg when the superficial femoral artery is occluded. The distal superficial femoral artery (*F*) is reconstituted via the collateral circulation.

and lies between the anterior and posterior tibial arteries. It provides branches to the calf muscles and is the nutrient artery to the fibula. Its more terminal branches can cross the ankle and anastomose with the plantar arch. The plantar arch is formed by the confluence of terminal branches from the posterior tibial artery with branches from the dorsalis pedis artery. The lateral and medial plantar branches are a continuation

of the posterior tibial artery. The plantar arch is formed by a continuation of the lateral plantar artery that joins the deep plantar branch of the dorsalis pedis artery. This deep arch courses underneath the metatarsals, giving off plantar metatarsal branches. The distal dorsalis pedis artery also gives off superficial branches that join the lateral tarsal branch, forming the equivalent of a superficial arch.

Anatomic Variants

Anomalies of the leg arteries are rare above the knee. A persistent sciatic artery can be seen in 0.03 percent of the population. The presence of this artery, originating from the internal iliac artery and extending to the popliteal, is normally associated with an underdeveloped

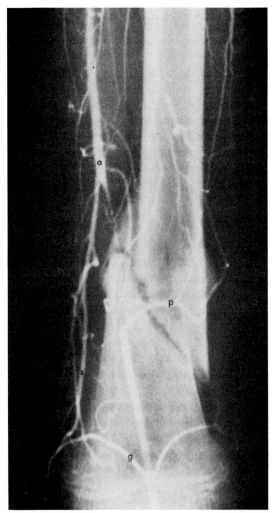

Figure 67-4. This late posttrauma arteriogram was done to evaluate the extent of arterial injury. The fractured femur has caused segmental occlusion of the superficial femoral artery (*a*). The collateral circulation is composed of the profunda femoris (*p*), the saphenous branch (*s*), and the medial genicular (*g*) arteries.

superficial femoral artery. There is also a strong association between persistent sciatic arteries and the presence of aneurysms in the gluteal region.[17a] On occasion, the profunda femoral artery can arise higher than expected near to the external iliac artery and take a medial course. Duplications of the superficial artery can also be seen. The presence of a saphenous artery that courses parallel with the saphenous vein has been reported in 0.02 percent of a large case series.[17b] The two variations most frequently encountered in the runoff branches involve the peroneal and anterior tibial arteries. Normally, the peroneal artery is a branch from a shared trunk with the posterior tibial artery (see Fig. 67-1). However, as a variant, it may rise from a shared trunk with the anterior tibial artery (Fig.

67-5). This configuration, which is a mirror image of the normal anatomy, may be present unilaterally or bilaterally.

The other common variation relates to the origin of the anterior tibial artery. This vessel usually originates from the popliteal artery at the level of the interosseous notch between the tibia and the fibula. As a variant, this vessel may arise more cephalad, near the knee joint or even above it (Fig. 67-6). In rare instances, the posterior tibial artery may be atrophic or nondeveloped, resulting in a two-vessel runoff.

Collateral Circulation

The collateral circulation, when pelvic or lower extremity arteries are occluded, involves the branches of the internal iliac artery (Fig. 67-7). This is part of the visceral collateral circulation because the internal iliac artery anastomoses with the mesenteric vessels (Fig. 67-8). The external iliac artery, via its deep circumflex iliac and inferior epigastric branches, also contributes to the collateral circulation of the leg (Fig. 67-9). This is part of the parietal collateral circulation. The internal iliac artery divides into an anterior and a posterior portion. The obturator and internal pudendal arteries, which are branches of the anterior division of the internal iliac artery, anastomose with the medial circumflex femoral branches of the profunda femoris artery. The superior and inferior gluteal arteries, which are posterior division branches, anastomose with the lateral circumflex femoral artery. The branches of the internal iliac artery are all paired, but only the obturator, internal pudendal, and lateral sacral arteries anastomose transversely with their contralateral partners. The posterior division branches, the superior and inferior gluteal arteries, anastomose only ipsilaterally.

The common and superficial femoral arteries are devoid of any branches that anastomose with the pelvic arteries. The profunda femoris artery, through its medial and lateral circumflex femoral branches, anastomoses extensively with the pelvic arteries. The profunda femoris artery also anastomoses freely with the popliteal artery branches around the knee via the descending lateral circumflex and the perforating branches. Thus, when the superficial femoral artery is occluded, the profunda femoris artery is the single most important vessel involved in the thigh collateral network between the pelvis and the lower leg (see Fig. 67-2).

At the knee level, when the popliteal artery is occluded, collateral circulation develops to reconstitute the distal runoff arteries. This circulation largely comprises small, unnamed branches from the medial and lateral genicular, popliteal, superficial femoral, and

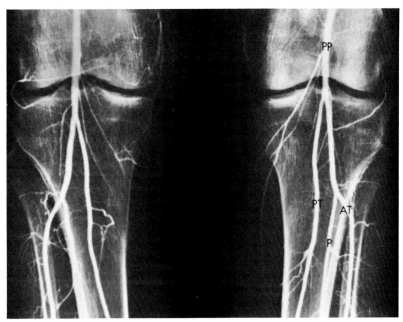

Figure 67-5. The origin of the distal runoff arteries is anomalous, bilaterally. Normally the posterior tibial (*PT*) and peroneal (*P*) arteries arise from a common trunk (see Fig. 67-1). In this anomaly there is a mirror image reversal of the normal, with the anterior tibial (*AT*) and peroneal arteries arising from a common trunk off the popliteal artery (*PP*).

Figure 67-6. The origin of the left anterior tibial artery (*AT*) is anomalous. The right anterior tibial artery arises normally at the proximal end of the interosseous membrane, whereas the left arises near the knee joint space. The posterior tibial (*PT*) and peroneal (*P*) arteries are normal bilaterally.

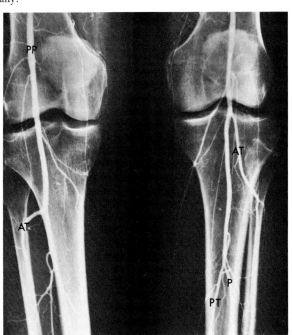

Figure 67-7. Multiple iliac artery occlusions with mainly visceral or left internal iliac branch artery collateral circulation reconstituting the right profunda femoris (*P*) and the left common femoral (*CF*), superficial femoral (*F*), and profunda femoris (*P*) arteries. The internal iliac branches that form the collaterals are the superior gluteal (*SG*), inferior gluteal (*IG*), obturator (*O*), lateral sacral (*LS*), and iliolumbar (*IL*). The profunda femoris (*P*) branches that complete the collateral circulation are the medial (*MC*) and lateral (*LC*) circumflex femoral arteries. The obturator (*O*) and lateral sacral (*LS*) arteries send branches across the pelvis to their counterparts on the contralateral side. *C1,* common iliac artery; *DIC,* deep iliac circumflex branch.

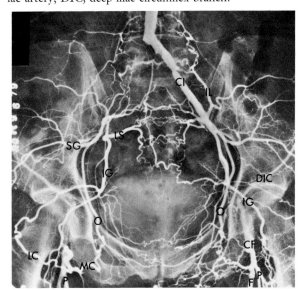

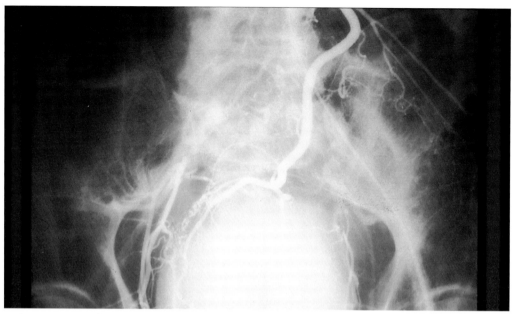

Figure 67-8. Arteriogram performed with a selective injection into the inferior mesenteric artery. A collateral branch communicates to the internal iliac artery (*arrow*). Flow is then directed into the external iliac artery. The underlying lesion is one of obstruction of the common iliac artery.

Figure 67-9. (A) Multiple iliac artery occlusions with both visceral and parietal collateral circulation. The right collaterals are visceral, the branches of the internal iliac artery (see Fig. 67-7 for abbreviations). The left collaterals are mainly parietal. *IP*, internal pudendal. (B) The right common iliac and internal iliac arteries are patent, and the remaining major pelvic vessels are occluded except for the reconstituted left common femoral artery. The left parietal collateral circulation comprises a lumbar artery (*L*) anastomosing with the deep iliac circumflex branch of the external iliac artery. The left superficial femoral and profunda femoris arteries are patent. The left internal iliac artery branches reconstitute only minimally. (See Fig. 67-7 for abbreviations.)

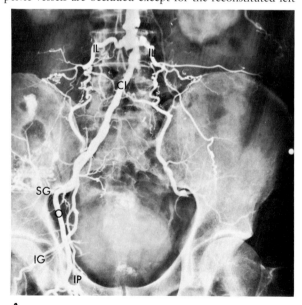

A

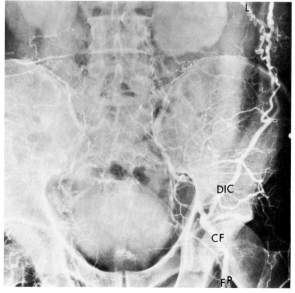

B

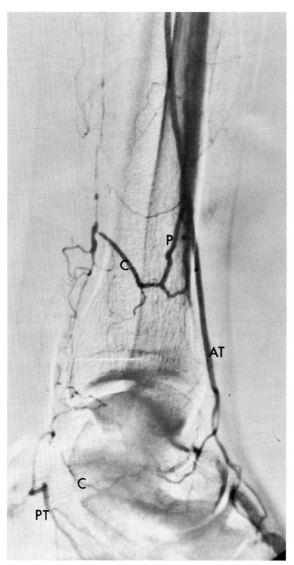

Figure 67-10. Subtraction film of the ankle in the oblique position demonstrates some of the unnamed collaterals (*C*) derived from the peroneal (*P*) and anterior tibial (*AT*) arteries. Only the distal posterior tibial artery (*PT*) reconstitutes via collateral circulation.

profunda femoris arteries (see Fig. 67-3). The level at which the popliteal artery is occluded helps to determine the source of the collaterals. More frequently at this site than elsewhere in the lower extremity, the collateral vessels are not particularly dilated and may not be very tortuous. Branches from the medial genicular arteries tend to reconstitute the posterior tibial artery, whereas the lateral genicular arteries reconstitute the anterior tibial artery.

At the ankle the peroneal artery may provide collateral circulation to both the anterior and posterior tibial arteries. When the posterior tibial artery is occluded at

its origin or elsewhere in the calf, its continuation into the foot may nevertheless still be patent; reconstitution occurs via a collateral from the peroneal artery just above the ankle joint. The posterior and anterior tibial arteries may also contribute to each other just below the ankle joint (Fig. 67-10).

Puncture and Catheterization

Catheter selection and catheter access vary with the type of angiography performed as well as with the type of arterial pathology being studied. For example, the intravenous digital arteriogram was very popular in the mid-1980s. Because large volumes of contrast needed to be injected as a short bolus, large-diameter catheters needed to be positioned either in the vena cava or in the right atrium.

Improvements in digital imaging techniques and the use of smaller-sized catheters, especially in digital subtraction arteriography, have helped in the trend toward outpatient studies[18] and encouraged more complex interventions.[19]

Retrograde Femoral Artery Approach

Percutaneous retrograde transfemoral catheterization is the common method for evaluating the aorta and lower extremity arteries. In 1953, when Seldinger[20] described the ingeniously simple technique of percutaneous catheterization, most major centers abandoned the translumbar technique. A 1975 review[21] describes the evolution of the various catheters, techniques, and angiographic equipment used in examining patients with obstructive peripheral vascular disease. The transfemoral catheter technique of arteriography facilitates examination of the aorta (for inflow disease) and permits serial filming of the pelvis, thigh, and runoff vessels in multiple views. These features are extremely important for complete evaluation of obstructive peripheral vascular disease.

The arterial puncture site for catheterization is determined according to the clinically symptomatic area and the presence of an accessible pulse. Puncture of the femoral artery is preferred because of the artery's proximity to the aorta and lower extremities and its superficial location in the inguinal area. If both femoral artery pulses are palpable, the least symptomatic extremity is selected for catheterization. Thus one can avoid such potential postcatheterization problems[22] as (1) a hematoma at the puncture site that could interfere with a subsequent bypass graft or further compromise the circulation to a partially ischemic leg, (2) the possibility that manual compression of the puncture site to prevent bleeding could induce further thrombosis of a partially compromised circulation, or (3) a folliculitis secondary to shaving of the groin on the same side that will have surgery.

Occasionally, the aorta or iliac arteries are found to be totally or subtotally occluded. Transfemoral catheterization with retrograde injection of contrast is another technique for demonstrating the lower extremity arteries. A small-diameter catheter (4 French) or sheath can be placed into the artery and attached to flexible tubing, which in turn is connected via a stopcock to the pressure injector. The major disadvantages of this technique are a lack of adequate contrast visualization of the proximal iliac arteries and abdominal aorta and the need to catheterize both femoral arteries to study the peripheral circulation in both legs. The problem of subtotal occlusion of the iliac artery on the side of arterial access may occasionally warrant more aggressive management once the diagnostic catheter crosses the lesion and occludes the lumen. Aggressive anticoagulation and possible angioplasty should be considered.

When catheterization is performed, sterile precautions are observed by the angiographer and his or her assistants. The previously shaved puncture site is cleansed with a suitable skin antiseptic solution (Betadine), and the area is draped with sterile towels. The femoral artery is punctured below the inguinal ligament to avoid potential retroperitoneal or scrotal hematomas after the procedure. The femoral puncture site is approximately 1 to 2 cm below the inguinal skin crease, or below an imaginary line drawn between the anterior superior iliac spine and the pubic eminence. Fluoroscopy can be used to confirm that needle entry into the common femoral artery will take place at the junction of the middle and proximal third of the femoral head. Local anesthesia at the puncture site is provided by the injection of 10 ml of 2 percent Xylocaine (lidocaine). It is important to infiltrate the femoral artery sheath on each side to minimize pain and avoid local arterial spasm.

A Seldinger-type needle is used to puncture the artery. The overlying skin is nicked with a scalpel blade to ease passage of the needle, and an attempt is made to traverse the artery by passing through both the anterior and posterior walls. The needle stylet is removed, and the blunt cannula is withdrawn until a strong, steady flow of blood spurts from the cannula. Frequently a slight popping sensation is felt as the blunt cannula is withdrawn just before the steady backflow of blood is observed. The forceful spurt of blood indicates that the blunt cannula tip is free in the vessel lumen and well situated so that the guidewire can be inserted. Unless strong spurts of blood in time with the cardiac cycle are observed, no attempt should be made to pass the guidewire into the artery. Gentle injection of contrast, once blood return is confirmed, can be used to determine the reason for the decreased inflow. It is important that the guidewire move easily into the artery with a minimum of force; otherwise complications at the puncture site may occur. Passage of the guidewire through the pelvic arteries and aorta may be observed fluoroscopically, and the wire should be in the abdominal aorta before a catheter is introduced. A single-wall entry can be done with an open-tip, bevel-shaped needle. Once blood return is confirmed, the needle needs to be advanced a few millimeters before the wire is introduced. This approach is favored in patients who have bypass grafts because the first lumen encountered is normally that of the graft.

Guidewires are available in a variety of sizes, constructions, and coatings. The basic wire that has proved to be extremely effective in femoral arteriography is a 0.035- or 0.038-inch stainless steel wire with a fixed core and a 3-mm J shape. Wires with a straight flexible tip of 10 cm or more are often used to navigate tortuous or diseased arteries. Guidewires with movable cores seem to have no particular advantage in the routine situation. Guidewires that offer torque control and a more flexible tip are increasingly used to navigate the tortuous and severely diseased artery.

A wide choice of catheters is commercially available for percutaneous transfemoral arteriography. Most angiographers base their selection on the principle of using a catheter with the smallest outer diameter that will deliver the desired amount of contrast without rupturing. The most popular catheters used for femoral arteriography are 4 or 5 French size and either polyethylene or Teflon in composition. The transition away from larger-diameter 6 or 7 French catheters started with a 1977 report[23] that 5 French catheters may be equally effective and possibly safer because their smaller diameter causes less lumen obstruction and decreases the incidence of hematoma formation.[24] All these catheters are of the end-hole variety and may be either straight with side holes or pigtail-shaped with side holes. A tip occluder was originally used with the straight end-hole catheter[25] but is not necessary because of improvements in catheter design. The purpose of the pigtail shape is to ensure that the bulk of the injected contrast will exit via the catheter's side holes rather than through the end hole. The contrast emerging from the side holes is more readily directed into the aortic branches. The usual length of the catheter used is 80 to 100 cm, because this is appropriate for the moving-tabletop technique of serial filming. After the catheter is inserted into the artery, it is regularly flushed during the procedure every 3 to 4 minutes with a heparinized saline solution to prevent clotting.

In elderly patients referred for examination, the iliac arteries are often tortuous and partially obstructed by arteriosclerotic lesions. Therefore, it may be impossible or extremely difficult to pass the guidewire retrograde through the iliac arteries into the abdominal aorta. A J guidewire[26] is used first in an attempt to traverse the sites of resistance. Alternate strategies include the use of J-shaped catheters,[27] curved wires that offer some amount of directional or "torque" control, and finally the combination of a curved catheter with a "floppy tip" wire. Combining catheter and wire permits the injection of a test dose of contrast material in the iliac artery and instant fluoroscopic visualization of the extent and degree of obstruction. This information allows the angiographer to decide whether, in the partially obstructed vessel, retrograde catheterization is possible from the particular femoral puncture site. When retrograde transfemoral catheterization is impossible, the examination is generally completed from the transaxillary approach.

The arteriography is concluded by withdrawing the catheter and applying digital pressure at the puncture site. Usually pressure applied for 10 to 15 minutes is sufficient to prevent bleeding or hematoma formation at the puncture site. This is particularly important in hypertensive patients and in those who may have a coagulopathy. The patient is kept at bedrest for 4 to 6 hours after the procedure. A new technique of percutaneous sealing with a fibrin plug promises to eliminate the need to compress the artery.[28]

Antegrade Femoral Artery Approach

The antegrade femoral approach has gained popularity with the increased performance of femoral, popliteal, and infrapopliteal interventions.[29] Either the Seldinger needle or the single-wall needle can be used. Some manipulation is often needed to facilitate access from the common femoral artery to the superficial femoral branch. This often requires a wire that can be directed—"torqued"—in a selected direction. An arterial sheath is normally left in place.

The procedure after removal of the catheter is similar to that used after the traditional retrograde approach. Care should be given to compressing the artery over the needle entry site, now located distal to the skin entry site.

Axillary or Brachial Artery Approach

When both femoral pulses are absent, the axillary artery, especially the left one, is a suitable site for percutaneous catheterization.[30-32] Alternatively, the brachial artery can be used. Both approaches have equal or slightly higher morbidity than the transfemoral approach.[33,34] This increase in complication rate is, in part, explained by the fact that these patients tend to have more severe peripheral arterial disease.[35] In addition, catheter size is more critical when the brachial artery approach is used.[10] Although the risks of axillary plexus injury are eliminated by the transbrachial approach, it is also associated with a higher risk of arterial injuries and thrombotic events.[12]

Less Common Approaches

Graft Puncture Approach

Some angiographers still fear puncturing aortofemoral, femorofemoral, or axillobifemoral prosthetic bypass graft and consider their presence a relative contraindication to transfemoral catheterization because this may lead to complications of thrombosis or local bleeding.

Direct catheter entry through synthetic bypass grafts can be done safely[36] and does not appear to be associated with an increased risk to the patient.[37-39] Two additional concerns were originally expressed. The first was the possibility of seeding the graft with bacteria, a major concern of the vascular surgeon in the 1970s and 1980s. This concern has not been borne out over the years. The second was the possibility of damaging either the graft or the catheter used to perform the study. Although graft ruptures were described when the early Dacron grafts were entered, more modern grafts—Dacron as well as polytetrafluoropropylene—do not seem susceptible to this problem. The use of the single-wall needle technique is favored because this decreases the risk of traversing the graft and then entering the diseased native artery. This can be somewhat disconcerting in cases of iliac artery occlusion.

Axillofemoral bypass grafts are easily entered because they lie in the subcutaneous tissues of the chest and abdomen. The entry site selected is usually proximal. A small sheath or catheter is normally placed pointing toward the graft origin so that reflux during a forceful injection will opacify the proximal anastomosis.

Translumbar Approach

Historically, translumbar aortography, introduced by dos Santos,[40] was the technique first employed. Direct needle puncture translumbar aortography remains an alternative to percutaneous peripheral artery catheterization, and a variation of this technique uses a catheter.[41,42] Although still done on occasion, it is now rarely needed. Although considered a safe approach, the use of computed tomography (CT) has shown that almost all patients have large periaortic hematoma following translumbar catheterization.[43,44] A small percentage of these actually cause clinical symptoms.

Popliteal Artery Approach

Direct access into the popliteal artery can be used to enter the femoropopliteal artery when attempts are made to recanalize the distal femoral or the proximal popliteal arteries.[45] The anatomic location of the artery[46] can be determined with the use of ultrasound imaging before or during the puncture.

Transvenous Approach

Placement of larger-diameter catheters for intravenous digital subtraction angiography is normally done through the basilic vein. On occasion, more central access through the internal jugular or common femoral veins can be chosen.[47] These approaches, popular in the early 1980s, have been replaced by more direct arterial access with smaller-diameter catheters.

Filming Equipment

Serial Filming

Aortogram

The diffuse nature of obstructive vascular disease makes it imperative that the abdominal aorta and its branches be examined as part of femoral arteriography. Thus potential inflow and the branch artery obstructions are certain to be visualized. When retrograde transfemoral catheterization is the method of approach, the catheter tip is positioned in the aorta at the T12-L1 interspace with the side holes opposite the renal arteries. Serial films are obtained in the anteroposterior and additional oblique or lateral positions, either simultaneously or successively. The lateral view often provides information not obvious in the anteroposterior view. Approximately 40 to 50 ml of contrast is injected, at a flow rate to 20 to 25 ml per minute, to opacify the abdominal aorta. Films are obtained at a rate of two per second for 2 to 4 seconds, one per second for 3 to 5 seconds, and one every 2 seconds for 6 to 8 seconds. Variations from this basic filming rate are determined by a test injection of contrast into the aorta with fluoroscopic observation of its rate of clearance. If the contrast clearance is more rapid than normal, the filming rate is increased; conversely, if it is slower, the rate is decreased.

The aortogram can be performed at the beginning of the study or may follow the "runoff" study.

Peripheral Runoff

The femoral arteriogram, particularly in obstructive vascular disease, must demonstrate the anatomic integrity of the leg circulation from the aorta to the ankles. The pelvic "station" is normally included as part of the evaluation of the more distal arteries. In most cases, however, additional oblique views of the iliac arteries are necessary.

Over the years, various pieces of angiographic equipment have been devised to demonstrate the physiologic circulation of injected contrast material as it flows from the aorta toward the ankles. To demonstrate the blood flow, various design configurations have been used in which the patient, the x-ray tube, or the films are moved.[21] The shifts are made singly or in combination, in a sequential manner, as the injected contrast moves through the circulation. The earliest pieces of equipment all depended on manual power to supply movement. Film cassettes of varying sizes, x-ray tables of unique design, and tube stands of exceptional heights all have been proposed and have given limited acceptance.

Most femoral arteriography employs an automatic serial film changer and a programmable moving tabletop with synchronized kilovoltage regulation.[48] The patient on the table moves over the film changer. The specific areas of interest—namely, the pelvis, thigh, knee, and runoff—are sequentially filmed automatically after a single injection of radiopaque contrast material.

For pelvic and lower extremity filming, the catheter is pulled down and positioned with the tip 4 cm above the aortic bifurcation, so that the side holes remain proximal to the bifurcation. The moving tabletop is programmed to stop serially and film the pelvic, thigh, knee, and runoff arteries. A single bolus of 60 to 90 ml of contrast, injected at a rate of 6 to 10 ml per second, is usually adequate to opacify the pelvic and leg arteries to the ankle. The contrast injection triggers the sequential filming and movement of the table. The film exposure rate is as follows: pelvis, one per second for 4 seconds; thigh, one per second for 3 seconds; knee, one per second for 4 seconds; and lower leg, one per second for 4 seconds. In some patients the pattern of their obstructive disease causes unequal circulation times between the two extremities; in these cases the standard filming sequence may fail to demonstrate adequately the anatomy of the two sides. In this event, the filming rate must be altered according to the observed flow and the nonvisualized circulation must be reexamined. Another strategy is to delay the onset of filming by a selected amount of time. In general, this delay can be calculated by measuring the arrival time of contrast in the popliteal artery segment following a short 5- to 10-ml bolus injection.

Digital Subtraction Imaging

Intraarterial Imaging

Intraarterial digital subtraction angiography is normally performed at a fixed station.[35,49] A preselected delay is chosen to minimize filming when there is no contrast present within the artery.[50] Imaging is conducted at a rate similar to that of a one-station "cut-film" angiogram.

For subtraction techniques, contrast is normally diluted 1:3. Volumes can also be reduced by a factor of 2 without compromising good-quality imaging. Image "masks" must be acquired before the contrast reaches the arterial segment in question. These are used as the background image to be subtracted from the contrast-containing image. Additional "late mask" images are acquired to compensate for possible patient motion.

Direct digital images mimic the "cut-film" arteriograms. Similar or slightly lower volumes of contrast—a function of device sensitivity—are injected. The images are digitized and acquired at the output of an imaging phosphor rather than exposed on a film emulsion. This leads to a significant cost savings during diagnostic studies as well as during interventions[7,9,51] without a significant loss of accuracy.[8] This type of imaging is normally done at one level or "station." Judicious timing of contrast table and patient motion with tracking of the bolus of contrast being injected creates a "digital runoff" study.[52] This approach requires greater technical skill than those mentioned previously.

Transvenous Imaging

This procedure is oriented to the outpatient.[53] The easiest access is the basilic vein of the arm, followed by the common femoral and jugular veins. The catheter is positioned centrally—in the superior vena cava or right atrium. Although large volumes of contrast are injected, only a small amount of markedly dilute material reaches the artery of interest.[54,55] Only a digital subtraction technique achieves sufficient contrast resolution to permit imaging of the peripheral arteries. Large delays (above 10 seconds) are needed because contrast must transit through the lungs into the left heart chambers and then to the peripheral arteries. The presence of vessel overlap requires that filming be done with multiple projections, which increases the number of injections dramatically. This type of study is decreasing in popularity. The major constraint is the amount of contrast necessary to achieve a study of diagnostic quality.[9]

Positioning

Peripheral Runoff

The principle of filming vessels in more than one view is well established in obstructive disease of the cerebral, coronary, and visceral circulations but is less well observed in peripheral vascular disease. Views of vessels in different planes generally offer additional information about the contour and lumen.

In general, the patient rests comfortably on his or her back. The legs are normally kept at a slight degree of internal rotation. The tube normally rotates when oblique and lateral views are needed. On older equipment, the patient must be positioned on top of a "wedge" of material if oblique views are needed.

Selected Projections

Native Arteries

When an aneurysm or obstructive lesion (Fig. 67-11) is present, a lateral view of the infrarenal aorta may demonstrate findings about the extent, location, and size of the lesion not available in the anteroposterior projection.[56–58] This is particularly important if bypass surgery is contemplated for a distal obstructive lesion. In that situation the severity of any inflow obstruction must be carefully assessed so that the blood flow is adequate to maintain graft patency.

Obstructive lesions in the pelvic arteries should also be viewed in more than one plane.[59,60] Unlike the aorta, in which the lateral view offers the best projection, the pelvic arteries are best studied in the oblique projection.[61] Initially a standard anteroposterior view of the pelvis should be obtained. If there is any suspicion of stenotic lesions in the iliac or common femoral arteries, the appropriate oblique view is filmed. It is not unusual that the anteroposterior view fails to separate the origins of the superficial and profunda femoris arteries at the bifurcation of the common femoral artery. An oblique view will separate the vessels and indicate the severity of any obstruction (Fig. 67-12). Similarly, the origin of the internal iliac artery may be inadequately visualized in the standard anteroposterior view and is better projected in the oblique (Fig. 67-13). Pelvic oblique views are valuable not only for imaging the native circulation but especially for evaluating bypass graft anastomoses (Figs. 67-14 and 67-15). The particular oblique projection used depends on

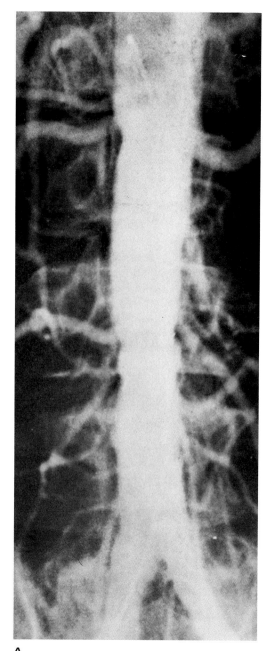

A

B

Figure 67-11. This patient has symptomatic peripheral vascular disease, a midline abdominal bruit, and diminished femoral artery pulses. (A) Anteroposterior view demonstrates only minimal arteriosclerotic changes of the abdominal aorta. (B) Lateral view reveals a large plaque extending into the lumen from the posterior wall (*dotted line*). This lesion causes inflow obstruction and was not appreciated in the anteroposterior view. There is also an associated celiac artery stenosis (*arrow*).

which vessel needs to be studied. The left posterior oblique (right anterior oblique) position is best for assessing the right common femoral bifurcation (superficial and profunda femoris arteries) and the bifurcation of the left common iliac (internal and external iliac) arteries. The reverse oblique projection, the right posterior oblique (left anterior oblique), best demonstrates the bifurcations in the opposite vessels. Thus the pelvic arteries are first studied in the anteroposterior projection, but, if any doubt remains about an inadequately visualized focal obstruction or bifurcation, the appropriate oblique view is obtained.

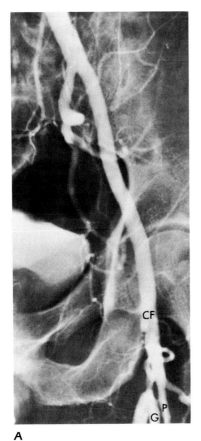

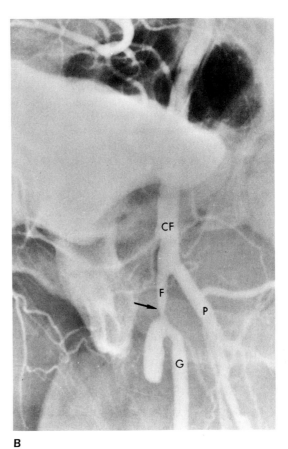

A　　　　　　　　　　**B**

Figure 67-12. Left femoropopliteal bypass graft. (A) Anteroposterior view does not clearly demonstrate any abnormality at the bifurcation of the common femoral artery (*CF*) into the graft (*G*) and profunda femoris artery (*P*). (B) Right posterior oblique view distinctly separates the origin of the graft (*G*) and profunda femoris artery (*P*). There is a definite proximal stenosis (*arrow*) of the occluded superficial femoral artery (*F*).

In the evaluation of obstructive lesions of the femoral, popliteal, and runoff arteries, the anteroposterior view generally suffices. It is often advantageous to obtain a simultaneous lateral view for better structural detail. A lateral view is useful for evaluating tumors and aneurysms in the thigh, knee, or calf area. At the ankle, the distal runoff arteries are best demonstrated when the feet are externally rotated because this rotation separates the vessels and sometimes moves them away from the dense cortex.[62]

Following Revascularization

Grafts. As mentioned, pelvic oblique views are especially valuable for evaluating bypass graft anastomoses (see Figs. 67-14 and 67-15). In general, the contralateral oblique projection to that used for the native artery will best demonstrate graft anastomoses to the common femoral artery. In addition, stenotic lesions either in the graft's conduit (vein grafts) or at the anastomoses can often be difficult to visualize unless additional oblique views are taken. These lesions are often asymptomatic[63] and can be focal or bandlike in appearance.

Percutaneous Angioplasty, Atherectomy, and Stent Placement. In general, a single projection is taken after an intervention in the femoral, popliteal, and infrapopliteal arteries. However, there is a question as to whether additional views are required when evaluating iliac lesions.

Selection of imaging technique plays a crucial role. Poorly performed digital arteriograms can mask lesions such as dissections. Additional views should generally be obtained whenever there is the slightest doubt about the results of an intervention.

Miscellaneous Approaches

In patients with aortic thrombosis or previous aortobifemoral bifurcation grafts, the left axillary artery approach to the abdominal aorta is used[30,31] rather than standard retrograde transfemoral catheterization. The patient with a peripheral artery aneurysm or an arterio-

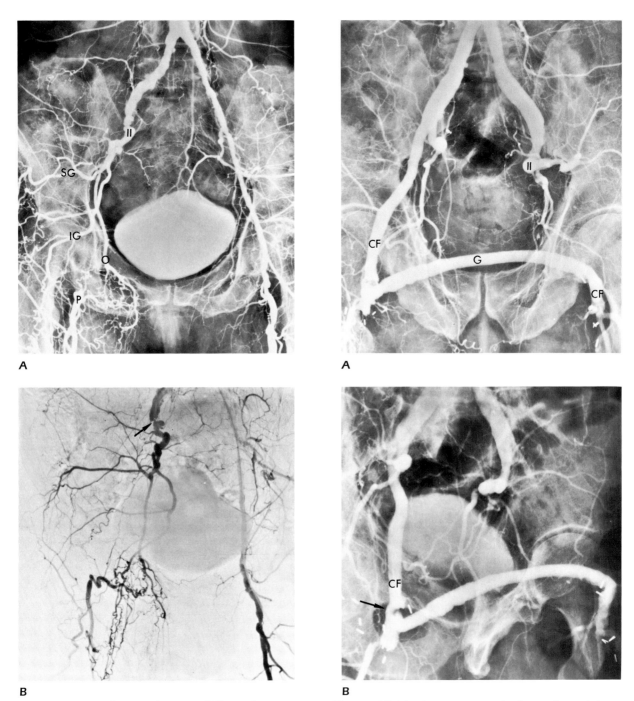

A

B

A

B

Figure 67-13. Occlusive right external iliac and common femoral disease and superficial femoral artery occlusion, same patient as in Figure 67-2. Reconstitution of the profunda femoris artery (*P*) to provide circulation to the leg depends on the collateral branches of the internal iliac artery (*II*). (A) Anteroposterior view shows arteriosclerotic changes at the origin of the internal iliac artery (see Fig. 67-7 for abbreviations). (B) Right posterior oblique view (subtraction) clearly shows the severe stenosis at the origin of the internal iliac artery (*arrow*).

Figure 67-14. An extraanatomic femorofemoral bypass graft was created to provide a blood supply to an ischemic left leg. The ischemia was secondary to occlusion of the left external iliac artery and inadequate collaterals from the internal iliac artery (*II*). (A) Anteroposterior view shows the patent graft (*G*) from the right to left common femoral artery (*CF*). (B) Left posterior oblique view shows the severe stenosis (*arrow*) of the right common femoral artery (*CF*). The stenosis was only questionable in the anteroposterior view.

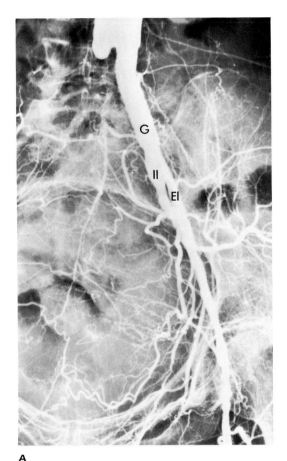

A

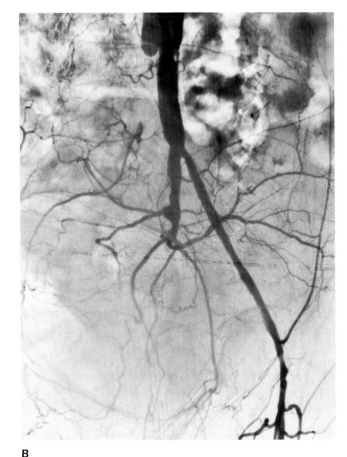

B

Figure 67-15. Because of an occluded right limb of an aortobiiliac bypass graft, a left-to-right femorofemoral bypass was contemplated in this patient to restore blood flow to the right leg. (A) Although the left graft limb (*G*) is patent, the bifurcation into the internal (*II*) and external (*EI*) arteries is overlapped and the vessel lumen size is uncertain. (B) Right posterior oblique view (subtraction) shows the distal anastomosis and bifurcation to be normal.

venous fistula will have an altered rate of blood flow at the site of interest. In this instance, the catheter is introduced on the same side as the lesion, and a change in the amount of contrast, rate of contrast injection, and filming is required. Because the low rate in an aneurysm is usually decreased, the injection and filming rates should be reduced. The reverse is true for an arteriovenous fistula. In both conditions, additional views to the standard anteroposterior projection may be helpful in demonstrating the lesions.

When a peripheral bone or soft tissue tumor is suspected, the femoral artery of the symptomatic leg is catheterized to enhance the degree of contrast filling in any tumor vessels. The catheter tip is positioned in the external iliac artery rather than at the aortic bifurcation. Magnification views of the tumor are helpful and should be obtained in more than one projection.

Special Techniques

Vasodilatation

In about 25 percent of all femoral arteriograms, the popliteal and particularly the distal runoff arteries (tibial and peroneal) are inadequately visualized for anatomic delineation.[64] The poor contrast visualization results from delayed or diminished blood flow to the lower leg. The decreased circulation may have a variety of causes, such as diminished cardiac output, vasoconstriction, a previous aortic bypass graft, an abdominal aortic aneurysm, and ectatic calcified arteries. Proximal obstruction in the aorta and iliac and superficial femoral arteries, as well as poor collateral circulation, compound the problem of diminished circulation.

The anatomic delineation of the distal runoff arter-

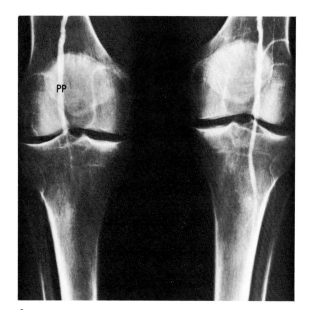

A

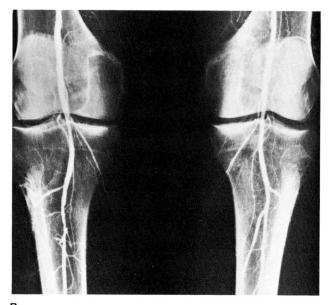

B

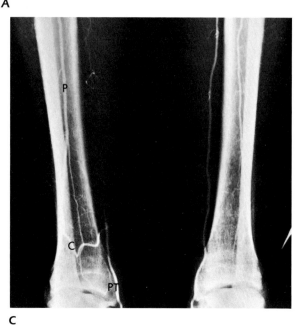

C

Figure 67-16. Combined lesion–occlusive peripheral vascular disease, involving the iliac and superficial femoral arteries, in the same patient as in Figure 67-7. (A) Initially the distal runoff arteries were not visualized; contrast demonstrated vessels only to the popliteal artery (*PP*) level at 11 seconds. (B) Following ischemic exercise the distal runoff vessels were seen at the knees and down to the ankles, at 7 seconds. The right posterior tibial artery is occluded. (C) The right posterior tibial artery (*PT*) reconstitutes at the ankle via a collateral (*C*) from the peroneal artery (*P*).

ies is important to determine the extent of the obstructive disease and the potential feasibility of revascularization to the popliteal and, more distally, to the peroneal or tibial arteries. To circumvent the problem of poor or absent visualization of the runoff arteries, two techniques have been used effectively: reactive hyperemia[65,66] and pharmacologic vasodilatation.[67,68] In both instances the blood flow to the popliteal artery and its branches is increased, augmenting the concentration of radiopaque contrast visualized in these vessels (Fig. 67-16). The pharmacologic agents used for this purpose are principally tolazoline hydrochloride

(Priscoline) and, more recently, the calcium channel blockers such as nifedipine. In general, vasoactive drugs have proved less effective than reactive hyperemia for enhancing contrast visualization of the distal runoff arteries. Their principal use is in patients with less severe peripheral arterial disease or in younger patients following trauma. These younger patients have marked vasoreactivity of their peripheral arteries. Severe vasoconstriction can be quickly induced and often requires a vasodilating agent to reverse it.

Reactive hyperemia is produced by ischemia alone or in conjunction with exercise. When ischemia is used, a blood pressure cuff is wrapped around the thigh and inflated to 150 mmHg for 5 to 7 minutes. Exercise may be added to the ischemia by actively or passively flexing and extending the foot (approximately 80–100 times) while the blood pressure cuff is inflated around the thigh. The addition of exercise causes more profound ischemia and consequently more reactive hyperemia. If an agent such as tolazoline is administered, imaging is normally conducted within the first minute of administering a short bolus. The calcium channel blockers are mostly used to prevent vasoconstriction from developing during the arteriographic examination.

If exercise-induced ischemia or ischemia alone is induced, the arteries are examined immediately after termination of exercise. One leg or both simultaneously may be examined this way, depending on how adequately the distal runoff has been demonstrated previously. In a report of 55 patients[64] with obstructive peripheral vascular disease who were studied after reactive hyperemia, excellent contrast visualization of the tibial and peroneal arteries was achieved in 50 patients (91 percent). It is worth noting that reactive hyperemia may be useful for enhancing visualization of the iliac and femoral arteries when proximal vessel obstruction diminishes blood flow to these areas. Why leg muscle ischemia results in hyperemia is not understood. Possible explanations for this phenomenon have included tissue anoxia, local carbon dioxide and lactic acid accumulation, the release of vasoactive polypeptides, and reduced venous pressure.

Angiography following Angioplasty

A complete peripheral arteriographic study is sometimes not obtainable before an interventional procedure is performed. Such is the situation when a catheter inadvertently placed across a critical iliac stenosis and obstructs flow. Withdrawal of the catheter may worsen the situation, but proceeding with the arteriogram may incite thrombosis or, at the very least, result in suboptimal visualization of the more distal runoff arteries. The intervention—angioplasty—is normally performed as quickly as possible and the arteriographic examination then proceeds. This scenario arises almost exclusively for subtotal or short-length occlusions of the iliac arteries.

Visualizing Distal Runoff Vessels

Strategies for visualizing the distal runoff branches and often the plantar arch include adopting digital subtraction techniques and, if needed, adding ancillary maneuvers such as hyperemia or even balloon occlusion arteriography.[69]

Patient Issues

Patient Preparation

The angiographer should examine all patients referred for arteriography (1) to evaluate the clinical need for the arteriogram, (2) to examine the patient's physical condition and palpate the lower extremity pulses, and (3) to obtain informed consent by explaining the procedure and its potential complications. A note is entered in the chart outlining the discussion of the procedure with the patient. In the general evaluation of the patient, associated conditions such as diabetes mellitus, hypertension, angina, blood dyscrasias, and previous allergic response to radiopaque contrast material should be assessed. In all patients, renal function must be determined before the procedure to ensure adequate contrast excretion of the contrast material. If the patient is receiving anticoagulant therapy or has a bleeding tendency, the appropriate clotting studies should be performed and any deficiency should be corrected before angiography to prevent postprocedure complications from hematomas or bleeding at the puncture site.

Premedication for the procedure usually involves moderate analgesia with either morphine or Demerol, to which is added Vistaril or a barbiturate, in doses appropriate for the patient's age and weight. The more recent trend has been to use short-acting morphine analogues such as fentanyl and shorter-acting hypnotics such as the benzodiazepine midazolam (Versed). These agents are normally administered at the time of arteriography and offer good analgesia.[70] Rarely is general anesthesia required except in children. Injected radiopaque contrast material may cause transient nausea and vomiting. To prevent particle aspiration, all solid foods are restricted for 4 to 6 hours before the procedure. However, clear liquids are encouraged so the patient does not become dehydrated. In diabetics receiving insulin or oral hypoglycemic agents, the medication dosage is adjusted to take into account the reduced caloric intake. The appropriate anatomic region for arterial puncture, inguinal or axillary, is shaved and readied for catheterization.

Contrast Agents

The injection of ionic contrast material during femoral arteriography is invariably painful for the patient. The perception of pain, of course, varies from patient to patient; some people find it excruciating, whereas others merely complain of an annoyance. Nevertheless, the fact that the majority of patients do experience a moderate to severe degree of pain motivates the search for an effective intraarterial anesthetic or a less painful contrast agent.

Several studies[48,71,72] have indicated that the intraarterial infusion of lidocaine is effective for diminishing the pain induced by the injection of ionic contrast agent. The perception of decreased pain was reported both subjectively and objectively, in particular, apparently, when analgesic premedication was given in conjunction with the intraarterial lidocaine infusion.[73]

Research on contrast material indicates that hypertonicity appears to be important in inducing pain during intraarterial injection.[74] Conray in an isoosmotic concentration has been shown to cause no pain when injected.[75]

The nonionic contrast materials are less painful during femoral arteriography than the ionic contrast agents.[76,77] This is but one of the reasons that a larger number of procedures are now being performed with nonionic materials. Although their cost is substantially greater than ionic materials, they have a lower rate of allergic reactions and may have less of an effect on renal function.[78–80] They also cause fewer systemic reactions such as blood pressure decreases and tachycardia than the ionic agents.

These arguments apply to the traditional cut-film arteriographic studies. The reliance on digital subtraction studies has decreased the need for "full-strength" contrast studies. In general, the ionic agents are diluted in fractions of 1:1 to 3:1 with saline and then used. The extent of the dilution depends on the sensitivity of the arteriographic device and the local blood flow.

Allergic reactions are less common during arteriography than after intravenous injections. Given a history of previous reactions, appropriate premedication with a steroid agent is recommended. In addition, the contrast agent is changed because it is believed that this will decrease the likelihood of a repeat, and possibly more severe, reaction.

Medications

The patient undergoing arteriography is normally given an anxiolytic agent and some form of analgesic. In both cases, there is a tendency to rely on shorter-acting agents because patients often undergo angiography as outpatients and should normally recover from their medication before their same-day discharge, typically on the same afternoon as the procedure.

A more traditional agent such as diazepam is better given by mouth or by the intramuscular route. Newer, shorter-acting agents such as midazolam can be given intravenously. This agent offers another advantage because it induces an amnesic response.

Morphine analogues or substitutes tend to have an effect for 4 to 6 hours following their administration. The shorter-acting fentanyl can be titrated to patient needs readily, and its effects will reverse within a couple of hours.[70,81]

Monitoring

The attention given to proper monitoring of patients during arteriography has increased over the last decade. Part of the motivation behind this trend is the need for a more rigorous monitoring of the quality of care to which the patient is subjected. Another driving force is the increasing referral of patients with severe coronary artery disease and peripheral arterial disease, often associated with pulmonary disease, to the interventional suite. Such patients with multiple risk factors definitely require careful monitoring during percutaneous interventions and can only benefit from the extra attention given to them during the diagnostic arteriogram.

Proper monitoring now includes frequent evaluation of vital signs, blood pressure, and cardiac rhythm and rate. There is also an increase in the use of infrared sensors for monitoring of peripheral oxygenation and more aggressive use of supplemental oxygen as needed. Evaluation of urine output and the extent of blood loss, if any, is also performed during more complex cases. The coagulation status can also be monitored more accurately with the aid of devices that display the results of an activated clotting time. A value above 160 seconds suggests that catheter withdrawal may be risky and that prolonged compression may be required. Alternatively, the catheter is exchanged for a sheath and the patient is monitored until catheter withdrawal is safely accomplished.

Patient monitoring does not cease with the end of the procedure. Subsequent evaluation for pulses, the presence of a hematoma, or even a suspected pseudoaneurysm is done for the first 24 hours. This may be done by telephone if the patient is managed on an outpatient basis.

Indications for Femoral Arteriography

The primary indication for arteriography is to evaluate patients with suspected arterial lesions. The evaluation of bone or soft tissue tumors of the lower extremities has decreased in demand unless an embolization procedure is being considered. The incidence of vascular lesions greatly exceeds that of tumors. Vascular lesions can be classified by etiology, as arteriosclerosis obliterans, emboli, aneurysms, thromboangiitis obliterans, trauma, arteriovenous fistulas, arteriovenous malformations, graft, and spasm. When management is chiefly surgical, by endarterectomy, resection, or bypass graft, preoperative arteriography is performed to accurately define the location and anatomic extent of the lesions.[82,83] It is principally performed before bypass grafting to ensure that the primary lesions are dealt with. On occasion, it has been performed in the operating room, where mixed results have been seen.[84,85] Great importance is given to the status of the runoff vessels so that the optimal site of the distal anastomosis is clearly identified.[62,86] In addition, the accurate delineation of arterial lesions, including their number and length, is given priority when a percutaneous procedure is considered.[87,88]

Atherosclerosis Obliterans

Baseline Evaluation

Arteriosclerotic obstructive lesions are by far the most common indications for aortofemoral arteriography. The etiology of these lesions is linked to factors such as hypercholesterolemia, dietary intake of saturated fatty acids, diabetes mellitus, heredity, obesity, and cigarette smoking, to name but the main ones. Arteriosclerotic lesions start as localized stenosing plaques affecting the intima or media that subsequently proceed to vessel occlusion.[89] These lesions in the lower extremities are most prevalent in older patients, with a peak incidence in the 60s and 70s. It is not unusual to encounter symptomatic patients with arteriosclerosis in the 50s and occasionally even in the 40s, but below this age it is rare. The ratio of men to women studied for symptomatic arteriosclerotic peripheral vascular disease is approximately 4:1. The prevalence of the disease process may, in fact, be underestimated in women.

The symptoms and signs encountered reflect ischemia in the extremity as a result of arterial obstruction. The symptomatic patient is aware of progressive or acute intermittent claudication as the chief presenting complaint. This cramping pain occurs most often in the calf muscles and is induced by exercise (walking) and relieved by rest. The pain may also occur in the thigh and buttock, depending on the site of the vascular obstruction. Pain at rest or nocturnal cramps are evidence of more severe disease and indicate a poor prognosis and possible imminent gangrene. The strength of the peripheral pulses is the physical finding of most significance in this disease. The pulses must be palpated and both sides compared from the aorta to the feet. The absence of pulse usually indicates a proximal obstruction. In some cases, collateral circulation secondary to an occlusion may be adequate to induce a weak pulse. Audible bruits, a palpable thrill, hair loss, temperature and color changes, and the degree of venous filling are other important physical findings in evaluating the extent of the vascular insufficiency.

The diffuse nature of the arteriosclerotic process ultimately leads to multiple sites of obstruction. However, arteriographic investigation has shown that most occlusion lesions are segmental. One of the most common sites of disease initially is the adductor canal portion[90] of the superficial femoral artery (Fig. 67-17). The continuous mechanical trauma to the vessel as it passes through the tendinous hiatus is generally credited with the early and frequent stenosis and occlusion at this site.[91] In terms of decreasing frequency, obstruction occurs in the superficial femoral artery, the distal runoff vessels, and the popliteal artery. The various patterns[90] of occlusive lesions encountered in the lower extremities have limited prognostic significance because there is such marked variability in the site and degree of disease.

The pattern of arteriosclerosis obliterans in the lower extremities is affected by diabetes mellitus. Especially in the runoff arteries, diabetic patients have a higher incidence of lesions and a more severe degree of obstruction than do nondiabetics.[90] Also, two-thirds of combined lesions of the femoral, popliteal, and runoff arteries occur in diabetic patients (Fig. 67-18). The profunda femoris artery likewise shows the effects of diabetes; this vessel is rarely obstructed, but, if stenosis or occlusion occurs, it is almost exclusively in diabetic patients.

In the evaluation of lower extremity occlusive vascular disease, the factor determining the suitability for revascularization is the condition of the inflow arteries (aorta and iliac vessels) and the distal runoff arteries (the terminal branches of the popliteal below the knee and more recently the pedal arch). Tandem lesions are common (Fig. 67-19). A report[83] of 321 extremities showed that 74 percent of the occlusions occurred as combined lesions, whereas 26 percent were isolated or involved only a single leg artery. In 27 percent of the occlusions there was associated obstructive aortoiliac disease.

Associated aortic branch artery lesions are also common in patients undergoing arteriography. The major indication for the abdominal aortogram remains confirming the absence of aortic disease such as stenosis or asymptomatic aneurysms. In addition, a history of hypertension, treated or not, suggests that renal artery lesions may be present. Combined aortic and iliac artery disease is less frequent than isolated lesions in either. The atherosclerotic process does not necessarily affect all vessels simultaneously; thus skipped areas of uninvolved vessels are common.

In general, the posterior aortic wall is more involved by arteriosclerosis than the anterior and lateral walls. This finding is partly explained by the fact that the lumbar artery origins fix the aorta at these sites and create local areas of boundary layer separation.[92] Occasionally lesions of the aorta are evident only in the lateral view because the obstructive process extends from the anterior or the posterior wall without affecting the lateral walls in the supine position.

Rarely, and with more severe disease, the aorta can have the appearance of an ''hourglass'' deformity with indentations in the aortic lumen roughly correspond-

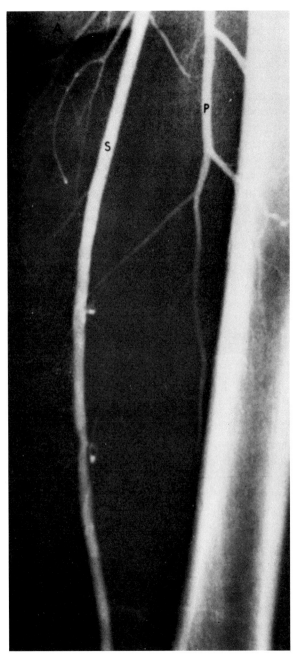 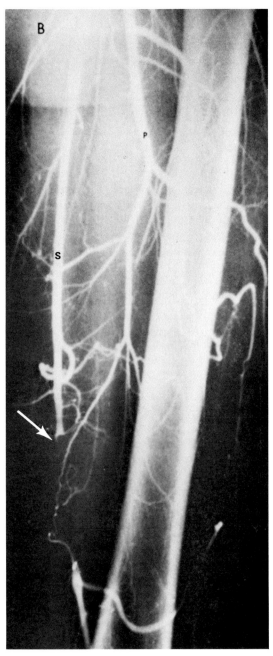

Figure 67-17. Typical early lesion of arteriosclerosis in the adductor canal region progressing from stenosis to occlusion. (A) Minimal segmental stenosis of the superficial femoral artery (*S*) at the tendinous hiatus in the adductor magnus muscle. *P*, profunda femoris artery. (B) Progression to segmental occlusion (*arrow*) with reconstitution of the popliteal artery, mainly via profunda femoris artery (*P*) branches.

ing to the level of the intervertebral disks. Possibly the aortic wall loses elasticity at these levels.

There is also a form of arteriosclerosis that is ectatic rather than constricting. The precise nature of this change is uncertain except that the media of the artery wall has lost its elastic lamina and the intima is less involved. The vessel may assume the appearance of a string of aneurysms, and the rate of the blood flow through the artery is sharply reduced. This appearance is most often seen in the superficial femoral arteries but has also been observed in the common iliac and common femoral arteries.

Grading of the extent of lesion severity focuses on the severity of the stenoses, their location, and their

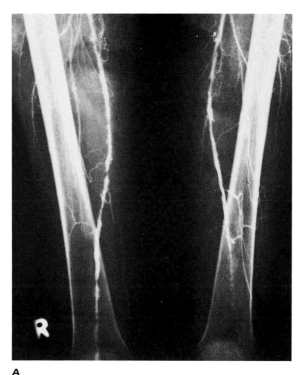

A

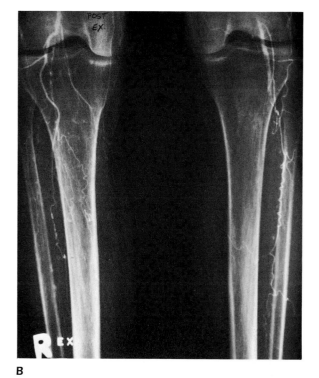

B

Figure 67-18. Adult onset of diabetes mellitus, with gangrenous toe changes in the left foot and associated occlusive arterial disease in the pelvis, thigh, and runoff vessels (same patient as in Fig. 67-9). (A) There are severe diffuse segmental stenoses in both superficial femoral arteries. The proximal left popliteal artery is not visualized. (B) The lack of any runoff arteries was seen only after ischemic exercise when vessel filling was maximal. The right and left popliteal arteries are occluded. There is minimal collateral artery filling, and none of the distal runoff arteries reconstitute because of the severity of the disease.

respective length. Solitary short focal lesions (Fig. 67-20) are likely to respond favorably to angioplasty.[87,88] Lesions above 50 percent diameter narrowing are normally considered to be significant.[86] Recent standards for the reporting of vascular lesions include disease categories such as 1 to 19 percent diameter narrowing and 20 to 49 percent. Occlusions are treated as such.

Revascularization

Bypass Grafts. Surgical revascularization is an attempt to restore adequate blood flow to an ischemic extremity to relieve clinical symptoms or prevent subsequent gangrene and amputation.[93,94] Revascularization employs two surgical techniques, endarterectomy and bypass grafting; the latter is more common.[36,95] Endarterectomy is usually limited to segmental occlusions of the aorta and the iliac arteries but may be extended to segmental occlusions of the superficial femoral and proximal popliteal arteries. When endarterectomy is used in the aorta, extreme care must be taken not to embolize atheromatous debris into the renal arteries.[96] Bypass grafts consist either of natural material such as autologous vein or of artificial woven

Dacron or Gore-Tex (polytetrafluoroethylene). The natural vein grafts are preferable because their patency rate is higher than that of artificial grafts.

Surgical revascularization of bilateral aortoiliac occlusions is best accomplished by introducing an aortobifemoral Dacron graft, rather than by endarterectomy.[97] It has been shown that even for unilateral aortoiliac occlusive disease a bilateral bifurcation graft is preferable to a unilateral one. In a 1973 study of 5-year patency rates, only 52 percent of unilateral grafts remained patent, whereas 78 percent of the bilateral bifurcation grafts were patent.[98] The main reasons for bypass graft failures are progression of the arteriosclerotic process distal to the graft, changes at the anastomosis[99] (false aneurysm, stricture, or infection) (Figs. 67-21; see also Fig. 67-12), and problems with the graft itself (incorrect caliber and length of kinks).[100,101] The late failure rate of either unilateral or bilateral aortic bifurcation grafts ranges from 10 to 28 percent.[102] Five-year patency rates are now in the range of 90 percent.

Extraanatomic grafts—namely, femorofemoral crossover (see Fig. 67-14) and axillofemoral by-

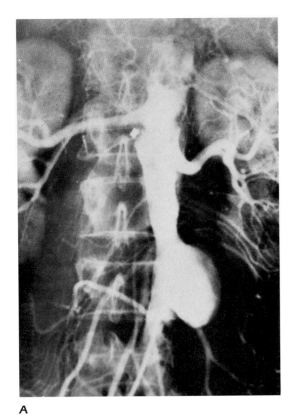

A

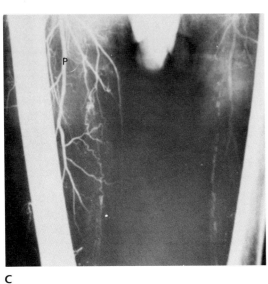

C

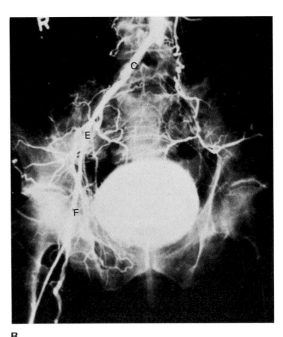

B

Figure 67-19. Severe symptoms of peripheral vascular insufficiency, particularly marked in the left leg. There is combined inflow obstruction with iliac artery occlusive lesions and an unsuspected aortic aneurysm. (A) The saccular aortic aneurysm is seen opposite the third lumbar vertebra. (B) The left common iliac, external iliac, and left common femoral arteries are occluded. A few left internal iliac artery branches reconstitute from the iliolumbar collateral vessel. The right common (*C*) and external (*E*) iliac arteries are patent, along with the common femoral artery (*F*). (C) In the thigh, the right profunda femoris artery (*P*) is patent and fills rapidly. The corresponding vessel on the left is poorly visualized; it was reconstituted by only the few internal iliac artery branches. Note the bilateral occlusions of the superficial femoral arteries and the calcifications in the walls of these vessels.

passes—are used mainly when one limb of an aortic bifurcation graft is occluded.[103,104] The crossover femorofemoral bypass graft was originally introduced for the poor-surgical-risk patient with unilateral iliac artery occlusion.[105] Because of its low operative risk, technical simplicity, and high graft patency rate, this procedure is favored when one limb of a bifurcation graft is occluded. A "steal phenomenon" may occur

in the donor limb after a femorofemoral bypass if a significant stenosis is present in the proximal iliac artery of the donor limb.[106]

In ischemic disease of the leg, the indications[107,108] for bypass grafting are (1) limb salvage as an alternative to amputation and (2) relief of severe claudication interfering with occupation or limiting activities in retirees. A femoropopliteal graft (Fig. 67-22) is the most popular for alleviating ischemic symptoms, but femorotibial or femoroperoneal bypass grafts are increasingly selected as viable alternatives. The femoropopliteal graft carries a lower complication rate than the other types of distal grafts.[108] The choice of a femoropopliteal bypass graft depends on patency of the popliteal artery and one distal branch, preferably a tibial artery.[108–110] Patency rate is readily related to the state of the runoff vessels, improving with the quality and number of tibioperoneal branches.[87,111] In general,

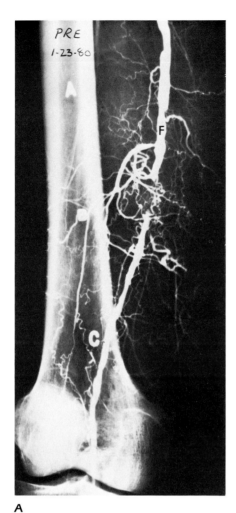

A

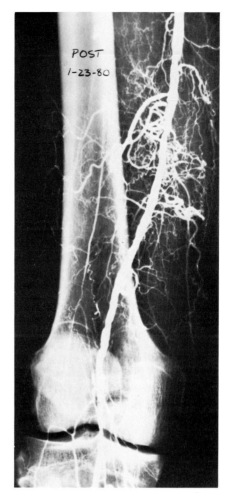

B

Figure 67-20. Percutaneous transluminal angioplasty offers an alternative to bypass grafting for revascularization in symptomatic vascular occlusive disease. (A) The prerecanalization study shows a 4-cm segmental occlusion of the superficial femoral artery (*F*) and distal vessel reconstitution. (B) After balloon dilatation the postrecanalization study shows restoration of luminal continuity.

patency rates of synthetic polytetrafluoroethylene (PTFE) grafts are much lower in the below-the-knee popliteal artery than for the above-knee grafts.

Autologous vein bypass grafts are increasingly favored for bypass operations. Of the two options, reversed grafts and in situ, it appears that the latter offer advantages in patency rates, especially for distal calf or pedal branch anastomoses.[112,113] These distal grafts (femorotibial and femoroperoneal) are mainly limb salvage procedures performed to avoid amputation.[114]

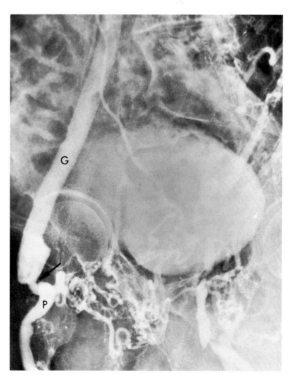

Figure 67-21. This patient had recurrent ischemic leg symptoms after an aortobifemoral graft (*G*). In the right posterior oblique view, a right distal anastomotic aneurysm and stenosis (*arrow*) at the origin of the profunda femoris artery (*P*) are evident. The right superficial femoral artery is occluded. The left limb of the bifurcation graft is occluded.

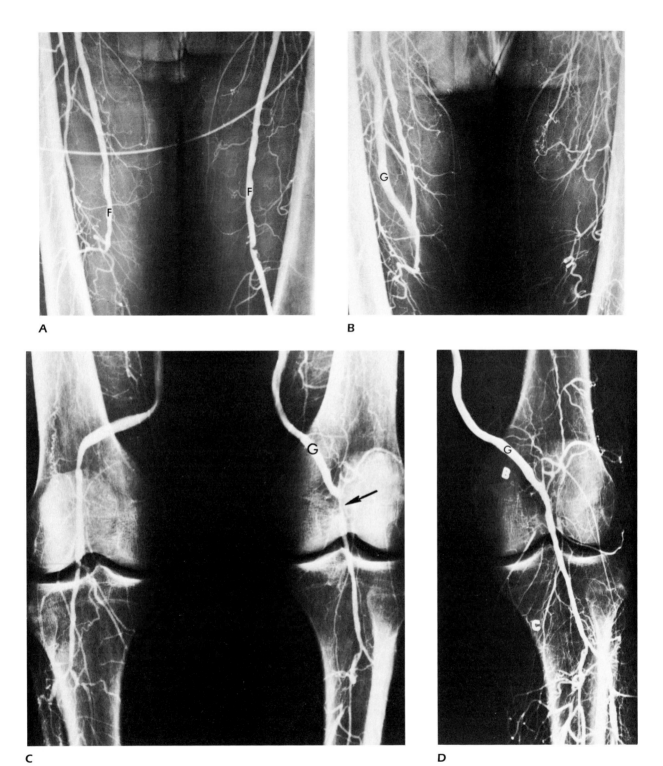

Figure 67-22. Typical problems of progressive arteriosclerotic peripheral ischemic disease and the complications of revascularization. (A) A patient was studied for right calf claudication. There was segmental occlusion of the right distal superficial femoral artery (*F*). The left distal superficial femoral artery (*F*) had severe segmental stenosis. (B) Six months later, the patient was reexamined for left calf claudication. A right femoropopliteal bypass (vein) graft (*G*) was patent. The left distal superficial femoral artery was totally occluded.

(C) Ten months later, there were recurrent ischemic symptoms in the left leg. A left femoropopliteal bypass (Gore-Tex, *G*) was patent but stenosed (*arrow*) at the distal anastomosis. The stenosis was probably secondary to fibrosis. The right femoropopliteal graft was patent. (D) The left graft (*G*) anastomotic stenosis was transluminally dilated with a balloon catheter. The lumen was restored to normal caliber, but by the following day the entire left femoropopliteal graft was thrombosed. A leg amputation was ultimately required.

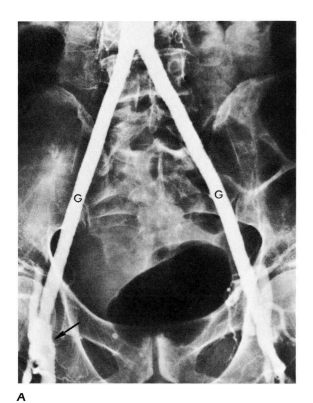

A

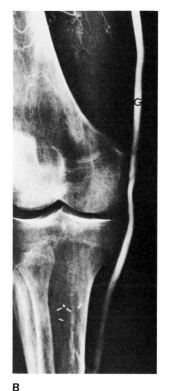

B

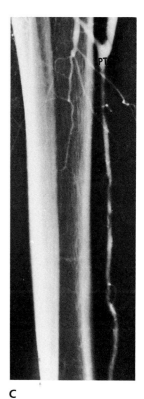

C

Figure 67-23. Multiple grafts may be required to restore adequate circulation in diffuse obstructive peripheral vascular disease. (A) An aortobifemoral bypass graft (*G*) was required because of bilateral common iliac artery occlusions. A right distal anastomotic aneurysm is evident (*arrow*). (B) In addition, the patient had occlusion of the right super- ficial femoral and popliteal arteries. A femoroposterior tibial bypass graft (*G*) was created. (C) The posterior tibial artery (*PT*) was the only patent distal runoff artery. The arterial lumen was diffusely irregular because of arteriosclerotic changes.

Both these grafts have higher rates of complications than a femoropopliteal graft.[115] Resorting to one of the more distal grafts is warranted only when the popliteal artery is occluded and a patent tibial or peroneal artery is demonstrated angiographically (Fig. 67-23). Diabetes mellitus influences the severity of obstructive disease in the distal runoff arteries. The incidence of distal runoff artery occlusion, tibial and peroneal, is higher in diabetic patients than in those with only uncomplicated arteriosclerosis. The weight of evidence[108,115] indicates that bypass grafts to the small-caliber runoff arteries preserve limb function and offer an alternative to amputation. Thus it is imperative that angiography clearly delineate the anatomic features of the distal runoff arteries down to the ankles[116] and, increasingly, to the pedal arch (Fig. 67-24).

Percutaneous Interventions. In the late 1970s, there was renewed interest in percutaneous transluminal angioplasty as a nonsurgical technique for restoring blood in obstructed pelvic and extremity arteries.[2,3] This technique, first described by Dotter and Judkins[117] in 1964, received a technologic boost by the development of an effective balloon catheter. The technique performs best for segmental stenoses of the pelvic and leg arteries and segmental occlusions of less than 4 to 7 cm in the superficial femoral or popliteal arteries (see Fig. 67-20) and less well in below-the-knee branches (Fig. 67-25). These indications may limit the applicability of the technique to approximately 25 to 30 percent of all patients with clinically symptomatic peripheral vascular disease.

The more aggressive strategies that emerged in the late 1980s broaden the range of percutaneous interventions.[118,119] Thrombolysis followed by angioplasty can now be used to treat longer iliac and femoropopliteal lesions. Irregular and long iliac lesions can also be managed by the placement of stents.[120,121] These appear to outperform angioplasty alone (Fig. 67-26) and offer patency rates similar to those of bypass surgery. More than ever, accurate delineation of the extent of arterial pathology is needed, not only to plan the appropriate intervention but also to help in documenting its therapeutic effectiveness.

Shared Issues. An increasing number of patients are

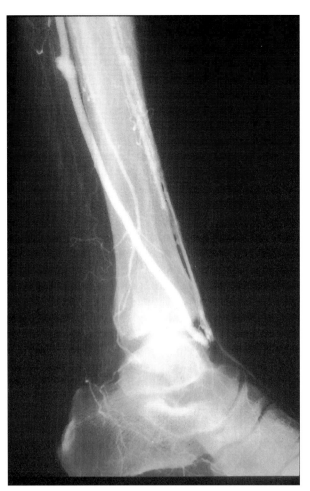

Figure 67-24. Vein bypass graft originating in the common femoral artery. The distal anastomosis to the dorsalis pedal artery is involved by a high-grade stenosis.

studied after one or more interventions. After bypass surgery, a patient can present with a developing lesion in the contralateral leg or in the same extremity. Lesions can develop at the inflow or outflow or can be linked directly to the placement of the bypass graft. Inflow and outflow lesions are easily handled with angioplasty or atherectomy. Lesions at the anastomoses or in the graft conduit, although they will respond acutely to percutaneous interventions,[122] might not show prolonged patency, especially after thrombolytic therapy.[123,124] Arteriographic access and the type of study being done are obviously related to the site of suspected pathology. If a lesion is already known to exist by noninvasive vascular imaging, a direct antegrade puncture may be all that is required to deal with the problem. If there are unexplained symptoms, a more formal complete arteriogram is often required in addition to pressure measurements.

Thromboembolism

Embolic obstruction, like thrombosis, may produce partial or complete arterial occlusion. Emboli are a common cause of acute arterial occlusion, and the diagnosis is usually inferred from the clinical history.[125,126] Atrial fibrillation, recurrent cardiac arrhythmias, myocardial infarction with mural thrombus, and bacterial endocarditis are the most common systemic conditions that predispose to peripheral arterial emboli. There is reason to believe that the incidence of embolic occlusion may be increasing as a result of improved cardiac care, an aging population, and more extensive use of prosthetic heart valves. Aortic aneurysms and atheromatous plaques may also cause embolization if a clot or plaque fragment breaks off and lodges distally.[127] Ulcerated atheromatous plaques, moreover, may shower cholesterol emboli into the small arteries of the leg, causing occlusion.[128] Emboli may obstruct a normal vessel but more frequently obstruct an already compromised arteriosclerotic artery. Newer techniques for managing emboli have increased the limb salvage rate and decreased the need for amputation. However, the mortality from arterial emboli remains high because of the seriousness of the predisposing cardiac disease that is nearly always present.[104,129]

The leg arteries, and specifically the superficial femoral artery, are the vessels most often occluded by emboli. In a series[130] of 203 embolectomies, 75 percent of the emboli lodged in the lower extremities, with 42 percent of these in the femoral artery. Additional vessels embolically occluded were as follows: iliac, 19 percent; popliteal, 14 percent; posterior tibial, 1 percent; and anterior tibial, 0.5 percent. The source of emboli in this series was mainly cardiac (78 percent) with cardiovascular surgery accounting for 7 percent; no etiology was established in 10 percent.

The success of therapy for acute embolic occlusion depends on the rapid recognition of the clinical problem and location of the obstruction. Arteriography is the most effective diagnostic procedure for confirming the clinical diagnosis, the extent of the occlusion, the degree of collateral circulation, and the condition of the distal circulation. The arteriographic appearance of embolic occlusion is fairly typical; a proximal curved margin reflects the nonopaque embolus protruding into the contrast-filled lumen (Fig. 67-27). In an acute occlusion there is usually little, if any, collateral circulation evident. The extent of collateral flow depends on the time interval between the occlusion and the arteriographic study, as well as on the presence of chronically obstructive arterial lesions.

Embolectomy, the treatment for embolic occlusion, should be performed as soon as possible after the

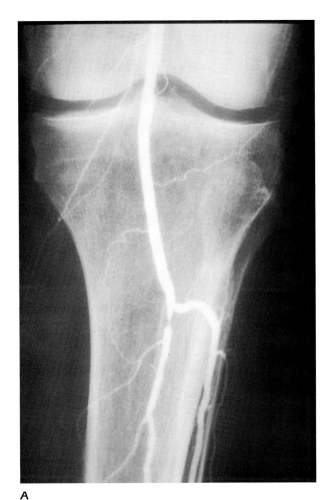 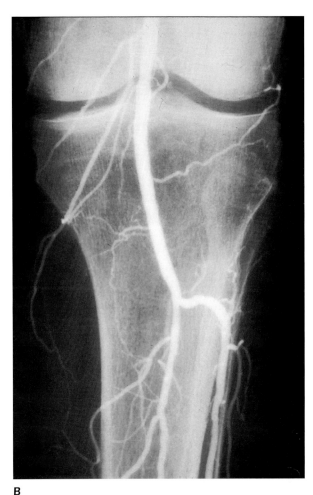

A   B

Figure 67-25. (A) Arteriogram showing a high-grade lesion of the tibioperoneal trunk (*arrow*). (B) A subsequent arteriogram taken after angioplasty shows resolution of the stenosis.

diagnosis is established.[131,132] The limb amputation rate is proportional to the time delay between acute occlusion and embolectomy. In two 1970s reports,[130,133] when embolectomy was performed within 24 hours, the amputation rate ranged from 0.1 to 4.4 percent, whereas after 24 hours the amputation rate ranged from 4.3 to 19.4 percent. It has been suggested that the longer the delay before embolectomy, the greater are the chances of thrombosis distal to the primary site of acute occlusion.[134] Embolectomy is now generally performed by the Fogarty technique using a balloon catheter.[135] The procedure can be performed under local anesthesia in the poor-surgical-risk patient and is both technically simple and effective. Following embolectomy in patients who survive, the limb salvage rate has been reported as high as 93 and 95 percent in two series of 163 and 300 patients, respectively.[130,133]

Alternatives such as aggressive thrombolytic therapy can also be used.[136] These cases are normally selected when there is apparent diffuse embolization and

compromise of the runoff vessels that could not be effectively dealt with by embolectomy.[137] As in the surgical cases, morbidity in this population is high. One of the advantages of the thrombolytic agents is believed to be their action in helping recanalize the smaller arterioles. To minimize the likelihood of hemorrhage, all sites of percutaneous arterial entry must be appropriately dealt with, more often by the insertion of arterial sheaths where a diagnostic catheter was used.

Aneurysms

Primary aneurysms of the lower extremity arteries are thought to be caused by arteriosclerosis obliterans.[138] However, there is the suggestion that primary aneurysm formation may have a genetic predisposition, possibly linked to elastin metabolism.[139] Secondary or acquired aneurysms may be caused by trauma, a bypass graft, mycotic infection, or a kinked vessel. Arteriosclerotic aneurysms in the lower extremity primarily

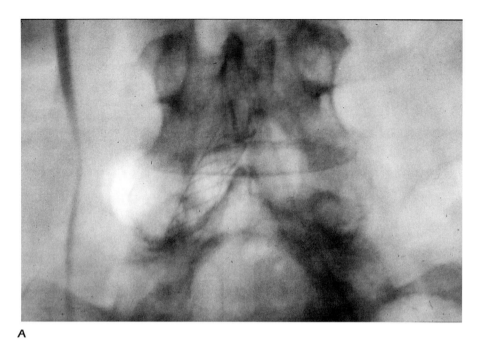

A

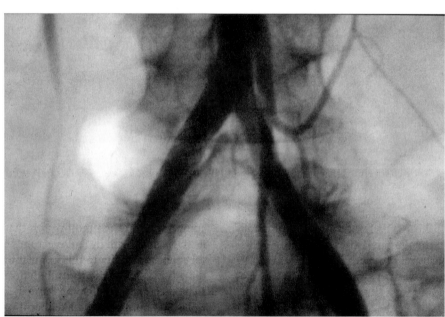

B

Figure 67-26. (A) Plain film showing a right iliac stent in the expected location. (B) The stent is faintly seen outlined against the contrast material on the arteriogram.

involve the popliteal artery; the superficial femoral and the distal runoff arteries are rarely involved with primary aneurysms, but acquired aneurysms are not infrequent in these vessels.[140]

A primary popliteal artery aneurysm presents clinically as a palpable mass behind the knee that usually does not pulsate because the lumen is clot-filled.[141, 142] The presence of pain depends on how rapidly the aneurysm expands or on the occurrence of wall dissec-

tion. Chronic lesions are often calcified, and both rim-like and amorphous patterns have been observed (Fig. 67-28). Approximately 30 to 50 percent of aneurysms occur bilaterally, although one side is usually larger than the other. Aneurysms are often saccular in type and usually filled with clot; thus little or no contrast enters the lumen (Fig. 67-29). It is important to assess the arterial patency distal to the aneurysm. The size of the aneurysm is difficult to evaluate if there are no arte-

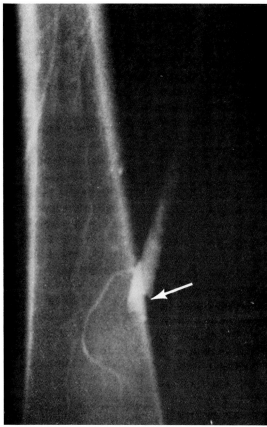

Figure 67-27. Atrial fibrillation and acute insufficiency due to an embolus in the right leg of a 62-year-old man. Note the smooth, curved, concave edge at the point of occlusion (*arrow*) and the minimal distal collateral circulation.

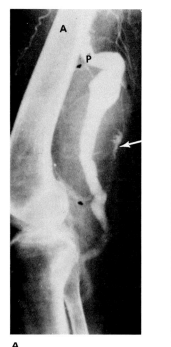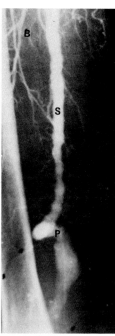

A   **B**

Figure 67-28. (A) Lateral view of a popliteal artery (*P*) aneurysm with amorphous (*arrow*) and rimlike (*arrowheads*) calcification. Note displacement of the surrounding vessels and lack of contrast filling of the aneurysm. (B) Anteroposterior view demonstrates the ectatic superficial femoral artery (*S*) and the extremely slow blood flow through the area.

Figure 67-29. Popliteal artery aneurysm with segmental occlusion of the distal superficial femoral (*S*) and popliteal (*P*) arteries. The saccular aneurysm (*arrowheads*) is much larger, although mostly clot filled, than the small fraction that contains contrast material (*arrow*).

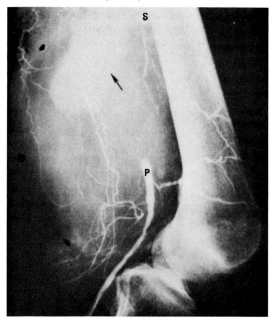

rial wall calcifications. Venous displacement with clinical symptoms of thrombophlebitis has been reported secondary to popliteal artery aneurysms.[143] The superficial femoral artery proximal to the aneurysm is often ectatic and has numerous small aneurysmal dilatations (see Fig. 67-28). Blood flow is normally very slow through the ectatic superficial femoral artery and further delayed through the aneurysm. Thus more contrast and a slower film rate than normal are needed to demonstrate these lesions. A later view of the aneurysm can often provide more information about the lesion than the standard anteroposterior view.

Superficial femoral artery aneurysms are more rarely encountered. These lesions are either saccular or fusiform, clot-filled, and usually unilateral. Whereas native common femoral artery aneurysms tend to be fusiform, anastomotic aneurysms at the common femoral artery secondary to a prosthetic graft are usually saccular. In general, common iliac artery aneurysms extend

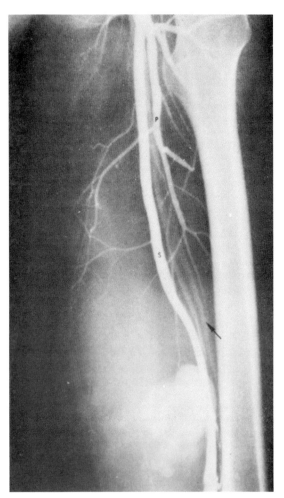

Figure 67-30. Acute traumatic arteriovenous fistula and false aneurysm caused by a stab wound. There is immediate venous filling (*arrow*) from the superficial femoral artery (*S*). Note that both the superficial femoral and profunda femoris (*P*) arteries are normal in caliber. There is contrast extravasation into the thigh in a false aneurysm with displacement and narrowing of the superficial femoral artery.

from fusiform infrarenal abdominal aortic aneurysms, although discrete saccular lesions can occur. The external and internal iliac arteries are rarely the site of primary aneurysms.[144]

Traumatic aneurysms or pseudoaneurysms (Fig. 67-30) are usually false aneurysms and are the result of arterial lacerations that disrupt all three layers of the artery wall. This is usually secondary to penetrating injury, but occasionally iatrogenic laceration due to surgery causes an aneurysm. Traumatic aneurysms may be associated with a traumatic arteriovenous fistula (see Fig. 67-30).

Thromboangiitis Obliterans (Buerger Disease)

Buerger disease, or thromboangiitis obliterans,[145] is a form of progressive arterial occlusive disease that characteristically occurs in young men. Symptoms are usually confined to the feet or lower legs. Pain at rest, mostly a burning sensation, is the main clinical feature and not exercise-induced intermittent claudication. Rest pain is often excessive when compared to the visible features of ischemia, and this element, too, is characteristic. Other findings are the strong association with smoking, involvement of the upper extremities, and recurrent thrombophlebitis. Intimal thickening with an inflammatory cell response and preservation of the media are associated with Buerger disease.[146]

Not all pathologists consider this pathologic lesion unique. Investigators have questioned the existence of thromboangiitis obliterans as a distinct disease entity.[147] In the literature, reports of specific arteriographic findings associated with this entity by some authors are denied by others.[148] The angiographic findings are indistinguishable from those observed with occlusion due to arteriosclerosis obliterans. Perhaps the only significant arteriographic feature is the preferential involvement of the tibioperoneal branches and the "corkscrew" appearance of collaterals (Fig. 67-31). There is often little or no evidence of any arteriosclerotic changes in the larger, more proximal arteries.

Trauma

Arteriography can make a significant contribution to the management of trauma patients.[149,150] This role can be broadened to the management of patients subjected to iatrogenic injury.[151]

Hemorrhage

Traumatic arterial injury of the pelvis and lower extremities, unless promptly recognized, can cause severe hemorrhage or ischemia and thus carries a high risk of death or loss of limb.[152] In the civilian population pelvic fracture is the major form of trauma responsible for massive extraperitoneal hemorrhage. It is generally impossible to determine clinically whether the source of bleeding is arterial or venous,[153] but the former is less responsive to fluid replacement. Inability to identify the bleeding source[1,154] causes the threat of fatal hemorrhage after pelvic trauma. Surgical exploration has been the traditional technique used in attempts to establish the bleeding site but is usually unsuccessful in the presence of massive hemorrhage.[155] If the tamponading effect of hemorrhage is disturbed

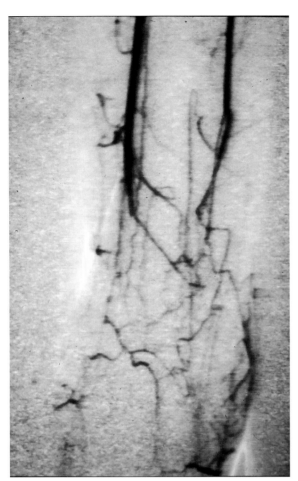

Figure 67-31. Distal arteriogram of the calf in a 40-year-old smoker. There are no lesions in the iliac, femoral, or popliteal arteries. Multiple occlusions and small collaterals are present. The presence of collaterals suggest a more chronic process than acute emboli. In such a young individual, this pattern of disease is typical of Buerger disease.

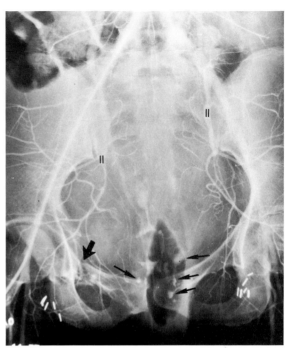

Figure 67-32. Massive hemorrhage resulting from acute traumatic injury to the pelvis. Arteriogram demonstrates contrast extravasation (*arrows*) originating from several internal iliac artery (*II*) branches, bilaterally. Note the fractured right superior pubic ramus (*thick arrow*) and the mass effect of the hemorrhage causing cephalad bowel displacement.

by surgical exploration, fatal hemorrhage and intraperitoneal rupture may be reactivated.[156] Even when successful, surgical exploration may result in sepsis. Despite these shortcomings, surgical ligation of the internal iliac artery, regardless of whether the bleeding site is identified, has been the accepted way to manage massive pelvic hemorrhage.[1,157] Blind ligation, without an established definite site of bleeding, is essentially a last-chance form of therapy. Its success has been variable[158,159] because the proximal ligation leaves numerous pelvic arterial collaterals free to rebleed.

Arteriography offers an alternative to surgery for both the diagnosis and management of massive pelvic hemorrhage.[156] The arteriogram can reveal the site of contrast extravasation and thus help to identify the individual vessels that are bleeding (Fig. 67-32). By studying the contralateral internal iliac artery, one can also identify the potential collaterals. With this information, the bleeding may be managed by surgical ligation of the appropriate arteries, by percutaneous transcatheter embolization,[156] or by balloon catheter tamponade.[160,161] Thus arteriography, if it is to be used, should be considered early in the evaluation of traumatic pelvic hemorrhage. In this context, it can diminish the mortality and morbidity of prolonged and massive hemorrhage.

Hemorrhage after delivery or pelvic surgery also responds well to arteriographically directed embolization.

Occlusion and Intimal Injuries

Arterial injury, such as laceration or contusion of the lower extremity vessels, is common, especially following penetrating or blunt injuries secondary to bullets (Fig. 67-33), stab wounds, or fractures.[162] Before the Korean War, the usual treatment for severe arterial injury in an extremity was vessel ligation and limb amputation.[163] The intent was to preserve life even if the extremity had to be sacrificed. Experience with arterial

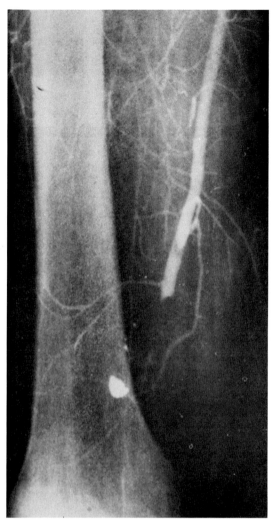

Figure 67-33. Acute traumatic injury with occlusion of the distal superficial femoral artery due to a bullet fragment. Note the lack of contrast extravasation, probably because of vessel spasm. Note also the early collateral vessel formation.

reconstruction during the Korean War, subsequently confirmed by civilian experience, has established this procedure as the treatment of choice for traumatic arterial injury. However, patient selection for arteriography may require that certain guidelines be followed.[164]

Arteries near the surface, fixed in position or adjacent to bone, are usually the ones most readily injured by the common mechanisms of trauma, namely, penetrating or blunt injury.[165] The distal superficial femoral artery is often the site of injury after fracture of the femur because of the vessel's proximity to the bone and its relatively fixed position in the adductor canal. Signs of arterial injury may not be evident at first, but ischemic symptoms may develop after the acute injury (see Fig. 67-4). Another frequently damaged vessel is the popliteal artery, behind the knee.[166,167] Because the

muscles of this region hold the artery fixed in position, a posterior dislocation of the knee may injure the vessel (Fig. 67-34). The anterior tibial artery, similarly, is easily injured as it passes through the interosseous membrane when the proximal tibia is fractured. The close approximation of the anterior tibial artery and bone in the distal portion of the leg makes this another site where the artery is readily injured.

Traumatic injury of the popliteal artery, although clinically similar to injury of the superficial femoral artery, differs from the latter in its response to surgical repair. Surgical repair of the injured popliteal artery more frequently results in amputation than repair of the superficial femoral artery.[168] Furthermore, penetrating injury to the popliteal artery has a better limb salvage rate than does blunt injury.

The clinical diagnosis of arterial injury in the lower extremities depends on recognizing the signs of acute ischemia distal to the traumatized site.[169] The signs and symptoms are pain, blanched skin, coldness to touch, loss of cutaneous sensation, absent motor function, and absent or faint arterial pulses. These findings usually are sufficient to give a strong suggestion of the diagnosis.[170] An arteriogram may be necessary to confirm and pinpoint the lesion before surgical repair as long as definitive therapy is not duly delayed. Because arterial spasm can mimic the clinical and arteriographic findings of severe arterial trauma, the diagnosis must be established by surgical exploration.[171]

The mechanism of arterial injury in the extremity vessels, regardless of cause, is postulated to involve either (1) overstretching, without transection, or (2) transection. An experimental trauma study[172] has indicated that the intima ruptures before either the medial or the adventitial layer. Arterial contusion may occur without transection and form an intramural hematoma, or the intima may dissect and form a flap. Transection of the wall generally results from penetrating injury by either a fractured bone fragment or an external object.[173]

All the potential mechanisms of arterial injury cause partial or complete vessel obstruction, and this threatens viability of the extremity. The *ischemic time* refers to the time elapsed before definitive repair of the arterial injury is attempted. It is a well-recognized fact that the longer the ischemic time, the greater the likelihood that arterial reconstruction will fail, necessitating amputation.[174] Chances of developing muscle contracture or atrophy are similarly increased. Ischemic times or delay before arterial reconstruction of more than 6 to 12 hours has been said to be critical.[163,174,175] However, the length of the ischemic time may be relative because additional factors such as the degree of associated soft tissue damage and the development of collateral circu-

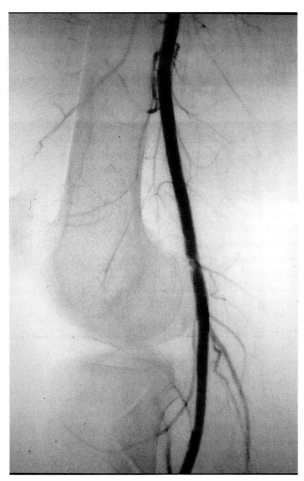

Figure 67-34. Arteriogram obtained following traumatic dislocation (not associated with a fracture) of the knee. The arterial wall injury, seen in the popliteal artery following reduction, causes a discrete intimal defect (*arrow*).

lation can influence the result. The techniques of surgical reconstruction for arterial injury include primary end-to-end anastomosis, patch angioplasty, and bypass grafts.

Arteriovenous Fistulas

An arteriovenous fistula is an abnormal communication between an adjacent artery and vein. It is either acquired or congenital in origin. Clinicians have long been fascinated by the lesion because of its pathophysiologic features. The following discussion focuses on acquired arteriovenous fistulas; the next section of this chapter considers the congenital variety of arteriovenous malformations.

Acquired fistulas almost always involve penetrating trauma from gunshot, stab wounds, shrapnel particles, fracture fragments, or catheterization. Gunshot and stab wounds account for about 50 percent of the lesions in most civilian reports.[176] Less common causes

are steel or glass splinters, iatrogenic injury in pelvic surgery[177] or intervertebral disk surgery, balloon thrombectomy,[178] and percutaneous arterial catheterization.[100] For a fistula to develop, the vascular injury must occur at a site where the artery and vein are in close proximity.[179] Most acquired fistulas occur in the extremities because adjacent arteries and veins are relatively close to the surface. The lower extremities are more frequently involved in both civilian and war injury–acquired fistulas, and the femoral artery is the single vessel most often affected.[176,180] At the fistula site there may be a localized, pulsatile soft tissue mass, but a palpable thrill, an audible bruit, and venous dilatation indicate the diagnosis (Fig. 67-35). In chronic fistulas, severe limb edema and pain may be evident.

The local features and systemic hemodynamic consequences of arteriovenous fistulas have been investigated in elegant work by Holman.[181,182] The pathophysiology of fistulas results from the excessive shunting of blood from the arterial to the venous circulation. There is marked increase in venous return to the heart, with consequent increased cardiac output, rapid pulse rate, and widened pulse pressure. The development of these systemic manifestations depends on the size of the artery involved and the length of time the fistula has been present. Thus a small fistula will probably not be hemodynamically significant, whereas a large fistula may result in congestive heart failure. The permanent or transient closure of an arteriovenous fistula causes an immediate, dramatic bradycardia. This is called the Branham sign[183] and is diagnostically useful because temporary digital compression of the fistula elicits bradycardia. The therapy for acquired arteriovenous fistulas is surgical closure to reverse the deleterious hemodynamic changes.

Screening tests such as radionuclide angiograms[184] have been replaced almost exclusively by ultrasound,[185] to the point that arteriography may be circumvented even if surgical intervention is contemplated. Arteriography is useful in more complex cases because it will demonstrate (1) the size and number of feeding arteries, (2) the collateral circulation, (3) the venous circulation distal to the fistula, (4) a possible aneurysm, and (5) the arterial circulation distal to the fistula.[186] In general, acquired fistulas (see Fig. 67-35) have a single feeding arterial branch that is markedly dilated. However, in multiple fragment injuries, several arterial feeders may be present. The multiple channels may be revealed only after one or more have been ligated in an attempt to ablate the fistula. The venous channels distal to the fistula become dilated because of the increased blood flow and direct exposure to arterial pressure. As competence of the venous valves becomes impaired because of the increased blood flow, retrograde

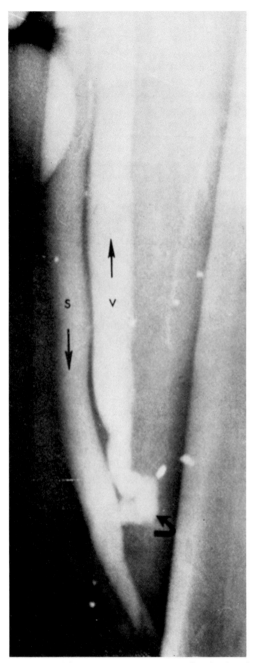

Figure 67-35. Traumatic arteriovenous fistula developed many years after the original injury by shrapnel fragments. There is immediate contrast filling of the dilated vein (*V*) through the shunt (*curved arrow*) from the dilated superficial femoral artery (*S*). The artery returns to normal caliber distal to the shunt.

venous flow may occur. A false aneurysm may form as a result of the initial arterial injury if there is extravasation of blood (see Fig. 67-30).

The arteriographic technique employed with fistulas must be altered to compensate for the rapid blood flow. Thus approximately 1.5 times the usual amount

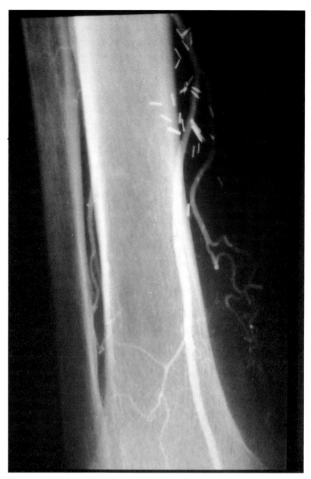

Figure 67-36. Arteriogram taken after a myocutaneous skin flap operation. The pedicle is anastomosed with the posterior tibial artery (*arrow*).

of contrast is injected as close to the fistulous site as possible, and the filming rate is increased so that two to three films per second are obtained for 4 to 5 seconds. Multiple projections are needed.

Skin and Bone Grafts

Arteriography is increasingly used to evaluate donor as well as recipient sites for potential skin flaps[187–189] or bone grafts.[190] This is generally done for myocutaneous free flaps where a muscle segment with its overlying skin is taken as a whole, with its blood supply, and transported to another portion of the body. An example of this is the myocutaneous flap placed over the shin with the distal thigh serving as a donor site.[191,192] Confirming the patency of the recipient arteries will help ensure successful placement of the graft and continued viability (Fig. 67-36). Fibular bone grafts are often harvested from the leg. In such cases, the blood supply to the extremity is studied to verify

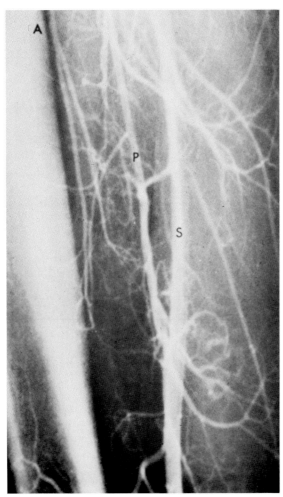 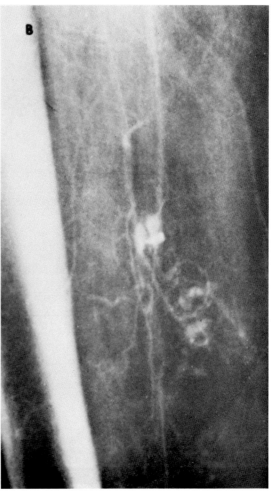

Figure 67-37. Congenital arteriovenous malformation of the capillary type with a biopsy diagnosis of cavernous hemangioma. (A) The lesion in the thigh receives its blood supply from the profunda femoris (*P*) and superficial femoral (*S*) arteries. Both vessels are normal in caliber. (B) Localized dilated contrast-filled spaces are observed late in the arterial phase, and no premature venous filling occurs.

that there are no anatomic variants—such as a solitary peroneal artery instead of posterior tibial and peroneal branches—that might compromise the donor site after the segment is removed.

Arteriovenous Malformations

Although congenital fistulas, like the acquired kind, may occur in any origin, the majority are located in the extremities. Congenital arteriovenous fistulas have been described by a confusing variety of names (*hemangioma simplex, angioma cavernosum, port-wine mark cirsoid aneurysm, congenital arteriovenous aneurysm,* and *racemose aneurysm*). Descriptive as these terms are, the underlying and unifying pathologic defect in this entity is the anomalous development of the

primitive vascular system. During early embryologic development future arteries and veins are poorly differentiated and normally communicate with each other. The potential for persistence of the communications exists, and at a more mature stage this persistence is abnormal. Hence this probably accounts for the clinical varieties of congenital fistulas designated as cirsoid aneurysms, arteriovenous malformations, or cavernous hemangiomas.

Szilagyi et al.[192a] suggest a classification of these lesions based on a correlation of their clinical and angiographic changes with the stages of embryologic development. Thus a simple cavernous hemangioma (Fig. 67-37) represents arrested development at the capillary network stage. Microfistulous and macrofistulous arteriovenous aneurysms are due to arrest at the reti-

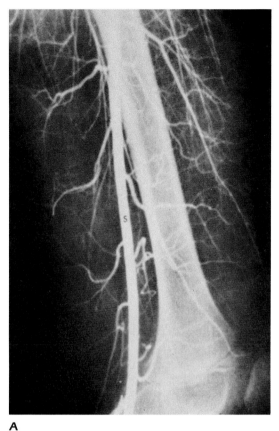

A

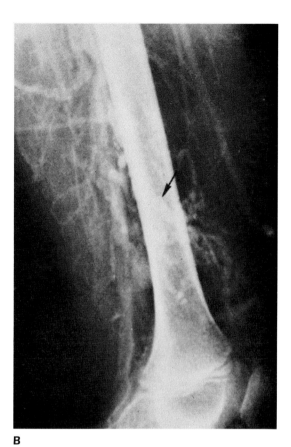

B

Figure 67-38. Congenital arteriovenous malformation of the venous type with a previous attempted excisional biopsy. (A) The superficial femoral artery (*S*) is not dilated, but its branches are more numerous than normal. Profunda femoris artery branches also supply the lesion. (B) In the venous phase the venous character of the lesion is evident from the numerous dilated, tortuous vessels (*arrow*).

form stage. Anomalous mature vascular channels result from maldevelopment at the stage of gross differentiation.

The terms *microfistula* and *macrofistula* designate whether the abnormal arteriovenous communication can be demonstrated by arteriography; only the macrofistulas are detectable by this technique. In any single patient a combination of hemangiomatous, microfistulous, and macrofistulous communications may be present because the different stages of embryologic development overlap.

Arteriography is very helpful for evaluating these lesions even when the clinical diagnosis may be obvious. Physical findings of a soft tissue swelling, with or without pigmentation, limb enlargement, prominent venous swelling, bruit, tenderness, and spontaneous bleeding, are all characteristic. Unlike acquired arteriovenous fistulas, the congenital variety seldom causes systemic hemodynamic changes. Arteriography is important to (1) define the site and extent of the arterial supply, (2) assess the feasibility of surgical extirpation,

and (3) help establish the adequacy of surgical resection. The common arteriographic feature in all these lesions is venous filling that is earlier than normal. The arterial vessels are not always dilated, but the veins usually are distended and complex. The lesions may be best appreciated in the venous or capillary phase of the injection (Fig. 67-38).

The therapy for congenital fistulas has been mainly surgical,[193] but permanent success resulting in a preserved, functioning extremity has been limited. The lack of success stems from the multiple sources of blood supply to the lesions. In the management of patients, there usually have been repeated attempts to eradicate the lesion by successive ligation of the feeding arteries. The result is finally limb amputation or recurrence of the lesion.

Transcatheter embolization is considered a therapeutic alternative or sometimes an adjunct to surgery for congenital fistulas.[194] Early clinical reports[195] mention Gelfoam, but the technique now relies on coils or other materials such as alcohol. In addition, the cutaneous abnormality is often directly injected with a sclerosing substance such as alcohol.[196]

The use of arteriography is especially critical for larger, deeper malformations in the pelvis.[197] A staged procedure with embolization followed by surgical exploration and ligation minimizes blood loss.

Spasm

Arterial spasm unrelated to severe arterial injury is a well-recognized entity in arteriography that may occur during or after the procedure.[198] It may be a response to the arterial trauma of catheterization, irritation of the vessel wall by the radiopaque contrast material, or a combination of both. Spasm is most often encountered in small-diameter vessels with a prominent muscle coat. Children and young adults are more prone to develop arterial spasm than older individuals because the latter may have fibrosis of the medial coat.[199] This phenomenon is demonstrated arteriographically as a localized narrowing of the artery with delayed blood flow distal to the site of spasm. Administration of calcium channel blockers can help alleviate the problem. Intraarterial injection of a vasodilator, Priscoline or nitroglycerine, may also reverse arterial spasm.

A distinctive arteriographic wave pattern (Fig. 67-39) has occasionally been observed in the superficial femoral, popliteal, pelvic, mesenteric, and other arteries throughout the body.[200] Various descriptive terms have been applied to this appearance, including *standing waves, stationary artery waves, beading, crenation, bamboo pattern,* and *string of pearls.* The phenomenon is not associated with any known pathologic process in the vessel at the site of the change. Fibrous dysplasia, a specific pathologic entity, has an arteriographic appearance similar to that of standing waves, but the two entities generally do not affect the same vessels. Standing waves usually disappear spontaneously.

The mechanisms responsible for the arterial standing wave pattern may include location in areas of decreased arterial flow—proximal to an occlusion or a severe tortuosity[201]—arterial spasm,[199,202] or purely physical factors such as pressure waves.[203] Another hypothesis accounts for both the physical and biologic mechanisms previously assumed and stresses the flow-pulse factor.[200]

Tumors

The tumors encountered in the lower extremity can be classified as tumors primary in bone, tumors primary in soft tissue, and metastatic lesions. Under the categories of bone and soft tissue tumors, malignant as well

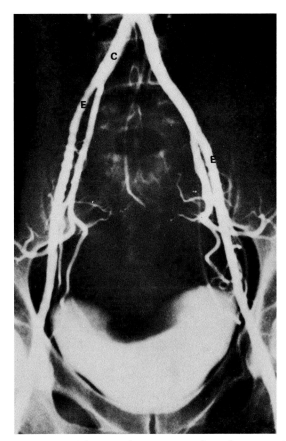

Figure 67-39. The typical appearance of standing waves in both external iliac arteries (*E*). The beaded pattern is more pronounced on the right. The common (*C*) and internal iliac arteries are normal.

as benign lesions should be considered. This chapter is confined mainly to malignant lesions because, in general, the benign tumors are avascular. Metastatic lesions may be subdivided into bone and soft tissue masses.

Although arteriography can be used to delineate these tumors,[204–206] it is rarely used to help in the differential diagnosis of tumors or for distinguishing malignant from benign lesions. However, arteriography can be of significant help in the management of these lesions. After identifying the feeding vessels to the tumor, it offers a map for percutaneous embolization.[207] The usual arteriographic finding of malignant tumors is increased vascularity consisting of tortuous, irregular vessels that do not gradually diminish in diameter (Fig. 67-40). The vessels may have altered diameters and appear to be beaded. Tumor stain or blush may be present, and the vascular pattern has an overall disorganized or chaotic appearance. Lakes of contrast filling due to dilated vascular spaces and early venous filling due to fine arteriovenous shunts may be observed.

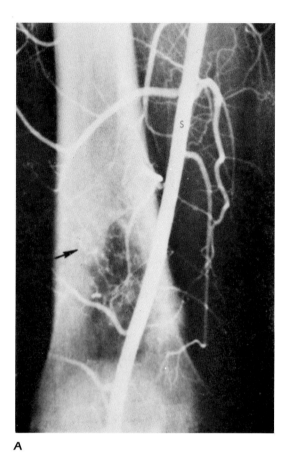

A

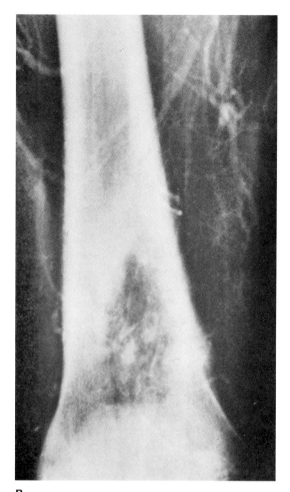

B

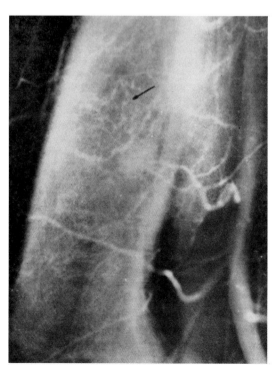

C

Figure 67-40. Osteogenic sarcoma of the femur. (A) The arterial phase demonstrates tumor vessels (*arrow*) in the area of the lytic bone lesion. The superficial femoral artery (*S*) is the main source of blood supply to the tumor. (B) There is early venous filling and a faint suggestion of tumor stain in the area of the lytic bone lesion. Note the periosteal elevation along the medial aspect of the femur. (C) Lateral view demonstrates the extent of the lesion and the chaotic pattern of the tumor vessels (*arrow*).

These findings are not specific to malignant lesions of bone and soft tissue. Some features may be present and then only to a varying degree. Furthermore, malignant tumors of the same histologic type do not necessarily exhibit the same arteriographic pattern (Figs. 67-41 and 67-42). Arteriographic interpretation also is complicated by benign tumors[208] and chronic inflammatory lesions,[209] which occasionally may stimulate the arteriographic appearance of a malignant tumor. Because of these limitations, arteriography plays a small role in the evaluation of lower extremity tumors. If done, either traditional film or digital imaging can be used.[210]

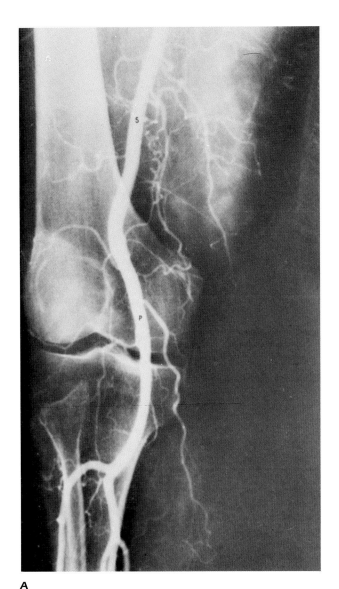

A

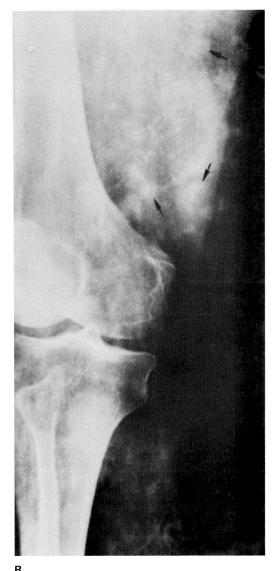

B

Figure 67-41. Malignant melanoma involving the lower leg thigh and inguinal nodes. (A) The superficial femoral artery (*S*) demonstrates numerous branches that supply multiple discrete melanomatous nodules in the soft tissues. *P*, popli-

teal continuation of superficial femoral artery. (B) In the capillary phase these nodules are hypervascular and vary in size (*arrows*).

Most osteogenic sarcomas display areas of increased vascularity (see Fig. 67-40) dispersed in relatively avascular zones, which help to identify these lesions. Chondrosarcomas vary greatly in their degree of vascularity and cover a spectrum from avascular to highly vascular malignancies. They sometimes show characteristic scalloped or wavy vessels. In the soft tissue malignancies of the lower extremity, the degree of vascularity has been said to serve as an index to the degree of their malignancy.[204,205] Fibrosarcomas,[211] like chondrosarcomas, vary markedly in the degree of their vascularity, but the more vascular tumors are highly

malignant. Liposarcomas (Fig. 67-43), rhabdomyosarcomas (Fig. 67-44), and synovial sarcomas may be quite vascular, but nothing characteristic distinguishes these lesions from one another.[205] Metastatic lesions to bone or soft tissue usually display the same characteristics as the primary lesion. Thus secondary lesions from the kidney (Fig. 67-45) and thyroid tend to be vascular because the primary lesions are hypervascular. Aggressive management of patients with these metastatic lesions includes the insertion of prosthesis in bones affected by metastases either following a fracture or in order to prevent one.[212,213] Hemorrhagic compli-

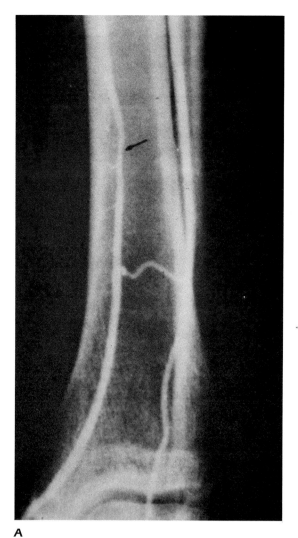

A

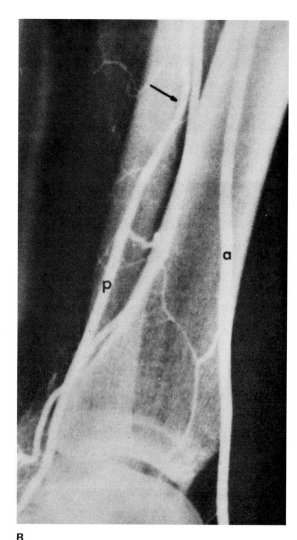

B

Figure 67-42. Malignant melanoma involving the foot and lower leg. (A) Anteroposterior view demonstrates a focal narrowing (*arrow*) of the posterior tibial artery. (B) Lateral view confirms this narrowing (*arrow*) of the artery (*p*) and shows localized displacement of the vessel. Tumor en-casement of the vessel by a melanomatous lesion causes the narrowing. Unlike the malignant melanoma in Figure 67-41, this lesion is not hypervascular. Note the normal anterior tibial artery (A).

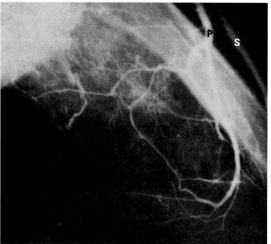

A

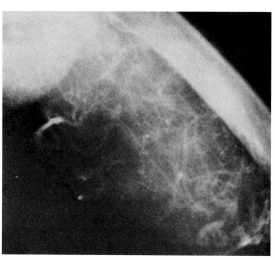

B

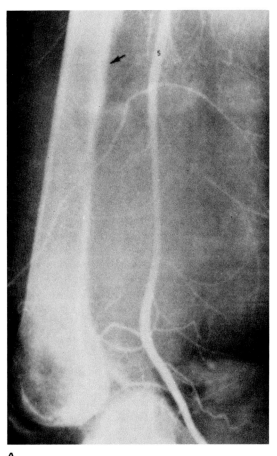

A

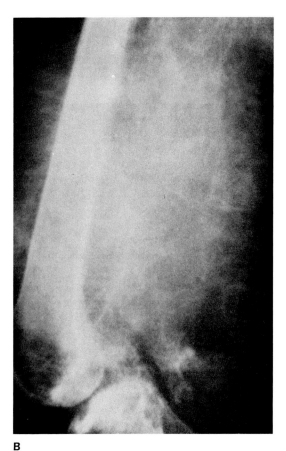

B

Figure 67-44. Rhabdomyosarcoma of the distal thigh causing a large soft tissue mass and bone involvement. (A) Arterial phase demonstrates a relatively hypovascular mass around which are stretched branches of the superficial femoral artery (*S*), which is compressed and displaced by the mass. There is cortical erosion (*arrow*) of the femur due to the tumor. (B) In the venous phase the chaotic nature of the vascularity is best appreciated, even though no distinct early venous filling is seen. A diffuse and uneven tumor stain is seen in different parts of the tumor.

cations are often seen in these cases. Preoperative arteriography and embolization, usually within 24 hours of the surgery, will decrease blood loss and help decrease the length of the surgical procedure.

Conclusion

Arteriography of the lower extremity remains an important diagnostic examination. It has changed in character, becoming more efficient as traditional film processing is replaced by digital technologies and inpa-

tient procedures become outpatient ones. More importantly, although its diagnostic role is decreasing because of the increased use of noninvasive technologies, it remains the critical element for the successful use of percutaneous vascular interventions.

Acknowledgments

Much of this chapter was prepared by Klaus M. Bron for Abrams' Angiography, 3rd ed. It has been revised and updated for the fourth edition by Joseph F. Polak.

◄ **Figure 67-43.** Liposarcoma of the thigh forming a large, firm, soft tissue mass. (A) The tumor is moderately vascular, supplied by branches of the profunda femoris artery (*P*) but not the superficial femoral artery (*S*). Irregular, fine tumor vessels and areas of tumor stain are evident. (B) There is early venous filling, and the veins are dilated and tortuous. The tumor was moderately well circumscribed.

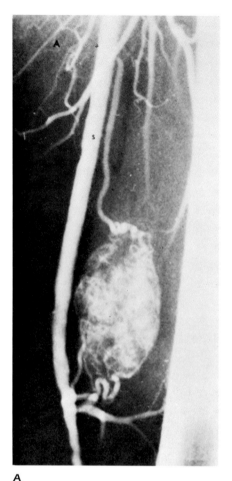

A

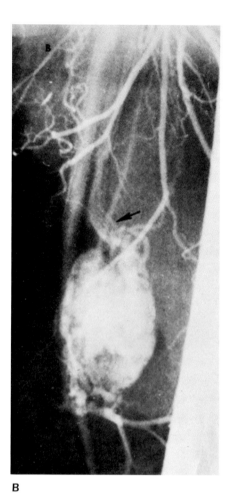

B

Figure 67-45. Metastasis from a renal cell carcinoma, clinically unsuspected and detected incidentally during arteriography for peripheral vascular disease. (A) The circumscribed hypervascular area derives its blood supply from the superficial femoral artery (*S*). The metastasis reflects the typical appearance of a primary renal cell carcinoma. (B) Tumor stain and early venous filling (*arrow*) are evident.

References

1. Braunstein PW, Skudder PA, McCarroll JR, et al. Concealed hemorrhage due to pelvic fracture. J Trauma 1964;4:832–838.
2. Gruntzig A, Kumpe DA. Technique of percutaneous transluminal angioplasty with the Gruntzig balloon catheter. AJR 1979;132:547–552.
3. Zeitler E, Gruntzig A, Schoop W, eds. Percutaneous vascular recanalization: technique, applications, clinical results. New York: Springer, 1978.
4. Sumner DS, Strandness DE. The relationship between calf blood flow and ankle blood pressure in patients with intermittent claudication. Surgery 1969;65:763–771.
5. Yao JST. Hemodynamic studies in peripheral arterial disease. Br J Surg 1970;57:761–766.
6. Darling RC, Raines JK, Brener BJ, et al. Quantitative segmental pulse volume recorder: a clinical tool. Surgery 1973;72:873–887.
7. Owen RS, Carpenter JP, Baum RA, Perloff LJ, Cope C. Magnetic resonance imaging of angiographically occult runoff vessels in peripheral arterial occlusive disease. N Engl J Med 1992;326:1577–1581.
8. Smith TP, Cragg AH, Berbaum KS, et al. Comparison of the efficacy of digital subtraction and film-screen angiography of the lower limb: prospective study in 50 patients. AJR 1992;158:431–436.
9. Kinnison M, Perler BA, White RI Jr, et al. Tailored approach for evaluation of peripheral vascular disease: intravenous digital subtraction angiography. AJR 1984;142:1205–1209.
10. Andersen PE Jr. Brachialis Seldinger puncture with use of introducer sheath. Br J Radiol 1985;58:777–778.
11. Berman HL, Katz SG, Tihansky DP. Guided direct antegrade puncture of the superficial femoral artery. AJR 1986;147:632–634.
12. Watkinson AF, Hartnell GG. Complications of direct brachial artery puncture for arteriography: a comparison of techniques. Clin Radiol 1991;44:189–191.
13. Anson BJ, Morris H. Human anatomy: a complete systematic treatise. 12th ed. New York: Blakiston, Division, McGraw-Hill, 1966.
14. Figge FHJ, Hild WJ. Sobotta/Figge atlas of human anatomy. 9th engl. ed. Baltimore: Urban & Schwarzenberg, 1977.
15. Strandness DEJ, ed. Collateral circulation in clinical surgery. Philadelphia: Saunders, 1969.
16. Friedenberg MJ, Perez CA. Collateral circulation in aorto-ilio-femoral occlusive disease: as demonstrated by a unilateral

percutaneous common femoral artery needle injection. AJR 1958;94:145–158.

17. Muller RF, Figley MM. The arteries of the abdomen, pelvis, and thigh: I. Normal roentgenographic anatomy. II. Collateral circulation in obstructive arterial disease. AJR 1957;77:296–311.

17a. Freeman MP, Tisnado J, Cho S-R. Persistent sciatic artery. Report of three cases and literature review. Brit J Radiol 1986;59:217–223.

17b. Nabatoff RA. Anomalies encountered during varicose vein surgery. Arch Surg 1978;113:586–588.

18. Millward SF, Marsh JI, Peterson RA. Outpatient transfemoral angiography with a two-hour observation period. Cardiovasc Intervent Radiol 1989;12:290–291.

19. Rogers WF, Kraft MA. Outpatient angioplasty. Radiology 1990;174:753–755.

20. Seldinger SI. Catheter replacement of the needle in percutaneous arteriography: a new technique. Acta Radiol 1953;39:368–376.

21. Wendth AJJ. Peripheral arteriography—an overview of its origins and present status. CRC Crit Rev Diagn Imaging 1975;6:369–401.

22. Lilly MP, Reichman W, Sarazen AAJ, et al. The role of extra-anatomic exclusion bypass in the treatment of disseminated atheroembolism syndrome. Ann Vasc Surg 1990;4:260–263.

23. Mani RL, Helms CA, Eisenberg RL. Use of a 5 French catheter with multiple side holes in abdominal aortography. Radiology 1977;123:233–234.

24. Cragg AH, Nakagawa N, Smith TP, et al. Hematoma formation after diagnostic angiography: effect of catheter size. J Vasc Intervent Radiol 1991;2:231–233.

25. Olin T. Studies in angiographic techniques. Stockholm: Hakan Ohlssons Boktryckeri, 1963.

26. Judkins MP, Kidd HJ, Frische LH, et al. Lumen-following safety J-guide for catheterization of tortuous vessels. Radiology 1967;88:1127–1130.

27. Baum S, Abrams HL. A J-shaped catheter for retrograde catheterization of tortuous vessels. Radiology 1964;83:436–437.

28. Ernst SM, Tjonjoegin RM, Schradrer R, et al. Immediate sealing of arterial puncture sites after cardiac catheterization and coronary angioplasty using a biodegradable collagen plug: results of an international registry. J Am Coll Cardiol 1993;21:851–855.

29. Sacks D, Summers TA. Antegrade selective catheterization of femoral vessels with a 4- or 5-F catheter and safety wire. J Vasc Intervent Radiol 1991;2:325–326.

30. Bron KM. Selective visceral and total abdominal arteriography via the left axillary artery in the older age group. AJR 1966;97:432–437.

31. Glenn JH. Abdominal aorta catheterization via the left axillary artery. Radiology 1975;115:227–228.

32. McIvor J, Rhymer JC. 245 transaxillary arteriograms in arteriopathic patients: success rate and complications. Clin Radiol 1992;45:390–394.

33. Field J, McIvor I, Greenhalgh RM. Transaxillary angiography: an acceptable approach when prefemoral angiography is not acceptable. Eur J Vasc Surg 1987;1:193–195.

34. Gritter KJ, Laidlaw WW, Peterson NT. Complications of outpatient transbrachial intraarterial digital subtraction angiography: work in progress. Radiology 1987;162:125–127.

35. Foley WD, Beres J, Smith DF, et al. I.V. and intraarterial hybrid digital subtraction angiography: clinical evaluation. AJR 1986;147:613–620.

36. Bell JW. Surgical treatment of chronic occlusion of the terminal aorta. Am Surg 1972;38:481–485.

37. Eisenberg RL, Mani RL, McDonald EJ Jr. The complication rate of catheter angiography by direct puncture through aortofemoral bypass grafts. AJR 1976;126:814–816.

38. Da Silva JR, Eckstein MR, Kelemouridis V, et al. Aortofemoral bypass grafts: safety of percutaneous puncture. J Vasc Surg 1984;1:642–645.

39. AbuRahma AF, Robinson PA, Boland JP. Safety of arteriography by direct puncture of a vascular prosthesis. Am J Surg 1992;164:233–236.

40. dos Santos R. Technique de l'aortographie. J Int Chir 1937;2:609–634.

41. Amplatz K. Translumbar catheterization of the abdominal aorta. Radiology 1963;81:927–931.

42. Riddervold HO, Seale DL. Translumbar aortography with Teflon catheters. Acta Radiol 1972;12:619–624.

43. Chuang VP, Fried AM, Chen CQ. Computed tomographic evaluation of para-aortic hematoma following translumbar aortography. Radiology 1979;130:711–712.

44. Amendola MA, Tisnado J, Fields WR, et al. Evaluation of retroperitoneal hemorrhage by computed tomography before and after translumbar aortography. Radiology 1979;133:401–404.

45. Hall P, Iyer SS, Dorros G. Successful thrombolysis of a chronically occluded femoropopliteal synthetic bypass graft via the popliteal approach: case report. Cardiovasc Intervent Radiol 1991;14:352–354.

46. Trigaux JP, Van Beers B, De Wisepelaere JF. Anatomic relationship between the popliteal artery and vein: a guide to accurate angiographic puncture. AJR 1991;157:1259–1262.

47. Hall JR, Hacking PM, Layzell T. Comparison of venous digital subtraction angiography and aortography in patients with peripheral vascular disease of the lower limbs. Clin Radiol 1985;36:315–319.

48. Agee OF, Kaude J. Arteriography of the pelvis and lower extremities with moving table technique. AJR 1969;107:860–865.

49. Takahashi M, Koga Y, Bussaka H, et al. The value of digital subtraction angiography in peripheral vascular diseases. Br J Radiol 1984;57:123–132.

50. Blakeman BM, Littooy FN, Baker WH. Intra-arterial digital subtraction angiography as a method to study peripheral vascular disease. J Vasc Surg 1986;4:168–173.

51. Brenot P, Raynaud A, Pernes JM, et al. Étude comparative de la réalisation des angioplasties iliaques en angiographie numérique et conventionnelle. Incidence sur les couts reels (consommables). J Radiol 1986;67:643–646.

52. Videl JL, Adam P, Lestrade M, et al. Technique d'angiographie numer i ponctioni arterielle femorale unilaterale et deplacement programs de la table d'examen. A propos de 56 cas. J Radiol 1986;67:41–45.

53. Schwarten DE. Percutaneous transluminal angioplasty of the iliac arteries: intravenous digital subtraction angiography for follow-up. Radiology 1984;150:363–367.

54. Burbank FH, Brody WR, Bradley BR. Effect of volume and rate of contrast medium injection on intravenous digital subtraction angiographic contrast medium curves. J Am Coll Cardiol 1984;4:308–315.

55. Wilson NM, Chan O, Thomas ML, et al. Intravenous digital subtraction angiography in the management of peripheral vascular disease. J Cardiovasc Surg 1991;32:747–752.

56. Eisenman JI, O'Loughlin BJ. Value of lateral abdominal aortography. AJR 1971;112:586.

57. Simon H, Fairbank JT. Biplane translumbar aortography for evaluation of peripheral vascular disease. Am J Surg 1977;133:447–452.

58. Thomas ML, Andress MR. Value of oblique projections in translumbar aortography. AJR 1972;116:187–193.

59. Sethi GK, Scott SM, Takaro T. Multiple-plane angiography for more precise evaluation of aortoiliac disease. Surgery 1975;78:154–159.

60. Ahovuo J, Lepantalo M, Kinnunen J et al. How many projections are really needed in angiographic assessment of the femoral bifurcation? Roentgenblaetter 1990;43:530–532.

61. McDonald EJ Jr, Malone JM, Eisenberg RL, et al. Arteriographic evaluation of the femoral bifurcation: value of the ipsilateral anterior oblique projection. AJR 1976;127:955–963.

62. Kozak BE, Bedell JE, Rösch J. Small vessel leg angiography for distal vessel bypass grafts. J Vasc Surg 1988;8:711–715.

63. Teeuwen C, Eikelboom BC, Ludwig JW. Clinically unsus-

pected complications of arterial surgery shown by post-operative digital subtraction angiography. Br J Radiol 1989;62:13–19.

64. Kahn PC, Boyer DN, Moran JM, et al. Reactive hyperemia in lower extremity arteriography: an evaluation. Radiology 1968;90:975–980.

65. Boijsen E, Dahn I. Femoral angiography during maximal blood flow. Acta Radiol 1965;3:543–553.

66. Wahren J, Cronestrand R, Juhlin-Dannfelt A. Leg blood flow during exercise in patients with occlusion of the iliac artery: pre- and postoperative studies. Scand J Clin Lab Invest 1963;32:257–263.

67. Erikson U. Peripheral arteriography during bradykinin induced vasodilation. Acta Radiol 1965;3:193–201.

68. Jacobs JB, Hanafee WN. The use of Priscoline in peripheral arteriography. Radiology 1967;88:957–960.

69. Cardella JF, Smith TP, Darcy MD, et al. Balloon occlusion femoral angiography prior to in-situ saphenous vein bypass. Cardiovasc Intervent Radiol 1987;10:181–187.

70. Holmes CM, Galletly DG. Midazolam/fentanyl: a total intravenous technique for short procedures. Anaesthesia 1982;37:761–765.

71. Gordon IJ, Westcott JL. Intra-arterial lidocaine: an effective analgesic for peripheral angiography. Radiology 1977;124:43–45.

72. Guthaner DF, Silverman JF, Hayden WG, et al. Intraarterial analgesia in peripheral arteriography. AJR 1977;128:737–739.

73. Nilsson P, Almen T, Golman K, et al. Addition of local anesthetics to contrast media: I. Effects on patient discomfort and hemodynamics in aortofemoral angiography. Acta Radiol 1987;28:209–214.

74. Lindgren P, Saltzman G-F, Tornell G. Vascular effects of metrizoate compounds, Isopaque Na and Isopaque Na/Ca/Mg. Acta Radiol Suppl (Stockh) 1967;270:44–57.

75. Eisenberg RL, Mani RL, Hedgcock MW. Pain associated with peripheral angiography: is lidocaine effective? Radiology 1978;127:109–111.

76. Almen T, Boijsen E, Lindell SE. Metrizamide in angiography: I. Femoral angiography. Acta Radiol 1977;18:33–38.

77. Gordon IJ, Skoblar RS, Chicatelli PD, et al. A comparison of iohexol and Conray-60 in peripheral angiography. AJR 1984;142:563–565.

78. Albrechtsson U, Hultberg B, Larusdottir H, et al. Nephrotoxicity of ionic and non-ionic contrast media in aortofemoral angiography. Acta Radiol 1985;26:615–618.

79. Lautin EM, Freeman NJ, Schoenfeld AH, et al. Radiocontrast-associated renal dysfunction: a comparison of lower-osmolality and conventional high-osmolality contrast media. AJR 1991;157:59–65.

80. Lautin EM, Freeman NJ, Schoenfeld AH, et al. Radiocontrast-associated renal dysfunction: incidence and risk factors. AJR 1991;157:49–58.

81. Cragg AH, Smith TP, Berbaum KS, et al. Randomized double-blind trial of midazolam/placebo and midazolam/fentanyl for sedation and analgesia in lower-extremity angiography. AJR 1991;157:173–176.

82. Foster JH. Arteriography: cornerstone of vascular surgery. Arch Surg 1974;109:605–611.

83. Haimovici H, Steinman C. Aortoiliac angiographic patterns associated with femoropopliteal occlusive disease: significance in reconstructive arterial surgery. Surgery 1969;65:232–240.

84. Kehler M, Albrechtsson U, Alwmark A, et al. Intra-operative digital angiography as a control of the in situ saphenous vein bypass grafts. Acta Radiol 1988;29:645–648.

85. Zatina MA, Schroder WB, Wilkerson DK, et al. Can intraoperative prebypass arteriography substitute for the preoperative arteriogram? Ann Vasc Surg 1991;5:143–149.

86. Rutherford RB, Flanigan DP, Gupta SK, et al. Suggested standards for reports dealing with lower extremity ischemia. J Vasc Surg 1986;4:80–94.

87. Hunink MGM, Magruder CD, Meyerovitz MF, et al. Risks and benefits of femoropopliteal percutaneous balloon angioplasty. J Vasc Surg 1993;17:183–194.

88. Johnston KW. Femoral and popliteal arteries: reanalysis of results of balloon angioplasty. Radiology 1992;183:767–771.

89. Brest AN, Moyer JH, eds. Atherosclerotic vascular disease: a hagnemann symposium. New York: Appleton-Century-Crofts, 1967.

90. Mavor GE. The pattern of occlusion in atheroma of the lower limb arteries: the correlation of clinical and arteriographic findings. Br J Surg 1956;43:352–364.

91. Lindbom A. Arteriosclerosis and arterial thrombosis in the lower limb: a roentgenological study. Acta Radiol Suppl (Stockh) 1950;80:1–80.

92. Glagov S, Zarins C, Giddens DP, et al. Hemodynamics and atherosclerosis: insights and perspectives gained from studies of human arteries. Arch Pathol Lab Med 1988;112:1018–1031.

93. Darling RC. Peripheral arterial surgery. N Engl J Med 1969;280:26–30.

94. Thompson JE, Garrett WV. Peripheral-arterial surgery. N Engl J Med 1980;302:491–503.

95. DeBakey ME, Crawford ES, Cooley DA, et al. Surgical considerations of occlusive disease of the abdominal aorta and iliac and femoral arteries: analysis of 803 cases. Ann Surg 1958;148:306–324.

96. Thurlbeck WM, Castleman B. Atheromatous emboli to the kidneys after aortic surgery. N Engl J Med 1957;257:442–447.

97. Hobson RW II, Rich NM, Fedde CW. Surgical management of high aortoiliac occlusion. Am Surg 1975;41:271–280.

98. Levinson SA, Levinson HJ, Halloran LG, et al. Limited indications for unilateral aortofemoral or iliofemoral vascular grafts. Arch Surg 1973;107:791–796.

99. Dennis JW, Littooy FN, Greisler HP, et al. Anastomotic pseudoaneurysms: a continuing late complication of vascular reconstructive procedures. Arch Surg 1986;121:314–317.

100. Christensen RD, Bernatz PE. Anastomotic aneurysms involving the femoral artery. Mayo Clin Proc 1972;47:313–317.

101. Szilagyi DE, Smith RF, Elliott JP, et al. Anastomotic aneurysms after vascular reconstruction: problems of incidence, etiology, and treatment. Surgery 1975;78:800–816.

102. Mozersky DJ, Sumner DS, Strandness DE. Long-term results of reconstructive aortoiliac surgery. Am J Surg 1972;123:503–509.

103. Brief DK, Alpert J, Parsonnet V. Crossover femoro-femoral grafts. Compromise or preference: a reappraisal. Arch Surg 1972;105:889–894.

104. Crawford FA, Sethi GK, Scott SM, et al. Femorofemoral grafts for unilateral occlusion of aortic bifurcation grafts. Surgery 1975;77:150–153.

105. Vetto RM. The treatment of unilateral iliac artery obstruction with a transabdominal, subcutaneous, femoro-femoral graft. Surgery 1962;52:342–345.

106. Trimble IR, Stonesifer GL Jr, Wilgis EFS, et al. Criteria for femoro-femoral bypass from clinical and hemodynamic studies. Ann Surg 1972;175:985–993.

107. Reichle FA, Tyson RR. Bypasses to tibial or popliteal arteries in severely ischemic lower extremities: comparison of long-term results in 233 patients. Ann Surg 1964;176:315–320.

108. Reichle FA, Tyson RR. Comparison of long-term results of 364 femoropopliteal or femorotibial bypasses for revascularization of severely ischemic lower extremities. Ann Surg 1975;182:449–455.

109. Menzoian JO, La Morte WW, Cantelmo NL, et al. The preoperative angiogram as a predictor of peripheral vascular run-off. Am J Surg 1985;150:346–352.

110. Kram HB, Appel PL, Shoemaker WC. Comparison of transcutaneous oximetry, vascular hemodynamic measurements, angiography, and clinical findings to predict the success of peripheral vascular reconstruction. Am J Surg 1988;155:551–558.

111. Procter AE, Cumberland DC. Peripheral angioplasty: empha-

sizing the need for complete visualization in lower limb angiography. Clin Radiol 1985;36:321–326.

112. Buchbinder D, Pasch AR, Verta MJ, et al. Ankle bypass: should we go the distance? Am J Surg 1985;150:216–219.
113. Friedman SG, Krishnasastry KV, Doscher W, et al. Lower extremity revascularization via the lateral plantar artery. Am Surg 1990;56:721–725.
114. Buchbinder D, Rollins DL, Semrow CM, et al. In situ tibial reconstruction: state-of-the-art or passing fancy? Ann Surg 1988;207:184–188.
115. Hallin RW. Femoropopliteal versus femorotibial bypass grafting for lower extremity revascularization. Am Surg 1976;42: 522–526.
116. Karacagil S, Almgren B, Bowald S, et al. A new method of angiographic runoff evaluation in femorodistal reconstructions: significant correlation with early graft patency. Arch Surg 1990;125:1055–1058.
117. Dotter CT, Judkins MP. Transluminal treatment of arteriosclerotic obstruction: description of a new technic and a preliminary report of its application. Circulation 1964;30:654–670.
118. Collins RH, Voorhees AB, Reemtsma K, et al. Efficacy of percutaneous angioplasty in lower extremity arterial occlusive disease. J Cardiovasc Surg 1984;25:390–394.
119. Graor RA, Whitlow PL. Transluminal atherectomy for occlusive peripheral vascular disease. J Am Coll Cardiol 1990;15: 1551–1558.
120. Palmaz JC, Richter GM, Noeldge G, et al. Intraluminal stents in atherosclerotic iliac artery stenosis: preliminary report of a multicenter study. Radiology 1988;168:727–731.
121. Gunther RW, Vorwerk D, Bohndorf K, et al. Iliac and femoral artery stenoses and occlusions: treatment with intravascular stents. Radiology 1989;172:725–730.
122. Kinnison ML, Perler BA, Kaufman SL, et al. In situ saphenous vein bypass grafts: angiographic evaluation and interventional repair of complications. Radiology 1986;160:727–730.
123. Belkin M, Donaldson MC, Whittemore AD, et al. Observations on the use of thrombolytic agents for thrombotic occlusion of infrainguinal vein grafts. J Vasc Surg 1990;11:289–294.
124. Whittemore AD, Donaldson MC, Polak JF, et al. Limitations of balloon angioplasty for vein graft stenosis. J Vasc Surg 1991;14:340–345.
125. Darling RC, Austen WG, Linton RR. Arterial embolism. Surg Gynecol Obstet 1967;124:106–114.
126. Weston TS. Arterial embolism of the lower limbs. Australas Radiol 1967;11:354–359.
127. Fisher DF Jr, Clagett GP, Brigham RA, et al. Dilemmas in dealing with the blue toe syndrome: aortic versus peripheral source. Am J Surg 1984;148:836–839.
128. Crane C. Atherothrombotic embolism to lower extremities in arteriosclerosis. Arch Surg 1967;94:96–101.
129. Takolander R, Bergquist D, Jonsson K, et al. Fatal thromboembolic complications at aorto-femoral angiography. Acta Radiol 1985;26:15–19.
130. Thompson JE, Sigler L, Raut PS, et al. Arterial embolectomy: a 20 year experience with 163 cases. Surgery 1970;67:212–220.
131. Levy JF, Butcher HRJ. Arterial-emboli: an analysis of 125 patients. Surgery 1970;68:968.
132. Stallone RJ, Blaisdell FW, Cafferata HT, et al. Analysis of morbidity and mortality from arterial embolectomy. Surgery 1969;65:207–217.
133. Fogarty TJ, Daily PO, Shumway NE, et al. Experience with balloon catheter technic for arterial embolectomy. Am J Surg 1971;122:231–237.
134. Linton RR. Peripheral arterial embolism: a discussion of the postembolic vascular changes and their relation to the restoration of circulation in peripheral embolism. N Engl J Med 1941;224:189–194.
135. Fogarty TJ, Cranley JJ, Krause RJ, et al. A method for extraction of arterial emboli and thrombi. Surg Gynecol Obstet 1971;116:241–244.
136. Weisman ID, Stanchfield WR Jr, Herzog CA, et al. Left ventricular thromboembolic occlusion of the popliteal artery treated nonoperatively with local urokinase infusion—a case report. Angiology 1988;39:179–186.
137. Goldberg L, Ricci MT, Sauvage LR, et al. Thrombolytic therapy for delayed occlusion of knitted Dacron bypass grafts in the axillofemoral, femoropopliteal and femorotibial positions. Surg Gynecol Obstet 1985;160:491–498.
138. Allen EV, Barker NW, Hines EA Jr. Peripheral vascular diseases. 3rd ed. Philadelphia: Saunders, 1962.
139. Sarkar R, Cilley RE, Coran AG. Abdominal aneurysms in childhood: report of a case and review of the literature. Surgery 1991;109:143–148.
140. Chan O, Thomas ML. The incidence of popliteal aneurysms in patients with arteriomegaly. Clin Radiol 1990;41:185–189.
141. Friesen G, Ivins JC, Janes JM. Popliteal aneurysms. Surgery 1962;51:90–98.
142. Wychulis AR, Spittell JAJ, Wallace RB. Popliteal aneurysms. Surgery 1970;68:942–952.
143. Sprayregen S. Popliteal vein displacement by popliteal artery aneurysms: report of 4 cases. AJR 1979;132:838–839.
144. Munk PL, Pitman RG, Chipperfield PM, et al. Iliac artery aneurysms arising in patients having had resections of abdominal aneurysms. Can Assoc Radiol J 1988;39:224–227.
145. Buerger L. The circulatory disturbances of the extremities, including gangrene, vasomotor and trophic disorders. Philadelphia: Saunders, 1924.
146. McKusick VA, Harris WS, Ottesen OE, et al. Buerger's disease: a distinct clinical and pathologic entity. JAMA 1962; 181:5–12.
147. Wessler S, Ming S-C, Gurewich V, et al. A critical evaluation of thromboangiitis obliterans: the case against Buerger's disease. N Engl J Med 1960;262:1149–1160.
148. Szilagyi DE, DeRusso FJ, Elliot JP Jr. Thromboangiitis obliterans: clinicoangiographic correlations. Arch Surg 1964;88: 824–835.
149. O'Gorman RB, Feliciano DV, Bitondo C, et al. Emergency center arteriography in the evaluation of suspected peripheral vascular injuries. Arch Surg 1984;119:568–573.
150. O'Gorman RB, Feliciano DV. Arteriography performed in the emergency center. Am J Surg 1986;152:323–325.
151. Smith SM, Galland RB. Late presentation of femoral artery complications following percutaneous cannulation for cardiac angiography or angioplasty. J Cardiovasc Surg 1992;33:437–439.
152. Bystrom JH, Dencker H, Jaderling J, et al. Ligation of the internal iliac artery to arrest massive haemorrhage following pelvic fracture. Acta Chir Scand 1968;134:199–202.
153. Miller WE. Massive hemorrhage in fractures of the pelvis. South Med J 1963;56:933–938.
154. Peltier LF. Complications associated with fractures of the pelvis. J Bone Joint Surg (Am) 1965;47:1060–1069.
155. Quinby WC Jr. Pelvic fractures with hemorrhage. N Engl J Med 1971;284:668–669.
156. Margolies MN, Ring EJ, Waltman AC, et al. Arteriography in the management of hemorrhage from pelvic fractures. N Engl J Med 1972;287:317–321.
157. Hauser CW, Perry JF Jr. Control of massive hemorrhage from pelvic fractures by hypogastric artery ligation. Surg Gynecol Obstet 1965;121:313–315.
158. Motsay GJ, Manlove C, Perry JF. Major venous injury with pelvic fracture. J Trauma 1969;9:343–346.
159. Ravitch MM. Hypogastric artery ligation in acute pelvic trauma. Surgery 1964;56:601–602.
160. Morrison KM, Ebraheim NA, Savolaine ER, et al. "Interventional angiography": a possible role in intraoperative balloon occlusion catheterization of lacerated pelvic arteries. J Orthop Res 1989;7:824–827.
161. Scalea TM, Sclafani SJA. Angiographically placed balloons for arterial control: a description of a technique. J Trauma 1991; 31:1671–1677.

162. Jebara VA, Haddad SN, Ghossain MA, et al. Emergency arteriography in the assessment of penetrating trauma to the lower limbs. Angiology 1991;42:527–532.

163. DeBakey ME, Simeone FA. Battle injuries of the arteries in World War II: an analysis of 2471 cases. Ann Surg 1946;123:534–579.

164. Dennis JW, Frykberg ER, Crump JM, et al. New perspectives on the management of penetrating trauma in proximity to major limb arteries. J Vasc Surg 1990;11:84–93.

165. Klingensmith W, Oles P, Martinez H. Fractures with associated blood vessel injury. Am J Surg 1965;110:849–852.

166. Kaufman SL, Martin LG. Arterial injuries associated with complete dislocation of the knee. Radiology 1992;184:153–155.

167. Treiman SG, Yellin AE, Weaver FA, et al. Examination of the patient with a knee dislocation: the case for selective arteriography. Arch Surg 1992;127:1056–1063.

168. Kelly GL, Eiseman B. Civilian vascular injuries. J Trauma 1975;15:507–514.

169. Applebaum R, Yellin AE, Weaver FA, et al. Role of routine arteriography in blunt lower-extremity trauma. Am J Surg 1990;160:221–225.

170. Blasier RB, Pape JM. Simulation of compartment syndrome by rupture of the deep femoral artery from blunt trauma. Clin Orthop 1991;266:214–217.

171. Nolan B, McQuillan WM. Acute traumatic limb ischaemia. Br J Surg 1965;52:559–565.

172. Bergan F. Traumatic intimal rupture of the popliteal artery with acute ischemia of the limb in cases with supracondylar fractures of the femur. J Cardiovasc Surg (Torino) 1963;4:300–302.

173. Norris CS, Zlotnick R, Silva WE, et al. Traumatic pseudoaneurysm following blunt trauma. J Trauma 1986;26:480–482.

174. Miller HH, Welch CS. Quantitative studies on the time factor in arterial injuries. Ann Surg 1949;130:428–438.

175. Kirkup JR. Major arterial injury complicating fracture of the femoral shaft. J Bone Joint Surg (Br) 1963;45:337–343.

176. Hewitt RL, Smith AD, Drapanas T. Acute traumatic arteriovenous fistulas. J Trauma 1973;13:901–906.

177. Gaylis H, Levine E, Van Dongen LGR, et al. Arteriovenous fistulas after gynecologic operations. Surg Gynecol Obstet 1973;137:655–658.

178. Gaspard DJ, Gaspar MR. Arteriovenous fistula after Fogarty catheter thrombectomy. Arch Surg 1972;105:90–92.

179. Creech O Jr, Gantt J, Wren H. Traumatic arteriovenous fistula at unusual sites. Ann Surg 1965;161:908–920.

180. Hewitt RL, Collins DJ. Acute arteriovenous fistulas in war injuries. Ann Surg 1969;169:447–449.

181. Holman E. The physiology of an arteriovenous fistula. Arch Surg 1923;7:64–82.

182. Holman E. Reflections on arteriovenous fistulas. Ann Thorac Surg 1971;11:176–186.

183. Branham HH. Aneurysmal varix of the femoral artery and vein following a gunshot wound. Int J Surg 1980;3:250–251.

184. Handa J, Handa H, Torizuka K, et al. Radioisotopic study of arteriovenous anomalies. AJR 1972;115:751–759.

185. Stephenson HE Jr, Lichti EL. Application of the Doppler Ultrasonic Flowmeter in the surgical treatment of arteriovenous fistula. Am Surg 1971;37:537–538.

186. Picus D, Totty WG. Iatrogenic femoral arteriovenous fistulae: evaluation by digital vascular imaging. AJR 1984;142:567–570.

187. May JWJ, Athanasoulis CA, Donelan MB. Preoperative magnification angiography of donor and recipient sites for clinical free transfer of flaps or digits. Plast Reconstr Surg 1979;64:483–490.

188. Katai K, Kido M, Numaguchi Y. Angiography of the iliofemoral arteriovenous system supplying free groin flaps and free hypogastric flaps. Plast Reconstr Surg 1979;63:671–679.

189. Gerlock AJ, Perry PE, Goncharenko V, et al. Evaluation of the dorsalis pedis free flap donor site by angiography. Radiology 1979;130:341–343.

190. Kaj R, Kauko S, Timo T, et al. Arteriography in evaluating vascularized bone graft in the hip joint. Australas Radiol 1988;32:251–256.

191. Harder T, Deroover M, Stark GB, et al. Angiography findings before and following transplantation of free myocutaneous flaps. Roentgenblaetter 1990;43:41–45.

192. Mialhe C, Brice M. A new compound osteo-myocutaneous free flap: the posterior iliac artery flap. Br J Plast Surg 1985;38:30–38.

192a. Szilagyi DE, Elliott JP, deRusso FJ, Smith RF. Peripheral congenital arteriovenous fistulas. Surgery 1965;57:61–80.

193. Fry WJ. Surgical considerations in congenital arteriovenous fistula. Surg Clin North Am 1974;54:165–174.

194. Zannetti PH, Sherman FE. Experimental evaluation of a tissue adhesive as an agent for the treatment of aneurysms and arteriovenous anomalies. J Neurosurg 1972;36:72–79.

195. Stanley RJ, Cubillo E. Nonsurgical treatment of arteriovenous malformations of the trunk and limb by transcatheter arterial embolization. Radiology 1975;115:609–612.

196. Yakes WF, Pevsner P, Reed M, et al. Serial embolizations of an extremity arteriovenous malformation with alcohol via direct percutaneous puncture. AJR 1986;146:1038–1040.

197. Van Poppel H, Claes H, Suy R, et al. Intraarterial embolization in combination with surgery in the management of congenital pelvic arteriovenous malformation. Urol Radiol 1988;10:89–91.

198. Wickbom I, Bartley O. Arterial "spasm" in peripheral arteriography using the catheter method. Acta Radiol 1957;47:433–448.

199. Lindbom A. Arterial spasm caused by puncture and catheterization: an arteriographic study of patients not suffering from arterial disease. Acta Radiol Suppl (Stockh) 1957;47:449–460.

200. Lehrer H. The physiology of angiographic arterial waves. Radiology 1967;89:11–19.

201. Theander G. Arteriographic demonstration of stationary arterial waves. Acta Radiol 1960;53:417–425.

202. Kohler R. Regular alternating changes in arterial width in lower limb angiograms. Acta Radiol 1965;3:529–542.

203. New PFJ. Arterial stationary waves. AJR 1966;97:448–449.

204. dos Santos R. Arteriography in bone tumours. J Bone Joint Surg (Br) 1950;32:17–29.

205. Lagergren C, Lindbom A. Angiography of peripheral tumors. Radiology 1962;79:371–377.

206. Margulis AR. Arteriography of tumors: difficulties in interpretation and the need for magnification. Radiol Clin North Am 1964;2:543–562.

207. Jonsson K, Johnell O. Preoperative angiography in patients with bone metastases. Acta Radiol 1982;23:485–489.

208. Margulis AR, Murphy TO. Arteriography in neoplasms of extremities. AJR 1958;80:330–339.

209. Cockshott WP, Evans KT. The place of soft tissue arteriography. Br J Radiol 1964;37:367–375.

210. Lee KR, Cox GG, Price HI, et al. Intraarterial digital subtraction arteriographic evaluation of extremity tumors: comparison with conventional arteriography. Radiology 1986;158:255–258.

211. Lagergren C, Lindbom A, Soderberg G. Vascularization of fibromatous and fibrosarcomatous tumors: histopathologic, microangiographic and angiographic studies. Acta Radiol 1960;53:1–16.

212. Bowers TA, Murray JA, Charnsangavej C, et al. Bone metastases from renal carcinoma: the preoperative use of transcatheter arterial occlusion. J Bone Joint Surg (Am) 1982;64:749–754.

213. Roscoe MW, McBroom RJ, St. Louis E, et al. Preoperative embolization in the treatment of osseous metastases from renal cell carcinoma. Clin Orthop 1989;238:302–307.

68

Venography

MICHAEL A. BETTMANN

The primary reason for evaluating the veins of the lower extremities, and to a lesser extent of the upper extremities, is to define clot in the deep veins. A secondary reason for studying the veins of the lower extremities is to determine the patency of valves and to precisely locate incompetent venous perforators. Rarely, venography is performed to establish the patency of veins prior to their use as arterial grafts. Of these three indications for venography, by far the most important historically has been the definition and delineation of thrombi.

Venography has long been considered the "gold standard" for defining thrombi for two reasons. First, the presence of thrombi in the veins of the lower extremity is a frequent occurrence, particularly in certain patient subsets,[1-3] and it is impossible to accurately make the diagnosis of deep vein thrombosis (DVT) on clinical grounds. Second, such thrombi, even in the total absence of clinical symptomatology, may propagate, embolize to the lungs, and prove fatal.[4,5] An accurate diagnostic method is therefore essential, and that has been the role of venography in the past. Noninvasive methods have more recently become the diagnostic tools of choice for the diagnosis of DVT. Both impedance plethysmography and ultrasound with Doppler have been shown to be sufficiently accurate when appropriately applied.[6,7] Lower extremity venography, however, remains an important diagnostic test for defining calf vein thrombi, for distinguishing acute from chronic DVT, and for confirming equivocal or confusing noninvasive findings. This chapter discusses the techniques, complications, and role of venography.

History

The injection of veins of the lower extremity was one of the earliest uses of both the new technology of clinical diagnostic radiology in general and of the use of contrast agents.[8] Many techniques were used, generally employing a cutdown to expose a dorsal pedal vein. In an attempt to develop a more accessible, less invasive technique, intraosseous venography was also used. This involved direct injection into the marrow cavity, generally in the medial malleolus of the ankle.[9]

The first contrast agent used clinically was sodium iodide, but because it caused pain and irritation of the venous endothelium, often leading to sclerotic changes, this agent was rapidly abandoned. All of the contrast agents which were subsequently developed for clinical use were used for venography, generally early in their clinical development. These included the mono-, di-, and tri-iodinated benzene rings. The history of the development of contrast agents was reviewed in superb detail by Grainger[10] and is discussed in Chapter 2.

Technique

Many techniques have recently been employed for venography of the lower extremity.[11-14] They include studies with and without tourniquets, simultaneous injection of the veins in both lower extremities, retrograde studies involving catheterization of the common femoral vein, and many variants of these approaches. Many of these techniques have specific uses.

The most common and logical approach is the technique initially developed in Sweden and later refined and well described by Rabinov and Paulin.[12] It depends on several key elements.

1. Only one leg is studied at a time. In most settings, venography is undertaken to define the presence or absence of thrombus, and in almost all cases, the treatment for DVT is the same regardless of whether thrombus involves one leg or two.

2. A tourniquet is not routinely used. Studies have shown that most thrombi that embolize begin in the muscular sinusoids of the calf.[5] These veins fill from the superficial venous system and drain into the deep veins of the high calf and thigh. If a tourniquet is effectively in place at the ankle while contrast material is injected into a foot vein, filling will be directly into the deep venous system, with little

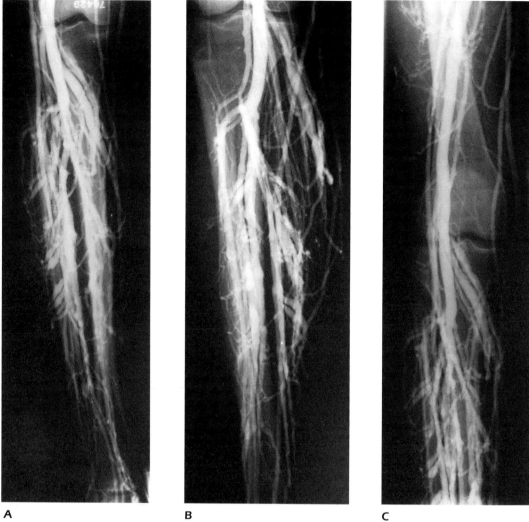

A   **B**   **C**

Figure 68-1. Normal leg venogram. (A) Lower leg, frontal view. (B) Lower leg, externally rotated view. The junction of the paired anterior tibial veins with the common posterior tibial-peroneal trunk is well seen. The popliteal vein, as is usually the case, is also duplicated. (C) Knee level, frontal view.

or no filling of the superficial system and of the muscular sinusoids, eliminating visualization of the latter to a substantial or complete extent.

3. A superficial vein on the dorsum of the foot is cannulated, preferably in the midfoot on the lateral aspect. Cannulation of a proximal dorsal pedal vein may lead to preferential filling of the greater saphenous vein (which is invariably located anterior to the medial malleolus), with consequent poor filling of the deep venous system. To encourage filling of the major venous channels in the foot and subsequently in the leg, the needle may be placed pointing toward the toes, particularly if a mid or proximal dorsal pedal vein is accessed.

4. The patient is elevated to 40 to 45 degrees reverse Trendelenburg (head up), and then contrast is slowly infused under fluoroscopic control. This is done because the venous system of the lower extremities may have a capacity of 700 milliliters or more.[12] Because of this large capacity and because filling may vary substantially among patients, the aim of contrast infusion is to allow mixing of the contrast with blood to achieve opacification of the veins. This is in contradistinction to arterial injections, where the aim is to essentially replace blood with contrast for brief periods of time. Further, venous filling may be altered significantly for various reasons: as a function of anatomy, of flow direction due to needle position, of the presence of thrombus, or of the existence of prior disease as manifest in occlusions or varicosities.

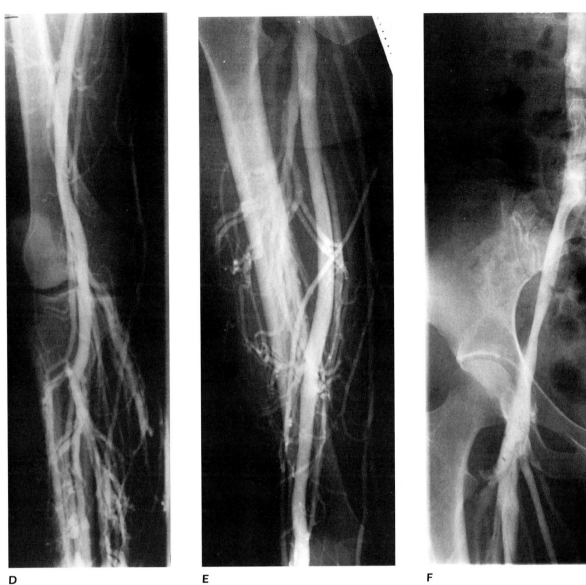

D   E   F

Figure 68-1 (continued). (D) Knee level, lateral view. (E) Thigh, frontal view. Note the medially positioned greater saphenous vein, the partially duplicated superficial femoral vein, and the profunda femoris vein, which fills from muscular veins of the thigh. (F) Frontal view demonstrates the common femoral vein, the external and common iliac veins, and the inferior vena cava.

The leg to be studied is kept in a dependent position with weight maintained on the contralateral leg, generally by having the patient place the contralateral leg on a box. It is important to ensure that the leg is relaxed throughout the procedure because muscular contraction rapidly leads to venous emptying. Contrast is slowly infused to visualize all major deep and superficial veins from the level of the ankle, or even foot, to at least the level of the external iliac vein and in general to the inferior vena cava. Once good filling is documented with fluoroscopic observation, overhead films are obtained: orthogonal views of the calf, the knee, and the thigh, and a single view of the pelvis

and inferior vena cava (Fig. 68-1). After the filming is completed, the patient is placed in a slight Trendelenburg position. Normal saline is infused at a slow rate for several minutes and the patient is asked to flex the muscles of the calf to encourage venous emptying.

Good filling of the ipsilateral external iliac and common iliac veins and of the inferior vena cava can generally be obtained by having the patient compress the common femoral vein and perform the Valsalva maneuver while the table is tilted into the Trendelenburg position; a film is then taken 4 to 6 seconds after release of compression and the Valsalva maneuver, while the patient is encouraging calf vein emptying by vigorous plantar flexion of the foot against pressure. This causes calf muscle contraction and rapid emptying from the muscular and deep veins of the calf (see Fig. 68-1F).

As in any radiographic study, it is important to use a contrast agent with an osmolality that is as low as possible to obtain good definition of the structures to be imaged. In venography, it has been shown that an iodine concentration of approximately 200 mg iodine/ml is ideal for this purpose.[15] In average patients, this concentration allows for accurate definition of all major veins, and the iodine content is low enough to avoid obscuring small clots. In certain settings, a higher iodine concentration, such as 300 mg/ml, may be advantageous, particularly in large patients and patients with a very high flow state, as may be encountered in the presence of cellulitis. In average patients, however, a higher iodine concentration may actually be disadvantageous, since it may hide small, nonocclusive clots.

Variations of this technique may be necessary, either when the deep system does not fill or when venography is used to define incompetent perforating veins. On routine venography, it is not rare to fail to visualize the deep venous system on initial infusion. Failure may be due to the position of the needle (with preferential filling of superficial veins), to chronic venous disease with old occlusion of much of the deep system, or to acute thrombosis of much or even all of the deep venous system. It is important to determine whether thrombus is acute or chronic, since anticoagulation is not generally necessary for old, healed venous thrombosis. If the deep system is not visualized, a tourniquet can be used to encourage deep filling. Since the aim is to visualize the deep system beginning in the calf, a tourniquet is applied at the level of the ankle. The most effective method is to use a blood pressure cuff of the appropriate size placed at the ankle. The cuff is inflated above venous pressure, generally to 40 or 50 mmHg, to allow even distribution of pressure. This approach is usually effective. Again, with fluoroscopic monitoring, suboptimal filling of the deep system may persist, and it may be necessary to further inflate the cuff to well above diastolic pressure. On occasion, it is necessary to reposition the needle to confirm that lack of filling is not due to malpositioning. As will be discussed, it is almost never impossible to define the deep system and to determine whether occlusions are acute or chronic.

The technique for defining incompetent perforating veins is somewhat different. Multiple thin tourniquets are placed on the lower leg from the level of the ankle, below the malleoli, to the low thigh at approximately 5-cm intervals. The contrast is then infused un-

der fluoroscopic control. The aim is to document specific sites at which there is reverse rather than normal flow, from the deep system to the superficial system. By using multiple tourniquets, one isolates the segments of the superficial system. Filling from the deep to superficial system at any given level therefore represents local incompetent perforators that are not filling from the superficial system more distally. When such filling is noted, it is marked on the skin with an indelible pen to indicate the specific level of the perforator that must be removed.

There is some controversy about the etiology of chronic venous stasis disease,[16-18] with some authors feeling that this condition is related not so much to incompetent perforating veins at the ankle and calf as to incompetent valves in the thigh. Incompetent veins in the calf may lead to uncomfortable varicosities and to nonhealing ulcers, symptoms that generally respond to local therapy. To examine for more significant chronic venous stasis disease, direct puncture of the common femoral vein is necessary, usually in antegrade fashion with a dilator pointing in a cephalad direction. The patient is then placed in reverse Trendelenburg, with head up, at 60 to 90 degrees. Contrast is infused under fluoroscopic control at a rate of 3 to 5 ml per second, a rate sufficient to fill the common femoral and external iliac veins. The presence or absence of retrograde flow, indicating an incompetent valve at the level of the common femoral vein, is then observed. If there is no retrograde flow, repeat infusion is done while the patient is performing a Valsalva maneuver to increase central venous pressure. If an incompetent vein is present, filling will occur into the superficial femoral vein in the thigh, and the extent of retrograde flow should be observed and noted. Retrograde flow at the knee, indicating an incompetent popliteal vein valve, is thought to be particularly important.

Venography of the upper extremity is generally carried out because of symptoms that suggest occlusion of the axillary or subclavian veins. This examination can be performed satisfactorily by using a small-bore scalp vein needle placed in a hand or forearm vein. A slow injection rate with digital imaging, if available, is generally satisfactory for visualization from the level of the antecubital fossa to the superior vena cava (Fig. 68-2).

Findings

The most important finding in venography is acute thrombus. Various criteria for acute DVT have been proposed, ranging from the classic "tram track" ap-

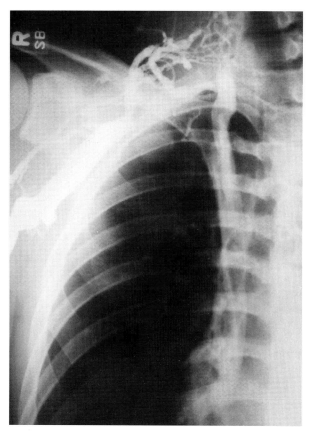

Figure 68-2. Upper extremity venogram, 22-year-old carpenter with effort thrombosis. The subclavian vein is acutely occluded (although no classic thrombus is seen) and empties via collaterals into the jugular and superior vena cava.

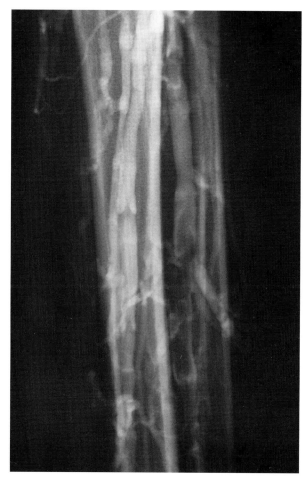

Figure 68-3. A 36-year-old woman with calf and chest pain 5 days after a craniotomy for a meningioma. Impedance plethysmography was normal, but a lung scan was interpreted as high probability. A venogram was performed to confirm the presence of venous thromboembolic disease. Film from calf venogram shows large, acute thrombus in the peroneal vein.

pearance to diversion of flow and nonfilling of the deep system. It cannot be overly stressed that the only finding that confirms DVT is a visualized venous thrombus (Fig. 68-3). As already noted, most thrombi that propagate begin in the muscular sinusoids of the calf (Fig. 68-4). Such thrombi can generally be visualized easily with careful technique including orthogonal views (Fig. 68-5). Isolated thrombi in muscular sinusoids, though rare, may occur. More often, thrombi are seen in more than one of the segments of the deep venous system (Fig. 68-6). It is particularly important to keep in mind that venography is the only available method that accurately depicts all calf and muscular venous thrombi. This again mandates very careful attention to detail, particularly in the calf.

Several other findings have been thought to indicate acute venous thrombosis, but none are reliable. Lack of filling of a specific vein may be associated with venous thrombosis but may also be the result of either faulty technique, with preferential filling of certain veins as compared to others, or of muscular contrac-

tion, which leads to rapid emptying of veins. Similarly, the presence of collaterals is sometimes thought to indicate chronic venous thrombosis. However, collaterals may be related to acute thrombosis and may be present, even acutely, as the result of extrinsic compression (Fig. 68-7). Collaterals may also be present because of chronic occlusion, but there may be superimposed acute thrombosis; one of the major risk factors for DVT is prior venous thrombosis. Underfilling due to extrinsic compression (Fig. 68-8) may be confused with DVT if only a single view is obtained or if the films are not carefully interpreted.

Certain findings are associated with prior venous thrombosis. Most notably, stringlike narrowing of vessels, with or without weblike scars (synechiae), indicate

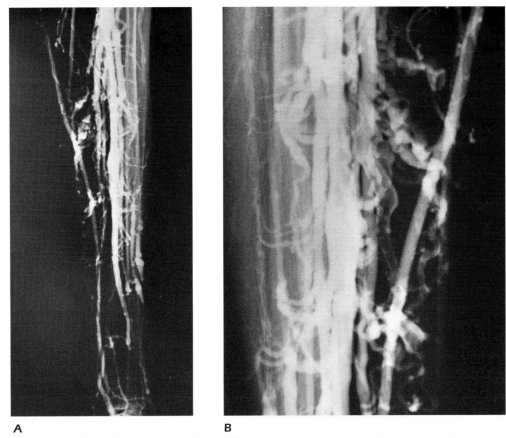

A   B

Figure 68-4. Frontal and coned-down views of the calf in a 45-year-old man with calf pain after direct trauma. (A) Frontal view shows no definite thrombi. (B) Spot film demonstrates clear filling defects, indicative of acute thrombi, in two muscular veins, without extension into the deep veins.

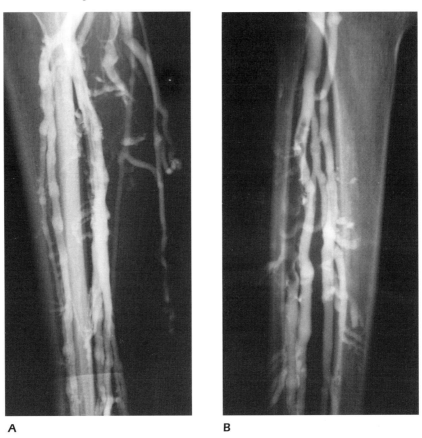

A   B

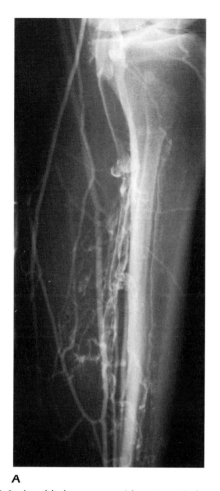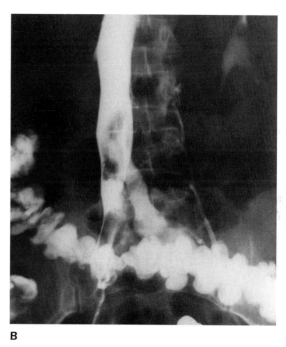

A　　　　　　　　　　　　　　　　　　**B**

Figure 68-6. An elderly woman with metastatic lung carcinoma and leg swelling. Separate foci of extensive thrombosis are seen in the calf (A) and iliac system and IVC (B).

that the patient has had venous thrombosis in the past (Fig. 68-9). Prominent varicosities, with preferential filling of the superficial veins and underfilling of the deep system, suggest prior venous thrombosis, although not strongly; varicosities are not a direct predictor of DVT. Acute or chronic deep vein changes may or may not be present in the presence of varicosities (Figs. 68-10 and 68-11).

Whenever venography is carried out, precise and reproducible technique must be used. This is an invasive procedure, and one that is now not routinely performed. If appropriately carried out, the accuracy is very high. However, findings may be subtle or, rarely, equivocal, and these difficulties can largely be obviated if very careful technique is always used.

Complications and Limitations

Contrast venography is limited only by technical factors and by complications. If properly performed on a cooperative patient, it allows for accurate and complete definition of the venous system of the lower extremity from the foot to the inferior vena cava. Problems may arise if venous access is difficult, if patients are markedly obese so that visualization of the venous system is difficult (particularly in the thigh or pelvis), or if the patient has cellulitis, in which case rapid flow may limit visualization. Visualization of the deep system may also be difficult in patients with marked varicosities, in whom the deep system is obscured by the varicosities (Figs. 68-11 and 68-12), or in patients

◄ **Figure 68-5.** Two views of the calf in a 44-year-old woman with calf tenderness 7 days after total abdominal hysterectomy. (A) No gross abnormalities are evident. (B) In an orthogonal view, extensive thrombosis is clearly present in a peroneal vein.

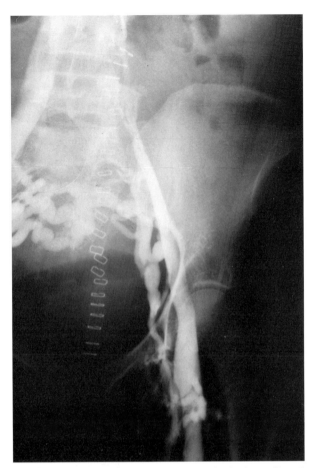

Figure 68-7. A 24-year-old woman with thigh swelling 2 days after a Cesarean section at term. The venogram demonstrates no evidence of acute or chronic DVT. Collaterals are present secondary to partial obstruction of the left common iliac vein by the previously gravid uterus. Note the cross-pelvic collaterals (via the hypogastric veins) as well as collaterals at the level of the left common femoral vein.

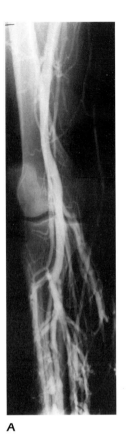 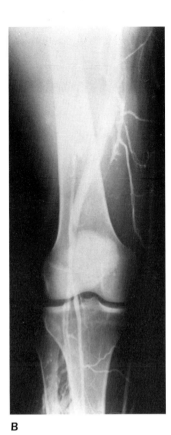

A   **B**

Figure 68-8. A 42-year-old man with high calf pain. Oblique (A) and frontal (B) views of a venogram demonstrate narrowing of the high popliteal vein due to extrinsic compression. Subsequent ultrasound demonstrated a Baker's cyst.

with extensive prior DVT, in whom precise delineation of the entire deep system may be difficult or even impossible. All of these situations, however, are unusual, and venography generally can completely delineate the deep venous system.

The complications of venography are essentially related to contrast agent administration. The only exceptions are vasovagal episodes related to needle placement or problems related to the patient's loss of position on the table. Contrast-related complications fall into two categories. First, any complications encountered with contrast use for other indications may also be encountered with venography. These include urticaria, bronchospasm, cardiopulmonary arrest, and renal failure. Whereas minor complications such as urticaria are common, more severe complications are very rare. Contrast-related renal failure with venogra-

phy, as with other uses, appears to occur essentially only in patients with underlying renal dysfunction and is related to the volume of contrast used as well as to the patients' state of hydration.

The second category, contrast complications that relate specifically to venography, are pain, the post-venography syndrome, and venous thrombosis. All are at least in part related to the osmolality of the contrast used, with what appears to be a threshold at the level of 800 to 1000 mOsm/kg. Many studies have been undertaken comparing high- and low-osmolality contrast agents for use in venography, and it is clear that the incidence and severity of pain are decreased as the osmolality of the contrast agents decreases.[15,19-24] It is also clear that there is a major difference between contrast agents used at an osmolality less than approximately 1000 mOsm and those of higher osmolality. Above this level, moderate and severe pain, by patient assessment, are frequent.[15] Below this level, both moderate and severe pain are unusual, and even mild discomfort is relatively rare.[15,19] Lowering the osmolality further appears to decrease the incidence of mild dis-

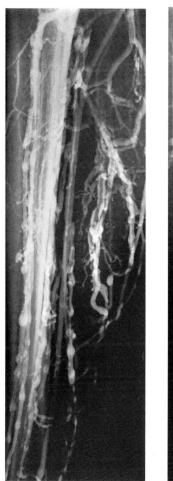
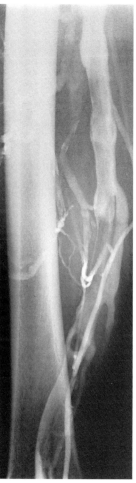

A

B

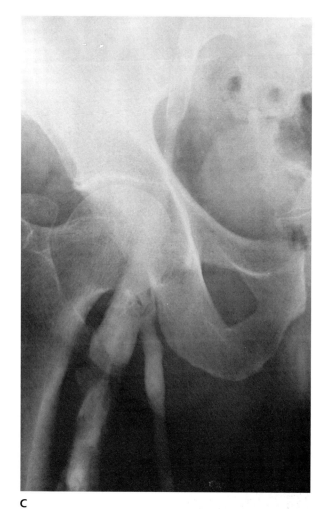

C

Figure 68-9. A 50-year-old man with a history of documented DVT and pulmonary embolism (PE) who presented with a clinical picture suggestive of recurrent PE. (A) The venogram demonstrates multiple muscular vein thrombi as well as marked irregularity of the deep veins in the thigh. Acute thrombus plus irregularity and narrowing due to scarring is seen in the superficial femoral vein (B) and external iliac vein (C).

comfort, but this is clearly a relatively minor factor in terms of patient care.[20]

The postvenography syndrome is characterized by the onset of pain and swelling in the high ankle and calf beginning 4 to 24 hours after venography. The symptoms are suggestive of superficial thrombosis, but thrombi can rarely be defined on repeat venography or confirmed by other studies. This syndrome is self-limited and resolves with symptomatic treatment.[19,21]

Figure 68-10. Two views of a normal deep venous system, with chronic changes in the greater saphenous vein (A) and prominent superficial varicosities (B).

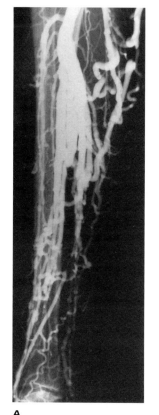
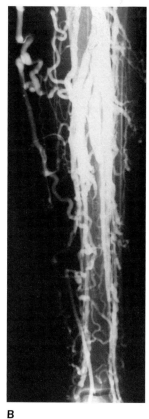

A

B

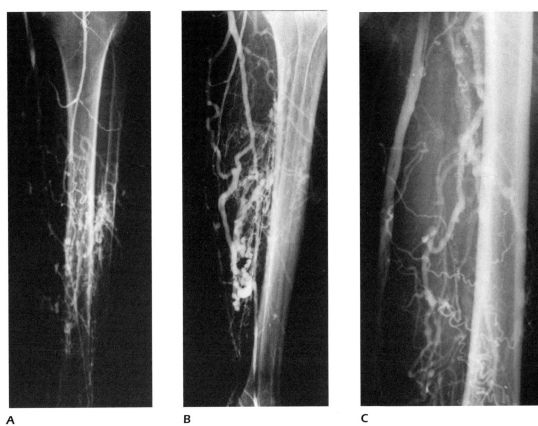

A   **B**   **C**

Figure 68-11. A 77-year-old woman with a history of prior DVT and recent right hip surgery, with left leg pain and swelling. Left leg venogram shows extensive chronic changes with no acute thrombi. Frontal (A) and lateral (B) views of the calf demonstrate varicosities and an absent popliteal vein. View of the thigh (C) shows a large greater saphenous vein, collateral filling of the profunda femoris, and no superficial femoral vein filling.

The most significant complication of venography is postvenographic thrombosis. Since venous thrombosis is impossible to diagnose accurately on clinical grounds, and since postvenographic thrombosis is almost invariably confined to the calf, the incidence of this complication in the literature varies fairly widely.[19-26] The variation is at least partly due to the various methods used for determining venous thrombosis. If objective criteria are used, such as ^{125}I fibrinogen scanning and repeat venography, the incidence of postvenographic thrombosis is as high as 27 percent when conventional high-osmolality contrast agents are used. Two-thirds of these thrombi are superficial.[19] If the osmolality of the contrast is lowered from the range of approximately 1400 mOsm to 1000 mOsm or less, the incidence falls to about 6 percent.[20] It is interesting to note that if one lowers the osmolality still further by using a low-osmolality contrast agent, the incidence of this complication does not decrease further.[20] To reiterate, if the osmolality is lowered from 1400 to 1000 mOsm by using a diluted conventional high-osmality contrast agent, severe pain is essentially completely eliminated. If the osmolality is lowered still

further, even moderate pain and much of the mild discomfort can be eliminated, and if the osmolality is lowered to 1000 mOsm, the incidence of postvenographic thrombosis decreases dramatically. If the osmolality is lowered further, however, there is no accompanying decrease in the incidence of this complication. As with other complications of iodinated contrast agents, then, the data suggest that low-osmolality contrast agents may contribute to a decrease in the incidence of minor complications but have little effect on the more important complications.[20]

The only additional complication of venography that is of concern is extravasation of contrast (Fig. 68-13). In most patients, if the amount of extravasation is limited, no more than minor local discomfort is likely to occur. This can be treated purely symptomatically, with wet soaks and elevation and analgesia. In certain patients, however, extravasation, particularly if substantial (greater than 25 ml), may have significant sequelae, ranging from pain to tissue loss that necessitates grafting or even amputation. Such complications are most likely to occur as a combination of increased volume of extravasate and poor tissue perfusion. Thus

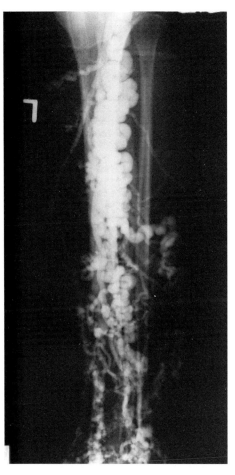

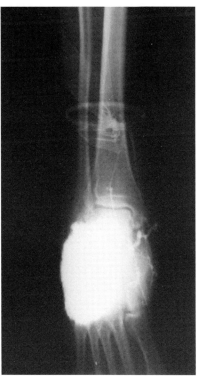

A

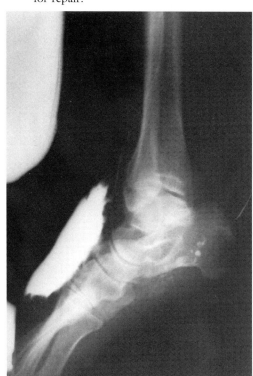

B

◄ **Figure 68-12.** A 45-year-old gravida 10, para 10 woman with left leg swelling 1 day postpartum. Single film of the calf from the left leg venogram demonstrates very extensive varicosities obscuring the deep system. Other views showed no evidence of acute DVT.

patients with severe peripheral arterial occlusive disease, particularly if combined with chronic venous stasis disease and/or complicated by severe diabetes, are at particular risk of this complication, and special care must be taken in such cases to avoid extravasation. Very young children also seem to be at particular risk of developing significant complications from extravasation. The most important single factor in regard to extravasation is limiting the amount. If a high-osmolality contrast agent is used, the patient is likely to feel discomfort with minimal extravasation. If a low-osmolality contrast agent is used, a larger amount of extravasation may occur before the onset of pain. It is not possible, therefore, to make a cogent argument for

Figure 68-13. An elderly woman with known peripheral arterial occlusive disease who presented with calf pain after prolonged bedrest. The venogram, attempted with an injection into a dorsal pedal vein, shows minor filling of superficial veins (A) and extensive extravasation in the foot (B). The patient experienced a skin slough that required skin grafting for repair.

the use of low-osmolality contrast agents on the basis of possible consequences of extravasation.

It is not clear what the optimal treatment for extravasation should be.[27-30] Animal studies using hot soaks followed by cold soaks or the reverse have failed to give definitive answers. Logic suggests that the best treatment for extravasation is, first, to be as careful as possible to limit extravasation, and if it occurs, to limit the amount. Second, elevation of the foot is likely to prove helpful. Third, cold soaks to initially limit the inflammatory response, followed by hot soaks to encourage perfusion and healing, appears to be a reasonable approach and has been effective in the author's practice. As with other significant complications of contrast agents, significant sequelae from extravasation must be kept in mind, but these occur very rarely.

Conclusion

Contrast venography remains an important technique with limited applicability, since it has been largely supplanted by ultrasound imaging with Doppler for the diagnosis of venous thrombosis. Ultrasound represents a true advance in medicine, being less expensive, more accessible, less morbid, and sufficiently accurate. Venography is primarily reserved for determining whether calf vein thrombosis is present and for defining valve patency, if ultrasound is either not available or is not definitive. With careful attention to technique, contrast venography is an accurate modality. Complications occur but can be minimized by using careful technique and a dilute, standard, high-osmolality contrast agent. Even with the use of ultrasound and such modalities as magnetic resonance angiography, venography is likely to remain an important, if infrequently used, angiographic tool.

References

1. Hume M, Sevitt S, Thomas DP. The incidence and importance of thromboembolism. In: Hume M, Sevitt S, Thomas DP, eds. Venous thrombosis and pulmonary embolism. Cambridge: Harvard University Press, 1970.
2. Coon WW, Willis PW, Keller JB. Venous thromboembolism and other venous disease in the Tecumseh Community Health Study. Circulation 1973;48:839–846.
3. Dalen JE, Alpert JS. Natural history of pulmonary embolism. Prog Cardiovasc Dis 1975;17:259–270.
4. Hull R, Hirsh J, Carter C, et al. Diagnostic efficacy of impedance plethysmography for clinically suspected deep-vein thrombosis: a randomized trial. Ann Intern Med 1985;102:21–28.
5. Nicolaides AN, Kakkar W, Field ES, Renney JTG. The origin of deep vein thrombosis: a venographic study. Br J Radiol 1971;44:653–663.
6. Hirsh J. Reliability of non-invasive tests for the diagnosis of deep vein thrombosis. Thromb Haemostasis 1991;65:221–222.
7. Lensing AWA, Prandoni P, Brandjes D, et al. Detection of deep vein thrombosis by real-time B-mode ultrasonography. N Engl J Med 1989;320:342–345.
8. Berberrich J, Hirsch S. Die Roentgenographische Darstellung der Arterien und Venen im lebenden Menschen. Klin Wochenschr 1923;2:2226–2234.
9. Arnoldi CC. A comparison between the phlebographic picture as seen in dynamic intraosseous phlebography and the clinical signs and symptoms of chronic venous insufficiency. J Cardiovasc Surg (Turin) 1961;2:184–192.
10. Grainger RG. Intravascular contrast media: the past, the present and the future. Br J Radiol 1982;55:1–18.
11. Lea Thomas M. Phlebography. Arch Surg 1974;104:145–151.
12. Rabinov K, Paulin S. Roentgen diagnosis of venous thrombosis in the leg. Arch Surg 1972;104:134–144.
13. Almen T, Nylander G. Serial phlebography of the normal leg during muscular contraction and relaxation. Acta Radiol 1962;57:264–278.
14. Lensing AWA, Bueller HR, Prandoni P, et al. Contrast venography, the gold standard for the diagnosis of deep vein thrombosis: improvement in observer agreement. Thromb Haemostasis 1992;67:8–13.
15. Bettmann MA, Paulin S. Lower limb phlebography: the incidence, nature and modification of undesirable side effects. Radiology 1977;122:101–104.
16. O'Donnell TF, Browse NL, Burnond KG, et al. Iliac vein thrombosis: a 10-year follow-up study. J Surg Res 1977;22:431–439.
17. Strandness ED Jr, Langlois T, Cramer M, Randlett A, Thiele BL. Long-term sequelae of acute venous thrombosis. JAMA 1983;250:1289–1292.
18. Gjores JE. The incidence of venous thrombosis and its sequelae in certain districts in Sweden. Acta Chir Scand 1956;206:11–88.
19. Bettmann MA, Salzman EW, Rosenthal D, et al. Reduction of venous thrombosis complicating contrast phlebography. Am J Roentgenol 1980;134:1169–1172.
20. Bettmann MA, Robbins A, Braun SD, Wetsner S, Dunnick NR, Finkelstein J. Comparison of the diagnostic efficacy, tolerance and complication rates of a nonionic and an ionic contrast agent for leg phlebography. Radiology 1987;165:113–116.
21. Albrechtsson U, Olsson CG. Thrombosis after phlebography: a comparison of two contrast media. Cardiovasc Radiol 1979;2:9–18.
22. Lensing AW, Prandoni P, Butler HR, Casara D, Cogo A, ten Cate JW. Lower extremity venography with iohexol: results and complications. Radiology 1990;177:503–505.
23. Stokes KR. Complications of diagnostic venography. Semin Intervent Radiol 1994;11:102–106.
24. Bettmann MA, Finkelstein J, Geller S. The use of iopamidol, a new nonionic contrast agent, in lower limb phlebography. Invest Radiol 1924;19:S225–S228.
25. Berge T, Bergquist D, Efsing HO, Hollbrook T. Local complications of ascending phlebography. Clin Radiol 1978;23:691–696.
26. Zeitler VE, Milbert L, Richter E-I, Ringelmann W, Strohm CH. Spezialle Komplicationen der Beinphlebographie. Rofo Fortschrift Geb Roentgenstr Neuen Bldgeb Verfahr 1983;138:670–677.
27. Cohan RH, Leder RA, Bolick D, et al. Extravascular extravasation of radiographic contrast media: effects of conventional and low osmolar agents in the rat thigh. Invest Radiol 1990;25:504–510.
28. Cohan RH, Dunnick NR, Leder RA, Baker ME. Extravasation of nonionic radiologic contrast media. Invest Radiol 1990;25:678–685.
29. Kim SH, Park JH, Kim YI, Kim CW, Han MC. Experimental tissue damage after subcutaneous injection of water-soluble contrast media. Invest Radiol 1990;176:65–67.
30. Sistrom CL, Gay SB, Peffley L. Extravasation of iopamidol and iohexol during contrast-enhanced CT: report of 28 cases. Radiology 1991;180:707–710.

69

Arteriography of the Upper Extremity

ARNOLD CHAIT

Although arteriography of the upper extremity is performed less frequently than lower extremity arteriography, the techniques are similar. The method of angiography via direct needle puncture, advocated in the last edition of this publication, has been all but replaced by catheter angiography since the availability of small-caliber catheters. For a diagnostic study, a catheter of 4 French outer diameter is adequate. With small-catheter angiography, iatrogenic damage to the accessed artery has been markedly reduced and the occurrence of brachial artery occlusion, large hematomas, and subintimal or perivascular injection, not uncommon with needle injections and with the use of larger catheters,[1] has all but disappeared. Local hematoma and pseudoaneurysm formation still occur[2] but with proper technique, rarely, and even when pseudoaneurysm does follow a catheterization procedure, it can often be handled without surgical intervention.[3] Larger catheters are often required for various cardiology procedures, with resultant greater incidence of vascular damage[4,5] when vascular access is via the brachial artery (Fig. 69-1); this has led, in part, to greater enthusiasm for access via the larger femoral artery by the majority of cardiologists.

Arterial access for upper extremity angiography may be via transfemoral catheterization with injection in the aortic arch for evaluation of the subclavian or innominate artery origin; for opacification of more distal arteries, selective catheterization of the subclavian artery and its branches can generally be readily performed from the same approach. Direct catheterization of the axillary or brachial artery for more direct access is also an option. The former approach has fallen out of favor because of potential brachial plexus injury, with a frequency variously reported to be between 0.4 and 9.5 percent unrelated to hematoma size, and has been generally replaced by a high brachial approach, even though there is some evidence that the incidence of neuropathy is not thereby reduced.[6] The brachial artery may also be entered at the antecubital space, but the vessel at this location is prone to spasm, which usu-

ally relents spontaneously or with the use of vasodilators (tolazoline, nitroglycerin); on occasion, however, spasm may lead to permanent occlusion. When using the direct brachial artery route, the angiographer must also be alert to the possibility that a runoff vessel arising in an anomalously high location may not be opacified by contrast material injected at the level of the elbow. A common anomaly is that of the radial artery originating from the brachial artery high in the upper arm, which occurs in 15 percent of the population (Fig. 69-2).[7-9] There have even been reports of aplasia of the radial artery.[10] Less frequently, there is a high origin of the ulnar artery. The advantage of direct brachial artery catheterization is that one can deliver contrast in close proximity to the area of interest, which results in better opacification, the use of lower volumes of contrast material, a shorter procedure time, and a shorter postprocedure observation period before ambulation. The last-mentioned advantage can be of major importance with the current increase in outpatient angiography. Angiography, and indeed angioplasty and other interventions, are now frequently performed safely on an outpatient basis, with significant cost savings.[11-13]

Recording may be performed either with standard serial filming, for most applications at a rate of two films per second, or with digital subtraction (or nonsubtraction) filming. Although the former technique produces studies of more exquisite detail, such detail is not required in most instances (compare Fig. 69-3 with Fig. 69-4), and digital recording offers real advantages in terms of patient comfort and decreased procedure time.[14] With the latter technique, dilute contrast yields adequate information and results in far less patient discomfort. Full-strength contrast injection in an upper extremity is often a painful experience; the addition of lidocaine to the injected contrast material has been advocated as a pain-reducing measure but has met with reports of mixed success. Low-osmolar contrast agents (ionic or nonionic) tend to be better tolerated than the standard high-osmolar agents. An

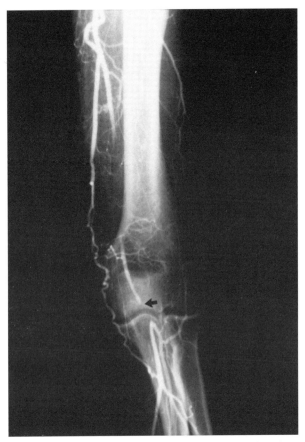

Figure 69-1. Iatrogenic injury. Short occlusion of the brachial artery (*arrow*) at site of catheterization with a large-diameter catheter, as well as at a more proximal location. This type of injury has become unusual with the use of smaller catheters.

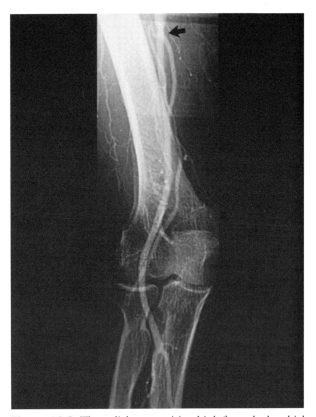

Figure 69-2. The radial artery arising high from the brachial artery (*arrow*) at a location likely to not be opacified from an injection site near the elbow, leading to a potential misdiagnosis of radial artery occlusion.

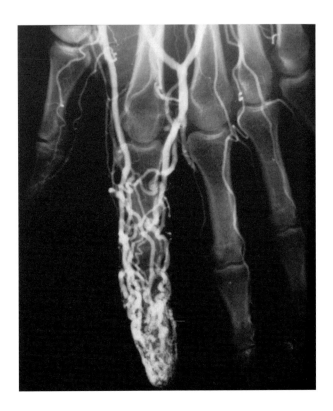

injection per filming sequence of 5 to 20 ml of contrast material containing 160 to 200 mg/ml of organically bound iodine usually suffices, depending on the location of the catheter. Warming of the hand has been advocated to promote vascular dilatation and optimal filling of small distal vessels.[15] Older techniques of promoting vasodilatation, such as general anesthesia, stellate ganglion blockade, and oral alcohol, have fallen into disuse.

Arteriography may be indicated in the workup of many unrelated conditions as an aid in their surgical, radiologic, or conservative management. Several examples follow.

Figure 69-3. Arteriovenous malformation of index finger, venous phase film-screen technique. The digital arteries of the uninvolved fingers are just beginning to fill, whereas the index finger is in deep venous phase.

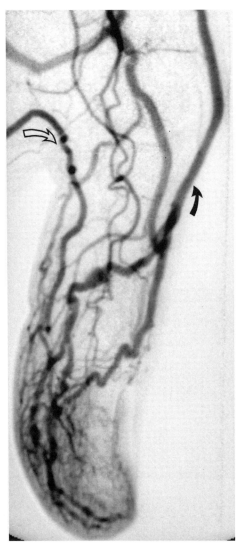

Figure 69-4. Arteriovenous malformation of thumb, digital subtraction technique (feeding artery, *open arrow*; draining vein, *solid arrow*). Resolution is inferior to that of Figure 69-3, but not critically so, even in these small digital vessels.

Penetrating Trauma

In the author's practice, the most common indication for arteriography of the upper extremity is penetrating trauma, that is, gunshot and knife wounds. These may lead to intimal injury (Fig. 69-5), vessel transection with or without extravasation of blood and the formation of pseudoaneurysm (Fig. 69-6), dissection, occlusion, thrombosis, or spasm (Fig. 69-7), arteriovenous fistula formation, and arterial displacement by hematoma.[16] Slow flow is often due to spasm induced by blast phenomenon, which may or may not relent with time or may be a result of compartment syndrome. Even significant injuries may not result in loss of pe-

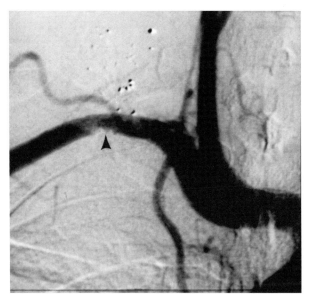

Figure 69-5. Proximity injury. Shotgun wound of neck with intimal injury to the subclavian artery (*arrowhead*) but with maintenance of peripheral flow and pulses.

ripheral pulses (see Figs. 69-5 and 69-6). There is considerable disagreement over the indications for angiography, let alone the need for urgency in performing angiography in cases of proximity injury, particularly when the pulses distal to the injury are not lost. With deficiencies in the distal pulses, or with the presence of a growing mass in the area of the injury with or without persistence of distal pulses, there can be no question of the indication for emergency angiography. Nevertheless, the early enthusiasm for emergency angiography in all cases of penetrating injury has been

Figure 69-6. Gunshot wound of axillary artery with transection and extravasation but maintenance of peripheral flow and pulses.

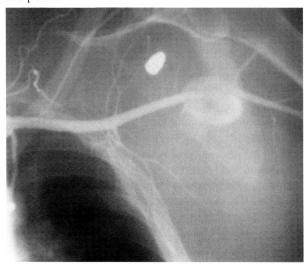

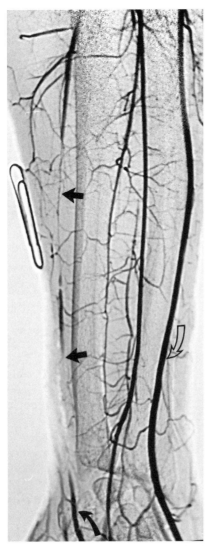

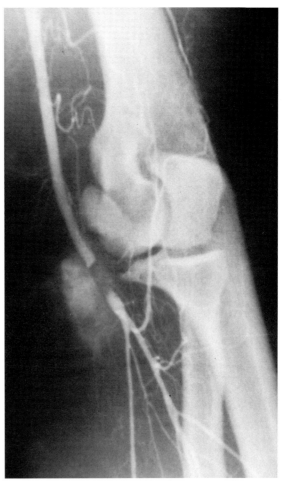

Figure 69-8. Transection of the brachial artery at the elbow during fracture dislocation of the ulna, resulting in extravasation and pseudoaneurysm but continued distal flow.

Figure 69-7. Proximity injury of forearm (knife wound) with generalized spasm and occlusions of the ulnar artery (*solid straight arrows*). Note the retrograde filling of the ulnar artery at the wrist (*curved arrow*) from the palmar arch.

largely replaced by a policy of observation in the absence of indication based on clinical findings.[17–23]

Iatrogenic injury resulting from catheterization of the brachial artery has been rarely seen since the introduction of small-caliber catheters (see Fig. 69-1).

Nonpenetrating Trauma

A less common use of angiography is in the diagnosis of vascular compromise in cases of closed trauma resulting from bone or joint injury. Fractures and dislocations can result in major arterial injury requiring surgical correction (Fig. 69-8).

Arteriography can also be useful in differentiating arterial damage due to repetitive trauma from other vascular diseases. Typical is the hypothenar hammer syndrome, which results from injury to the ulnar artery where it passes over the hamate bone as a result of repeated blows struck to the area during occupational or recreational activity. Arteriographic findings include very localized vascular irregularities or occlusions, sometimes progressing to aneurysm formation and distal embolization and resulting in painful digital ischemia.[24–26]

Arteriosclerosis

Symptomatic arteriosclerosis is a much less common condition in the upper extremities than it is in the lower extremities, and arteriography is rarely indicated

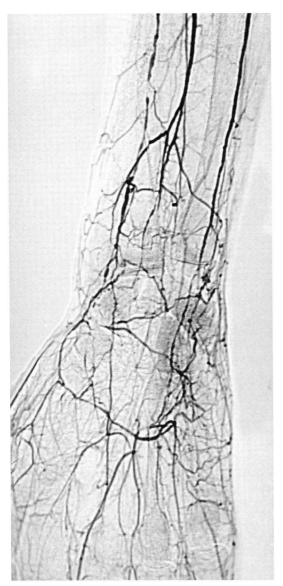

Figure 69-9. Arteriosclerosis in long-standing diabetes; extensive sclerotic, stenotic, and occlusive disease of the small vessels of the wrist and hand.

in its evaluation. Even arteriographically apparent vascular deficiencies are usually overcome by collateral flow; however, in cases of severe ischemia in which corrective surgery is contemplated, arteriography may be required. The manifestations of this condition vary widely but generally involve the proximal (see Fig. 69-16A) rather than the distal arteries,[16,27,28] and there is often intimal calcification. In the accelerated atherosclerosis of diabetes, distal involvement occurs as well (Fig. 69-9) and can threaten the patency of dialysis fistulas.

Raynaud's Phenomenon

Raynaud's phenomenon is an idiopathic vasospastic condition of the small vessels of the extremities that occurs most frequently in young women and is more often symptomatic in the upper than in the lower extremities.[16,28] Symptoms include pain, paresthesias, pallor, cyanosis, and rubor, and are precipitated by cold. When not associated with other disease, the condition is usually referred to as *primary Raynaud's phenomenon* or *Raynaud's disease*. When associated with collagen vascular disorders such as scleroderma, systemic lupus erythematosis, or rheumatoid arthritis, it is generally termed *secondary Raynaud's phenomenon*. The arteriographic findings are those of spasm with slow flow and poor opacification of the distal small vessels. Angiography following injection of vasodilators (e.g., tolazoline) can lead to dramatic improvement in rapidity of flow as well as visualization of small distal arteries (Fig. 69-10).

Buerger's Disease

Buerger's disease (thromboangiitis obliterans) is a painful bilateral vascular disease of young men, more commonly affecting the lower extremities than the upper and often associated with thrombophlebitis. In one study, it accounted for 9 percent of patients with ischemic ulcers of the fingers.[29] It may be difficult to distinguish from arteriosclerosis angiographically, with the diagnosis depending in part on its occurring at a young age in a male smoker, because there is a strong association with tobacco usage. Its angiographic recognition depends on absence of calcification, a distal rather than a proximal predilection with segmental occlusions in the palmar arches and the digital arteries, occlusion of the radial and ulnar arteries with preservation of the interosseous artery, and typically corkscrew collaterals bridging the areas of occlusion (Fig. 69-11).[27]

Arteriovenous Malformations

Arteriovenous malformations of congenital origin are caused by a local deficiency of capillary development. There is a diffuse network of innumerable collaterals, the malformation "nidus," fed by enlarged arteries and drained by large veins (see Figs. 69-3 and 69-4). Therapy, short of amputation, must consist of obliteration of the nidus. Any surgical approach less than this is doomed to failure and recurrence in a very short time. Ligation of the large feeding arteries is a tempo-

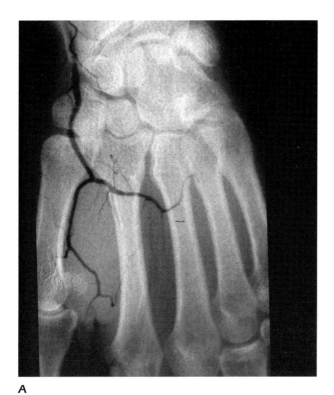

A

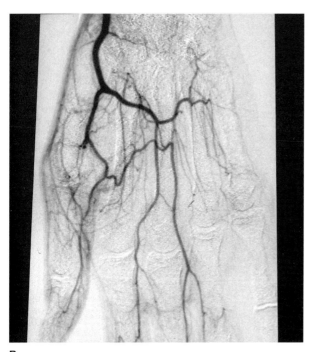

B

Figure 69-10. Raynaud's disease. (A) Angiographic exposure made 23 seconds after contrast injection in the brachial artery via a transfemoral catheterization. Contrast has just arrived at the deep palmar arch. (B) Angiographic exposure made at the same sitting as (A), 5 seconds after contrast injection immediately following the intraarterial injection of 25 mg of tolazoline. The distal spasm has largely relented, but occlusive disease of the digital arteries remains evident.

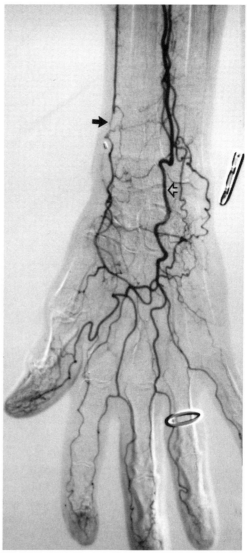

Figure 69-11. Buerger's disease. Note occlusions of the radial artery at the wrist (*solid arrow*) and of the ulnar artery, as well as deficiency of the superficial palmar arch. The interosseous artery (*open arrow*) remains widely patent and is the main vascular supply of the hand. The corkscrew collaterals seen here at the wrist are said to be typical of this condition.[27]

rizing matter at best; the residual nidus acts as a sump, and collateral feeders are recruited from multiple adjacent sources (Fig. 69-12).[30] Magnetic resonance imaging (MRI) may have a role in pretherapeutic evaluation and decision making.[31] Transcatheter embolization is a more logical approach than is surgery to this challenging problem,[32,33] but here too, occlusion must be of the nidus and not of the feeding arteries. There has been some success with the injection of liquid polymers into the nidus. Previous surgical ligations may make access of the embolic material to the nidus impossible and preclude success.

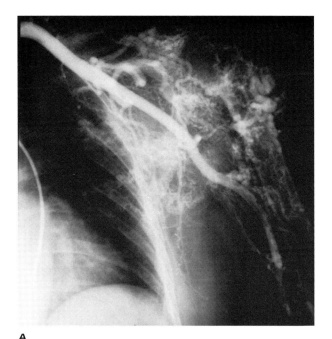

A

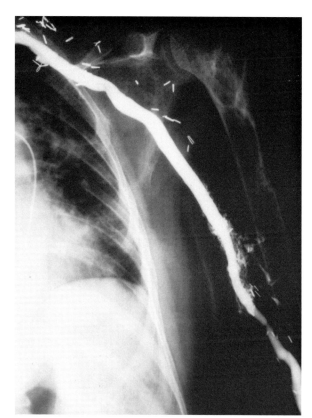

B

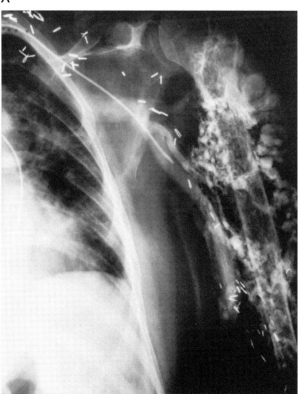

C

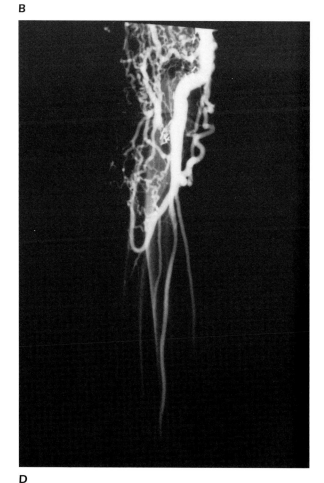

D

Figure 69-12. Arteriovenous malformation of the shoulder. (A) Initial arteriogram, before surgical intervention, demonstrates this large lesion to be fed principally by branches of the axillary and subclavian arteries. (B) Many years, many operations, and many arteriograms later, this exposure during the early arterial phase of the arteriogram demonstrates the axillary and subclavian arteries to have been skeletonized. (C) A later exposure during the same arteriogram as (B). The malformation continues to fill, is even larger than on the initial presurgical angiogram (A), and the draining veins have enlarged. (D) Arterial supply has been recruited from below the elbow as shown, and also from the intercostal arteries, the thyrocervical trunk, and from vessels as remote as the internal and external carotid arteries.

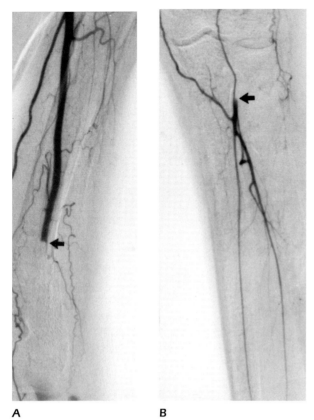

A   **B**

Figure 69-13. (A) Sharp cutoff of contrast column in the brachial artery above the elbow (*arrow*), typical for embolism, in this case originating in the left ventricle. (B) Reconstitution of brachial artery just below the elbow (*arrow*). Even in acute occlusions, collaterals are usually adequate to reconstitute distal vessels.

Embolization

Digital ischemia may be due to embolic occlusion in up to one-third of cases and may mimic primary distal disease.[34] For that reason, arteriograms designed to demonstrate distal disease must include the proximal vessels as well. Care must also be taken to demonstrate, where possible, arterial reconstitution distal to the occlusion (Fig. 69-13) so that proper management, surgical or endovascular, may be planned. Lytic therapy is often the procedure of choice (Fig. 69-14).[35] Emboli may be related to arteriosclerotic disease of large arm arteries or to thoracic outlet syndrome, but in most cases they originate in the heart.

Thoracic Outlet Obstruction

Concerning the entity of thoracic outlet syndrome, there is considerable confusion and disagreement over its anatomic basis, the implications of angiographic findings, and the indications and results of surgery.[36–39] Only 1 percent of cases of thoracic outlet syndrome involve the subclavian artery; a slightly greater percentage are venous-related, and 97 percent have a neurologic basis. It can be difficult to separate an arterial cause of symptoms of arm and hand pain and paresthesias from a neurologic etiology. Furthermore, it is extremely difficult to determine the clinical significance of subclavian artery narrowing demonstrated on angiography with the extremity stressed because some degree of narrowing can be produced in the asymptomatic patient with the arm hyperabducted (Fig. 69-15). The production of complete occlusion on arteriography makes the diagnosis more acceptable.

The anatomic basis for arterial compromise is most often compression of the subclavian artery between a cervical rib and the clavicle; other sites of compression may be between the scalenus anticus tendon and the scalenus medius tendon, or at the costoclavicular space due to a prominent subclavius muscle; the axillary artery may be compressed between the coracoid process and the pectoralis tendon.[16,40] Typical symptoms resulting from compression of the subclavian artery consist of cramping, pain, and pallor of the arm, and more often of the hand. Most frequently, symptoms are precipitated by trauma. In addition to the symptoms produced by direct vascular compromise, subclavian artery compression can lead to poststenotic aneurysm formation. Thrombus can line the poststenotic aneurysm and result in distal embolization. It is the author's practice to perform arteriography with the involved extremity at rest as a baseline, and then in the position that reproduces symptoms. The classical Adson maneuver has not been successful in our hands in eliciting arterial compromise. There is a high rate of recurrence following first rib resection and scalenectomy, reportedly as high as 15 to 20 percent.[37]

Subclavian Steal

A stenosis or occlusion of the subclavian artery (generally atherosclerotic) proximal to the origin of the vertebral artery, with resultant decreased pressure in this vessel distal to the lesion, will cause lack of filling of the vertebral artery in an antegrade direction. Flow may occur from the contralateral vertebral artery,

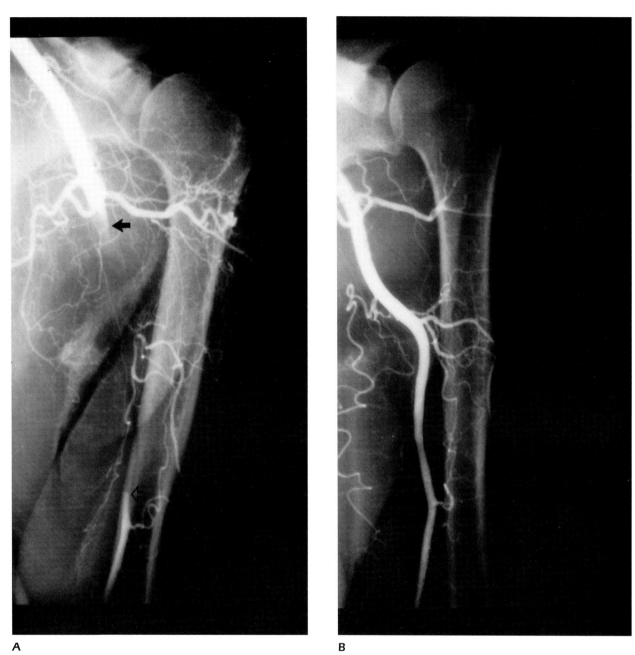

A

B

Figure 69-14. (A) High brachial artery occlusion (*solid arrow*), with reconstitution of the brachial artery above the elbow (*open arrow*). (B) Reestablishment of patency after lytic therapy.

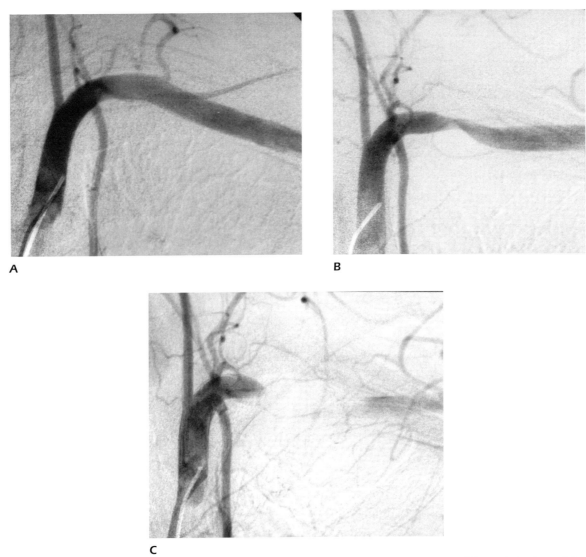

Figure 69-15. (A) Left subclavian artery of normal diameter with the arm in neutral position. (B) Narrowing of the left subclavian artery of the same patient as (A) with the arm in partial abduction. (C) Maximal hyperabduction of the left arm results in occlusion of the subclavian artery and reproduction of symptoms.

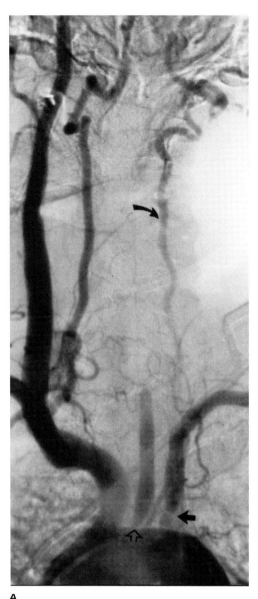

A

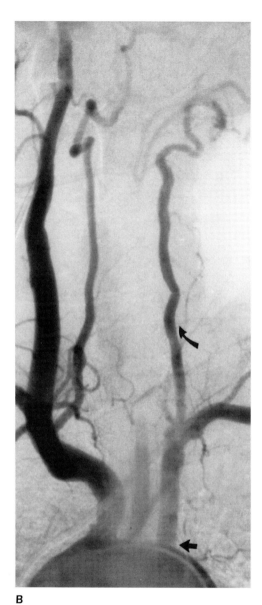

B

Figure 69-16. (A) Subclavian steal. The left subclavian artery is stenotic at its origin (*solid straight arrow*), leading to retrograde flow in the left vertebral artery (*curved solid arrow indicating direction of flow*) filling from the basilar artery. (Note also incidental occlusion of the left common carotid artery, low in the neck.) (B) After percutaneous transluminal angioplasty, the left subclavian artery origin (*straight solid arrow*) is of normal caliber, and flow in the left vertebral artery is in an antegrade direction (*curved solid arrow indicating direction of flow*).

through the basilar artery, and then in a retrograde direction through the ipsilateral vertebral artery into the brachial artery distal to the stenosis (Fig. 69-16A). Blood will be "stolen" from the basilar circulation, with resultant symptoms of basilar insufficiency, the so-called subclavian steal syndrome.[41] This lesion is often amenable to correction by means of transluminal angioplasty (see Fig. 69-16B).

Bone and Soft Tissue Tumors

Tumors of bone and soft tissue, both benign and malignant, primary and metastatic, have in the past been studied angiographically for diagnosis, for purposes of tumor staging, and for surgical and chemotherapeutic planning. With the availability of computed tomographic and magnetic resonance and nuclear medicine imaging, angiography is of diagnostic value only on those rare occasions when these modalities do not adequately demonstrate the relationships of the tumor to adjacent vascular structures.[42,43] Angiography continues to have a place in the planning and conduct of intraarterial chemotherapy.[44]

References

1. McCollum CH, Mavor E. Brachial artery injury after cardiac catheterization. J Vasc Surg 1986;4:355–359.
2. Feild JR, Lee L, McBurney RF. Complications of 1000 brachial arteriograms. J Neurosurg 1972;36:324–332.
3. Skibo L, Polak JF. Compression repair of a postcatheterization pseudoaneurysm of the brachial artery under sonographic guidance. Am J Roentgenol 1993;160:383–384.
4. Cragg AH, Nakagawa N, Smith TP, et al. Hematoma formation after diagnostic angiography: effect of catheter size. J Vasc Intervent Radiol 1991;2:231–233.
5. Kresowik TF, Khoury MD, Miller BV, et al. A prospective study of the incidence and natural history of femoral vascular complications after percutaneous transluminal coronary angioplasty. J Vasc Surg 1991;13:328–335.
6. Smith DC, Mitchell DA, Peterson GW, et al. Medial brachial fascial compartment syndrome: anatomic basis of neuropathy after transaxillary arteriography. Radiology 1989;173:149–154.
7. Keller FS, Rösch J, Dotter CT, et al. Proximal origin of radial artery: potential pitfall in hand angiography. Am J Roentgenol 1980;134:169–170.
8. McCormack LJ, Cauldwell EW, Anson BJ. Brachial and antebrachial patterns: a study of 750 extremities. Surg Gynecol Obstet 1953;96:43–54.
9. Machleder H. Vaso-occlusive disorders of the upper extremity. Curr Probl Surg 1988;25:1–67.
10. Odero A, Chierichetti F, Canidio E, et al. Aplasia of the radial artery. Cardiovasc Surg 1993;1:270–272.
11. Lemarbre L, Hudon G, Coche G, et al. Outpatient peripheral angioplasty: survey of complications and patients' perceptions. Am J Roentgenol 1987;148:1239–1240.
12. Saint-Georges G, Aube M. Safety of outpatient arteriography: a prospective study. Am J Roentgenol 1985;144:235–236.
13. Adams PS Jr, Roub LW. Outpatient angiography and interventional radiology: safety and cost benefits. Radiology 1984;151:81–82.
14. Picus D, Hicks ME, Darcy MD, et al. Comparison of nonsubtracted digital angiography and conventional screen-film angiography for the evaluation of patients with peripheral vascular disease. J Vasc Intervent Radiol 1991;2:359–364.
15. Rösch J, Antonovic R, Porter JM. The importance of temperature in angiography of the hand. Radiology 1977;123:323–326.
16. Gomes A. Diagnostic and interventional angiography. In: Machleder HI, ed. Vascular disorders of the upper extremity, 2nd rev. ed. Mt Kisco, NY: Futura, 1989:59–99.
17. Rose SC, Moore EE. Angiography in patients with arterial trauma: correlation between angiographic abnormalities, operative findings, and clinical outcome. Am J Roentgenol 1987;149:613–619.
18. Itani KMF, Burch JM, Spjut-Patrinely V, et al. Emergency center arteriography. J Trauma 1992;32:302–307.
19. Weaver FA, Yellin AE, Bauer M, et al. Is arterial proximity a valid indication for arteriography in penetrating extremity trauma? A prospective analysis. Arch Surg 1990;125:1256–1260.
20. Smyth SH, Pond GD, Johnson PL, et al. Proximity injuries: correlation with results of extremity arteriography. J Vasc Intervent Radiol 1991;2:451–456.
21. Reid JDS, Redman HC, Weigelt JA, et al. Wounds of the extremities in proximity to major arteries: value of angiography in the detection of arterial injury. Am J Roentgenol 1988;151:1035–1039.
22. Kaufman JA, Parker JE, Gillespie DL, et al. Arteriography for proximity of injury in penetrating extremity trauma. J Vasc Intervent Radiol 1992;3:719–723.
23. Rose SC, Moore EE. Emergency trauma angiography: accuracy, safety, and pitfalls. Am J Roentgenol 1987;148:1243–1246.
24. Conn J Jr, Bergan JJ, Bell JL. Hypothenar hammer syndrome: post traumatic digital ischemia. Surgery 1970;68:1122–1128.
25. Pineda CJ, Weisman MH, Bookstein JJ, et al. Hypothenar hammer syndrome: form of reversible Raynaud's phenomenon. Am J Med 1985;79:561–570.
26. Vayssairt M, DeBure C, Cormier J-M, et al. Hypothenar hammer syndrome: seventeen cases with long-term follow-up. J Vasc Surg 1987;5:838–843.
27. Erlandson EE, Forrest ME, Shields JJ, et al. Discriminant arteriographic criteria in the management of forearm and hand ischemia. Surgery 1981;90:1025–1036.
28. Castaneda-Zuniga WR, Amplatz K. Raynaud's syndrome. In: Teplick JG, Haskin ME, eds. Surgical radiology. Philadelphia: Saunders, 1981:1556–1557.
29. Mills JL, Friedman EI, Taylor LM, et al. Upper extremity ischemia caused by small artery disease. Ann Surg 1987;206:521–528.
30. Lawdahl RB, Routh WD, Vitek JJ, et al. Chronic arteriovenous fistulas masquerading as arteriovenous malformations: diagnostic considerations and therapeutic implications. Radiology 1989;170:1011–1015.
31. Cohen JM, Weinreb JC, Redman HC. Arteriovenous malformations of the extremities: MR imaging. Radiology 1986;158:475–479.
32. Gomes AS, Busuttil RW, Baker JD, et al. Congenital arteriovenous malformations: the role of transcatheter embolization. Arch Surg 1983;118:817–825.
33. Stanley RJ, Cubillo E. Nonsurgical treatment of arteriovenous malformations of the trunk and limb by transcatheter arterial embolization. Radiology 1975;115:609–612.
34. Maiman MH, Bookstein JJ, Bernstein EF. Digital ischemia: angiographic differentiation of embolism from primary arterial disease. Am J Roentgenol 1981;137:1183–1187.
35. Widlus DM, Venbrux AC, Benenati JF, et al. Fibrinolytic therapy for upper-extremity arterial occlusions. Radiology 1990;175:393–399.
36. Roos DB. Thoracic outlet syndrome: update 1987. Am J Surg 1987;154:568–573.
37. Sanders RJ, Haug CE, Pearce WH. Recurrent thoracic outlet syndrome. J Vasc Surg 1990;12:390–400.
38. Roos DB. Overview of thoracic outlet syndromes. In: Machleder HI, ed. Vascular disorders of the upper extremity, 2nd rev. ed. Mt Kisco, NY: Futura, 1989:155–177.
39. Lang EK. Thoracic outlet syndrome. In: Teplick JG, Haskin ME, eds. Surgical radiology. Philadelphia: Saunders, 1981:1269–1278.
40. Makhoul RG, Machleder HI. Developmental anomalies at the thoracic outlet: an analysis of 200 consecutive cases. J Vasc Surg 1992;16:534–545.
41. Reivich M, Holling HE, Roberts B, et al. Reversal of blood flow through the vertebral artery and its effect on cerebral circulation. N Engl J Med 1961;265:878–885.
42. Voegeli E, Fuchs WA. Arteriography in bone tumors. Br J Radiol 1976;49:407–415.
43. Pettersson H, Gillespy T III, Hamlin DJ. Primary musculoskeletal tumors: examination with MR imaging compared with conventional modalities. Radiology 1987;164:237–241.
44. Soulen MC, Weissmann JR, Sullivan KL. Intraarterial chemotherapy with limb-sparing resection of large soft-tissue sarcomas of the extremities. J Vasc Intervent Radiol 1992;3:659–663.

70

Angiography of Dialysis Shunts

ARNOLD CHAIT

Reliable long-term vascular access for hemodialysis became a reality with the development of the endogenous side-of-radial-artery-to-side-of-cephalic-vein anastomosis described by Brescia and Cimino in 1966,[1] usually placed in the nondominant upper extremity. In most situations this anastomosis, or the modification of side of artery to end of vein, remains the initial access of choice (Figs. 70-1 through 70-4).[2] The reported longevity of these fistulas varies widely; one report of a 4-year secondary patency rate of 57 percent appears typical.[3] In about 30 to 40 percent of cases, a Brescia-Cimino shunt fails to develop adequately[2] and a radial artery or brachial artery anastomosis to a more proximal vein may be created. As initially successful distal shunts inevitably fail, more proximal shunts must be created, often from the brachial artery to brachial, subclavian, or axillary veins. Other commonly constructed alternatives are either straight or U grafts of polytetrafluoroethylene (PTFE; Figs. 70-5 and 70-6), with an expected short-term longevity somewhat less and a long-term longevity significantly less than that of a primary fistula. When all access sites, including those in the lower extremities, have been exhausted in patients who are not candidates for renal transplantation, the only viable alternatives are peritoneal dialysis or dialysis via venous catheter access, both unattractive for the long term. The responsibility for preserving fistulas for as long as possible is therefore a weighty one shared by the nephrologist, the vascular surgeon, and the vascular-interventional radiologist.

Complications experienced with autogenous fistulas, PTFE grafts, and the less frequently used bovine heterografts, human umbilical vein grafts, autogenous saphenous vein grafts, and synthetic Dacron grafts, include thrombosis, infection, aneurysm and pseudoaneurysm, hemorrhage, tears, stenoses, venous hypertension, and ischemia of the involved extremity, the latter sometimes due to an arterial "steal." Contrast fistulagrams are the primary method of demonstrating most of these problems. Recent reports of fistula examination by means of color Doppler[4,5] suggest that this modality shows promise for screening purposes, although it has yet to achieve the sensitivity of angiography.

Technique

Angiography of dialysis fistulas is generally performed on an outpatient basis, often on the day of the patient's visit for dialysis. No preparation is required, nor is sedation usually necessary. If angiography immediately follows dialysis, one of the needles placed for dialysis may be used for angiography. More commonly, angiographic access is initiated in the Special Studies suite. The patent fistula is readily palpated, and the direction of flow is determined by momentary digital compression of the fistula and noting on which side of the compressing finger flow is obliterated. Because infection is one of the feared complications associated with these fistulas, strict aseptic technique must be observed. A 21-gauge butterfly needle is adequate for angiography and is placed percutaneously via a single wall puncture near the arterial end of the fistula, in either an upstream or downstream direction. Every effort must be made to traumatize these fistulas as little as possible, and because catheterization is usually not required, it is best avoided. The arterial end of the fistula is selected for needle entry so that as much of the fistula as possible is readily opacified on initial contrast injection.

Filming may be performed on a standard rapid film changer, but digital subtraction (or nonsubtraction) recording offers several advantages.[5,6] Although there may be some degradation of spatial resolution even with modern digital systems, enhanced contrast resolution more than compensates, and interfering bone images, particularly in the forearm, can be eliminated with subtraction. The study is accomplished much more rapidly with digital recording, and, importantly, the need for filming in multiple obliquities when superimposed blood vessels, arteries, or veins interfere can be immediately appreciated and accomplished (Figs. 70-2 and 70-7). Dilute contrast material may be

1767

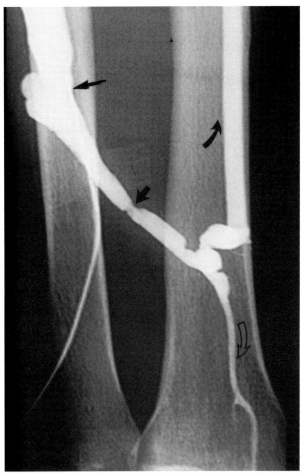

Figure 70-1. Arterial anastomosis of modified Brescia-Cimino type (i.e., side of radial artery to end of cephalic vein) demonstrated by contrast injection during momentary proximal graft occlusion. (*Curved open arrow,* radial artery distal to the anastomosis; *curved solid arrow,* radial artery proximal to the stenosis; *narrow straight arrow,* aneurysm or pseudoaneurysm within the fistula; *broad straight arrow,* stenosis in the fistula.) The stenosis is proximal to the needle entry site, and neither it nor the arterial anastomosis would have been demonstrated without filming during proximal graft occlusion. Note the relative diameters of the radial artery proximal and distal to the anastomosis; the artery proximal to the anastomosis typically increases in diameter, often markedly.

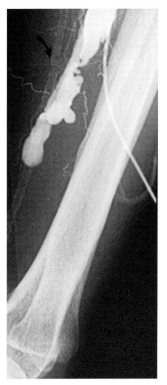 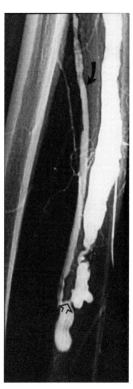

A **B**

Figure 70-2. (A) Brescia-Cimino fistula. Initial injection into the venous limb of the fistula during proximal occlusion. Venous stenoses and aneurysms are demonstrated, but the feeding radial artery is obscured by the overlapping vein. The *arrow* indicates the calcified ulnar artery, not involved in the fistula. There is no distal flow through the radial artery. In the absence of ischemia, adequate distal perfusion must be assumed to occur through the ulnar artery. (B) Filming in an oblique projection is required to demonstrate the opacified radial artery (*solid arrow*) unobscured by the cephalic vein. The artery is generally sclerotic and calcified, occludes at the anastomosis, and does not supply the hand. Note too the critical venous stenosis (*open arrow*) not demonstrated in (A).

used and volume kept to a minimum. Contrast injections of 5 to 15 ml per filming sequence at an injection rate of 2 to 3 ml per second usually suffice.

Using a large image intensifier, preferably one of 14- or 16-inch diameter, filming is performed in four or five steps, with separate injections, from the needle entry site through the superior vena cava. Refilming may then be accomplished, as desired, using a more magnified mode over areas of question or of disease,

in the necessary obliquities. Finally, the arterial anastomosis and the fistula proximal to the needle tip are opacified by filming during contrast injection while the fistula above the needle entry site is momentarily occluded. This may be accomplished by using a tourniquet or a blood pressure cuff inflated above fistula systolic pressure and released immediately after completion of filming. Should neither technique be successful in accomplishing retrograde flow through the arterial anastomosis, digital compression may be used with the lead-protected compressing finger outside the direct beam and the operator making use of accepted radiation safety procedures. Should this too fail to demonstrate the arterial anastomosis, catheterization of the fistula and contrast injection through an occlud-

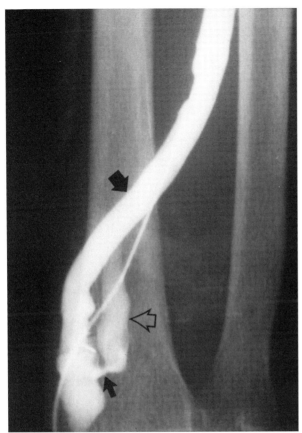

Figure 70-3. Brescia-Cimino fistula. The arterial anastomosis is critically stenotic (*small solid arrow*). As is generally the case, the feeding artery (*open arrow*) is broadened in diameter and is occluded distal to the anastomosis. Perfusion of the hand must be through the ulnar artery. The venous limb of the fistula (*broad solid arrow*) is widely patent.

ing balloon catheter with side holes below the balloon is an acceptable alternative to direct arterial catheterization.

Contrast injection may be done by hand with the operator well protected by the usual leaded garments and lead shield and distanced from the radiation source by a length of connecting tubing. If one is confident of proper needle placement, injection may be performed with an automatic injector.

Patients are usually referred for angiography when warning signs are appreciated in the dialysis suite. The most common indicator of impending occlusion is related to an outflow problem manifested by an increase in venous dialysis pressure or increased recirculation.[2,7,8] There is evidence of a positive correlation between the severity of the stenosis and graft pressure. Other reasons for referral include a nonmaturing fistula, clinically observed results of venous hypertension, palpated aneurysms, decreased thrill in the fistula, and ischemia of the hand.

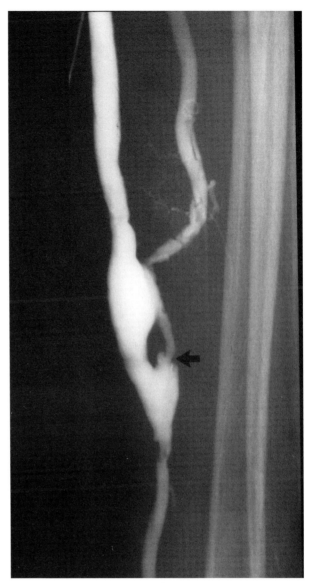

Figure 70-4. Brescia-Cimino fistula. The arterial anastomosis is only mildly narrowed (*arrow*), but the radial artery, both proximal and distal to the anastomosis, is markedly atherosclerotic and narrowed.

Complications

Problems routinely demonstrated angiographically occur at the following sites.

The Feeding Artery

Although arterial problems are relatively infrequent, they do occur in this often diabetic population; the arterial walls are often calcified, and atherosclerotic stenoses can jeopardize the fistula as well as the extremity distal to the fistula (see Figs. 70-2 and 70-4).

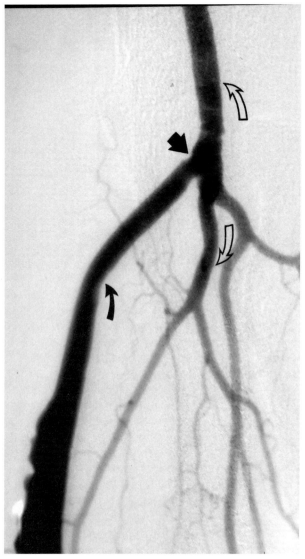

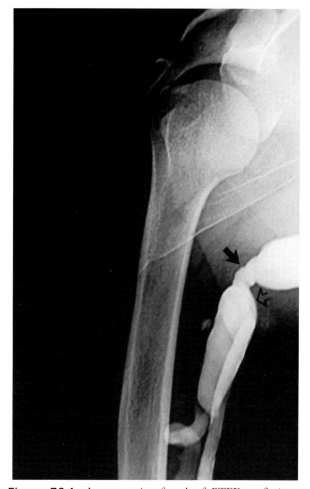

Figure 70-6. Anastomosis of end of PTFE graft (*open arrow*) to side of axillary vein. Note the stenosis of the axillary vein just distal to the anastomosis (*solid arrow*); the anastomosis is not stenotic.

Figure 70-5. Anastomosis of side of brachial artery (*open arrows*) to end of PTFE graft (*closed curved arrow*). Note the minor stenosis at the anastomosis (*closed straight arrow*) and aneurysms within the graft. Distal arterial flow is maintained.

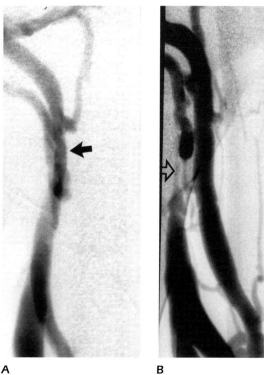

Figure 70-7. Venous outflow remote from a forearm fistula. On this anteroposterior projection, a critical stenosis of the main outflow (brachial) vein is obscured by an overlying adjacent vein (*arrow*). (B) A slight obliquity demonstrates the critical stenosis (*arrow*).

A   B

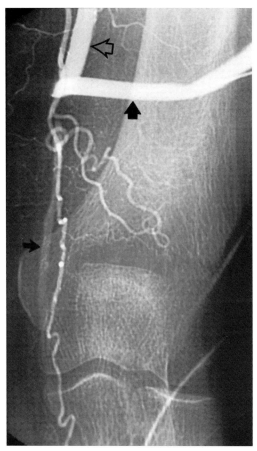

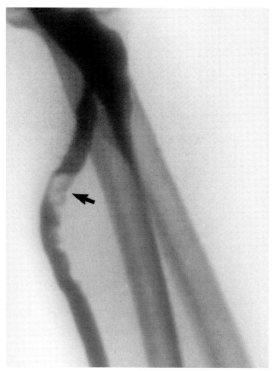

Figure 70-9. Significant, but as yet nonoccluding, clot (*arrow*) in body of fistula. Immediate intervention is required.

Figure 70-8. A brachial artery stenosis distal to the anastomosis has proceeded to occlusion (*open arrow*, artery; *large solid arrow*, graft). Perfusion of the extremity is maintained, although diminished, via collateral reconstitution of the brachial artery distal to the occlusion (*small solid arrow*).

The Arterial Anastomosis

Problems with the arterial anastomosis are much more infrequent than those at the venous anastomosis, but stenoses do occur at this site as well and can be devastating to the longevity of the fistula. The arterial anastomosis and the artery proximal and distal to it can be adequately visualized on injection of the fistula during proximal compression as described above, usually without the need to resort to direct arteriography (Figs. 70-1 through 70-5 and 70-8).

The Body of the Fistula

1. Thrombotic occlusion of a fistula in the absence of stenosis may be related to hypotension, hypovolemia, a hypercoagulable state, or, infrequently, to excessive compression exerted while achieving hemostasis after removal of the needles placed during

a hemodialysis session. For this last reason, great care must also be exercised during puncture site compression after fistulography. Thrombosis may be corrected by surgical embolectomy or by local lytic therapy.[9,10] On occasion, nonoccluding clot may be demonstrated on fistulography (Fig. 70-9); immediate intervention will avert occlusion of the fistula, and perhaps uncover an underlying stenosis.

2. Stenoses occur in the bodies of endogenous vein grafts (Fig. 70-10) as well as in PTFE grafts, in which frequent needle punctures may significantly disrupt the graft material (Fig. 70-11).

3. Aneurysms and pseudoaneurysms occur commonly, the former more frequently in endogenous fistulas (see Fig. 70-10) and the latter in PTFE grafts (Fig. 70-12) as the material deteriorates with time and is distorted with repeated needle trauma. As an attempt to delay such pseudoaneurysm formation, it is recommended that puncture sites be continuously alternated.

4. Puncture sites may leak intermittently and, rarely, profusely. Although it is difficult to demonstrate the site of such a leak angiographically outside a bleeding episode, its location is usually evident clinically and can be inferred from the angiographic appearance (Fig. 70-13).

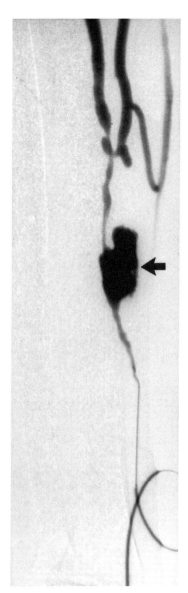

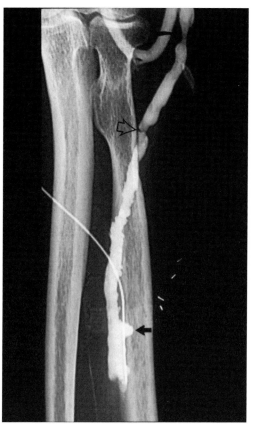

Figure 70-11. Multiple stenoses (*curved solid arrow* and *open arrow*) and aneurysm (*solid straight arrow*) in forearm fistula. Note also the multiple mural irregularities caused by multiple punctures during dialysis.

Figure 70-10. Aneurysm (*arrow*) in fistula that has otherwise become diffusely stenotic, almost to occlusion. This fistula cannot be salvaged.

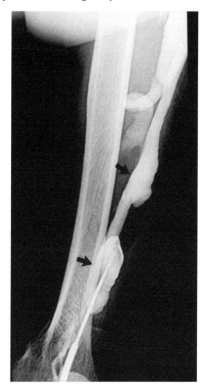

Figure 70-12. Typical pseudoaneurysms (*arrows*) in PTFE graft. Note the large dialysis needle placed directly into one of these aneurysms. This was a frequent access site during dialysis, and doubtless, over time, the pseudoaneurysm resulted from continued damage to the prosthetic material.

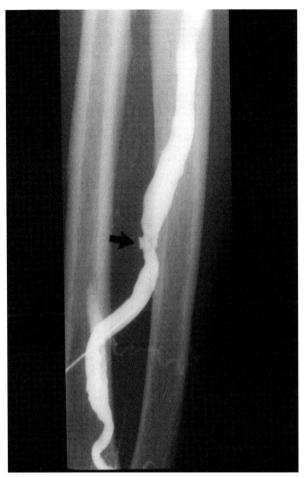

Figure 70-13. Fistulagram in a patient who had frequent significant hemorrhages from her fistula. The *arrow* indicates the site of previous bleeds, occluded spontaneously and intermittently by clot.

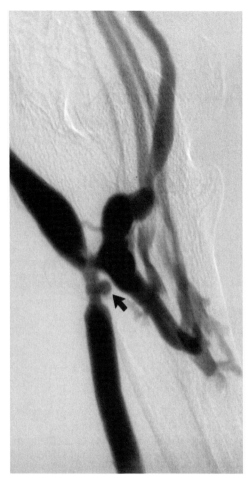

Figure 70-14. An unusual aneurysm (*arrow*) within an area of focal stenosis at the venous anastomosis of a PTFE graft. The etiology of this lesion is not clear, but it will respond to angioplasty. Note collateral retrograde flow.

The Venous Anastomosis

The most common problems are related to stenoses at the venous anastomosis (Figs. 70-14 through 70-16), most often due to intimal hyperplasia, and leading frequently to thrombosis. If these stenoses are to be detected and corrected before the occurrence of thrombosis, fistulas must be continuously evaluated at the time of dialysis. Fortunately, these venous anastomotic stenoses are generally amenable to correction by endovascular techniques, most commonly transluminal angioplasty.[11-13] There have also been reports of successes with atherectomy[14] and intravascular stenting.[15] An unusual lesion that the author has seen several times and for which the etiology remains obscure is an aneurysm within a stenosis at the venous anastomosis of a PTFE graft (see Fig. 70-14). This lesion responds to angioplasty as well as any other venous anastomotic stenosis. Whichever therapeutic course is decided on,

it is of great importance that it be promptly instituted, preferably during the same visit on which the diagnostic study uncovers the fistula-threatening lesion. On more than one occasion a fistula has occluded only days after the angiographic demonstration of a treatable lesion, while the patient was waiting for a scheduled angioplasty (see Fig. 70-15). Restenosis after balloon angioplasty does occur, but it may be months or years before there must be reintervention, and then a repeat angioplasty is often the management of choice, preserving proximal sites for potential use as eventually required (see Fig. 70-16).

The Outflow Veins

For reasons not completely understood, but doubtless related to the arterial pressures to which they are subjected, stenoses of outflow veins remote (often quite remote) from the fistula frequently occur, resulting in

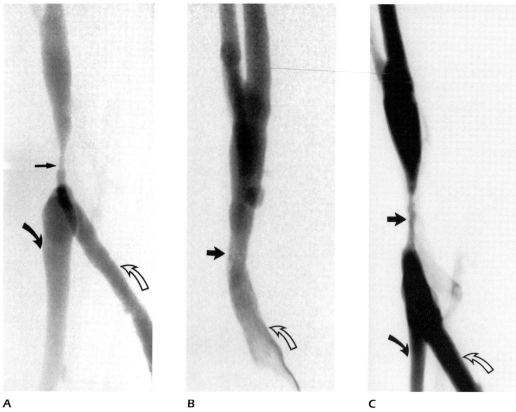

A   B   C

Figure 70-15. (A) This fistula (*open arrow*) is patent, but there is a tubular stenosis at the venous anastomosis (*small arrow*). Outflow continues, but there is retrograde flow through a collateral vein (*solid curved arrow*), suggesting that the stenosis is of hemodynamic significance. (B) Satisfactory result of angioplasty (*solid arrow*) and no collateral flow. (The *curved arrow* indicates the body of the fistula.)

(C) Restenosis at 10 months (*solid straight arrow*). The fistula (*open curved arrow*) remains patent, but there is again retrograde flow into a collateral vein (*closed curved arrow*). A repeat angioplasty was scheduled for later in the same week, but the fistula occluded in the interim. This case emphasizes the need for prompt correction of stenoses of this severity.

Figure 70-16. (A) Stenosis at venous anastomosis (*arrow*). (B) Satisfactory result of transluminal angioplasty (*arrow*). (C) Some restenosis (*arrow*) at 11 months, but still markedly improved over (A). Repeat angioplasty may be performed as required.

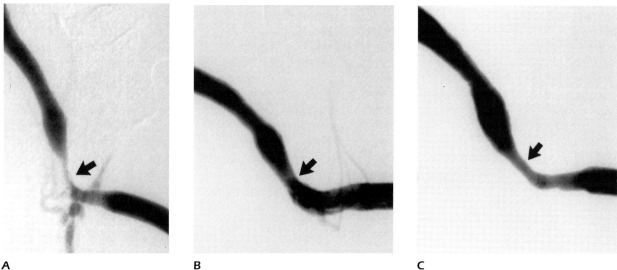

A   B   C

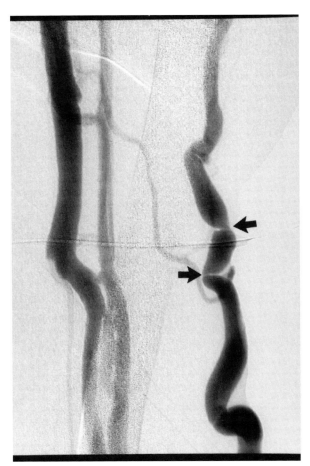

Figure 70-17. Several focal stenoses (*arrows*) of the outflow vein, probably at valvular sites.

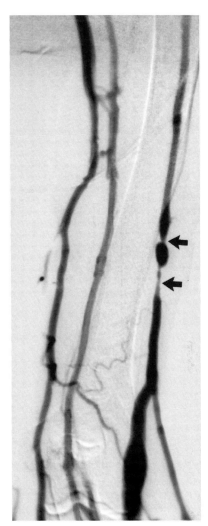

Figure 70-18. Severe stenoses (*arrows*) of outflow vein remote from the fistula.

part from intimal hyperplasia and/or valve damage (Figs. 70-7, 70-17, and 70-18). Indeed, even veins not in the direct outflow of the fistula may participate in this stenotic process.

The outflow vein may occlude completely and the graft nonetheless remain patent, draining through collaterals (Fig. 70-19). Despite its patency, such a graft is no longer adequate for dialysis and must be revised.

The outflow vein may remain patent, but efficient drainage may be compromised by extrinsic pressure, either by fibrosis in an area of previous surgery or by compression at a site of arm flexion (Fig. 70-20).

The outflow vein may not "mature" adequately and may remain small in caliber with a poorly palpable thrill. This may result from poor inflow or, as the author has seen on occasion, from an unfortunate anatomic situation, such as a venous bifurcation very close to the arterial anastomosis reducing arterialized flow into the main venous drainage channel (Fig. 70-21).

Stenosis of the subclavian vein and innominate vein may be due to the previous placement of access cathe-ters or temporary dialysis catheters in these locations, with resultant vascular damage (Figs. 70-22 through 70-24). It has been suggested, with justification, that patients who have had such access catheters previously placed on the side of proposed fistula construction should have a venogram performed before surgery.[16] Indeed, venography has been advocated before the creation of all fistulas[17] but is generally felt not to be required before placement of first-time fistulas in an extremity not previously used for access. Venography may also be useful in an extremity in which a new fistula must be created after initial fistula failure. Venography may demonstrate that an extremity may not be used for access because of central venous occlusion (see Fig. 70-24), or venography may indicate that access must be specifically restricted to basilic or to cephalic outflow (see Fig. 70-23).

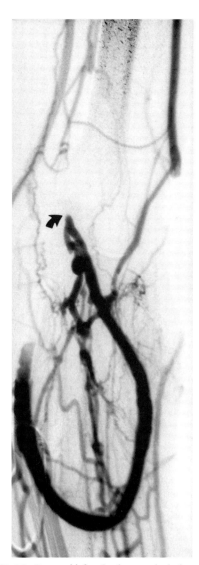

Figure 70-19. Patent U fistula, but occluded outflow vein (*arrow*). Despite the patency of the fistula, it must be revised.

Venous hypertension as a consequence of central venous stenosis or occlusion may lead to extensive edema and the development of often large varices.[18–20] A particularly distressing form of venous hypertension that occurs in 4 percent of Brescia-Cimino anastomoses at the wrist results from arterialization of the cephalic venous system in the hand and consequent ulcerations, the so-called sore thumb syndrome.[20]

The Extremity Distal to the Fistula (Arterial Steals and Occlusion of Arterial Outflow)

"Steal" syndromes have been reported in 8 percent of autogenous antecubital fistulas and in 1 percent of radiocephalic wrist fistulas.[20] When they occur, they

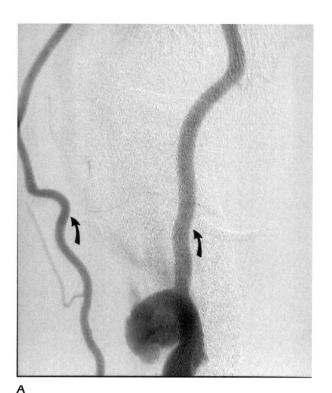

A

B

Figure 70-20. (A) Initial central outflow is through large collateral veins (*arrows*). (B) Several seconds later, the main outflow vein opacifies but is extrinsically compressed as it crosses the antecubital fossa (*arrow*).

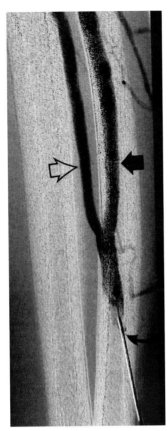

Figure 70-21. The venous limb of a Brescia-Cimino fistula above the angiographic needle (*curved arrow*) divides low in the forearm into two branches of near-equal diameter. Arterial pressure is dissipated between the large side branch (*open arrow*) and the main outflow vein (*solid arrow*), which does not mature. Correction would consist of ligating the side branch.

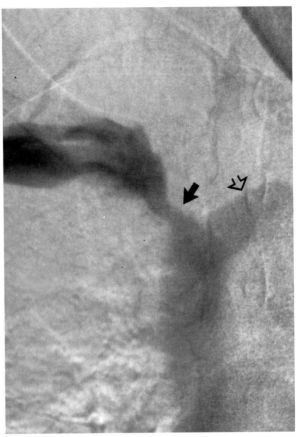

Figure 70-22. Stenosis of the right innominate vein (*solid arrow*), the site of a previously placed and subsequently removed temporary dialysis catheter. This lesion should be amenable to angioplasty, and perhaps stenting. Note the reflux into the left innominate vein (*open arrow*) of normal caliber.

Figure 70-23. Occlusion of right axillary vein (*straight solid arrow*) with central reconstitution (*open arrow*). Venous flow from the arm is intact through the cephalic vein (*curved arrow*), which drains into the subclavian vein central to the occlusion. In such a situation, care must be taken to place the fistula in the cephalic, and not the basilic, system.

Figure 70-24. The occluded segment of the left subclavian vein (*arrow*) includes the entry site of the cephalic vein; in this situation, this left upper extremity may not be used for fistula construction.

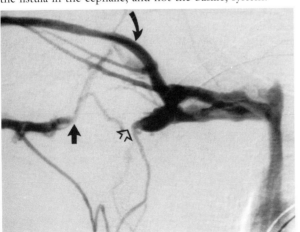

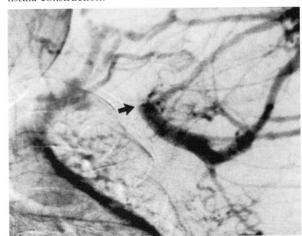

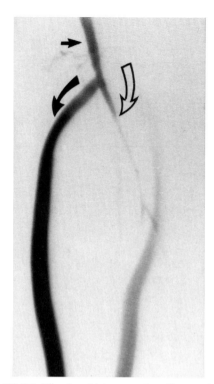

Figure 70-25. The brachial artery (*small arrow*) supplies this U (PTFE) fistula (*curved solid arrow*). Arterial flow to the hand (*open arrow*) is through an extremely stenotic brachial artery distal to the anastomosis, with resultant ischemia of the forearm and hand.

can threaten the viability of the extremity. Demonstration of a suspected steal is the only situation in which a direct arteriogram need be performed in the evaluation of a dialysis fistula. Distal ischemia occurs when blood flow through the artery feeding the fistula flows only or principally through the fistula and does not adequately perfuse the hand because resistance in the fistula is much lower than that in the often diseased outflow arteries (Fig. 70-25). Exacerbation of a "steal" may occur through a radial-artery-to-cephalic-vein fistula when there is excessive flow into the cephalic vein from the radial artery with flow to the hand predominantly through the ulnar artery, across the palmar arch, and then retrograde through the radial artery and again into the fistula, effectively "stealing" both radial and ulnar blood from the hand and resulting in distal ischemia. Corrective action usually consists of ligation of the radial artery distal to the shunt, or some form of surgical banding of the fistula to increase resistance within it.

Nonetheless, occlusion of the radial artery distal to the arterial anastomosis can generally be tolerated because of continued hand perfusion through the ulnar artery and palmar arch. However, when construction of a fistula above the origins of the runoff arteries re-

sults in the occlusion of the brachial artery, severe ischemia may result even though there is reconstitution of distal vessels via collaterals (see Fig. 70-8).

References

1. Brescia MJ, Cimino JE, Appel K, et al. Chronic hemodialysis using venipuncture and a surgically created arteriovenous fistula. N Engl J Med 1966;275:1089–1092.
2. Fan P-Y, Schwab SJ. Vascular access: concepts for the 1990s. J Am Soc Nephrol 1992;3:1–11.
3. Mehta S. Statistical summary of clinical results of vascular access procedures for hemodialysis. In: Sommer BJ, Henry ML, eds. Vascular access for hemodialysis: II. Precept Press, 1991:145–156.
4. Middleton WD, Picus DD, Marx MV, et al. Color Doppler sonography of hemodialysis vascular access: comparison with angiography. AJR 1989;152:633–639.
5. Dousset V, Grenier N, Douws C, et al. Hemodialysis grafts: color Doppler flow imaging correlated with digital subtraction angiography and functional status. Radiology 1991;181:89–94.
6. Picus D, Hicks ME, Darcy MD, et al. Comparison of nonsubtracted digital angiography and conventional screen-film angiography for the evaluation of patients with peripheral vascular disease. J Vasc Intervent Radiol 1991;2:359–364.
7. Gaylord GM, Taber TE. Long-term hemodialysis access salvage: problems and challenges for nephrologists and interventional radiologists. J Vasc Intervent Radiol 1993;4:103–107.
8. Sullivan KL, Besarab A, Dorrell S, et al. The relationship between dialysis graft pressure and stenosis. Invest Radiol 1991;27:352–355.
9. Valji K, Bookstein JJ, Roberts AC, et al. Pharmacomechanical thrombolysis and angioplasty in the management of clotted hemodialysis grafts: early and late clinical results. Radiology 1991;178:243–247.
10. Brunner MC, Matalon TAS, Patel SK, et al. Ultra rapid urokinase in hemodialysis access occlusion. J Vasc Intervent Radiol 1991;2:503–506.
11. Gordon DH, Glanz S, Butt KM, et al. Treatment of stenotic lesions in dialysis access fistulas and shunts by transluminal angioplasty. Radiology 1982;143:53–58.
12. Gmelin E, Winterhoff R, Rinast E. Insufficient hemodialysis access fistulas: late results of treatment with percutaneous balloon angioplasty. Radiology 1989;171:657–660.
13. Hunter DW, Castaneda-Zuniga WR, Coleman CC, et al. Failing arteriovenous dialysis fistulas: evaluation and treatment. Radiology 1984;152:631–635.
14. Vorwerk D, Guenther RW. Removal of intimal hyperplasia in vascular endoprostheses by atherectomy and balloon dilatation. AJR 1990;154:617–619.
15. Gunther RW, Vorwerk D, Bohndorf K, et al. Venous stenoses in dialysis shunts: treatment with self-expanding metallic stents. Radiology 1989;170:401–405.
16. Surratt RS, Picus D, Hichs ME, et al. The importance of preoperative evaluation of the subclavian vein in dialysis access planning. AJR 1991;156:623–625.
17. Harasawa H, Yamazaki C, Kobayashi M, et al. Utility of venography in shunt surgery on hemodialyzed patients. Nephron 1991;57:167–174.
18. Bhuta K, Rajdeo H. Recognition and management of venous hypertension complicating hemodialysis access. In: Sommer BG, Henry ML, eds. Vascular access for hemodialysis: II. Precept Press, 1991:229–236.
19. Butt KMH, Friedman EA, Kountz SL. Angioaccess. Curr Probl Surg 1976;13:28–32.
20. Guthrie CR, Wilson SE. Complications of vascular access. In: Machleder HI, ed. Vascular disorders of the upper extremity. Mt Kisco, NY: Futura, 1989:131–152.

71

Angiography of Bones, Joints, and Soft Tissues

CHARLES J. TEGTMEYER
DAVID J. SPINOSA
ALAN H. MATSUMOTO

Establishing the exact diagnosis of certain bone and soft tissue tumors remains one of the most perplexing problems in medicine. Often there is considerable delay in the diagnosis because specific clinical symptoms are lacking. The radiologic examination is a critical step in the diagnosis of these lesions. However, because bone continually reacts to local and systemic changes in its environment by either removing or laying down mineralized matrix, the changes depicted on plain radiographs may be misleading and difficult to interpret.

The pathologist plays a crucial role in the diagnosis of these lesions. Because these tumors are relatively uncommon, however, most pathologists do not have many opportunities to examine them. The problem is further complicated because much of the biopsy material submitted for examination is inadequate: either the biopsy site is inappropriate or the biopsy specimen does not accurately represent the lesion. It has been repeatedly emphasized that close cooperation among the radiologist, pathologist, and surgeon is necessary to arrive at a correct diagnosis in these difficult lesions.

Although angiography is a well-established procedure in the evaluation of other neoplasms, it has not gained wide acceptance in the diagnosis of bone tumors—perhaps because the angiographic pattern does not allow an exact diagnosis to be made. However, the same can be said for the clinical, histologic, and other radiographic examinations of these lesions. The advent of CT and MRI have further limited the role of angiography in the evaluation of neoplasms. Nevertheless, if the limitations of angiography are understood and the procedure is used properly in conjunction with other diagnostic studies, it can play a valuable role in the diagnosis of bone and soft tissue lesions.

Vascular Anatomy

A knowledge of the vascular anatomy is necessary to understand the findings made at angiography. Current knowledge of the vascular supply of the bones is based on the observations of Doan,[1] Drinker et al.,[2] Tilling,[3] and Trueta.[4]

The long bones have three sources of arterial blood: (1) nutrient arteries supplying the diaphysis and epiphysis, (2) the periosteal and perichondrial arteries, and (3) the metaphyseal and epiphyseal vascular systems. The nutrient arteries enter the diaphysis to supply the medullary cavity. There are extensive anastomoses between the nutrient arteries and the metaphyseal vessels. The nutrient arteries also anastomose with the rich periosteal blood supply, which perforates the compact bone to enter the haversian system. Branches from the vascular supply of the surrounding muscles and tendons also perforate the bone to supply the epiphyseal and metaphyseal portions of the bone. Although the epiphyseal and metaphyseal systems are separate, they anastomose with each other across the epiphyseal cartilage except for a short period of time during the development of the femoral head in the child. The venous drainage of the long bones is similar in distribution to the arterial blood supply.

Enlarged arteries are often seen coursing through the muscles and other soft tissues surrounding tumors. These vessels supply the soft tissue tumors and feed the periosteal and perichondrial arteries that constitute the main blood supply in most bone lesions.[5] Depending on the location of the lesion, the metaphyseal and epiphyseal vessels may also contribute to the vascular supply of the tumor. The nutrient artery usually does not contribute a significant, angiographically visible blood supply to the tumor. If the tumor breaks out of the bone, the vessels supplying the surrounding tissue feed the tumor.

Technique

The percutaneous Seldinger technique is employed to introduce the catheter into the vascular tree. The angiographic demonstration of bone and soft tissue tumors is markedly improved when the catheter is directed with the arterial flow in the antegrade position.[6] Catheters with the appropriate shape are then used to select the major vessels supplying the region of the tumor.

The pelvis and upper thigh are studied using 4 or 5 French catheters. The contralateral femoral artery is used to approach these lesions. Either the aortic bifurcation or the common iliac artery is injected. Using a shepherd's crook type of catheter, the contralateral common iliac artery is selected. With this angiographic run as a map, the catheter is placed selectively in the major vessel supplying the tumor or as close to this vessel as possible. As with all angiographic studies, the contrast medium should be injected as near the lesion as is feasible. Selective injections are then made into the vessels supplying the tumor, usually the internal or distal external iliac artery. Filling of the adjacent overlying vessels is thereby eliminated, aiding in the interpretation of the angiograms. This is a particularly necessary step in the pelvis. Injections are also repeated in different projections to delineate the entire extent of the tumor. If entry into the upper thigh is desired, a tight J-shaped guidewire can be passed into the common femoral or superficial femoral artery and the catheter can be advanced over the wire.

Lesions in the distal lower extremity are usually studied by entering the ipsilateral common femoral artery with an antegrade puncture. The antegrade puncture is easier to perform if a large sponge pad or blanket roll is placed under the patient's buttocks to hyperextend the hips. The small catheters used (5 French) can be easily advanced into the popliteal artery.

For lesions of the upper extremity, the femoral approach is ordinarily employed. A 5 French Cook HIH catheter can usually be advanced over a tight J-shaped guidewire into the brachial artery. A retrograde high brachial artery approach can also be used. This approach makes it easy to select the branches of the subclavian and axillary arteries. A 5 French catheter with a small C-shaped curve at the tip is used.

Visualization of both the arterial and venous circulations is desirable in all cases because the venous phase

of the arteriogram often provides extremely valuable information. The radiographs should be obtained initially at two films per second for 3 seconds, then one film per second for 10 seconds followed by films every 2 seconds for a total of 26 seconds. After the first run, the angiographic program can be tailored to the circulation of the individual lesion.

Depending on the size of the patient, 5 to 12 ml of contrast material is injected per second for 4 to 5 seconds. The average injection rate into the common iliac artery is 8 to 10 ml per second for a total of 40 ml of contrast material. The axillary and femoral arteries require 7 to 8 ml per second for a total of 30 to 40 ml of contrast material.

Subtraction radiographs are extremely valuable in bone and soft tissue tumors. By eliminating the superimposed bones and the tumoral calcifications, they permit a more thorough evaluation of the vascular pattern. When the diagnosis is in doubt, magnification radiographs may also be helpful because they can enhance the visualization of tiny vessels.

Digital subtraction angiography plays an important role in the angiographic workup of bone and soft tissue tumors because it defines the anatomy and the local vascular relationships to the lesion. Cut film, however, is unsurpassed in defining the anatomic detail of the tumor.

Pharmacoangiography is important for the enhancement of bone and soft tissue tumors. Ekelund et al.[7] compared the effects of a vasoconstrictor (angiotensin) and a vasodilator (tolazoline) in 18 patients with bone and soft tissue tumors and concluded that angiotensin was more effective. Angiotensin is administered by diluting 10 to 15 mg in 10 ml of normal saline and injecting it slowly through the catheter at a rate of 5 ml per second. The angiogram is repeated 15 to 45 seconds later. Many investigators,[1,6] however, feel that tolazoline (Priscoline) is more effective. A total of 25 to 50 mg of Priscoline is diluted in 10 ml of normal saline and infused slowly through the catheter. The amount depends on the size of the patient and the area studied. An injection of Omnipaque 300 is made 30 seconds later with the catheter in the antegrade position, with its tip as close to the lesion as possible. Subsequent contrast injections can be supplemented by 12.5 mg of Priscoline before each angiographic run.

Several points must be borne in mind when pharmacoangiography is employed. It is important to obtain a standard angiographic run before augmenting the angiography with vasoactive drugs. If a retrograde injection is performed, increasing the injection rate produces reflux into proximal vessels and does not improve the quality of the angiogram. Because Priscoline increases the intravascular volume and decreases the circulation time, a higher injection rate and a higher total volume are required.[6]

Angiographic Appearance of Tumors

The evaluation of the arteriogram is based on visualization of the entire circulation throughout the lesion. The arteries supplying the tumor need to be adequately opacified, and the film program should be long enough to visualize the capillary phase and the venous drainage.

Malignant Tumors

The angiographic picture of malignancy is a composite of several of the following factors:

1. Neovascularity
2. Pooling or laking of contrast material
3. Tumor stain or blush
4. Encasement and occlusion of vessels
5. Extension of the tumor outside the bone
6. Displacement of vessels
7. Arteriovenous shunts
8. Large abnormal draining veins
9. Tumor invasion of veins
10. Abnormal course of veins

Neovascularity

The term *neovascularity* or *pathologic vessel* has been defined by Strickland[8] as a vessel that is "deployed seemingly without purpose, keeps to no set course and shows no progressive diminution in calibre." Histologically, such a tumor vessel is a primitive vascular channel often consisting only of an endothelial layer surrounded by a connective tissue sheath, hence its irregular course and caliber.

The presence of neovascularity is the single most important finding upon which the differentiation between benign and malignant is based.[9] Abnormal vascularity, however, may also be present in certain benign lesions,[10] including giant-cell tumors, aneurysmal bone cysts, osteoblastomas, and Paget disease. Benign nerve sheath tumors and certain hemangiomas may also exhibit abnormal vascularity. Fortunately, most of these lesions can be differentiated by their clinical and plain film appearances.

Pooling or Laking of Contrast Material

Ill-defined accumulation of contrast material may be seen in a malignant lesion, resulting from neovascular vessels that end their haphazard journey in amorphous spaces within necrotic tissue.[8] The amorphous spaces often retain contrast material well into the venous phase of the arteriogram. This angiographic finding is another expression of the abnormal vascularity seen in tumors and is a reliable sign of malignancy.

Tumor Stain or Blush

Diffuse staining of the tumor by contrast material is a nonspecific finding. The presence of a tumor blush by itself does not indicate malignancy. There is a small group of benign bone lesions that have a tendency to retain contrast material: giant-cell tumors, aneurysmal bone cysts, osteoid osteomas, and osteoblastomas. This finding, however, is of great value in assessing the size of the tumor, and it may indicate that the tumor has broken out of the bone.

Encasement and Occlusion

Encasement or occlusion of vessels is seen in malignant tumors. Although atherosclerosis may also cause stenoses and occlusions of vessels, an abrupt termination of an otherwise normal artery in the area of a bone or soft tissue tumor is a frequent indicator of malignancy.

Tumor Extension

Extension of the tumor outside the confines of the bone is a reliable sign of malignancy that is not seen in benign hypervascular lesions unless a fracture is present. Fractures occasionally cause bizarre-appearing hypervascularity.[11] Angiography, however, does not always define the complete intraosseous extent of the tumor, and skip metastases within the bone are not always seen.[11]

Displacement of Vessels

The displacement of vessels is an indication of the anatomic extent of the tumor. This information is important if a radical local resection is contemplated because the surgeon will know whether he or she will have to deal with these vessels. The degree of vascularity is also important in the preoperative assessment because it gives some indication of the blood loss to be expected.

Arteriovenous Shunts

Early opacification of the veins draining the tumor is an expression of rapid blood flow through the tumor. Opacified veins during the arterial phase of the arteriogram indicate arteriovenous shunting and an abnormal microcirculation. This is not, however, a specific sign of malignancy. If prolonged injections are used, venous filling can be seen and arteries remain opacified; therefore, only the early phase of the study is helpful for identifying arteriovenous shunting.

Large Abnormal Draining Veins

Large abnormal draining veins are also seen in hypervascular lesions. These veins often encircle the tumors and are helpful in defining their extent. The identification of these major venous drainage pathways is important to facilitate early ligation and prevent tumor embolization during surgery.[11]

Tumor Invasion of Veins

Direct invasion of the veins by the tumor may sometimes be seen. When present, this is a sign of malignancy.

Abnormal Course of Veins

Strickland[8] described another venous sign of malignancy: the presence of straight veins coursing at right angles to the normal flow of venous blood. This finding is more frequent in metastatic tumors than in primary lesions.

Differentiation Between Benign and Malignant Tumors

Arteriography is of considerable assistance in distinguishing between benign and malignant bone tumors. It must be remembered that the angiographic picture of malignancy is a composite of signs, all of which will not be present in any one tumor. Nevertheless, more than one sign of malignancy is usually present in a given tumor. Strickland[8] found angiographic evidence of malignancy in all but 2 of the 33 malignant bone tumors he examined. Voegeli and Uehlinger[9] examined 100 bone tumors with angiography and concluded that the use of angiographic studies as a supplement to plain film radiography increased the diagnostic accuracy in differentiating a benign from a malignant lesion by approximately 25 percent.

If the definitive angiographic signs of malignancy are present, it can be reasonably assumed that the lesion is malignant. However, the converse is *not* true, because a small number of malignant tumors, especially those that do not breach the cortex,[12] fail to demonstrate any of the angiographic signs of malignancy. Therefore, a normal arteriogram does not entirely rule out a malignancy.

Benign bone neoplasms usually do not deviate from the normal angiographic appearance. The vessels may be displaced by the bulk of the tumor, and in some instances a tumor stain or blush and hyperemia are present. It is important to remember that a tumor stain or blush is not a specific sign of malignancy.

Furthermore, one often cannot distinguish among the individual types of bone tumors using the angiographic picture alone. This is not surprising considering the difficult diagnostic problem bone tumors cause the plain film radiographer, pathologist, and clinician.

Extent of Tumors

Although angiography's role in determining the extent of bone and soft tissue tumors has diminished since the advent of CT and MRI, it can provide reliable information on this subject. It accurately demonstrates the soft tissue extension of tumors.[13] It also defines the most suitable site for biopsy because the highly vascularized areas within a particular tumor correspond to its most malignant areas, and necrotic areas within the tumor, which appear as hypovascular areas, can be avoided. In addition, newer surgical techniques for tumors of the limb require assessment of the status of the neurovascular bundle. Limb salvage procedures are precluded when there is encasement of the major vessels to the distal limb.[14]

Inflammatory Lesions of Bone

Osteomyelitis

In osteomyelitis, the invading organism may attack the bone directly from an infected wound, a penetrating injury, or a contaminated fracture or may gain access by hematogenous spread from a distant infection. Hematogenic osteomyelitis is the most common form and is predominantly a disease of infants and children. The most frequent infecting organism is *Staphylococcus aureus,* less commonly *Streptococcus,* and least commonly other organisms.

The plain film radiologic findings are well known. The primary locus of osteomyelitis in children is the metaphysis. Early changes are first noted in the soft tissue. The changes in the bone usually take 2 weeks to develop, and then small osteolytic areas appear in the metaphysis. Periosteal elevation occurs as the infection spreads and new bone is laid down. At this stage the infection often mimics neoplastic lesions. If treatment is delayed, the changes of chronic osteomyelitis will ensue.

The angiographic picture of osteomyelitis parallels the progress of inflammatory changes. These changes are seen first in the surrounding soft tissue and later in the bone. Hyperemia is observed, and the arteries and veins appear more numerous and are dilated. Rapid circulation is noted throughout the area of infection. The arteries are tortuous but have regular lumina and show none of the variations in caliber that characterize pathologic vessels.[15] The small contrast-filled vascular lakes often seen in malignancy are not present.[16]

Chronic osteomyelitis is usually accompanied by a normal angiographic picture, although occasionally hyperemia is seen.

Brodie Abscess

Brodie abscess, an often painful lesion usually found near the end of a long bone, frequently presents as a round or oval radiolucent area with a sclerotic rim. It has a radiographic appearance similar to that of an osteoid osteoma, but angiography can easily differentiate the lesions because a Brodie abscess is avascular,[5,17] whereas an osteoid osteoma is highly vascular.[17,18]

Bone Tumors of Cartilaginous Origin

Benign Tumors

Chondroblastomas

Chondroblastoma or Codman tumor is a rare benign tumor of cartilaginous origin with a predilection for the epiphyses. The lesion usually occurs in the second decade of life and is more common in men than in women, with a ratio of 2:1.

Roentgenographically, the lesion appears as a radiolucent defect involving the epiphysis, and a thin sclerotic margin is often present. The lesion originates in the epiphysis but may enlarge and involve the metaphysis (Fig. 71-1A). CT scanning demonstrates the matrix mineralization and an intact cortex. MRI signal characteristics are nonspecific for chondroblastoma.

Experience with the angiographic patterns of chondroblastoma is limited. Yaghmai[5] reported the angiographic findings in five cases. The arteries supplying the lesions arose from the surrounding soft tissue, and his cases exhibited a low degree of vascularity with a faint tumor stain. The authors have obtained an angiogram of one completely avascular chondroblastoma. However, chondroblastomas may exhibit hypervascularity.[19] The vessels supplying the lesion may be extremely tortuous, but they appear to taper normally (see Fig. 71-1B and C) and do not have the irregular course of malignancy.

The plain film differential diagnosis of chondroblastomas includes giant-cell tumors. Angiographically, however, the entities are easily separated. The giant-cell tumor has intense hypervascularity and a prolonged intense blush that is not seen in chondroblastomas.

Chondromyxoid Fibromas

Chondromyxoid fibroma is a benign bone tumor, apparently derived from cartilage-forming connective tissue, that contains chondroid, myxoid, and fibrous elements. It occurs predominantly in the lower limb but may occur elsewhere, including the flat bones. Although it may be found at any age, its peak incidence is in the second and third decades.

The radiographs usually suggest a benign process. In the long bones, the lesion is likely to be eccentrically situated in the metaphysis. It is visualized as a sharply outlined radiolucent defect that thins the cortex and that may contain trabeculae. Angiographically, the lesion is avascular and has a benign appearance.[5]

Osteochondromas

The osteochondroma is the most common benign neoplasm of bone. It is a cartilage-capped bony protuberance composed of osseous and chondroid elements. The lesion is usually located at the metaphysis, particularly in the long bones around the knee. However, it can involve any bone that develops from cartilage.

CT scanning reliably demonstrates cortical continuity between the affected bone and the osteochondroma. MRI is particularly helpful in evaluating the contiguity of the marrow between the host bone and the lesion.[20] It also can evaluate the thickness of the cartilaginous cap more accurately than CT and can better demonstrate the relationship to adjacent structures.

Vascular complications resulting from osteochondromas are not rare, particularly in the area of the knee. Because of the size and location, osteochondromas may damage the popliteal artery or vein. Both thrombosis[21] and pseudoaneurysms[22] have been reported in the popliteal artery. Angiography reveals that osteochondromas, because of their size, may displace vessels. However, the tumor does not exhibit hypervascularity or abnormal vessels (Fig. 71-2).[23]

Enchondromas

An enchondroma is a benign cartilaginous neoplasm located within the medullary cavity of a bone. It is poorly vascularized and reveals no abnormal vessels.[24]

Malignant Tumors

Chondrosarcomas

Chondrosarcoma is a malignant bone tumor of cartilaginous origin, arising either in bone (primary type) or from a preexisting cartilaginous lesion (secondary type). Central chondrosarcomas arise in the interior of

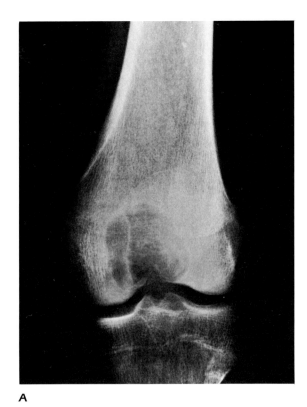

A

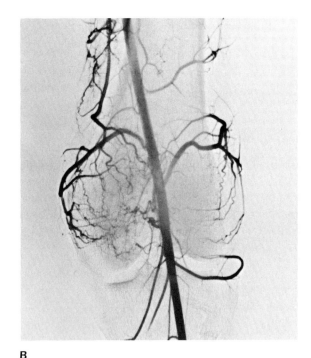

B

Figure 71-1. Chondroblastoma of the distal femur in a 14-year-old boy with a 6-month history of knee pain. (A) The plain film demonstrates a well-demarcated destructive lesion involving the epiphysis and distal metaphysis. (B) The subtraction film of the arteriogram demonstrates increased vascularity in the area of the tumor. Branches of the genicular arteries supply the tumor. (C) The lateral subtraction film shows the marked tortuosity of the vessels supplying the tumor.

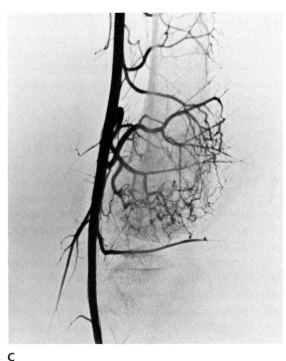

C

the bone. Peripheral chondrosarcomas develop on the surface of the bone as a protruding mass. Chondrosarcoma is the second most common primary malignant bone tumor, if myeloma is excluded. The lesions usually occur in the fourth, fifth, and sixth decades of life;

when the tumor occurs in childhood, it carries a grave prognosis.

Peripheral chrondrosarcoma presents a distinct appearance radiographically. It is usually a large lobulated mass projecting from a flat or long bone. It is invariably calcified.

Central chondrosarcomas are more difficult to diagnose because they often present as benign-appearing radiolucent defects in the bone that contain calcification. This is one bone tumor that may appear completely benign roentgenographically. If the lesion progresses, it will become less well defined and eventually penetrate the cortex.

CT scanning can evaluate the matrix mineralization and the integrity of the involved cortex. Cortical destruction, a wide zone of transition, and a changing margin are signs signaling malignant transformation. CT can also evaluate the soft tissue component of the lesion; however, this is best done with MRI. An inhomogeneous signal due to fibrous bands weaving through cartilaginous lobules is believed to be characteristic of chrondrosarcoma.[25]

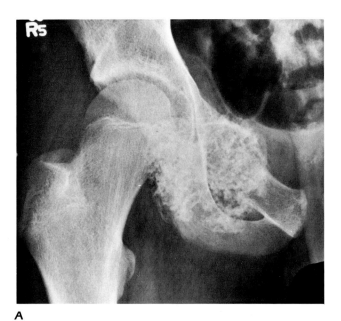

A

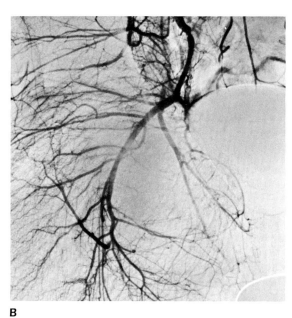

B

Figure 71-2. Osteochondroma of the pubic bone in a 15-year-old boy with a slowly enlarging mass. (A) A well-defined lesion containing extensive irregular calcification is present in the pubic bone. (B) The normal-appearing vessels are displaced by the lesion. No hypervascularity or neovascularity is present.

Figure 71-3. Low-grade chondrosarcoma of the pubic bone in a 61-year-old man. The lesion had been present for 9 years. (A) A huge mass arises from the pubic ramus near the symphysis. It contains amorphous calcification. (B) The hypovascular lesion displaces the surrounding normal vessels.

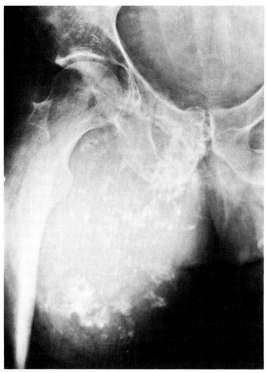

A

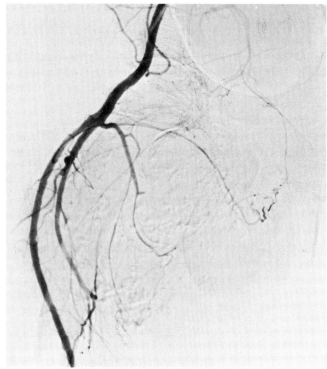

B

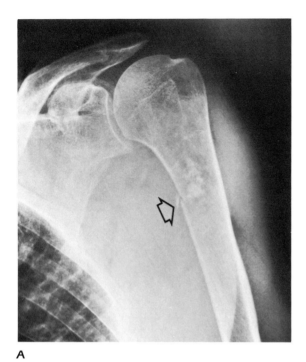

A

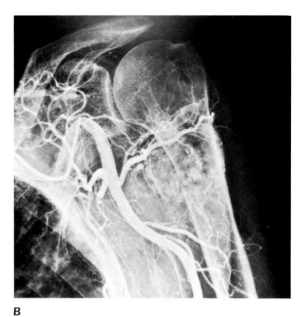

B

Figure 71-4. Chondrosarcoma of the humerus in a 73-year-old man. The patient related his shoulder pain to a fall on his left shoulder 7 weeks previously. (A) An ill-defined lytic defect containing flocculent calcification is present in the humerus. A pathologic fracture is seen (*arrow*). (B) The arteriogram exhibits abnormal vascularity and a tumor blush. The neoplasm extends into the surrounding soft tissue. (C) The pooling of contrast material within the tumor persists into the venous phase. Abnormal veins are seen draining the lesion.

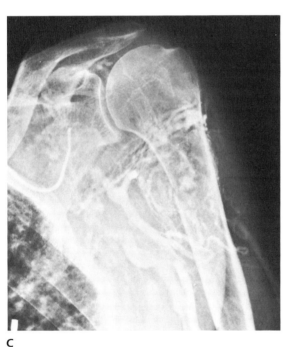

C

The angiographic pattern of chrondrosarcomas is varied, ranging from normal to hypervascular.[23] Large tumors may be hypovascular, exhibiting only displacement of the normal surrounding arteries (Fig. 71-3). At the other end of the spectrum, the tumor may exhibit florid neovascularity, and large abnormal veins may be seen draining the tumor (Fig. 71-4). The lesion may display a tumor stain (Fig. 71-5), but this is not a prominent feature. Despite the varied angiographic pattern, angiography contributes valuable information in the evaluation of chondrosarcomas. Lagergren et al.[26] demonstrated a relationship between the degree of vascularity and the degree of differentiation of the tumor. The highly vascular tumors are poorly differentiated and have a poor prognosis (Fig. 71-6). The most vascular area of the tumor corresponds to the most aggressive portion of the tumor. This is the area that should be subjected to biopsy. The displacement of surrounding normal vessels, the peripheral reactive vascularity, and the neovascularity all contribute to defining the extent of the lesion. Therefore, angiography usually accurately delineates the extent of the tumor (see Figs. 71-4 and 71-6).[11]

It is important to remember that the lack of abnormal vascularity does not completely rule out malignancy in chondroid tumors. Some slow-growing chrondrosarcomas will have a deceptively normal vascular pattern.

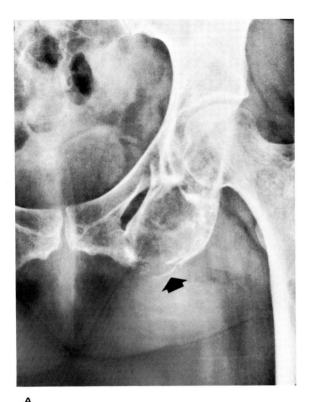

A

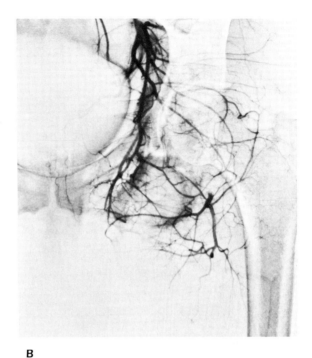

B

Figure 71-5. Chondrosarcoma of the ischium in a 33-year-old woman with a 5-month history of pain and tenderness in the left buttock. (A) There is an osteolytic lesion in the ischium. The cortex is expanded, and a fracture is seen (*arrow*). (B) The arteriogram exhibits a faint blush around the periphery of the lesion in the arterial phase. (C) The venous phase again shows the tumor blush at the margins of the lesion (*open arrows*). The tumor can be seen extending through the fracture site into the soft tissue (*solid arrow*).

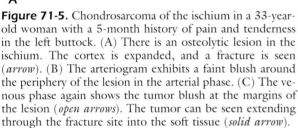

C

Bone Tumors of Osteoblastic Origin

Benign Tumors

Osteoid Osteomas

Osteoid osteoma is a small, painful, benign neoplasm of bone. It is a not uncommon entity. Ninety percent of the patients are below the age of 25 years, and it is more prevalent in men than in women, with a ratio of 2:1.

Osteoid osteoma has been observed in nearly all the bones of the body. Ordinarily, however, it affects the diaphysis of the tibia and femur. Radiographically, the changes are related to the central nidus and its location. The tumor usually presents as a small, radiolucent intracortical nidus less than 1 cm in size surrounded by a dense area of sclerosis. The nidus may contain calcium or may be completely radiolucent. In

this situation, the diagnosis is obvious; however, the lesion does not always present the classic roentgenographic picture. The surrounding dense sclerosis may obscure the central nidus, or, if the lesion is located in cancellous bone, relatively little sclerosis may be present. Occasionally, when the osteoid osteoma is

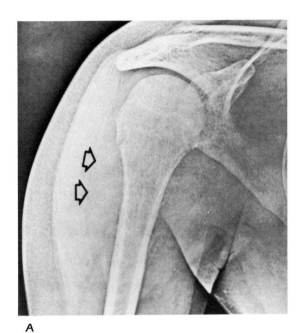

A

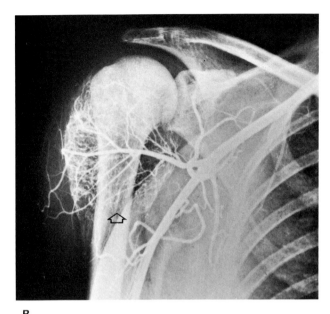

B

Figure 71-6. A poorly differentiated chondrosarcoma of the humerus in a 20-year-old woman. The patient presented with a 3-month history of pain and swelling in the shoulder. (A) The xerogram shows displacement of the soft tissue (*arrows*). However, the bone appears normal. (B) The florid neovascularity clearly outlines the extent of the tumor. Vertical streaks of contrast material are seen within the medullary cavity (*arrow*), indicating the origin of the tumor. The patient developed pulmonary metastases 7 months after primary resection of the tumor.

located adjacent to a joint, it lacks the classic roentgenographic findings and instead appears as a synovitis.[18,27]

Computed tomography can often demonstrate the nidus. The characteristic findings include a mineralized center within a well-defined lytic lesion with surrounding reactive sclerosis.[28] Gadolinium-enhanced MRI demonstrates the prominent vascularity of the lesion.

Angiography can be extremely helpful when the diagnosis is in doubt. The findings at angiography are characteristic.[17,18,29] A small vessel with an irregular lumen supplies a circumscribed highly vascular area in bone. An intense circumscribed blush appears early in the arterial phase and persists into the late venous phase (Figs. 71-7 and 71-8). This pattern easily allows for differentiation from osteomyelitis, Brodie abscess, and stress fractures, which lack the intense vascular blush seen in osteoid osteoma.

Osteoblastomas

Benign osteoblastoma is a rare neoplasm of bone. The lesion is similar to osteoid osteoma in histologic appearance and in age incidence but differs in size, location, and roentgenographic appearance. The tumor principally affects the vertebrae and the bones of the limbs. It has an affinity for the vertebral arch, chiefly in the transverse and spinous processes, although the bodies may also be affected. In the tubular bones, the lesion is eccentrically located in the metaphysis or shaft.

The radiographic features are not distinctive, and lesions vary in size and density, ranging from 2 to 12 cm in size. The lesion is expansile and readily breaks the cortex. The soft tissue component may be surrounded by a thin calcific shell. There is usually no periosteal reaction.

The roentgenograms are often misleading, and angiography may be helpful. The angiographic pattern of osteoblastomas, however, has not been clearly defined. Yaghmai[30] reported the angiographic features of one lesion, stating that it contained mild hypervascularity. On the other hand, osteoblastomas may be extremely vascular and exhibit an intense tumor stain (Fig. 71-9). This is not surprising because of the lesion's histologic similarity to osteoid osteoma.

Malignant Tumors

Osteosarcomas

Osteosarcoma is a malignant bone tumor characterized by the predominant production of osteoid matrix by tumor cells. Osteosarcomas have been subdivided, on the basis of histologic pattern, into many types: sclerosing, osteolytic, medullary, and telangiectatic.

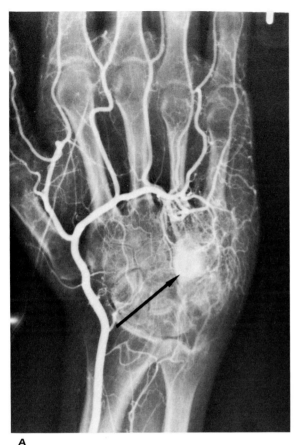

A

B

Figure 71-7. Osteoid osteoma of the hamate in a 29-year-old man complaining of increasing pain, swelling, and limitation of motion of the left wrist of 18 months' duration. (A) The arterial phase shows an intense circumscribed vascular blush in the hamate (*arrow*). (B) The venous phase of the arteriogram (subtraction film) shows the persistence of the blush (*arrow*). (From O'Hara JP III, Tegtmeyer C, Sweet DE, et al. Angiography in the diagnosis of osteoid-osteoma of the hand. J Bone Joint Surg (Am) 1975;57:163. Used with permission.)

However, this classification is of little prognostic significance. Osteosarcoma is the most common primary tumor of bone, multiple myeloma excluded. The lesion usually occurs in the second decade of life. It is more often found in men than in women, with a ratio of 2:1. Osteosarcomas occurring in older age groups are usually associated with a preexisting bone disorder such as Paget disease, postirradiated bone, or osteochondromas.

The metaphyseal area of long bones is by far the most common site of origin of osteosarcoma. It occurs most often in the lower end of the femur, upper end of the tibia or femur, and upper humerus.

The radiographic picture of osteosarcoma is usually a combination of bone destruction (lysis), bone formation (increased density), and periosteal reaction (periosteal new bone formation). Osteosarcomas produce a Codman triangle due to subperiosteal bone formation that is simulated by the advancing tumor. The tumor may present a roentgenographic picture ranging from very dense to (rarely) a purely osteolytic lesion.

When present, a coexisting soft tissue mass is an important sign of malignancy. MRI is a sensitive method for evaluating this involvement and for demonstrating the extension into adjacent tissues, which is important for local staging of the lesion.

Although the varied tissue components of osteosarcomas create a spectrum of vascular architecture, osteosarcomas are usually hypervascular.[31] The vessels supplying the tumor may be enlarged. Neovascularity and hypervascularity are invariably present (Fig. 71-10).[30] Subtraction films are helpful in evaluating the vascular pattern in sclerotic osteosarcomas (Fig. 71-11). A tumor stain is usually present (Fig. 71-12). Encasement of the vessels is often seen (see Fig. 71-10). A vascular sunburst pattern with small vessels running perpendicular to the shaft of the bone may be seen in some cases.[32]

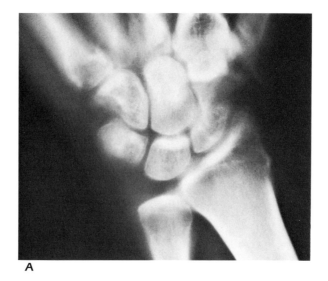

A

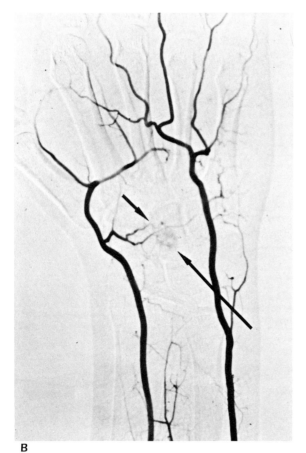

B

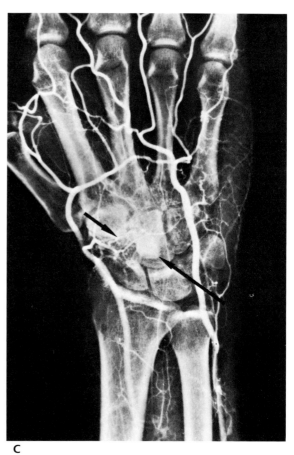

C

Figure 71-8. Osteoid osteoma of the capitate bone in a 28-year-old man suffering from pain in the right wrist for the previous 2 years. (A) A magnified tomogram of the wrist demonstrates sclerosis of the distal part of the wrist with a suggestion of a lucent area abutting the area of sclerosis. (B) A subtraction roentgenogram of the early arterial phase demonstrates a small irregular vessel (*short arrow*) supplying a vascular lesion in the capitate (*long arrow*). (C) The angiogram in the later arterial phase again shows the irregular vessel (*short arrow*). The intense persistent blush of the lesion is clearly seen (*long arrow*). (From O'Hara JP III, Tegtmeyer C, Sweet DE, et al. Angiography in the diagnosis of osteoid-osteoma of the hand. J Bone Joint Surg (Am) 1975;57:163. Used with permission.)

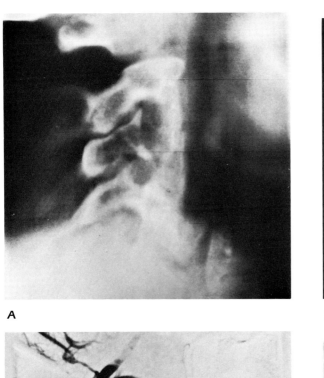

A

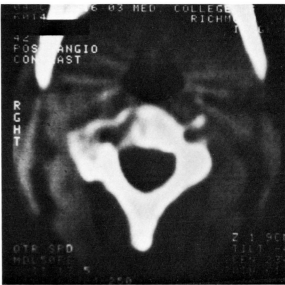

B

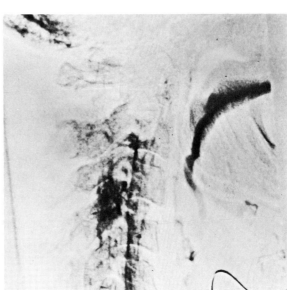

C

D

Figure 71-9. Osteoblastoma of the cervical spine in a 42-year-old woman who complained of right arm pain. (A) A tomogram of the cervical spine demonstrates an expansile lytic lesion involving the posterior elements of the third cervical vertebra. (B) A CT scan shows the expansion and thin-ning of the lateral mass and pedicle of the third cervical vertebra. (C) The vertebral angiogram reveals a highly vascular lesion supplied by tortuous vessels. (D) A persistent intense tumor blush is present. (Courtesy of Frederick S. Vines, M.D.)

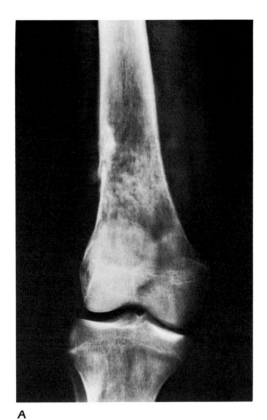

A

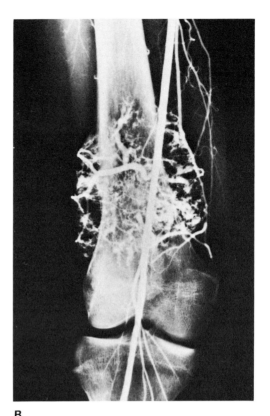

B

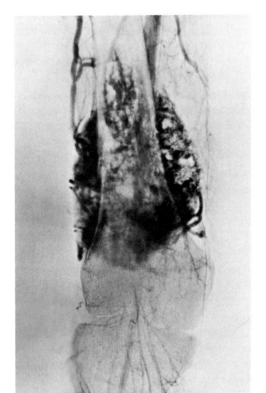

C

Figure 71-10. Osteosarcoma of the distal femur in a 15-year-old girl. (A) A destructive mixed lesion is seen in the distal femur. Soft tissue calcification is present on the lateral side of the femur. (B) The arteriogram exhibits considerable neovascularity, and encasement of some vessels is seen. (C) An intense tumor blush is present, and abnormal veins demonstrate the extension of the tumor into the soft tissue on both the medial and lateral aspects of the bone.

Early-draining veins are present in most of the tumors. The veins are usually dilated and often displaced by the tumor (see Fig. 71-10). The tumor may invade the veins, causing obstruction of the venous flow.

Most, if not all, osteosarcomas penetrate the cortex and invade the surrounding soft tissues before they are discovered.[5,19] This greatly aids in the angiographic diagnosis of malignancy because the abnormal vascularity in the surrounding soft tissue is readily visualized even when the plain film findings are subtle or nonexistent (Fig. 71-13).

Angiography is extremely helpful in osteosarcomas. It demonstrates that the tumor is malignant, delineates the best site for biopsy, and accurately depicts the degree of soft tissue extension. However, skip areas within the medullary canal are not always detected.[11] Computed tomography may prove to be helpful in detecting these skip metastases, but experience is limited.[33]

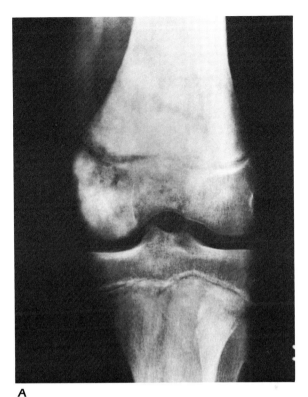

A

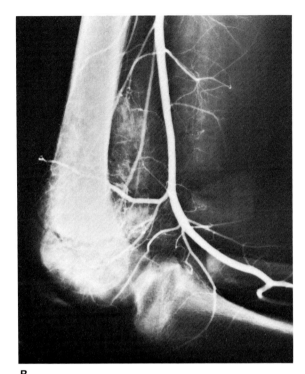

B

Figure 71-11. Osteosarcoma of the distal femur in a 13-year-old boy with intermittent leg pain of several years' duration. (A) A sclerotic lesion is noted in the metaphysis, and it appears to have crossed the epiphyseal plate—an unusual situation. (B) The arteriogram demonstrates the lesion in the distal femur and surrounding soft tissue. (C) The subtraction film enhances the visualization of the vessels, clearly showing the involvement of the epiphysis and the soft tissue extension.

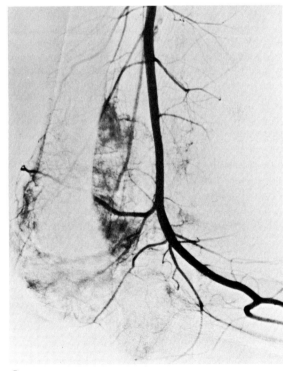

C

Bone Tumors of Marrow Origin

Plasma Cell Myelomas

Plasma cell (multiple) myeloma is a primary malignant tumor of bone characterized by a neoplastic proliferation of plasma cells of the bone marrow. It is the most common primary malignant bone tumor. Although the age range is from 25 to over 80 years, 75 percent of the patients are between the ages of 50 and 70 years. The most frequently involved bones are the vertebra, rib, skull, pelvis, and femur.

Radiographically, multiple myeloma is usually a destructive lesion, although it may uncommonly be partly or dominantly sclerotic. The hallmark of the disease is the sharply circumscribed "punched-out" lesion. The lesions are usually multiple, and in such cases the diagnosis is obvious.

Unlike with metastatic disease, there is little or no

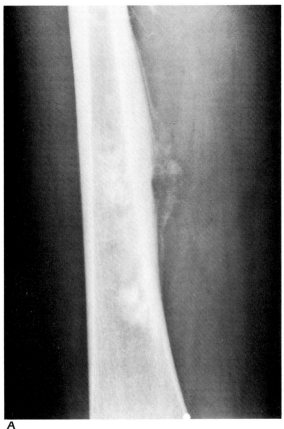

A

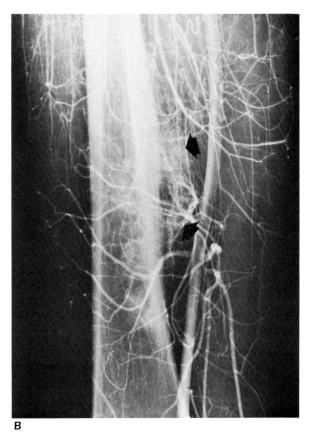

B

Figure 71-12. Osteosarcoma involving the diaphysis of the femur in a 14-year-old girl with a 1-month history of thigh pain. (A) A sclerotic lesion is present in the femur, and a small amount of periosteal new bone formation is seen form-

ing a Codman triangle. (B) The magnification film shows the tumor blush more marked in the area of the periosteal new bone formation (*arrows*). This is the most active area of the tumor and the best site for biopsy.

osteoblastic activity, so that radionuclide scanning is frequently not helpful. MRI is the most sensitive study to identify neoplastic involvement of bone marrow.[34,35] Findings include a nonspecific pattern of decreased signal on T1-weighted images and bright signal intensity on T2-weighted images.[35-37] Although MRI is sensitive in detecting involved bone, confirmatory tests such as immune and serum electrophoresis and ultimately bone biopsy are required for a specific diagnosis. Uncommonly, the disease may appear as a solitary focus. In this situation angiography may be helpful.

The angiographic findings in myeloma have been described by Laurin et al.[38] In their review of 10 cases, 9 were found to be solitary on admission, and all of the lesions exhibited various degrees of hypervascularity. The arteries were slightly enlarged in most cases. Neovascularity was present in 9 of the 10; in the other case, the arterial detail was obscured by an intense vascular blush. A diffuse tumor blush was present in all instances, and subtraction films were of help in dem-

onstrating the blush. Early venous filling was observed in 9 cases. Soft tissue extension of the tumor, which was present in all cases, helped differentiate the lesions from benign hypervascular lesions. In addition to the 10 hypervascular cases just cited, an isolated instance of hypovascular multiple myeloma has been described.[5]

Ewing Sarcomas

Ewing sarcoma is an uncommon primary malignant tumor of the bone that apparently arises from immature reticulum cells of the bone marrow. It is the fourth most prevalent primary malignant bone tumor. Ewing sarcoma is mainly a tumor of youth and adolescence, usually occurring between the ages of 5 and 30 years. It is more frequent in men than in women, with a ratio of 2:1.

Ewing sarcoma has occurred in almost all the bones of the body. The tubular bones are most likely to be

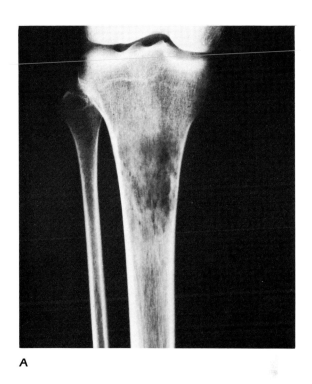

A

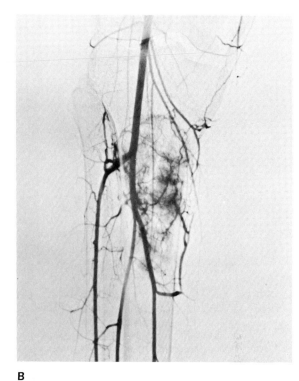

B

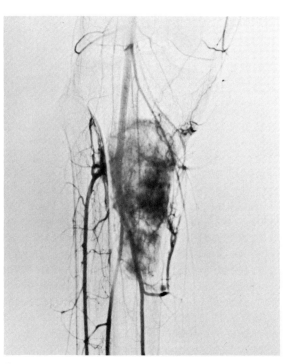

C

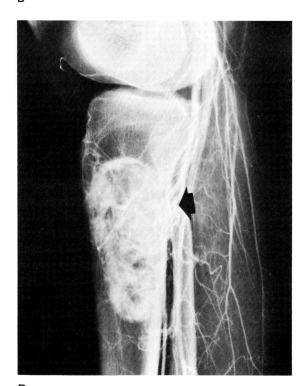

D

Figure 71-13. Osteosarcoma of the proximal tibia in a 27-year-old woman complaining of leg pain of 4 weeks' duration. (A) A radiolucent destructive lesion with a permeative pattern is present in the proximal tibia. (B) The arterial phase reveals some neovascularity. (C) An intense tumor stain is present. (D) The lateral film clearly shows extension of the lesion outside the bone (*arrow*) although this was not apparent on the plain films. The biopsy was interpreted as indicating a giant-cell tumor. However, because of the arteriogram, the tissue was reviewed by a consultant, who considered the tumor to be an osteosarcoma.

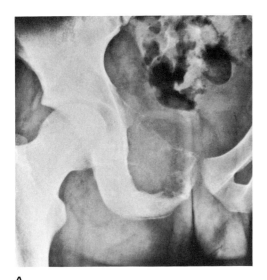

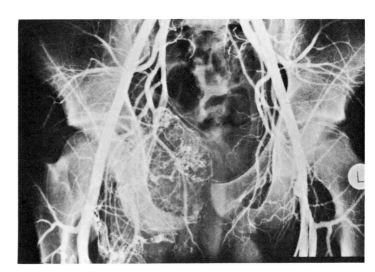

A   **B**

Figure 71-14. Ewing sarcoma of the pubic bone in a 16-year-old boy with a 1-month history of a lump in his groin. (A) The plain radiograph of the pelvis revealed a large lytic lesion destroying the right pubic bone. (B) The pelvic arteriogram demonstrates a large hypervascular tumor extending into the soft tissues. (C) Arteriography, with magnification, exhibits florid neovascularity, displacement of the surrounding vessels, and arteriovenous shunting. Extension of the tumor into the veins is seen (*arrow*).

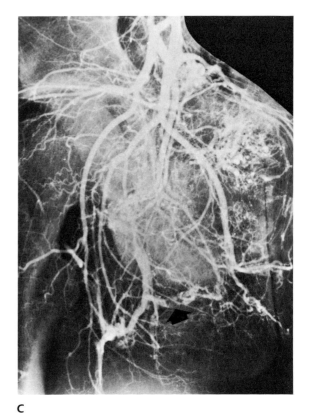

C

involved in younger patients, but in patients over the age of 20 the flat bones are the most frequent sites. Although the tumor classically involves the diaphyses, it may affect the metaphyses or epiphyses.

The radiographic picture is that of a rapidly growing tumor with destructive and reparative processes going on simultaneously. In the long bones, cortical destruction may be associated with "onionskin" lamination of the periosteum. In the flat bones, mottled destruction is associated with patchy sclerosis.

CT scanning defines the pattern of bone destruction and can identify soft tissue involvement. However, MRI clearly depicts the extent of the lesion. On T1-weighted images, Ewing sarcoma is of low signal intensity, contrasting with the high signal of uninvolved marrow. On T2-weighted images, the lesion is hyperintense to bone.[39] The cellular regions of the tumor enhance on T1-weighted images following the administration of gadolinium, separating the sarcoma from peritumoral edema.

The degree of vascularity, as depicted by angiography, varies in Ewing sarcomas, but most of these tumors have a sparse vascular bed.[5,16] A faint tumor stain is often visualized in the late capillary phase. Circumscribed avascular regions, representing areas of tumor necrosis, are likely to be present. Figure 71-14 demonstrates a Ewing sarcoma with unusually intense vascularity. Ewing sarcoma tends to penetrate the cortex, and a soft tissue component usually accompanies the tumor. The extension of the tumor is usually well delineated by arteriography (see Fig. 71-14). Neovascularity is often visible at the periphery of the tumor, and encasement of small vessels may be seen. Displacement of adjacent major vessels is often present.

Reticulum Cell Sarcomas

Reticulum cell sarcoma of bone is an isolated focus of this disease that apparently arises from the medullary cavity. The tumor has been reported in almost every bone in the body; however, it has a predilection for the long bones. It is a tumor of adults.

Radiographically, reticulum cell sarcoma appears as a destructive lesion, often with little periosteal response. The angiographic findings are similar to those of Ewing sarcoma.[5] In the early stages of the tumor, angiography may appear deceptively innocent.[8]

Bone Tumors of Uncertain Origin

Giant-Cell Tumors

Giant-cell tumor is an uncommon, aggressive tumor that develops within bone and apparently arises from the mesenchymal cells of the connective tissue framework. Microscopically, the lesion is composed of a moderately vascularized stoma, plump spindle- or ovoid-shaped cells, and regularly interspersed giant cells. Because these multinucleated giant cells are almost ubiquitous in bone lesions, many tumors must be differentiated from giant-cell tumors. Giant-cell tumors are rare before the age of 20 or after the age of 55, and are more common in females than in males. These tumors have a tendency to recur if they are not completely removed. The incidence of malignancy is estimated at about 20 percent. A review of reported giant-cell tumors, however, failed to reveal any known metastases at the time of original diagnosis.[19] Therefore, complete removal is essential.

Roentgenographically, the lesion appears as an osteolytic lesion, with an indistinct margin in the epiphyseal end of a long bone. The tumor begins as an eccentric lesion but may progress to involve the entire diameter of the bone. There is an absence of periosteal new bone formation and reactive bony sclerosis. The tumor invariably arises in the epiphysis and secondarily involves the metaphysis. The classic appearance is that of a radiolucent expansile lesion, and a light trabeculation is often present. CT and MRI are complementary to plain films. CT best evaluates the integrity of the cortical rim of bone around the lesion.[40,41] MRI helps define subchondral breakthrough and extension of the tumor into the joint.[42] Giant-cell tumors have a propensity for the distal femur, proximal tibia, and distal radius, but the lesion has been reported in almost all the tubular bones and many of the flat bones as well.

The angiographic appearance of giant-cell tumors has been described in several series.[5,43–46] The tumors are usually hypervascular (Fig. 71-15). The blood supply is derived primarily from the surrounding tissue, and the vessels are dilated. A prominent arterial network is present on the surface of the tumors, and these vessels often have a corkscrew appearance. Abundant neovascularity and an intense blush are present. Early venous filling takes place in about 20 percent of the tumors. Venous pooling may also be seen, as well as vessel encasement and occlusion. The synovial tissue in the vicinity of the tumor may look hyperemic at angiography, causing occasional confusion with extraosseous extension of the tumor.[47] Approximately 10 percent of the tumors are avascular or hypovascular.[5,46] The avascular lesions are often necrotic or hemorrhagic or have been previously treated.

Angiography has an important role in the preoperative evaluation of giant-cell tumors. It accurately depicts the intraosseous extent of the tumor and defines the extraosseous extent in 89 percent of patients.[46] This is of particular importance in view of the high recurrence rate of the tumor and its ability to become malignant after treatment.

Aneurysmal Bone Cysts

Aneurysmal bone cyst is an uncommon benign lesion of bone consisting of blood-filled spaces and solid areas containing spindled stroma, osteoid, and multinucleated giant cells. The lesions are most frequent in the second and third decades, although 78 percent of the patients are less than 20 years old. The lesion is more prevalent in women than men. It may involve almost any bone but has a predilection for the long bones, particularly the femur, and the spine. The majority of aneurysmal bone cysts in the long bones are located in the metaphysis, but they may extend into the epiphysis.

The classic appearance is that of an osteolytic, eccentric, expansile lesion that causes marked ballooning of a paper-thin cortex. Fine trabeculation is present within the lesion.

CT scanning can demonstrate fluid-fluid levels in some aneurysmal bone cysts.[48] However, this finding is not specific to aneurysmal bone cysts and can be seen in other benign and malignant lesions as well.[49] MRI findings are also nonspecific, giving variable signal characteristics of the fluid-fluid levels.[50,51]

The angiographic findings in aneurysmal bone cysts have been described in several reports.[5,45,52–54] These cysts are generally less vascular than giant-cell tumors. Although the arteries supplying them may be somewhat increased in size, the arterial network seen on their periphery is not as prominent as in the giant-cell tumor. A peripheral blush of contrast material may be

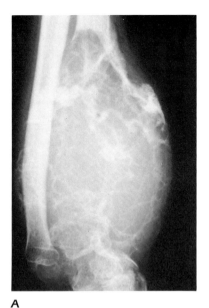
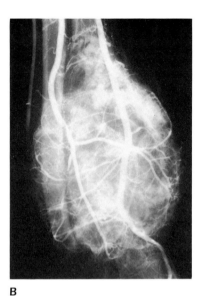
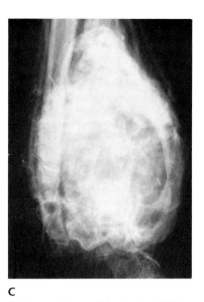

A   B   C

Figure 71-15. Giant-cell tumor in a 29-year-old man complaining of pain and swelling of 5 years' duration. (A) The plain film reveals a large, expansile, multiloculated bone lesion. (B) The arteries supplying the tumor are increased in size and draped around the periphery of the lesion. (C) An intense nonhomogeneous blush is present within the tumor. (From Yaghmai I. Angiography of bone and soft tissue lesions. New York: Springer, 1979. Used with permission.)

present, and often areas of contrast blush are interspersed with areas of no vascularity.

Some aneurysmal bone cysts are highly vascular, and differentiating them from giant-cell tumors is impossible.[5,45,54,55] However, a poorly vascularized tumor devoid of arteriovenous fistulas and soft tissue invasion is probably an aneurysmal bone cyst.

Bone and Soft Tissue Tumors of Fibrous Tissue Origin

Tumors of fibrous tissue origin may originate in either soft tissue or bone, and may spread to involve the adjacent structures. For this reason, they are discussed together. Fibrous histiocytomas are also included here because of their microscopic and radiographic similarity to fibrous tissue tumors.

Benign Tumors

Nonossifying Fibromas

Nonossifying fibroma is a benign bone lesion derived from fibrous tissue that usually occurs between the ages of 8 and 20. It is commonly located in the shaft of a long bone.

Radiographically, the lesion presents as an ovoid radiolucent defect with scalloped, sclerotic edges. A nonossifying fibroma generally has a typical plain film appearance, and CT, MRI, and angiography are very seldom indicated. The interosseous forms of fibroma have a benign angiographic appearance.[45,56,57]

Soft tissue fibromas have a slight hypervascularity, but the vessels look normal.[57]

Desmoid Tumors

The desmoid tumor is a benign fibrous tumor that usually arises in the soft tissue. On rare occasions, it may arise as a primary bone tumor. Although the tumor is benign, it is locally invasive. CT and MRI can define the integrity of the cortex, the amount of containment by periosteum, and the extent of soft tissue invasion.[58,59]

Angiographically, no abnormal vessels are seen; however, the tumor may displace the adjacent vessels. The vascularity is usually normal,[57] but a faint blush may occasionally be present (Fig. 71-16).

Malignant Tumors

Fibrosarcomas

Fibrosarcomas are malignant tumors arising from the fibrous elements either in the medullary cavity of bone or in the soft tissue. They are relatively rare bone tumors that have a predilection for the long bones, particularly about the knee. Fibrosarcoma of the bone occurs at any age but is most common in the second,

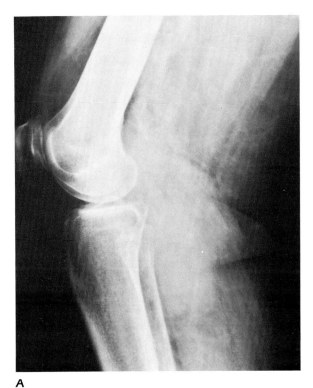

A

Figure 71-16. Desmoid tumor of upper calf in a 51-year-old woman. (A) The plain film demonstrates a soft tissue mass in the upper calf. The bones have a normal appearance.

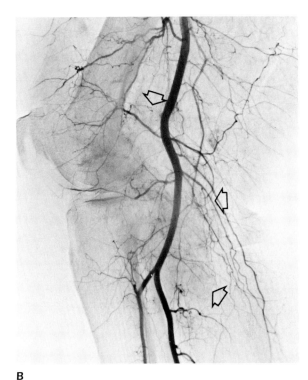

B

(B) The arteriogram shows displacement of the popliteal artery by the tumor (*arrows*). A faint blush is present, but there are no abnormal vessels.

third, and fourth decades. When it arises in preexisting lesions, such as Paget disease, it occurs in older patients. Soft tissue fibrosarcomas usually occur in children or young adults.

Roentgenographically, the tumor most often originates eccentrically in the metaphysis of a long bone; less commonly it may arise in a periosteal location. It appears as a destructive lesion, and it is not unusual for the tumor to erode through the cortex into the soft tissue. A bone sequestrum may be present. The margin of the lesion is poorly defined, and reactive bone formation is sparse.

MRI is helpful in defining the intraosseous and extraosseous extent of the tumor and its anatomic relationship to nearby structures. Although signal intensity is typically described as low on T1-weighted images and high signal on T2-weighted images, atypical signal characteristics are found with varying degrees of fibrous tissue and cellularity within the tumor.[60–63]

Fibrosarcomas of bone and soft tissue origin exhibit varying degrees of vascularity. Some have a highly vascular appearance (Fig. 71-17), and others are poorly supplied with vessels. However, fibrosarcomas usually have increased vascularity when compared to the surrounding tissue.[57,64] The degree of hypervasculariza-

tion and the degree of malignancy in fibrosarcomas show good correlation; a highly malignant tumor is usually richly supplied by vessels.[57,64,65] Furthermore, in fibrosarcomas of nonhomogeneous vascularity, the areas of the tumor showing the greatest vascularity are the most malignant.[64] Displacement of the major arteries and veins is a frequent finding. Encroachment and invasion of the major vessels are seen more often in fibrosarcomas than in other malignant tumors of bone. Yaghmai[57] studied 35 malignant fibrosarcomas by angiography and demonstrated neovascularity in every instance. Osseous fibrosarcoma often breaches the cortex to invade the soft tissue (Fig. 71-18).

Fibrosarcomas reveal considerable variability in their angiographic appearance, and slow-growing fibrosarcomas may look deceptively innocent, especially in the early stage.[8,9]

Malignant Fibrous Histiocytomas

Malignant fibrous histiocytoma is a malignant tumor of probable histiocytic origin.[66,67] It may arise either as a primary lesion in the bone or as a lesion in the soft tissue. A host of labels has been applied to the tumors, depending on their location and predominance of fibrous, histiocytic, or xanthomatous elements. The

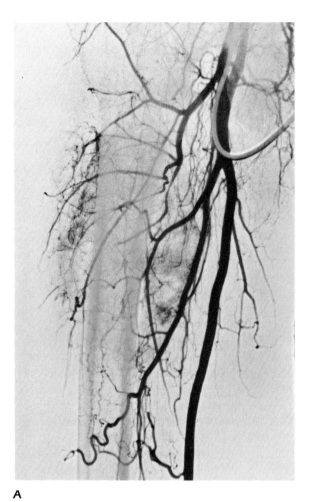

A

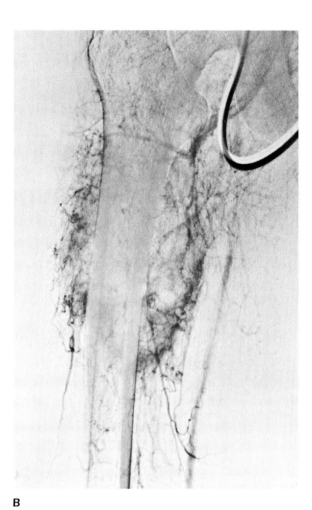

B

Figure 71-17. Fibrosarcoma of the thigh in a 63-year-old man. (A) The early arterial phase reveals a large hypervascular mass in the soft tissue of the right thigh. (B) The late arterial phase exhibits florid neovascularity, early venous drainage, and an avascular center in the lower portion of the tumor.

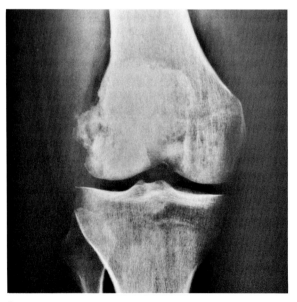

A

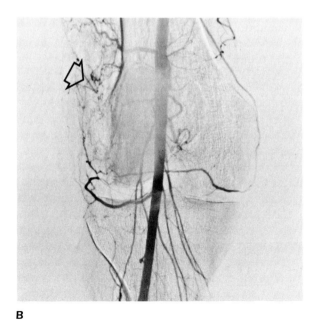

B

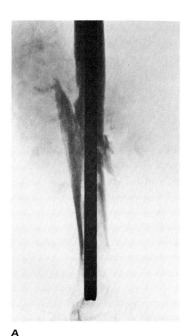

A

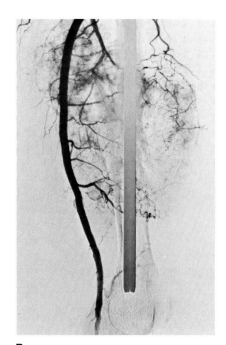

B

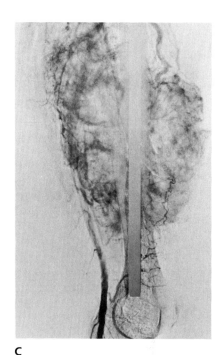

C

Figure 71-19. Malignant fibrous histiocytoma of the femur in a 69-year-old man. The patient sustained a fracture of his femur when he was kicked by a cow, and an intramedullary rod was inserted. Three weeks later he developed pain in his thigh. Lung metastases were present 6 months later. (A) An intramedullary rod is seen in place through a fracture in the femur. A large soft tissue mass is apparent. (B) The superficial femoral artery is displaced by a hypervascular mass containing fine neovascularity. (C) A diffuse blush is seen, arteriovenous shunts are present, and large veins drain the tumor.

tumors may occur at any age, but the typical age is 55 years.

Soft tissue tumors are found most often in the extremities and the chest wall. Radiographically, the soft tissue masses are usually well defined and lack distinguishing features. The roentgenographic appearance, when the bone is involved, is that of a malignant process. The osseous lesions are frequently purely osteolytic.

Marked destruction is seen in the form of motheaten and permeative patterns. An ill-defined margin is often present. Extension into the soft tissue and pathologic fractures are often seen. MRI features are not unlike those of fibrosarcoma, and MRI plays a similar role in defining tumor extent and anatomic relationships.

Malignant fibrous histiocytomas of the bone are usually hypervascular and exhibit a diffuse capillary blush (Fig. 71-19). Hudson et al.[68] found neovascularity in 6 of the 10 patients with primary bone ma-

lignant fibrous histiocytoma whom they studied angiographically. Laking of contrast material and arteriovenous shunts may also be present. Displacement of vessels is often found.

Soft tissue fibrous histiocytomas have a similar angiographic appearance. A circumscribed hypervascular mass is observed (Fig. 71-20). Neovascularity, early-draining veins, and displacement or encasement of vessels may also be present.[69]

Bone and Soft Tissue Lesions of Vascular Origin

Benign Lesions

Hemangiomas

There is confusion in the literature concerning the classification of hemangiomas, partly because of the problem of nomenclature. It is difficult to determine

◄ **Figure 71-18.** Fibrosarcoma of the distal femur in a 43-year-old man. The patient gave a 2½-year history of knee pain, beginning after minor trauma. He was originally treated for infection by his local physician. (A) An irregular destructive lesion is present in the distal femur, and the cortex is destroyed. (B) The small vessels are displaced (*arrow*), demonstrating the soft tissue extension of the tumor. A faint tumor blush is seen.

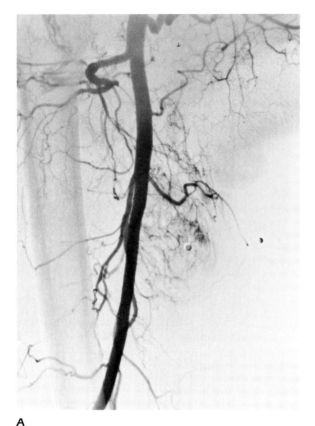

A

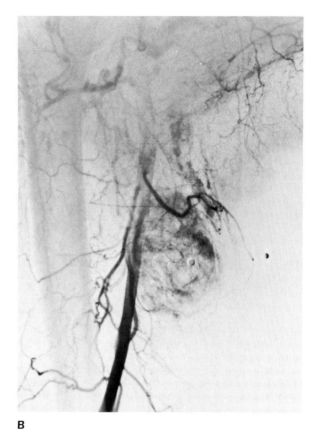

B

Figure 71-20. Recurrent malignant fibrous histiocytoma of the upper arm in a 60-year-old man. The original tumor had been excised 3 years previously. (A) A circumscribed hyper-vascular mass is demonstrated in the soft tissue of the upper arm. (B) An intense blush, fine neovascular vessels, and early-draining veins are present.

whether hemangiomas are true neoplasms or congenital malformations. They are not considered true neoplasms despite the fact that they infiltrate and have the potential to grow. They may be designated as congenital hamartomas, representing mesodermal rests of basal formative tissue. Hemangiomas may occur primarily in the bone or soft tissue. They all have abnormal arteriovenous communications.

Hemangiomas can be grouped into four categories: (1) capillary hemangiomas, (2) cavernous hemangiomas, (3) venous hemangiomas, and (4) arteriovenous malformations. Capillary hemangiomas are composed of capillary loops that tend to spread outward in a "sunburst" pattern. Cavernous hemangiomas are aggregations of larger thin-walled vessels and sinusoidal blood spaces. The shunts in these lesions are probably at the level of the arterioles and small veins. Both these lesions lack smooth muscle cells in the vessel walls. Venous hemangiomas have thickened walls containing muscle cells. The vascular malformation is another subcategory of hemangioma consisting of abnormal arteriovenous communications, resulting from a fail-

ure of differentiation of the common embryologic anlage into artery and vein.

Osseous hemangiomas are rather uncommon lesions. They are found in patients of all ages but are more prevalent in the fifth decade of life. Hemangiomas occur most frequently in the vertebrae, skull, and long bones, but they also occur in the jaws.

Radiographically, hemangioma of the spine is usually a single lesion, although two or more vertebral bodies may be involved. There is a slight loss of bone density of the vertebral body. The hallmark is a vertical-striped pattern, the "corduroy cloth" appearance. CT reveals the classic "polka dot" appearance that is pathognomonic for vertebral body hemangioma. MRI characteristics of classic asymptomatic vertebral body hemangioma have been described as increased signal on T1- and T2-weighted images.[70] Compression of the vertebra causes loss of the characteristic picture. Most hemangiomas of the spine are asymptomatic, but occasionally spinal cord compression is present.

Hemangiomas of the skull and flat bones usually exhibit a round area of rarefaction with central reticulations assuming a "honeycomb" appearance. The striations may be exaggerated or may extend at right angles from the bone, giving a sunburst pattern. In the extremities hemangiomas may appear as well-circumscribed lytic lesions with scattered trabeculae coursing through them. Sometimes the bony contour is expanded. If the trabecular pattern is not evident, identification of hemangiomas may be difficult and they may simulate malignancy.

Hemangiomas usually involve the soft tissues. These lesions are the most common tumors of skeletal muscles and are second only to lipomas as the most common soft tissue tumors of the extremities.[71] They are frequently associated with overlying skin abnormalities. On the plain radiographs, hemangiomas may demonstrate phleboliths, periosteal elevation, cortical thinning, osteoporosis, and bone loss due to lysis or erosion. Enlargement of the adjacent bone may also be present.

MRI can be helpful in determining the extent of the soft tissue and intramuscular involvement. Signal characteristics of soft tissue hemangiomas have been extensively described.[72,73]

The angiographic appearance of hemangiomas has been described in several series.[5,71,74-76] A continuum of angiographic patterns exists. The hemangioma may be very vascular with coarse, irregular, enlarged arteries and pooling of contrast material, and arteriovenous shunting may be found (Fig. 71-21). In the osseous form, dilated vascular spaces may be encountered, or

the lesion may exhibit only a heavy, even tumor stain (Fig. 71-22). Many hemangiomas show fine-caliber arteries with smooth walls and orderly distribution with some staining in the area. Pooling of contrast may be seen (Fig. 71-23) but is not necessarily present. Arteriovenous malformations may be localized (Fig. 71-24)[77] or diffuse (Fig. 71-25). The feeding arteries are enlarged and moderately tortuous. The smaller vessels are numerous and markedly tortuous. There is a rapid circulation, with essentially simultaneous visualization of the arteries and veins. In large lesions, the shunts may not be seen in all parts of the limb. A striking feature is the considerable dilatation of the veins.

Venous malformations are only occasionally visualized at arteriography. Venography demonstrates multiple large saccular or varicose veins.

Arteriography is helpful as a preoperative diagnostic examination because it defines the source of the vascular supply to the hemangioma and delineates the extent of the lesion better than clinical examination. However, it is difficult to ascertain whether the entire lesion has been shown by angiography.[74] MRI is useful in depicting the full extent of the lesion, including the relationship of the lesion to surrounding muscle and associated structures. The formation is useful because defining the extent of the lesion is a particularly vexing problem at surgery. Angiography can also detect local recurrences (see Fig. 71-21), and it distinguishes arteriovenous malformations from other types of hemangiomas. However, benign hemangiomas occasionally

Figure 71-21. Recurrent hemangioma in the heel of a 26-year-old woman. Early (A) and late (B) arterial phases show numerous enlarged tortuous vessels with early visualization of the veins.

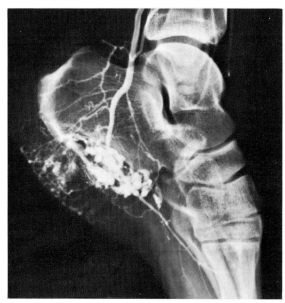

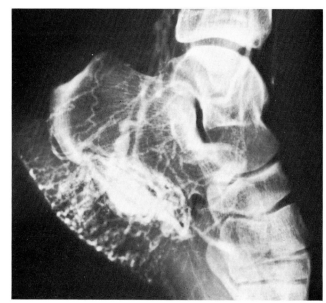

A

B

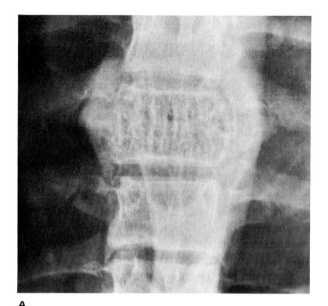

A

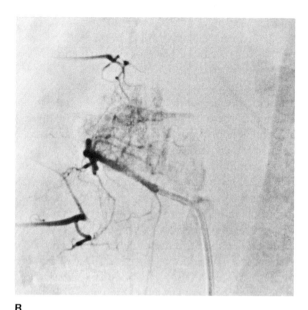

B

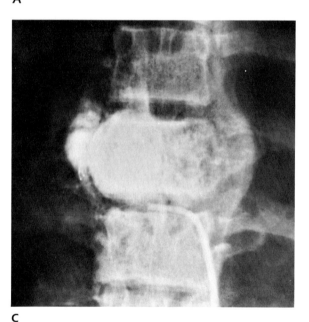

C

Figure 71-22. Hemangioma of a dorsal vertebra in an asymptomatic 14-year-old girl. (A) The typical striated appearance of a vertebral body hemangioma is present. Note the accompanying paravertebral mass. (B) A selective injection of an intercostal artery reveals early opacification of the vertebral body. (C) The late phase shows a diffuse blush of contrast material in the vertebral body and adjacent soft tissue. Injection of the opposite intercostal artery revealed a similar opacification of the other half of the vertebral body and adjacent paravertebral mass.

exhibit the angiographic characteristics of malignant vascular tumors.[75] In this situation, a specific diagnosis of a benign hemangioma can be made only if the hypervascular tumor was noted in early life and if it is associated with skin abnormalities.

Hemangiopericytomas

Hemangiopericytoma is a rare vascular tumor originating from Zimmermann pericytes, which are found surrounding the capillaries. The tumor is usually encapsulated and is believed to be benign. However, it is difficult to predict the biologic behavior of the tumor from the histologic appearance. Microscopically, ma-

lignant tumors cannot be separated from benign tumors.

Since the only prerequisite for the tumor is the presence of capillaries, it occurs in the soft tissues and very rarely in bone. The lesions occur at any age but are most common in the fifth decade of life.

Radiographically, hemangiopericytoma presents as a homogeneous mass. It is often well demarcated. Calcification is occasionally noted in the mass and may take the form of spicules or whorls. There may be local erosion of the bone caused by pressure.

Primary hemangiopericytoma of bone is rare. When present, it arises in the medullary canal, causing expansion and associated destruction. CT and MRI have failed to distinguish benign from malignant lesions.[78] Hemangiopericytoma is a hypervascular tumor.[79–82] There may be displacement of the major arteries by the mass. The arteries feeding the tumor may form a pedicle[82] and then branch and encircle the tumor. Numerous tortuous vessels are present in the tumor. A very dense, prolonged, uniform tumor stain or blush is characteristic (Fig. 71-26).

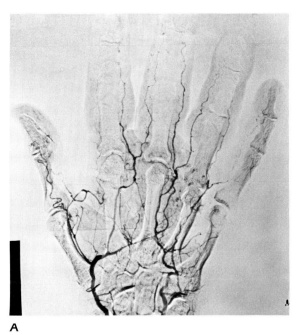

A

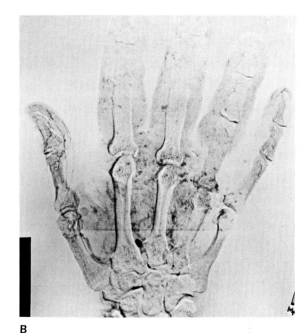

B

Figure 71-23. Hemangioma of the hand in a 53-year-old man. The patient's hand had had a lifelong bluish discoloration, but the hand had become more swollen and numb

in the past 5 months. (A) The arterial phase exhibits slight tortuosity of the arteries. (B) Small circular pools of contrast material are seen in the venous phase.

Figure 71-24. Arteriovenous malformation of the third metacarpal in a 19-year-old woman. (A) The plain film shows multiple "punched-out" radiolucent holes in the head of the metacarpal. (B) Multiple enlarged tortuous arter-

ies are seen, with dense opacification of the metacarpal head. Immediate opacification of the enlarged draining veins is seen. (Courtesy of Frank McCue, M.D.)

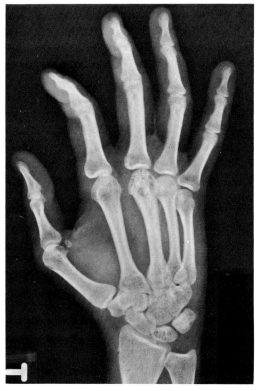

A

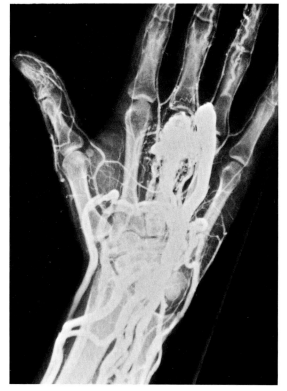

B

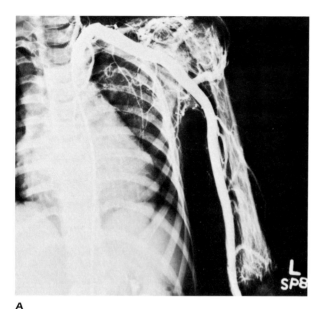

A

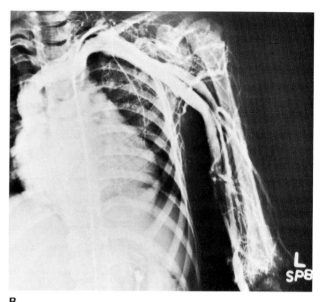

B

Figure 71-25. Diffuse arteriovenous malformation of the left arm in a 5½-year-old girl. The lesion had been present since birth, and three surgical procedures had been per-

formed on it. (A) Enormous arteries supply the diffuse lesion, which occupies the entire left arm. (B) Early venous drainage is demonstrated through greatly enlarged veins.

Figure 71-26. Hemangiopericytoma in a middle-aged man with a slowly enlarging mass in his left neck. A well-demarcated hypervascular lesion containing tortuous vessels is present. A homogeneous blush is seen throughout the tumor.

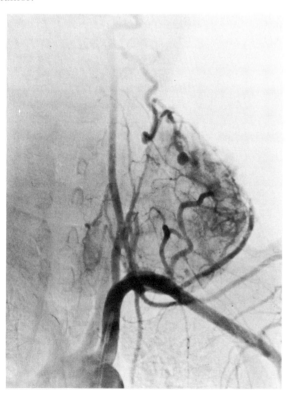

Malignant Lesions

Hemangioendotheliomas (Angiosarcomas)

Hemangioendotheliomas are rare vascular tumors that may occur in either soft tissue or bone but more often affect the soft tissue. There is no valid histologic criterion to differentiate hemangioendotheliomas from angiosarcomas, and they are considered the same tumor.[83,84] The tumors may occur at any age. In the soft tissue, they present as a mass. Any bone may be affected, but the femur, tibia, and vertebrae are most commonly involved. Any portion of the bone may be affected, and a third of the cases are multicentric.

Radiographically, the lesions are seen to produce osteolytic destructive zones with various amounts of marginal sclerosis and, in some cases, expansion of the cortex. Periosteal reaction is often lacking. Trabeculae may cause a "soap bubble" appearance in low-grade tumors. The more anaplastic lesions produce indistinct margins, and the trabeculae are absent. The CT and MRI appearances of these lesions are nonspecific.

The angiographic features of the tumor are highly irregular, tortuous arteries with pooling of contrast material.[5,75,85] Arteriovenous shunts and encasement of vessels are usually present. These changes are seen in both osseous and soft tissue tumors.

Metastatic Tumors in Bone and Soft Tissue

Metastatic cancer is the most prevalent malignant tumor of bone. The usual routes of spread are through the arterial and venous systems; lymphatic spread in bone is rare. All malignant tumors may metastasize to the bones, and any of the bones in the body may be involved. The sites of greatest predilection, however, are the vertebrae, pelvis, ribs, skull, sternum, and the upper ends of the femur and humerus. Roentgenographically, metastases to bone are divided into osteolytic, osteoblastic, and mixed varieties, depending on the dominant radiographic features of the lesion.

The common osteolytic metastases include neuroblastoma in the child, carcinoma of the lung in the adult male, and carcinoma of the breast in the adult female. Carcinoma of the thyroid and kidney are also common osteolytic lesions. Although mammary carcinoma usually produces lytic destructive lesions, it may produce mixed lesions or lesions that show bone production. Metastatic squamous cell carcinoma is usually osteolytic. Lytic metastases are often ill defined and poorly marginated. Periosteal reaction is rare.

The common osteoblastic metastases include carcinoma of the prostate and mucinous carcinomas. Carcinoma of the urinary bladder and carcinoid tumors also cause osteoblastic metastases. Radiographically, ill-

Figure 71-27. Metastatic renal cell carcinoma of the left shoulder in a 46-year-old man. The patient presented with left shoulder pain as the first clinical manifestation of his disease. (A) A lytic destructive lesion is evident in the glenoid. (B and C) Arteriography reveals a highly vascular lesion with an intense tumor blush. (D) A selective renal arteriogram demonstrates the primary renal cell carcinoma (*solid arrows*). A metastatic deposit is shown in the adrenal gland (*open arrow*).

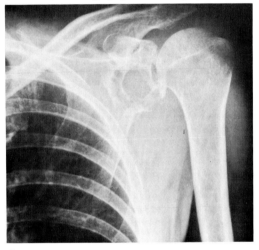

A

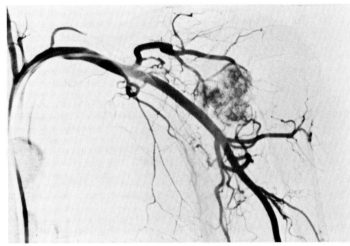

B

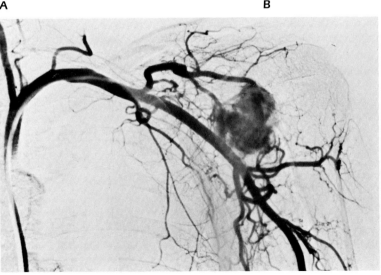

C

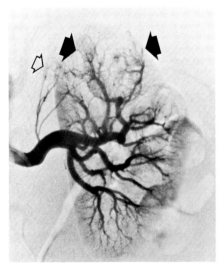

D

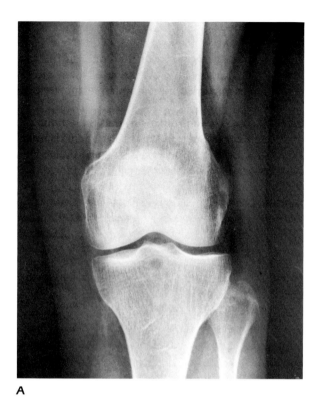
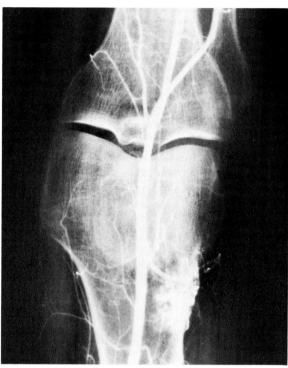

A   B

Figure 71-28. Metastatic renal cell carcinoma in the right femur of a 54-year-old woman. (A) The plain film of the right femur has a normal appearance. (B) A hypervascular lesion is shown in the metaphysis.

defined areas of radiodensity are seen. These may indicate loss of the bony architecture. Periosteal reaction may be present.

Metastases are particularly evident with MRI of the marrow cavity and later involve the cortical and trabecular bone. Focal lesions are typically low signal on T1-weighted images and high signal on T2-weighted images. Even though MRI is nonspecific, it is sensitive for determining the extent of disease and localizing individual lesions.

Most metastatic lesions have the same vascular characteristics that are exhibited by their primary tumor.[5,8] Yaghmai[5] states that in the early stages, when the cortex is intact, the lesion reveals practically no vascularity. It is important to remember, however, that 50 percent of the mineral content must disappear before the radiographic changes can be visualized (Fig. 71-27). Metastases may be manifest before, at the same time as, or after the primary tumor is discovered. The first clinical manifestation of cancers of the kidney (Fig. 71-28), lung, and pancreas is often at the site of metastasis. Marked hypervascularity is frequently seen in renal carcinomas (see Figs. 71-27 and 71-28) and thyroid carcinomas.[86] Bronchial carcinomas (Fig. 71-29), gastrointestinal carcinomas, and melanomas may also be very vascular. Angiography, however, cannot distinguish with certainty between the different types of metastases, nor can it distinguish a primary osseous or soft tissue tumor from a secondary growth.

Lesions of Synovial Origin

Benign Lesions

Pigmented Villonodular Synovitis

Pigmented villonodular synovitis is an uncommon lesion characterized by diffuse proliferation of the synovial lining and connective tissue strata of the synovium with numerous villous projections. The etiology is unknown; the lesion may be inflammatory or may be of histiocytic origin.[66] It may be present at any age but is most often found in young adults. The knee and hip are the most commonly involved joints, but other joints are also affected.

Radiographic manifestations of this condition are usually nonspecific, consisting of diffuse soft tissue swelling or a lobular soft tissue mass with occasional superficial erosion and cystic changes in the adjacent bones. Calcification is not present.

Hemosiderin deposition results in focal areas of marked signal loss on T2-weighted images when MRI

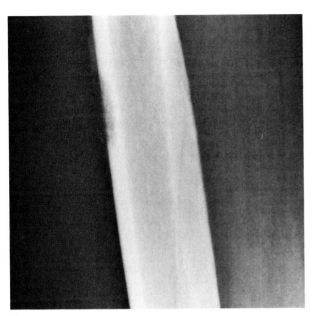

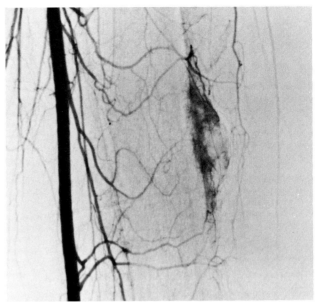

A

B

C

Figure 71-29. Metastatic bronchial carcinoma in a 53-year-old woman who complained of pain and swelling in the thigh. (A) A destructive lytic lesion is seen in the cortex of the femur. Periosteal reaction is present. (B and C) Arteriography demonstrates a hypervascular lesion that involves the cortex and extends into the soft tissue. Prominent veins are seen draining the lesion.

is performed. This finding combined with bony erosions seen on both sides of the joint and a joint effusion are characteristic of pigmented villonodular synovitis.[87-89]

The literature contains only a few reports describing the angiographic findings in villonodular synovitis.[5,24,86,90] The lesions are hypervascular, and the surrounding arteries and veins may be stretched around the mass. A diffuse blush may be seen in the synovium, and early opacification of the veins is sometimes present.

Malignant Lesions

Synovial Sarcomas

Synovial sarcoma is a rare malignant tumor that arises from the synovial membrane of joints. It may occur at any age but is most frequent between the ages of 20 and 40 years. It is more common in men than in women. The tumor is usually located near a joint, and the lower extremities, especially the knees, are most often involved. The tumor metastasizes to the lungs and also to the regional lymph nodes.

Radiographically, a soft tissue mass is present; it may be quite large, and lobulation of the mass may be seen. Amorphous calcification may be present in the mass. The adjacent bones may exhibit pressure erosion with sharp margins and reactive scleroses or direct invasion of the bone with destructive changes.

Angiographically, synovial sarcomas are seen to be hypervascular lesions.[86,90-92] Neovascularity may be present (Fig. 71-30). However, the lesions may contain multiple irregular vessels that cannot definitely be considered classic neovascularity.[91] A tumor blush or stain is observed, and early-draining veins may be seen but are not invariably present. Angiography demonstrates the malignant nature of the tumor. It is also

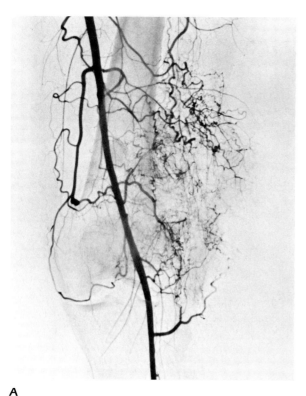

A

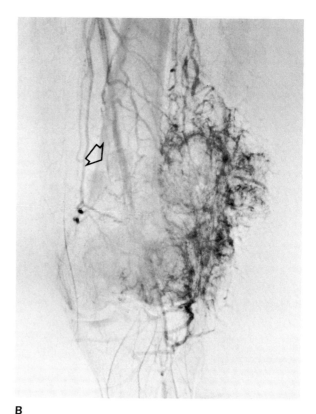

B

Figure 71-30. Synovial sarcoma of the knee in a 40-year-old woman who complained of swelling in the distal thigh of 4 months' duration. (A) A hypervascular lesion containing neovascularity is present in the distal thigh. (B) The late arterial phase reveals a diffuse nonhomogeneous blush. Early-draining veins are seen. Popliteal lymph nodes (*arrow*) are opacified by the contrast material.

accurate not only in delineating the gross extent of the soft tissue tumor but also in defining its exact anatomic orientation.[93] This can be of critical aid to the operating surgeon if radical resection is performed.[94]

Soft Tissue Tumors

Plain films may yield some information regarding the nature and extent of soft tissue tumors.[92] Irregular amorphous calcium suggests malignancy, and dense well-defined calcium suggests a benign process. Phleboliths indicate the presence of a hemangioma. Changes in the adjacent bones may provide clues. Bony overgrowth and deformity suggest a benign lesion, whereas periosteal new bone formation and bony destruction indicate a malignant process. If the interface of the tumor with the soft tissue is well defined, the lesion is probably benign. An indistinct margin is consistent with malignancy or inflammation. Tumors that may appear radiolucent include lipomas, hamartomas, and teratomas.

MRI has generally replaced CT scanning as the primary noninvasive method of evaluating soft tissue tumors, with the exception of lesions suspected of containing subtle calcification or ossification. In these cases, CT scanning can be more helpful. MRI provides useful information about the extent of tumor and the relationship of the lesion to nearby structures. It also provides information regarding characteristics of tissues within the lesion. However, MRI has not been successful in accurately determining benign from malignant lesions. In general, benign tumors are expected to be small, well circumscribed, and to have homogeneous signal characteristics. Malignant tumors tend to be large, inhomogeneous, and poorly marginated.[95] Therefore, local staging is the primary information obtained from MRI studies at this time.

The value of angiography in soft tissue tumors has been described in several series.[86,91,92,96–102] However, it is important to correlate the angiographic findings with the clinical findings and with the plain film appearance.

The angiographic pattern of benign soft tissue tu-

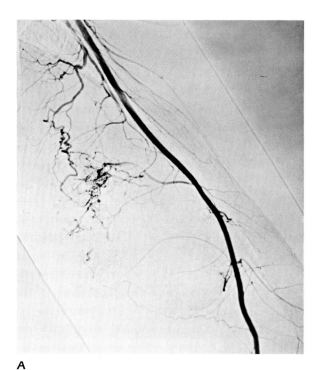

A

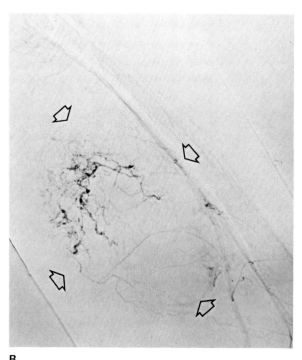

B

Figure 71-31. A malignant neurofibrosarcoma of the thigh in a 17-year-old girl. (A) A large oval mass displaces the superficial femoral artery and surrounding soft tissue vasculature. (B) The extent of the mass becomes more apparent in the later arterial phase (*arrows*). Extensive neovascularity is present in one area of the lesion. The remainder of the lesion is relatively avascular.

mors is usually one of avascularity and stretching or displacement of vessels around the tumor mass. Exceptions to this rule are lesions of vascular origin. Glomus tumors are highly vascular, are characterized by enlarged feeding vessels, and exhibit an intense blush. Early venous filling is often seen.[86] Hemangiomas have already been discussed.

Tumors of nerve origin are also an exception. Although benign nerve tissue tumors may be avascular, they may contain very tortuous vessels or neovascularity.[103] Angiography often cannot distinguish between a benign nerve sheath tumor and a malignant one (Fig. 71-31) with certainty, although the presence of vascular encasement usually indicates a malignant tumor.

Malignant tumors of the soft tissue are in most cases more abundantly vascularized than the adjacent soft tissues (Fig. 71-32). The highly malignant tumors show an intense vascularity. Neovascularity, pooling of contrast material, a tumor blush, encasement, and arteriovenous shunts may also be present. Tumors demonstrating neovascularity are frankly malignant or have a propensity to local recurrence and metastases even though they have the histologic picture of a benign lesion. Sharp delineation of the borders of the mass

favors the diagnosis of neoplasm. Hemangiomas and inflammatory lesions do not have sharp margins. Liposarcomas, myxofibrosarcomas, rhabdomyosarcomas, mesenchymal sarcomas, and malignant fibrous histiocytomas are usually highly vascular. Fibrosarcomas are often highly vascular, but a few are poorly supplied with vessels[104]; the highly vascular tumors are the most malignant.[57,64] Angiography does not distinguish one sarcoma from another. This is of little consequence, however, because, despite differences in histogenesis, analysis of the rates of local recurrence and metastasis of these sarcomas reveals that their rates are almost the same.[94] The exceptions are low-grade fibrosarcomas and grade I liposarcomas (Fig. 71-33). These tumors are poorly vascularized and are locally invasive but do not usually metastasize.

The angiogram provides a fairly clear impression of the size of the tumor and its relationship to the surrounding tissues.[86] It can also demonstrate unsuspected satellite lesions.[91] This helps the surgeon decide what type of surgery should be performed, whether amputation or radical excision.[94] If arteriography shows that a major vessel is displaced or that a nonexpendable bone is involved, amputation is preferable.[94]

Angiography can aid in the selection of a biopsy

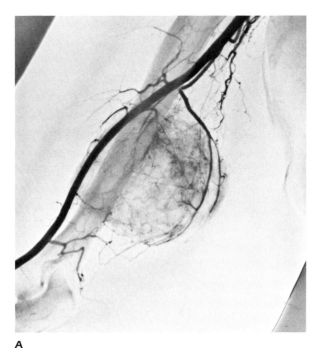

A

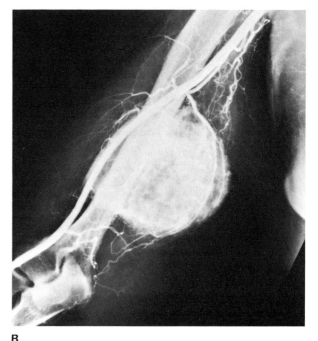

B

Figure 71-32. A pleomorphic high-grade sarcoma in the soft tissues of the upper arm of a 62-year-old woman. The mass had been present for 6 months. (A) A circumscribed

mass containing neovascularity displaces the brachial artery. (B) The late arterial phase reveals an intense homogeneous blush.

Figure 71-33. An atypical intramuscular lipoma, grade I liposarcoma, in the upper leg of a 58-year-old man. The tumor had been present for many years and was slowly enlarging. The plain film demonstrated a radiolucent mass in the thigh. The vessels are displaced by the mass (*arrows*), but no abnormal vascularity is evident.

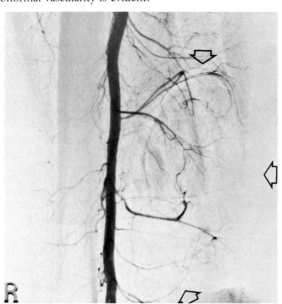

site, delineate the vascular supply of the lesion, and detect local recurrences.[91] Angiography is of most value when the surgeon and the angiographer confer during the procedure and when questions posed by the surgeon are answered during the angiographic procedure.

Myositis Ossificans

Myositis ossificans circumscripta is a reactive lesion occurring in the soft tissues, at times near bone and periosteum. The lesion is characterized by fibrous, osseous, and cartilaginous proliferation and metaplasia. A history of trauma can be obtained in most cases, but in a certain number of patients no antecedent injury can be elicited. Localized myositis ossificans occurs most often in children and young adults. The lesion has a predilection for areas prone to trauma. It arises in the large muscle groups, in and around the elbow, thigh, buttocks, shoulder, and calf.

Although there are many unanswered questions concerning its pathogenesis, the microscopic evolution of the lesion has been well documented.[105] It is important to understand the stages of myositis ossificans when interpreting the histology, plain films, and angiograms. Three stages of maturation are recognized. The developing lesion also demonstrates three zones of maturation, and if this is not recognized the lesion is easily mistaken for a malignancy. The maturation proceeds inward from the periphery, the central area being the last to ossify. CT can identify this zonal pattern of mineralization and aid in the early diagnosis of myositis ossificans when plain films are still nonspecific.[106]

The first stage is one of a rapidly developing soft tissue mass. There is usually no evidence of calcification. During this time of tissue necrosis and regeneration, angiography may show a hypervascular mass.[107]

The second or active stage begins in the second week and continues for 12 to 14 weeks. In the first 3 to 6 weeks, the microscopic zonal pattern of maturation that is characteristic of the entity develops. The plain films exhibit faint calcification, and periosteal reaction is present if the underlying bone is injured. At 6 to 8 weeks, the lacy pattern of new bone is sharply circumscribed about the periphery and may have an eggshell-like appearance. The angiographic features during the active stage are characterized by hypervascularity and a poorly defined stain in the mass.[86,108–110] The criteria for malignancy (neovascularity, pooling of contrast material, and arteriovenous shunting) are usually absent, allowing the diagnosis of a benign process to be established.[109,110] However, a disturbing hypervascular pattern with markedly irregular vessels may be seen during this stage.[92] It is important to review the

clinical history and the plain films before intepreting the angiograms.

The third stage is the healing stage, which usually begins at around 16 weeks and lasts 5 to 6 months. The lesion gradually shrinks in size and may persist as a hard mass or undergo almost total regression. Occasionally in this stage myositis ossificans will take on the appearance of an exostosis (Fig. 71-34). Angiographic findings in this stage are variable. The pattern is less vascular than in the active stage and may be normal (see Fig. 71-34).

Embolization of Bone and Soft Tissue Tumors

Transcatheter selective arterial embolization of bone and soft tissue tumors has been used in several clinical situations. It has served as an adjunct to surgery to control inoperative bleeding.[111] It has been used in hemangiomas either for palliation[112] or to decrease intraoperative blood loss[113,114] and lessen the chance of recurrence.[114] It has also been employed to relieve chronic pain in patients with pelvic tumors.[111,115]

In 1975 Feldman et al.[111] first succeeded in alleviating the pain of a patient with metastasis to the right ilium by embolizing the branches of the right internal

Figure 71-34. Posttraumatic exostosis, myositis ossificans, in a 27-year-old man who sustained an injury 8 months before these films were obtained. (A) A calcified mass is seen extending from the pubic bone (*arrows*). (B) The arteriogram exhibits a normal vascular pattern.

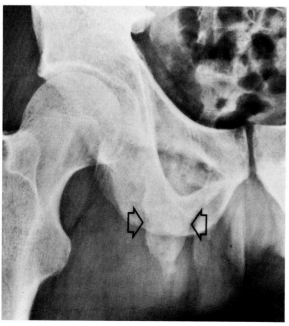

A

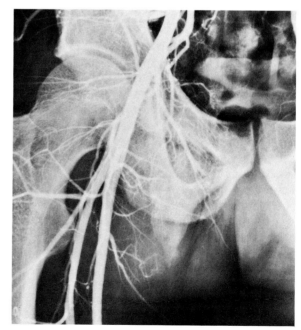

B

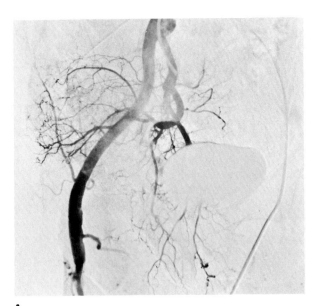

A

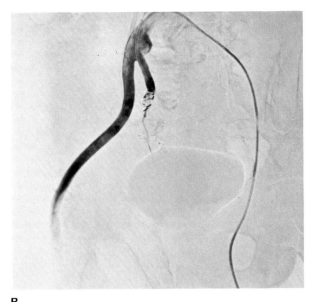

B

Figure 71-35. Recurrent chondrosarcoma of the pelvis in a 66-year-old man with persistent pain following irradiation. (A) A large hypervascular lesion is present in the iliac bone. The tumor extends into the soft tissue. (B) The right internal iliac artery is totally occluded after selective embolization with Gelfoam particles and the insertion of Gianturco coils. One week after the procedure the patient experienced a marked decrease in his pain.

iliac artery and the fourth lumbar artery. The relief of pain lasted until the patient's death 2½ months later. These authors also described the successful use of preoperative embolization with Gelfoam to decrease intraoperative blood loss in a man with large giant-cell tumors of both fibulas.

Wallace et al.[115] reported the use of therapeutic arterial occlusion of the internal iliac artery for symptomatic relief of pain. They were successful in eight of nine patients.

The embolization of pelvic tumors is performed by first obtaining selective arteriograms to accurately delineate the vascular supply to the lesion (Fig. 71-35). The vascular supply to these neoplasms is frequently through the internal iliac artery; additional blood supply may originate from the lower lumbar, the middle sacral, the circumflex iliac, and the external pudendal arteries. The major vessels of supply are embolized first with 2 × 3 mm particles, followed by Gianturco coils to occlude the vessels permanently (see Fig. 71-35). Subselective catheterization can be performed using a Tracker catheter for more localized lesions.

The patients will experience severe pain requiring

narcotics, beginning shortly after embolization and subsiding in 3 to 7 days. Temperature elevation ranging from 38.8 and 39.8°C will occur, subsiding in 72 to 96 hours. If a persistent sacral artery is present on the side to be embolized, the procedure is contraindicated because embolization of this artery may result in sacral nerve injury and footdrop.

Embolization with particles has been successfully employed in the treatment of hemangiomas. It has been used to control pain associated with a peripheral hemangioma[116] and to decrease the size of a hemangioma and control a persistent left-to-right shunt.[112] Voigt et al.[114] reported the use of Gelfoam embolization in 10 patients with deforming vascular malformations in the craniofacial area. The procedure allowed reconstructive surgery to be carried out with decreased blood loss, and good cosmetic results were obtained. No recurrences were seen, but the follow-up was short, only 6 to 9 months.

When tortuous vessels supplying an arteriovenous malformation are present or direct intravascular access is difficult (such as in some hemangiomas or previously treated lesions by surgery or embolization), direct

Figure 71-36. Palliative treatment of venous hemangioma in a 16-year-old male complaining of swelling and pain in the right forearm with exertion. (A) Venous phase of the upper extremity arteriogram demonstrates extensive venous hemangioma. (B) Direct injection of venous hemangioma.

(C) Three-month follow-up with MRI shows an extensive ▶ soft tissue and muscle hemangioma, although symptoms have diminished. (D) Follow-up venogram approximately 2½ years later demonstrates significant reduction in the hemangioma, although it is still present.

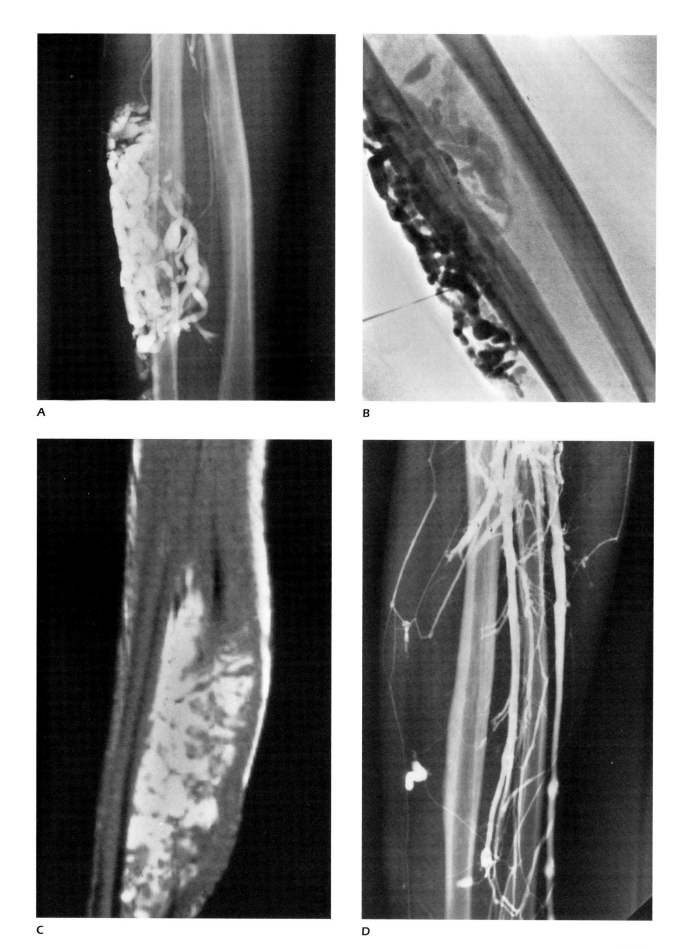

A

B

C

D

1815

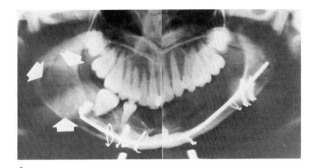

A

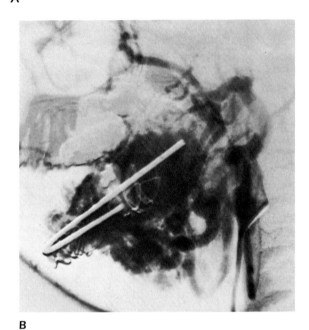

B

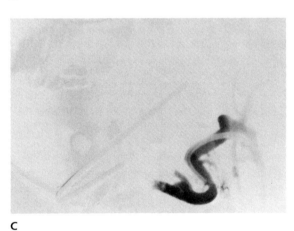

C

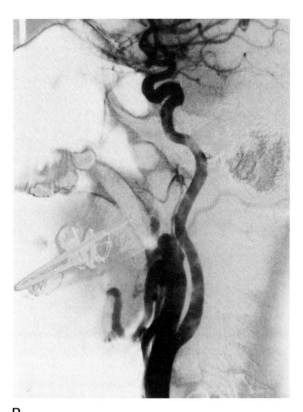

D

Figure 71-37. Recurrent hemangioma in a 12-year-old girl who presented with loosening of the teeth. (A) Panorex shows the sequelae of the previous resection of the left mandible at age 2. A large multilocular radiolucent defect is seen in the right mandible (*arrows*). (B) A selective right external carotid angiogram shows a large hypervascular hemangioma involving the soft tissue and bone of the right jaw. (C) A selective injection of the facial artery demonstrates complete occlusion of the artery following transcatheter embolization with Gelfoam. (D) A common carotid arteriogram shows absence of filling of the hemangioma after selective embolization of the feeding vessels. The patient did well for 6 months and then developed bleeding from the gums. The soft tissue hemangioma appeared well controlled; the hemangioma within the mandible was the source of the hemorrhage. (From Tegtmeyer CJ, Keats TE. The mouth, tongue, jaws and salivary glands. In: Teplick JG, Haskin ME, eds. Surgical radiology: a complement in radiology imaging to the Sabiston-Davis-Christopher Textbook of Radiology. Philadelphia: Saunders, 1981. Used with permission.)

puncture of the symptomatic lesion can be performed.[117]

A Chiba needle is inserted directly into the arteriovenous malformation or hemangioma. Contrast is then injected into the Chiba needle to confirm position within the targeted vessels. A proximal tourniquet can be applied to provide proximal stasis in the lesion. The arteriovenous malformation or hemangioma is embolized with a particulate agent or absolute alcohol.[118] Alcohol is then injected in 1- to 2-ml volumes until flow is occluded (Fig. 71-36).

The surgery for deforming hemangiomas of the craniofacial region is difficult, and recurrences are not uncommon. Embolization before surgery may be very helpful (Fig. 71-37). Gelfoam embolization usually

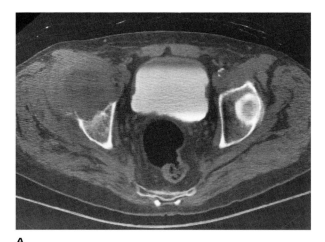

A

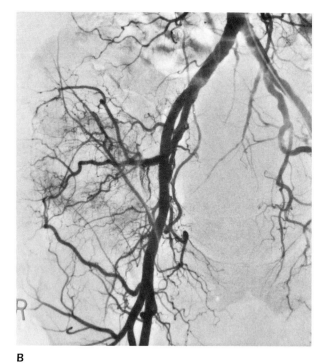

B

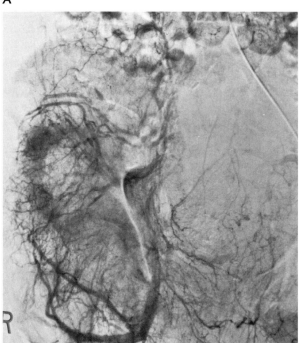

C

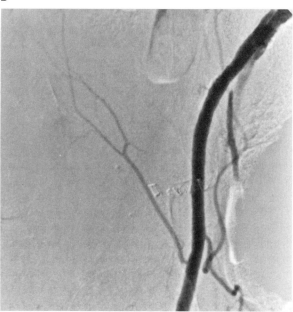

D

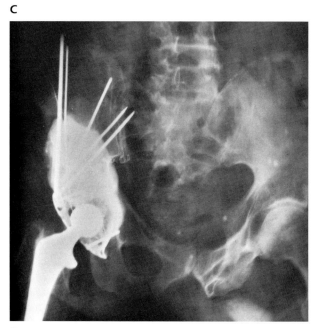

E

Figure 71-38. A 77-year-old man with metastatic lung cancer and metastases to the right ilium and femur. The patient was complaining of severe hip pain. (A) CT scan shows a large mass involving the right ilium. (B) Arterial phase of angiogram demonstrates extensive neovascularity in the right ilium. Florid vascularity of the tumor is noted. (C) Venous phase shows extent of tumor. (D) Postembolization arteriogram. (E) Follow-up study demonstrates reconstruction of the right hip. Despite the extensive vascular nature of this tumor, less than 300 ml of blood was lost at surgery. (Courtesy of Christopher Zielinski, M.D.)

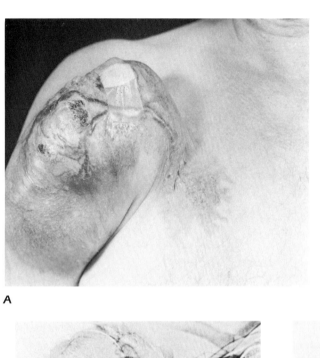

A

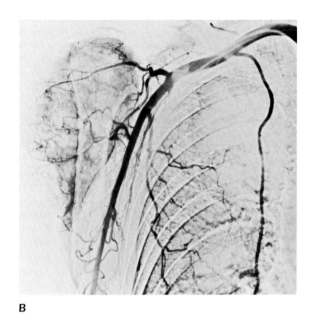

B

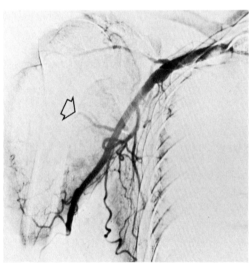

C

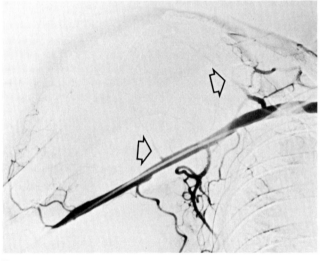

D

Figure 71-39. Recurrent liposarcoma in a 61-year-old man. (A) The huge tumor of the shoulder is seen with large vessels coursing across the surface of the lesions. (B) A hypervascular mass is present, which contained florid neovascularity and a tumor stain. (C) The embolization procedure was performed in stages. The circumflex humeral artery (*arrow*) was occluded with Gelfoam. (D) Two weeks later, the branch of the thoracicoacromial artery supplying the tumor was occluded (*upper arrow*). The occluded circumflex artery is again seen (*lower arrow*). After this occlusion the patient experienced intense pain. Surgery was subsequently performed with minimal blood loss.

provides only temporary relief, however, because of the breakdown of the Gelfoam and the formation of new collateral vessels. Therefore, if surgery is contemplated, it should take place shortly after embolization for optimum results.

Vascular metastases can also be treated with embolization preoperatively to help control intraoperative blood loss (Fig. 71-38).

The embolization of soft tissue tumors may result in severe, prolonged muscle pain if acute muscle ischemia takes place. The pain usually subsides in a week, without permanent sequelae, but its severity can be distressing for the patient and unnerving for the angiographer. Doppman and Di Chiro[119] reported two cases with this complication, and the authors have encountered it in one patient in whom a recurrent sarcoma of the shoulder was embolized (Fig. 71-39).

Cautious use of embolization seems indicated in certain situations: for palliation of pain in patients with inoperable tumors, preoperatively to decrease blood loss during resection, and in hemangiomas to decrease blood loss and help prevent recurrences. It may also be helpful in hemangiomas to relieve symptoms and decrease the size of the lesion when resection is not contemplated.

Acknowledgments

We want to extend our gratitude to Shirley Yowell, Sherry Deane, and Geelee Tegtmeyer for their help in preparing this chapter.

References

1. Doan CA. The circulation of the bone-marrow. Contrib Embryol 1992;14:27.
2. Drinker CK, Drinker KR, Lund CC. The circulation in the mammalian bone-marrow. Am J Physiol 1922;62:1.
3. Tilling G. The vascular anatomy of the long bones: a radiological and histological study. Acta Radiol Suppl (Stockh) 1958; 161:1.
4. Trueta J. The normal vascular anatomy of the human femoral head during growth. J Bone Joint Surg (Br) 1957;39:358.
5. Yaghmai I. Angiography of bone and soft tissue lesions. New York: Springer, 1979.
6. Hawkins IF Jr, Hudson T. Priscoline in bone and soft-tissue angiography. Radiology 1974;110:541.
7. Ekelund L, Laurin S, Lunderquist A. Comparison of a vasoconstrictor and vasodilator in pharmacoangiography of bone and soft-tissue tumors. Radiology 1977;122:95.
8. Strickland B. The value of arteriography in the diagnosis of bone tumours. Br J Radiol 1959;32:705.
9. Voegeli E, Uehlinger E. Arteriography in bone tumors. Skeletal Radiol 1976;1:3.
10. Viamonte M Jr, Roen S, LePage J. Nonspecificity of abnormal vascularity in the angiographic diagnosis of malignant neoplasms. Radiology 1973;106:59.
11. Hudson TM, Haas G, Enneking WF, et al. Angiography in the management of musculoskeletal tumors. Surg Gynecol Obstet 1975;141:11.
12. Steckel RJ. Usefulness of extremity arteriography in special situations. Radiology 1966;86:293.
13. Yaghmai I, Shamza AZ, Shariat S, et al. Value of arteriography in the diagnosis of benign and malignant bone lesions. Cancer 1971;27:1134.
14. Mitty HA, Hermann G, Abdelwahab IF. Role of angiography in limb-tumor surgery. RadioGraphics 1991;11:1029–1044.
15. Lagergren C, Lindbom A, Soderberg G. Hypervascularization in chronic inflammation demonstrated by angiography: angiographic, histopathologic, and microangiographic studies. Acta Radiol 1958;49:441.
16. Halpern M, Freiberger RH. Arteriography as a diagnostic procedure in bone disease. Radiol Clin North Am 1970;8:277.
17. Lindbom A, Lindvall N, Soderberg G, et al. Angiography in osteoid osteoma. Acta Radiol 1960;54:327.
18. O'Hara JP III, Tegtmeyer C, Sweet DE, et al. Angiography in the diagnosis of osteoid-osteoma of the hand. J Bone Joint Surg (Am) 1975;57:163.
19. Spjut HJ, Dorfma HD, Fechner RE, et al. Tumors of bone and cartilage. Atlas of tumor pathology. 2nd series, fasc. 5. Washington, DC: Armed Forces Institute of Pathology, 1971.
20. Lee JK, Yao L, Wirth CR. MR imaging of solitary osteochondromas: report of eight cases. AJR 1987;149:557.
21. Han SK, Henein MHG, Novin N, et al. An unusual arterial complication seen with a solitary osteochondroma. Am Surg 1977;43:471.
22. Gomez-Reino JH, Radin A, Gorevic PD. Pseudoaneurysm of the popliteal artery as a complication of an osteochondroma. Skeletal Radiol 1979;4:26.
23. Yaghmai I. Angiographic features of chondromas and chondrosarcomas. Skeletal Radiol 1978;3:91.
24. Steinbach HL. Angiography of bones and joints. In: Abrams HL, ed. Angiography. 2nd ed. Boston: Little, Brown, 1971.
25. Giudici MA, Moser RP, Kransdorf MJ. Cartilaginous bone tumors. Radiol Clin North Am 1993;31(2):237–295.
26. Lagergren C, Lindbom A, Soderberg G. The blood vessels of chondrosarcomas. Acta Radiol 1961;55:321.
27. Sherman MS. Osteoid osteoma associated with changes in an adjacent joint: report of two cases. J Bone Joint Surg 1947; 29:483.
28. Bloem JL, Kroon HM. Osseous lesions. Radiol Clin North Am 1993;31(2):261–278.
29. Lateur L, Baert AL. Localisation and diagnosis of osteoid osteoma of the carpal area by angiography. Skeletal Radiol 1977;2:75.
30. Yaghmai I. Angiographic features of osteosarcoma. AJR 1977;129:1073.
31. Lagergren C, Lindbom A, Soderberg G. The blood vessels of osteogenic sarcomas: histologic, angiographic and microradiographic studies. Acta Radiol 1961;55:161.
32. Rittenberg GM, Schabel SI, Vujic I, et al. The vascular "sunburst" appearance of osteosarcoma: a new angiographic finding. Skeletal Radiol 1978;2:243.
33. de Santos LA, Bernardino ME, Murray, JA. Computed tomography in the evaluation of osteosarcoma: experience with 25 cases. AJR 1979;132:535.
34. Daffner RH, Lupetin AR, Dash N, et al. MRI detection of malignant infiltration of bone marrow. AJR 1986;146:353.
35. Fruehwald FXJ, Tscholakoff D, Schwaiglofer B, et al. Magnetic resonance imaging of the lower vertebral column in patients with multiple myeloma. Invest Radiol 1988;29:193.
36. Majumber S, Thomasson D, Shimakawa A, et al. Quantitation of the susceptibility difference between trabecular bone and bone marrow. Experimental studies. Magn Reson Med 1990; 22:111.
37. Steiner RM, Mitchell DG, Rao VM, et al. Magnetic resonance imaging of the bone marrow. In: Bloem J, Sartoris DJ, eds. MRI and CT of the musculoskeletal system. Baltimore: Williams & Wilkins, 1992:108.
38. Laurin S, Akerman M, Kindblom L-G, et al. Angiography in myeloma (plasmacytoma): a correlated angiographic and histologic study. Skeletal Radiol 1979;4:8.
39. Essli KD, Quiogue T, Moser RP. Ewing's sarcoma. Radiol Clin North Am 1993;31(2):325.
40. Hudson TM, Schiebler M, Springfield DS, et al. Radiology of giant cell tumors of bone: computed tomography, arthrotomography, and scintigraphy. Skeletal Radiol 1984;11:85.
41. Moser RP, Kransdorf MJ, Gilkey FW, et al. Giant cell tumor of the upper extremity. RadioGraphics 1990;10:83.
42. Herman SD. Megarzadeh M, Bonadkarpour A, et al. The role of magnetic resonance imaging in giant cell tumor of bone. Skeletal Radiol 1987;16:635.
43. Gunterberg B, Kindblom L-G, Laurin S. Giant-cell tumor of bone and aneurysmal bone cyst: a correlated histologic and angiographic study. Skeletal Radiol 1977;2:65.
44. Laurin S. Angiography in giant cell tumors. Radiologe 1977; 17:118.
45. Lundstrom B, Lorentzon R, Larsson SE, et al. Angiography in giant-cell tumours of bone. Acta Radiol 1977;18:541.
46. Prando A, de Santos LA, Wallace S, et al. Angiography in giant-cell bone tumors. Radiology 1979;130:323.
47. de Santos LA, Prando A. Synovial hyperemia in giant cell tumor of bone: angiographic pitfall. AJR 1979;133:281.
48. Hudson TM. Fluid levels in aneurysmal bone cysts: a CT feature. AJR 1984;141:1001.
49. Tsai JC, Dalinka MK, Fallon MD, et al. Fluid-fluid level: a

non-specific finding in tumors of bone and soft tissue. Radiology 1990;175:779.

50. Beltran J, Simon DC, Levy M, et al. Aneurysmal bone cysts: MR imaging at 1.5 T. Radiology 1986;158:689.
51. Monk PL, Helms CA, Hold RG, et al. MR imaging of aneurysmal bone cysts. AJR 1989;153:99.
52. de Santos LA, Murray JA. The value of arteriography in the management of aneurysmal bone cyst. Skeletal Radiol 1978; 2:137.
53. Fuhs SE, Herndon JH. Aneurysmal bone cyst involving the hand: a review and report of two cases. J Hand Surg 1979; 4:152.
54. Lindbom A, Soderberg G, Spjut HJ, et al. Angiography of aneurysmal bone cyst. Acta Radiol 1961;55:12.
55. Ring SM, Beranbaum ER, Madayag MA, et al. Angiography of aneurysmal bone cyst. Bull Hosp Joint Dis 1972;33:1.
56. Voegeli E, Fuchs WA. Arteriography in bone tumours. Br J Radiol 1976;49:407.
57. Yaghmai I. Angiographic features of osteosarcoma. AJR 1977;124:57.
58. Crim JR, Gold RH, Mirra JM, et al. Desmoplastic fibroma of bone: radiographic analysis. Radiology 1989;172:827.
59. Gebhardt MC, Campbell CJ, Schiller AL, et al. Desmoplastic fibroma of bone: a report of eight cases and review of the literature. J Bone Joint Surg (Am) 1985;87:732.
60. Hudson TM, Stiles RG, Monson DK. Fibrous lesions of bone. Radiol Clin North Am 1993;31(2):279.
61. Bloem JL, Taminiav AHM, Eulderink F, et al. Radiographic staging of primary bone sarcoma: MR imaging, scintigraphy, angiography, and CT correlation with pathologic examination. Radiology 1988;169:805.
62. Pettersson H, Gillespy T, Hamlin DJ, et al. Primary musculoskeletal tumors: examination with MR imaging compared with conventional modalities. Radiology 1987;164:237.
63. Sundaram M, McLeod RA. MR imaging of tumor and tumor-like lesions of bone and soft tissues. AJR 1990;155:817.
64. Lagergren C, Lindbom A, Soderberg G. Vascularization of fibromatous and fibrosarcomatous tumors: histopathologic, microangiographic and angiographic studies. Acta Radiol 1960;53:1.
65. Dibbelt W. Uber die Blutgefasse der Tumoren. Arb Pathol Anat Bakt 1912;8:114.
66. Feldman F, Lattes R. Primary malignant fibrous histiocytoma (fibrous xanthoma) of bone. Skeletal Radiol 1977;1:145.
67. Feldman F, Norman D. Intra- and extraosseous malignant histiocytoma (malignant fibrous xanthoma). Radiology 1972; 104:497.
68. Hudson TM, Hawkins IF Jr, Spanier SS, et al. Angiography of malignant fibrous histiocytoma of bone. Radiology 1979; 131:9.
69. Yaghmai I. Malignant giant cell tumor of the soft tissue: angiographic manifestations. Radiology 1976;120:329.
70. Ross JS, Masarykk TJ, Modic MT, et al. Vertebral hemangiomas: MR imaging. Radiology 1987;165:165.
71. Bliznak J, Staple TW. Radiology of angiodysplasias of the limb. Radiology 1974;110:35.
72. Buetow PC, Kransdorf MJ, Moser RP, et al. Radiographic appearance of intramuscular hemangiomas with emphasis on MR imaging. AJR 1990;154:563.
73. Cohen EK, Kressel HY, Perosio T, et al. MR imaging of soft tissue hemangiomas: correlation with pathologic findings. AJR 1988;150:1079.
74. Bartley O, Wickbom I. Angiography in soft tissue hemangiomas. Acta Radiol 1959;51:81.
75. Levin DC, Grodon DH, McSweeney J. Arteriography of peripheral hemangiomas. Radiology 1976;121:625.
76. Pochaczevsky R, Sussman R, Stoopack J. Arteriovenous fistulas of the maxillofacial region. J Can Assoc Radiol 1972;23: 201.
77. Scottie D, Edeiken J, Madan V. Arteriovenous malformation of the hand with involvement with bone. Skeletal Radiol 1978;2:151.
78. Conway WF, Hayes CW. Miscellaneous lesions of bone. Radiol Clin North Am 1993;31(2):339.
79. Ayella RJ. Hemangiopericytoma. Radiology 1970;97:611.
80. De Villiers DR, Farman J, Campbell JAH. Pelvic haemangiopericytoma: preoperative arteriographic demonstration. Clin Radiol 1976;18:318.
81. Joffe N. Haemangiopericytoma: angiographic findings. Br J Radiol 1960;33:614.
82. Yaghmai I. Angiographic manifestations of soft-tissue and osseous hemangiopericytomas. Radiology 1978;126:653.
83. Dahlin DC. Bone tumors: general aspects and data on 6,221 cases. 3rd ed. Springfield, IL: Charles C Thomas, 1978.
84. Unni KK, Ivins JC, Beabout JW, et al. Hemangioma, hemangiopericytoma, and hemangioendothelioma (angiosarcoma) of bone. Cancer 1971;27:1403.
85. Srinivasan CK, Patel MR, Pearlman HS, et al. Malignant hemangioendothelioma of bone: review of the literature and report of two cases. J Bone Joint Surg (Am) 1978;60:696.
86. Lagergren C, Lindbom A. Angiography of peripheral tumors. Radiology 1962;79:371.
87. Jalinek JS, Kransdorf MJ, Utz JA, et al. Imaging of pigmented villonodular synovitis with emphasis on MR imaging. AJR 1989;152:337.
88. Kiottal RA, Vogler JB, Matamoros A, et al. Pigmented villonodular synovitis: a report of MR imaging in two cases. Radiology 1987;163:551.
89. Manelbaum BR, Grant TT, Hartzman S, et al. The use of MR to assist in diagnosis of pigmented villonodular synovitis of the knee joint. Clin Orthop 1988;231:135.
90. Probst FP. Extra-articular pigmented villonodular synovitis affecting bone: the role of angiography as an aid in its differentiation from similar bone-destroying conditions. Radiologe 1973;13:436.
91. Levin DC, Watson RC, Baltaxe HA. Arteriography in diagnosis and management of acquired peripheral soft-tissue masses. Radiology 1972;103:53.
92. Martel WM, Abell MR. Radiologic evaluation of soft tissue tumors: a retrospective study. Cancer 1973;32:352.
93. Murray JA. Synoval sarcoma. Orthop Clin North Am 1977; 8:963.
94. Simon MA, Enneking WF. The management of soft-tissue sarcomas of the extremities. J Bone Joint Surg (Am) 1976; 58:317.
95. Greenfield GB, Arrington JA, Kodryk BT. MRI of soft tissue tumors. Skeletal Radiol 1993;22:77.
96. Finck EJ, Moore TM. Angiography for mass lesions of bone, joint and soft tissue. Orthop Clin North Am 1977;8:999.
97. Herzberg DL, Schreiber MH. Angiography in mass lesions of the extremities. AJR 1971;111:541.
98. Kindblom L-G, Merck C, Svendsen P. Myxofibrosarcoma: a pathologico-anatomical, microangiographic and angiographic correlative study of eight cases. Br J Radiol 1977;50: 876.
99. Margulis AR, Murphy TO. Arteriography in neoplasms of extremities. AJR 1958;80:330.
100. Rosenberg JC. The value of arteriography in the treatment of soft tissue tumors of the extremities. J Int Coll Surg 1964; 41:405.
101. Stanley P, Miller JH. Angiography of extremity masses in children. AJR 1978;130:1119.
102. Templeton AW, Stevens E, Jansen C. Arteriographic evaluation of soft tissue masses. South Med J 1966;59:1255.
103. Dunnick NR, Castellino RA. Arteriographic manifestations of ganglioneuromas. Radiology 1975;115:323.
104. Cockshott WP, Evans KT. The place of soft tissue arteriography. Br J Radiol 1964;37:367.
105. Ackerman LV. Extra-osseous localized non-neoplastic bone and cartilage formation (so-called myositis ossificans): clinical and pathological confusion with malignant neoplasms. J Bone Joint Surg (Am) 1958;40:279.
106. Kransdorf MJ, Jelinek JS, Moser RP. Imaging of soft tissue tumors. Radiol Clin North Am 1993;31(2):359.

107. Gronner AT. Muscle necrosis simulating a malignant tumor angiographically: case report. Radiology 1972;103:309.

108. Goldman AB. Myositis ossificans circumscripta: a benign lesion with a malignant differential diagnosis. AJR 1976;126:32.

109. Hutcheson J, Klatte EC, Kremp R. The angiographic appearance of myositis ossificans circumscripta: a case report. Radiology 1972;102:57.

110. Yaghmai I. Myositis ossificans: diagnostic value of arteriography. AJR 1977;128:811.

111. Feldman F, Cassarella WJ, Dick HM, et al. Selective intraarterial embolization of bone tumors: a useful adjunct in the management of selected lesions. AJR 1975;123:130.

112. Stanley RJ, Cubillo E. Nonsurgical treatment of arteriovenous malformations of the trunk and limb by transcatheter arterial embolization. Radiology 1975;115:609.

113. Hemmy DC, McGee DM, Armbrust FH, et al. Resection of a vertebral hemangioma after preoperative embolization: a case report. J Neurosurg 1977;47:282.

114. Voigt K, Schwenzer N, Stoeter P. Angiographic, operative, and histologic findings after embolization of craniofacial angiomas. Neuroradiology 1978;16:424.

115. Wallace S, Granmayeh M, de Santos LA, et al. Arterial occlusion of pelvic bone tumors. Cancer 1979;43:322.

116. Mitty HA, Kleiger B. Partial embolization of large peripheral hemangioma for pain control. Radiology 1978;127:671.

117. Doppman JL, Peusner P. Embolization of arteriovenous malformations by direct percutaneous puncture. AJR 1983;140:773.

118. Yakes WF, Pevsner P, Reed M, et al. Serial embolization of an extremity arteriovenous malformation with alcohol via direct percutaneous puncture. AJR 1986;146:1038.

119. Doppman JL, Di Chiro G. Paraspinal muscle infarction: a painful complication of lumbar artery embolization associated with pathognomonic radiographic and laboratory findings. Radiology 1976;119:609.

72

Peripheral Vascular Magnetic Resonance Angiography

RICHARD A. BAUM
JEFFREY P. CARPENTER

The workup of a patient with peripheral vascular disease includes both invasive and noninvasive imaging. Usually patients with mild disease undergo noninvasive testing, whereas those with advanced disease proceed to contrast angiography, which provides a road map prior to revascularization. Many noninvasive imaging techniques have been introduced as potential replacements for contrast angiography. Intravenous digital subtraction angiography and Doppler ultrasound were both hailed as possible alternatives for the aortogram and runoff study. In each case it quickly became apparent that these modalities alone were not sufficient to plan surgical or angiographic interventions.[1]

The recent introduction of peripheral vascular magnetic resonance angiography (PVMRA) has been greeted with similar euphoria. However, unlike its predecessors, PVMRA has been shown to be more sensitive than contrast angiography in visualizing patent vessels in the leg and foot.[2-5] Although this modality is still in its infancy, in some centers it has already replaced contrast angiography as the primary imaging tool in evaluating patients with peripheral vascular ischemia.[6] As the role of PVMRA continues to evolve, it becomes increasingly apparent that the real question to ask is not *if* MRA will replace contrast angiography but *when* this will occur.

Noninvasive Peripheral Vascular Imaging

For more than 30 years contrast arteriography has been the "gold standard" for the diagnostic evaluation of the peripheral vascular system. If performed with care, contrast arteriography is a safe and valuable procedure in the identification and treatment of peripheral arterial occlusive disease. However, arterial puncture and intravascular contrast delivery have well-described complications.[7-9] In attempts to eliminate the need for this invasive procedure, many noninvasive tests have been introduced over the years to evaluate the peripheral arterial tree in symptomatic patients. Physical examination, pulse volume recordings, segmental pressure measurements, and duplex Doppler ultrasound are all useful for localizing regions of disease, but none can reliably or consistently provide the precise morphologic information that is required for revascularization planning. Thus, as already mentioned, the workup of the patient with severe symptomatic peripheral occlusive disease still requires an aortogram and runoff examination to provide an anatomic road map prior to surgical or percutaneous intervention.[10] To date, the ideal noninvasive imaging technique that could replace conventional contrast arteriography has remained elusive.

Magnetic Resonance Angiography

Magnetic resonance imaging (MRI), first introduced in 1979, has contributed to the revolution that has occurred in diagnostic imaging. Every organ system has benefited from its high resolution and multiplane capabilities. Modifications in both software and hardware have occurred almost daily since this modality was introduced. Low-field-strength resistive systems, which were common only a decade ago, are now obsolete antiques. Today high-field-strength superconducting magnets and body-specific surface coils are the norm.

The ability of MRI to image flowing blood was not first apparent. In fact, flowing blood initially was a nuisance, producing many artifacts and degrading image quality. Much time was spent developing techniques to suppress this "flow artifact." These same techniques have since been modified to maximize rather than minimize imaging of the cardiovascular system.[11-13]

1822

Although magnetic resonance angiography (MRA) is not a new technique, it has only been recently applied to the peripheral vascular system.[14-16] This is surprising, because the peripheral vascular system is perfectly suited for MRA, there being no cardiac or respiratory motion and favorable flow dynamics. For the most part, blood flow is unidirectional, traveling from cephalad to caudad. In addition, flow in patients with advanced peripheral vascular disease is monophasic. These patients have no reversal of flow during diastole as do normal patients. Because of this dampening of the arterial pulse waveform, PVMRA can image patients with advanced disease far better than patients without disease. Indeed, the worst patient to image is the "normal volunteer."

PVMRA is a recent advance in noninvasive vascular imaging. Innovations in magnetic resonance hardware and software allow the peripheral arteries and veins to be visualized with great detail. Results of comparison studies in the diagnosis of atherosclerotic peripheral vascular disease indicate that the accuracy of PVMRA exceeds that of contrast arteriography, especially in identifying and localizing distal runoff vessels in the leg and foot (Fig. 72-1).[2-4] This information has been used by interventional radiologists and vascular surgeons to plan revascularization and as an aid in limb salvage. Combined with standard spin-echo imaging and surface coils, MRA can also image the blood vessel itself. High-resolution MR imaging of vessels following angioplasty reveals morphologic changes and injury in the walls. This information can be used in follow-up and may provide clues to the puzzle of restenosis.[17]

Peripheral Vascular MRA Techniques

Many MRA techniques have been effectively used for peripheral vascular imaging. Technique selection is generally based on institutional preference and variations in MR field strengths and scanners (Table 72-1). Regardless of the technique or field strength, all MRA has the same imaging goals. Spins from stationary tissues are minimized while spins from flowing blood are maximized.

Two-dimensional time of flight (2D-TOF) was the

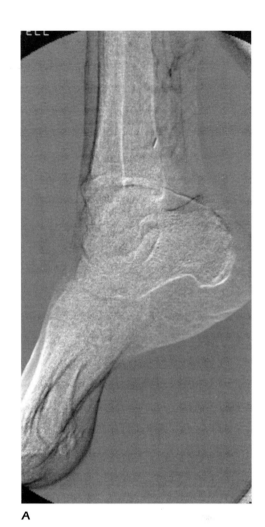

A

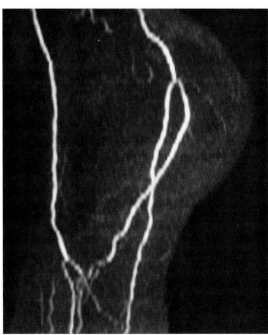

B

Figure 72-1. Angiographically occult runoff vessels. (A) Intraarterial digital subtraction angiography of the left foot shows numerous collaterals; however, no named runoff vessels are seen entering the foot. (B) Peripheral vascular MRA in the same patient demonstrates patent pedal vessels.

Table 72-1. Typical Protocol for Two-Dimensional (2D) Time-of-Flight (TOF) Magnetic Resonance Imaging

Feature	Body Part Imaged	
	Pelvis	Leg
Field strength	1.5 T	1.5 T
Coil	Body	Extremity
Pulse sequence	2D-TOF	2D-TOF
Slice thickness	2.5 mm	2.0 mm
Saturation band	Inferior	Inferior
Repetition time	33 msec	33 msec
Echo time	7.7 msec	7.7 msec
Field of view	28 cm	16 cm
Flip angle	60 degrees	60 degrees
Patient position	Supine	Supine

From Baum RA, Carpenter JP. Magnetic resonance angiography in peripheral arterial disease. In: Beltran J. Current review of MRI. Philadelphia: Current Medicine, 1995. Used with permission.

first imaging sequence to routinely visualize lower extremity vasculature (Fig. 72-2) and is still the standard to view the popliteal, tibial, and pedal arteries. This robust technique uses very short repetition times (TR) and echo times (TE) to suppress stationary spins from soft tissue while moving spins (flowing blood) produce flow-related enhancement. Blood traveling perpendicular to the imaging plane has maximum signal intensity, whereas stationary soft tissue has minimal signal intensity. The major advantage of 2D-TOF is its ability to visualize slowly flowing blood. It has been shown to be more sensitive than contrast angiography in identifying patent tibial and pedal vessels. Disadvantages include the numerous flow-related artifacts produced and the long imaging times. Artifacts occur most frequently in the aorta and iliac vessels, where turbulent and retrograde flow is common. Since flow in the extremities is from cephalad to caudad, axial 2D-TOF imaging produces maximum flow-related enhancement. Problems arise in the foot, where pedal vessels course ventral and lie parallel to the axial imaging slice. These vessels produce little if any flow-related enhancement. Fortunately, this limitation is easily rectified by plantar-flexing the foot and realigning the pedal vessels perpendicular to the imaging slice (Fig. 72-3).

Saturation bands are easily applied to selectively image the arteries or veins. They are placed superior (to suppress arteries) or inferior (to suppress veins) to the imaging plane. After a series of axial images are acquired, "maximum intensity pixel" (MIP) algorithm produces multiple three-dimensional projection images from the volume of imaged data. 2D-TOF therefore acquires axial and projectional images, both of which are used in vascular diagnosis. Axial images are

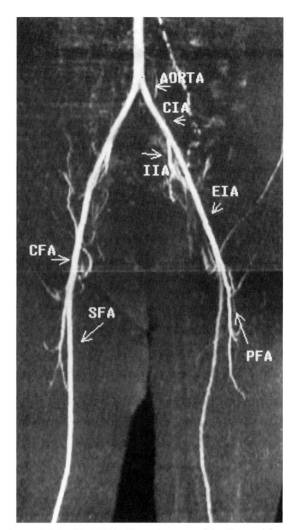

Figure 72-2. 2D-TOF MR angiogram of the iliac and femoral vessels, from which a 3D MR angiogram is produced using MIP reconstruction. The aorta, iliac, and femoral arteries are all identified. This is a three-dimensional projectional image, which can be rotated or viewed in any projection. *CIA,* common iliac artery; *IIA,* internal iliac artery; *EIA,* external iliac artery; *CFA,* common femoral artery; *SFA,* superficial femoral artery; *PFA,* profunda femoris artery.

extremely valuable in identifying vessels and in defining relationships of arteries and veins to surrounding soft tissues. Reformating the source images on computer workstations and independent consuls can yield additional views. This valuable three-dimensional information is not available from conventional projection arteriography and requires a thorough knowledge of cross-sectional vascular anatomy.

Axial Angiography

Vascular radiologists and surgeons are unaccustomed to viewing the peripheral arteries in cross section (Fig. 72-4). Axial images are extremely valuable in identi-

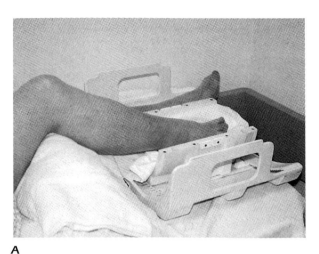

A

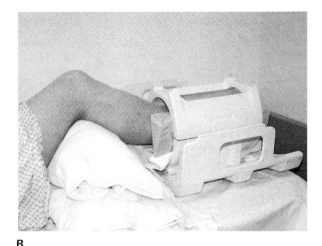

B

Figure 72-3. MRA of the foot. To minimize in-plane flow, the foot is positioned in the extremity coil with (A) the toes planar-flexed and (B) the knees supported on pillows. (From

Baum RA, Carpenter J. Magnetic resonance angiography in peripheral arterial disease. In: Current review of MRI. Philadelphia: Current Medicine, 1995. Used with permission.)

fying vessels and defining the relationships of arteries and veins relative to the surrounding soft tissues. Such practical cross-sectional anatomic information is not available from projectional contrast angiography. A meticulous review of cross-sectional images is required when reviewing peripheral vascular MR angiograms.

The advantage of viewing vascular pathology in cross section is demonstrated best with aortic dissections. Axial imaging with CT, MRI, or transesophageal echo allows intimal flaps to be visualized with far greater detail than with projectional angiography. This

is also the case when examining the peripheral vascular system. Identifying vessels and the relationships of peripheral vessels to surrounding soft tissues, as well as assessing intimal injury, is easily accomplished with axial 2D-TOF imaging (Fig. 72-5). Even though soft tissue signal is suppressed on MRA, enough anatomic detail is present to easily and accurately identify soft tissue structures. Unfortunately, vascular radiologists are unaccustomed to viewing the peripheral arteries in this manner, and familiarity with cross-sectional vascular anatomy is essential for the proper interpretation of MR angiograms.

Figure 72-4. Axial image from a 3D-TOF MR angiogram. An axial image from a 2D-TOF angiogram of the leg demonstrates cross-sectional axial anatomy. The posterior tibia (*PT*), the peroneal artery (*PE*), and the anterior tibial artery (*AT*) are all easily identified from their cross-sectional anatomic locations.

Figure 72-5. Popliteal dissection on MRA. Multiple 2D-TOF axial images are obtained through the popliteal artery after a percutaneous angioplasty. A spiral intimal dissection is seen (*bright signal*) forming a crescent. (From Baum RA, Carpenter J. Magnetic resonance angiography in peripheral arterial disease. In: Current review of MRI. Philadelphia: Current Medicine, 1995. Used with permission.)

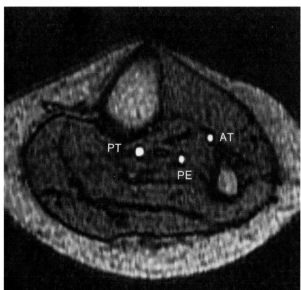

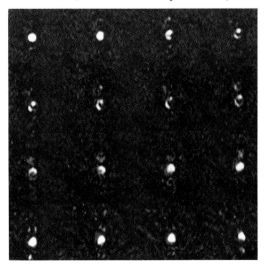

Cross-sectional Vascular Anatomy

The common iliac arteries bifurcate into internal and external iliac arteries just anterior to the sacroiliac joint (Fig. 72-6). On axial imaging, the internal iliac arteries can be seen coursing posteriorly and inferiorly until they divide into anterior and posterior divisions. Smaller branches of the anterior and posterior trunks can also be routinely identified on MRA (Fig. 72-7). The external iliac artery travels ventrally and laterally along the psoas muscle until it enters the thigh midway between the anterior superior iliac spine and the symphysis pubis. The ureter and ovarian vessels are seen crossing the midportion of the external iliac artery on cross-sectional imaging, and care must be taken not to misidentify flow in these structures for pathology.

The common femoral artery lies anterior and medial to the femoral head and the iliopsoas muscle and lateral to the pectineus muscle. Immediately after the femoral bifurcation the deep femoral artery travels dorsally to lie just posterior to the femur between the adductor magnus, the adductor longus, and the vastus medialis muscles. The superficial femoral artery travels along the thigh between the sartorius, the vastus medialis, and the adductor longus muscles (Figs. 72-8 and 72-9).

The popliteal artery is posterior to the distal femur and anterior to the semimembranous muscle (Fig. 72-10). The anterior tibial artery courses between the triangular anterior tibialis muscle and the lateral surface of the tibia anterior to the interosseous membrane.

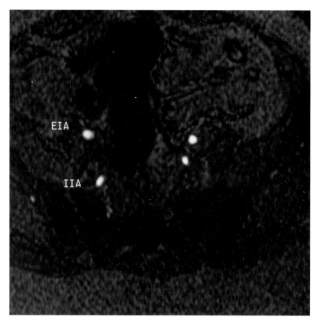

Figure 72-7. Iliac artery bifurcation on cross-sectional MRA. The external iliac arteries (*EIA*) and the internal iliac arteries (*IIA*) are demonstrated on this 2D-TOF angiogram.

The peroneal artery lies posterior to the interosseous membrane between the tibia and fibula. The posterior tibial artery courses along the dorsal surface of the tibia

Figure 72-8. Cross section of the upper thigh. An anatomic drawing demonstrates the relationship of the superficial and deep femoral arteries to soft tissue structures in the upper thigh. (From Moore KL. Clinically oriented anatomy, 3rd ed. Baltimore: Williams & Wilkins, 1992. Used with permission.)

Figure 72-6. The common iliac arteries (*CIA*) are identified on this 2D-TOF cross-sectional MR angiogram.

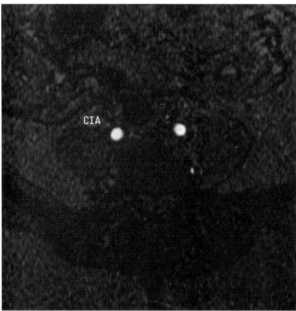

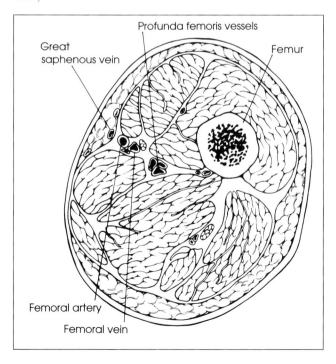

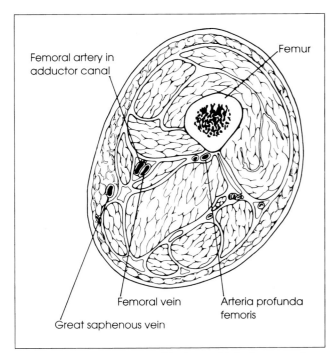

Figure 72-9. Cross section of the lower thigh. An anatomic drawing demonstrates the relationship of vascular structures to soft tissues in the lower thigh. (From Moore KL. Clinically oriented anatomy, 3rd ed. Baltimore: Williams & Wilkins, 1992. Used with permission.)

Figure 72-11. Cross section of the leg. The anterior tibial, posterior tibial, and peroneal arteries are shown in their cross-sectional anatomic locations in the midleg. (From Moore KL. Clinically oriented anatomy, 3rd ed. Baltimore: Williams & Wilkins, 1992. Used with permission.)

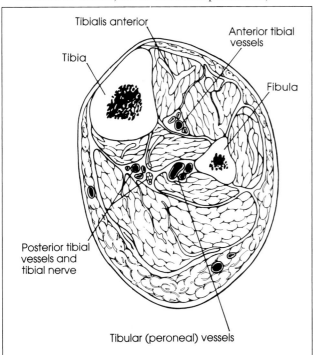

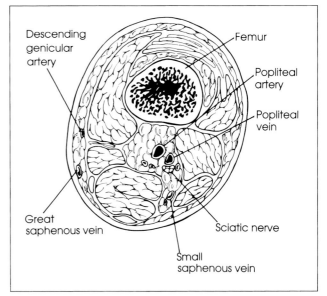

Figure 72-10. Cross section of the knee. An anatomic drawing demonstrates the relationship of the popliteal artery to soft tissue structures just above the knee joint. (From Williams PL, Warwick R, eds. Gray's anatomy, 3rd ed. Baltimore: Williams & Wilkins, 1992. Used with permission.)

next to the flexor digitorum longus muscle (Figs. 72-11 and 72-12).

In the foot the dorsalis pedis artery lies anterior to the talus, and the posterior tibial artery courses along the medial portion of the cuboid and calcaneus (Fig.

Figure 72-12. Cross section just above the ankle. This anatomic drawing shows the relationship of the distal anterior tibial, peroneal, and posterior tibial arteries just above the ankle joint. (From Williams PL, Warwick R, eds. Gray's anatomy, 3rd ed. Baltimore: Williams & Wilkins, 1992. Used with permission.)

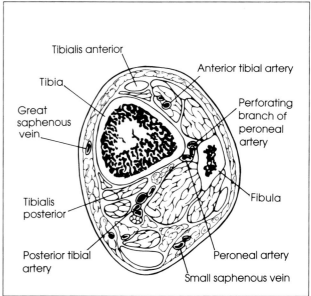

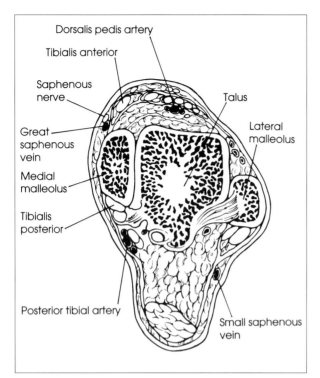

Figure 72-13. Cross section of the foot. An anatomic drawing demonstrates the relationship of the dorsalis pedis and posterior tibial arteries to the soft-tissue structures at the level of the lateral malleolus. (From Williams PL, Warwick R, eds. Gray's anatomy, 3rd ed. Baltimore: Williams & Wilkins, 1992. Used with permission.)

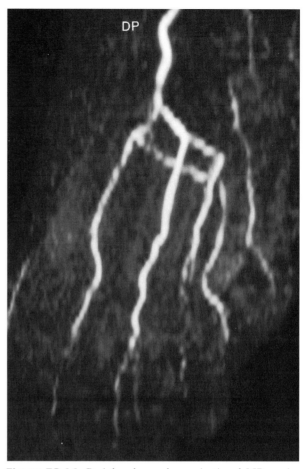

Figure 72-14. Peripheral vascular projectional MR angiogram demonstrates the termination of the dorsalis pedis artery into several digital vessels, which can be seen running into the toes of the foot.

72-13). The medial and lateral plantar arteries are routinely imaged along the medial surface of the foot. With the extremity coil and small fields of view, even small digital arteries can be seen in the toes (Fig. 72-14).

Artifacts

As with any imaging modality, it is important to understand the pitfalls of technique and interpretation. This is especially true with MRA, where artifacts can simulate occlusive disease. A recent study showed learning effects with the interpretation of MR angiograms. The accuracy of MRA interpretation increased consistently during a 6-month multicenter trial as readers became more familiar with techniques and artifacts.[18]

Metallic artifacts are commonly encountered in patients with peripheral occlusive disease. Surgical clips and prosthetic joints are the most common offenders and may produce large signal voids on the axial 2D-TOF images (Fig. 72-15). Superficial clips from saphenous vein harvesting rarely produce signal voids large

enough to preclude MRA imaging; however, prosthetic hip and knee joints pose a significant problem. Signal voids eliminate flow-related enhancement from adjacent arteries and veins and on projection MIP images mimic stenosis and occlusion.

Horizontal banding is related to the saturation bands, which allow for selective imaging of the arteries or veins. Blood flow temporally reverses direction, and saturated spins enter the imaging slice. This phenomenon is seen most often when imaging veins or in arteries with triphasic flow (Fig. 72-16). Horizontal banding appears as stripes across otherwise normal arteries (Fig. 72-17). Banding is easily corrected by positioning the saturation band further from the imaging slice.

Patient motion is a common problem encountered in all MRI and is particularly troublesome with MRA and MR venography. Reconstruction projection images require exact alignment of the 2D-TOF axial images. It is important to recognize motion artifacts because they mimic stenoses and occlusions (Fig. 72-18).

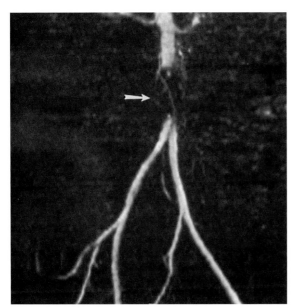

Figure 72-15. Metallic artifact. Projectional 2D-TOF MR angiogram of the distal aorta and iliac arteries shows a signal void (*arrow*) simulating occlusion of the distal aorta. This artifact is caused by a metal Palmaz aortic stent.

Reviewing the axial images or reimaging the area in question can alleviate this imaging obstacle.

Phase ghosting occurs when the pulse sequence timing does not match the periodicity of blood flow

Figure 72-17. Banding artifact. 2D-TOF MR angiogram of a normal volunteer shows multiple banding defects (*arrows*) involving all of the iliac and femoral vessels.

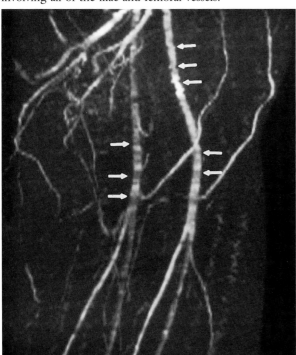

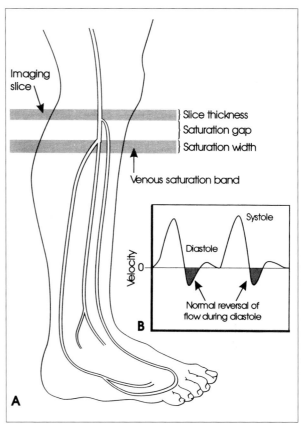

Figure 72-16. Banding artifact. (A) Peripheral vascular MRA imaging slice is above the venous saturation band. (B) The patient's reversal of flow during diastole causes spins that have already been saturated to enter the imaging slice. (From Baum RA, Carpenter J. Magnetic resonance angiography in peripheral arterial disease. In: Current review of MRI. Philadelphia: Current Medicine, 1995. Used with permission.)

(Fig. 72-19). The true vessel is surrounded by ghost vessels that occur at regularly spaced intervals in the phase-encoding direction. This common artifact can be minimized by cardiac gating (at the expense of imaging time) or by using postprocessing reconstruction techniques that use seeded reconstruction algorithms.

In-plane flow artifacts occur when blood flow is parallel to the imaging slice (Fig. 72-20). In the peripheral vascular system this most commonly occurs at the origin of the anterior tibial artery and in tortuous iliac vessels. Signal dropoff mimics stenoses or occlusions. A careful review of axial images will confirm the patency of affected vessels.

MRA Using Gadolinium

Recently, intravenous gadolinium has been used to eliminate flow artifacts caused by turbulent and retrograde flow in the aorta and iliac vessels. Contrast is

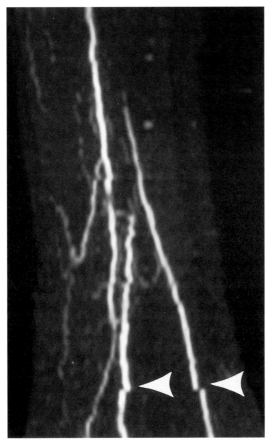

Figure 72-18. Motion artifact. This patient has moved during his TOF MR angiogram. A sharp step-off can be seen involving both reconstituted tibial vessels (*arrowheads*). These pseudostenoses should not be mistaken for true stenotic vessels.

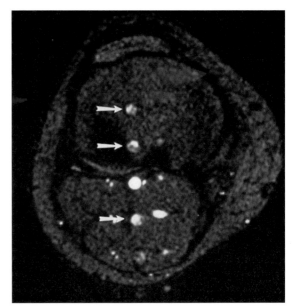

Figure 72-19. Phase ghosting. Actual image from a 2D-TOF MR angiogram of the knee demonstrates severe phase ghosting of the popliteal artery. Many ghost images (*arrows*) are identified in the phase-encoded direction.

injected through a peripheral intravenous line, and scanning is begun after a 15- to 30-second delay from initiation of the bolus. As with contrast angiography, care must be taken so that images are acquired during the arterial phase of the contrast bolus. Imaging is in the coronal plane during a single 20-second breath hold. The signal intensity of the resultant images is a result of the increase in T1 relaxation times from gadolinium rather than flow-related enhancement. This

Figure 72-20. In-plane flow. (A) A peripheral vascular MR angiogram fails to reveal the femoral-to-femoral bypass graft shown on (B), the contrast angiogram, because the blood is flowing in the plane of the axial TOF image. (From Baum

RA, Carpenter J. Magnetic resonance angiography in peripheral arterial disease. In: Current review of MRI. Philadelphia: Current Medicine, 1995. Used with permission.)

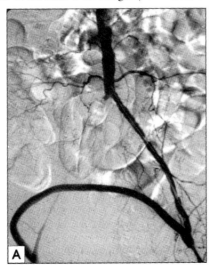

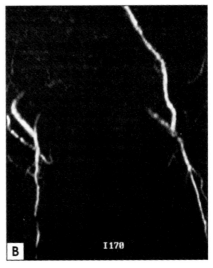

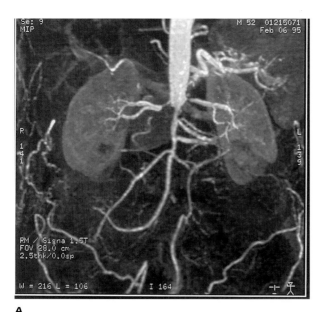
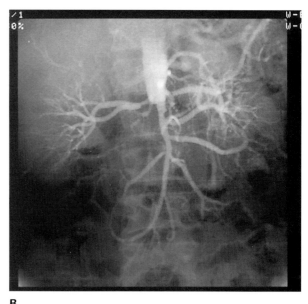

A   **B**

Figure 72-21. (A) Gadolinium-enhanced 3D-TOF MR angiogram shows an aortic occlusion just below the level of the renal arteries. This image was obtained during a single breath hold. (B) Comparison angiogram obtained via the left brachial artery.

eliminates most flow-related artifacts and dramatically increases resolution (Fig. 72-21).

Comparison Between PVMRA and Contrast Angiography

As with the introduction of any new imaging technique, comparisons must be made with existing modalities. Investigators have compared PVMRA and contrast angiography in patients with severe peripheral vascular disease (Fig. 72-22). Early investigations have shown that PVMRA can serve as a powerful noninvasive tool that provides imaging of the peripheral vascular system comparable to conventional contrast arteriography. Because PVMRA is performed differently in the pelvis than in the leg, these studies may be separated into those comparing inflow and those comparing runoff vessels.

PVMRA of Runoff Vessels

Advances in surgical technique and instrumentation make infrapopliteal bypass procedures an effective method of maintaining limb viability in patients with advanced disease. It has never been more important to accurately identify and characterize peripheral occlusive disease in the leg and foot. Small reconstituted vascular segments, once only a curiosity, are now com-

monly used as target vessels during vascular reconstruction.

MRA of the leg and foot has been shown to be more sensitive than conventional contrast arteriography in identifying tibial and pedal vessels, which can be used for distal bypass procedures. This is especially true in patients with severe atherosclerotic disease who have multiple segmental occlusions (Fig. 72-23). In these patients, contrast material must traverse one or more capillary beds before entering the leg and foot. High resistance to flow, as well as dilution by unopacified blood, may prevent contrast from being delivered in sufficient concentration to be visualized radiographically.[16,19-20] Even with intraarterial digital subtraction angiography, delivery of contrast to the distal leg and foot can sometimes be extremely difficult. MRA requires only the presence of flowing blood to produce vascular imaging, whereas x-ray examinations require delivery of contrast. In a comparative study evaluating runoff vessels in 71 patients, Carpenter and colleagues reported that 18 percent of vessels identified on MRA were occluded at contrast arteriography. The surgical management plan was modified in 8 percent of patients who were evaluated based on new information gained from the MRA.[21] This was validated by a large multicenter trial completed in January 1995.[18]

PVMRA of the Aortoiliac System

The evaluation of patients with peripheral vascular disease requires accurate characterization of inflow as well

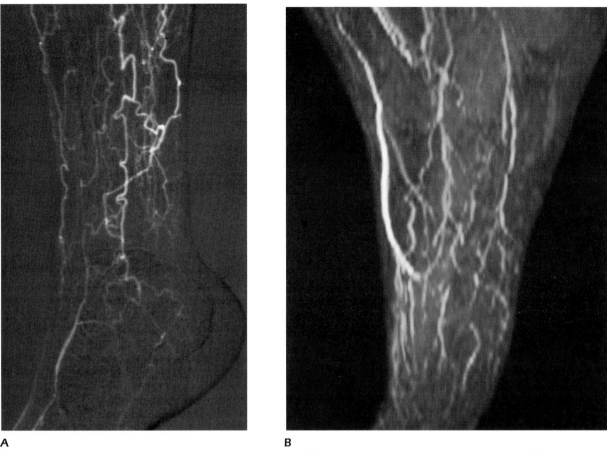

A   B

Figure 72-22. An intraarterial digital subtraction angiogram (A) compared to a 2D-TOF MR angiogram (B).

Figure 72-23. Angiographically occult runoff vessels. Intraarterial digital subtraction angiograms demonstrate (A) a long segmental iliac occlusion and (B) no distal runoff in the foot. (C) A 2D-TOF peripheral vascular MR angiogram shows three vessels descending down the leg and into the foot. (From Baum RA, Carpenter J. Magnetic resonance angiography in peripheral arterial disease. In: Current review of MRI. Philadelphia: Current Medicine, 1995. Used with permission.)

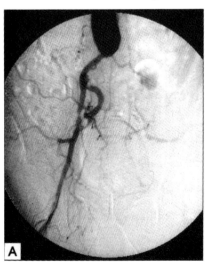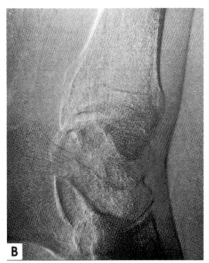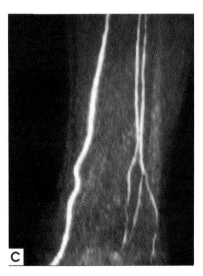

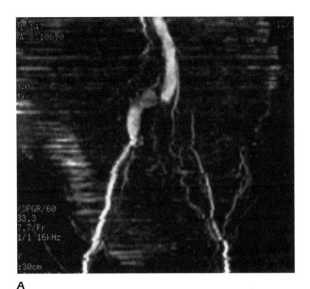

A

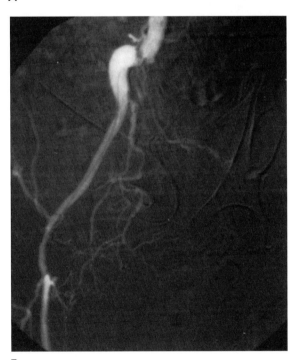

B

Figure 72-24. Overestimation of occlusive disease on 2D-TOF imaging. (A) A 2D-TOF MR angiogram viewed in the anteroposterior MIP projection shows an occlusion just distal to the aortic bifurcation. (B) The comparison conventional arteriogram shows this area to contain a severe stenosis. This loss of signal was caused by turbulent flow and is a limitation of 2D-TOF imaging.

as runoff vessels. Many obstacles must be overcome to image the aorta, iliac, and femoral vessels in these patients. Tortuosity of vessels, turbulent flow, and pulsatility all contribute to loss of signal and degradation of images when standard 2D-TOF techniques are used (Fig. 72-24). In addition, because the body coil is used

to image the aortoiliac vessels, large fields of view are required, further limiting resolution. Thus, because of differences in coils and technique, PVMRA has been shown to be superior to contrast arteriography in identifying and characterizing peripheral vessels below the adductor canal but not as sensitive in imaging the aortoiliac and femoral vessels.

Recently, contrast-enhanced 3D-TOF imaging has emerged as a rapid and sensitive method of imaging the aorta, iliac, and femoral vessels. In addition to its being faster, artifacts are far less of a problem when 3D- rather than 2D-TOF is used. As advances in hardware and software continue, most of the current limitations of aortoiliac imaging will disappear.

Pitfalls of PVMRA

Long examination times remain the bottleneck preventing widespread use of peripheral vascular MRA. The examination time for performing a 2D-TOF MRA of the aorta through the distal pedal arteries approximates 2 hours, and most of this time is spent in repositioning the patient and coils. Patients with severe disease, manifested by rest pain or ischemic tissue loss, present to the hospital at all hours, and emergent imaging is required in these patients to plan revascularization. Most busy MRA centers lack the flexibility to accommodate 2-hour emergency studies of the peripheral vascular system.

The introduction of gadolinium-enhanced 3D-TOF imaging has drastically decreased imaging times, with an entire MR aortogram and runoff taking less than an hour to perform. In this technique, 3D-TOF imaging of the aorta, iliac, and femoral arteries is combined with 2D-TOF imaging of the legs. The total examination time averages 45 minutes. The examinations can be further streamlined if the patient arrives in the department with a working intravenous line. As MRA technology improves with the further reduction of echo and repetition times as well as the introduction of leg-length surface coils, the time required to complete the examination will no doubt continue to decrease.

When to Use PVMRA

Many factors must be evaluated before a patient is referred for PVMRA. Most importantly, the facility must have the expertise to properly perform and interpret MR angiograms. This is best accomplished in a center in which there is close collaboration between the interventional radiologist, the MRA radiologist, and the

Table 72-2. Imaging Algorithm

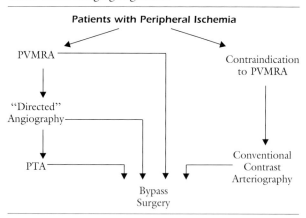

vascular surgeon. As with any other noninvasive vascular imaging modality, PVMRA needs to be compared to the current gold standard contrast angiography. Institutional validation is imperative before this tech-

nique should be used to guide surgeons and interventional radiologists.

At the authors' institution (Table 72-2) the most common indication for PVMRA is the initial evaluation in patients with limb-threatening ischemia. Patients presenting to the emergency department or vascular surgery clinic with severe peripheral ischemia are referred for PVMRA. Revascularization plans are then formulated by an interventional radiologist and vascular surgeon. If an operative plan can be established based on the PVMRA findings, a surgical procedure is performed without conducting a conventional contrast arteriogram. "Directed" angiography is performed if more diagnostic information is required than was provided by the PVMRA or if endovascular proce-

Figure 72-25. "Directed" angiography. (A) 2D-TOF MR angiogram of the popliteal artery demonstrates a severe stenosis. An antegrade puncture is made of the ipsilateral femoral artery. (B) The stenosis is confirmed. (C) A percutaneous transluminal angioplasty is performed.

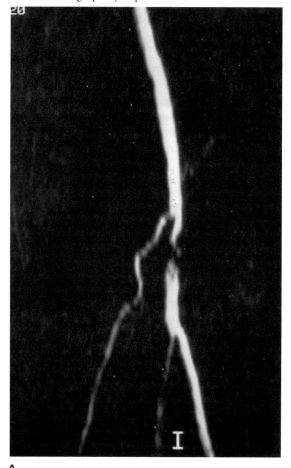

A

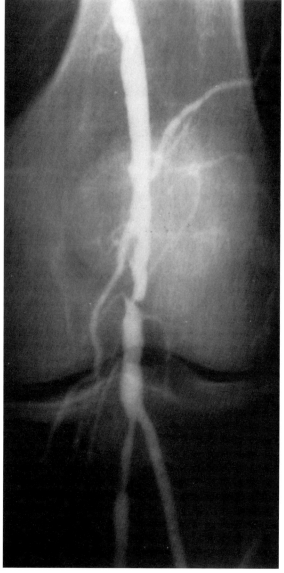

B

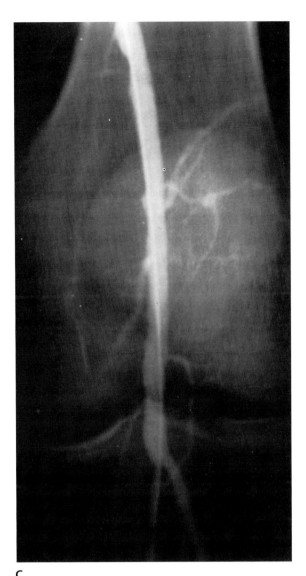

C

Figure 72-25 (continued).

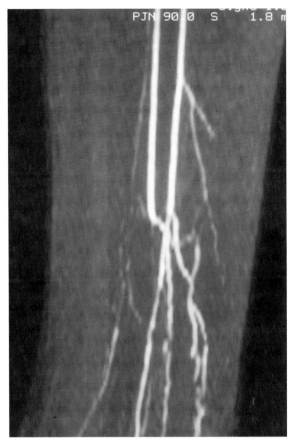

Figure 72-26. 2D-TOF MR angiogram in acute ischemia. An abrupt cutoff of both tibial vessels is identified in the mid-calf in this patient with new-onset atrial fibrillation in a mottled left foot.

dures are deemed possible. Rather than performing a complete aortogram and runoff examination, one "directs" the angiography to those areas in which PVMRA was not considered satisfactory because of pulsatility artifacts, tortuosity of vessels, metallic artifacts, or turbulent flow, or when angiography is considered a prerequisite to percutaneous intervention (Figs. 72-25 and 72-26). This approach has been shown to be cost-effective.[22]

In summary, surgical or angiographic interventions may be performed in patients presenting with severe peripheral occlusive disease if PVMRA is used as the primary imaging approach. In a few centers PVMRA has already successfully replaced the traditional aortogram and runoff examination as the initial imaging modality in patients with severe arterial occlusive dis-

ease. Minor technical and more substantial practical limitations must still be overcome before it gains widespread acceptance. However, it is clear that in the not-too-distant future PVMRA will be standard procedure in the workup of patients with peripheral ischemia. Contrast angiography will be reserved only for those patients who are to undergo percutaneous interventions or have contraindications to MRI.

References

1. Ricco J-B, Pearce WH, Yao JST, et al. The use of operative prebypass arteriography and Doppler ultrasound recordings to select patients for extended femoral-distal bypass. Ann Surg 1983;198:646–653.
2. Owen RS, Carpenter JP, Baum RA, Perloff LJ, Cope C. Magnetic resonance imaging of angiographically occult runoff vessels in peripheral arterial occlusive disease. N Engl J Med 1992; 326:1577–1581.
3. Carpenter JP, Owen RS, Baum RA, et al. Magnetic resonance angiography of peripheral runoff vessels. J Vasc Surg 1992;16: 807–815.

4. McCauley TR, Monib A, Dickey KW, et al. Peripheral vascular occlusive disease: accuracy and reliability of time-of-flight MR angiography. Radiology 1994;192:351–357.

5. Owen RS, Baum RA, Carpenter JP, Holland GA, Cope C. Symptomatic peripheral vascular disease: selection of imaging parameters and clinical evaluation with MR angiography. Radiology 1993;187:627–635.

6. Carpenter JP, Baum RA, Holland GA, Barker CF. Peripheral vascular surgery with magnetic resonance angiography as the sole preoperative imaging modality. J Vasc Surg 1994;20:861–871.

7. Hessel SJ, Adams DF, Abrams HL. Complications of angiography. Radiology 1981;138:273–281.

8. Waugh JR, Sacharias N. Arteriographic complications in the DSA era. Radiology 1992;182:243–246.

9. Shehadi WH, Toniolo G. Adverse reactions to contrast media: a report from the Committee on Safety of Contrast Media of the International Society of Radiology. Radiology 1980;137:299–302.

10. Moneta GL, Yeager RA, Antonovic R, et al. Accuracy of lower extremity arterial duplex mapping. J Vasc Surg 1992;15:275–284.

11. Herfkins RJ, Higgins CB, Hricak H, et al. Nuclear magnetic resonance imaging of the cardiovascular system: normal and pathologic findings. Radiology 1983;147:749–759.

12. Edelman RR, Mattle HP, Atkinson DJ, Hoogewoud HM. MR angiography. AJR 1990;154:937–946.

13. Kaufman L, Crooks LE, Sheldon PE, Hricak H, Herfkens R, Bank W. The potential impact of nuclear magnetic resonance imaging on cardiovascular diagnosis. Circulation 1983;67:251–257.

14. Yucel EK, Kaufman JA, Geller SC, Waltman AC. Atherosclerotic occlusive disease of the lower extremity: prospective evaluation with two-dimensional time-of-flight MR angiography. Radiology 1993;187:637–641.

15. Cambria RP, Yucel EK, Brewster DC, et al. The potential for lower extremity revascularization without contrast arteriography: experience with magnetic resonance angiography. J Vasc Surg 1993;17:1050–1057.

15a. Scheibler ML, Listerud J, Baum RA, et al. Magnetic resonance arteriography of the pelvis and lower extremities. Magn Reson Q 1993;9(3):152–187.

16. Patel PR, Semel L, Clauss RH. Extended reconstruction rate for limb salvage with intraoperative prereconstruction angiography. J Vasc Surg 1988;7:531–537.

17. Hertz SM, Baum RA, Owen RS, Holland GA, Logan DR, Carpenter JP. Comparison of magnetic resonance and contrast arteriography in peripheral arterial stenosis. Amer J Surg 1993;166(2):112–116.

18. Baum RA, Rutter CM, Sunshine JH, et al. Multicenter trial to evaluate vascular magnetic resonance angiography of the lower extremity. JAMA 1995;274:875–880.

19. Flanigan DP, Williams LR, Keifer T, et al. Prebypass operative angiography. Surgery 1982;92:627–633.

20. Scarpato R, Gembarowicz R, Farber S, et al. Intraoperative prereconstruction arteriography. Arch Surg 1981;92:627–633.

21. Carpenter JP, Owen RS, Holland GA, et al. Magnetic resonance angiography of the aorta, iliac and femoral arteries. Surgery 1994;116:17–23.

22. Yin D, Baum RA, Carpenter JP, et al. Cost-effectiveness of MR angiography in cases of limb-threatening peripheral vascular disease. Radiology 1995;194:755–764.

73

MR Venography in the Detection of Venous Thrombosis

GEORGE A. HOLLAND
MARYELLYN GILFEATHER

Epidemiology

Deep venous thrombosis (DVT) is a major cause of morbidity and mortality, with an estimated 1 to 5 million cases each year in the United States.[1-4] Complications from recurrent DVT include venous insufficiency and postphlebitic syndrome.[5-10] The serious complications of DVT are pulmonary artery hypertension and death due to embolization of thrombi to the pulmonary arteries. There are an estimated 700,000 to 900,000 cases of significant and symptomatic pulmonary emboli (PE)[11-14] and 125,000 to 200,000 deaths from pulmonary emboli annually in the United States.[3,4,11,15-18] In 75 to 95 percent of cases, the sources of pulmonary emboli are DVTs of the veins of the pelvis and lower extremities.[1-3,17-26]

The seriousness of thromboembolic disease is further underscored by an epidemiologic study in elderly patients. Kniffin et al. reviewed a random sample of 5 percent of enrollees of Medicare claims in the United States from 1986 to 1989. The authors identified 8923 cases of DVT and 7174 cases of PE. They reported a 1-year mortality rate of 21 percent for DVT and 39 percent for PE.[27] These high mortality rates are probably secondary to serious concomitant medical conditions in many of these patients.

The predisposing factors for the development of DVT were described by Virchow in 1860.[28] The risk factors he described were endothelial damage, venous stasis, and hypercoagulability of blood. These risk factors can also occur in younger patients, and thromboembolic disease poses a significant health problem to younger patients with the following conditions: young women on oral contraceptives,[29-32] pregnant women,[33-36] trauma victims,[37,38] general surgery patients,[24,39-43] orthopedic surgery patients,[35,44-49] cardiac patients,[50-54] hypercoagulable patients (polycythemia, dysproteinemia, abnormal clotting factors),[52,55] bed-ridden patients,[56-60] and oncology patients.[61-65]

The vast majority of PE from DVT are silent, and the incidence of PE in patients with DVT ranges from 15 to 53 percent. Moser and LeMoine reported that 0 out of 12 patients with below-the-knee DVT had PE, but that 8 out of 15 patients with above-the-knee DVT had PE by ventilation perfusion (V/Q) scan.[21] Only 1 of these patients was symptomatic. However, separate studies by Lotke et al. and Nielsen et al. demonstrated no significant difference between the incidence of PE from DVT below the knee or above the knee.[66,67] Lotke et al. reported a 17 percent (103 out of 602) incidence of PE based on pre– and post–lower extremity total joint arthroplasty V/Q scans in 602 patients and postoperative venograms in 920 patients. Only 5 (0.8 percent) of these patients with PEs were symptomatic, and there were only 2 deaths (0.2 percent). They concluded from this study of 920 joint arthroplasty patients that larger proximal clots had a greater likelihood of having a high probability V/Q scan, but that the size of the clot that is clinically significant was undetermined.[66] Dorfman et al. reported that 17 out of 45 (35 percent) patients with above-the-knee DVT had occult or clinically silent PE as evidenced by high probability V/Q scans.[68]

Clinicians have attempted to prevent DVT and resultant pulmonary emboli by identifying patients at increased risk for developing thromboembolic disease and by placing them on prophylactic regimens.[26,52,69-71] However, because of reports of failure of prophylactic regimens and significant complications with high-dose heparin, many of these authors also suggest routine surveillance for DVT to reduce the risk of fatal PE.[72-77] Therefore, objective diagnostic studies are important for the prompt and accurate diagnosis of pelvic and lower extremity DVT.

Patients who are diagnosed with PE or who have abnormal but not high-probability V/Q scans need to be assessed for DVT.[78-80] Patients who survive a PE are at greater risk for a subsequent PE.[81] Additional pulmonary emboli pose a threat to a patient's health and life. Treatment of patients diagnosed with PE is primarily directed at preventing subsequent PE by treating DVT. Appropriate therapy of the DVT depends on the clinical setting, size, and location of the thrombus. The therapies include long-term anticoagulation,[52,82] filter placement,[83–86] or, less commonly, lysis[87–91] or thrombectomy.[82,90,92–96]

A variety of algorithms have been proposed for managing patients with thromboembolic disease. After studying 1564 patients, Hull et al. have suggested that patients with adequate cardiorespiratory reserve who have abnormal but not high-probability V/Q and who have no evidence of DVT by noninvasive studies do not require therapy.[97,98] Others have also advocated a variation of this approach to managing patients with abnormal, non-high-probability V/Q scans.[99–102] Although Hull's approach may be controversial because of some failures of these noninvasive studies,[103,104] a safer, more rational approach to the treatment of patients with thromboembolic disease can be made when a careful accurate study of the venous system is available. For example, filter placement in the infrarenal inferior vena cava for PE prophylaxis is of little value to the patient with left gonadal vein or upper extremity vein thrombosis.

Clinical Diagnosis

Clinical diagnosis of deep venous thrombosis is insensitive and nonspecific.[20,105–116] Most DVTs are clinically silent.[20,24,66,107,108,117] An autopsy series of 2427 hospitalized patients from the Mayo Clinic reported that over 70 percent of DVTs were clinically occult and that premortem diagnostic tests for thromboembolic disease were performed in only 22 percent of patients. Thromboembolic disease was not considered by the clinician even at the time of death in 51 percent of the 92 cases of autopsy-proven fatal pulmonary emboli.[118] The lack of symptoms and signs from DVT is probably due to nonocclusive clot,[100,119–122] duplicated (20 percent) or triplicated (2 percent) venous systems, fenestration of the superficial femoral vein (8 percent), and the rich collateral drainage of the venous system.[123] Among the patients with symptoms in the lower extremities, 33 to 50 percent of patients present with the classical symptoms of calf discomfort, venous distention, and pain on dorsiflexion of the foot (Homan sign).[115,124,125] When symptoms and findings are attributed to DVT, the clinical diagnosis by objective tests is correct in less than 50 percent of the cases.[112,115,117,126–128] In addition, DVT may be bilateral in 14 to 35 percent of cases.[117,129] Clot is identified in the asymptomatic leg and not the symptomatic leg in as many as 36 percent of patients with symptoms.[117]

Despite the well-reported failings of the clinical diagnosis of DVT, 18 percent of patients discharged from 16 hospitals in Massachusetts were discharged with a final diagnosis of thromboembolic disease without undergoing any objective studies.[130,131] These patients were treated for thromboembolic disease based on clinical diagnosis alone. The consequence of a false-positive diagnosis of DVT is needlessly exposing the patient to risks of anticoagulation.[132] A false-negative diagnosis exposes the patient to the numerous complications of DVT, including fatal PE. Therefore, accurate and objective methods for the diagnosis of thromboembolic disease is extremely important for the proper management of patients.

Diagnosis

Ascending Contrast Venography

Most authors consider the ascending contrast venographic technique described by Rabinov and Paulin[133] to be the "gold standard" for the diagnosis of DVT.[104,106,134–139] A postmortem study compared conventional contrast venography with anatomic venous dissections performed at autopsy and reported an 89 percent sensitivity and 97 percent specificity for venographic detection of DVT.[140] However, there are problems with this "gold standard." For example, 5 to 10 percent of patients are unable to have the study because of failure to gain intravenous access.[66,136,137] Even when performed, the studies may be technically inadequate in 3 to 5 percent of patients.[104,141] Even when diagnostic studies are obtained, observers disagree about the presence or absence of clot on contrast venography in 9 to 22 percent of cases.[76,142–144] Conventional venography does not routinely visualize the deep pelvic or deep femoral veins, both of which are large potential sources of thromboemboli. Finally, this technique is costly and invasive, and intravascular contrast agents are responsible for complications in 0.04 to 0.22 percent of cases.[145] The multiple associated complications of venography include pain, skin necrosis,[146] postvenographic thrombophlebitis, contrast-induced renal failure,[147] anaphylactoid reaction to contrast, and, very rarely, death.[112,148–159]

Noninvasive Studies

Because of the complications of conventional venography, many investigators have attempted to develop noninvasive methods of diagnosing DVT. These studies include blood tests (e.g., D-dimer), impedance plethysmography (IPG), radionuclide venography, a variety of ultrasound techniques, computed tomography

(CT),[160,161] and magnetic resonance imaging (MRI) techniques.

Impedance plethysmography, which has been widely used for the diagnosis of DVT, relies on decreased electrical impedance as the leg becomes engorged with blood. Proximal venous obstruction interferes with the characteristic increased impedance when the tourniquets or cuffs are released. However, nonocclusive clot or extensive collateral circulation may prevent venous engorgement and lead to false-negative studies.[162] In addition, IPG cannot distinguish between intrinsic and extrinsic causes of venous obstruction. IPG will not detect clot in the internal iliac or gonadal veins.

Initially, there was a great deal of enthusiasm for IPG because of early reports that showed greater than 90 percent sensitivity and specificity.[163,164] Later studies demonstrated poorer results in the calf but claimed IPG to be efficacious when used in combination with radionuclide venograms, ultrasound, or serial IPG.[126,165,166] Cardella et al. reported less satisfactory results, with a specificity of 72 percent.[167] Another study investigating the utility of IPGs in screening for DVT in 381 patients was prematurely terminated because of 4 documented deaths from PE due to misdiagnosed proximal DVT.[103] Other studies have reported IPG's sensitivity for diagnosing DVT at less than 70 percent even with ^{125}I fibrinogen.[122,168] A recent review of the literature confirmed the poor sensitivity of IPG.[169]

Duplex ultrasound is currently considered by many authors to be the noninvasive technique of choice.[58,100,105,170] However, this technique is extremely operator-dependent, as evidenced by the reported range of sensitivities of 38 to 99 percent.[104,121,162,165,171–174] Ultrasound has a sensitivity of 38 to 67 percent for the diagnosis of DVT in high-risk asymptomatic patients.[104,121,139,174–176] A multicenter study involving seven large medical centers compared venography with duplex, compression, and color Doppler ultrasound for the diagnosis of DVT in both thighs of 385 consecutive patients 10 days after knee or hip total joint arthroplasty. Technically adequate conventional venograms were available in only 319 of the 385 patients, and DVT was identified in 25 percent (80 out of 319) of the patients tested. The DVTs were above the knee in 26 percent of the patients (21 out of 80). Compression, duplex, and color Doppler ultrasound of the proximal veins in the thigh had a sensitivity of 38 percent, a specificity of 92 percent, and a positive predictive value of 26 percent.[104] Similar findings were reported by another group that examined both thighs with compression, duplex, and color Doppler ultrasound in 100 asymptomatic patients who had craniot-

omies. Above the knee, DVT was identified in 13 percent of patients (13 out of 100) by venography. Ultrasound detected only 5 out of 13 DVTs and had 4 false positives, for a sensitivity of 38 percent and a positive predictive value of 56 percent.[121] From the data from these studies, ultrasound does not appear to be a sensitive test for routine screening of asymptomatic patients at increased risk for thromboembolic disease or for evaluating patients with abnormal but not high-probability V/Q scans. In addition, ultrasound does not routinely visualize the deep pelvic or profunda femoris veins, both of which are large potential sources of thromboemboli.[177]

Magnetic Resonance Imaging Diagnosis

The ability of MRI to evaluate blood flow[178–183] and to detect deep venous thrombosis with cross-sectional, spin-echo (SE) imaging has been previously reported.[184,185] With the SE technique, blood flow is typically hypointense or dark and clot appears as intermediate signal intensity or gray (Fig. 73-1). However, SE is unreliable for the routine diagnosis of clot because slow-flowing blood may mimic an intravascular tumor or clot and appear as gray or intermediate signal.[180,181] Therefore, a flow-sensitive technique termed *low-flip-angle gradient-echo imaging* is often used to evaluate arteries and veins. When combined with a "walking presaturation pulse," this technique can suppress signal from vessels with blood flowing in a given direction (e.g., superior-to-inferior for arteries in the lower extremities when a superior presaturation pulse is used).[179,186] Early MR venography (MRV) was performed using cross-sectional gradient-echo images of the venous system, but no projectional images were produced.[187–189] Although these studies reported sensitivities and specificities in the veins above the knee greater than 90 percent, cross-sectional MRV has not gained wide clinical acceptance for the diagnosis of DVT. The reasons for this limited clinical acceptance may be due in part to the multiple cross-sectional images, flow artifacts, the lack of projectional images, and low sensitivity below the knee of 70 to 80 percent.

In contrast to these cross-sectional techniques, projectional MRV requires maximizing signal from the moving spins of flowing blood in the veins while suppressing signal from the stationary spins in the surrounding soft tissues. A large body of literature exists on MR arteriography using two-dimensional time-of-flight magnetic resonance angiography (2D-TOF MRA).[182,190–197] In comparison, only the initial experiences with projectional MRV in small numbers of patients have recently been reported.[198–200] Unlike the arterial system, the venous system is characterized

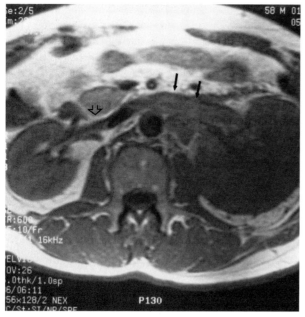

A

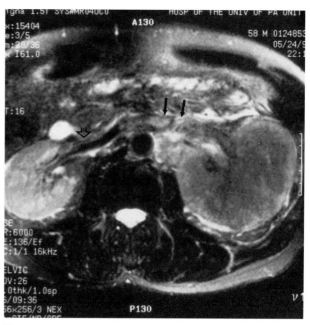

B

Figure 73-1. Left renal vein thrombosis in a 58-year-old man with renal cell carcinoma. (A) Transaxial T1-weighted spin-echo image (TR/TE 600/10 milliseconds) through the abdomen reveals an increased intermediate signal within an enlarged left renal vein (*black arrows*). The left kidney is enlarged, and there is a perihilar node secondary to renal cell carcinoma. There is hypointense signal from rapidly flowing blood in the inferior vena cava and aorta. However, the distal right renal vein has intermediate signal (*open arrow*) due to slow flow and inadequate saturation. The vein was patent on flow-sensitive gradient-echo imaging (not shown here) and on the T2-weighted fast spin-echo image. (B) T2-weighted fast spin-echo (FSE) image performed with fat saturation (TR/TE 136/6000 milliseconds) in the same patient. The left renal vein thrombus is hyperintense on this image. Flowing blood in the right renal vein, inferior vena cava, and aorta is hypointense. Although FSE is less sensitive to slow flow or in-plane flow, as seen in the right renal vein, this case demonstrates the lack of specificity in intermediate signal on spin-echo imaging. For arrows, see (A).

by (1) low pressures, (2) high capacitance, (3) thin-walled compressible vessels, (4) slower rates of flow, (5) variations in the rates and direction of flow, and (6) multiple collaterals. These differences from arterial flow require adjusting imaging parameters to optimize projectional MRV. Flow-related enhancement (FRE) depends on a complex relationship between slice thickness, flip angle, repetition time (TR), and flow rate. In general, thinner slices, lower flip angle, and longer TR allow for improved sensitivity to slow flow. However, if the TR is too long, there will not be any difference between the signal intensity of stationary tissue and flowing blood. Slices that are too thin will not have enough tissue in the imaged volume to provide enough signal for imaging with a given receiver coil. In addition, there is marked variation of the direction of venous flow due to respiration. These variables were systematically altered and optimized for a 30- to 45-minute MRV examination (Fig. 73-2).[200,201] The 2D-TOF protocol used spoiled gradient-echo imaging, and the optimized parameters were as follows:

Scanner	1.5 Tesla
TR/TE	33–45/7 milliseconds (minimum echo time available)
Field of view	26–28 cm
Matrix	256 × 128
Slice thickness	2.0–2.5 mm (0.7-mm overlap between slices)
Plane	Axial
Receiver bandwidth	32 kHz
Coil	Body coil or multicoil array if available
Saturation band	Superior walking saturation band spaced 8 cm from the imaging slice
Average	1 signal average
Flow compensation	On

This MRV technique was used to study 126 venous systems that had conventional ascending venography. Axial 2D-TOF images were reconstructed into projection MR venograms with a maximum intensity projec-

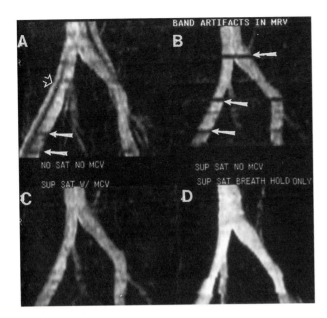

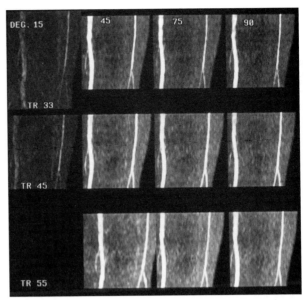

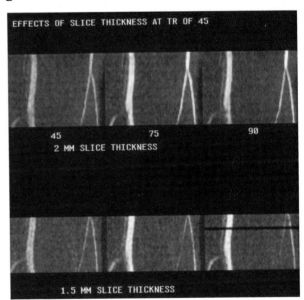

Figure 73-2. MRV optimization. (A to D) Effects of saturation bands and respiration on 2D-TOF MRA in a single volunteer. (A) No saturation bands were used in this 2D-TOF pelvic MR angiogram. Both arteries and veins are visualized. The parameters were flip angle 45 degrees, TR/TE 33/7 milliseconds, 2.5-mm slice thickness, 28-cm field of view, and matrix 256 × 128. The right iliac artery is free of significant artifacts (*open arrow*). The right iliac vein has a series of hypointense horizontal bands (*arrows*) due to slow flow produced by expiration. (B) The study was repeated with a "walking" superior presaturation band. The same parameters were used in this 2D-TOF MR venogram. The superior saturation band was applied 5 mm superior to the imaging plane. This walking superior saturation band suppresses the arterial signal and results in an MR venogram. However, the spacing of 5 mm between the saturation band and imaging plane leads to increased horizontal hypointense bands because of saturated venous blood entering the imaging plane during expiration. This effect is improved or eliminated with increased spacing between the saturation band and the imaging plane or with breath-hold imaging. (C) The MRV was repeated, but with the spacing of the superior saturation band applied 80 mm superior to the imaging plane instead of 5 mm. Note the decreased horizontal banding when compared with the previous image. (D) The MRV was repeated with the same parameters as in (B), but the images were acquired in multiple breath holds. Note the lack of horizontal banding despite a 5-mm spacing of the superior saturation pulse from the imaging plane. In addition, there is marked increased signal intensity during breath holding because of the more constant venous flow rates during apnea. Variations in flow rate during image acquisition lead to decreased signal due to amplitude modulation. (E) Effects of varying flip angle and repetition time (TR) on MRV of tibial vein of a normal volunteer. The slice thickness is 2.9 mm. The columns denote the degree of flip angle used, and the rows are the TR used in milliseconds. The best contrast-background ratio was obtained with a 45-millisecond TR and a 45- to 75-degree flip angle. (F) Effects of slice thickness and flip angle with a fixed TR of 45 milliseconds. The first row was obtained with a slice thickness of 2.0 mm and the second row with a slice thickness of 1.5 mm. Flip angles of 45, 75, and 90 degrees were used. The best MR venogram in terms of contrast-background ratio is the image with a 1.5-mm slice thickness and a 90-degree flip angle; however, the vessels with in-plane flow are best seen with a 45-degree flip angle at the same slice thickness.

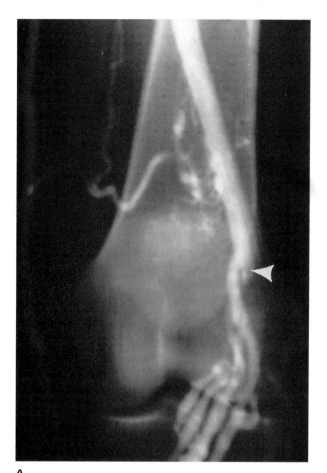

A

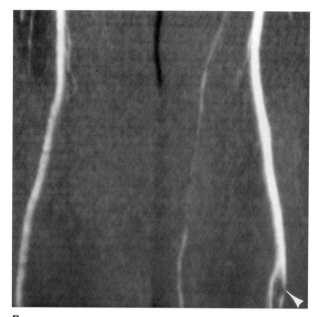

B

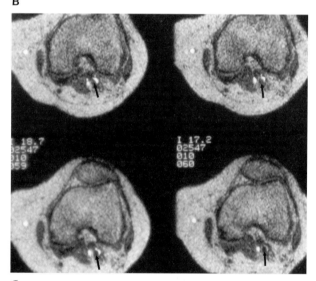

C

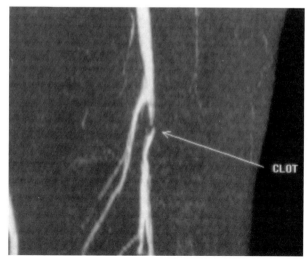

D

Figure 73-3. A 55-year-old woman with swelling of the left calf. (A) Ascending contrast venogram at the level of the knee fails to opacify the popliteal vein, presumably secondary to DVT (*arrowhead*). There is reconstitution of the popliteal vein by muscular branches approximately at the level of the adductor canal. The saphenous vein is seen medially. (B) MR venogram of both lower extremities at approximately the level of the knee and midthigh performed with 2D-TOF (axial slices 2.5-mm thick, TR/TE 33/7 milliseconds, flip angle 45 degrees). Frontal projection reveals a normal-appearing popliteal vein and superficial femoral vein on the right. On the left lower extremity, a muscular branch is seen, as well as faint visualization of the saphenous vein medially. A portion of the popliteal vein is poorly seen, secondary to a DVT (*arrowhead*). (C) Four contiguous transverse axial source images from 2D-TOF MRV. These images of the left lower extremity reveal hypointense signal or a dark area in the left popliteal vein, representing acute clot (*arrow*), with hyperintense signal from flowing blood in the popliteal vein. The muscular branch is also seen, and the saphenous vein is seen medially. (D) Higher-resolution frontal projection image of the knee was performed with an extremity coil and the same parameters, except that a 16-cm instead of a 26-cm field of view was used. The higher resolution improves evaluation of the saphenous vein, which is better seen on these images than on the body coil images in previous figures. The popliteal vein clot (*arrow*) and muscular branches are again demonstrated.

tion (MIP). The criterion for an MR diagnosis of acute DVT was

1. a central signal void with surrounding hyperintense signal on five contiguous axial 2D-TOF images,
2. no flow-related enhancement identified in the vessel in question and multiple collaterals on MRV images on 2D-TOF, or
3. an enlarged vessel with increased signal on the spin-echo images with no flow-related enhancement of the vessel in question on the source 2D-TOF images.

Deep venous thrombosis can be accurately diagnosed by MRV (Figs. 73-3, 73-4, and 73-5). The clots appear hypointense or dark when compared with flowing blood.[189,202–206]

Projections of MRVs are useful in demonstrating collaterals, in providing a general road map of the venous anatomy, and in identifying chronic disease with a small number of images. These MIP images are use-ful in communicating with referring clinicians, but all DVTs were identified on the source and reformatted images. The MIP reconstructions completely or partially obscured nonocclusive clot in 35 percent of cases[202,207] because of the way in which the MIP algorithm reconstructs axial or source images into a projection image. The MIP reconstructed image is produced by computer-generated parallel rays that trace through each axial source image. The brightest pixel along each ray is the value of the pixel on the projected image.[208] Therefore, when hypointense clot is completely surrounded by bright hyperintense flowing blood, it is the bright pixels representing the flowing blood that are projected and the information of the hypointense pixels is lost in the MIP reconstructed image.[209] An alternative reconstruction technique described by Listerud, termed *summation of intensities following soft thresholding* (SIST), is less prone to this problem (Fig. 73-6; see also Fig. 73-5).[209] Unless or until better reconstruction algorithms are developed and are commercially available, axial or reformatted images must be carefully scrutinized.

Figure 73-4. Proximal DVT involving a right lower extremity in a 65-year-old woman. (A) MR venogram performed with 2D-TOF imaging of both lower extremities from the level of the adductor canal to the level of the inferior vena cava. The left superficial femoral vein and profunda femoris veins are well seen, as are the hypogastric, external, and common iliac veins. There is left iliac artery compression on the common iliac vein. On the right, only a small segment of the common iliac vein is visualized (*arrowheads*). None of the named deep veins are seen in the right lower extremity, and multiple collaterals are identified. Marked edema was seen on the axial images (not shown). Ascending venography did not identify the proximal extent of the thrombus. (B) A descending venogram was performed at the time of filter placement. On the right, the venogram confirms the occlusion of the internal and external iliac veins and the proximal extent of thrombus (*arrows*) in this patient, as was identified on the MRI study. A caval filter was placed following this study.

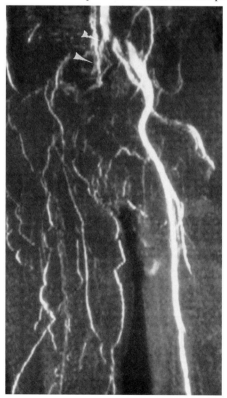

A

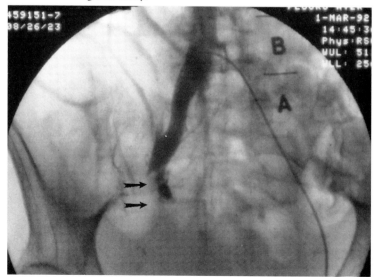

B

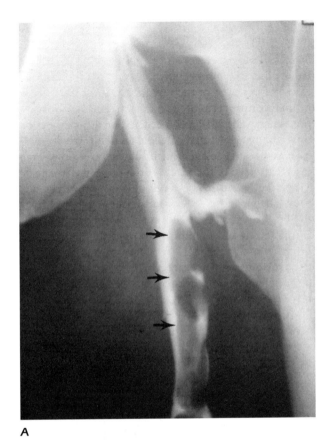

A

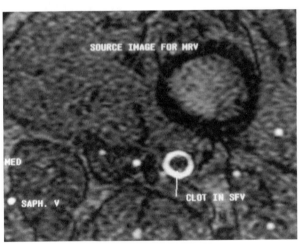

D

B   **C**

Figure 73-5. DVT in the superficial femoral vein obscured by maximum intensity projection (MIP) image. (A) Descending venogram reveals the proximal extent of the clot at the level of the superficial femoral vein immediately below the level of the profunda femoris vein. The proximal extent was not defined on ascending venography but was correctly demonstrated on MRI. (B) MIP image of an MRV performed in the same patient reveals several hypointense areas within the superficial femoral vein. However, these appear to be isolated, and the extent of the clot is not well appreciated. The clot is obscured in part by the MIP. (C) Another projection algorithm performed on the same MRV data using summation of intensities following soft thresholding. This image reveals the free-floating clot (*arrows*) with better detail than the MIP and more closely resembles the appearance of the venogram. Hypointense signal is seen to the left of the vein secondary to subcutaneous fat. (D) Axial source image of the 2D-TOF MR venogram demonstrates a hypointense signal in the superficial femoral vein (*arrow*). The clot is completely surrounded by hyperintense signal from flowing blood. For this reason, the MIP failed to demonstrate a clot in this region. No ray can be drawn through the vessel, which does not encounter hyperintense signal, and this hyperintense signal is what is projected on an MIP. The dark clot is obscured.

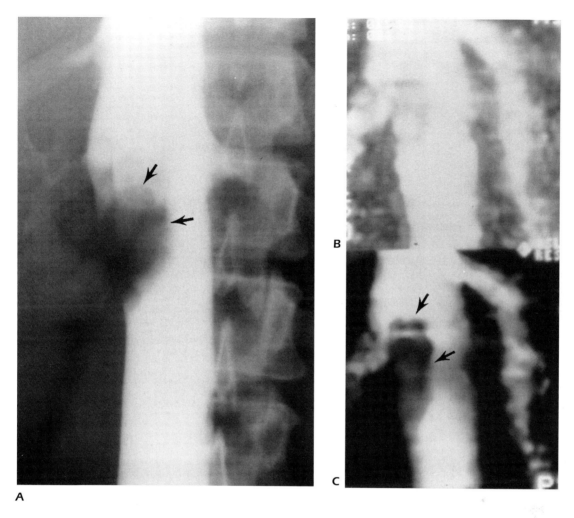

Figure 73-6. Inferior vena caval filling defect in a 45-year-old woman secondary to an intravascular leiomyoma. (A) A cavogram was performed on a 45-year-old patient following a hysterectomy for fibroids. At the time of hysterectomy, a leiomyoma was identified extending into the right gonadal vein. The cavogram reveals a filling defect within the inferior vena cava on the right secondary to the leiomyoma (*arrows*). (B) MIP of a small segment of an MR venogram obscures the hypointense tumor thrombus. These projection images obscure the leiomyoma. (C) Summation of signal intensity reconstruction of the same data set, which better demonstrates the hypointense signal from the intravascular leiomyoma (*arrows*). Following oophorectomy the tumor regressed over a 3-year period. Typically these tumors require resection because they tend to grow and may embolize.

The profunda femoris veins were identified to their first branch in 216 out of 220 deep femoral veins examined by MRV (98 percent). The internal iliac veins were visualized to their first branch in 196 out of 220 in the supine position (89 percent). All external and common iliac veins examined were visualized by MRV (Fig. 73-7).

Effects of positioning were demonstrated when 24 patients who had abnormalities noted on the supine MRV had repeat images in the prone or prone oblique position. There was improved visualization of the hypogastric veins in 23 out of 24 cases when they were not demonstrated in the supine position. Altered positioning eliminated flow artifacts resembling clot, which accounted for 4 out of 5 false positives (Figs. 73-8 and 73-9). About 8 percent of patients were noted to have abdominal and pelvic venous anomalies, such as duplicated inferior vena cava, retroaortic renal veins, azygous continuation, or anomalous drainage of the internal iliac veins. The anomalous internal iliac vein drained into the contralateral common iliac vein or were duplicated in about 2 percent of cases (Fig. 73-10).[202,203] Knowledge of these anomalies can be important for assessing patients for potential pelvic DVT or for placing filters.

MRV reliably visualizes the profunda femoris and pelvic veins, which are large potential sources for emboli or varices that no other conventional technique

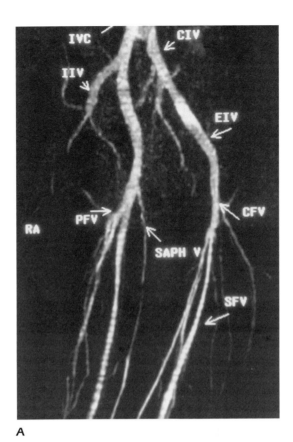

A

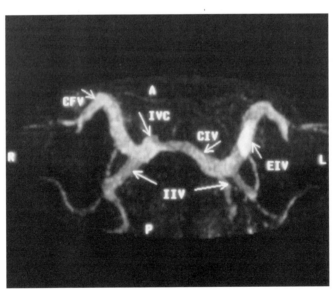

B

Figure 73-7. Normal MR venogram. Evaluation of hypogastric veins and profunda femoris veins. (A) Oblique projection image of an MR venogram demonstrating normal venous anatomy. On the right is the inferior vena cava (*IVC*) and the internal iliac vein (IIV). On the left is a duplicated internal iliac venous system: *CIV*, common iliac vein; *EIV*, external iliac vein. The profunda veins (*PFV*) are seen bilaterally. The saphenous veins (*SAPH V*) are also seen in both lower extremities. The superficial femoral veins (*SFV*) are seen bilaterally and are normal. (B) Axial projection of the same patient. Note the duplicated internal iliac vein on the left.

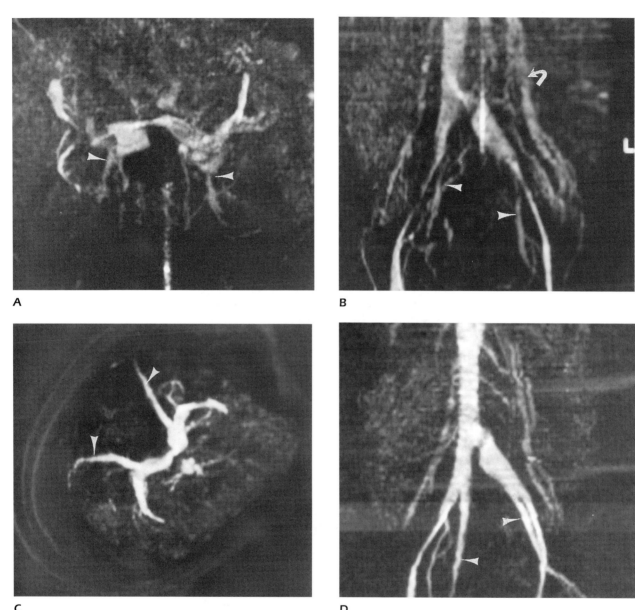

Figure 73-8. Effects of positioning on MRV in a postpartum patient. (A) Supine MR venogram, axial projection, reveals diminutive hypogastric veins bilaterally (*arrowheads*). (B) Supine MR venogram, frontal projection of the same patient, reveals decreased flow and small hypogastric veins. The external iliac veins bilaterally appear compressed (*arrowheads*). The possibility of DVT was considered in this patient. The gonadal vein on the left is enlarged (*curved arrow*). (C) Axial projection of the same patient, who was reimaged in the prone decubitus position. Padding was placed under the abdomen to avoid compression of the venous structures by the large postpartum uterus. The internal and external iliac veins are much better demonstrated (*arrowheads*) than in the previous images. (D) Prone oblique MR venogram, frontal projection. The internal and external iliac veins appear normal, and the gonadal veins are less well seen on these images because of preferential blood flow through the iliac veins (*arrowheads*). The uterine compression of the iliac veins and compression of the gluteal veins were relieved with the altered positioning.

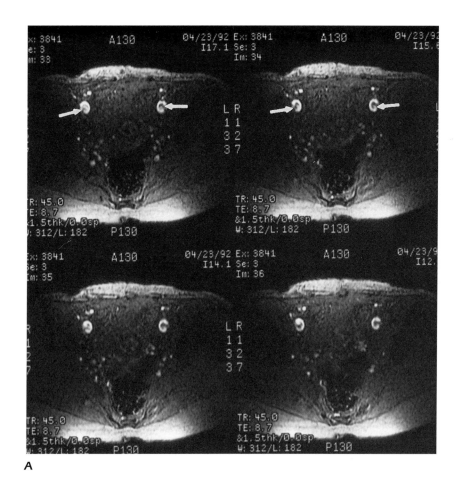

A

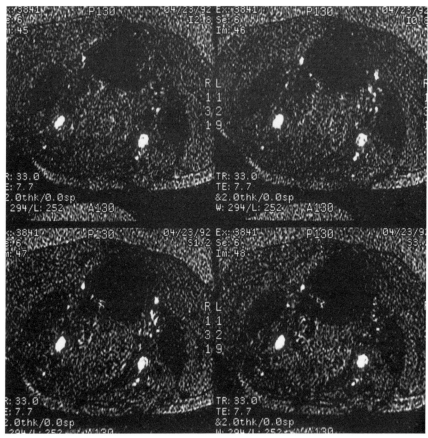

B

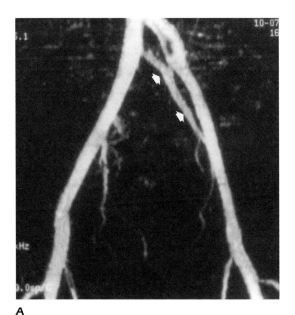

A

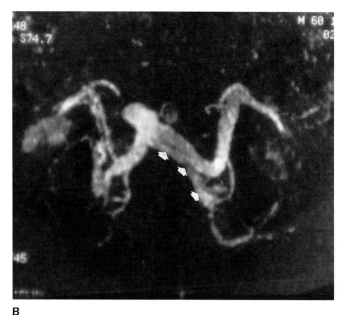

B

Figure 73-10. Anomalous internal iliac vein. (A) Frontal oblique projection of an MR venogram in the pelvis reveals a small duplicated right internal iliac vein. The left internal iliac vein drains into the right common iliac vein (*arrows*).

No other hypogastric vein on the left is identified. (B) Axial projection of an MR venogram demonstrating an anomalous left internal iliac vein draining into the right common iliac vein (*arrows*).

can routinely image (Figs. 73-11 and 73-12).[202] MRV can visualize these vessels because it detects flow. However, conventional contrast venography does not typically detect these vessels because it depends on the opacification of a vascular lumen with contrast, and contrast is not delivered to the vascular beds drained by the profunda femoris or hypogastric veins during an ascending contrast venogram. Contrast is injected into a dorsal vein of the foot and drains into the calf veins to the popliteal and then the superficial femoral veins. Unopacified blood from the thigh drains into the profunda femoris vein and then into the superficial femoral vein, diluting the contrast in the common femoral vein. The dilution of contrast is repeated again when the external iliac vein receives unopacified blood draining from the hypogastric veins to form the common femoral vein. The profunda femoris and hypogastric veins can therefore only be studied with descending venography using retrograde injection via catheter. However, this is rarely done because it is more invasive and does not evaluate large areas of venous anatomy. Ultrasound does not reliably evaluate these areas be-

cause they cannot be compressed and are too distant for the use of high-frequency probes, and bowel gas interferes with visualization of the pelvic veins.

A potential problem with MRV is the imaging of patients with implanted metallic devices. Over 190 patients following hip arthroplasty have been successfully studied with MRV and conventional contrast venography, with sensitivities of 100 percent and specificities of 98 percent.[198,202,203] Although 2D-TOF may have short segments of signal void in the region of a metallic prosthesis because of dephasing from distortion of the magnetic field (B_0), these areas were successfully imaged with SE and fast spin-echo (FSE) sequences. These sequences are much less prone to B_0 artifact than standard gradient-echo techniques and ruled out DVT in these small areas.[210] Alternatively, fast gradient-echo sequences with extremely short echo times of less than 2 milliseconds can also be used to image some of these patients. The shorter echo time is less prone to B_0 artifact because there is less time for dephasing produced by inhomogeneity in the magnetic field (Fig. 73-13).[211]

◄ **Figure 73-9.** Effects of positioning on MRV in a postpartum patient. (A) Four contiguous source images obtained in the supine position show bilateral hypointensities in the common femoral and external iliac veins (*arrows*), initially misdiagnosed as clot. Following bilateral venograms, which were normal, the patient was reimaged with MRI. These re-

peat images revealed the same filling defects the following day. The hypointensities persisted despite the use of single-dose gadolinium, multicoil imaging, and the use of smaller pixel size. (B) When the patient was placed in a prone oblique position, the hypointense pseudothrombi were eliminated.

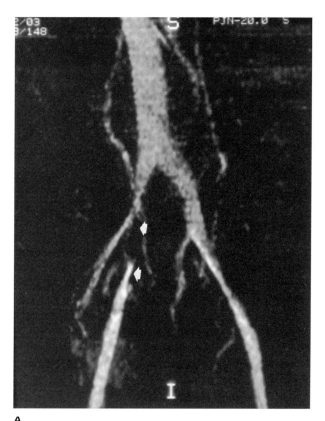

A

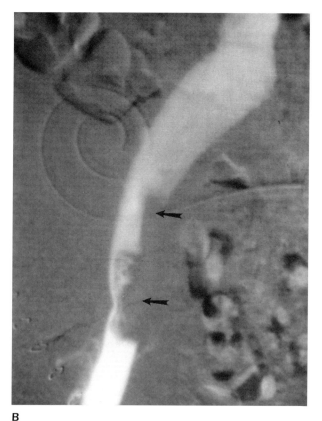

B

Figure 73-11. Right external iliac vein thrombus in a peritoneal dialysis patient with an intermediate probability ventilation perfusion scan. (A) Frontal projection MR venogram reveals a signal void in the right external iliac vein, which represented an isolated pelvic vein DVT (*arrows*). (B) Venogram performed via a right common femoral venous injection confirms the MRV diagnosis of a clot isolated in the right external iliac vein (*arrows*).

Figure 73-12. MRV of perirectal varices before and after a transjugular intrahepatic portosystemic shunt (TIPS) procedure. (A) Axial projection of an MR venogram reveals the external iliac vein (*EIV*) on the right and left and also the common iliac vein (*CIV*). The inferior vena cava was not visualized on these images. The internal iliac vein (*IIV*) is seen draining a large hyperintense tangle of perirectal varices. The patient was bleeding profusely from these perirectal varices secondary to portal hypertension and underwent a TIPS procedure to control the bleeding. (B) Repeat MR venogram 24 hours after the TIPS procedure reveals a marked decrease in the perirectal varices. MRV allows for noninvasive imaging of the pelvic veins, which are not normally imaged by interventional techniques.

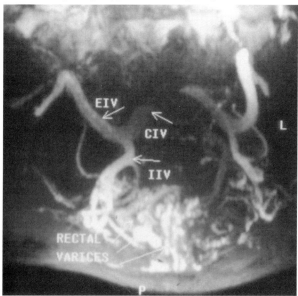

A

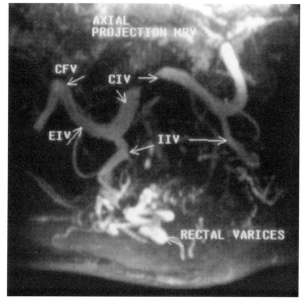

B

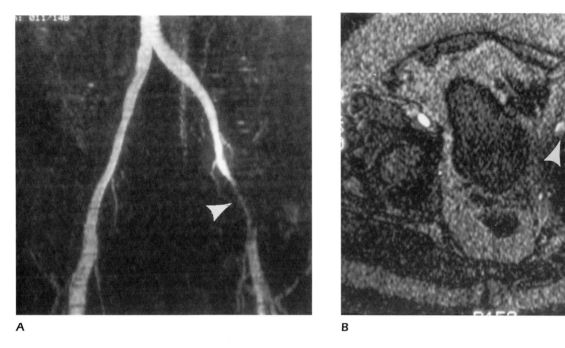

A

B

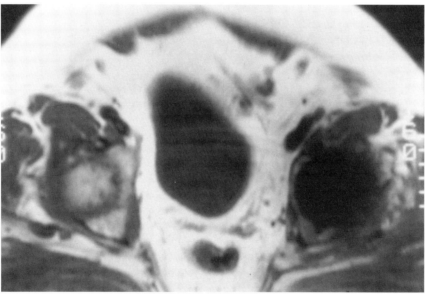

C

Figure 73-13. MRV in a patient following a right hip arthroplasty. (A) MR venogram, MIP image performed with 2D-TOF, reveals a pseudonarrowing of the left common femoral and external iliac veins (*arrowhead*) due to B₀ artifact from the hip prostheses. However, this diagnosis cannot be made from the projection images, and the source images must be scrutinized. (B) Axial source image from the same patient reveals a hypointensive dark region in the area of the left hip secondary to the prosthetic joint. Although there is hypointense signal in the common femoral vein (*arrowhead*), there is still signal demonstrating a normal common femoral vein. However, in some cases the artifact is so severe that it completely obscures the vein. (C) Spin-echo imaging performed in the same patient (TR/TE 300/13 milliseconds) is much less susceptible to the metallic artifacts because of the refocusing 180-degree pulses used. There is minimal artifact from the hip prostheses, and both artery and vein on the left are well seen.

Patients with intravascular filters can be successfully imaged with MRV at 1.5 Tesla for clot superior to the filter or for inferior vena cava occlusion.[201,212,213] Most of the filters currently in use produce minimal artifact, and the individual struts or wires can often be seen with MRI. The percutaneously placed Greenfield filter, which contains beta-3 titanium alloy, has the least artifact.[214] The Simon nitinol filter, Amplatz (MP32-N) filter, Vena Tech (LGM) filter[215] produce minimal artifact.[201,214,216,217] However, devices composed of stainless steel alloys, such as the Bird's Nest filter and the early Greenfield filter, produce significant B_0 artifact and dephasing, resulting in a large black area around the filter.[214] Watanabe et al. reported similar problems of imaging the Bird's Nest filter and Gianturco coils.[218] This does not preclude imaging these patients, but evaluation in or near the filter will be limited. There are no reports to date of caval perforation or migration of filters associated with imaging patients or animals with these filters in place.

Some patients have relative or absolute contraindications to MRI. These include patients with implanted pacemakers, implanted defibrillators, implanted intracochlear devices, intraorbital metallic foreign bodies, and intracranial aneurysm clips. Patients with relative contraindications include pregnant women, patients with shrapnel, and patients with thermodilution Swan-Ganz catheters. Unstable patients who can be transported for angiographic procedures can be imaged with MRI in the hospital if there is adequate MRI-compatible monitoring equipment and experienced medical staff available to monitor the patient. Most claustrophobic patients can be imaged if adequately sedated and monitored.

MRI Characterization of Thrombus

Early work by Gomori et al. demonstrated the ability of MRI to image intracranial bleeds with varying signal intensity on spin-echo imaging.[219-222] Some investigators have reported some success in imaging experimental clots in vitro and in the veins of dogs.[223,224] Others have been less successful in differentiating acute from chronic intravascular clot based on signal characteristics.[225] Many of the differences observed in vitro for intravascular clot may be due to experimental artifact,[226] since some investigators have failed to reliably differentiate acute from chronic intravascular clot based on signal intensity alone.[188,202,204,227-229] Both acute and chronic thrombus are dark or hypointense on MRV relative to flowing blood when the parameters described previously are used.[189,201-204,206,230] Acute clot can be differentiated from chronic clot on the basis of perivascular edema and nonretracted thrombus.[188,202] Other techniques such as magnetization transfer may be useful in differentiating chronic from acute clot.[228,229]

Several pitfalls may result in false-positive results with MRV. Yousem et al. described hyperintense-appearing clot that was indistinguishable from flowing blood in the venous sinuses of the head on gradient-echo images.[231] However, the parameters that were used differed from the 2D-TOF MRV parameters. The authors have seen only one case of intermediately increased signal in a clot, but it was still hypointense relative to flowing blood. Very slow or turbulent flow can be confused with clot.

Remedies for differentiating flow artifacts from clot include altered positioning, magnetic tagging techniques,[232] or gadolinium DTPA–enhanced fast 3D-spoiled gradient-echo techniques (see Figs. 73-9 and 73-10).[211]

In some cases MRI can differentiate bland thrombus from tumor thrombus. Both tumor and bland thrombus appear dark on gradient-echo images; however, after intravascular contrast (gadolinium DTPA) tumor thrombus may enhance (Figs. 73-14 through 73-17).[233-235] Arterial signal has also been detected in tumor thrombus by ultrasound[236] and has been described as subtle enhancement in tumor thrombus with CT.[237] The diagnostic criterion for tumor thrombus is

1. uniform enhancement,
2. an enhancement pattern similar to the primary tumor, or
3. tumor invading beyond the vessel wall.

Lack of enhancement or extravascular extension does not exclude the diagnosis of tumor thrombus. An example is a poorly vascular nonaggressive tumor such as a vascular leiomyoma (see Fig. 73-6). Bland thrombus does not enhance (see Fig. 73-14), but chronic bland thrombus may develop channels through the thrombus. Contrast percolating through these channels will produce heterogeneous irregular strands of enhancement. This is a potential pitfall, since similar enhancement patterns may be seen with some tumor thrombus.

Evaluation of Renal and Portal Venous Systems

One of the main uses of renal MRI has been to evaluate the intravascular extent of tumor thrombus for the staging of renal cell carcinoma.[238] For this purpose MRI was shown to be equal to cavography.[239,240] It was

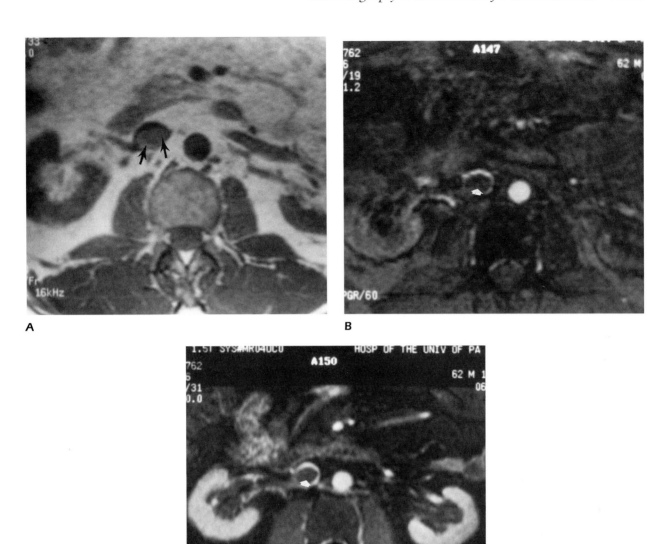

Figure 73-14. Bland thrombus in inferior vena cava. (A) T1-weighted spin-echo (TR/TE 383/10 milliseconds) image through the kidneys reveals an area of intermediate signal intensity in the inferior vena cava (*arrows*), representing thrombus. There is a small rim of hypointense signal around it caused by rapid flow. The aorta is a normal-appearing hypointense signal void. The signal in the inferior vena cava could be due to slow flow or to tumor thrombus. (B) Single axial image from a 2D-TOF acquisition without saturation reveals hyperintense signal in the aorta and a crescentic region of hyperintense signal in the inferior vena cava representing thrombus (*arrow*). Bland thrombus can-not be differentiated from tumor thrombus on these images. (C) Following the injection of gadolinium DTPA, repeat axial images were obtained with a fat-saturated spoiled gradient-echo sequence. The kidneys are now enhanced, and there is hyperintense signal in both the aorta and the inferior vena cava. A crescentic area of increased signal is seen in the inferior vena cava, with a central signal void extending into the renal vein on the right representing bland thrombus (*arrow*). The lack of enhancement within the thrombus is suggestive but not diagnostic of bland thrombus. The failure to see enhancement within a thrombus does not exclude a diagnosis of tumor thrombus.

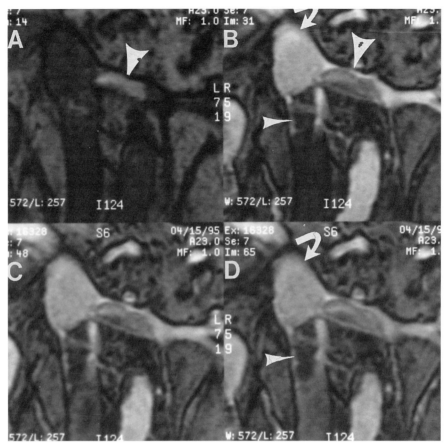

Figure 73-15. Bland thrombus and tumor thrombus in a patient with renal cell carcinoma. (A) Unenhanced coronal gradient-echo image reveals hyperintense signal in the right renal vein (*arrowhead*). The inferior vena cava is otherwise hypointense, as is a small portion of the aorta, because of the saturation effects of this sequence. (B) Arterial and early venous phase following the intravenous injection of 40 ml of gadolinium shows hyperintense signal in the aorta. The left renal vein thrombus is hypointense to the surrounding blood (*large arrowhead*). There is no evidence of enhancement when compared to the precontrast study. An enhancing mass is seen within the inferior vena cava (*curved arrow*), which represents tumor thrombus from the right kidney. The right renal vein is not visualized on these images. Inferior to the enhancing mass is hypointense signal surrounded by enhanced blood in the IVC representing bland thrombus (*small arrowhead*). (C and D) Images from the same patient obtained later to ensure that no enhancement was identified within the regions of bland thrombus. Only a small portion of the right kidney is visualized on these images.

more sensitive than CT or cavography for the detection and evaluation of proximal extent of tumor thrombus in 20 patients with surgical correlation (see Figs. 73-14 through 73-16).[241]

MRI can evaluate portal venous flow rates and direction in patients with portal hypertension.[242–245] In

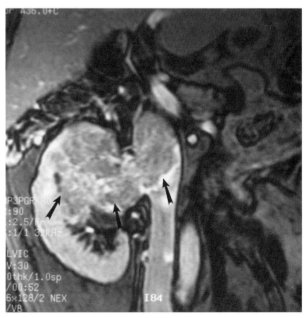

Figure 73-16. Tumor thrombus. Coronal image following the injection of 20 ml of gadolinium DTPA reveals hyperintense signal in the kidney. There is a large heterogeneously enhancing mass in the upper pole of the right kidney representing a renal cell carcinoma. The mass is seen extending into a dilated renal vein and inferior vena cava (*arrows*).

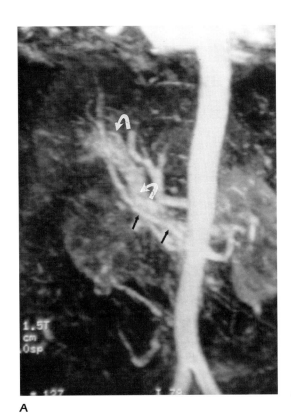

A

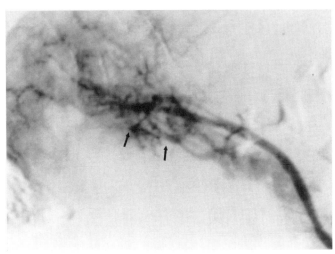

B

Figure 73-17. Pre-TIPS evaluation reveals a hepatocellular carcinoma with arterial venous shunting. (A) Ultrafast 3D spoiled gradient-echo MR angiogram (30-second acquisition, TR/TE 4.8/1.1 milliseconds) performed after 60 ml of intravenous gadolinium DTPA. The study reveals arterial venous shunting into the portal vein due to an unsuspected hepatocellular carcinoma (*curved arrows*). There is a replaced right hepatic artery (*arrows*). (B) Digital subtraction angiogram confirmed the diagnosis of a hepatocellular carcinoma and arterial venous shunting into the portal vein (*arrows*).

addition, MRI can evaluate portal venous patency and determine the presence of varices, which are difficult to evaluate with other imaging techniques. MRI may be helpful in assessing patients before or after a transjugular intrahepatic portosystemic shunt (TIPS) procedure.[202,246–249] In addition, it can be used for staging hepatocellular carcinoma and detecting tumor thrombus (see Figs. 73-12, 73-17, and 73-18).[250–253]

Figure 73-18. Portal venous hypertension. (A) Oblique projection of an ultrafast 3D spoiled gradient-echo MR angiogram (30-second acquisition, TR/TE 4.8/1.1 milliseconds) performed after 60 ml of intravenous gadolinium DTPA. Study reveals shunting of contrast to the spleen, evidenced by the marked splenic enhancement with no evidence of hepatic enhancement in the early portal phase (*arrow* = portal vein). The caudate lobe is the only portion of the liver with appreciable enhancement (*thin arrowhead*). Multiple varices are seen in the paraesophageal and splenic hilar region (*short arrowheads*). (B) Frontal projection of the same patient.

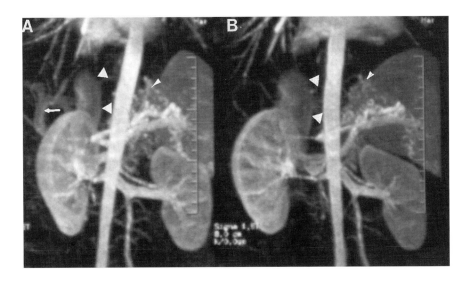

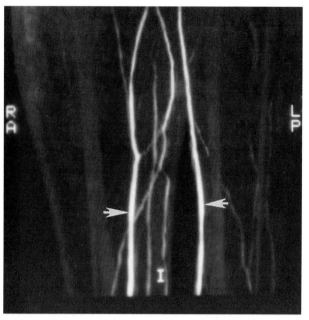

A

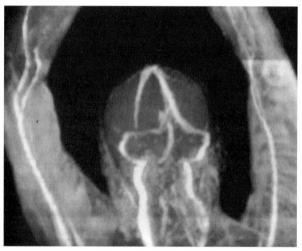

B

Figure 73-19. Mapping of the arm and saphenous veins for potential graft material. (A) Bilateral lower extremity imaging from the ankle to the knee performed in a head coil. The extremities were heated and an MR venogram was performed without the use of tourniquets. The saphenous veins are seen bilaterally (*arrows*). (B) MR venogram of the upper extremities performed in a patient with arms over the head. A single saturation band was applied over the heart to eliminate arterial flow. The veins in both arms are well visualized, as are the jugular veins and the sinuses within the calvarium.

Venous Mapping for Evaluating Vein Vascular Grafts

Identifying veins for potential graft material in bypass surgery has been performed in the legs and upper extremities with 2D-TOF MRV (Fig. 73-19).[254]

MRV of the Brachiocephalic Veins

Brachiocephalic veins have become a more common source for pulmonary emboli because of the use of central venous catheters.[123] In addition, evaluation of these vessels for intravenous access has become important for patients who require long-term chemotherapy, hyperalimentation, or antibiotics. Finn et al. and Erdman et al. have reported sensitivities of over 90 percent for 2D-TOF MRV of the brachiocephalic veins.[188,255] However, these techniques require 6 to 10 minutes per acquisition, and it is often necessary to perform both axial and sagittal acquisitions to achieve saturation effects on veins with in-plane flow.

New MRV Techniques: Contrast MRV

Creasy et al. described the use of gadolinium-enhanced 3D-gradient MR angiography.[256] The authors have used a faster version of this technique to image both arteries and veins.[211] This technique is less susceptible to signal dropout from turbulent flow or from metallic B_0 artifact because of the markedly reduced echo time of conventional 2D-TOF, from 7.0 to 1.1 milliseconds. In addition, the technique better visualizes vascular structures with slow flow because it depends on the presence of contrast only (Figs. 73-17, 73-18, and 73-20). It does not have the problems of saturating flow within vessels that are in the same plane of acquisition, and it has minimal pulsation artifact from cardiac motion. This technique can be performed in 10- to 30-second acquisitions to evaluate the brachiocephalic veins (Fig. 73-21). Because of saturation effects on vessels with flow in the same plane of acquisition with 2D-TOF, the same study with 2D-TOF may require two separate acquisitions in the axial and sagittal planes of 6 to 9 minutes each. Three-dimensional MRV can be performed with less contrast than 3D MRA if the venous system to be studied is cannulated and injected with 20 ml of gadolinium DTPA diluted with 40 ml of 0.9 percent saline. Full-strength gadolinium will produce T_2 shortening and cause the intravascular signal to be dark.

Summary

1. MRV is an accurate, noninvasive method for diagnosing deep venous thrombosis in the veins of the thigh and pelvis. The pelvis and both lower extremities can be studied in 30 to 45 minutes. This is

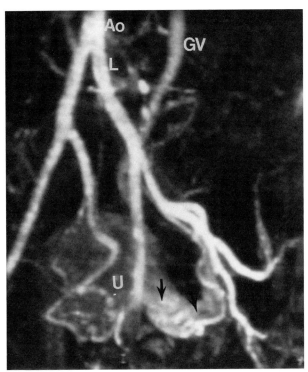

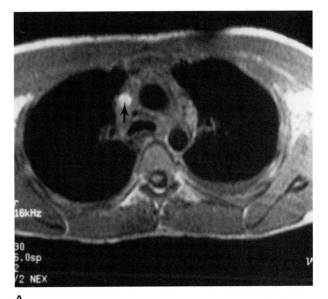

A

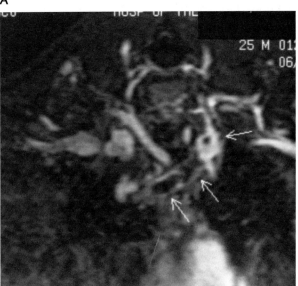

B

Figure 73-20. Varicocele in a woman demonstrated with an ultrafast 3D spoiled gradient-echo angiogram performed after the injection of 60 ml of gadolinium DTPA. The aorta (*Ao*) and iliac vessels (*L*, common iliac artery) are well seen. There is a large tangle of vessels in the broad ligament on the left representing a varicocele (*arrows*) and early visualization of a large left gonadal vein (*GV*). The uterus is enhancing normally (*U*). 2D-TOF images failed to demonstrate the varicocele, but saturation bands did confirm occasional retrograde flow in the gonadal vein with Valsalva maneuvers. This varicocele was felt to be the source of emboli in a patient with a patent foramen ovale and two embolic strokes that occurred during sexual intercourse.

Figure 73-21. Subclavian vein and superior vena cava thrombosis. (A) Transaxial cardiac gated T1-weighted image through the chest reveals hyperintense signal in the superior vena cava (*arrow*) secondary to thrombosis in a patient with protein C deficiency. Signal voids are seen in the ascending and descending aorta for comparison. (B) Coronal reformatted image from an ultrafast 3D spoiled gradient-echo image (after 60 ml of gadolinium) reveals hypointense thrombus extending from the subclavian vein into the brachiocephalic vein (*arrows*). The study was performed in 30 seconds.

important because clot is bilateral in 14 to 30 percent of cases.

2. MRV reliably demonstrates the internal iliac and deep femoral veins, both of which are large potential sources of emboli and are not evaluated with ultrasound or contrast venography.

3. Projectional MRV provides an overview of anatomy and collaterals with a small number of images. However, the maximum intensity projection technique obscures clots. Therefore, axial images must be carefully scrutinized.

4. MRV with spin-echo imaging can be performed in patients with prosthetic joints.

5. Inflow and compression are significant potential pitfalls that may be alleviated with altered positioning.

6. MRV can better demonstrate proximal extent of clot than can ascending contrast venography.

7. MRV can be used for assessing veins for possible graft material.

8. MRV with gadolinium can differentiate bland from tumor thrombus.

9. MRV with gadolinium-enhanced 3D fast spoiled gradient-echo imaging is a more rapid method of imaging the central veins for DVT and varices than 2D-TOF.

References

1. Freiman DG, Suyemoto J, Wesseler S. Frequency of pulmonary thromboembolism in man. N Engl J Med 1965;290: 1278–1286.
2. Schuman LM. The epidemiology of thromboembolic disorders: a review. J Chronic Dis 1965;18:815–845.
3. Atik M. Venous thrombotic disease. In: Moore WS, ed. Vascular surgery: a comprehensive review. 2nd ed. Orlando: Grune & Stratton, 1986:1043–1091.
4. Roberts HJ. Controversies and enigmas in thrombophlebitis and pulmonary embolism: perspectives on alleged overdiagnosis. Angiology 1980;31:686–699.
5. Johnson BF, Manzo RA, Bergelin RO, Strandness D Jr. Relationship between changes in the deep venous system and the development of the postthrombotic syndrome after an acute episode of lower limb deep vein thrombosis: a one- to six-year follow-up. J Vasc Surg 1995;21:307–312.
6. Lohr JM, Kerr TM, Lutter KS, Cranley RD, Spirtoff K, Cranley JJ. Lower extremity calf thrombosis: to treat or not to treat? [published erratum appears in J Vasc Surg 1992;15(2): 323]. J Vasc Surg 1991;14:618–623.
7. Meissner MH, Manzo RA, Bergelin RO, Markel A, Strandness D Jr. Deep venous insufficiency: the relationship between lysis and subsequent reflux. J Vasc Surg 1993;18:596–605.
8. Meissner MH, Manzo RA, Bergelin RO, Strandness D Jr. Venous diameter and compliance after deep venous thrombosis. Thromb Haemostasis 1994;72:372–376.
9. Monreal M, Martorell A, Callejas JM, et al. Venographic assessment of deep vein thrombosis and risk of developing postthrombotic syndrome: a prospective study. J Intern Med 1993;233:233–238.
10. van Bemmelen PS, Bedford G, Beach K, Strandness D Jr. Functional status of the deep venous system after an episode of deep venous thrombosis. Ann Vasc Surg 1990;4:455–459.
11. Harmon B. Deep vein thrombosis: a perspective on anatomy and venographic analysis. J Thorac Imaging 1989;4:15–19.
12. Anderson F Jr, Wheeler HB, Goldberg RJ, et al. A population-based perspective of the hospital incidence and case-fatality rates of deep vein thrombosis and pulmonary embolism: the Worcester DVT study. Arch Intern Med 1991;151: 933–938.
13. Dalen JE, Paraskos JA, Ockene IS, Alpert JS, Hirsh J. Venous thromboembolism: scope of the problem. Chest 1986;89: 370S–373S.
14. Dalen JE, Alpert JS. Natural history of pulmonary embolism. Prog Cardiovasc Dis 1975;17:257–270.
15. Giuntini C, Di Ricco G, Marini C, Melillo E, Palla A. Pulmonary embolism: epidemiology. Chest 1995;107:3S–9S.
16. Freiman DG. The pathology of pulmonary embolism and venous thrombosis. In: Frantoni J, Wessler S, eds. Prophylactic therapy of deep vein thrombosis and pulmonary embolism. U.S. Department of Health, Education, and Welfare Publ. no. 965. Bethesda: NIH, 1975;420:11–17.
17. Smith GT, Dexter L, Dammin GJ. Post-mortem quantitative studies in pulmonary embolism. In: Sasahara AA, Stein M, eds. Pulmonary embolus disease. New York: Grune & Stratton, 1965:120–130.
18. Frantoni J, Wessler S. Prophylactic therapy of deep vein thrombosis and pulmonary embolism. U.S. Department of Health, Education, and Welfare Publ. no. 76-866. Bethesda: NIH 1975;420:127–136.
19. Godleski JJ. Pathology of deep venous thrombosis and pulmonary embolism. In: Goldhaber SZ, ed. Pulmonary embolism and deep venous thrombosis. Boston: Saunders, 1985:11–25.
20. Sandler DA, Martin JF. Autopsy proven pulmonary embolism in hospital patients: are we detecting enough deep vein thrombosis? J Roy Soc Med 1989;82:203–205.
21. Moser KM, LeMoine JR. Is embolic risk conditioned by location of deep venous thrombosis? Ann Intern Med 1981;94: 439–444.
22. Ramsay LE. Impact of venography on the diagnosis and management of deep vein thrombosis. Br Med J Clin Res Ed 1983;286:698–699.
23. Lindblad B, Sternby NH, Bergqvist D. Incidence of venous thromboembolism verified by necropsy over 30 years. Br Med J 1991;302:709–711.
24. Lindblad B, Eriksson A, Bergqvist D. Autopsy-verified pulmonary embolism in a surgical department: analysis of the period from 1951 to 1988. Br J Surg 1991;78:849–852.
25. Sevitt S, Gallagher N. Venous thrombosis and pulmonary embolism: a clinico-pathological study in injured and burned patients. Br J Surg 1961;48:475–489.
26. Salzman EW. Heparin for prophylaxis of venous thromboembolism. Ann NY Acad Sci 1989;556:371–377.
27. Kniffin W Jr, Baron JA, Barrett J, Birkmeyer JD, Anderson F Jr. The epidemiology of diagnosed pulmonary embolism and deep venous thrombosis in the elderly. Arch Intern Med 1994;154:861–866.
28. Virchow R, Chance F, trans. In: Cellular pathology. New York: Dewitt, 1860.
29. Ansell JE. Oral anticoagulant therapy—50 years later. Arch Intern Med 1993;153:586–596.
30. Badaracco MA, Vessey MP. Recurrence of venous thromboembolic disease and use of oral contraceptives. Br Med J 1974;1:215–217.
31. Breckwoldt M, Wieacker P, Geisthovel F. Oral contraception in disease states. Am J Obstet Gynecol 1990;163:2213–2216.
32. Drill VA. Oral contraceptives and thromboembolic disease. JAMA 1972;221:602–603.
33. Kierkegaard A. Incidence and diagnosis of deep vein thrombosis associated with pregnancy. Acta Obstet Gynecol Scand 1983;62:239–243.
34. Rutherford SE, Phelan JP. Deep venous thrombosis and pulmonary embolism in pregnancy. Obstet Gynecol Clin North Am 1991;18:345–370.
35. Brabeck MC. Ambulatory management of thromboembolic disease during pregnancy with continuous infusion of heparin. JAMA 1987;257:1790–1791.
36. Demers C, Ginsberg JS. Deep venous thrombosis and pulmonary embolism in pregnancy. Clin Chest Med 1992;13:645–656.
37. Buerger PM, Peoples JB, Lemmon GW, McCarthy MC. Risk of pulmonary emboli in patients with pelvic fractures. Am Surg 1993;59:505–508.
38. Dorfman GS, Froehlich JA, Cronan JJ, Urbanek PJ, Herndon JH. Lower-extremity venous thrombosis in patients with acute hip fractures: determination of anatomic location and time of onset with compression sonography. AJR 1990;154: 851–855.
39. Olin JW, Graor RA, O'Hara P, Young JR. The incidence of deep venous thrombosis in patients undergoing abdominal aortic aneurysm resection. J Vasc Surg 1993;18:1037–1041.
40. Bounameaux H, Huber O, Khabiri E, Schneider PA, Didier D, Rohner A. Unexpectedly high rate of phlebographic deep venous thrombosis following elective general abdominal surgery among patients given prophylaxis with low-molecular-weight heparin. Arch Surg 1993;128:326–328.
41. Cisek LJ, Walsh PC. Thromboembolic complications following radical retropubic prostatectomy: influence of external sequential pneumatic compression devices. Urology 1993;42: 406–408.
42. Freiman DG. Surgical conditions as risk factors in the development of venous thrombosis. Milbank Mem Fund Q 1972; 50:60–70.
43. Hamilton MG, Hull RD, Pineo GF. Venous thromboembolism in neurosurgery and neurology patients: a review. Neurosurgery 1994;34:280–296.
44. Seagroatt V, Tan HS, Goldacre M, Bulstrode C, Nugent I, Gill L. Elective total hip replacement: incidence, emergency readmission rate, and postoperative mortality. Br Med J 1991; 303:1431–1435.
45. Parmet JL, Berman AT, Horrow JC, Harding S, Rosenberg

H. Thromboembolism coincident with tourniquet deflation during total knee arthroplasty. Lancet 1993;341:1057–1058.

46. Kraay MJ, Goldberg VM, Herbener TE. Vascular ultrasonography for deep venous thrombosis after total knee arthroplasty. Clin Orthop Relat Res 1993;286:18–26.

47. Dalldorf PG, Perkins FM, Totterman S, Pellegrini V Jr. Deep venous thrombosis following total hip arthroplasty: effects of prolonged postoperative epidural anesthesia. J Arthroplasty 1994;9:611–616.

48. Brach BB, Moser KM, Cedar L, Minteer M, Convery R. Venous thrombosis in acute spinal cord paralysis. J Trauma 1977;17:289–292.

49. Haake DA, Berkman SA. Venous thromboembolic disease after hip surgery: risk factors, prophylaxis, and diagnosis. Clin Orthopaed Relat Res 1989;242:212–231.

50. Dunkman WB. Thromboembolism and antithrombotic therapy in congestive heart failure. J Cardiovasc Risk 1995;2:107–117.

51. Kierkegaard A, Norgren L. Venous function of the leg during atrial arrhythmias. Vasa 1990;19:296–300.

52. Coffman JD. Deep venous thrombosis and pulmonary emboli: etiology, medical treatment, and prophylaxis. J Thorac Imaging 1989;4:4–7.

53. Doig RG, O'Malley CJ, Dauer R, McGrath KM. An evaluation of 200 consecutive patients with spontaneous or recurrent thrombosis for primary hypercoagulable states. Am J Clin Pathol 1994;102:797–801.

54. Kakkar VV. Venous thrombosis after myocardial infarction. Lancet 1972;1:258–259.

55. Ginsburg KS, Liang MH, Newcomer L, et al. Anticardiolipin antibodies and the risk for ischemic stroke and venous thrombosis. Ann Intern Med 1992;117:997–1002.

56. Dittmer DK, Teasell R. Complications of immobilization and bed rest: 1. Musculoskeletal and cardiovascular complications. Can Family Physician 1993;39:1428–1432.

57. Kierkegaard A, Norgren L, Olsson CG, Castenfors J, Persson G, Persson S. Incidence of deep vein thrombosis in bedridden non-surgical patients. Acta Med Scand 1987;222:409–414.

58. Murphy TP, Cronan JJ. Vascular ultrasound in the intensive care unit. Crit Care Clin 1994;10:341–363.

59. Moser KM, LeMoine JR, Nachtwey FJ, Spragg RG. Deep venous thrombosis and pulmonary embolism: frequency in a respiratory intensive care unit. JAMA 1981;246:1422–1444.

60. Hoyt DB, Swegle JR. Deep venous thrombosis in the surgical intensive care unit. Surg Clin North Am 1991;71:811–830.

61. Goldhaber SZ, Buring JE, Hennekens CH. Cancer and venous thromboembolism. Arch Intern Med 1987;147:216.

62. Nordstrom M, Lindblad B, Bergqvist D, Kjellstrom T. A prospective study of the incidence of deep-vein thrombosis within a defined urban population. J Intern Med 1992;232:155–160.

63. Prandoni P, Lensing AW, Buller HR, et al. Deep-vein thrombosis and the incidence of subsequent symptomatic cancer. N Engl J Med 1992;327:1128–1133.

64. Cheruku R, Tapazoglou E, Ensley J, Kish JA, Cummings GD, al-Sarraf M. The incidence and significance of thromboembolic complications in patients with high-grade gliomas. Cancer 1991;68:2621–2624.

65. Kakkar VV. Prevention and management of venous thrombosis. Br Med Bull 1994;50:871–903.

66. Lotke PA, Steinberg ME, Ecker ML. Significance of deep venous thrombosis in the lower extremity after total joint arthroplasty. Clin Orthopaed Relat Res 1994;299:25–30.

67. Nielsen HK, Husted SE, Krusell LR, Fasting H, Charles P, Hansen HH. Silent pulmonary embolism in patients with deep venous thrombosis: incidence and fate in a randomized, controlled trial of anticoagulation versus no anticoagulation. J Intern Med 1994;235:457–461.

68. Dorfman GS, Cronan JJ, Tupper TB, Messersmith RN, Denny DF, Lee CH. Occult pulmonary embolism: a common occurrence in deep venous thrombosis. AJR 1987;148:263–266.

69. Broaddus C, Matthay MA. Pulmonary embolism: guide to diagnosis, treatment, and prevention. Postgrad Med 1986;79:333–337, 340–343.

70. Paiement GD, Wessinger SJ, Harris WH. Cost-effectiveness of prophylaxis in total hip replacement. Am J Surg 1991;161:519–524.

71. Hull RD, Raskob GE. Prophylaxis of venous thromboembolic disease following hip and knee surgery. J Bone Joint Surg (Am) 1986;68:146–150.

72. Gallerani M, Manfredini R, Moratelli S. Non-haemorrhagic adverse reactions of oral anticoagulant therapy. Int J Cardiol 1995;49:1–7.

73. Wheeler HB, Anderson F Jr. Prophylaxis against venous thromboembolism in surgical patients. Am J Surg 1991;161:507–511.

74. Stein PD, Hull RD. Relative risks of anticoagulant treatment of acute pulmonary embolism based on an angiographic diagnosis vs a ventilation/perfusion scan diagnosis. Chest 1994;106:727–730.

75. Carter CJ. The natural history and epidemiology of venous thrombosis. Prog Cardiovasc Dis 1994;36:423–438.

76. Pellegrini V Jr, Langhans MJ, Totterman S, Marder VJ, Francis CW. Embolic complications of calf thrombosis following total hip arthroplasty. J Arthroplasty 1993;8:449–457.

77. Persson AV, Davis RJ, Villavicencio JL. Deep venous thrombosis and pulmonary embolism. Surg Clin North Am 1991;71:1195–1209.

78. Stein PD, Hull RD, Saltzman HA, Pineo G. Strategy for diagnosis of patients with suspected acute pulmonary embolism. Chest 1993;103:1553–1559.

79. Kruit WH, de Boer AC, Sing AK, van Roon F. The significance of venography in the management of patients with clinically suspected pulmonary embolism. J Intern Med 1991;230:333–339.

80. Henry JW, Relyea B, Stein PD. Continuing risk of thromboemboli among patients with normal pulmonary angiograms. Chest 1995;107:1375–1378.

81. Monreal M, Lafoz E, Ruiz J, Callejas JM, Arias A. Recurrent pulmonary embolism in patients treated because of acute venous thromboembolism: a prospective study. Eur J Vasc Surg 1994;8:584–589.

82. Hold M, Bull PG, Raynoschek H, Denck H. Deep venous thrombosis: results of thrombectomy versus medical therapy. Presented at the 5th European-American Symposium on Venous Diseases, Vienna, Austria, Nov. 7–11, 1990. Vasa 1992;21:181–187.

83. Mohan CR, Hoballah JJ, Sharp WJ, Kresowik TF, Lu CT, Corson JD. Comparative efficacy and complications of vena caval filters. J Vasc Surg 1995;21:235–245.

84. Sullivan TM, Martinez BD, Lemmon G, Clark PM, Schwartz RA, Bondy B. Clinical experience with the Greenfield filter in 193 patients and description of a new technique for operative insertion. J Am Coll Surg 1994;178:117–122.

85. Kaufman JA, Geller SC. When to use an inferior vena cava filter. AJR 1995;164:256–257.

86. Becker DM, Philbrick JT, Selby JB. Inferior vena cava filters: indications, safety, effectiveness. Arch Intern Med 1992;152:1985–1994.

87. Semba CP, Dake MD. Iliofemoral deep venous thrombosis: aggressive therapy with catheter-directed thrombolysis. Radiology 1994;191:487–494.

88. Tarry WC, Makhoul RG, Tisnado J, Posner MP, Sobel M, Lee HM. Catheter-directed thrombolysis following vena cava filtration for severe deep venous thrombosis. Ann Vasc Surg 1994;8:583–590.

89. Comerota AJ, Aldridge SC. Thrombolytic therapy for deep venous thrombosis: a clinical review. Can J Surg 1993;36:359–364.

90. Comerota AJ, Aldridge SC, Cohen G, Ball DS, Pliskin M, White JV. A strategy of aggressive regional therapy for acute iliofemoral venous thrombosis with contemporary venous thrombectomy or catheter-directed thrombolysis. J Vasc Surg 1994;20:244–254.

91. Goldhaber SZ, Polak JF, Feldstein ML, Meyerovitz MF, Creager MA. Efficacy and safety of repeated boluses of urokinase in the treatment of deep venous thrombosis. Am J Cardiol 1994;73:75–79.

92. Kniemeyer HW, Grabitz K, Buhl R, Wust HJ, Sandmann W. Surgical treatment of septic deep venous thrombosis. Surgery 1995;118:49–53.

93. Block P, Schandevyl W, Cham B, et al. Recurrent pulmonary embolism: importance, diagnosis, management and prevention. Acta Chir Belg 1986;86:109–117.

94. Scheeren TW, Hopf HB, Peters J. Intraoperative thrombolysis with rt-PA in massive pulmonary embolism during venous thrombectomy. Anaesthesiol Intensivmed Notfallmed, Schmerzther 1994;29:440–445.

95. Shimokawa S, Toyohira H, Iwamura H, et al. Pulmonary embolectomy for massive pulmonary embolism. Nihon Kyobu Geka Gakkai Zasshi 1995;43:191–195.

96. Willens HJ, Ciraldo R, Vuoto T, Kessler KM. Combined pulmonary embolectomy and right atrial thromboembolectomy guided by transesophageal echocardiography. Am Heart J 1995;130:180–182.

97. Hull RD, Raskob GE, Ginsberg JS, et al. A noninvasive strategy for the treatment of patients with suspected pulmonary embolism. Arch Intern Med 1994;154:289–297.

98. Hull RD, Raskob GE, Coates G, Panju AA, Gill GJ. A new noninvasive management strategy for patients with suspected pulmonary embolism. Arch Intern Med 1989;149:2549–2555.

99. Beecham RP, Dorfman GS, Cronan JJ, Spearman MP, Murphy TP, Scola FH. Is bilateral lower extremity compression sonography useful and cost-effective in the evaluation of suspected pulmonary embolism? AJR 1993;161:1289–1292.

100. Wells PS, Ginsberg JS. DVT and pulmonary embolism: choosing the right diagnostic tests for patients at risk. Geriatrics 1995;50:29–32.

101. Killewich LA, Nunnelee JD, Auer AI. Value of lower extremity venous duplex examination in the diagnosis of pulmonary embolism. J Vasc Surg 1993;17:934–938.

102. Lotke PA, Ecker ML, Alavi A, Berkowitz H. Indications for the treatment of deep venous thrombosis following total knee replacement. J Bone Joint Surg (Am) 1984;66:202–208.

103. Prandoni P, Lensing AW, Buller HR, et al. Failure of computerized impedance plethysmography in the diagnostic management of patients with clinically suspected deep-vein thrombosis. Thromb Haemostasis 1991;65:233–236.

104. Davidson BL, Elliott CG, Lensing AW. Low accuracy of color Doppler ultrasound in the detection of proximal leg vein thrombosis in asymptomatic high-risk patients: the RD Heparin Arthroplasty Group. Ann Intern Med 1992;117:735–738.

105. Bendayan P, Boccalon H. Cost effectiveness of non-invasive tests including duplex scanning for diagnosis of deep venous thrombosis: a prospective study carried out on 511 patients. Vasa 1991;20:348–353.

106. Weinmann EE, Salzman EW. Deep-vein thrombosis. N Engl J Med 1994;331:1630–1641.

107. Harris WH, Salzman EW, Athanasoulis C, et al. Comparison of 125I fibrinogen count scanning with phlebography for detection of venous thrombi after elective hip surgery. N Engl J Med 1975;292:665–667.

108. Sevitt S, Gallagher NG. Prevention of venous thrombosis and pulmonary embolism in injured patients: a trial of anticoagulant prophylaxis with phenindione in middle aged and elderly patients with fractured necks of the femur. Lancet 1959;2:981–989.

109. Salzman EW. Venous thrombosis made easy. N Engl J Med 1986;314:847–848.

110. Nicolaides AN, Kakkar VV, Field ES, Renney JT. The origin of deep vein thrombosis: a venographic study. Br J Radiol 1971;44:653–663.

111. Sigel B, Felix W Jr, Popky GL, Ipsen J. Diagnosis of lower limb venous thrombosis by Doppler ultrasound technique. Arch Surg 1972;104:174–179.

112. Hull R, Hirsh J, Sackett DL, et al. Clinical validity of a negative venogram in patients with clinically suspected venous thrombosis. Circulation 1981;64:622–625.

113. Hull R, Hirsh J, Sackett DL, Powers P, Turpie AG, Walker I. Combined use of leg scanning and impedance plethysmography in suspected venous thrombosis: an alternative to venography. N Engl J Med 1977;296:1497–1500.

114. Wells PS, Hirsh J, Anderson DR, et al. Accuracy of clinical assessment of deep-vein thrombosis. Lancet 1995;345:1326–1330.

115. Cranley JJ, Canos AJ, Sull WJ. The diagnosis of deep venous thrombosis: fallibility of clinical symptoms and signs. Arch Surg 1976;111:34–36.

116. Haeger K. Problems of acute deep venous thrombosis: I. The interpretation of signs and symptoms. Angiology 1969;20:219–223.

117. Lohr JM, Hasselfeld KA, Byrne MP, Deshmukh RM, Cranley JJ. Does the asymptomatic limb harbor deep venous thrombosis? Am J Surg 1994;168:184–187.

118. Morgenthaler TI, Ryu JH. Clinical characteristics of fatal pulmonary embolism in a referral hospital. Mayo Clin Proc 1995;70:417–424.

119. Bauer G. A venographic study of thrombo-embolic problems. Acta Chir Scand Suppl 1940;61:1–75.

120. Anderson DR, Lensing AW, Wells PS, Levine MN, Weitz JI, Hirsh J. Limitations of impedance plethysmography in the diagnosis of clinically suspected deep-vein thrombosis. Ann Intern Med 1993;118:25–30.

121. Jongbloets LM, Lensing AW, Koopman MM, Buller HR, Cate JW. Limitations of compression ultrasound for the detection of symptomless postoperative deep vein thrombosis. Lancet 1994;343:1142–1144.

122. Ginsberg JS, Wells PS, Hirsh J, et al. Reevaluation of the sensitivity of impedance plethysmography for the detection of proximal deep vein thrombosis. Arch Intern Med 1994;154:1930–1933.

123. Ferris EJ, George W. Holmes Lecture. Deep venous thrombosis and pulmonary embolism: correlative evaluation and therapeutic implications. AJR 1992;159:1149–1155.

124. Kakkar VV, Howe CT, Nicolaides AN, Renney JT, Clarke MB. Deep vein thrombosis of the leg: is there a "high risk" group? Am J Surg 1970;120:527–530.

125. Kakkar VV, Renney JT, Nicolaides AN. Prophylaxis of venous thrombosis. Br Med J 1970;2:540.

126. Hull R, Hirsh J, Sackett DL, et al. Replacement of venography in suspected venous thrombosis by impedance plethysmography and 125I-fibrinogen leg scanning: a less invasive approach. Ann Intern Med 1981;94:12–15.

127. Kakkar VV, Howe CT, Flanc C, Clarke MB. Natural history of postoperative deep-vein thrombosis. Lancet 1969;2:230–232.

128. Vine HS, Hillman B, Hessel SJ. Deep venous thrombosis: predictive value of signs and symptoms. AJR 1981;136:167–171.

129. Curley FJ, Pratter MR, Irwin RS, et al. The clinical implications of bilaterally abnormal impedance plethysmography. Arch Intern Med 1987;147:125–129.

130. Anderson FA, Forcier A, Pathwardhan NA, Wheeler HB. Utilization of objective testing for venous thromboembolism: a community-wide study. J Vasc Tech 1989;13:117–118.

131. Anderson F Jr, Wheeler HB, Goldberg RJ, Hosmer DW, Forcier A, Patwardhan NA. Physician practices in the prevention of venous thromboembolism. Ann Intern Med 1991;115:591–595.

132. Brathwaite CE, Mure AJ, O'Malley KF, Spence RK, Ross SE. Complications of anticoagulation for pulmonary embolism in low risk trauma patients. Chest 1993;104:718–720.

133. Rabinov K, Paulin S. Roentgen diagnosis of venous thrombosis in the leg. Arch Surg 1972;104:134–144.

134. Ramchandani P, Soulen RL, Fedullo LM, Gaines VD. Deep

vein thrombosis: significant limitations of noninvasive tests. Radiology 1985;156:47–49.

135. Hull R, Hirsh J, Sackett DL, Stoddart G. Cost effectiveness of clinical diagnosis, venography, and noninvasive testing in patients with symptomatic deep-vein thrombosis. N Engl J Med 1981;304:1561–1567.

136. Redman HC. Deep venous thrombosis: is contrast venography still the diagnostic "gold standard"? Radiology 1988; 168:277–278.

137. Rose SC, Zwiebel WJ, Murdock LE, et al. Insensitivity of color Doppler flow imaging for detection of acute calf deep venous thrombosis in asymptomatic postoperative patients. J Vasc Intervent Radiol 1993;4:111–117.

138. Lensing AW, Buller HR, Prandoni P, et al. Contrast venography, the gold standard for the diagnosis of deep-vein thrombosis: improvement in observer agreement. Thromb Haemostasis 1992;67:8–12.

139. Wells PS, Lensing AW, Davidson BL, Prins MH, Hirsh J. Accuracy of ultrasound for the diagnosis of deep venous thrombosis in asymptomatic patients after orthopedic surgery: a meta-analysis. Ann Intern Med 1995;122:47–53.

140. Lund F, Diener L, Ericsson JL. Postmortem intraosseous phlebography as an aid in studies of venous thromboembolism: with application on a geriatric clientele. Angiology 1969; 20:155–176.

141. Cogo A, Lensing AW, Prandoni P, Hirsh J. Distribution of thrombosis in patients with symptomatic deep vein thrombosis: implications for simplifying the diagnostic process with compression ultrasound. Arch Intern Med 1993;153:2777–2780.

142. McLachlan MS, Thomson JG, Taylor DW, Kelly ME, Sackett DL. Observer variation in the interpretation of lower limb venograms. AJR 1979;132:227–229.

143. Kilpatrick TK, Lichtenstein M, Andrews J, Gibson RN, Neerhut P, Hopper J. A comparative study of radionuclide venography and contrast venography in the diagnosis of deep venous thrombosis. Aust N Z J Med 1993;23:641–645.

144. Bounameaux H, Prins TR, Schmitt HE, Schneider PA. Venography of the lower limbs: pitfalls of the diagnostic standard. The ETTT Trial Investigators. Invest Radiol 1992;27:1009–1011.

145. Katayama H, Yamaguchi K, Kozuka T, Takashima T, Seez P, Matsuura K. Adverse reactions to ionic and nonionic contrast media: a report from the Japanese Committee on the Safety of Contrast Media. Radiology 1990;175:621–628.

146. Spigos DG, Thane TT, Capek V. Skin necrosis following extravasation during peripheral phlebography. Radiology 1977; 123:605–606.

147. Parfrey PS, Griffiths SM, Barrett BJ, et al. Contrast material–induced renal failure in patients with diabetes mellitus, renal insufficiency, or both: a prospective controlled study. N Engl J Med 1989;320:143–149.

148. Cohan RH, Dunnick NR. Intravascular contrast media: adverse reactions. AJR 1987;149:665–670.

149. Arndt RD, Grollman J Jr, Gomes AS, Bos CJ. The heparin flush: an aid in preventing post-venography thrombophlebitis. Radiology 1979;130:249–250.

150. Thomas ML, Briggs GM, Kuan BB. Contrast agent–induced thrombophlebitis following leg phlebography: meglumine ioxaglate versus meglumine iothalamate. Radiology 1983; 147:399–400.

151. Bettmann MA, Paulin S. Leg phlebography: the incidence, nature and modification of undesirable side effects. Radiology 1977;122:101–104.

152. Bettmann MA, Robbins A, Braun SD, Wetzner S, Dunnick NR, Finkelstein J. Contrast venography of the leg: diagnostic efficacy, tolerance, and complication rates with ionic and nonionic contrast media. Radiology 1987;165:113–116.

153. Laerum F, Holm HA. Postphlebographic thrombosis: a double-blind study with methylglucamine metrizoate and metrizamide. Radiology 1981;140:651–654.

154. Laerum F, Dehner LP, Rysavy J, Amplatz K. Double blind evaluation of the effects of various contrast media on extremity veins in the dog. Acta Radiol 1987;28:107–113.

155. Hessel SJ, Adams DF, Abrams HL. Complications of angiography. Radiology 1981;138:273–281.

156. Golman K, Almen T. Contrast media–induced nephrotoxicity: survey and present state. Invest Radiol 1985;20:S92–S97.

157. Golman K, Cederholm C. Contrast medium–induced acute renal failure: can it be prevented? Invest Radiol 1990;25: S127–S128.

158. Lea Thomas M, Briggs GM, Keeling FP. Iohexol and meglumine iothalamate in phlebography of the leg: comparison of the tolerance. Acta Radiol Suppl (Stockh) 1983;366:54–57.

159. Shehadi WH, Toniolo G. Adverse reactions to contrast media: a report from the committee on safety of contrast media of the International Society of Radiology. Radiology 1980;137: 299–302.

160. Witlin AG, Sibai BM. Postpartum ovarian vein thrombosis after vaginal delivery: a report of 11 cases. Obstet Gynecol 1995;85:775–780.

161. West WM, Brown E. Computed tomography of the calves: a screening procedure in the diagnosis of unilateral thrombosis of the deep veins of the lower limbs. West Indian Med J 1992; 41:150–151.

162. Lensing AW, Prandoni P, Brandjes D, et al. Detection of deep-vein thrombosis by real-time B-mode ultrasonography. N Engl J Med 1989;320:342–345.

163. Benedict K Jr, Wheeler HB, Patwardhan NA. Impedance plethysmography: correlation with contrast venography. Radiology 1977;125:695–699.

164. Comerota AJ, Cranley JJ, Cook SE, Sipple P. Phleborheography—results of a ten-year experience. Surgery 1982;91:573–581.

165. Naidich JB, Feinberg AW, Karp-Harman H, Karmel MI, Tyma CG, Stein HL. Contrast venography: reassessment of its role. Radiology 1988;168:97–100.

166. Hull RD, Hirsh J, Carter CJ, et al. Diagnostic efficacy of impedance plethysmography for clinically suspected deep-vein thrombosis: a randomized trial. Ann Intern Med 1985;102: 21–28.

167. Cardella JF, Young AT, Smith TP, et al. Lower-extremity venous thrombosis: comparison of venography, impedance plethysmography, and intravenous manometry. Radiology 1988; 168:109–112.

168. Moser KM, Brach BB, Dolan GF. Clinically suspected deep venous thrombosis of the lower extremities: a comparison of venography, impedance plethysmography, and radiolabeled fibrinogen. JAMA 1977;237:2195–2198.

169. Kearon C, Hirsh J. Factors influencing the reported sensitivity and specificity of impedance plethysmography for proximal deep vein thrombosis. Thromb Haemostasis 1994;72:652–658.

170. Cronan JJ. Venous thromboembolic disease: the role of US. Radiology 1993;186:619–630.

171. Appelman PT, De Jong TE, Lampmann LE. Deep venous thrombosis of the leg: US findings. Radiology 1987;163: 743–746.

172. Dorfman GS, Cronan JJ. Venous ultrasonography. Radiol Clin North Am 1992;30:879–894.

173. Day TK, Fish PJ, Kakkar VV. Detection of deep vein thrombosis by Doppler angiography. Br Med J 1976;1:618–620.

174. Woolson ST, Pottorff G. Venous ultrasonography in the detection of proximal vein thrombosis after total knee arthroplasty. Clin Orthopaed Relat Res 1991;273:131–135.

175. Fernandez-Canton G, Lopez Vidaur I, Munoz F, Antonana MA, Uresandi F, Calonge J. Diagnostic utility of color Doppler ultrasound in lower limb deep vein thrombosis in patients with clinical suspicion of pulmonary thromboembolism. Eur J Radiol 1994;19:50–55.

176. Agnelli G, Radicchia S, Nenci GG. Diagnosis of deep vein thrombosis in asymptomatic high-risk patients. Haemostasis 1995;25:40–48.

177. Cronan JJ, Leen V. Recurrent deep venous thrombosis: limitations of US. Radiology 1989;170:739–742.

178. Singer JR. Blood flow rates by nuclear magnetic resonance measurements. Science 1959;130:1652.

179. Keller PJ, Drayer BP, Fram EK, Williams KD, Dumoulin CL, Souza SP. MR angiography with two-dimensional acquisition and three-dimensional display: work in progress. Radiology 1989;173:527–532.

180. Axel L. Blood flow effects in magnetic resonance imaging. AJR 1984;143:1157–1166.

181. Bradley WJ, Waluch V, Lai K, Fernandez E, Spalter C. The appearance of rapidly flowing blood on magnetic resonance images. AJR 1984;143:1167–1174.

182. Axel L, Morton D. MR flow imaging by velocity-compensated/uncompensated difference images. J Comput Assist Tomogr 1987;11:31–34.

183. Wehrli FW, Shimakawa A, Gullberg GT, MacFall JR. Time-of-flight MR flow imaging: selective saturation recovery with gradient refocusing. Radiology 1986;160:781–785.

184. Hricak H, Amparo E, Fisher MR, Crooks L, Higgins CB. Abdominal venous system: assessment using MR. Radiology 1985;156:415–422.

185. Choyke PL, Kressel HY, Axel L, et al. Vascular occlusions detected by magnetic resonance imaging. Magn Reson Med 1985;2:540–554.

186. Felmlee JP, Ehman RL. Spatial presaturation: a method for suppressing flow artifacts and improving depiction of vascular anatomy in MR imaging. Radiology 1987;164:559–564.

187. Spritzer CE, Sussman SK, Blinder RA, Saeed M, Herfkens RJ. Deep venous thrombosis evaluation with limited-flip-angle, gradient-refocused MR imaging: preliminary experience. Radiology 1988;166:371–375.

188. Erdman WA, Jayson HT, Redman HC, Miller GL, Parkey RW, Peshock RW. Deep venous thrombosis of extremities: role of MR imaging in the diagnosis. Radiology 1990;174:425–431.

189. Evans AJ, Sostman HD, Knelson MH, et al. 1992 ARRS Executive Council Award. Detection of deep venous thrombosis: prospective comparison of MR imaging with contrast venography. AJR 1993;161:131–139.

190. Carpenter JP, Owen RS, Holland GA, et al. Magnetic resonance angiography of the aorta, iliac, and femoral arteries. Surgery 1994;116:17–23.

191. Carpenter JP, Baum RA, Holland GA, Barker CF. Peripheral vascular surgery with magnetic resonance angiography as the sole preoperative imaging modality. J Vasc Surg 1994;20:861–871.

192. Owen RS, Baum RA, Carpenter JP, Holland GA, Cope C. Symptomatic peripheral vascular disease: selection of imaging parameters and clinical evaluation with MR angiography. Radiology 1993;187:627–635.

193. Yucel EK. Magnetic resonance angiography of the lower extremity and renal arteries. Semin Ultrasound CT MRI 1992;13:291–302.

194. Yucel EK, Kaufman JA, Geller SC, Waltman AC. Atherosclerotic occlusive disease of the lower extremity: prospective evaluation with two-dimensional time-of-flight MR angiography. Radiology 1993;187:637–641.

195. Owen RS, Carpenter JP, Baum RA, Perloff LJ, Cope C. Magnetic resonance imaging of angiographically occult runoff vessels in peripheral arterial occlusive disease. N Engl J Med 1992;326:1577–1581.

196. Cambria RP, Yucel EK, Brewster DC, et al. The potential for lower extremity revascularization without contrast arteriography: experience with magnetic resonance angiography. J Vasc Surg 1993;17:1050–1057.

197. Caputo GR, Masui T, Gooding GA, Chang JM, Higgins CB. Popliteal and tibioperoneal arteries: feasibility of two-dimensional time-of-flight MR angiography and phase velocity mapping. Radiology 1992;182:387–392.

198. Carpenter JP, Holland GA, Baum RA, Owen RS, Carpenter JT, Cope C. Magnetic resonance venography for the detection of deep venous thrombosis: comparison with contrast venography and duplex Doppler ultrasonography. J Vasc Surg 1993;18:734–741.

199. Edelman RR, Wentz KU, Mattle H, et al. Projection arteriography and venography: initial clinical results with MR. Radiology 1989;172:351–357.

200. Holland GA, Owen RS, Carpenter JP, et al. Optimization of MR venography in the veins of the pelvis and lower extremities. Magn Reson Med 1992 (abstract): 3104.

201. Teitelbaum GP, Ortega HV, Vinitski S, et al. Optimization of gradient-echo imaging parameters for intracaval filters and trapped thromboemboli. Radiology 1990;174:1013–1019.

202. Holland GA, Baum RA, Carpenter JP, Owen RS, Scheibler MS, Cope C. Prospective evaluation of MR venography in the detection of deep venous thrombosis in the veins of the pelvis and lower extremities. Radiology 1992;185:277.

203. Foster SA, Holland GA, Lotke PA, Baum RA, Cope C, Steinberg ME. Prospective comparison of MR venography with contrast venography in patients with lower extremity joint replacement. Radiology 1994;193:323.

204. Erdman WA, Weinreb JC, Cohen JM, Buja LM, Chaney C, Peshock RM. Venous thrombosis: clinical and experimental MR imaging. Radiology 1986;161:233–238.

205. Erdman WA, Parkey RW. MR imaging of deep venous thrombosis. AJR 1990;155:897.

206. Spritzer CE, Norconk J Jr, Sostman HD, Coleman RE. Detection of deep venous thrombosis by magnetic resonance imaging. Chest 1993;104:54–60.

207. Anderson CM, Saloner D, Tsuruda JS, Shapeero LG, Lee RE. Artifacts in maximum-intensity-projection display of MR angiograms. AJR 1990;154:623–629.

208. Laub G. Displays for MR angiography. Magn Reson Med 1990;14:222–229.

209. Listerud J. First principles of magnetic resonance angiography. Magn Reson Q 1991;7:136–170.

210. Tartaglino LM, Flanders AE, Vinitski S, Friedman DP. Metallic artifacts on MR images of the postoperative spine: reduction with fast spin-echo techniques. Radiology 1994;190:565–569.

211. Holland GA, Baum RA, Danehy E, Carpenter JP, Cope C, Axel L. MR angiography of the aortoiliac system: prospective comparison of contrast enhanced 3D and 2D time-of-flight techniques. J Vasc Intervent Radiol 1995;6:4–5.

212. Grassi CJ, Matsumoto AH, Teitelbaum GP. Vena caval occlusion after Simon nitinol filter placement: identification with MR imaging in patients with malignancy. J Vasc Intervent Radiol 1992;3:535–539.

213. Teitelbaum GP, Ortega HV, Vinitski S, et al. Low-artifact intravascular devices: MR imaging evaluation. Radiology 1988;168:713–719.

214. Teitelbaum GP, Bradley W Jr, Klein BD. MR imaging artifacts, ferromagnetism, and magnetic torque of intravascular filters, stents, and coils. Radiology 1988;166:657–664.

215. Kiproff PM, Deeb ZL, Contractor FM, Khoury MB. Magnetic resonance characteristics of the LGM vena cava filter: technical note. Cardiovasc Intervent Radiol 1991;14:254–255.

216. Kim D, Edelman RR, Margolin CJ, et al. The Simon nitinol filter: evaluation by MR and ultrasound. Angiology 1992;43:541–548.

217. Simon M, Athanasoulis CA, Kim D, et al. Simon nitinol inferior vena cava filter: initial clinical experience. Work in progress. Radiology 1989;172:99–103.

218. Watanabe AT, Teitelbaum GP, Gomes AS, Roehm J Jr. MR imaging of the bird's nest filter. Radiology 1990;177:578–579.

219. Gomori JM, Grossman RI, Bilaniuk LT, Zimmerman RA, Goldberg HI. High-field MR imaging of superficial siderosis of the central nervous system. J Comput Assist Tomogr 1985;9:972–975.

220. Gomori JM, Grossman RI, Goldberg HI, Zimmerman RA, Bilaniuk LT. Intracranial hematomas: imaging by high-field MR. Radiology 1985;157:87–93.

221. Gomori JM, Grossman RI, Yu-Ip C, Asakura T. NMR relaxation times of blood: dependence on field strength, oxidation state, and cell integrity. J Comput Assist Tomogr 1987;11: 684–690.

222. Gomori JM, Grossman RI, Hackney DB, Goldberg HI, Zimmerman RA, Bilaniuk LT. Variable appearances of subacute intracranial hematomas on high-field spin-echo MR. AJR 1988;150:171–178.

223. Rapoport S, Sostman HD, Pope C, Camputaro CM, Holcomb W, Gore JC. Venous clots: evaluation with MR imaging. Radiology 1987;162:527–530.

224. Stuhlmuller JE, Scholz TD, Olson JD, Burns TL, Skorton DJ. Magnetic resonance characterization of blood coagulation in vitro: effect of platelet depletion. Invest Radiol 1991;26:343–347.

225. Blackmore CC, Francis CW, Bryant RG, Brenner B, Marder VJ. Magnetic resonance imaging of blood and clots in vitro. Invest Radiol 1990;25:1316–1324.

226. Bass J, Sostman HD, Boyko O, Koepke JA. Effects of cell membrane disruption on the relaxation rates of blood and clot with various methemoglobin concentrations. Invest Radiol 1990;25:1232–1237.

227. Bass JC, Hedlund LW, Sostman HD. MR imaging of experimental and clinical thrombi at 1.5 T. Magn Reson Imaging 1990;8:631–635.

228. Gomori JM, Grossman RI, Asakura T, et al. An in vitro study of magnetization transfer and relaxation rates of hematoma. AJNR 1993;14:871–880.

229. Mittl R Jr, Gomori JM, Schnall MD, Holland GA, Grossman RI, Atlas SW. Magnetization transfer effects in MR imaging of in vivo intracranial hemorrhage. AJNR 1993;14:881–891.

230. Wu JJ, MacFall JR, Sostman HD, Hedlund LW. Clot-blood contrast in fast gradient-echo magnetic resonance imaging. Invest Radiol 1993;28:586–593.

231. Yousem DM, Balakrishnan J, Debrun GM, Bryan RN. Hyperintense thrombus on GRASS MR images: potential pitfall in flow evaluation. AJNR 1990;11:51–58.

232. Hatabu H, Gefter WB, Axel L, et al. MR imaging with spatial modulation of magnetization in the evaluation of chronic central pulmonary thromboemboli. Radiology 1994;190:791–796.

233. Delany SG, Doyle TC, Bunton RW, Hung NA, Joblin LU, Taylor DR. Pulmonary artery sarcoma mimicking pulmonary embolism. Chest 1993;103:1631–1633.

234. Bressler EL, Nelson JM. Primary pulmonary artery sarcoma: diagnosis with CT, MR imaging, and transthoracic needle biopsy. AJR 1992;159:702–704.

235. Rafal RB, Nichols JN, Markisz JA. Pulmonary artery sarcoma: diagnosis and postoperative follow-up with gadolinium-diethylenetriamine pentaacetic acid–enhanced magnetic resonance imaging. Mayo Clin Proc 1995;70:173–176.

236. Pozniak MA, Baus KM. Hepatofugal arterial signal in the main portal vein: an indicator of intravascular tumor spread. Radiology 1991;180:663–666.

237. Quinn SF, Erickson S. Neovascularity in venous extension of renal cell carcinoma: CT and arteriographic evaluation. South Med J 1988;81:1010–1012.

238. Amendola MA, King LR, Pollack HM, Gefter W, Kressel HY, Wein AJ. Staging of renal carcinoma using magnetic resonance imaging at 1.5 Tesla. Cancer 1990;66:40–44.

239. Horan JJ, Robertson CN, Choyke PL, et al. The detection of renal carcinoma extension into the renal vein and inferior vena cava: a prospective comparison of venacavography and magnetic resonance imaging. J Urol 1989;142:943–947.

240. Pritchett TR, Raval JK, Benson RC, et al. Preoperative magnetic resonance imaging of vena caval tumor thrombi: experience with 5 cases. J Urol 1987;138:1220–1222.

241. Goldfarb DA, Novick AC, Lorig R, et al. Magnetic resonance imaging for assessment of vena caval tumor thrombi: a comparative study with venacavography and computerized tomography scanning. J Urol 1990;144:1100–1103.

242. Applegate GR, Thaete FL, Meyers SP, et al. Blood flow in the portal vein: velocity quantitation with phase-contrast MR angiography. Radiology 1993;187:253–256.

243. Burkart DJ, Felmlee JP, Johnson CD, Wolf RL, Weaver AL, Ehman RL. Cine phase-contrast MR flow measurements: improved precision using an automated method of vessel detection. J Comput Assist Tomogr 1994;18:469–475.

244. Burkart DJ, Johnson CD, Reading CC, Ehman RL. MR measurements of mesenteric venous flow: prospective evaluation in healthy volunteers and patients with suspected chronic mesenteric ischemia. Radiology 1995;194:801–806.

245. Kuo PC, Li K, Alfrey EJ, Jeffrey RB, Garcia G, Dafoe DC. Magnetic resonance imaging and hepatic hemodynamics: correlation with metabolic function in liver transplantation candidates. Surgery 1995;117:373–379.

246. Muller MF, Siewert B, Stokes KR, et al. MR angiographic guidance for transjugular intrahepatic portosystemic shunt procedures. J Magn Reson Imaging 1994;4:145–150.

247. Lomas DJ, Britton PD, Alexander GJ, Calne RY. A comparison of MR and duplex Doppler ultrasound for vascular assessment prior to orthotopic liver transplantation. Clin Radiol 1994;49:307–310.

248. Eustace S, Buff B, Kruskal J, et al. Magnetic resonance angiography in transjugular intrahepatic portosystemic stenting: comparison with contrast hepatic and portal venography. Eur J Radiol 1994;19:43–49.

249. Katz JA, Rubin RA, Cope C, Holland G, Brass CA. Recurrent bleeding from anorectal varices: successful treatment with a transjugular intrahepatic portosystemic shunt. Am J Gastroenterol 1993;88:1104–1107.

250. Ohtomo K, Itai Y, Furui S, Yoshikawa K, Yashiro N, Iio M. MR imaging of portal vein thrombus in hepatocellular carcinoma. J Comput Assist Tomogr 1985;9:328–329.

251. Mathieu D, Guinet C, Bouklia-Hassane A, Vasile N. Hepatic vein involvement in hepatocellular carcinoma. Gastrointest Radiol 1988;13:55–60.

252. Mitani T, Nakamura H, Murakami T, et al. Dynamic MR studies of hepatocellular carcinoma with portal vein tumor thrombosis. Radiat Med 1992;10:232–234.

253. Glassman MS, Klein SA, Spivak W. Evaluation of cavernous transformation of the portal vein by magnetic resonance imaging. Clin Pediatr 1993;32:77–80.

254. Carpenter JP, Holland GA, Baum RA, Riley CA. Preliminary experience with magnetic resonance venography: comparison with findings at surgical exploration. J Surg Res 1994;57: 373–379.

255. Finn JP, Zisk JH, Edelman RR, et al. Central venous occlusion: MR angiography. Radiology 1993;187:245–251.

256. Creasy JL, Price RR, Presbrey T, Goins D, Partain CL, Kessler RM. Gadolinium-enhanced MR angiography. Radiology 1990;175:280–283.

74

Technique and Complications of Lymphangiography

WALTER A. FUCHS

Radiologic demonstration of lymph vessels and lymph nodes is mainly achieved only by direct lymphangiography, which is performed by injecting contrast material directly into the lymph vessels, lymph nodes, or occasionally lymph cysts. Indirect lymphangiography is used solely in animal experimentation. The contrast agents in this technique are introduced outside the lymphatic system either orally or by injection into subcutaneous tissue, muscle, joints, serous cavities, or solid organs. No contrast agent for indirect lymphangiography of the human body exists. Therefore, clinical lymphangiography demonstrates only those lymph vessels and nodes connected with the subcutaneous lymphatics of the extremities. Radiologic investigation of the lymphatic systems of the internal organs remains outside the range of diagnostic possibilities.

Clinical Lymphangiography

Clinical lymphangiography is performed essentially according to the direct technique of Kinmonth,[1,2] in which injection of contrast material is preceded by the subcutaneous injection of a vital dye. The dye facilitates visualization of the lymph vessels during the surgical cutdown for their direct puncture.[3]

Instruments

Several types of needles and catheters are used for puncture of the lymphatic vessel. Automatic injectors have been constructed for the slow and continuous injection of the viscous oily contrast material. The quantity injected is automatically adjusted to the prevailing pressure within the lymph vessels to avoid accidental rupturing of a lymph vessel. Injection by hand, or by a simple injector that uses weights, cannot precisely control the injection pressure and is therefore not ad-

visable. The contrast agent is kept at body temperature.

Vital Staining

Lymph vessels are stained by the subcutaneous injection of vital dye to make possible their visualization and dissection. Only the lymphatics absorb the dye and become visible through the skin as fine, greenish-blue streaks a few minutes after injection. A 1 percent dye solution is prepared by diluting one part of 2 percent patent blue-violet with an equal part of 2 percent procaine without epinephrine. The sites of injection are the interdigital webs, in which a great number of lymphatics find their source. Active or passive movements of the extremity or region injected increase lymph flow and speed up dye absorption.

Surgical Dissection

The vital dye injection sites are swabbed with skin disinfectant, and the subcutaneous injections are made. When the subcutaneous lymph vessels are sufficiently stained to be recognized as fine, greenish-blue streaks through the skin, the procedure may be started (Fig. 74-1). The area of incision is chosen at a place in which the stained lymphatics are clearly seen. A local anesthetic is injected subcutaneously, and a superficial transverse incision (2–4 cm long) is made. The subcutaneous lymphatics become visible as fine, greenish-blue vessels within the subcutaneous tissue. They are lifted with curved forceps, and the adherent fat and fibrous tissue are stripped away (Fig. 74-2). Complete stripping is essential for a successful puncture; it ensures that the needle tip will lie in the lumen of the vessel and not in surrounding tissue. A loop of silk thread is then placed around the vessel near the proximal border of the incision, and the lymphatic is pulled upward slightly by the silk, thereby producing a fold that obstructs the vessel.

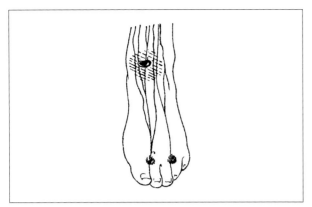

Figure 74-1. Interdigital injection of a vital dye using local anesthesia and a transverse incision of the skin.

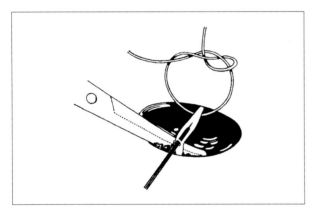

Figure 74-3. A silk loop is placed around the lymphatic and pulled upward to obstruct and dilate the vessel. The lymphatic is stretched by curved forceps and is punctured by the needle on the edge of the forceps. The stylet is withdrawn.

The tip of the puncture needle is placed exactly over the upper edge of the curved forceps and introduced into the lumen of the vessel with a gentle rotating movement (Fig. 74-3). The needle is carefully set down, the curved forceps is removed, and a silk knot is tightened over the needle (Fig. 74-4). A soft polyethylene tube that has been filled with contrast agent is then connected to the needle by means of a Luer-Lok and to the syringe that has been placed in position on the automatic injector.

After the injection is completed, the incision is cleaned of any traces of oil by copious irrigation with sterile saline. Antiseptic powder is applied, and the skin is closed with interrupted sutures. The stitches are removed 10 days later. Following the injection of oily contrast material, the patient should remain in the horizontal position for about 1 to 2 hours. The patient should remain in bed until the next day, and ambulatory patients should be driven home.

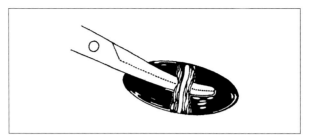

Figure 74-2. A lymph vessel is lifted up with curved forceps, and the adherent fat and fibrous tissue are stripped away.

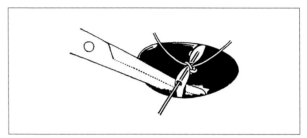

Figure 74-4. The blunt needle tip is advanced within the vessel, and a silk knot is tightened over the rough part of the needle.

Radiographic Technique

The radiographic technique includes routine exposures of the inguinal, iliac, and aortic areas immediately after the contrast injection (filling phase) and 24 hours later (storage phase). A standard chest film is also taken with the second series to demonstrate whether lung changes have been caused by the contrast material. The standard 90-kV exposure is correct when the structure of the lymph nodes is shown in good detail.

Preliminary screening with an image intensifier and television may become necessary in special cases to observe the extent of filling obtained. Laminography is very valuable as a supplementary method to distinguish between fused and superimposed lymph nodes.[4] In obese patients and in the event of the superimposition of bony structures, the lymphangiographic pattern of lymph nodes is demonstrated in detail. Direct roentgenographic magnification with an x-ray tube combining a high x-ray output with a fine focal spot produces very sharp images at two or three times linear magnification.[5,6] Logetronic detail enhancement by the photographic technique yields additional definition of the structural pattern of lymph nodes because small details are accentuated. The subtraction technique cannot be applied for lymphangiography because it is difficult to obtain roentgenograms of identical position, both before the investigation and after the lymph nodes are contrast-filled.

Foot Lymphangiography

Vital Staining

Subcutaneous injection of 1 to 2 ml of 1 percent dye solution is made into each of the first and fourth interdigital webs. The anteromedial and anterolateral subcutaneous lymphatics are thus demonstrated.

Surgical Dissection

The region of the first metatarsal bone is usually the most appropriate site for incision because the anteromedial lymphatics are easily dissected.

Contrast Injection

For adults, a 5- to 7-ml injection is used on each side in bilateral visualization. The unilateral injection dose is 8 to 10 ml with provision made for some contralateral filling of the aortic lymph nodes. For children, 1 to 4 ml is sufficient to fill the entire retroperitoneal lymph system unilaterally. The injection rate is set at 0.1 to 0.15 ml per minute at a pressure of 1.4 atm.

Radiographic Technique

Films of the lower extremities are required only in cases of edema after malignant invasion. The following routine exposures are made twice, immediately after injection and 24 hours later: inguinal and pelvic region, anteroposterior and right and left oblique films; thoracic duct and thoracic region, anteroposterior and lateral films; upper abdominal region, lateral projection (optional); and standard chest roentgenogram (24 hours only).

Cavography combined with *urography* is routinely performed by some investigators simultaneously with the 24-hour roentgenography. A bilateral femoral venous injection of 20 ml each of a water-soluble contrast agent is used. The rationale for doing this combined study is to demonstrate lymph node disease within the upper lumbar (aortic) region compressing the inferior vena cava, and to investigate stasis or dislocation of the ureter by malignant disease.

Arm Lymphangiography

Vital Staining

Injection of 0.5 ml of the 1 percent dye solution is made into each of the interdigital webs of the hand.

Surgical Dissection

The group of lymphatics demonstrated (i.e., either the radial or the ulnar group) corresponds to the side of the carpus chosen as the site for incision and injection.

Contrast Injection

For demonstration of the lymph vessels and nodes of the upper extremity and axilla, 4 to 5 ml of oily contrast material is required. The speed of injection should not exceed 0.1 ml per minute to prevent rupture of the delicate lymph vessels.

Radiographic Technique

The following routine exposures are made twice, immediately after injection and 24 hours later: forearm, anteroposterior and lateral films; upper arm, anteroposterior and lateral films; axillary and supraclavicular regions, anteroposterior and right and left oblique films with an angle of 25 degrees; and standard chest roentgenogram.

Contrast Material and Vital Dyes

Vital Dyes

The standard dye for direct lymphangiography is patent blue-violet, which is injected intradermally or subcutaneously. Patent blue-violet is a triphenylmethane dye with the molecular weight of 1159.4. Alphazurine 2 G is a blue dye, similar to patent blue-violet, which has been frequently used in the United States. The prepared dye solution should be made sterile by autoclaving in sealed ampules. Other dyes that have been used are Evans blue, brilliant blue, direct sky blue, and Prontosil rubrum. An 11 percent water solution of patent blue-violet is isotonic with body fluids, and 0.2 to 0.5 ml, diluted in 1.5 to 3.0 ml of 1 percent procaine or other local anesthetic, is injected subcutaneously in the web space between toes or fingers. The patent blue-violet is then absorbed and transported from the tissue, mainly by the lymphatics, and is excreted in the urine. The blue coloration progressively clears from the injected area and is essentially gone at 2 weeks.

Contrast Material

Oily contrast material is far superior to the water-soluble media for visualizing the lymph nodes and lymph vessels because it does not diffuse through the wall of the lymphatics. Therefore, detailed opacification of lymph nodes distant from the injection site is achieved. Water-soluble organic iodide contrast agents are now seldom used for lymphangiography because they diffuse rapidly from lymph vessels and nodes and thus obscure details of structure. The standard contrast agent used for lymphangiography is an iodized oil known commercially as Ethiodol in the United States and as Lipiodol Ultra-Fluid in Europe.[7,8]

Ethiodol is synthesized from the natural oil of poppy seeds and consists of the iodized glyceryl esters of oleic, linolenic, palmitic, and stearic acids.[9] It is yellow and has a specific gravity of 1.280 at 15°C. The viscosity is 53.6 centipoises at 20°C and 30.2 centipoises at 37°C. The iodine content is 37 percent. Stored in closed ampules and protected from light, Ethiodol is stable. Progressive liberation of iodine takes place when it is heated or in contact with air. Decomposition is indicated by discoloration. Solutions of contrast agent with a darker color should never be used.

Ethiodol injected directly into a peripheral lymphatic fills the lymph vessels and nodes. The opaque material remains in the nodes for several months. The oily contrast material is phagocytized by polynuclear giant cells and metabolized by esterases to sodium iodine. After the oily substance is eliminated from the nodes, the foreign-body reaction subsides. Sodium iodine is excreted mainly by the kidneys, but the pancreas, liver, and salivary glands also take part in its elimination.[10] Contrast medium in excess of that retained in the nodes enters the systemic veins via the thoracic duct or lymphaticovenous communications. From the great veins it passes into the lung capillaries. Some of the contrast material is removed via the pulmonary circulation. The macrophages in the alveolar spaces phagocytize parts of the agent, which is later removed by the sputum. With increase of the administered dose, the lung becomes a less efficient filter for the oily particles, and the amounts reaching other organs such as the liver, spleen, kidneys, and bone marrow are greater.

Complications of Lymphangiography

Wound Infection

Wound infection is rare after lymphangiography when adequate cleansing of the skin, strict aseptic technique, and careful dressing of the wound are carried out. Lymphangiitis is uncommon but may occasionally be observed in preexisting lymphedema. Slight swelling of the extremity rarely occurs. Delayed wound healing is seen as a result of excessive skin tension because of

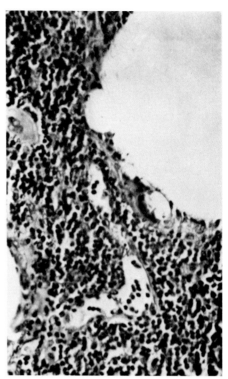

Figure 74-5. Foreign-body reaction. Granulation tissue with inflammatory cell infiltration and giant cells surround oil droplets.

movement. Extravasation of the oily contrast material from the lymph vessels is related to excessive injection pressure and is common in lymphatic obstruction.[11]

Foreign-Body Reaction

Foreign-body reaction and considerable dilatation of the marginal and intermediary sinuses occur within a few hours after lymphangiography.[12,13] The number of giant cells increases until the 14th day after administration of the contrast material. Granulation tissue and inflammatory cell infiltration surround oil droplets of various sizes (Fig. 74-5). The increased size of lymph nodes observed on the lymphangiogram in the first days after contrast injection can be attributed to the dilatation of the sinuses filled with contrast material and to the foreign-body reaction. A significant decrease in phagocytic reaction is observed after 3 to 6 weeks, and the foreign-body reaction subsides almost completely within 12 to 15 months. Small, circumscribed areas of fibrosis and scar reaction in the marginal sinuses and fibrous encapsulation of oil droplets may be observed as irreversible changes. These structural alterations of the lymph nodes are too minute to be demonstrated by lymphangiography. When the nodes have been examined by a second lymphangiography several months later, no change in the structural pattern of normal lymph nodes and no impairment of lymph circulation have been encountered.

Spread or Extension of a Neoplasm

The question of whether lymphangiography causes a neoplasm to spread has not been conclusively answered. A few clinical and experimental observations indicate the possibility of propagation of tumor cells by lymphangiography, but very extensive clinical experience with this method gives strong evidence that lymphangiography with oily contrast material does not increase the number of metastases.

Sensitivity Reactions to Contrast Media and to Iodine

Sensitivity reactions are very rare, occurring with an incidence of approximately 0.1 percent.[11,14] Dermatitis and erythematous skin reactions have been observed.[15] Sialadenitis is occasionally encountered and is considered to be a hypersensitivity of the salivary gland to iodine. Corticoids and antihistamines are used to treat these reactions. Adverse reactions to the blue dye are infrequent; the incidence is 1 in 700 examinations.[11,14] A few cases of nonfatal anaphylactic reactions to patent blue-violet have been reported.[16]

Lung Complications

Lung complications of lymphangiography are caused by embolism of the iodized oil into the pulmonary

Figure 74-6. Pulmonary oil embolism. Reticular deposits of oily substance are visible.

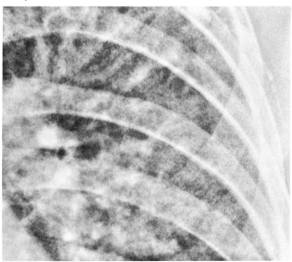

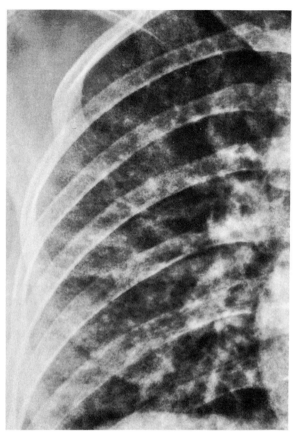

Figure 74-7. Chemical pneumonia. Miliary deposits of oily contrast substance and bronchopneumonic infiltration 5 days after lymphangiography.

capillaries.[11,14,12–24] After each lymphangiogram oily contrast material not retained in the lymph nodes enters the venous circulation. Miliary or reticular deposits of oily substance in the lungs are visible on the roentgenograms within 24 hours after injection in about 10 percent of the patients (Figs. 74-6 and 74-7). Most of these patients have neither clinical symptoms nor respiratory impairment, but scintiscanning of the lungs after the injection of a radioactive tracer material shows that lung embolization has occurred in every case.

No significant impairment of ventilation is observed as a result of lymphangiography. Wedging of the small lipid particles temporarily decreases the capillary bed available for diffusion of gases.[21,23] The maximum decrease in diffusing capacity ranges between 12 and 60 percent and is noted between 3 and 72 hours. Recovery time may vary from 21 to 256 hours. The decreased diffusing capacity is due to the decrease in capillary blood volume, which is between 28 and 60 percent of normal.

Twenty-four hours after lymphangiography the oily

contrast material is not found exclusively in the capillary bed of the lung but is scattered in the interstitial tissue of the lung. The oily substance leaves the lung partially via the vascular system. Lipid material also traverses the capillary endothelium into the interstitial tissue and later into the alveolar spaces, in which it is phagocytized by macrophages that are later expectorated. Reactive granulation tissue within the alveolar walls and areas of focal atelectases due to small infarctions are frequently encountered. These histologic inflammatory reactions subside within a few months after lymphangiography. The mechanical vascular occlusive phase, which sometimes causes acute symptoms, is followed in some patients by a chemical phase. In the chemical phase a lung response may develop that consists of edematous and inflammatory changes as a reaction to the fatty acids released by hydrolysis. The fatty acids damage the vessel endothelium and alveolar membranes, causing hemorrhage and exudation.[11] The chemical phase is marked by fever, hemoptysis, and varying degrees of respiratory distress.

Radiographic investigations demonstrate the change of the finely stippled pattern of uncomplicated oil embolism to massive bronchopneumonic infiltration in the perihilar and basal areas (see Fig. 74-7). Clinical and radiologic symptoms usually disappear within 10 to 14 days, and the patient returns to normal without residual effects.

In a survey of 32,000 lymphangiograms, in approximately 0.5 percent of cases serious pulmonary complications were reported.[14] They included hemoptysis, infarction, edema, and pneumonia. Because lung complications are clearly related to oily contrast material embolism, the amount of oil reaching the lungs must be kept to a minimum. The dosage of oily material injected in the adult patient has been reduced from 10 to 15 ml for each leg to 5 to 6 ml. Low dosage is appropriate in cases of irradiation fibrosis of lymph nodes because only small amounts of contrast material are retained in these nodes. The same dosage applies to lymphatic obstruction because oily material enters the lung by way of lymphaticovenous anastomoses.

Pulmonary function tests are necessary in every patient with a history of pulmonary disease, prior radiation therapy to the chest, or metastatic neoplasm or lymphoma in the lung.[21,23] In poor-risk patients unilateral left lymphangiography completed by vena cavography is the safest procedure. General anesthesia should not be administered in the immediate postlymphangiography period because lung diffusion is diminished. The aims of treatment of lung complications due to acute vascular obstruction are to improve oxygenation of blood and to maintain blood circulation.[11] Dyspnea, tachypnea, tachycardia, and cyanosis require

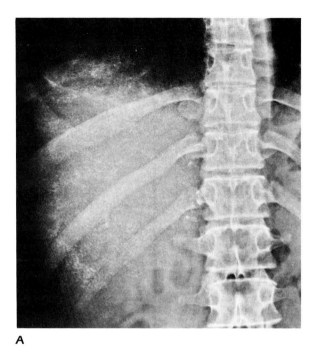

A

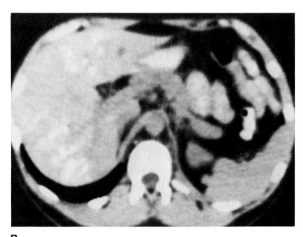

B

Figure 74-8. Hepatic oil embolism. (A) Reticular deposits of oily material visible in the portal venous system. (B) High-density deposits of oily contrast substance demonstrated at CT.

immediate administration of oxygen. Digitalis should be given parenterally in case of heart failure. Hypotension and shock must be treated. Intermittent positive pressure respiration may be needed. Intravenous administration of ethyl alcohol is advised to block the activity of lipase. Low-molecular-weight dextran is recommended to combat the sludging phenomenon of the blood.

Hepatic Oil Embolism

Hepatic oil embolism is rarely a cause of complications of lymphangiography (the incidence is approximately

0.2 percent).[11,25,26] Severe lymphatic obstruction in the common iliac and lower aortic region and occlusion of the pelvic veins must be present to shunt the oily contrast material through lymphaticovenous anastomoses and then via a venous collateral circulation into the portal venous system. The complication does not produce symptoms. Finely stippled deposits of oily material are seen radiographically (Fig. 74-8). Hepatic oil embolism occurs in all lymphangiography, but impairment of hepatic function has not been observed.[27]

Cerebral Oil Embolism

Cerebral oil embolism has been reported in a few cases as a complication of lymphangiography.[11,28–31] When excessive doses of oily material reach the venous circulation, the lung does not retain all of it and embolisms of oily material reach the brain.

Fever and pain in the back and groin, weakness, headache, unpleasant taste sensations, and nausea are transitory symptoms requiring no medication. Iodine sialitis and thyroiditis have been reported. Hemolytic crisis and thrombocytopenic purpura may be attributed to the oily material used in lymphangiography.

Cardiovascular Reactions

Such complications as hypertensive crisis and hypotensive reaction have been observed in a few cases.[11,22]

The incidence of fatal cases is generally extremely low. However, most patients examined by lymphangiography are frequently critically ill, and therefore caution has to be applied to prevent major complications.

References

1. Kinmonth JB. Lymphography in man: a method of outlining lymphatic trunks at operation. Clin Sci Mol Med 1952;11:13.
2. Kinmonth JB, Taylor GW, Kemp Harper R. Lymphangiography: a technique for its clinical use in the lower limb. Br Med J 1955;1:940.
3. Fuchs WA. Investigation techniques. In: Fuchs WA, Davidson JW, Fischer HW, eds. Lymphography in cancer. New York: Springer, 1969.
4. De Roo T, Thomas P, Kropholler RW. The importance of tomography for the interpretation of the lymphographic picture of lymph node metastases. AJR 1965;94:924.
5. Ditchek T, Scanlon GT. Direct magnification lymphography. JAMA 1967;199:654.
6. Love RW, Takaro T. Lymphangiography with direct roentgenographic magnification: new application for an old technique. Radiology 1966;87:123.
7. Fischer HW. Experiences in seeking an Ethiodol emulsion for lymphography. Invest Radiol 1966;1:29.
8. Fischer HW. Contrast media. In: Fuchs WA, Davidson JW, Fischer HW, eds. Lymphography in cancer. New York: Springer, 1969.
9. Guerbet M. Étude expérimentale de la toxicité du Lipiodol ultrafluide par voie intraveineuse ou lymphatique. J Radiol Electrol Med Nucl 1964;45:887.
10. Koehler PR, Meyers WA, Skelly JF, Schaffer B. Body distribution of Ethiodol following lymphangiography. Radiology 1964;82:866.
11. Fischer HW. Complications. In: Fuchs WA, Davidson JW, Fischer HW, eds. Lymphography in cancer. New York: Springer, 1969.
12. Oehlert W, Weissleber H, Gollasch D. Lymphogramm und histologisches Bild normaler und pathologischer veränderter Lymphknoten. ROEFO 1966;104:751.
13. Ravel R. Histopathology of lymph nodes after lymphangiography. Am J Clin Pathol 1966;46:335.
14. Koehler PR. Complications of lymphography. In: Viamonte M, Koehler PR, Witte M, Witte C, eds. Progress in lymphology. Stuttgart: Thieme, 1970. Vol. II.
15. Redman HC. Dermatitis as a complication of lymphangiography. Radiology 1966;86:323.
16. Kopp WL. Anaphylaxis from alphazurine 2G during lymphography. JAMA 1966;198:200.
17. Bron KM, Baum S, Abrams HL. Oil embolism in lymphangiography: incidence, manifestations and mechanism. Radiology 1963;80:194.
18. Clouse ME, Hallgrimsson J, Wenlund DE. Complications following lymphography with particular reference to pulmonary oil embolization. AJR 1966;96:972.
19. Desprez-Curely JP, Bismuth V, Langier A, Descamps J. Accidents et incidents de la lymphographie. Ann Radiol (Paris) 1962;5:577.
20. Dolan PA. Lymphography: complications encountered in 522 examinations. Radiology 1966;86:876.
21. Fraimow W, Wallace S, Lewis P, Greening RR, Cathcart RT. Changes in pulmonary function due to lymphangiography. Radiology 1965;85:231.
22. Fuchs WA. Complications in lymphography with oily contrast media. Acta Radiol 1962;57:427.
23. Gold WM, Youker J, Anderson S, Nadel JA. Pulmonary function abnormalities after lymphangiography. N Engl J Med 1965;273:519.
24. Sokol GH, Clouse ME, Kotner LM, Sewell JB. Complications of lymphangiography in patients of advanced age. AJR 1977;128:43.
25. Bodie JF, Linton DS Jr. Hepatic oil embolization as a complication of lymphangiography. Radiology 1971;99:317.
26. Chavez GM, Picard J, Davis D. Liver opacification following lymphangiography; pathogenesis and clinical significance. Surgery 1968;63:564.
27. Fuchs WA, Preisig R, Bucher H. Liver function after lymphography. In: Viamonte M, Koehler PR, Witte M, Witte C, eds. Progress in lymphology. Stuttgart: Thieme, 1970. Vol. II.
28. Jay JC, Ludington JC. Neurologic complications following lymphangiography: possible mechanisms and a case of blindness. Arch Surg 1973;106:863.
29. Jochem W, Buchelt L. A case of cerebral embolism after lymphography. Radiology 1969;93:711.
30. Nelson B, Rush EA, Takasugi M, Wittenberg J. Lipid embolism to the brain after lymphography. N Engl J Med 1965;273:1132.
31. Rasmussen KE. Retinal and cerebral fat emboli following lymphography with oily contrast media. Acta Radiol 1970;10:199.

75

Normal Radiologic Anatomy of the Lymphatics and Lymph Nodes

WALTER A. FUCHS

Normal Structural Roentgen Anatomy

Although the basic topographic anatomy of lymph vessels and lymph nodes in the inguinal, pelvic, lumbar, and axillary regions is constant, there is considerable variation in the size, shape, number, and structure of the lymph nodes. Normal lymph nodes vary between 1 and 30 mm in diameter, depending on the functional load, constitutional elements, and age. They may be round, oval, elongated, or bean-shaped with a slight indentation at the hilar region. Lymph nodes consist of lymphatic tissue, which is connected with the lymphatic circulation by afferent and efferent lymphatics (Figs. 75-1 and 75-2).[1-4] The sinus system of the lymph nodes includes the marginal sinus, situated close to the lymph node capsule of fibrous tissue, and extensions of the marginal sinus, the intermediate sinuses, which converge toward the hilus, where they unite to form the terminal sinuses. The lymphatic tissue is formed by a netlike stroma of reticular fibers and both free and fixed reticulohistiocytic, lymphatic, and plasmatic cells. Myeloid and mast cells are also present. Loose lymphatic tissue, consisting of a meshwork of reticular fibers and reticulohistiocytic cells, fills the sinuses, which are the main channels for lymph circulation.[5,6]

The diffuse lymphatic tissue of the nodes is formed by a dense network of reticular fibers and uniformly distributed cells of the lymphatic group. The nodular lymphatic tissue of the lymph nodes includes follicles, which are rounded, and dense accumulations of predominantly lymphatic cells embedded in a very loose reticular stroma. The diffuse lymphatic tissue is arranged into a rather compact cortex, and a medulla, which consists of a coarse network of medullary cords. The cortex is divided into lymphatic lobules by trabeculae of dense connective tissue arising from the capsule. The lymph follicles, which are not permanent structures, are localized predominantly in the cortex but may also be found in the medullary cords. The functions of the nodules are lymph filtration and cell production, chiefly of lymphatic and plasma cells. Depending on the functional state of the lymph node, primary and secondary nodules may be present. These differ in that the primary follicle has a more uniform structure whereas the secondary follicle contains a so-called germinal center.

In lymphangiography the filling phase immediately after injection of a contrast medium demonstrates both lymph vessels and lymph nodes (Fig. 75-3A).[7-10] Contrast medium enters a node through the numerous afferent lymphatics joining its marginal lymph sinus, passes through the medullary sinuses in streaks, and leaves the lymph node by way of efferent lymphatics from the hilus. Generally, there are more afferent than efferent lymphatics. Often the contrast medium first passes directly from the afferent to the efferent lymph vessels of a lymph node without demonstrating the entire sinus system. Then gradually, as more contrast material enters the node, the entire sinus system is visualized. Direct connections between efferent lymphatics of a lymph node and afferent lymphatics of other nodes are frequently observed.

During the storage phase, which is 2 to 24 hours after injection, the contrast material leaves the lymph vessels and accumulates in the lymph nodes (see Fig. 75-3B). Contrast filling of the lymph vessels for more than 24 hours must generally be regarded as a sign of impaired lymphatic circulation. The oily contrast agent is retained as drops in the lymph nodes by the network of fibrous and reticulohistiocytic cells.[2] Intracellular deposits of contrast medium are rare because reabsorption of the fluid takes place very slowly. The major portion of the contrast material remains embedded in the meshwork of the reticulum cells, which phagocytize it for about 5 to 9 months. The marginal sinus of the nodes and the peripheral parts of the intermediary sinuses are most densely filled with contrast fluid. Small

1871

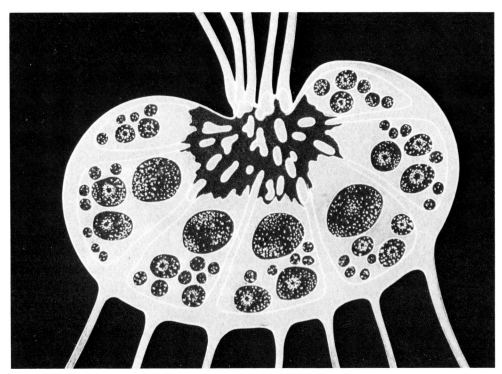

Figure 75-1. Schematic representation of structural lymph node anatomy.

structural changes in the lymph nodes may be obscured by an excessive amount of contrast medium within the sinuses. The follicular lymphatic tissue of the nodes is not penetrated by oily contrast agent. Small, round filling defects of varied sizes corresponding to the different lymph follicles lead to a fine homo-

Figure 75-2. Lymphographic storage pattern of normal lymph nodes.

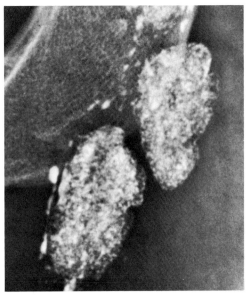

geneous, reticular appearance.[11] In the medullary parts without nodules, however, the distribution may appear to be irregular.

The size of lymph nodes and vessels as determined by lymphangiography tends to decrease in old age, but size depends more on the functional state than on age.[12] With the same qualification in mind, it is generally found that children and young women have fine, delicate lymphatics.

Fibrolipomatosis is considered a manifestation of the normal physiologic involution of the lymph nodes. It is characterized by the replacement of the central parts of the lymph nodes by connective and fatty tissue.[7,8,10,13] Lymphatic structures are left only in the periphery of the nodes. The intermediary sinuses traversing the fibrolipomatous tissue stay intact (Fig. 75-4A). Lymphography results in a large central filling defect permeated by the intermediary sinuses, because only the reticular meshwork of the lymphatic tissue is able to retain the contrast substance (see Fig. 75-4B). Consequently, careful analysis of the radiographic pattern of the intermediary sinuses during the lymphographic filling phase is of paramount importance in the diagnostic evaluation of filling defects.

Involutive changes are very common in inguinal and axillary lymph nodes, because they are the primary regional lymph node groups of the extremities, and

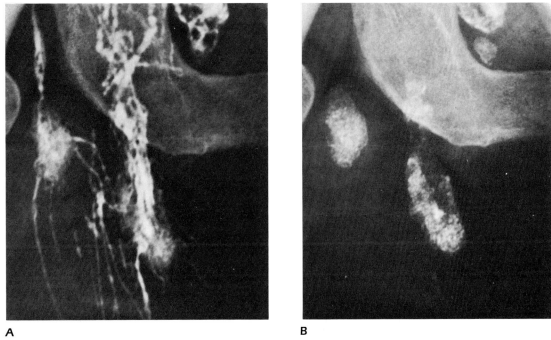

A   B

Figure 75-3. Normal inguinal lymph nodes. (A) Filling phase. (B) Storage phase.

therefore are most often affected by inflammatory lesions. The external iliac and the aortic node groups at the level of L1-L2 manifest similar, but less extensive, involutive changes. Fibrolipomatosis is more pronounced in patients of the middle and older age groups.

Figure 75-4. Fibrolipomatosis of inguinal lymph nodes. (A) Filling phase. (B) Storage phase.

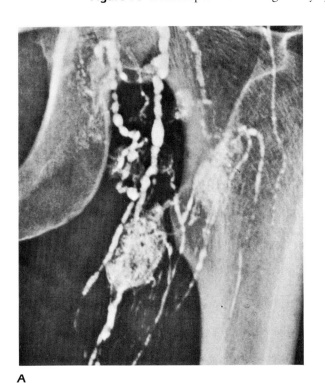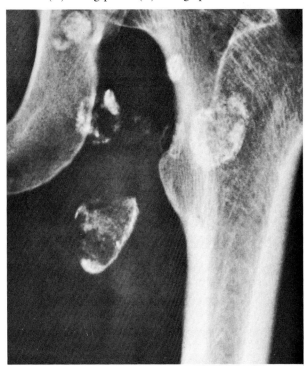

A   B

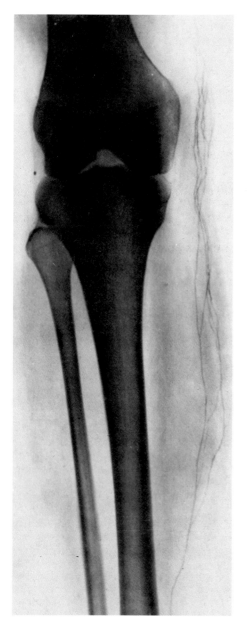

Figure 75-5. Anteromedial group of subcutaneous lymphatics.

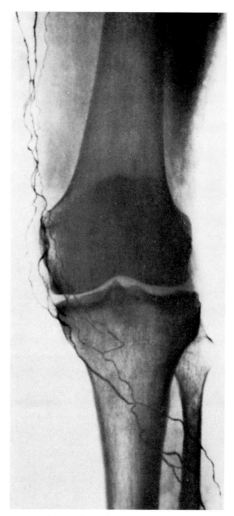

Figure 75-6. Anterolateral group of subcutaneous lymphatics.

Topographic Anatomy

Lower Extremity

The lymphatics of the lower extremities[9,14–17] consist of a subcutaneous prefascial and a deep subfascial lymph system. The lymph from the capillary network of the skin and the subcutis drains through delicate lymphatics into groups of larger, longitudinal lymph vessels situated above the fascia. They are closely connected with the largest subcutaneous veins. The deep subfascial lymph vessels collect the lymph from the muscles, fascia, and joints. The valves in lymphatics direct the flow, contrary to veins, from the deep to the superficial lymphatic system. At present, lymphangiography as a routine procedure can outline only the prefascial lymphatics.

According to their relationship to the veins, the lymph vessels of the leg are divided into an anterior vena saphena magna group and a posterior vena saphena parva group. The anterior group is composed of a medial and a lateral bundle of lymphatics. The anteromedial group follows a straight and almost parallel course on the medial side of the leg and comprises 5 to 6 vessels in the lower leg and 10 to 20 vessels in the thigh (Fig. 75-5).

The vessels of the anterolateral group of lymphatics, five to six in number, course distally on the peroneal side of the leg and cross in a wide curve toward the medial side at the level of the knee, where they become

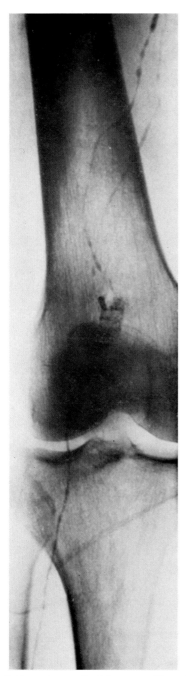

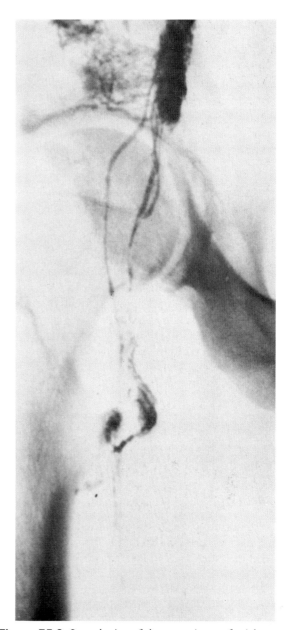

Figure 75-8. Lymphatics of the posterior prefascial group connected with deep inguinal lymph nodes and intermediate and lateral external iliac lymph nodes.

Figure 75-7. Posterior prefascial group of lymphatics connected with two popliteal lymph nodes.

of large diameter and tortuous (Fig. 75-6). Above the knee these lymphatic trunks are always situated medially in close connection with the great saphenous vein until they join the superficial inguinal lymph nodes.

The posterior prefascial lymphatic group, which accompanies the lesser saphenous vein, consists of only one to three prefascial collecting trunks that reach one to three subfascial lymph nodes in the popliteal region

(Fig. 75-7). The latter nodes are connected to the deep inguinal or iliac nodes by subfascial lymphatics, which follow the deep blood vessels on the medial aspect of the thigh (Fig. 75-8). The collecting subcutaneous prefascial lymph vessels branch dichotomously as they course proximally. Despite this division, they retain equal diameters of about 0.75 to 1.0 mm. Normally, there are no anastomoses among the various superficial groups of vessels.

Inguinal Region

The lymph nodes of the inguinal region[9,12–14,17–21] are subdivided into a superficial and a deep group (Figs. 75-9 and 75-10). The superficial inguinal lymph nodes are separated into a superior and an inferior group. On the lymphangiogram the perineal and genital groups of superior superficial inguinal lymph nodes are rarely demonstrated because these nodes are very seldom connected with afferent lymphatics from the lower extremity. The crural group of superior superficial inguinal lymph nodes is situated cranially in the inguinal region and cannot be differentiated on the lymphangiogram from the deep inguinal lymph nodes. The configuration of both groups is similar—round and small. Afferent and efferent lymphatics do not provide a distinction between two groups. For this reason the superior superficial inguinal lymph nodes receiving afferent lymphatics from the right and the deep inguinal nodes have been grouped together.

The most cranial of the deep inguinal nodes is the largest and most constant. It is situated in the inguinal fossa close to the lacunar ligament and medial to the femoral vein in intimate relationship with the medial external iliac lymph nodes. The inferior superficial inguinal lymph nodes (subinguinal lymph nodes) localized around the hiatus saphenus are regularly filled with contrast material because their afferent lymphatics drain the lymph from the lower extremity.

Pelvic Region

According to their relationship to the iliac blood vessels, the lymph nodes of the pelvic region[9,12–14,17–23] are divided into the external, internal, and common iliac node groups (Fig. 75-11).

The external iliac lymph nodes are situated along the external iliac artery and vein and are continuous with the inguinal lymph nodes (Figs. 75-12 and 75-13). They are subdivided into the lateral, intermediate, and medial external iliac node groups, which are connected by numerous lymphatics. The lateral external iliac lymph node chain is localized along the lateral aspect of the external iliac artery within a cleft formed by the artery with the psoas muscle. The medial external iliac lymph node group is positioned medial and dorsal to the external iliac vein near the pelvic wall and between the external iliac artery and the obturator nerve.

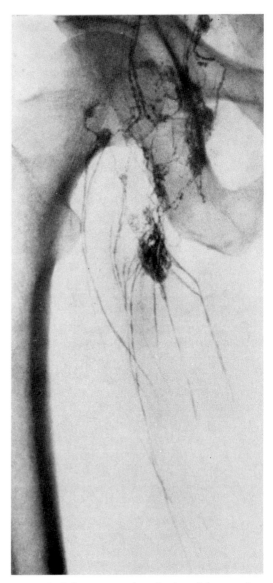

Figure 75-9. Subcutaneous lymphatics of the anterior medial group enter inferior superficial inguinal (subinguinal) lymph nodes and deep inguinal lymph nodes.

The common iliac lymph nodes are arranged along the common iliac vessels and are a direct continuation of the lateral, intermediate, and medial node groups of the external iliac area (see Figs. 75-12 and 75-13). The lateral iliac lymph nodes are situated at the lateral aspect of the common iliac artery and on the inner margin of the psoas muscle. Their afferent lymphatics arise from the lateral external iliac lymph nodes. The

Figure 75-11. Topographic roentgenographic anatomy of the inguinal and iliac lymph nodes (oblique projection). (From ▶ Fuchs WA. Normal anatomy. In: Fuchs WA, Davidson JW, Fischer HW, eds. Lymphography in cancer. New York: Springer, 1969. Used with permission.)

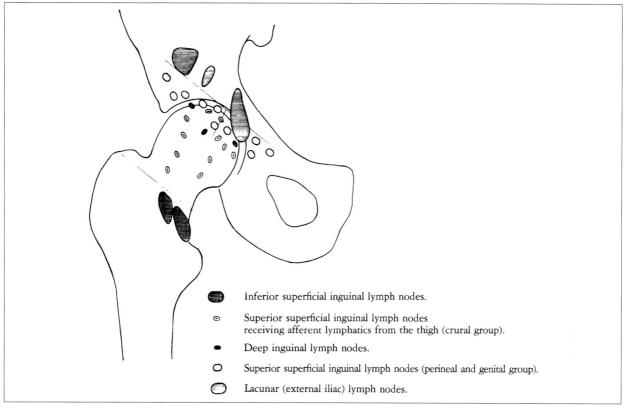

Figure 75-10. Topographic anatomy of the inguinal lymph nodes. (From Fuchs WA. Normal anatomy. In: Fuchs WA, Davidson JW, Fischer HW, eds. Lymphography in cancer. New York: Springer, 1969. Used with permission.)

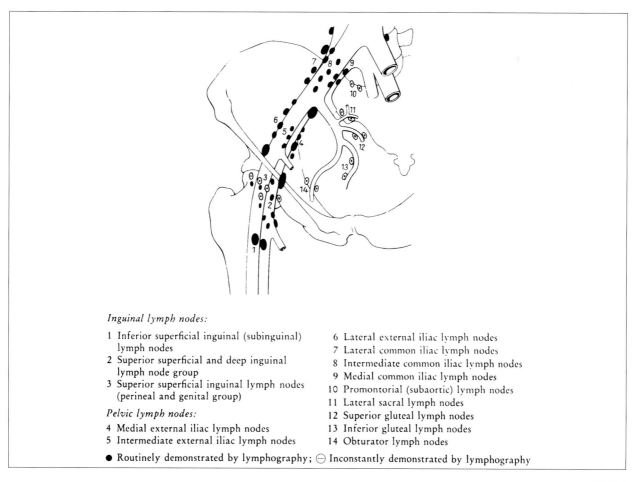

Inguinal lymph nodes:

1 Inferior superficial inguinal (subinguinal) lymph nodes
2 Superior superficial and deep inguinal lymph node group
3 Superior superficial inguinal lymph nodes (perineal and genital group)

Pelvic lymph nodes:

4 Medial external iliac lymph nodes
5 Intermediate external iliac lymph nodes

6 Lateral external iliac lymph nodes
7 Lateral common iliac lymph nodes
8 Intermediate common iliac lymph nodes
9 Medial common iliac lymph nodes
10 Promontorial (subaortic) lymph nodes
11 Lateral sacral lymph nodes
12 Superior gluteal lymph nodes
13 Inferior gluteal lymph nodes
14 Obturator lymph nodes

● Routinely demonstrated by lymphography; ⊖ Inconstantly demonstrated by lymphography

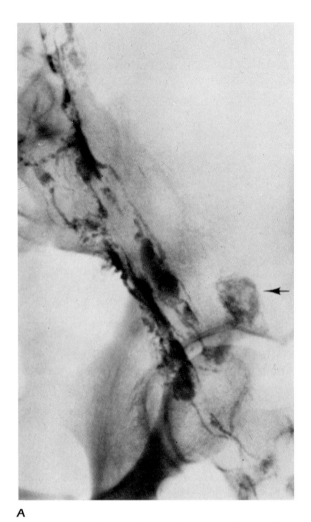

A

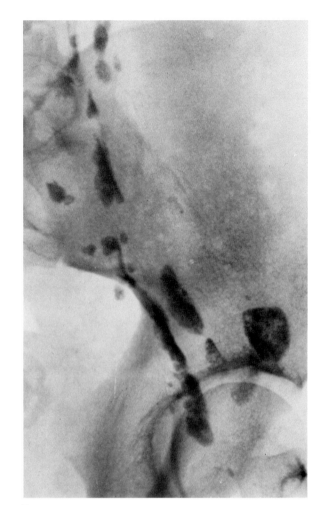

B

Figure 75-12. The lateral (*arrow*), intermediate, and medial external iliac lymph node chains connected by numerous lymphatics. (A) Filling phase. (B) Storage phase.

efferent lymphatics reach the lateral aortic lymph nodes on the corresponding side. The intermediate common iliac lymph nodes are found on the posterior aspect of the common iliac artery and vein and are continuous with the intermediate external iliac lymph node group. The medial common iliac lymph nodes are localized on the medial aspect of the common iliac artery and vein. The lymphatics and nodes of both sides form a triangular arrangement.

All lymph nodes situated within the region of supply of the internal iliac artery and its branches make up the internal iliac lymph nodes, also called hypogastric lymph nodes (see Fig. 75-13).[21,22,24] According to their relation to parietal and visceral arterial branches, they are divided into parietal and visceral lymph node groups. The parietal lymph node group is composed

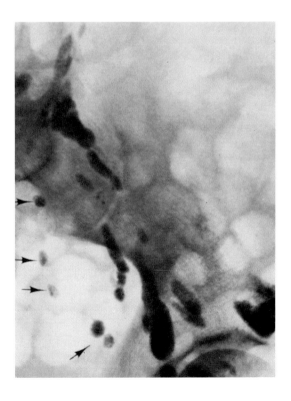

Figure 75-13. Contrast filling of multiple parietal internal iliac lymph nodes: superior (*left arrows*) and inferior gluteal nodes (*bottom arrow*), lateral sacral nodes (*top arrow*), and fusion of the medial external iliac nodes.

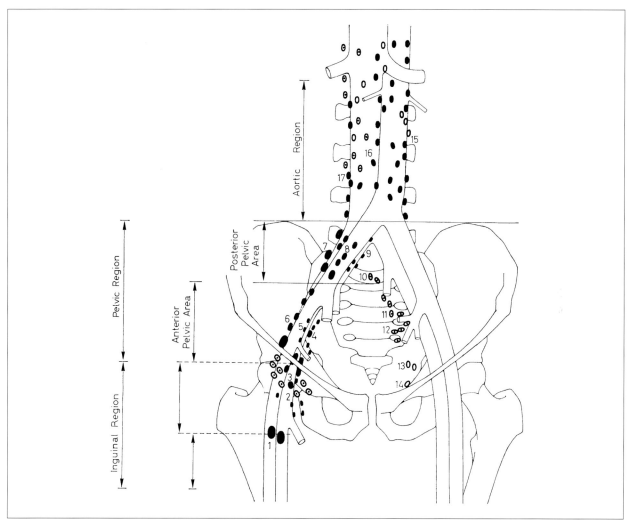

Figure 75-14. Topographic roentgenographic anatomy of the inguinal, iliac, and aortic lymph nodes (anteroposterior projection). *1,* inferior superficial inguinal (subinguinal) lymph nodes; *2,* superior superficial (crural group) and deep inguinal lymph node group; *3,* superior superficial inguinal lymph nodes (perineal and genital group); *4,* medial external iliac lymph nodes; *5,* intermediate external iliac lymph nodes; *6,* lateral external iliac lymph nodes; *7,* lateral common iliac lymph nodes; *8,* intermediate common iliac lymph nodes; *9,* medial common iliac lymph nodes; *10,* promontorial (sub- aortic) lymph nodes; *11,* lateral sacral lymph nodes; *12,* superior gluteal lymph nodes; *13,* inferior gluteal lymph nodes; *14,* obturator lymph nodes; *15,* left aortic lymph nodes; *16,* preretroaortic lymph nodes; *17,* right aortic lymph nodes. ● Routinely demonstrated by lymphangiography; ☉ facultatively demonstrated by lymphangiography. (From Fuchs WA. Normal anatomy. In: Fuchs WA, Davidson JW, Fischer HW, eds. Lymphography in cancer. New York: Springer, 1969. Used with permission.)

of the superior and inferior gluteal lymph nodes and the lateral, sacral, and obturator lymph nodes, which are occasionally contrast-filled by foot lymphangiography. The visceral lymph nodes are only partially connected with the visceral arterial branches and are situated close to the related organs. They comprise the vesical, rectal, and parauterine lymph node groups. The internal iliac lymph nodes, which are not contrast-filled by foot lymphangiography, receive lymph from the joints and muscles of the pelvis and from the organs in the pelvic region, the upper third of the vagina, uterus, ovaries, prostate, vesicular gland and urinary

bladder, and areas of the penis and the rectum. They are connected to the common iliac and aortic node group by efferent lymphatics.

Lumbar (Aortic) Region

The lumbar lymph nodes[9,12-14,19-21] are situated on the anterior aspect of the lumbar vertebrae and around the abdominal aorta and inferior vena cava. Anatomically they are divided into the right intermediate and left lumbar node groups (Fig. 75-14). In the lymphangiogram only one intermediate and two lateral lymph

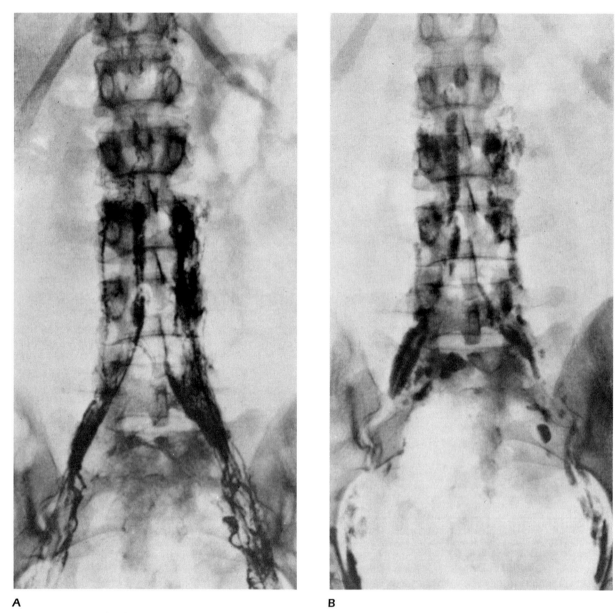

A   **B**

Figure 75-15. Lumbar lymph nodes, development of the three aortic lymph node chains. (A) Filling phase. (B) Storage phase.

node chains are discernible (Fig. 75-15): the exact position of the preaortic and retroaortic node groups in relation to the abdominal aorta cannot be determined on roentgenograms. Unilateral injection of contrast material leads to retrograde contrast filling of the common iliac lymph nodes of the contralateral side in about half the cases, which therefore may not be interpreted as a pathologic finding. Visualization of contralateral lymph nodes at the level of the fourth to fifth lumbar vertebrae by anastomosing lymphatics is also observed in about 50 percent of normal lymphangiograms.

The right lumbar lymph nodes, situated on the right side of the abdominal aorta, are grouped according to their relation to the inferior vena cava into the precaval, interaorticocaval, retrocaval, and laterocaval nodes. In the lymphangiogram they are projected upon the right aspect of the vertebral bodies and up to 2 cm further laterally. The number of right lumbar lymph nodes that are contrast-filled by lymphangiography is considerably smaller than that of the other two lumbar node chains (Fig. 75-16). This is in contrast to anatomic findings, which show the right lumbar lymph node group comprising the greatest number of nodes.

In 70 percent of cases the upper border of the right lymph nodes filled with contrast material reaches the level of the third lumbar vertebra or below, in about 20 percent it reaches the second lumbar vertebra, and in only 10 percent does it reach the first lumbar vertebra.

The intermediate lumbar lymph nodes (preaortic and retroaortic lymph nodes) are projected onto the vertebral bodies of the lumbar spine in lymphangiography. Contrast filling of the intermediate lymph nodes is considerably more frequent than is found with the right lumbar lymph node group. It reaches the level of the first lumbar vertebra in 50 percent of cases and the second lumbar vertebra in 40 percent. In only 10 percent is the upper border of this chain situated at or below the third lumbar vertebra.

The left lumbar lymph nodes are situated between the psoas muscle and the abdominal aorta and form a chain of 5 to 10 nodes. On the lymphangiogram they are projected onto the left lateral aspect of the lumbar spine and up to 2 cm further laterally. They receive afferent lymphatics from the lateral common iliac lymph nodes and are connected to the other aortic lymph node chains. Radiologically the left lumbar lymph node group is the most constant of all lumbar node groups and comprises the largest number of contrast-filled nodes. Clustering of lymph nodes is seen below the left renal artery and vein. It reaches the level of the first and second lumbar vertebrae in about 90 percent of cases and the level of the third lumbar vertebra in 10 percent.

Contrast filling of lumbar lymphatics and lumbar lymph nodes on the dorsal aspect of the lumbar fossa is a rare variation.

Upper Extremity

In the forearm and arm[9,17,24] the subcutaneous lymphatics are divided into a medial ulnar (basilic) group and a lateral radial (cephalic) group.

The ulnar group of lymphatics drains primarily the third, fourth, and fifth finger and the ulnar side of the hand and forearm (Fig. 75-17). The majority of these lymph channels run along with the basilic vein to the cubital region. Above this point they follow the medial border of the biceps muscle to reach the prefascial axillary lymph nodes. One to two lymphatics may accompany the basilic vein through the deep fascia and join the deep subfascial lymph vessels of the upper arm.

The radial group of lymphatics drains the first and second digits and the radial side of the hand and forearm. These lymphatics are situated on the lateral side of the wrist and join the cephalic vein in the forearm.

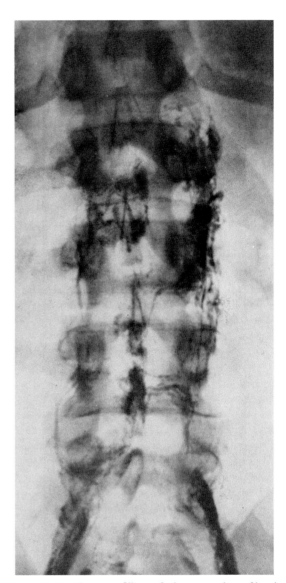

Figure 75-16. Contrast filling of a large number of lumbar nodes situated at the level of the left renal blood vessels. There is sparse filling of the right lumbar nodes above the fourth lumbar vertebra.

They follow the vein to the level of the olecranon, at which point most of them curve medially to enter the lateral group of axillary lymph nodes. A few lymphatics continue with the cephalic vein to reach the infraclavicular lymph nodes. The collecting lymphatics from the deltoid region pass over the anterior and posterior axillary folds to end in axillary lymph nodes. The skin of the scapular region is drained by lymph vessels that end in the subcapsular groups of axillary nodes or follow the transverse cervical vessels to the interior deep cervical lymph nodes. The deep lymph channels of the arm follow the muscles, vessels, and nerves and end at the lateral axillary lymph nodes. They are less numer-

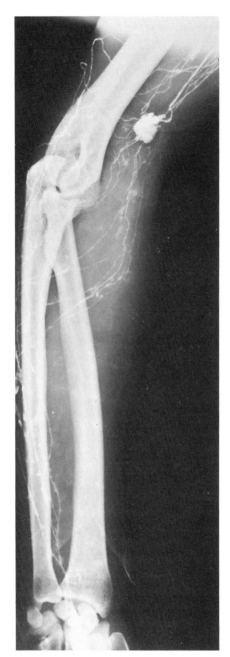

Figure 75-17. Ulnar group of lymphatics. Lymph channels follow the basilic vein and the medial border of the biceps muscle. Contrast filling of cubital lymph node.

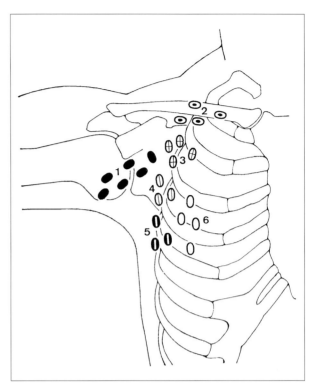

Figure 75-18. Topographic roentgenographic anatomy of the axillary lymph nodes. *1*, lateral axillary lymph nodes; *2*, supraclavicular lymph nodes; *3*, apical axillary lymph nodes; *4*, central axillary lymph nodes; *5*, posterior or subscapular axillary lymph nodes; *6*, anterior or pectoral axillary nodes. (From Fuchs WA. Normal anatomy. In: Fuchs WA, Davidson JW, Fischer HW, eds. Lymphography in cancer. New York: Springer, 1969. Used with permission.)

ous than the superficial vessels, with which they communicate at intervals. A few deep lymph nodes are connected with the deep lymphatic system.

Axillary Region

The axillary lymph nodes[9,17,24] are the first regional nodes of the whole upper limb and are divided into five groups (Fig. 75-18).

The lateral axillary group is situated medial and posterior to the axillary vein. The afferent lymphatics of this group drain the lymph of the entire upper extremity, except for the regions drained by radial subcutaneous vessels following the cephalic vein. The efferent vessels join the central and apical axillary lymph nodes or the inferior deep cervical lymph nodes.

The anterior or pectoral group of axillary lymph nodes is located along the inferior border of the lesser pectoral muscle near the lateral thoracic vessels. The afferent lymphatics of this group drain the skin and muscles of the anterior and lateral walls of the thorax, the abdominal wall above the umbilicus, and the central and lateral areas of the mammary gland. The efferent lymph vessels enter the central and apical axillary node group.

The posterior or subcapsular axillary lymph nodes are placed along the lower margin of the posterior wall of the axilla close to the axillary vessels. The afferent lymphatics of this group drain the skin and muscles of the lower part of the neck and of the dorsal aspect of the body as far inferiorly as the iliac crests. The efferent lymphatics enter the apical and central groups of axillary nodes.

The central axillary lymph node group is situated near the base of the axilla. The group has no drainage area of its own but receives efferent lymphatics from most of the other axillary lymph node groups. The efferent lymphatics of the group enter the apical axillary lymph nodes.

The apical axillary lymph nodes are situated within the apex of the axilla medial to the axillary vein, dorsal to the superior portion of the lesser pectoral muscle, and cranial to the superior margins of the pectoral muscles. The only direct territorial afferents of this group are those that accompany the cephalic vein. The nodes receive efferent lymphatics from all the other axillary lymph node groups. The efferent vessels of the apical axillary group unite to form the subclavian trunk, which opens either directly into the junction of the internal jugular and subclavian veins or into the jugular lymphatic trunk. On the left side the subclavian trunk may enter the thoracic duct directly. A few efferents of the apical axillary lymph nodes are usually connected with inferior deep cervical nodes.

Lymphangiography by injection of contrast material into a lymph vessel of the radial or ulnar group of lymphatics in the forearm demonstrates only a few lymph nodes of the lateral axillary group (Fig. 75-19). Complete contrast filling of all lateral axillary lymph nodes is not achieved because each lymphatic of the forearm may enter a different node. The efferent lymphatics of the contrast-filled lateral axillary lymph nodes drain into a few nodes of the central and apical groups of axillary nodes. From the apical axillary node group, efferent lymphatics are demonstrated, uniting to form the subclavian trunk. Occasionally, some supraclavicular and deep cervical lymph nodes are filled with contrast material.

Thoracic Duct

The frequency of lymphographic demonstration of the thoracic duct varies.[9,25–32] It depends on the amount of contrast material, the timing of the films, and the positioning of the patient.

On the basis of its embryologic development, the thoracic duct is subdivided into abdominal, thoracic, and cervical sections.

The *abdominal section of the thoracic duct* is formed by the union of the two lumbar trunks, originating from the efferent lymphatics of the upper lumbar lymph nodes and the intestinal trunk, which collect the lymph from the gastrointestinal tract. The intestinal trunk is not a constant finding, because the efferent

Figure 75-19. Axillary lymphangiogram. Contrast filling of lateral, central, and apical axillary lymph nodes.

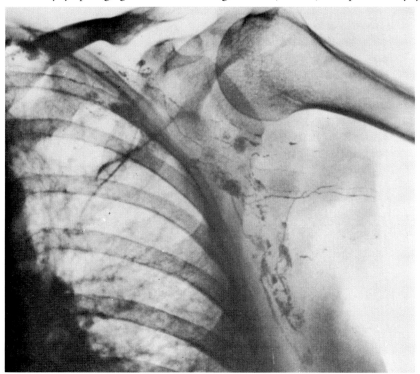

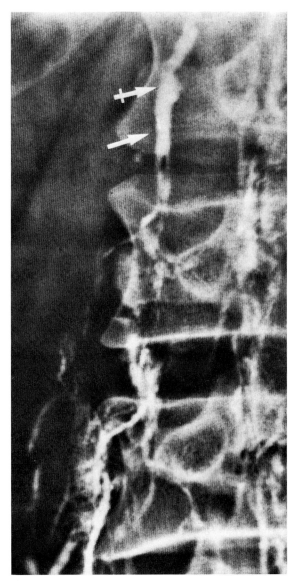

Figure 75-20. Solitary lumbar trunk (*arrow*) in continuous connection with the fusiform cisterna chyli (*barred arrow*).

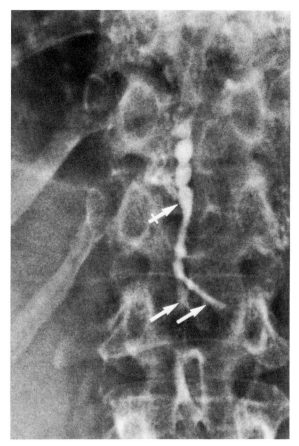

Figure 75-21. Two lumbar trunks (*arrows*) entering the beadlike cisterna chyli (*barred arrow*).

lymphatics of the abdominal organs usually unite to form a few larger lymph vessels, which enter the thoracic duct or one of the lumbar trunks directly. Extensive variations of the abdominal section of the thoracic duct are encountered. The entry of trunks into the thoracic duct is most frequently localized between T12 and L2, but it may be situated between T11 and L3-L4. The cisterna chyli, an ampullaceous enlargement of the thoracic duct at its origin, was found mainly when the origin of the thoracic duct was low. Large reticular lymph trunks, but no cisterna chyli, are frequently observed (40–50 percent), particularly when the origin of the thoracic duct is close to T11. Rare configurations are ampullaceous dilatation of the

lumbar trunks and numerous anastomosing small lymphatics. A beadlike appearance of the lower thoracic duct may be found, especially in cases of low origin. The configuration of the cisterna chyli may be conical, ampullaceous, fusiform, or moniliform.

Lumbar trunk *visualization by lymphography* occurs in about 25 percent of cases. In the lymphogram, lumbar trunks are demonstrated as large, oblique lymph vessels, with medially directed courses originating from several small efferent lymphatics. Topographic localization and configuration of the *lumbar trunks* are variable because of partial contrast filling. A single lumbar trunk (Fig. 75-20) or two lumbar trunks (Figs. 75-21 and 75-22) as well as three lumbar trunks (Fig. 75-23) are commonly found; a reticular configuration of the lumbar trunks is demonstrated occasionally (5 percent of cases). In 30 percent the lumbar trunks are situated at L1, in 39 percent at L2, and in 15 percent at L3. In a few cases, the beginning of the thoracic duct is found to be above T12 or below L4. The diameter of the lumbar trunks varies between 1 and 6 mm, with an average of 2 mm.

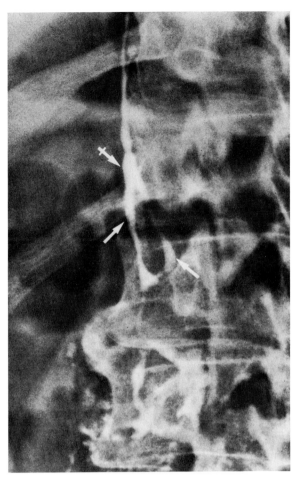

Figure 75-22. Two lumbar trunks (*arrows*) in connection with the conical cisterna chyli (*barred arrow*).

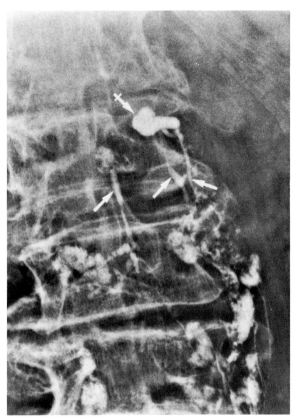

Figure 75-23. Three lumbar trunks (*arrows*) entering the ampullaceous cisterna chyli (*barred arrow*).

On the lymphogram, the cisterna chyli is recognized as a large lymph trunk situated between T12 and L3 and formed by the union of the lumbar trunks from which the thoracic duct originates. Its size is definitely larger than that of all the surrounding vessels. In 30 to 80 percent of cases the cisterna chyli is visualized by lymphography. It is mainly situated at the level of T12 (10 percent), L1 (40–50 percent), and L2 (30–40 percent). The cisterna chyli is usually projected over the vertebral bodies. Its configuration may be reticular, ampullaceous (see Fig. 75-23), conical (see Fig. 75-22), or fusiform (see Fig. 75-20) with about equal frequency. Its diameter ranges between 2 and 16 mm, with an average of 4 to 6 mm.

Contrast filling of retrocrural lymph nodes situated dorsal to the diaphragmatic crura is observed in about half the cases. These lymph nodes are situated at the level of T12 and L1 (Fig. 75-24).

The topographic anatomy of the *thoracic section of the thoracic duct* shows considerable variation. After passage through the diaphragm at the aortic opening, the first part of the thoracic section of the thoracic duct is situated, in 60 percent of cases, in the posterior mediastinum, on the right side of the aorta. Continuing at about the level of T5-T6, the thoracic duct crosses obliquely to the left dorsal to the thoracic aorta. It leaves the thoracic cavity between the left subclavian artery and the esophagus. In the older age group, four types of anatomic variations are observed: left-sided duct in 36 percent of cases, midline position in 20 percent, oblique course in 17 percent, and right-sided duct in 6 percent. Because of the close connection of the two structures, the topographic-anatomic position of the thoracic duct depends largely on that of the thoracic aorta. With increasing age the elongation of the aorta, due to arteriosclerosis, causes a displacement of the thoracic duct from the right side toward the midline and the left. In addition, the elongation of the aortic arch leads to elongation or angulation of the thoracic duct. The presence of a hemithoracic duct, situated on the left side of the main trunk of the thoracic duct, is rather frequent. Numerous narrow lymphatic channels that course away from the main trunk

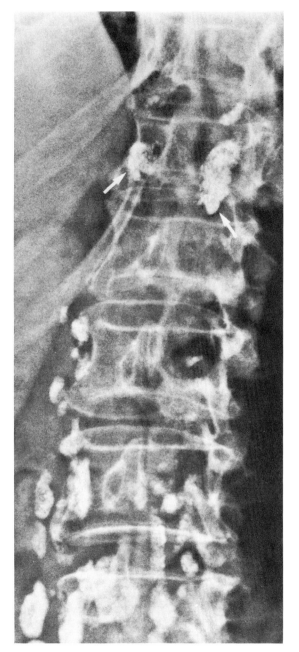

Figure 75-24. Contrast filling of several retrocrural lymph nodes at the level T10-T11 (*arrows*).

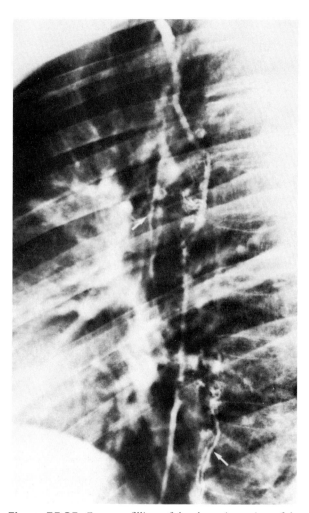

Figure 75-25. Contrast filling of the thoracic section of the thoracic duct and several small concomitant lymph trunks (*arrows*) and posterior mediastinal lymph nodes.

for short distances, often to nodes alongside, and then return to the thoracic duct are occasionally observed. Duplication of the thoracic duct, with one duct situated on each side of the thoracic aorta, is another rare anatomic variation. Cranially, both trunks may join together.

The thoracic section of the thoracic duct is frequently connected with posterior mediastinal lymph nodes. Efferent lymph vessels of the thoracic wall, the

heart, and the mediastinum enter the thoracic section of the thoracic duct. On *lymphograms,* the thoracic section of the thoracic duct is filled with contrast material in about 75 percent of cases. The upper part of the thoracic duct is visualized most frequently, and the entire thoracic duct is demonstrated in only about 10 percent of cases.

The thoracic section of the thoracic duct may divide into a caudal subsection, situated between the diaphragm and T3, and a cranial subsection reaching the supraclavicular region (Fig. 75-25). This subdivision is important, because the thoracic duct is projected onto the vertebral bodies up to the region of T3. In about two-thirds of the cases, the lower subsection of the thoracic duct is situated to the left of the midline (see Fig. 75-27). In one-third its position is median, and only in rare cases is it projected to the right of the midline. The upper subsection of the thoracic duct,

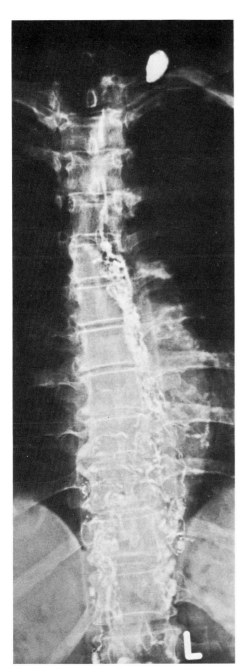

Figure 75-26. Netlike configuration of the thoracic duct.

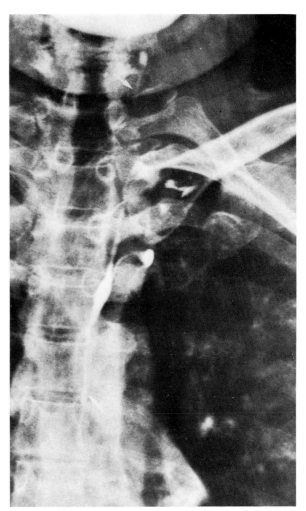

Figure 75-27. Left lateral position of the thoracic duct. Triple entering of the cervical section into the external jugular (*arrow*) and subclavian vein.

above T3, is mainly localized on the left side. Duplication of the thoracic duct is present in 1 case out of 10 (see Fig. 75-29). Very seldom, both lymph trunks are situated to the left of the midline, or separate trunks on each side of the midline are recognized. When present, partial duplication of the thoracic duct is observed predominantly in the lower thoracic section of the thoracic duct. A reticular configuration of the thoracic duct is seen in about 20 percent of cases (Fig. 75-26),

but only rarely is the entire thoracic section reticular. The largest diameter of the thoracic section of the thoracic duct is usually measured at the level of T2. In most instances, the maximum diameter ranges between 4 and 6 mm. Posterior mediastinal lymph nodes connected with the thoracic duct are demonstrated in 15 percent of cases at the level of T4-T8 (see Fig. 75-30). In 4 percent of cases retrosternal lymph nodes situated in the anterior mediastinum, arising from the thoracic duct with netlike lymphatics, are contrast-filled by lymphography. In 4 percent of cases lymph nodes of the hilar region of the lungs are demonstrated, and in 6 percent paratracheal lymph nodes are demonstrated.

The *cervical section of the thoracic duct* runs through the left upper thoracic aperture toward the subclavian triangle to enter the veins. In only one-fourth of the

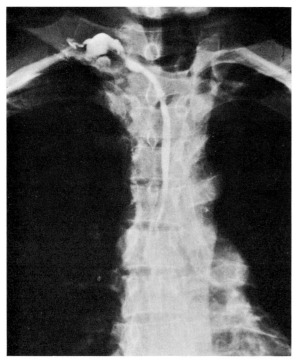

Figure 75-28. Right-sided ampullaceous entering of the thoracic duct.

Figure 75-29. Bilateral entering of the netlike cervical section of the thoracic duct.

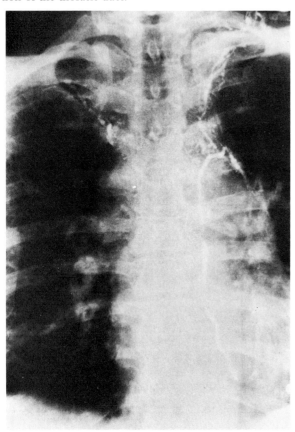

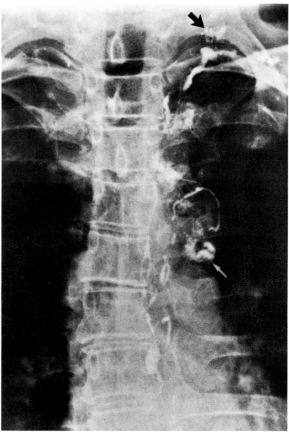

Figure 75-30. Contrast filling of posterior mediastinal (*white arrow*), retrosternal (*black arrow*), and bilateral supraclavicular lymph nodes.

Figure 75-31. Contrast filling of supraclavicular and axillary lymph nodes from thoracic duct (pulmonary oil embolism).

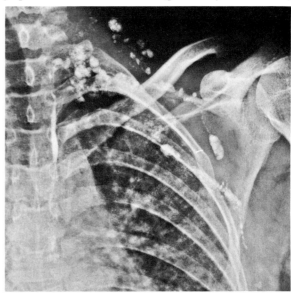

cases is a single channel present. In half the cases a double channel is observed. Multiple branching, accompanied by multiple entry points, may also be seen. The thoracic duct may enter the internal jugular vein, the venous angle, and either the subclavian or the innominate vein. An ampullaceous dilatation of the terminal part of the thoracic duct containing one or two valves is observed in 50 percent of cases.

The cervical part of the thoracic duct is frequently connected with cervical and supraclavicular lymph nodes by numerous lymphatics with a bidirectional flow. The left subclavian and left mediastinal trunks—collecting the lymph from the left thorax, the left arm, and the cervical region—enter the cervical section of the thoracic duct. On the right side, identical lymphatic trunks are in direct connection with the venous system, or in rare cases with a right lymphatic duct. On *lymphograms* the cervical section of the thoracic duct is demonstrated in 65 to 90 percent of patients. In 90 percent of cases it enters the venous system on the left side (Fig. 75-27); in about 3 percent on the right side (Fig. 75-28); and in 5 percent bilaterally (Fig. 75-29). In about 50 percent of cases only one lymph trunk is present; in 25 percent two branches of the cervical section of the thoracic duct are encountered; and in 25 percent three or more lymphatic vessels. An ampullaceous configuration at the terminus of the thoracic duct is observed in half the patients. Usually, there is only a single ampullaceous trunk, and rarely two or three ampullaceous trunks are present. Supraclavicular lymph nodes are visualized in about half of all lymphograms. They are generally situated on the left side (40 percent) and in only about 5 percent of cases on the right side. Occasionally (2 percent), lymph nodes are demonstrated within both the left and right supraclavicular regions (Fig. 75-30).

In about 2 percent of cases left axillary lymph nodes are filled with contrast material (Fig. 75-31). Left cervical lymph nodes are visualized on 3 percent of lymphograms. Rarely is a single right cervical lymph node demonstrated by lymphography. Contrast filling of the supraclavicular, cervical, axillary, paravertebral, mediastinal, and pulmonary hilar lymph nodes is of clinical significance. Visualization of these lymph nodes is not a definitive sign of collateral circulation and is therefore not a sign of a pathologic condition. All these nodes, which are closely connected with the thoracic duct, are necessarily demonstrated by lymphography when they are the last regional lymph nodes of the system, draining the abdominal retroperitoneal organs and the lower extremities. In cases of malignant tumors in these areas, metastatic spread into these node groups must be considered. Cancer cells within the thoracic duct are relatively frequent. Malignant cells are likely to migrate into these lymph node groups connected with the thoracic duct. Cancer metastases in the supraclavicular lymph nodes are frequently demonstrated by lymphography. Cancer metastases in paravertebral, tracheobronchial, and anterior mediastinal lymph nodes occur occasionally in later stages of the disease.

References

1. Bargmann W. Histologie und mikroskopische Anatomie des Menschen. 7th ed. Stuttgart: Thieme, 1977.
2. Bourquin J. Histologische Grundlagen des Lymphadenogramms. Radiologe 1968;8:150.
3. Leiber B. Der menschliche Lymphknoten: Anatomie, Physiologie und Pathologie nach Ergebnissen der Vergleichenden Klinischen und histologischen Zytodiagnostic. Munich-Berlin: Urban & Schwarzenberg, 1961.
4. Lennert K. Handbuch der speziellen pathologischen Anatomie und Histologie. Berlin: Springer, 1960.
5. Tjernberg B. Lymphography: an animal study on the diagnosis of V × 2 carcinoma and inflammation. Acta Radiol Suppl (Stockh) 1962:214.
6. Yoffey JM, Courtice FC. Lymphatics, lymph and lymphoid tissue. 2nd ed. Cambridge: Harvard University Press, 1956.
7. Ditchek T, Blahut RJ, Kittleson AC. Lymphadenography in normal subjects. Radiology 1963;80:175.
8. Fischer HW, Lawrence MS, Thornbury JR. Lymphography of the normal adult male. Radiology 1962;78:399.
9. Fuchs WA. Normal anatomy. In: Fuchs WA, Davidson JW, Fischer HW, eds. Lymphography in cancer. New York: Springer, 1969.
10. Fuchs WA, Böök-Hederström G. Inguinal and pelvic lymphography. Acta Radiol 1961;56:340.
11. Van Pernis PA. Variations of the thoracic duct. Surgery 1949; 28:806.
12. Fuchs WA, Pfammatter Th. Die topographische Röntgenanatomie der inguinalen und retroperitonealen Lymphknoten. Radiologe 1970;10:262.
13. Kolbenstvedt A. Normal lymphographic variation of lumbar, iliac and inguinal lymph vessels. Acta Radiol 1974;15:662.
14. Barthels P. Das Lymphgefässystem. In: von Bardeleben K, ed. Handbuch der Anatomie des Menschen. Jena: Fischer, 1909.
15. Jacobsson S, Johansson S. Normal roentgen anatomy of the lymph vessels of upper and lower extremities. Acta Radiol 1959;51:321.
16. Kaindl FK, Mannheimer E, Pfleger-Schwarz L, Thurnher B. Lymphangiographie und Lymphadenographie der Extremitäten. Stuttgart: Thieme, 1960.
17. Rusznyak I, Földi M, Szabo G. Physiologie und Pathologie des Lymphkreislaufs. Jena: Fischer, 1957.
18. Cunéo B, Marcille M. Topographie des ganglions iliopelviens. Bull Soc Anat 1901;76:653.
19. Herman PG, Benninghoff DL, Nelson JH, Mellins HZ. Roentgen anatomy of the ilio-pelvic-aortic lymphatic system. Radiology 1963;80:182.
20. Wirth W. Zur Röntgenanatomie des Lymphsystems der inguinalen pelvinen und aortalen Region: 1. ROEFO 1966;105: 441. 2. ROEFO 1966;105:636.
21. Wirth W, Kubik S. Lymphographic roentgen anatomy. In: Viamonte M, Rüttimann A, eds. Atlas of lymphography. Stuttgart: Thieme, 1980.
22. Kubik, S. Die normale Anatomie des Lymphsystems unter besonderer Berücksichtigung der Sammelgebiete der Lymphknoten der unteren Körperhälfte. Strahlentherapie (Sonderb) 1969;69:8.

23. Rosenberger A, Abrams HL. Radiology of the thoracic duct. AJR 1971;111:807.
24. Jossifow GM. Das Lymphgefässystem des Menschen. Jena: Fischer, 1930.
25. Baltaxe HA, Constable WC. Mediastinal lymph node visualization in the absence of intrathoracic disease. Radiology 1968; 90:94.
26. Fuchs WA, Galeazzi R. Die Röntgenanatomie des Ductus thoracicus. Radiologe 1970;10:180.
27. Idanov DA. Anatomie du canal thoracique et des principaux collecteurs lymphatiques du tronc chez l'homme. Acta Anat (Basel) 1959;37:35.
28. Kubik S. Lagevarianten, Lage- und Formveränderungen der Pars thoracalis des Ductus thoracicus. ROEFO 1975;122:1.
29. Poirier P. Traité d'Anatomie Humaine. Paris: Masson, 1898.
30. Rouvière H. Anatomie des lymphatiques de l'homme. Paris: Masson, 1932.
31. Weissleder H. Das pathologische Lymphangiogramm des Ductus thoracicus. ROEFO 1964;101:573.
32. Wirth W, Frommhold H. Der Ductus thoracicus und seine Variationen: lymphographische Studie. ROEFO 1970;112: 450.

76

The Thoracic Duct

GEORGE A. HOLLAND
ALEXANDER ROSENBERGER

*T*he growing recognition of the importance of the lymphatic system and thoracic duct in circulatory physiology, metastatic changes, and immunologic processes has led to an increased interest in the study of their anatomy, physiology, and pathology. The thoracic duct is the central collecting trunk of all the lymph vessels of the body, with the exception of those of the right side of the head and neck, the right upper limb, the right hemithorax, the right side of the heart, and the convex surface of the liver.[1] The first description of the thoracic duct in man is attributed to Pecquet in 1651; by the end of the eighteenth century the gross anatomy of the thoracic duct had been thoroughly explored.

In order to have a better understanding of the anatomy and anatomic variations of the thoracic duct, a succinct review of the development of the lymph system is necessary. In the human embryo six lymph sacs can be found from which lymph vessels are derived: two paired jugular and posterior lymphatic sacs and two unpaired ones, namely, the retroperitoneal sac and the cisterna chyli. There are two opinions as to the origin of these lymph sacs. According to the first, lymphatic spaces develop from the mesenchyma, forming capillary plexuses from which the lymph sacs are derived. The second theory connects the lymph vessels to the venous system; it considers the lymphatics as offshoots from the endothelium of the veins, forming plexuses. These plexuses lose their connection with the veins and are transformed into lymph sacs. The lymph vessels originate from the lymph sacs. With the exception of the cisterna chyli, the lymph sacs are transformed in a later stage into lymph nodes.[1]

In the embryo the thoracic duct is a paired structure formed by an anastomotic outgrowth of the jugular sac and the cisterna chyli; there are numerous transverse connections between the two sides. The jugular sac lies at the junction of the subclavian vein with the anterior cardinal vein. The cisterna chyli lies anterior to lumbar vertebrae L3–L4. In embryonic life numerous valves can be present in the thoracic duct. They appear about the fifth month but may disappear prior to birth.

Anatomy of the Thoracic Duct

The anatomy of the thoracic duct is quite variable. The thoracic duct begins at the upper end of the cisterna chyli, usually at the height of the 12th thoracic vertebra. It originates from the union of three roots, the right and left lumbar trunk and the intestinal trunk; these trunks can meet at an identical site or successively.

With the aorta on its left and the azygos vein on its right, the thoracic duct enters the thoracic cavity through the aortic hiatus of the diaphragm (Fig. 76-1). It courses anterior and to the right of the dorsal spine in the posterior mediastinum. At about the fifth thoracic vertebra level it turns to the left side of the spine. At about the height of the third thoracic vertebra it leaves the aortic arch and lies between the mediastinal pleura and the left side of the esophagus. In its course upward it arches forward above the dome of the pleura between the left common carotid artery and the left subclavian artery to reach about the level of the seventh cervical vertebra, the anteriorly situated left internal jugular vein, or the junction of the latter with the left subclavian vein. Before entering the veins it usually receives the lymph coming from the jugular, mammary, and subclavian trunks draining the lymph from their respective regions, whereas the left bronchomediastinal trunk can open separately into the great veins. In the neck the arch of the thoracic duct lies 3 to 4 cm above the clavicle, anterior to the vertebral vessels, sympathetic trunk, and thyrocervical vessels. In its course the thoracic duct collects lymph vessels from lumbar, posterior intercostal, posterior mediastinal lymph nodes, and the esophagus.

The slightly right-to-left sweep of the thoracic duct in the thorax is easily explained by its phylogenesis.

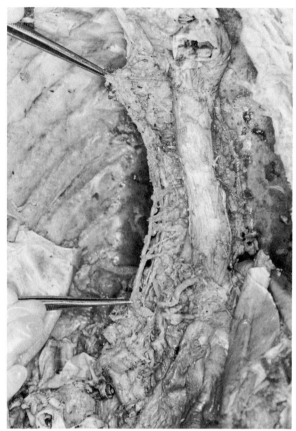

Figure 76-1. Anatomic preparation of the entire thoracic duct. Because of removal of the mediastinal organs, the duct lies lateral to the spine in its course. In the middle part a network of small channels is present, giving the duct a plexuslike appearance.

Originally a paired structure with numerous transverse anastomoses, in its ultimate form it is an unpaired structure, its caudal part belonging to the embryonic right vessel and its cranial portion to the left vessel, whereas the middle part originates from the transverse anastomoses.

Radiologic Studies of the Thoracic Duct

In vivo the thoracic duct can be studied by cannulation of the duct in the neck and retrograde injection of contrast material under operative conditions.[2,3] Lymphangiography with oily contrast material based on the principles of Kinmonth[4] represents a physiologic way to study the thoracic duct. Briefly this technique consists of identification and cannulation of a superficially situated lymph vessel on the dorsum of the foot and slow injection of the oily contrast material into the ves-

sel. When satisfactory opacification of the thoracic duct is achieved, controlled by television-monitored fluoroscopy or radiographs, the morphology of the thoracic duct is studied by anteroposterior, lateral, and oblique radiographs of the chest. The cross-sectional anatomy of the contrast-filled thoracic duct as seen on computed tomography (CT) has been studied (Fig. 76-2).[5]

The functional aspects of the flow of opacified lymph in the thoracic duct may be visualized by cine or 70-mm camera technique.[6] Studies are done during quiet and deep respiration, apnea, and the Valsalva maneuver. Posture changes from the recumbent to the upright position and their influence on lymph flow can be studied in this way as well.

Radiologic Anatomy of the Thoracic Duct

The thoracic duct can be divided into abdominal, thoracic, and cervical segments. The landmarks used in the radiologic description are sometimes different from those mentioned in the anatomic study.

Abdominal Segment

The abdominal part of the thoracic duct consists of the cisterna chyli and a short segment of the duct below the diaphragm.

The cisterna chyli is formed by the confluence of the two lumbar trunks draining the lymph of the lower extremities, pelvis, and abdominal organs and the intestinal trunk carrying the lymph from the gastrointestinal tract.[7,8] In the lymphangiogram only the lumbar trunks can be visualized, usually as 2-mm-wide vessels originating from the confluence of small lymph vessels and coursing in an oblique fashion upward to reach the cisterna chyli or the opposite vessel (Fig. 76-3). The union of the lumbar trunks usually lies at the level of T12–L2.[7] The intestinal trunk is demonstrated only in experimental lymphangiography or (seldom) in the presence of lymphatic obstruction, in which case it serves as a collateral pathway.

The cisterna chyli is the initial saclike dilated portion of the thoracic duct. It may have various shapes[9]: round, oval, commalike, linear, beaded, inverted V, or inverted Y (Fig. 76-4). The size of the cisterna also shows a wide range of variations: 2 to 16 mm in width in lymphangiography[7] and 5 to 7 cm in length.[10] These measurements were made on radiographs, which reproduce static aspects of the cisterna chyli, whereas cine studies[6] have demonstrated different calibers in

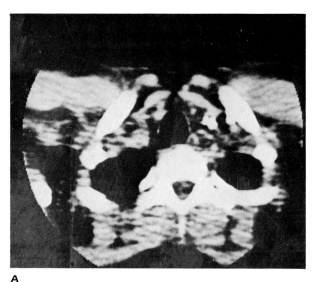

A

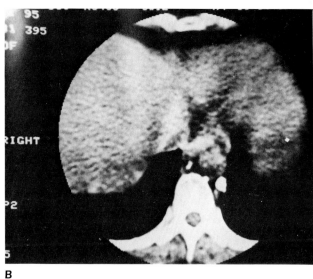

B

Figure 76-2. Computed tomography study of the contrast-filled duct. (A) Cervical portion of the duct. The point of emptying into the great veins is well seen. (B) Visualization of the abdominal portion of the duct at the level of the diaphragmatic crura. Some lymph nodes opacified by contrast material are also delineated.

Figure 76-3. Lumbar trunks and cisterna chyli. The lumbar trunks are converging toward the cisterna chyli, which overlies the midline of the spine at L2. The caliber of the latter is larger than that of the thoracic duct above it and the lumbar trunks below it.

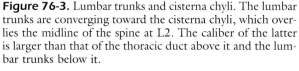

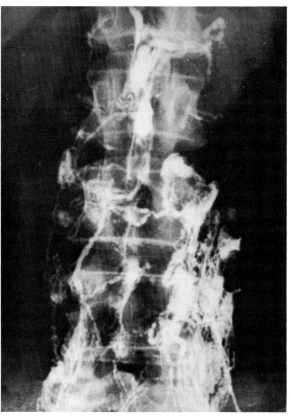

the same individual depending on the state of relaxation or contraction of the cisterna.

The location of the cisterna may be anywhere between T12 and L3[7,10–12]; in 77 percent of cases, it lies in the midline anterior to the vertebral column. In the series by Rosenberger et al.,[13] it was situated at the height of T12 in 36 percent of cases and at L2 in the rest.

Thoracic Segment

The thoracic portion of the thoracic duct is the segment from the entrance of the duct into the thoracic cavity through the aortic hiatus to an arbitrary point where the duct lies between the esophagus and the aortic arch.

The thoracic duct as visualized in lymphangiographic studies[7,8,10,14] courses at the midline of the spine or slightly to the right of it. At the height of T5–T6 it changes its course progressively to the left of the spine (Fig. 76-5A). At the level of the carina the duct crosses the main left bronchus as viewed in the anteroposterior radiograph and ascends parallel but dorsal to the left lateral wall of the trachea (see Fig. 76-5A). Over the dorsal aspect of the aortic arch it turns ventrally as seen in the lateral chest radiograph to course toward the thoracic inlet (see Fig. 76-5B).

The duct can be visualized in its entire length during the lymphangiographic studies in the minority of the cases (about 7 percent).[7] Usually only certain parts of it can be illustrated, the lower segments being demonstrated less often than the cranial portions.

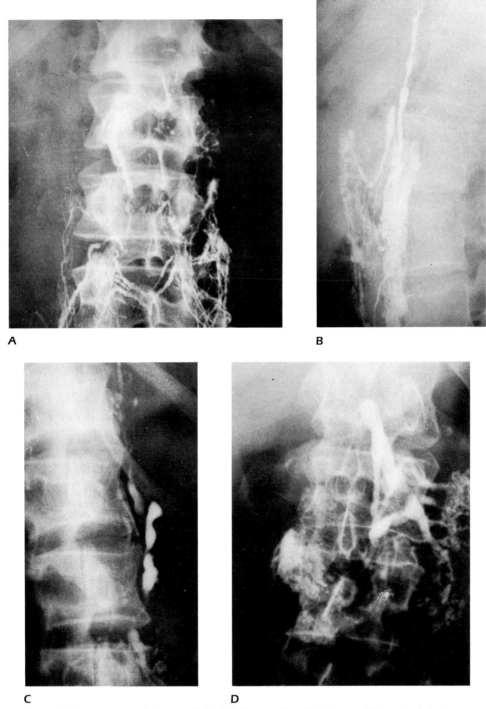

Figure 76-4. Various shapes of cisterna chyli. (A) Commalike. (B) Linear. (C) Beaded. (D) Inverted Y.

Figure 76-6. Cervical portion of the thoracic duct. (A) The cervical portion is formed by one channel arching above the ▶ clavicle. (B) Numerous glands surrounding the terminal portion of the duct. Note also the opacification of the right duct.

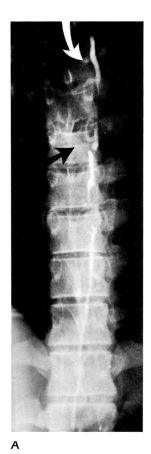
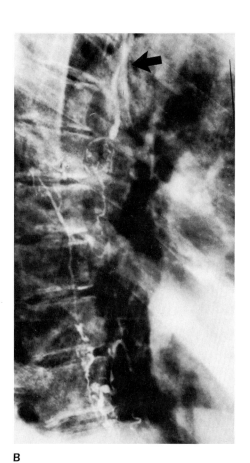

A   B

Figure 76-5. Thoracic part of the thoracic duct opacified by contrast material in the whole length. (A) Anteroposterior view, showing progressive course of the duct from right to left. At the level of the left main bronchus (*black arrow*) it reaches the left side of the spine and ascends parallel to the left wall of the trachea (*white arrow*). The distance between the duct and the tracheal wall should not exceed 1 cm. (B) Lateral view of a double thoracic duct. The anterior channel (*arrow*) is the main carrier of the lymph.

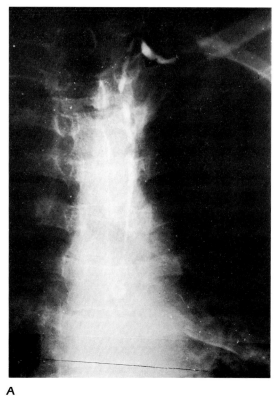
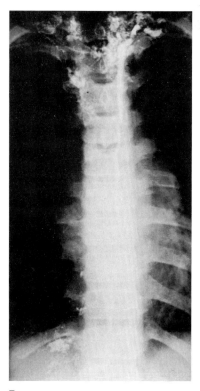

A   B

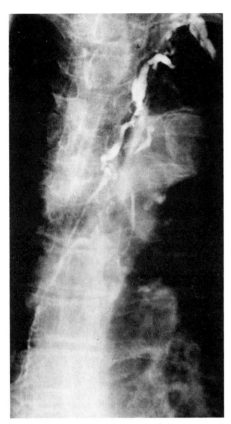

Figure 76-7. Ampullalike dilatation of the terminal portion of the thoracic duct. Below this level doubling of the thoracic duct is visible.

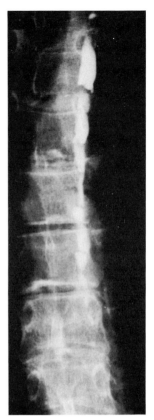

Figure 76-8. Beaded appearance given by numerous valves in the upper half of the duct. The valves of the thoracic duct are bicuspid. They may vary in number (see Fig. 76-5A), and their visualized size depends on whether they are opening or closing.

The width of the duct varies on average between 2 and 6 mm, but diameters between 0.5 and 12.0 mm[15] have been described. This great range in visualization of different parts of the thoracic duct as well as the variations in the caliber is related to many factors: quantity of contrast material injected, tonus of the duct, positioning of the patient, timing of the radiographs, and individual differences.

Cervical Segment

The cervical portion of the thoracic duct is the terminal part of the duct between the thoracic inlet and the point of its emptying into the large veins of the neck. In the anteroposterior radiograph the duct turns cranially and slightly to the left, resembling an inverted J (Fig. 76-6A); it either courses parallel to the clavicle or arches 2 to 3 cm above it. Sometimes this terminal part has a more vertical course (Fig. 76-6B).

The highest portion of the duct in the neck lies at C6–T2,[14] but during coughing it may move upward.[15] The cervical segment is visualized in 65 to 90 percent of lymphangiograms.[7,8] The duct terminates in various

fashions; there may be a single duct (25 percent), or it can divide into two to four channels, which open separately or reunite before entering the veins. Three channels have been found in 15 percent of cases, and four channels in 6 percent of cases. These figures are in striking contrast to reports in anatomic dissections, in which one terminal was found in 90 percent of cases.[16] Sometimes an ampullalike dilatation of the cervical portion of the duct can be observed (Fig. 76-7). The cervical portion of the duct empties into the left great veins of the neck in 92 to 95 percent, on the right side in 2 to 3 percent, and bilaterally in 1.0 to 1.5 percent (see Fig. 76-6A).[7,8,10]

In 60 percent of patients the duct empties into the internal jugular vein. In the remaining cases the site of emptying may be the subclavian vein (15 percent), between the external and internal jugular veins (7 percent), in the angle between the external jugular and subclavian veins (2.5 percent), and in the innominate vein (1.5 percent).

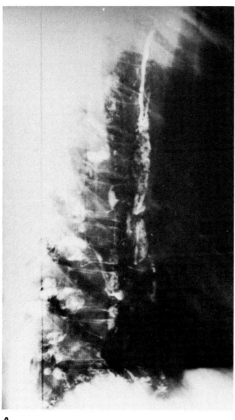
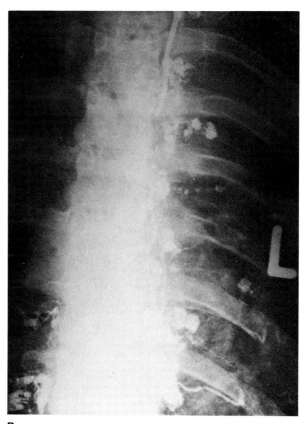

A　　　　　　　　　　　　　　　**B**

Figure 76-9. Filling of posterior mediastinal nodes and intercostal vessels. These structures can be seen in 20 percent of the studies. (A) Lateral view of a thoracic duct with filling of numerous posterior mediastinal glands. (B) Filling of intercostal lymph vessels mainly in the left lower half of the thorax.

Valves

Bicuspid valves can be seen in the course of the thoracic duct, their function being to ensure unidirectional flow of the lymph. In the lymphangiogram the open valve resembles a fish mouth; the closed valve produces a localized bulging of the lateral contour of the duct, giving it a beaded appearance (Fig. 76-8). The function of the valve can be studied in cine or rapid-filming studies.[6] As to the number of valves present in the duct, findings differ widely, but all agree that they are more numerous in the upper portion. One valve at least is always present in the high upper cervical segment.

Lymph Nodes Along the Thoracic Duct

Filling of lymph nodes in the supraclavicular area around the terminal portion of the duct (one of which is the Virchow-Troisier node[17]) can be seen in the large majority of lymphangiograms and is a normal finding.

Filling of lymph nodes in the posterior mediastinum (Fig. 76-9A) and along the posterior intercostal vessels (see Fig. 76-9B) emptying into the duct can be seen in 20 percent of studies. In exceptional cases filling of middle mediastinal, carinal (Fig. 76-10A), hilar (Fig. 76-10B), and anterior mediastinal lymph nodes (Fig. 76-11) can occur.

Filling and visualization of these nodes probably represent a normal finding and are due to bidirectional flow in the lymph channels connecting these nodes with the thoracic duct. The pathologic architecture of mediastinal lymph nodes as visualized by lymphangiography has the same implications as elsewhere in the body.

Variations in the Thoracic Duct

The thoracic duct is subject to many variations; Rouvière[9] remarks that articles dealing with duct variations are more numerous than those devoted to its normal anatomy.

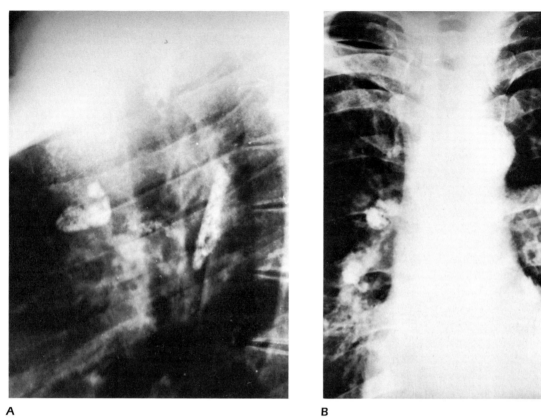

A   B

Figure 76-10. Filling of middle mediastinal nodes and hilar nodes. (A) Lateral view illustrating filling of middle mediastinal lymph nodes. (B) Filling of hilar nodes. In this case the hilar nodes are bilateral, a finding that is more the exception than the rule.

The variations in the appearance of the thoracic duct can be explained by its embryologic development. In the absence of lumbar trunks the lymph vessels form a netlike structure, thereafter uniting to form the duct.[7] In the absence of the cisterna chyli the lumbar trunks may ascend to a higher level before uniting (Fig. 76-12). Most variations in the aspect of the thoracic duct occur in its thoracic portion (40 percent).[2] The crossing of the duct from right to left at the height of T5-T6 may be abrupt instead of progressive. In some cases the entire course of the duct may be left-sided or right-sided. There are different opinions about the multiplicity of the channels in the duct in the thoracic segment. Whereas anatomists state[18] that doubling occurs only above the level of T5-T6, lymph-angiographic studies[7,14,19] have shown two or three channels at every level in about 10 percent of cases. Double thoracic ducts can terminate in a single duct at the level of the third to eighth thoracic vertebra (Fig. 76-13). Bilateral superior mediastinal thoracic ducts (Fig. 76-14; see also Fig. 76-5B) are not necessarily related to double ducts at lower levels. In 3 percent of cases, many small lymph vessels arise from the

lower portion of the duct and reach the duct again higher up. The large number of anastomoses between them can give the duct a plexuslike appearance. Wide variations in the number and site of emptying of the thoracic duct in its cervical portion are well known

Figure 76-11. Filling of a group of anterior superior mediastinal lymph nodes.

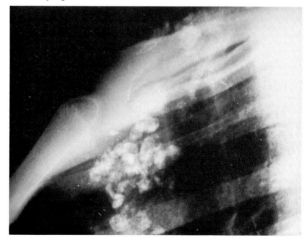

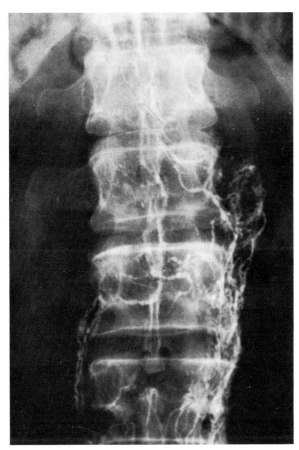

Figure 76-12. In the absence of the cisterna chyli the lumbar trunks form a netlike structure and reach up to the level of the body of L1.

from anatomic and lymphangiographic studies. The knowledge of these variations is most important to clinicians, for the cervical portion of the duct is easily subject to trauma and to surgical manipulation.

Functional and Experimental Aspects of the Thoracic Duct

The role of lymph circulation is to return tissue-fluid proteins and large molecules from the interstitial space to the bloodstream. Fat from the intestine enters the lymph too, giving it a milky appearance. The constituents of lymph are similar to those of plasma, but the protein content of lymph is lower, reflecting the permeability of functionally different blood-lymph barriers.[20,21] The main sources of the proteins in the lymph are the liver and the intestine. The coagulation properties of lymph are lower than the coagulation properties of blood.[20,22] The flow rate of thoracic duct lymph is about 1 ml per minute, and the pressure of lymph is

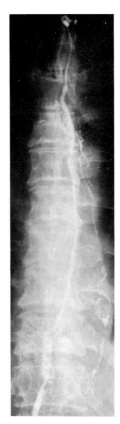

Figure 76-13. Doubling of the thoracic duct up to the level of T4.

about 11 cm H_2O. About 1500 to 2400 ml of lymph empties into the venous system daily.[23] Lymphatic production and flow are greatly influenced by diet. Ingesting long-chain fatty acids or water increases lymph flow in the thoracic duct. It is estimated that 60

Figure 76-14. Doubling of cervical portion of the thoracic duct with filling of lymph nodes around the two channels.

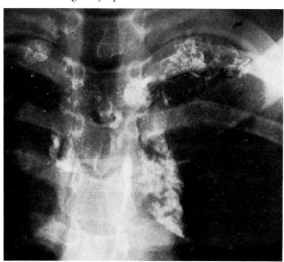

percent of ingested fat passes into the lymphatics.[24,25] Ingesting medium-chain triglycerides, protein, and carbohydrates has little effect on lymphatic production or flow. Medium-chain triglycerides are absorbed directly into the portal venous circulation.[26] Starvation and parenteral nutrition markedly decrease flow of clear lymph.[27,28]

Flow of lymph[29] depends on formation of tissue fluid, movement of tissue fluid into the lymphatics, and factors that move the lymph along the lymphatic vessels. The flow of lymph in the thoracic duct is a passive phenomenon, depending on lymph formation and distensibility of the duct. Factors influencing lymph flow in the thoracic duct are residual pressure from the pumping action of the heart, active and passive movement of the muscular system,[9] suction effect of the negative intrathoracic pressure, movements of the diaphragm, and, possibly, transmitted pulsations from the great intrathoracic vessels.[19] The flow in the duct, as shown in animal observation and in man, is rhythmic, the valves ensuring a unidirectional stream. Cine and 70-mm camera radiologic studies are very useful for observing these phenomena.[6,9,19,30] The thoracic duct possesses an autonomic innervation that causes relaxation and contraction of the duct, thus influencing lymph propulsion.[31]

The thoracic duct functions as the major pathway of immunologically active lymphocytes and proteins to blood; pathogenic microorganisms may also be transported by the duct. Many experimental studies concerned with the immunologic aspects of the thoracic duct have been carried out.[32,33]

Cannulation and drainage of the thoracic duct for 10 to 14 days can deplete the body of a large portion of the circulating T lymphocytes.[34,35] Such depletion leads to immunosuppression and was used clinically as a technique for prolonging allograft survival.[36] This technique is no longer done because of limited patency of the thoracic duct cannula, infection, prolonged hospitalizations, and improvements in immunosuppressive drugs.

Radiologic Aspects of the Abnormal Thoracic Duct

The major pathologic conditions of the thoracic duct are manifested clinically by chylothorax, chyloperitoneum, and rarely as mediastinal or neck masses. Chylothorax is most commonly due to malignant or iatrogenic etiologies. The clinical manifestation of a chylothorax depends on the variable anatomy of the thoracic duct and the location of obstruction or injury

of the duct. Rupture of the thoracic duct above the fifth or sixth thoracic vertebra usually results in a left-sided chylothorax; injury below this level often results in a right-sided chylothorax. Bilateral chylothoraces may result from these injuries or secondary to chyloperitoneum, which can gain access to the pleural space via diaphragmatic lymphatic or congenital diaphragmatic defects.[37] Chronic loss of proteins, lymphocytes, and lipids from leaking chyle can pose a serious nutritional problem and cause immunosuppression.[36,38–40] In addition, the large volume of chylous effusion may cause severe respiratory compromise.[41–43]

Diagnosis of chylothorax is usually made by a combination of chest radiographs and by examination of pleural fluid obtained from thorocentesis or from chest tube drainage. The appearance of the fluid depends on the nutritional state of the patient.[44,45] On gross inspection, typically chylous effusions are odorless, milky, or turbid fluids that do not clear on centrifugation. However, one reported that only 50 percent of chylous effusions were milky and 12 percent were serous or serosanguineous.[46] On microscopic inspection and cell count there are no bacteria, and lymphocytes are the predominant cell type. On chemical analysis the fluids are characterized by high triglyceride content and low cholesterol levels. Triglyceride levels greater than 110 mg/dl is highly suggestive, whereas levels less than 50 mg/dl virtually rule out the diagnosis of chylothorax. The presence of chylomicrons by lipoprotein analysis is indicative of chylous effusion.[46] Chylothorax is distinguished from pseudochylothorax by the presence of cholesterol crystals in the latter. These crystals are chronic pleural effusions usually caused by rheumatoid arthritis or tuberculosis.[44,47]

The etiologies of chylothorax were reviewed from nine separate series involving a total of 191 patients.[48] The article reported that 72 percent (138) of the cases were of nontraumatic origin. Malignancy accounted for 45 percent (87) of all cases, and lymphoma was the most common malignancy, responsible for 37 percent (70). Twenty-seven percent (41) were due to nonmalignant causes; 26 of these cases were termed idiopathic, and 15 were due to miscellaneous etiologies, including benign tumors, lymphangioleiomyomatosis,[49] protein-losing enteropathy, regional ileitis, reticular hyperplasia, pleuritis, cirrhosis, thoracic aortic aneurysm, severe congestive heart failure, mitral valvular diseases,[50] venous thrombosis of the superior vena cava and subclavian veins, lupus, filariasis, lymphadenopathy, tuberculosis, sarcoidosis, amyloidosis, and congenital disorders.[47]

Posttraumatic chylothorax accounted for 28 percent (52) of cases. Surgery was the cause for most of the posttraumatic chylothoraces, accounting for 25 percent (48) of cases.[48] Chylothorax has been reported as complicating intrathoracic procedures with an estimated incidence of 0.24 to 0.5 percent.[51–53] Repairs of coarctation of the aorta and esophagectomies are the two intrathoracic surgeries with the highest reported incidences of chylothorax; the incidence of chylothorax following esophagectomy is 3 to 9 percent.[51,54] Coronary artery bypass grafting is rarely complicated by chylothorax.[55,56] Extrathoracic surgeries such as neck dissections,[57,58] abdominal aortic aneurysm repair,[59] and transabdominal vagotomy have very rarely been complicated by chylothorax.[60] Other traumatic etiologies of chylothorax include gunshot wounds, stab wounds, blunt trauma, and motor vehicle accidents.[47]

The management of chylothorax varies depending on the etiology and the clinical condition of the patient. Conservative therapy is usually attempted first. This consists of chest tube drainage combined with attempts to decompress the lymphatics by decreasing the flow and production of lymph. Decreased lymphatic production can be accomplished by changing from fat-restricted oral diets to diets with medium-chain triglycerides, which do not enter the thoracic duct,[26] or with parenteral nutrition.[45] If this fails, after 1 to 4 weeks surgical intervention may be needed.[42] Open thoracotomy and ligation of the thoracic duct can be performed if conservative therapy fails or if the patient is too nutritionally depleted to undergo a trial of conservative therapy.[38,39] Ligation may be guided by preoperative lymphangiography, which will identify the anatomy of the duct and may identify the location of the leak. Preoperative administration of lipophilic dye or cream may assist in locating the site of lymphatic leak.[61,62] Ligation of the duct may not be effective in patients with malignancy and is usually unnecessary in posttraumatic cases or in infants. When conservative measures fail in infants or the terminally ill, pleuroperitoneal shunts may be attempted. Other interventions include pleurodesis or pleurectomy.[42,48,63,64]

Congenital Disorders

Congenital chylothorax is one of the most common causes of pleural effusion in the neonatal period. It is typically associated with birth trauma and developmental lymphatic anomalies as seen in neonates with either Down or Noonan syndrome. It has also been associated with maternal polyhydramnios, tuberous sclerosis, congenital lymphangiectasia, and Gorhman syndrome.[41,65,66]

Malformations and variations of congenital origin have already been mentioned. It is presumed that in some cases of Noonan syndrome[67] the pulmonary lymphangiectasis may be caused by interruption of the thoracic duct.[68] Congenital defects, stenosis, or atresia of the thoracic duct is presumed to cause bilateral hydrochylothorax, thus leading to bilateral pulmonary hypoplasia in neonates.[69]

Inflammation

Tuberculosis and syphilis can cause changes in the lymphatic vessels; theoretically, therefore, similar changes should occur in the thoracic duct. However, there is no radiologic documentation of inflammatory lesions of the thoracic duct.

Tumors

Masses involving the thoracic duct are rare and typically benign. The lesions include cysts, lymphangiomas, and lymphatic aneurysms. These lesions may present as mediastinal or even supraclavicular neck masses.[70–72] Diagnosis can be made by fine-needle aspiration with biochemical analysis. The natural history of these lesions remains unknown.[72]

The thoracic duct is the main pathway of lymph drainage for the organs below the diaphragm to the lesser circulation. It is a known fact that the incidence of lung metastases from primary tumors below the diaphragm is higher than from suprathoracic tumors.[73]

Secondary involvement of the thoracic duct can occur by embolization of malignant cells arrested in the thoracic duct or by invasion from contiguous structures.

Mediastinal Masses

Mediastinal masses can cause displacement, kinking, tortuosity, and obstruction of the thoracic duct, according to the site and the size of the mass. A useful radiologic measurement for evaluating the presence of a mediastinal mass is the distance between the thoracic duct and the left wall of the trachea in the anteroposterior radiograph. The distance should not exceed 10 mm (see Fig. 76-5A)[10]; a wider separation points toward a mediastinal mass. Computed tomography of the thoracic duct is an additional method for evaluating mediastinal masses.[5]

Obstruction

Intrinsic or extrinsic pathology may lead to obstruction of the thoracic duct (Fig. 76-15). Extrinsic obstruction can be caused by mediastinal masses[74] or mediastinal fibrosis. Pathology inside the duct may be due to filariasis[19] or metastasis.[73]

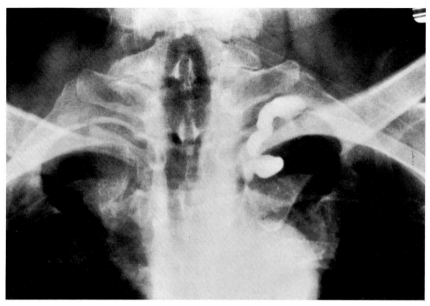

Figure 76-15. Partial obstruction of the thoracic duct at the venous angle.

The suspicion of thoracic duct obstruction should arise if lymphangiography reveals a sharp cutoff of the contrast medium in the course of the duct associated with dilatation distal to it, visualization of lymphatic collaterals such as an intestinal trunk, lymphaticovenous communications,[10,75,76] and delayed emptying. Because of the known variety in the radiologic appearance of the normal thoracic duct, the size of the duct, visualization of intercostal lymphatics, or filling of mediastinal lymph nodes as a single criterion for thoracic duct obstruction is inadequate.

New Imaging Techniques of the Thoracic Duct

Noninvasive imaging of the thoracic duct has been reported with nuclear medicine and magnetic resonance imaging (MRI). Lymphoscintigraphy can be used to evaluate patients with lymphedema and to determine the level of obstruction or leak.[77,78] This technique avoids the complications of lymphangiography, but it lacks anatomic detail and has missed frank lacerations placed in animal models. In addition, some surgeons prefer lymphangiography prior to ligation of the thoracic duct for chylothorax.[61,62,78]

Magnetic resonance lymphangiography has been reported in animals and in humans. Several studies have reported promising results with using supramagnetic contrast agents to differentiate nodes involved with tumor from inflammatory nodes.[79–82] Two reports have described the MRI signal characteristics of Lipiodol and of lymph nodes following a lymphangiogram.[83,84] Both described hyperintense signal on T2-weighted images. This increased signal could lead to an erroneous diagnosis of an inflammatory node or a node involved with tumor. There was discrepancy between the two papers on the appearance on T1-weighted scans. Buckwalter and coworkers described increased signal on T1-weighted images, and Harvard and others reported intermediate signal intensity.[83,84] Hyperintense signal or intermediate signal of nodes on

Figure 76-17. Percutaneous cannulation of the cisterna chyli in a dog. (A) Frontal projection of a canine abdomen following a lymphangiogram. The cisterna chyli was identified and a 16-gauge, 10-cm-long stainless steel needle was percutaneously placed into the abdomen to serve as a guide. A 20-cm-long, 21-gauge spinal needle was inserted through the 16-gauge blunt cannula. Under fluoroscopic guidance the cisterna chyli was punctured with the 21-gauge needle. (B) Frontal projection of the same canine abdomen reveals a 0.016-cm soft platinum-tipped mandrel guidewire (Cook, Inc.) overlying the vertebral bodies. The guidewire is located within the thoracic duct. (C) Right anterior oblique projection of the same dog after dilating the tract. The cisterna chyli was cannulated with a 3 French catheter advanced over the guidewire, and the thoracic duct was completely opacified with 60 percent ionic iodinated contrast medium. (Images courtesy of Dr. Constantin Cope.) ▶

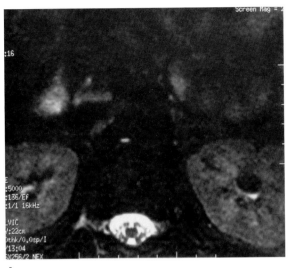

A

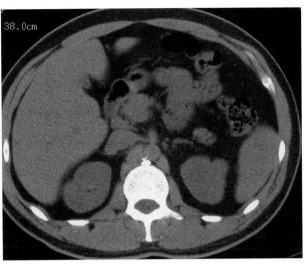

B

Figure 76-16. (A) Transaxial heavily T2-weighted MR image reveals a hyperintense signal immediately anterior to the vertebral body and to the right of the aorta, representing the cisterna chyli. The echo time is 136 milliseconds and the repetition time is 5000 milliseconds, with fat saturation to suppress soft tissue signal. Fluid appears hyperintense in the thoracic duct or cisterna chyli and in the cerebral spinal fluid surrounding the cord. (B) Transaxial CT scan of the same patient in the same anatomic location was performed several hours after a lymphangiogram. No intravenous contrast was used. Note the hyperintense signal of the duct immediately to the right of the aorta and anterior to the vertebral body. This confirms the findings of the location of the duct on MRI.

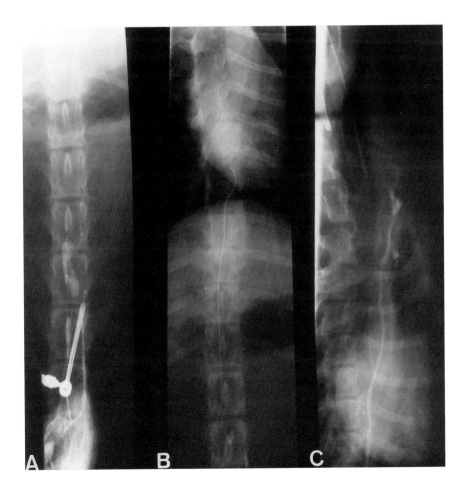

T1-weighted scans decreases the normal contrast between nodes and fat, which is hyperintense on T1-weighted images. The authors have noted similar hyperintense signal on T1- and T2-weighted scans with Ethiodol. In addition, fat signal can be selectively suppressed without decreasing the signal from Ethiodol. This allows for improved visualization of the hyperintense nodes and the lymphatic vessels if they contain Ethiodol at the time of the scan. Although termed *lymphangiography,* these MRI techniques were used to evaluate and characterize lymph nodes and not lymphatic vessels.[83,84]

The natural contrast of MRI allows for the noninvasive imaging of the cisterna chyli and the thoracic duct. The lymphatics are hypointense or intermediate signal intensity on T1-weighted images. On heavily T2-weighted images with fat suppression the lymphatics appear hyperintense. MR lymphangiograms can be performed using this T2 scanning technique and using maximum intensity projection of images performed in the coronal plane. Slow-flowing blood in small veins may have a similar appearance but can be differentiated from lymphatic vessels with scans performed following intravenous gadolinium injections or with flow-sensitive gradient-echo images (Fig. 76-16).

Direct Cannulation and Interventions

Recently two minimally invasive techniques involving the thoracic duct have been reported. The first technique is successful thoracoscopic ligation of the thoracic duct, which has been performed in 16 patients and the results published in four separate reports.[85–88] The second technique is direct cannulation of the thoracic duct, which has been reported in three separate animal studies.[89–91] Lymphangiography often incompletely opacifies the thoracic duct.[92] Cope's direct cannulation[90] allowed for improved visualization of the thoracic duct in 13 of 13 pigs without subsequent evidence of vascular or lymphatic injury at necropsy. This technique is depicted in Figure 76-17. Because only one-limb lymphangiography is required, the dose of Ethiodol is reduced and thus the potential for pulmonary complications due to oil embolization. This percutaneous technique allows for possible stenting or embolization of the duct for treatment of chylothorax or chyloperitoneum.

References

1. Gray's anatomy. 35th ed. Philadelphia: Saunders, 1973:168, 727.
2. Dumont AE, Witte MH. Clinical usefulness of thoracic duct cannulation. Adv Intern Med 1969;15:51.
3. Ellis FG. Technique for intermittent collection of thoracic duct lymph. Surgery 1966;60:1251.
4. Kinmonth JB. Lymphangiography by radiological methods. Clin Radiol 1955;6:217.
5. Adler BO, Rosenberger A. Computerized tomography of the thoracic duct: an anatomic study. Cardiovasc Intervent Radiol 1981;4:224.
6. Adler BO, Rosenberger A. Observations on physiological aspects of the thoracic duct with 70 mm camera. Unpublished data.
7. Fuchs WA, Galeazzi RL. Die Röntgenanatomie des Ductus thoracicus. Radiologe 1970;10:180.
8. Wirth W, Fromhold H. Der Ductus thoracicus und seine Variationen: Lymphographische Studie. ROEFO 1970;112:450.
9. Rouvière H. Anatomie des Lymphatiques de l'Homme. Paris: Masson, 1932.
10. Rosenberger A, Abrams HL. The thoracic duct. In: Abrams HL ed. Angiography. 2nd ed. Boston: Little, Brown, 1971.
11. Kausel HW, Reeve TS, Stein AA, Alley RD, Stranahan A. Anatomic and pathologic study of the thoracic duct. J Thorac Cardiovasc Surg 1957;34:631.
12. Zhdanov DA. Anatomie du canal thoracique et des principaux collecteurs lymphatiques du tronc chez l'homme. Acta Anat (Basel) 1959;37:20.
13. Rosenberger A, Adler O, Abrams H. The thoracic duct: structural, functional and radiologic aspects. CRC Crit Rev Radiol Sci 1972;3:523.
14. Hidden G, Florent J. Étude radioanatomique du canal thoracique opacifié par lymphographie pédieuse. J Chir (Paris) 1966;91:373.
15. Pomerantz MJ, Herdt JR, Rockoff SD, Ketcham AS. Evaluation of the functional anatomy of the thoracic duct by lymphangiography. J Thorac Cardiovasc Surg 1963;46:568.
16. Greenfield J, Gottlieb MI. Variation in the terminal portion of the human thoracic duct. Arch Surg 1956;73:955.
17. Negus D, Edwards JM, Kinmonth JB. Filling of cervical and mediastinal nodes from the thoracic duct and the physiology of Virchow's node; studies by lymphography. Br J Surg 1970;57:267.
18. Van Permis PA. Variations of the thoracic duct. Surgery 1949;26:806.
19. Rocca-Rosetti S, Marrocu F, Cossu F, Sulis E. La lymphographie dans l'étude de la morphophysiologie systeme du canal thoracic. J Belge Radiol 1965;48:306.
20. Rusznyak I, Foldi M, Szabo G. Lymphatics and lymphatic circulation. 2nd Engl. ed. New York: Pergamon, 1967.
21. Bergström K, Werner B. Proteins in human thoracic lymph: studies on distribution of some proteins between lymph and blood. Acta Chir Scand 1966;131:413.
22. Chrobák L, Bartós V, Brzek V, Hnízdová D. Coagulation properties of human thoracic duct lymph. Am J Med Sci 1967;253:69.
23. MacFarlane JR, Holman CW. Chylothorax. Am Rev Respir Dis 1972;105:287–291.
24. Williams KR, Buford TH. The management of chylothorax. Ann Surg 1964;160:131–140.
25. Beesone LN, Ferguson TB, Buford TH. Chylothorax. Ann Thorac Surg 1971;12:527–550.
26. Hashim SA, Roholt HB, Babayan VK, Van Itallie TB. Treatment of chyluria and chylothorax with medium chained triglycerides. N Engl J Med 1964;270:756–761.
27. Sasoon CS, Light RW. Chylothorax and pseudochylothorax. Clin Chest Med 1985;6:163–167.
28. Robinson CLN. The management of chylothorax. Ann Thorac Surg 1985;39:90–95.
29. Hall JG. Flow of lymph. N Engl J Med 1969;281:720.
30. Weissleder H. Das pathologische Lymphangiogramm der Ductus thoracicus. ROEFO 1964;101:573.
31. Vajda J. Innervation of lymph vessels. Acta Morphol Acad Sci Hung 1966;14:197.
32. Fitts CT, Williams AV, Graber CD, Artz CP, Hargerst TS.

Thoracic duct lymph: its significance in dialysis and immunology. Surg Clin North Am 1969;49:533.

33. Graber CD, Fitts CT, Williams AV, Artz CP, Othersen HB. Recovery of immune responsiveness after cessation of thoracic duct drainage in calves and men. Ann Surg 1970;171:241.

34. Canafax D, Ascher NL. Cyclosporine immunosuppression. Clin Pharmacol 1983;2:515.

35. Bach FH, Sachs DH. Transplantation immunology. N Engl J Med 1987;317:489.

36. Starzl TE, Weil R, Koep LJ, et al. Thoracic duct fistula and renal transplantation. Ann Surg 1979;190:474–486.

37. Lowe DK, Fletcher WS, Horowitz IJ, Hyman HD. Management of chylothorax secondary to lymphoma. Surg Gynecol Obstet 1972;135:35–38.

38. Fairfax AJ, McNabb WR, Spiro SG. Chylothorax: a review of 18 cases. Thorax 1986;41:880–885.

39. Orringer MB, Bluett M, Deeb GM. Aggressive treatment of chylothorax complicating transhiatal esophagectomy without thoracotomy. Surgery 1985;104:720–726.

40. Breaux JR, Marks C. Chylothorax causing reversible T-cell depletion. J Trauma 1988;28:705–707.

41. Allen SJ, Koch SM, Tonnesen AS, Bowman-Howard M, Khalil K. Tracheal compression caused by traumatic thoracic duct leak. Chest 1994;106(1):296–297.

42. Marts BC, Naunheim KS, Fiore AC, Pennington DG. Conservative versus surgical management of chylothorax. Am J Surg 1992;164(5):532–535.

43. Pennington DW, Warnock ML, Stulbarg MS. Chylothorax and respiratory failure in Kaposi's sarcoma. West J Med 1990;152:421–422.

44. Sasoon CS, Light RW. Chylothorax and pseudochylothorax. Clin Chest Med 1985;6:163–167.

45. Robinson CLN. The management of chylothorax. Ann Thorac Surg 1985;39:90–95.

46. Staats BA, Ellefson RD, Budhan LL, Dines DE, Prakash UB, Offord K. The lipoprotein profile of chylous and nonchylous pleural effusions. Mayo Clin Proc 1980;55:700–704.

47. Light RW. Pleural diseases. Philadelphia: Lea & Febiger, 1990: 269–281.

48. Valentine VG, Raffin TA. The management of chylothorax. Chest 1992;102:586–591.

49. Taylor JR, Ryu J, Colby TV, Raffin TA. Lymphangioleiomyomatosis: clinical course in 32 patients. N Engl J Med 1990;323:1254–1260.

50. Brenner WI, Bernard HB, Reed GE. Chylothorax as a manifestation of rheumatic heart mitral stenosis. Chest 1978;73:672–673.

51. Higgins CB, Mulder DG. Chylothorax after surgery for congenital heart disease. J Thorac Cardiovasc Dis 1971;61:411–418.

52. Cevese PG, Vecchioni R, D'Amico DF, Cordiano C, Biasiato R, Favia G, et al. Postoperative chylothorax: 6 cases in 2,500 operations, with a survey of the world literature. J Thorac Surg 1985;40:542–545.

53. Furguson MK, Little AG, Skinner DB. Current concepts in the management of postoperative chylothorax. Ann Thorac Surg 1985;40:542–545.

54. Dougenis D, Walker WS, Cameron EW, Walbaum PR. Management of chylothorax complicating extensive esophageal resection. Surg Gynecol Obstet 1992;174(6):501–506.

55. Chaiyaroj S, Mullerworth MH, Tatoulis J. Surgery in the management of chylothorax after coronary artery bypass with left internal mammary artery. J Thorac Cardiovasc Surg 1994; 108(6):1155–1156.

56. Smith JA, Goldstein J, Oyer PE. Chylothorax complicating coronary artery by-pass grafting. J Cardiovasc Surg 1994;35(4):307–309.

57. Jabbar AS, al-Abdulkareem A. Bilateral chylothorax following neck dissection. Head & Neck 1995;17(1):69–72.

58. La Hei ER, Menzie SJ, Thompson JF. Right chylothorax following left radical neck dissection. Aust N Z J Surg 1993;63(1):77–79.

59. Williams R, Vetto J, Quinones-Baldrich W, Bongard FS, Wilson SE. Chylous ascites following abdominal aortic surgery. Ann Vasc Surg 1991;5(3):247–252.

60. Roy PH, Carr DT, Payne WS. The problem of chylothorax. Mayo Clin Proc 1967;42:457–467.

61. Kohnoe S, Takahashi I, Kawanaka H, Mori M, Okadome K, Sugimachi K. Combination of preoperative lymphangiography using Lipiodol and intraoperative lymphangiography using Evans Blue facilitates the accurate identification of postoperative chylous fistulas. Surgery Today 1993;23(10):929–931.

62. Sachs PB, Zelch MG, Rice TW, Geisinger MA, Risius B, Lammert GK. Diagnosis and localization of laceration of the thoracic duct: usefulness of lymphangiography and CT. AJR 1991; 157(4):703–705.

63. Paes ML, Powell H. Chylothorax: an update. Br J Hosp Med 1994;51(9):482–490.

64. Nakano A, et al. OK-432 chemical pleurodesis for the treatment of persistent chylothorax. Hepato-Gastroenterology 1994;41(6):568–570.

65. Tie ML, Poland GA, Rosenow EC III. Chylothorax in Gorham's syndrome: a common complication of a rare disease. Chest 1994;105(1):208–213.

66. Harvey JG, Houlsby W, Sherman K, Gough MH. Congenital chylothorax: report of a unique case associated with "H"-type tracheo-oesophageal fistula. Br J Surg 1979;66:485–487.

67. Noonan JA, Walters LR, Reeves JT. Congenital pulmonary lymphangiectasia. Am J Dis Child 1970;20:314.

68. Baltaxe JA, Lee JG, Ehlers KH, Engle MA. Pulmonary lymphangiectasia demonstrated by lymphangiography in 2 patients with Noonan's syndrome. Radiology 1975;115:149.

69. Swischuk LE, Richardson CJ, Nichols MM, Ingman MJ. Bilateral pulmonary hypoplasia in the neonate. AJR 1979;133: 1057.

70. Okabe K, Miura K, Konishi H, Hara K, Shimizu N. Thoracic duct cyst of the mediastinum. Scand J Thorac Cardiovasc Surg 1993;27(3–4):175–177.

71. Livermore GH, Kryzer TC, Patow CA. Aneurysm of the thoracic duct presenting as an asymptomatic left supraclavicular neck mass. Otolaryngol Head Neck Surg 1993;109(3):530–533.

72. Wax MK, Treloar ME. Thoracic duct cyst: an unusual supraclavicular mass. Head & Neck 1992;14(6):502–505.

73. Celis A, Kuthy J, del Castillo E. The importance of the thoracic duct in the spread of malignant disease. Acta Radiol 1956;45: 169.

74. Wallace S, Jackson L, Dodd GD, Greening RR. Lymphatic dynamics in certain abnormal states. AJR 1964;91:1187.

75. Edwards JM, Kinmonth JB. Lymphovenous shunts in man. Br Med J 1969;4:579.

76. Escobar-Prieto A, Gonzalez G, Templeton AW, Cooper BR, Palacios E. Lymphatic channel obstruction: patterns of altered flow dynamics. AJR 1971;113:366.

77. Stewart G, Gaunt JI, Croft DN, Browse DL. Isotope lymphography: a new method of investigating the role of the lymphatics in chronic limb edema. Br J Surg 1985;72:90.

78. Hodges CC, Fossum TW, Komkov A, Hightower D. Lymphoscintigraphy in healthy dogs and dogs with experimentally created thoracic duct abnormalities. Am J Vet Res 1992;53(6): 1048–1053.

79. Vassallo P, Matei C, Heston WD, McLachlan SJ, Koutcher JA, Castellino RA. AMI-227-enhanced MR lymphography: usefulness for differentiating reactive from tumor-bearing lymph nodes. Radiology 1994;193(2):501–506.

80. Anzai Y, et al. Initial clinical experience with dextran-coated super paramagnetic iron oxide for detection of lymph node metastases in patients with head and neck cancer. Radiology 1994; 192:617–618.

81. Wagner S. Benign lymph node hyperplasia and lymph node metastases in rabbits. Animal models for magnetic resonance lymphography. Invest Radiol 1994;29(3):364–371.

82. Weissleder R, Heautot JF, Schaffer BK, Nossiff N, Papisov MI, Bogdanov A Jr, Brady TJ. MR lymphography: study of a high-

efficiency lymphotropic agent. Radiology 1994;191(1):225–230.

83. Harvard AC, Collins DJ, Guy RL, Husband JE. Magnetic resonance behaviour of Lipiodol. Clin Radiol 1992;45(3):198–200.

84. Buckwalter KA, Ellis JH, Baker DE, Borello JA, Glazer GM. Pitfalls in MR imaging after lymphangiography. Radiology 1986;161:831–832.

85. Kent RB III, Pinson TW. Thoracoscopic ligation of the thoracic duct. Surg Endosc 1993;7(1):52–53.

86. Mihalka J, Burrows FA, Burke RP, Javorski JJ. One-lung ventilation during video-assisted thoracoscopic ligation of a thoracic duct in a three-year-old child. J Cardiothorac Vasc Anes 1994; 8(5):559–562.

87. Zoetmulder F, Rutgers E, Baas P. Thoracoscopic ligation of a thoracic duct leakage. Chest 1994;106(4):1233–1234.

88. Graham DD, McGahren ED, Tribble CG, Daniel TM, Rodgers BM. Use of video-assisted thoracic surgery in the treatment of chylothorax. Ann Thorac Surg 1994;57(6):1507–1512.

89. Frank WL, Stuhldreher D, Muchnik S, Ray P, Guinan P. A new technique for the cannulation of the rat thoracic duct. Lab Anim Sci 1992;42(5):526–527.

90. Cope C, Kensey KR. Percutaneous thoracic duct cannulation. J Vasc Intervent Radiol 1994;5:33.

91. Cope C. Percutaneous thoracic duct cannulation: feasibility study in swine. J Vasc Intervent Radiol 1995;6(4):561–566.

92. Cox SJ, Kinmonth JB. Lymphangiography of the thoracic duct: a new technique for improving visualization. J Cardiovasc Surg 1975;16:120–122.

77

Lymphangiopathies

WALTER A. FUCHS

Lymphedema

Lymphedema is caused by an abnormal increase in the interstitial fluid associated with lymphatic insufficiency. A distinction is made between lymphedema secondary to a well-defined cause and primary lymphedema.

Primary Lymphedema

In primary lymphedema a number of different etiologies may be described from the standpoints of radiologic and clinical features, sex incidence, familial tendencies, age of onset, and associated deformities.[1]

Congenital lymphedema includes Milroy disease,[2] a rare hereditary abnormality of the lymph system. Lymphedema may be present at birth or may develop during puberty or adolescence. The disease is believed to be predominantly inherited and female sex–linked. The form known as Meige disease occurs chiefly in women with onset in adolescence and is considered to be female sex–linked.[3] In Turner syndrome primary lymphedema is associated with dysgenesis of the ovaries and other deformities. The testicular feminization syndrome is a subvariety of this group associated with primary amenorrhea and lymphedema.

Nonhereditary congenital lymphedema is much more frequent. Lymphedema praecox is the most common form of primary lymphedema and is found mainly in women.[4,5] It is caused by congenitally anomalous lymphatics, but lymphedema does not develop until between the ages of 9 and 25 years. Injury, surgery, or other forms of trauma or stress lead to insufficiency of the lymph circulation, primarily within the malformed lymph trunks. In lymphedema tarda symptoms appear after the age of 35 years.

Lymphangiopathia obliterans is another cause of primary lymphedema.[6] It is characterized by a pronounced proliferation and hyaline degeneration of the intima of the lymph vessels. This process causes progressive narrowing of the lumen with ultimate occlusion. The disorder occurs chiefly in young women. Its etiology is not known, but it is assumed to be a degenerative vascular process. At first it is limited to one extremity, but the contralateral limb becomes involved some years later. Differentiation between congenital hypoplasia of the lymphatics and obliterative lymphangiopathy can be established only by histologic examination.

The radiologic signs in primary lymphedema are hyperplasia and hypoplasia.[7-10] In hyperplasia the lymph vessels are dilated and tortuous (Fig. 77-1; see Figs. 77-4A and B and 77-11A). The varicosity may be confined to a section of a lymph trunk, or it may involve larger regions of the lymph system. Dermal backflow is often associated with hyperplasia and is due to contrast filling of dermal lymphatics caused by valvular insufficiency. Retrograde filling of interstitial lymphatics is also frequently observed. In hypoplasia the lymph vessels are fewer and smaller than normal. Sometimes subcutaneous lymph trunks cannot be found, and the term *aplasia* is then used (Fig. 77-2). If blue dye is injected subcutaneously, it will spread rapidly in the dermal plexus of the dorsum of the foot and ankle. In some cases a solitary lymph trunk is observed, which is usually dilated and tortuous (Fig. 77-3).

Chylous reflux designates the condition in which the direction of chyle flow from the intestines is abnormal because of congenital abnormalities or disease of the lymphatic system.[1,11,12] Dysplasia of the lymphatic system, congenital insufficiency of lymphatic valves, atresia of lymph vessels, traumatic laceration of lymphatic structures, and obstruction due to inflammatory or malignant lesions are the major causes of chylous reflux. Proximal to the obstruction of lymph flow, the lymphatics are severely dilated. Their valves become incompetent, with consequent lymph flow. The intralymphatic pressure is considerably increased, and lymph vessels may rupture, with subsequent fistula formation.

Chylous edema is the result of retrograde flow of the intestinal lymph to the pelvis, genitals, and lower limbs (Fig. 77-4C). It leads to vessel dilatation and tortuosity in both the superficial and deep lymphatics.

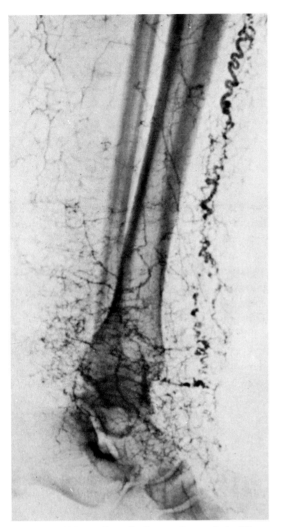

Figure 77-1. Primary lymphedema—hyperplasia. There are numerous dilated and tortuous lymphatics and dermal backflow.

Progressive dilatation of the dermal lymphatics causes formation of chyloderma. Rupture of the vesicles results in chylorrhea. In rare cases of long-standing lymphedema, sarcomatous degeneration occurs (Stewart-Treves syndrome).[13] Lymphangiomatosis of the bone may be due to incompetent lymphatic valves.[14,15] Retrograde lymph flow from the pelvic region gradually leads to cystlike areas of bone destruction, which vary in size and contain oily contrast material after lymphangiography (Fig. 77-5).

Secondary Lymphedema

Secondary lymphedema is due to inflammatory lesions of the lymphatic and venous systems as well as to trauma, parasite invasion, tumor infiltration, surgical excision, or radiotherapy.[1,16–18]

Inflammatory Lesions

In lymphangiitis, lymphangiography reveals multiple occlusions of otherwise normal lymph channels (Fig. 77-6). Peripheral to the occlusions the lymph vessels are distended and tortuous and often show backflow into dermal and intestinal lymphatics. Generally, many more lymphatics are contrast-filled than normal lymphangiograms show. Frequently a diffuse or localized extravasation of contrast agent is seen. Histologic examination shows inflammation, with a dense, perivascular cellular infiltration.

In the venous postthrombotic syndrome the prefascial lymphatics may exhibit certain changes after obliterative inflammations of the deep venous system. The contrast material flows in a retrograde direction into very fine lymphatics that join the major lymphatic channels. In chronic venous ulceration, the opaque material enters into the dermal lymph plexus and is

Figure 77-2. Primary lymphedema—aplasia. There is dermal backflow of the vital dye after subcutaneous injection. No subcutaneous lymphatics were found at dissection.

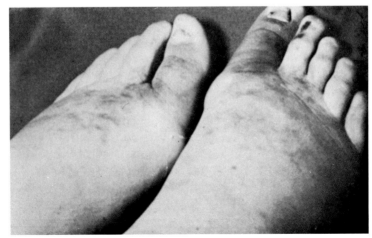

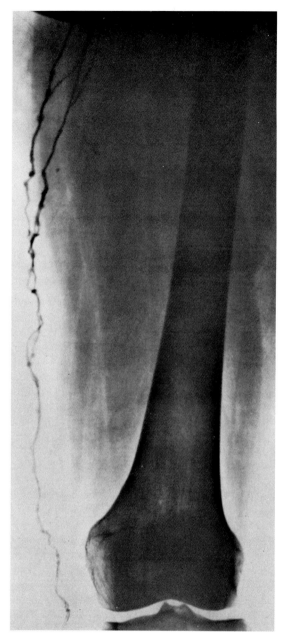

Figure 77-3. Primary lymphedema—hypoplasia. There is a solitary dilated and tortuous lymph trunk.

seen at the periphery of the ulcers as minute deposits of contrast medium.

Filariasis

Filariasis, due to infection with *Wuchereria bancrofti*, is the most frequent cause of secondary lymphedema and one of the most common diseases in the world.[1,19,20] Stenosis and complete obstruction of the lymphatics by inflammatory and sclerotic processes or by the parasite itself, as well as extensive collateral circulations and dermal backflow, are observed. Inflam-

matory reaction occurs in the regional lymph nodes but does not block lymph flow.

Noninflammatory Lesions

Malignant infiltration of lymph vessels and lymph nodes is a major cause of obstruction of lymph flow and secondary lymphedema. Details of pathogenesis and radiologic appearance are discussed in Chapter 79.

Postoperative Lymphedema

Experimental animal studies indicate that regeneration of lymph vessels occurs approximately 20 days after surgical incision. In lymphangiography, extravasation of contrast material into the operation site is observed (Fig. 77-7; see Figs. 77-12 and 77-13).[1,21,22] Regeneration of lymphatics progresses from afferent lymph vessels. In cases of large incisions, repair proceeds via direct regeneration from the major lymph trunks. Collaterals bypassing the operation area are encountered when not all anatomic connections have been interrupted (Fig. 77-7B). Lymphaticovenous anastomoses develop to restore the balance of lymph flow. Complete repair of lymphatic circulation is achieved usually between 2 and 11 months postoperatively but will be retarded by infection, venous alterations, and irradiation.

Irradiation Fibrosis

The sensitivity of the lymphatics to irradiation is low. Slight changes in the lymph vessel wall occur when doses of 40 Gy are applied. A high dosage of 150 Gy is necessary to alter the lymphatic circulation significantly.[23] The impairment of lymphatic circulation due to irradiation is primarily consequent to scar formation in adjacent, highly radiosensitive connective tissue. No alterations of the lymphatic circulation occur in the normal or slightly altered lymphatic system when a therapeutic radiation dose is applied (Fig. 77-8). Small, delicate lymph vessels and small lymph nodes with structural patterns still intact are encountered. The small irradiated lymph nodes are not able to retain large amounts of contrast material. Irradiation of lymph nodes and lymph vessels extensively infiltrated by malignant disease frequently causes partial or complete obstruction of the lymph vessel because of necrosis and secondary scar formation within the connective tissue (Fig. 77-9). Formation of a collateral circulation follows. Complete fibrosis and replacement of the lymphatic tissue make visualization of the lymph nodes impossible by lymphangiography. Secondary inflammations seem to play an important role in producing these obstructive fibrotic changes.

Text continues on page 1915

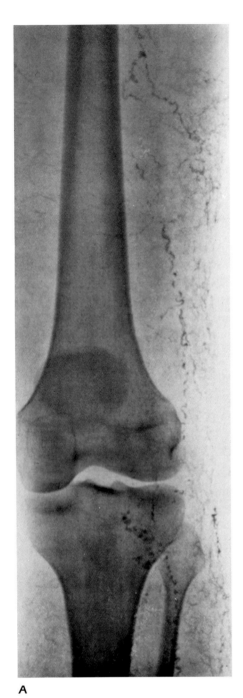

A

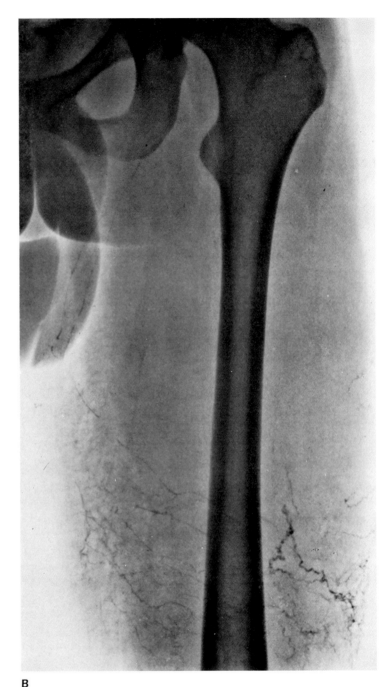

B

Figure 77-4. Primary lymphedema—chylous reflux. (A and B) Hyperplasia of the dilated, tortuous lymphatics in the left lower leg and thigh. (C) Chylous reflux. Contrast material fills the contralateral lymph nodes and lymphatics of the scrotum. There is dysplasia of the retroperitoneal lymphatic system.

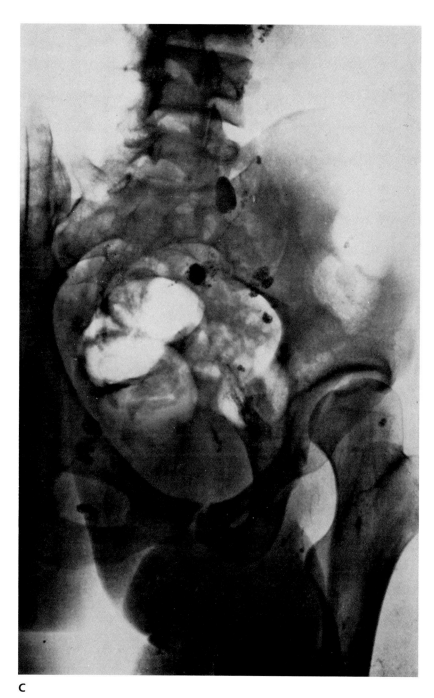

C

Figure 77-4 (continued).

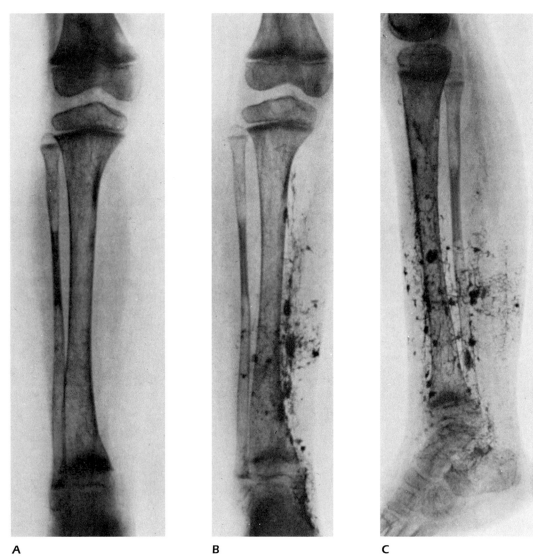

A   **B**   **C**

Figure 77-5. Lymphangiomatosis of the bone. (A) Cystlike areas of bone destruction. The areas are irregular in shape and vary in size within the tibia and fibula. (B and C) Lymphangiography. Primary lymphedema with hyperplasia of the lymphatics and extravasation of contrast material. (D and E) Accumulation of oily substance within the cystlike areas in the calcaneus. The diagnosis was confirmed by biopsy of the fibula 10 days after lymphangiography.

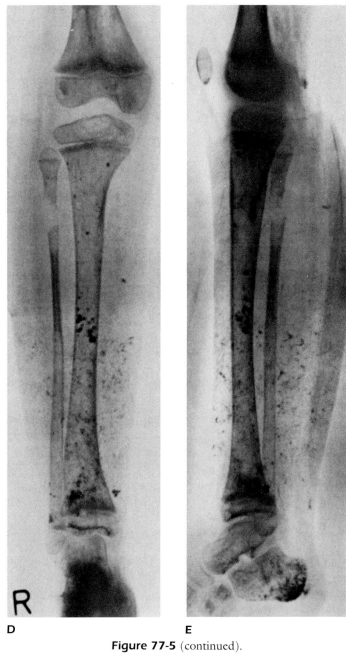

Figure 77-5 (continued).

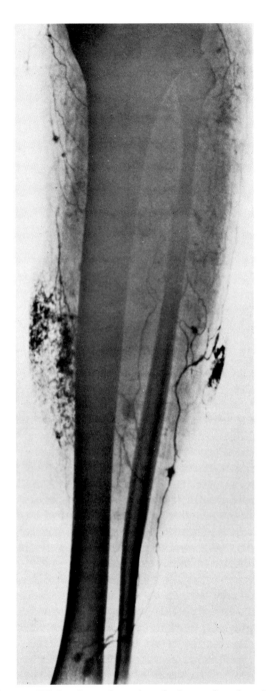

Figure 77-6. Secondary lymphedema—lymphangiitis. There is obstruction of numerous subcutaneous lymphatics, extensive collateral circulation, and dermal and interstitial backflow.

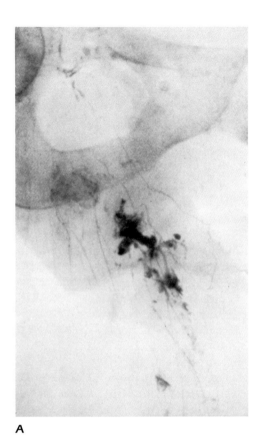

A

Figure 77-7. Postoperative lymphedema. (A) Extravasation of contrast material into the operation area, new formation of efferent lymphatics, and collateral circulation 3 months after inguinal lymphadenectomy. (B) Scar formation in the axilla after surgery and radiotherapy of breast cancer. Newly formed lymphatics traverse the area of operation. Collateral circulation is via the cephalic lymphatic chain.

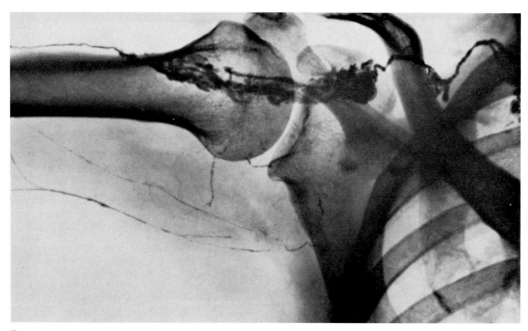

B

Figure 77-7 (continued).

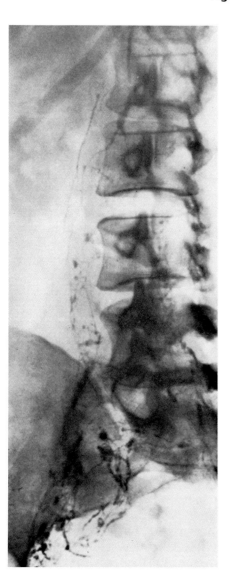

Retroperitoneal Fibrosis

Idiopathic retroperitoneal fibrosis is a relatively uncommon clinical entity. The etiology of this disease is still unknown, but it is considered to be a hypersensitivity or autoimmune phenomenon.[24,25] Lymphangiography reveals complete or partial obstruction of the lymphatic circulation (Fig. 77-10B).[26–29] Collateral lymphatics within the pelvic and inferior aortic region are contrast-filled. Fibrotic induration of the retroperitoneal connective tissue leads to external compression of the lymphatics. The lymph vessels superior to the fourth lumbar vertebra are usually not visualized, and irregular filling defects within the iliac and aortic lymph nodes may be observed. Cavography demonstrates dislocation, compression, and complete obstruction of the inferior vena cava and pelvic veins, and the end result is an extensive collateral circulation. Urography shows urinary stasis with dilatation of the ureters and hydronephrosis (see Fig. 77-10A). Computed tomography demonstrates a retroperitoneal mass lesion obliterating the vascular contours and extending toward the ureters (Fig. 77-10C). In structure and density it cannot be differentiated from malignant disease.

Figure 77-8. Irradiation fibrosis. Multiple fine lymphatics and lymph nodes after radiotherapy of Hodgkin disease with 7500 rad.

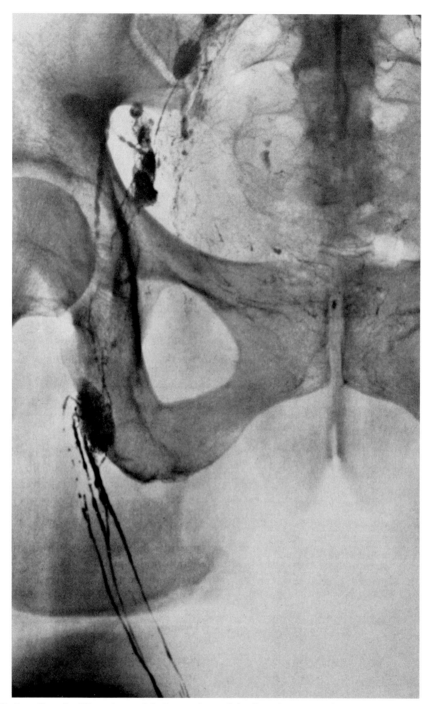

Figure 77-9. Irradiation fibrosis. There is partial obstruction of the lymphatic circulation leading to collaterals within the pelvic area 3 years after radiotherapy (60 Gy) of a carcinoma of the uterine corpus.

Figure 77-10. Retroperitoneal fibrosis. (A) Low lumbar obstruction of the right ureter. (B) Partial obstruction of the lymphatic ▶ and venous circulation. (C) Prevertebral mass lesion surrounding the abdominal aorta and inferior vena cava (*arrowheads*). *MP*, psoas muscle.

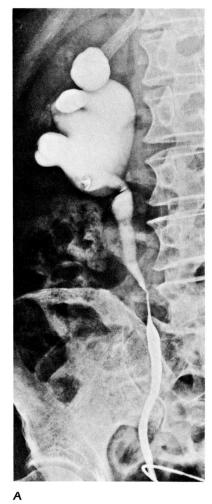

A

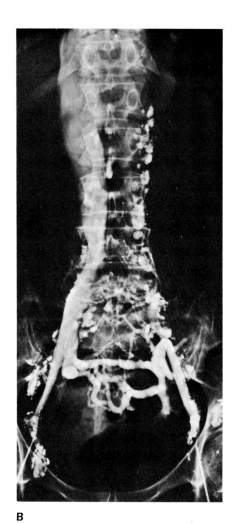

B

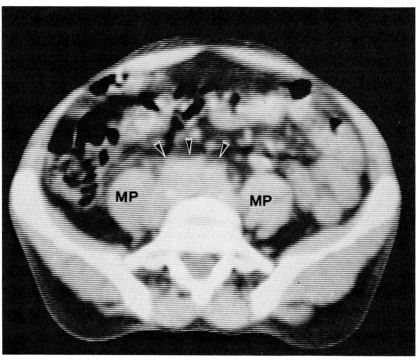

C

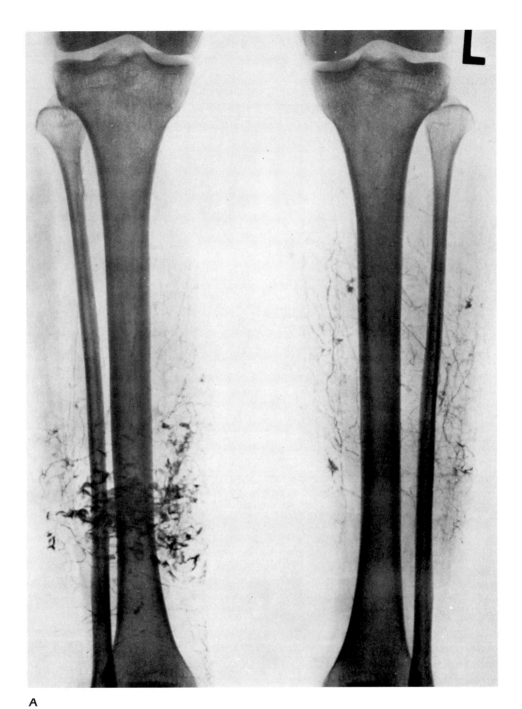

A

Figure 77-11. Primary lymphedema, chyloretroperitoneum, and chylothorax due to congenital abnormalities and secondary obstruction of lymph flow. This 28-year-old woman was operated on for valvular pulmonary stenosis and atrial septal defects. (A) Primary lymphedema of both legs. There are numerous fine interstitial and dermal lymphatics. (B) Bilateral extravasation of contrast material into the retroperitoneal space and dilatation of the thoracic duct. There is no chyluria. (C) Effusion of contrast medium along the peribronchial sheaths into the right pleural cavity and into the mediastinum. Fine intrapulmonary, mediastinal, and supraclavicular lymphatics act as collaterals. The severe dilatation of the thoracic duct was due to obstruction caused by an inflammatory reaction after insertion of a catheter into the subclavian vein during extracorporeal circulation.

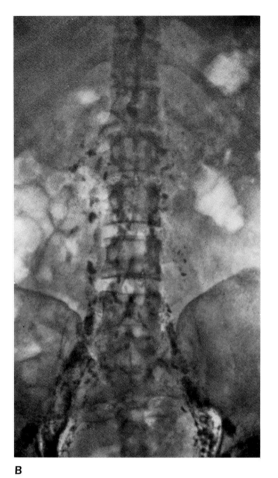

B

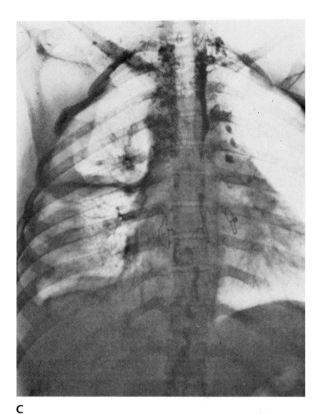

C

Figure 77-11 (continued).

Lymph Fistula

Chyloperitoneum

The presence of chyle in the peritoneal cavity is due to congenital atresia in the newborn or to obstruction of the lymphatic circulation in the adult.[1,11,30,31] Malignant tumors are the most frequent cause of chyloperitoneum. The compression or obliteration of lymph channels may occur at any point between the abdominal wall and the entry of the thoracic duct into the venous system. Dilatation of the lymph trunks and valve insufficiency lead to reversal of lymph flow. Extravasation of contrast material into the peritoneal cavity and the retroperitoneal area may be demonstrated by lymphangiography (Fig. 77-11B). Traumatic rupture, inflammatory adenopathies, pancreatic lesions, and thrombosis of the subclavian vein are occasionally responsible for chylous effusion.

Lymphointestinal Fistula

Exudative enteropathy may be related to congenital abnormalities of the intestinal lymph channels. Diffuse dilatation of the lymphatics of the intestinal mucosa, called *intestinal lymphangiectasis,* then occurs.[32-37] Blockage of the lymph circulation by tumor, pancreatitis, or constrictive pericarditis has been reported as a direct cause of exudative enteropathy. When the site of obstruction is situated in the thoracic duct or retroperitoneal area, lymphangiography demonstrates interruption, stasis, and even reversal of lymph flow. Fistulas into the intestines may occasionally be visualized. If the obstacle is confined to the visceral lymph channels, the lymphangiogram appears normal. The cause of chylous effusion is valve insufficiency due to either malformation, mainly malignant, or inflammatory obstruction. Occasionally, the fistula is acquired after injury. Chylous disease occurs when the lymphatic circulation is decompensated and all collateral channels are exhausted.

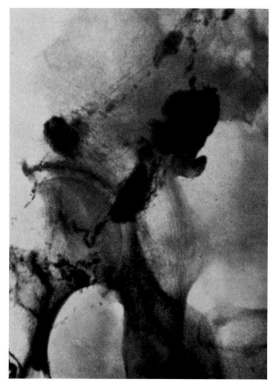

Figure 77-12. Postoperative lymphocyst 4 months after lymphadenectomy in carcinoma of the uterine cervix. Drainage of the operation area is by efferent lymphatics.

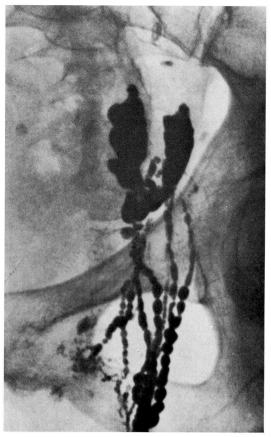

Figure 77-13. Postoperative lymphocyst 10 days after lymphadenectomy in carcinoma of the uterine cervix. Interruption of the lymph circulation and dilatation of the afferent lymphatics are seen.

Chyluria

The common etiology of chyluria is filariasis. Lymphangiography demonstrates unilateral or bilateral renal lymphatic reflux and multiple lymphocalyceal fistulas related to obstruction of lymph flow at the origin of the thoracic duct.[19,20,38-41] Lymphedema of the legs and genital organs is found invariably as a manifestation of general invasion of the lymphatic system by the parasite.

Chylothorax

Trauma is the most frequent cause of effusion of lymph in the pleural cavities. It results from penetrating trauma and injury to the thoracic duct by operative or diagnostic procedures.[31,42] Spontaneous chylothorax is related to blockage of the thoracic duct by malignant tumor and inflammatory and parasitic disease, as well as to congenital malformations.[43] Lymphangiography makes it possible to determine the anatomic site and the type of laceration. It permits differentiation between congenital malformations and acquired conditions. In the presence of an obstruction, lymphangiography shows dilatation of the thoracic duct and effusion of contrast material along the peribronchial

sheaths into the pleural cavity and mediastinum (see Fig. 77-11C).

Lymphocele

Lymphocyst formation is a complication of lymphadenectomy.[44-46] The lymphatics that have been cut continue to pour lymph into the space left at the site of operation. If the lymph drainage from the operation area is not readily reestablished by the proliferation of new lymphatics, cyst formation occurs (Figs. 77-12 and 77-13). The cyst may be demarcated, or it may continue to fill, extending beyond the operation site. It can persist for months or years. Preoperative irradiation probably contributes to lymphocyst formation, and irradiation delays its absorption. Lymphangiography provides a direct method of diagnosing lymphocysts because they are more densely filled with contrast material than the structured lymph nodes. Lympho-

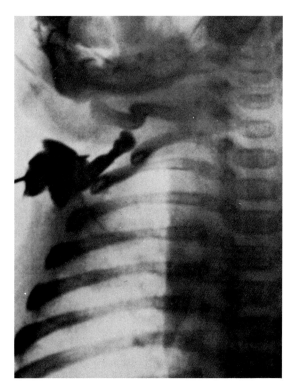

Figure 77-14. Cavernous lymphangioma in the right axillary region. There is partial contrast filling by direct puncture; no efferent lymphatics are seen.

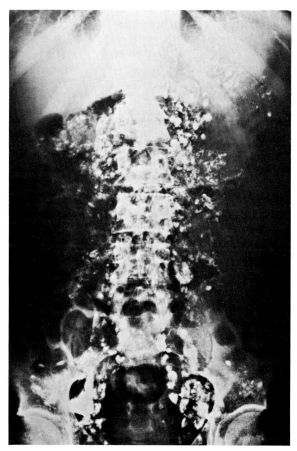

Figure 77-15. Lymphangiomyomatosis with numerous multicystic lesions within the retroperitoneum.

cysts remain densely opaque when only traces of residual contrast medium are left in the lymph nodes. By enlarging and compressing adjacent structures, lymphocysts can cause pelvic pain, urinary symptoms, alterations in bowel habits, and edema of the external genitalia and extremities. It is important that lymphocysts be recognized as such and not confused with recurrent malignancies, so that the patient can be appropriately treated. Traumatic lymphocysts occur rarely and only are localized to the area traumatized.

Lymphogenic Neoplasm

Cavernous lymphangioma and cystic hygroma originate from a peripheral sequestration of primary lymphatic cavities.[47] In children they constitute 6 percent of all benign tumors. *Cavernous lymphangioma* consists of multiple cavities lined with endothelium and surrounded by fibrous tissue. *Cystic hygroma* contains larger cavities lined with endothelium and filled with clear or hemorrhagic fluid. These lymphatic cavities are localized in the face, neck, mediastinum, and axillae. Because they are sequestered from lymph flow, lymphangioma and hygroma are only rarely demonstrable by

intravascular lymphangiography but may be visualized by direct puncture (Fig. 77-14). Mesenteric and retroperitoneal cysts induce symptoms by compression of the digestive and urinary tracts. Sudden rupture results in an acute abdomen.

Lymphangiomyomas are congenital and usually occur in women in the retroperitoneum or mediastinum (Fig. 77-15).[48] Lymphography demonstrates multicystic lesions, chylothorax, and chylous ascites.

Lymphangiosarcoma (Stewart-Treves syndrome) represents a malignant degeneration in primary or secondary lymphedema, usually following radical mastectomy.[13]

References

1. Kinmonth JB. The lymphatics: diseases, lymphography and surgery. London: Arnold, 1972.
2. Milroy WF. An undescribed variety of hereditary oedema. NY Med J 1892;56:505.
3. Meige H. Dystrophie oedémateuse héréditaire. Presse Med 1898;6:341.

4. Kinmonth JB, Taylor GW, Tracy GD, Marsh JD. Primary lymphoedema. Br J Surg 1957;45:1.

5. Taylor GW. Chronic lymphoedema. Br J Surg 1967;54:898.

6. Kaindl F, Mannheimer E, Pfleger-Schwarz L, Thurnher E. Lymphangiographie und Lymphadenographie der Extremitäten. Stuttgart: Thieme, 1960.

7. Gough MH. Primary lymphoedema: clinical and lymphangiographic studies. Br J Surg 1966;53:917.

8. Jacobsson S, Johansson S. Lymphangiography in lymphedema. Acta Radiol 1962;57:81.

9. Kinmonth JB, Taylor GW. Lymphatic circulation in lymphedema. Ann Surg 1954;139:129.

10. de Roo T. The value of lymphography in lymphedema. Surg Gynecol Obstet 1967;124:755.

11. Bismuth V, Bourdon R. Les ascites chyleuses de l'adulte: apport de la lymphographie (5 cas). J Radiol Electrol Med Nucl 1964;45:413.

12. Kinmonth JB, Taylor GW. Chylous reflux. Br Med J 1964;1:529.

13. Stewart FW, Treves N. Lymphangiosarcoma in postmastectomy lymphedema: a report of six cases in elephantiasis chirurgica. Cancer 1948;1:64.

14. Nixon GW. Lymphangiomatosis of bone demonstrated by lymphangiography. AJR 1970;110:582.

15. Winterberger AR. Radiographic diagnosis of lymphangiomatosis of bone. Radiology 1972;102:321.

16. Collette JM. La lymphographie dans les lymphostases acquises. Ann Radiol (Paris) 1958;1:211.

17. Fuchs WA, Rüttimann A, del Buono MS. Zur Lymphographie bei chronisch-sekun-dären Lymphödemen. ROEFO 1960;92:608.

18. Gregl A, Kienle J. Lymphangiographie beim peripheren Lymphödem. ROEFO 1966;105:622.

19. Akisada M, Tani S. Filarial chyluria in Japan: lymphography, etiology, and treatment in 30 cases. Radiology 1968;90:311.

20. Rajaram PC. Lymphatic dynamics in filarial chyluria and prechyluric state: lymphographic analysis of 52 cases. Lymphology 1970;3:114.

21. Abbes M. Les altérations de la circulation lymphatique après amputation du sein. Ann Chir 1966;20:660.

22. Tsangaris NT, Yutzy CV. Lymphangiographic study of postmastectomy lymphedema. Surg Gynecol Obstet 1966;123:1228.

23. Engeset A. Irradiation of lymph nodes and vessels: experiments in rats, with reference to cancer therapy. Acta Radiol Suppl (Stockh) 1964;229:1.

24. Kerr WS, Suby HI, Vickert A, Praley P. Idiopathic retroperitoneal fibrosis: clinical experiences with 15 cases, 1956–1967. J Urol 1968;99:575.

25. Wagenknecht LV. Retroperitoneale Fibrosen. Stuttgart: Thieme, 1978.

26. Beltz L, Lymberopoulos S. Die retroperitoneale Fibrose. Urologe A 1966;5:276.

27. Clouse ME, Fraley EF, Litwin SB. Lymphangiographic criteria for diagnosis of retroperitoneal fibrosis. Radiology 1964;83:1.

28. Haertel M, Bollmann J, Vock P, Zingg E. Computertomographie und retroperitoneale Fibrose (Morbus Ormond). ROEFO 1979;131:504.

29. Virtama P, Helfia T. Lymphography and cavography in retroperitoneal fibrosis. Br J Radiol 1967;40:231.

30. Camiel MR, Benninghoff DL, Herman RG. Chylous ascites with lymphographic demonstration of lymph leakage into the peritoneal cavity. Gastroenterology 1964;47:188.

31. Nix JT, Albert M, Dugas JE, Wendt DL. Chylothorax and chylous ascites: a study of 302 selected cases. Am J Gastroenterol 1957;28:40.

32. Amos JAS. Multiple lymphatic cysts of the mesentery. Br J Surg 1969;46:588.

33. Desprez-Curely JP, Bismuth V, Bourdon R. Hypoprotéinémie idiopathique et stéatorrhé: démonstration radiographique d'une fistule intestinale. Ann Radiol (Paris) 1958;1:744.

34. Leonidas JC, Kopel FB, Danese CA. Mesenteric cyst associated with protein loss in the gastrointestinal tract: study with lymphangiography. AJR 1971;112:150.

35. Oh C, Danese CA, Dreiling DA, Elmhurst MD. Chylous cysts of mesentery. Arch Surg 1967;94:790.

36. Pomerantz M, Waldmann TA. Systemic lymphatic abnormalities associated with gastrointestinal protein loss secondary to intestinal lymphangiectasia. Gastroenterology 1963;45:703.

37. Servelle M, Rouffilange F, Andrieux J, Soulie J, Sequin P, de Leersnider D. Lymphographie des chylifères intestinaux. Semin Hop Paris 1968;44:881.

38. Bernageau J, Bismuth V, Desprez-Curely JP, Bourdon R. La lymphographie dans les chyluries. J Radiol Electrol Med Nucl 1964;45:529.

39. Koehler R, Chiang TC, Lin CT, Chen KC, Chen KY. Lymphography in chyluria. AJR 1968;102:455.

40. Picard JD. La lymphographie au cours de chyluries (à propos de 30 observations). J Urol Nephrol (Paris) 1967;73:671.

41. Servelle M, Turiaf J, Rouffilange F, Scherer G, Perrot H, Frentz F, Turpyn H. Chyluria in abnormalities of the thoracic duct. Surgery 1963;54:536.

42. Althaus U, Fuchs WA. Chylothorax nach kardiovaskulären Eingriffen. Schweiz Med Wochenschr 1972;102:44.

43. Freundlich IM. The role of lymphangiography in chylothorax: a report of six nontraumatic cases. AJR 1975;125:617.

44. Dodd GD, Rutledge F, Wallace S. Postoperative pelvic lymphocysts. AJR 1970;108:312.

45. Parker JJ, Schmutzler KJ. Chylous lymphocyst. Radiology 1971;98:569.

46. Weingold AB, Olivo E, Marino J. Pelvic lymphocyst: diagnosis and management. Arch Surg 1967;95:304.

47. Castellino RA, Finkelstein S. Lymphographic demonstration of a retroperitoneal lymphangioma. Radiology 1975;115:355.

48. Kruglik GD, Reed JC, Daroca PJ. RPC from the AFIP. Radiology 1976;120:583.

78

Benign Lymph Node Disease

WALTER A. FUCHS

Involutive Changes

Fibrolipomatosis, a manifestation of the normal physiologic involution of the lymphatic system,[1] is characterized by the complete replacement of the central parts of the lymph nodes by connective and fatty tissue (Fig. 78-1). Lymphatic structures are left only in the periphery of the nodes, as incomplete cortical margins, and consequently the lymphangiographic appearance of those nodes is characterized by large central filling defects. The intermediary sinuses are preserved and are therefore contrast-filled during the filling phase of lymphography (Fig. 78-2). Fibrolipomatosis is most common in the inguinal and axillary lymph nodes because they are the primary regional node groups of the extremities and are the nodes most often affected by inflammatory lesions. The external iliac lymph nodes and the lymph node groups at the level of the first to second lumbar vertebrae manifest similar but less extensive involutive changes. Fibrolipomatosis is more pronounced in patients of the middle and older age groups.

Reactive Hyperplasia

Reactive hyperplasia is characterized histologically by a proliferative process in which histioreticular and lymphocytic cells may take part. Hyperplasia may involve the medulla and cortex separately, but medullary and follicular hyperplasia may also be present simultaneously. The lymphangiographic node pattern of reactive hyperplasia is similar to that of a nonspecific hyperplasia inflammatory reaction. The large follicles and the wide sinuses give rise to larger, evenly distributed, filling defects (Fig. 78-3). The lymph circulation is not impaired.[2]

Reactive hyperplasia is encountered in regional lymph nodes of primary tumors or of operation sites and should be regarded as a reactive change induced by inflammatory toxic products and metabolic agents of tumor cells. The presence of reactive hyperplasia in regional lymph nodes of a primary tumor implies the presence of a defense mechanism within these nodes.

Inflammatory Disease

The classification of inflammatory reactions of lymph nodes is best made on the basis of morphologic change and not on the basis of etiology. The cellular reactions are not specific, even though they may be characteristic of a certain group of agents. In lymphangiography, the observed patterns are necessarily less specific. The morphologic alterations distinguished are hyperplastic inflammatory changes, granulomatous epithelial cell changes, and abscess-forming and necrotizing changes.

Hyperplastic Inflammatory Changes

The characteristic histologic changes of inflammatory reactions in lymph nodes are generalized hyperplasia of the lymphatic tissue with consequent node enlargement and new follicle formation.[2] The newly formed follicles cause filling defects that alter the structural pattern seen in the lymphadenogram. The number and size of the follicles vary from node to node, depending on the degree of the inflammatory reaction. This variation in turn produces marked variations in the structural lymphangiographic architecture of the nodes.

The lymphangiographic pattern of an inflamed node resembles that of an enlarged node.[3] However, a great variety of structural patterns in hyperplastic inflammatory disease are encountered. Large follicles and wide sinuses produce large filling defects within coarse, opaque strands. An increase in follicle size will loosen up the storage pattern, which always presents a regular, harmonious structure. In some cases, extensive filling defects by very large follicles may dominate the lymphadenogram (Fig. 78-4).

The storage phase of the lymphadenogram is most often characterized by a reticular pattern in which contrast droplets are localized within small sinuses. When

1923

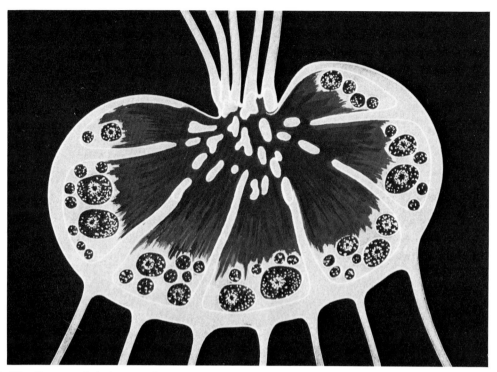

Figure 78-1. Fibrolipomatosis (schematic drawing). There is extensive fibrolipomatous replacement of centrally located lymphatic tissue leading to central filling defects. The marginal lymphatic tissue is contrast-filled.

sinuses are wide, coarse droplets within them may dominate the lymphadenogram. Hyperplastic inflammatory changes of lymph nodes occur as nonspecific reactive phenomena in general infectious disease, infectious mononucleosis, measles and other viral infections, and syphilis,[4] as well as in rheumatic arthritis, ankylosing spondylitis,[5] and psoriatic arthropathy.

Figure 78-3. Reactive hyperplasia. The inguinal and external iliac lymph nodes are enlarged and show a homogeneous storage pattern.

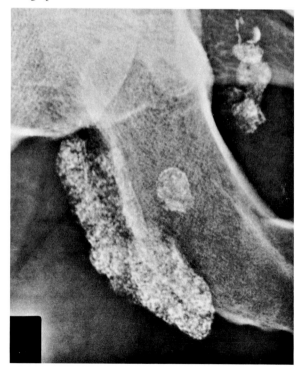

Figure 78-2. Fibrolipomatosis of the inguinal lymph nodes. (A) Filling phase with an intact intermediary sinusoidal system. (B) Storage phase with a contrast-filled marginal sinus system.

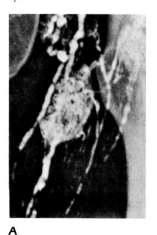
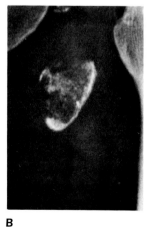

A   **B**

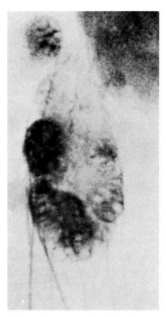

Figure 78-4. Chronic hyperplastic inflammatory reaction. The inguinal lymph nodes are enlarged and have large follicular filling defects.

Granulomatous Epithelioid Cell Inflammatory Changes

Granulomatous epithelioid cell reactions are encountered in chronic inflammatory diseases of widely varying etiology[6]: tuberculosis, sarcoidosis, toxoplasmosis, brucellosis, syphilis, histoplasmosis, coccidioidomycosis, tularemia, leprosy, blastomycosis, Crohn disease, and parasitic diseases.

In *tuberculosis,* filling defects of various sizes in enlarged lymph nodes are the structural alterations of the lymphangiographic pattern that are most often encountered.[6–9] The multiple well-demarcated central and marginal filling defects are due to the tuberculous granuloma (Fig. 78-5). The pathologic lymph nodes are slightly enlarged and are situated predominantly within the lumbar area. These changes are nonspecific and may resemble malignancy.[10] Calcifications within lymph nodes may occasionally be recognized. The lymphatic circulation may be impaired.

The lymphangiographic pattern of *sarcoidosis* has been described as similar to that of malignant lymphoma.[6,7,11,12] The pattern of enlarged lumbar lymph nodes manifests structural loosening because of lacunar filling defects and droplike deposits of contrast material (Fig. 77-6). Lymphatic obstruction is extremely rare. Brucellosis, syphilis, and leprosy have been seen to produce the same type of lymphangiographic pattern as has nonspecific inflammation.

Histoplasmosis is reported to produce lymph node

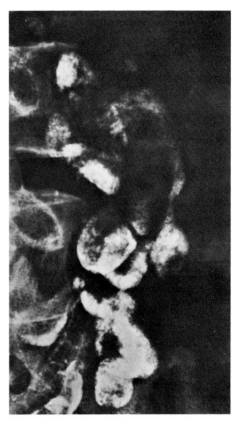

Figure 78-5. Tuberculosis. The common left iliac and aortic lymph nodes are enlarged and show large central filling defects and loosening of the storage pattern.

involvement that is also similar in appearance to that of malignant lymphoma.[13] The lymphangiographic pattern of toxoplasmosis is also that of a nonspecific hyperplastic reaction.

In *Bancroft filariasis,* signs of reactive inflammatory reaction are observed in the early stages of the disease. Poor opacification of the lymph nodes is observed in the later stages of filariasis, when permanent chyluria and stasis of the lymph circulation caused by extensive fibrosis are present.

The lymphangiographic findings in *Whipple disease* are general enlargement of the iliac and aortic lymph nodes, filling defects, and loosening of the structural pattern.[3]

Abscess-Forming and Necrotizing Changes

Abscess-forming and necrotizing changes develop in inguinal lymphogranuloma (Nicolas-Favre disease), lymphogranuloma venereum, cat-scratch disease, and abscess-forming lymphadenitis.

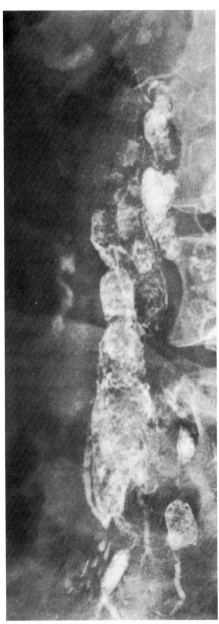

Figure 78-6. Sarcoidosis. The common iliac and lumbar lymph nodes are enlarged and show structural loosening because of lacunar filling defects.

Radiation Fibrosis

Irradiation of the lymph nodes causes the alteration and destruction of lymphocytes, even when small doses are used. However, repopulation with lymphocytes from the circulating blood is a continuous process.[14,15]

Circumscribed necrosis occurs when high radiation doses are applied and additional vascular and inflammatory lesions are present. The sensitivity of the lymphatics to irradiation is comparatively small.[14]

The lymphogram does not demonstrate alterations of the lymphatic circulation in the normal or the slightly altered lymphatic system when a therapeutic radiation dose is applied.[1,16]

Small, delicate lymph vessels and small lymph nodes with intact macroscopic structural patterns are encountered; they are not able to retain normal amounts of contrast material.

References

1. Fuchs WA. Benign lymph node disease. In: Fuchs WA, Davidson JW, Fischer HW, eds. Lymphography in cancer. New York: Springer, 1969.
2. Tjernberg B. Lymphography. Acta Radiol Suppl (Stockh) 1962;214:1.
3. Viamonte M. Lymphography in inflammatory conditions. In: Rüttimann A, ed. Progress in lymphology. Stuttgart: Thieme, 1967.
4. Bergstrom JF, Navin JJ. Luetic lymphadenitis: lymphographic manifestations simulating lymphoma. Radiology 1973;106:287.
5. Fournier AM, Denizet D, Delagrange A. La lymphographie dans la spondylarthrite ankylosante. J Radiol Electrol Med Nucl 1969;50:773.
6. Rauste J. Lymphographic findings in granulomatous inflammations and connective tissue diseases. Acta Radiol Suppl (Stockh) 1972;317.
7. Albrecht A, Taenzer V, Nickling H. Lymphographische Befunde bei Sarkoidose und Lymphknotentuberkulose. ROEFO 1967;106:178.
8. Bétroulières P, Lamarque JL, Ginestie JF, Combes C. Étude des aspects lymphographiques de la tuberculose ganglionnaire. J Radiol 1968;49:1.
9. Bussat PL, Béboux JM, Petite J, Wettstein P. Lymphography in a patient with nonreactive tuberculosis. AJR 1966;98:436.
10. Parker BR, Blank N, Castellino RA. Lymphographic appearance of benign conditions simulating lymphoma. Radiology 1974;111:267.
11. Silver HM, Tsangaris NT, Eaton DM. Lymphedema and lymphography in sarcoidosis. Arch Intern Med 1966;117:712.
12. Strickstrock KH, Weissleder H. Lymphographische Diagnose und Differentialdiagnose bei der Sarkoidose. ROEFO 1968;108:576.
13. Walter JF, Sodeman TM, Cooperstock MS, Bookstein JJ, Whitehouse WM. Lymphangiographic findings in histoplasmosis. Radiology 1975;114:65.
14. Lenzi M, Bassani G. The effect of radiation on the lymph and on the lymph vessels. Radiology 1963;80:814.
15. Sherman JO, O'Brien PH. Effect of ionizing irradiation on normal lymph vessels and lymph nodes. Cancer 1967;20:1851.
16. Ludvik W, Wachtler F, Zaunbauer W. Veränderungen am Lymphogramm durch Operation und ionisierende Strahlen. ROEFO 1969;110:307.

79

Malignant Metastatic Disease

WALTER A. FUCHS

Formation of Cancerous Metastases

Lymph node metastases are formed by emboli of small groups of cancer cells that reach the marginal sinuses via afferent lymphatics. Tumor cells are deposited in close proximity to the entry points of the afferent lymph vessels and in the intermediary sinuses. Because malignant cells from a primary tumor reach a regional lymph node by way of numerous afferent lymphatics, multiple foci of malignant growth may implant in the periphery of the node (Fig. 79-1A). With increasing growth of the malignant cell formation, irregular destruction of the marginal area of the affected lymph node occurs. Further malignant infiltration of the node leads to compression of the lymphatic tissue, destruction of the capsule, and obliteration of the intermediary sinus. In advanced stages, the entire lymph node is infiltrated, and the afferent lymphatics are obstructed (Fig. 79-1B). Lymph flow is blocked, and a collateral circulation develops.[1]

Metastases from a cancerous organ do not necessarily implant in the primary regional lymph nodes of the organ. Malignant infiltration may occur in only secondary and tertiary regional node groups. Primary regional lymph nodes may be bypassed via direct anastomoses between afferent and efferent lymphatics. Some of the major lymphatic channels may not be linked directly with the primary regional nodes, and some of the intermediate sinuses in lymph nodes may be so large that they do not act as filters. Malignant metastases to nonregional lymph node groups may also occur when lymphatic vessels are obstructed. Consequent dilatation of the afferent lymphatics renders their valves defective and leads to retrograde flow, collateral lymph circulation, and atypical metastatic spread.

Principles of Lymphographic Diagnosis

The lymphographic symptoms of malignant metastatic spread comprise as *direct diagnostic signs* nodal filling defects and lymph node enlargement, whereas obstruction of the lymphatic circulation and displacement of adjacent lymph nodes and lymphatics are considered *secondary indirect symptoms*. This triple combination of (1) large marginal filling defects, (2) enlargement of the lymph node, and (3) lymph stasis may be called the *metastatic triad*.[2–5]

Nodal Filling Defects

Tumor metastases will appear as filling defects, since malignant tissue is impervious to oily contrast material. Malignant metastatic foci may, however, be recognized as such only if they produce filling defects that differ in size and shape from those of the follicles. Areas of neoplastic growth must therefore be larger than the largest follicle in a particular node before lymphographic recognition becomes possible. The minimum size of malignant cellular deposits recognizable by lymphography is considered to be within the range of 2 to 10 mm, with an average of 5 mm (Fig. 79-2; see Figs. 79-14 and 79-15). Lymph follicles become enlarged by *inflammation* and *reactive hyperplasia*, conditions that in the case of carcinoma occur concomitantly within the regional lymph nodes. The defects due to nonspecific inflammation reaction appear larger, but they retain their form and regular distribution throughout the node.[1] With increasing size of the tumor foci, compression and then obstruction of the marginal and the intermediate sinus take place. The filling defects become irregular in shape but are well demarcated in the case of direct infiltration; they are more regular if invasion is less prominent. The destruction of the sinus system, leading to permanent filling defects in the filling and retention phase of the lymphogram, is a diagnostic feature (see Figs. 79-2, 79-5, and 79-14) of particular importance for differentiation from filling defects due to *fibrolipomatosis*, in which the marginal and intermediary sinus system stays intact. *Granulomatous inflammatory alterations* within a lymph node may produce identical changes, since destruction of the lymphatic structure by granu-

1927

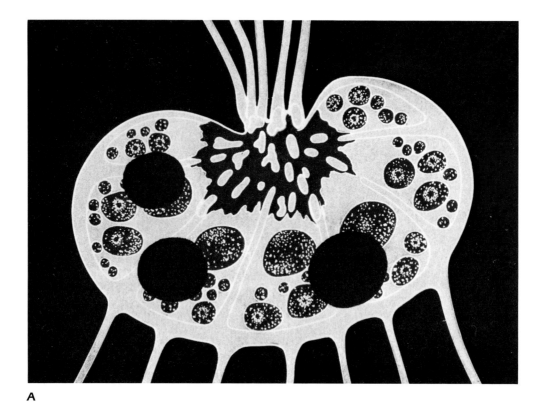

A

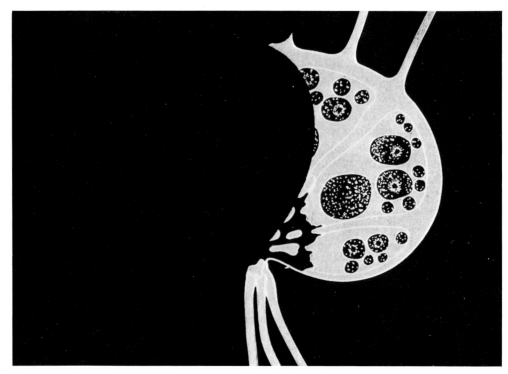

B

Figure 79-1. Formation of cancer metastases. (A) Multiple foci of malignant growth implanted in the periphery of the nodes destroying the sinus system. (B) Advanced malignant metastatic invasion with destruction of lymphatic tissue and blockage of afferent lymphatics.

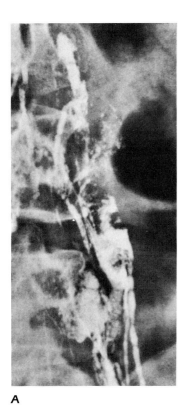
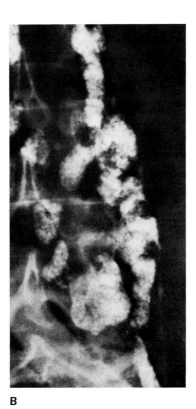
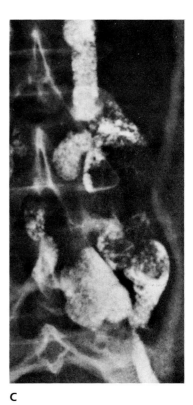

A   **B**   **C**

Figure 79-2. Cervical carcinoma of the uterine cervix stage II, showing small marginal and central filling defects within normal-size lumbar lymph nodes. (A) Filling phase showing the destruction of the sinus system. (B) Storage phase. (C) Follow-up study after 3 months showing increase in node size and large filling defects due to malignant metastatic deposits.

lation tissue takes place. Well-demarcated marginal and central filling defects and obliteration of the sinus system are then observed on the lymphogram, identical with the findings produced by malignant deposits.[1]

The genesis of cancer metastases leads to their peripheral deposition in a node, whereas filling defects of fibrolipomatosis are predominantly situated in the hilar region. Malignant growth tends to infiltrate the entire lymph node, obstructing the lymphatic circulation and displacing the remaining lymphatic tissue toward the periphery of the node (see Figs. 79-4 through 79-6, 79-8, and 79-12).

The *demarcation* of regular and irregular filling defects due to malignant deposits is well defined, whereas the defects of fibrolipomatosis are somewhat unevenly delineated. On the combined evidence of localization, contour appearance, and, particularly, the presence or absence of obstruction of the intermediate and marginal sinuses, the distinction between fibrolipomatosis and neoplastic disease is made reliably in most cases. However, interpretation of inguinal lymph nodes and the most caudally situated external iliac and axillary lymph nodes may be difficult because involutive changes in these node groups are common findings. Tangential projections, tomography, and follow-up

studies will help to confirm doubtful lymphographic diagnoses.

Follow-up studies at short regular intervals are of great diagnostic importance in doubtful cases because the lymphographic diagnosis becomes significantly more accurate by comparing the size and structure of suspicious lymph nodes (see Figs. 79-2 and 79-15). Lymph nodes that were previously normal or did not show conclusive pathologic findings may enlarge and develop central and marginal filling defects due to metastatic foci. Alteration of form, increase in the size of the lymph nodes, and displacement or separation of contrast-filled lymphatic tissue indicate the presence of malignant disease. A slight but definite increase in size, with a subsequent gradual decrease, is observed in normal lymph nodes; it is due to reactive inflammatory changes induced by the oily contrast material. Comparative analysis of follow-up roentgenograms taken at intervals of 2 weeks for periods as long as 6 months is necessary for careful evaluation.

Second-look lymphography by reinjection of contrast material becomes necessary if an inadequate amount of contrast material is present within the lymph nodes at the time of follow-up.

Differentiation between certain histologic types of

carcinoma on the basis of the topographic arrangement of filling defects caused by metastatic foci within lymph nodes is not possible because the process of malignant metastatic spread into regional lymph nodes is independent of the histologic type of a malignant tumor. However, the growth rate of the malignant tissue depends on its histologic structure, and a degree of differentiation on the basis of the growth rate should be possible. Measurement of the time it takes for the node size to double yields additional information on the biologic behavior of certain types of carcinoma (see Figs. 79-2 and 79-14). The number of malignant cell deposits within a lymph node may be another important factor influencing the lymph node architecture and facilitating diagnosis. In malignant melanoma, central filling defects within enlarged lymph nodes are frequent findings, not commonly seen in other histologic types of lymph node metastases (see Fig. 79-16).[6,7] The central position of the defects may be explained by the fact that the number of tumor cells invading the lymphatic system is quite large. The numerous malignant cell groups not only are deposited within the marginal sinuses of a lymph node but may invade the entire node, leading to large central filling defects seen in the lymphogram. Malignant metastatic spread of testicular tumors in aortic lymph nodes often causes a particular lymphographic finding: diffuse multifocal infiltration of the lymphatic tissue due to neoplastic disease (see Figs. 79-7 through 79-9). In the early stages of the metastatic process, the malignant tissue produces marked loosening of the lymphatic structure within the lymph nodes, which have still preserved their basic structural appearance. The lymphographic findings then closely resemble those of primary malignant lymphoma. With increasing tumor growth the entire lymph node is invaded by malignant tissue, and only displaced remainders of the lymphatic tissue are visualized by lymphography.

Size and Shape of Lymph Nodes

The size of lymph nodes affected by cancer spread is generally increased, particularly in fast-growing tumors. However, the affected nodes may remain normal in size (see Figs. 79-2 and 79-13). The degree of malignant involvement must be considerable before the size and shape of a lymph node are altered. The size of lymph nodes shows a good deal of variation. Normal-sized inguinal and iliac lymph nodes may measure up to 3 cm in diameter, and aortic lymph nodes may have a maximum length of 4 cm but with a width never exceeding 1.5 cm. Parietal internal iliac lymph nodes are normally small and when enlarged may still be smaller than nodes in other regions. It is important to compare the size of the questionable lymph node with the size of the corresponding contralateral lymph node group. The evaluation of enlargement thus requires substantial experience.

Dislocation and Absence of Lymph Vessels and Lymph Nodes

Dislocation of lymph vessels and lymph nodes is of limited value in the diagnosis of malignant metastatic disease. It may be regarded as a reliable indirect diagnostic sign only if malignant invasion of lymph nodes is simultaneously observed (see Figs. 79-6, 79-7A, and 79-8). The reason is that great anatomic variations of the lymph system and the dislocation of lymph vessels and lymph nodes are associated with tortuous arteriosclerotic arteries in the elderly patient. Topographic boundary lines to localize certain groups of lymphatics and lymph nodes are of equally limited significance.

The absence of a node or a node group that is usually filled with contrast material is without diagnostic significance because the lymphatic system is subject to innumerable variations. Additional signs of lymph flow obstruction must be present before such "empty regions" may be considered pathologic findings. This is particularly the case for the aortic area, where numerous connections between the various node groups are present.

Obstruction of the Lymphatic Circulation

Lymph stasis is visualized on the lymphogram as dilated afferent lymphatics, which remain contrast-filled after injection. Node groups distal to the site of obstruction are not demonstrated when blockage is complete (Fig. 79-3; see Fig. 79-11). A stenosis of the vessel just before the occlusion is also a common finding. Impeded flow results in increased intralymphatic pressure, and extravasation of contrast medium may occur during injection. In addition, a collateral circulation bypassing the obstruction develops, so that lymph vessels appear that are not normally visible (Fig. 79-3). The collaterals are contrast-filled by a reversed flow, consequent on the process of lymph stasis, with vessel dilatation and the resulting valve insufficiencies. Collateral lymph flow in perivascular fibrous sheaths and perineural sheaths is occasionally observed. However, differentiation of these conditions from simple extravasation may be difficult. A persistent contrast filling of a few solitary lymph vessels up to 24 hours after contrast injection may not be attributable to lymph stasis (see Fig. 79-11). The only conclusive symptom of lymphatic obstruction is abrupt nonfilling of lymphatics immediately following contrast injection, together with contrast filling of collateral lymphatics. Dilatation

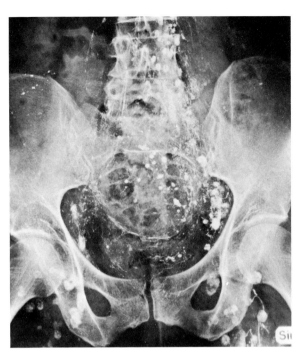

Figure 79-3. Recurrent carcinoma of the uterine cervix. There is extensive obstruction of the lymphatic circulation within the iliac and lower aortic area due to recurrent malignancy following surgery and radiotherapy. Also shown are retroperitoneal and perivesical collaterals and metastatic lower left aortic lymph nodes.

of the lymphatics, change of vessel caliber with incomplete filling of lymph vessels, and extravasation of contrast material may be due to technical shortcomings and are therefore not diagnostic. Obstruction of lymph vessels and development of collaterals occur in more advanced cases of malignant metastatic spread and are therefore less frequently observed.

The *topographic anatomy of collateral lymphatic circulation* is determined by the topographic-anatomic localization of lymphatic obstruction. The extent of collateral flow depends mainly on the degree of lymphatic obstruction. Blockage of a subcutaneous lymph vessel group in the *lower extremity* leads to the formation of collaterals in unaffected areas. Obstruction of the lymph vessels of the saphena magna region introduces lymphatic collaterals in the saphena parva region and vice versa. Additional cutaneous, subcutaneous, interstitial, and deep collateral lymphatics are commonly filled with contrast material. Obstruction of the lymph flow in the *inguinal region* will cause collaterals via subcutaneous lymphatics in the thigh, in the outer genital organs (scrotum, vulva), across the perineum to the opposite side, and in lymphatics of the lateral and medial aspects of the anterior abdominal wall. Interruption of the lymphatic circulation in one of the *external iliac lymph node chains* leads to collateral circulation via the remaining nonobstructed external iliac lymphatics (see Fig. 79-3). Lymph vessels situated medially in the pelvic region serve as collaterals to the contralateral side. Lymph vessels of the urinary bladder, uterus, and rectum may also act as collaterals. Laterally situated collateral lymphatics of the lower lumbar region are frequently observed. Extravasation of contrast agent into the abdominal cavity and the lumen of pelvic organs may occasionally be demonstrated by lymphography. In rare cases direct collaterals to the axillary region are found. In subtotal and total blockage of the lymphatic circulation in the common iliac lymph node group, retroperitoneal lymph vessels and nodes in the parietal lumbar region act as collaterals. Aortic lymph nodes distal to the obstruction site may then be contrast-filled via these particular groups of lymphatics (see Fig. 79-3).

Obstruction of the *aortic lymph vessels and nodes* produces collateral circulation to lymph vessels of the contralateral side (see Fig. 79-6). The unaffected lymph nodes situated distal to the malignant infiltration are usually filled with contrast medium. Because of the numerous physiologic connections between the aortic lymph node chains, the lymph nodes invaded by malignant growth are easily bypassed. Lymphography may then not demonstrate blocked infiltrated lymphatics, and collateral circulation will not be demonstrated as such. The numerous anatomic variations of contrast-filled aortic lymph nodes lead to further difficulties of interpretation. False-negative lymphographic findings due to unrecognized tumor-induced nonfilling of lymph nodes must therefore be taken into account.

Obstruction of the *thoracic duct* leads to dilatation of the cisterna chyli and the lumbar trunks (see Fig. 79-9A). Valvular insufficiency develops, and reflux of lymph may occur to the intestinal, pleural, peritoneal, renal, and hepatic lymphatics, with consequent chylothorax, chylous ascites, and chyluria.[8] Lymphography demonstrates extravasation of contrast material into the pleural and peritoneal cavities and to the renal pelvis. Contrast filling of collateral intercostal lymph channels and axillary lymphatics is occasionally observed. Lymphaticovenous anastomoses to the inferior and superior vena cava and the portal venous system frequently occur. The mechanism of collateral circulation in obstruction of the thoracic duct has been studied experimentally by ligation of the thoracic duct in dogs. The results of the investigations reproduce exactly the pathophysiologic data observed in malignant obstruction of the thoracic duct and resemble those seen in congenital lymphatic malformation.

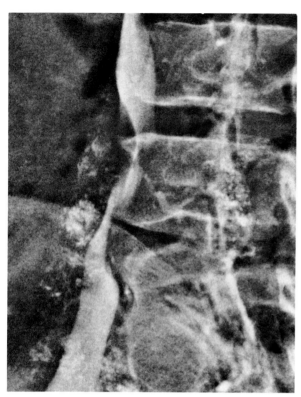

Figure 79-4. Carcinoma of the corpus uteri stage II, showing filling defects by metastatic deposits within the right common iliac lymph nodes. Compression and indentation of the right common iliac vein are due to enlarged metastatic lymph nodes.

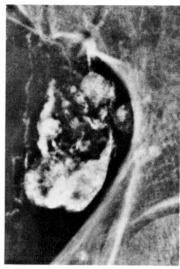

Figure 79-5. Carcinoma of the vagina. Marginal and central filling defects are obstructing the sinus system within enlarged medial external iliac lymph nodes due to malignant metastases. The afferent lymphatics are partially obstructed.

Clinical Indications for Lymphangiography

The clinical indication for lymphography in epithelial malignancies is the detection of malignant metastatic spread to regional lymph nodes—that is, N staging.[9] The proved presence of malignant lymph node metastases dramatically affects both the therapeutic approach and the prognostic outlook in every type of malignant neoplasm. Therefore, radiologic and cyto-histologic diagnosis of malignant metastatic deposits within lymph nodes is of paramount importance.

Gynecologic Tumors

The treatment of *carcinoma of the uterine cervix* depends not only on the continuous extension of the primary tumor but also on the discontinuous fashion of metastatic spread to regional lymph nodes (see Fig. 79-2). Consequently, lymphography gives important information concerning the planning of both the surgical and the radiotherapeutic approach.[3,10–14] Since

therapeutic measures rely mainly on the degree of lymphatic metastatic spread to the regional lymph nodes, it is evident that lymphography must be done prior to all therapeutic interventions.

In about 15 to 25 percent of all cases in clinical stages I and II, lymphatic metastatic spread can be demonstrated by lymphography, which may show that tumor infiltration is more advanced than could be judged by clinical investigations. In clinical stage III disease, malignant lymph node metastases are demonstrated by lymphography in about 30 to 50 percent of patients.

Two-thirds of all pathologic lymphograms show tumor spread in the external iliac lymph nodes only. In 15 percent, metastatic spread is exclusively localized in the aortic lymph nodes at the level of L4–L5, a group of lymph nodes that is normally not excised at retroperitoneal lymphadenectomy. In 10 percent of all cases, lymphatic metastatic spread is demonstrated in both the iliac and the aortic lymph nodes.

Carcinoma of the corpus uteri shows, contrary to general opinion, a relatively high percentage of lymph node metastases as demonstrated by lymphography— 10 to 20 percent in clinical stages I and II and 20 to 40 percent in clinical stage III disease. Malignant metastatic spread most commonly occurs to the aortic (lumbar) and common iliac lymph nodes (Fig. 79-4).[3,4]

In *carcinoma of the vulva and vagina*, false-negative lymphographic findings are relatively frequent. The first regional lymph node group in the inguinal region, the medial superior superficial inguinal lymph nodes, is not demonstrated by lymphography. Furthermore, fibrolipomatosis and chronic inflammation make the diagnostic evaluation of the inguinal lymph nodes rather difficult. The indication for lymphography is the necessity to evaluate the external iliac lymph nodes prior to surgery and radiotherapy, in which case pathologic lymphographic findings may be expected in about one-third of the patients (Fig. 79-5).[3,4,15]

In *malignant tumors of the ovaries,* lymphatic metastatic spread is more common than is generally thought (Fig. 79-6). Because of the high frequency of positive lymphographic findings, clinical stages I, II, and III are changed into clinical stage IV in 40 to 50 percent of the cases. These data demonstrate clearly the need for lymphography for accurate staging in this type of tumor.[3,4,15–17] However, negative lymphographic findings are sometimes in sharp contrast to the large-sized primary tumors, which themselves lead to a dislocation of the lymph vessels and lymph nodes.

Tumors of the Genitourinary Tract

In *malignant testicular tumors,* the clinical indications for lymphography are well established.[3,4,18–21] The first regional lymph nodes of the testicles are the aortic (lumbar) lymph nodes at the level of L2–L3 (Figs. 79-7 and 79-8). Thus they cannot be investigated by clinical methods, and lymphography should be performed in all cases for the classification of the tumor stage. Cavography is routinely undertaken as an additional method because lymphography does not show all aortic lymph nodes, particularly those that are not situated in the vicinity of the inferior vena cava. False-negative lymphographic findings occur in about one-third of cases. The frequency of lymphographic metastatic spread increases with increased malignancy of the neoplastic disease (Fig. 79-9). Positive lymphographic findings are observed in about 30 percent of cases of seminoma, 40 percent of teratocarcinoma, 60 percent of embryonal carcinoma, and 80 percent of choriocarcinoma.[19]

The indications for lymphography in *carcinoma of the penis* are acceptable only if a diagnostic evaluation of the external iliac lymph nodes is necessary prior to lymphadenectomy or radiotherapy (Fig. 79-10).[3] This limitation must be attributed to the fact that the first regional lymph node groups, the medial superior superficial inguinal lymph nodes, are not demonstrated by lymphography, and that fibrolipomatosis and chronic inflammation often render the lymphographic interpretation very difficult.

With *carcinoma of the prostate* the lymphographic findings have shown that lymphatic metastatic spread is much more common than was previously thought

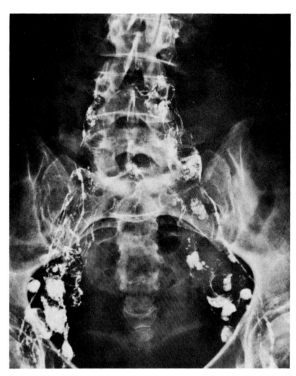

Figure 79-6. Ovarian carcinoma. The extensive metastatic deposits within the enlarged bilateral aortic lymph nodes are obstructing the afferent lymphatic circulation.

(Fig. 79-11). Metastases are demonstrated lymphographically in more than 50 percent of cases.[3,18,22–26] In clinical stage I, pathologic lymphograms are relatively rare, whereas the frequency of positive lymphographic findings in stage II is about 40 percent and in stage III up to 75 percent. Skeletal metastases are as frequent in patients with lymph node metastases as in those without.

In *malignant tumors of the urinary bladder,* lymphography is not indicated in the presence of superficial tumors limited to the mucosa and submucosa, because malignant spread to regional lymph nodes then seldom occurs. When malignant invasion of the muscular structures has been demonstrated, or even perivesical infiltration clinically diagnosed, malignant metastases in regional lymph nodes are common.[3,4,18] Lymphography will then demonstrate metastatic foci within the external iliac lymph nodes in more than one-third of cases (Fig. 79-12). If lymphatic metastatic spread is demonstrated by lymphography, no radical surgery, including cystectomy and lymphadenectomy, or aggressive radiotherapy need be performed because the survival rate is not altered by these invasive measures.

In *malignant renal tumors* the surgical approach, and particularly the prognosis of the disease, may be altered by the presence and extent of lymphatic meta-

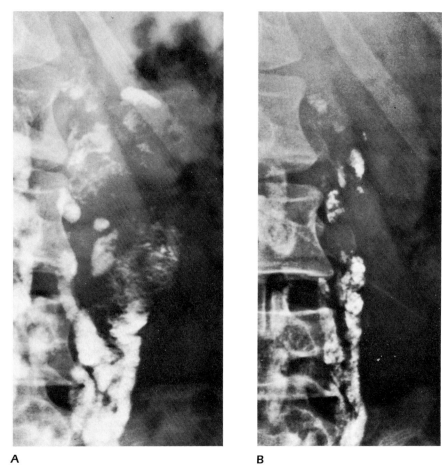

A   B

Figure 79-7. Seminoma of the left testicle. (A) Metastatic spread to enlarged left aortic lymph nodes containing extensive filling defects. (B) Follow-up study after adequate radiotherapy showing marked reduction of lymph node size.

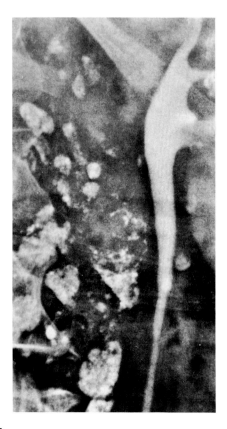

Figure 79-8. Embryonal carcinoma of the left testicle. The multiple confluent filling defects within enlarged left aortic lymph nodes are due to metastatic deposits.

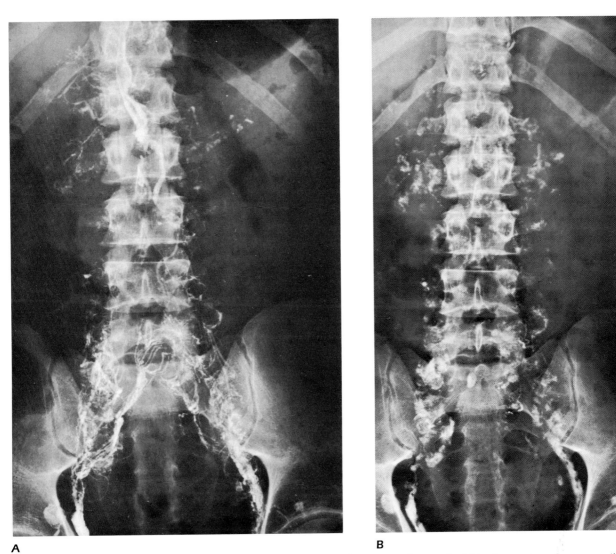

A **B**

Figure 79-9. Choriocarcinoma of the right testicle. There is extensive metastatic spread within the aortic and common iliac lymph nodes, moderate obstruction of other lymphatic circulation, and partial blockage of the cisterna chyli. (A) Filling phase. (B) Storage phase.

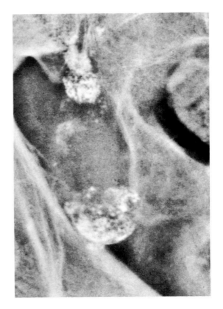

Figure 79-10. Carcinoma of the penis. The malignant metastases within enlarged medial external iliac lymph nodes contain extensive confluent filling defects.

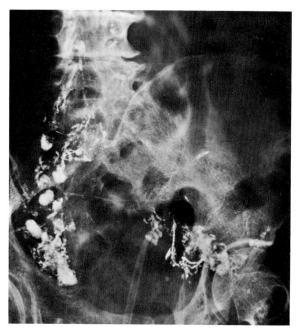

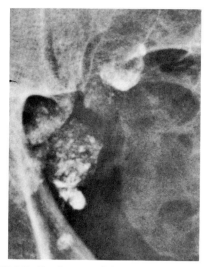

Figure 79-12. Carcinoma of the urinary bladder, showing confluent filling defects due to metastatic deposits within enlarged external iliac lymph nodes.

Figure 79-11. Carcinoma of the prostate. Obstruction of the lymphatic circulation is due to extensive metastatic spread to the left and right iliac lymph nodes. Stasis of afferent lymphatic circulation is demonstrated.

static spread. In the advanced stages of the malignancy, positive lymphographic findings within the regional aortic lymph nodes may be expected in 30 to 40 percent of cases (Fig. 79-13). Sympathicoblastoma of the *adrenal gland* has a high frequency of lymph node metastases.[7,27] The great extent of lymphatic involvement explains the relatively poor prognosis of most of the cases.

Malignant Tumors of the Gastrointestinal Tract

There is no clinical indication for lymphography in malignant tumors of the gastrointestinal tract, with the possible exception of carcinoma of the rectum. In all other anatomic localizations of malignant tumors of the gastrointestinal tract lymphography does not demonstrate the regional lymph node groups.[3]

In rectal carcinoma, metastatic spread to the regional lymph nodes demonstrated by lymphography is mainly observed in cases with clinically advanced tumor infiltration (Fig. 79-14). Consequently, since lymphography seems to give no additional diagnostic

Figure 79-13. Carcinoma of the left kidney. There is extensive metastatic spread within multiple enlarged left aortic lymph nodes containing numerous filling defects. The lymphatic circulation is partially obstructed.

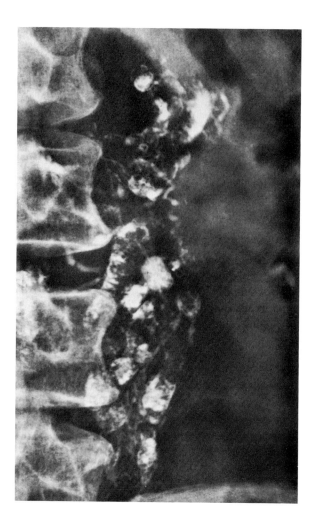

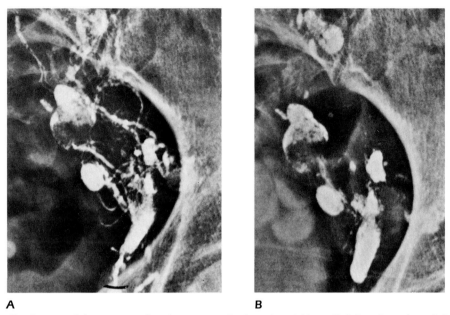

A   B

Figure 79-14. Carcinoma of the rectum, showing metastatic deposits within a slightly enlarged medial external iliac lymph node. Large confluent marginal filling defects are destroying the sinus system. (A) Filling phase. (B) Storage phase.

Figure 79-15. Melanoma of the right thigh. (A) Inguinal lymph node with fibrolipomatosis and small marginal filling defect destroying the sinus system. (B) Follow-up study 4 months later shows massively enlarged lymph nodes due to progressive growth of malignant tissue.

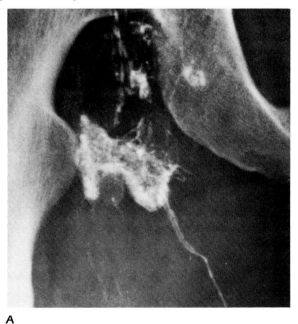 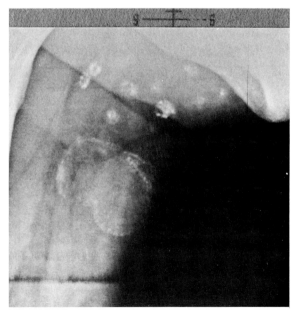

A   B

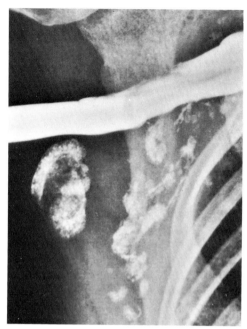

Figure 79-16. Melanoma of the right forearm. The sharply demarcated large central filling defect within an enlarged axillary lymph node is due to tumor metastases.

information that would influence the therapeutic approach in a given patient, its clinical indications are questionable.

Carcinoma of the Breast

In carcinoma of the breast there is no indication for lymphographic investigations. Lymphography of the upper extremity demonstrates only a few lymph nodes within the axillary region. In the case of lymphedema of the upper extremity, differentiation between postsurgical and postirradiation changes and recurrence of malignant tumor is not possible.

Neoplasms of the Skin

In *malignant melanoma* a clinical indication for lymphography is present only if the primary tumor is situated within an area where lymphography may demonstrate the regional lymph nodes (Figs. 79-15 and 79-16).[4,6,7,28] Accurate knowledge of the topographic anatomy is therefore of particular importance. Filling defects caused by chronic inflammation and involution may lead to an inconclusive diagnosis. The lymphographic findings may, however, facilitate the evaluation of prognosis in a particular patient, since a threefold difference in the survival rate is observed in cases of negative or positive findings.[6,29]

Lymph node metastases of *skin carcinoma* are again demonstrated by lymphography only when the regional lymph nodes are within the drainage area of the dissected lymph vessel. Because the regional lymph nodes of the skin are often affected by inflammatory and involutive changes, lymphographic diagnosis is likely to be inconclusive.

References

1. Tjernberg B. Lymphography: an animal study on the diagnosis of V × 2 carcinoma and inflammation. Acta Radiol Suppl (Stockh) 1962;214.
2. Fuchs WA. Lymphographie und Tumordiagnostik. Berlin: Springer, 1965.
3. Fuchs WA. Diagnosis of cancer metastases. In: Fuchs WA, Davidson JW, Fischer HW, eds. Lymphography in cancer. Berlin: Springer, 1969.
4. Viamonte M, Rüttimann A, Gerteis W, Bismuth V, Desprez-Curely JP. Metastatic disease. In: Viamonte M, Rüttimann A, eds. Atlas of lymphography. Stuttgart: Thieme, 1980.
5. Wiljasalo M. Lymphographic differential diagnosis of neoplastic diseases. Acta Radiol Suppl (Stockh) 1965;247.
6. Fischer B, Göthlin J, Fuchs WA. Die Lymphographie beim malignen Melanom. ROEFO 1974;121:224.
7. Rauste J, Tallroth K, Wiljasalo M. Lymphographic changes caused by lymph node metastases in carcinoma of the suprarenal glands. Lymphology 1976;9:19.
8. Takashima T, Benninghoff DL. Lymphatic venous communications and lymph reflux after thoracic duct obstruction: an experimental study in the dog. Invest Radiol 1966;1:188.
9. Dunnick NR, Castellino RA. Lymphography in patients with suspected malignancy or fever of unexplained origin. Radiology 1977;125:107.
10. Benninghoff DL, Herman PG, Nelson JH. Clinicopathologic correlation of lymphography and lymph node metastases in gynecological neoplasms. Cancer 1966;19:885.
11. Fuchs WA, Seiler-Rosenberg G. Lymphography in carcinoma of the uterine cervix. Acta Radiol 1975;16:353.
12. Ginaldi S, Wallace S, Jing BS, Bernardino ME. Carcinoma of the cervix: lymphangiography and computed tomography. AJR 1981;136:1087.
13. Kolbenstvedt A. Lymphography in the diagnosis of metastases from carcinoma of the uterine cervix stages I and II. Acta Radiol 1975;16:81.
14. Piver MS, Wallace S, Gastro JR. The accuracy of lymphangiography in carcinoma of the uterine cervix. AJR 1971;111:278.
15. Parker BR, Castellino RA, Fuks ZY, Bagshaw MA. The role of lymphography in patients with ovarian cancer. Cancer 1974;34:100.
16. Athey PA, Wallace S, Jing B-S, Gallagher HS, Smith JD. Lymphography in ovarian cancer. AJR 1975;123:106.
17. Markovits P, Bergiron C, Chauvel CH, Castellino RA. Lymphography in the staging, treatment planning, and surveillance of ovarian dysgerminomas. AJR 1977;128:835.
18. Cosgrove MD, Metzger CK. Lymphangiography in genitourinary cancer. J Urol 1975;113:93.
19. Fuchs WA, Girod M. Lymphography as a guide to prognosis in malignant testicular tumours. Acta Radiol 1975;16:305.
20. Jonsson K, Ingemansson S, Ling L. Lymphography in patients with testicular tumours. Br J Urol 1973;45:548.
21. Maier JG, Schamber DT. The role of lymphangiography in the diagnosis and treatment of malignant testicular tumors. AJR 1972;114:482.
22. Castellino RA, Ray G, Blank N, Govan D, Bagshaw M. Lymphography in prostatic carcinoma: preliminary observation. JAMA 1973;223:877.

23. Loening SA, Schmidt JD, Brown RC, Hawtrey CE, Fallon B, Culp DA. A comparison between lymphangiography and pelvic node dissection in the staging of prostatic cancer. J Urol 1977; 117:752.

24. Sherwood T, O'Donoghue EPN. Lymphograms in prostatic carcinoma: false-positive and false-negative assessments in radiology. Br J Radiol 1981;54:15.

25. Spellmann MC, Castellino RA, Ray GR, Pistenna DA, Bagshaw MA. An evaluation of lymphography in localized carcinoma of the prostate. Radiology 1977;125:637.

26. Zingg EJ, Fuchs WA, Héritier P, Göthlin J. Lymphography in carcinoma of the prostate. Br J Urol 1974;46:549.

27. Musumeci RE, Fossati-Bellani F, Damascelli B, Uslengh C, Bonadonna G. Usefulness of lymphography in childhood neoplasia. Cancer 1972;29:51.

28. Cox KR, Hare W, Bruce T. Lymphography in melanoma: correlation of radiology with pathology. Cancer 1966;19:637.

29. de Roo T. Lymphangiographic studies in a series of 55 patients with malignant melanoma. Lymphology 1973;6:6.

30. Veronesi U, Cascinelli N, Preda F. Prognosis of malignant melanoma according to regional metastases. AJR 1971;111:301.

80

Malignant Lymphomas

RONALD A. CASTELLINO

Bipedal lymphography (LAG) is most commonly used in evaluating patients with *malignant lymphomas,* which are primary malignancies of lymph nodes. This term encompasses the distinct clinical and pathologic entity of Hodgkin disease, as well as the heterogeneous group of disorders collectively termed the non-Hodgkin lymphomas. Although the malignant lymphomas share many common features, there are profound differences in pathology, clinical presentation, patterns of disease involvement, response to therapy, and prognosis. As with other imaging studies, interpretation is greatly enhanced when integrated with an understanding of the pathophysiology of the disease entity under consideration.[1,2] The following points should be kept in mind when interpreting a lymphogram in a patient with a known diagnosis of malignant lymphoma.

Histopathologic Classification

Hodgkin Disease

A modification of the Lukes-Butler classification for Hodgkin disease is given in Table 80-1. The histologic subtypes are listed with increasingly unfavorable histologies (i.e., lymphocyte predominance is the most favorable histology, whereas lymphocyte depletion carries the worst prognosis). The majority of patients have nodular sclerosis histology (70–85 percent of all newly diagnosed patients), in which there is typically large amounts of fibrous tissue within involved lymph nodes. This accounts for the frequent irregular and/or discrete filling defects within opacified lymph nodes, which at times can mimic the "typical" appearance of the "rim sign" seen on lymphography in nodes involved by metastasis from epithelial carcinomas (e.g., prostate, cervix).

Non-Hodgkin Lymphoma

The current classification of non-Hodgkin lymphomas is based on the NIH Working Formulation,[3] which is compared to the prior Rappaport classification in Table 80-2. On low-power microscopy, the non-Hodgkin lymphomas may involve lymph nodes with multiple nodules of tumor within the node, the so-called *follicular* pattern, or the tumor may irregularly infiltrate portions of the node in a *diffuse* pattern. Once the gross morphology is identified at low-power microscopy, the characteristics of the malignant cell are evaluated at high-power microscopy. The malignant cells in the non-Hodgkin lymphomas have a varied appearance at light microscopy, and some morphologically resemble histiocytes. However, immunochemistry has shown that the vast majority of these large cells that resemble histiocytes (or the prior so-called reticulum cells) are in fact "transformed" lymphocytes. Therefore, in the NIH Working Formulation, the cells are described by their size and appearance rather than by their cell line of origin: that is, small cell (with cleaved or uncleaved nuclei) or large cell.

In general, indolent tumors are of the follicular appearance and contain small cells, whereas the more aggressive tumors have a diffuse histology and contain large cells. The more indolent follicular lymphomas frequently are more widespread (at a more advanced stage) at presentation, so that multiple node groups are involved. In comparison, the diffuse non-Hodgkin lymphomas, as well as Hodgkin disease, frequently involve one or several node groups, whereas others are spared.

Table 80-1. Rye Classification of Hodgkin Disease

Histologic Findings	Proportion (%)
Lymphocytic predominance	5–10
Nodular sclerosis	50–80
Mixed cellularity	15–40
Lymphocytic depletion	5–10
Unclassified	<5

From Castellino RA. Hodgkin disease: practical concepts for the diagnostic radiologist. Radiology 1986;159:305–310. Used with permission.

Table 80-2. Relationship Between Histologic Classifications of non-Hodgkin Lymphoma

Working Formulation	Rappaport Classification	Proportion (%)
Low grade		
Small lymphocytic (diffuse)	Lymphocytic, well differentiated	3.60
Follicular, small cleaved cell	Nodular lymphocytic, poorly differentiated	22.50
Follicular, mixed (small and large) cell	Nodular mixed (histiocytic and lymphocytic)	7.70
Intermediate grade		
Follicular, large cell	Nodular histiocytic	3.80
Diffuse, small cleaved cell	Diffuse lymphocytic, poorly differentiated	6.90
Diffuse, mixed (small and large) cell	Diffuse mixed (histiocytic and lymphocytic)	6.70
Diffuse, large cell	Diffuse histiocytic	19.70
High grade		
Large cell, immunoblastic	Diffuse histiocytic	7.90
Lymphoblastic	Lymphoblastic	4.20
Small noncleaved cell	Diffuse undifferentiated, Burkitt and non-Burkitt	5.00
Miscellaneous		
Composite	Composite	~12.00
Mycosis fungoides	Mycosis fungoides	
Histiocytic	Histiocytic	
Extramedullary plasmacytoma	Extramedullary plasmacytoma	
Unclassifiable	Unclassifiable	
Other	Other	

From Castellino RA. The non-Hodgkin lymphomas: practical concepts for the diagnostic radiologist. Radiology 1991;178:315–321. Used with permission.

Lymph Node Patterns of Involvement

Hodgkin Disease

Hodgkin disease progresses in an orderly fashion from one lymph node group to the next contiguous group. Knowledge of this orderly progression is helpful when interpreting lymphograms, because "skip metastases" are extremely uncommon at the time of initial presentation. Since most patients present with neck and/or mediastinal lymphadenopathy, the lymph nodes at highest risk for involvement that are opacified at lymphography are the upper paraaortic and/or paracaval nodes (Figs. 80-1 and 80-2). In the less common presentation of inguinal disease, the contiguous exter-

Figure 80-1. A 27-year-old woman with newly diagnosed nodular sclerosing Hodgkin disease from a cervical lymph node biopsy. Staging lymphogram demonstrates a normal-size lymph node that is partially replaced (*arrows*) and that was interpreted as representing involvement by lymphoma. The adjacent opacified nodes appear architecturally unre-markable. At staging laparotomy, tumor was histologically shown in this lymph node, as well as in the resected spleen and splenic hilar nodes. (From Castellino RA. Abdominal and pelvic lymph node imaging. In: Margulis AR, ed. Diagnostic Radiology 1979. Gooding, CA: Univ. of California, 1979:867–884.)

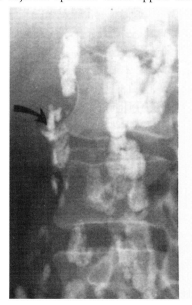
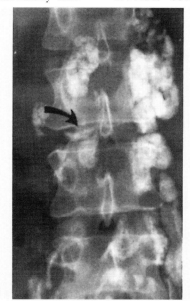
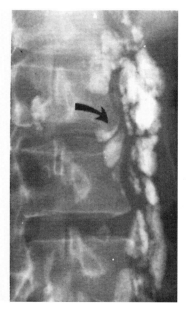

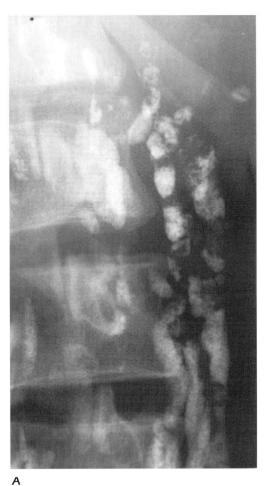

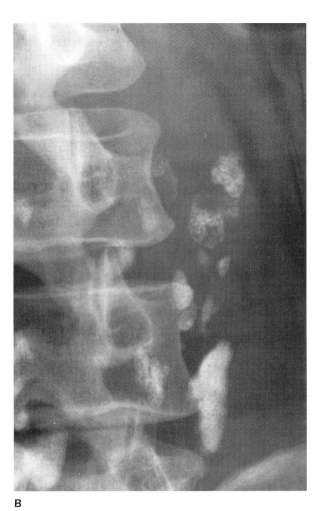

A

B

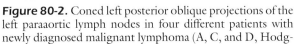

Figure 80-2. Coned left posterior oblique projections of the left paraaortic lymph nodes in four different patients with newly diagnosed malignant lymphoma (A, C, and D, Hodg- kin disease; B, follicular non-Hodgkin lymphoma). Note the compelling architectural abnormalities in the normal-size to slightly enlarged lymph nodes.

nal iliac lymph node group is at highest risk. Thus min- imal departures from a normal appearance in the nodes at highest risk deserve consideration for possible involvement whereas similar minimal architectural ab- normalities in nodal groups that are not contiguous with sites of known disease can usually be dismissed.

Non-Hodgkin Lymphoma

As noted above, in the *follicular* non-Hodgkin lymphomas, there is often widespread involvement of nodal groups at initial presentation. On lymphogra- phy, this usually is manifest as abnormalities of all opacified nodes. Importantly, in the follicular non- Hodgkin lymphomas, the relative degree of involve- ment (architectural distortion) often appears similar in all nodal groups (Fig. 80-3). This can create differen-

tial diagnostic problems in trying to distinguish early, widespread involvement by non-Hodgkin lymphoma from generalized, nonspecific reactive follicular hyper- plasia (as noted below). The other lymphomas, includ- ing Hodgkin disease and the diffuse non-Hodgkin lymphomas, can also involve all nodes opacified at lymphography. However, when this occurs there is usually evidence of greater involvement of one lymph node group compared to another, reflecting the pro- gression of disease from one contiguous lymph node site to the next. In the *diffuse* non-Hodgkin lympho- mas, although there is also a strong tendency to spread by contiguity, there are frequent exceptions to this concept so that architectural abnormalities that are suspicious for involvement in nodes not contiguous to known sites of disease should be interpreted with cau- tion.[4]

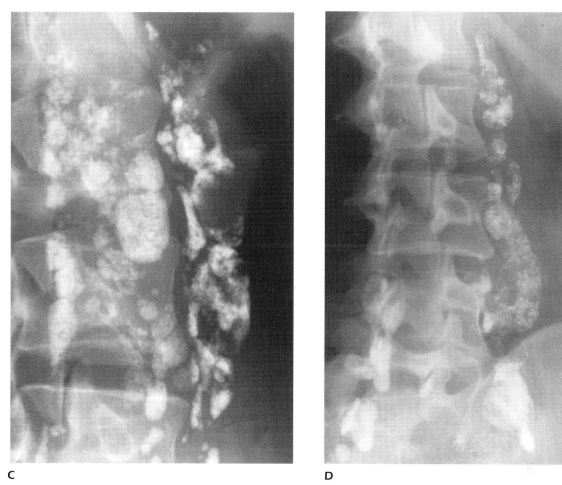

C

D

Figure 80-2 (continued).

Differential Diagnosis

Although architectural abnormalities noted on lymphography are sensitive in depicting structural abnormalities within lymph nodes, the etiology for the structural alteration can be varied (Fig. 80-4). Thus distortion of the usual lymph node internal architecture by any process that destroys or compromises portions of the lymph node (and particularly the sinusoidal network within the lymph node, in which the Ethiodol droplets are trapped) will produce corresponding abnormalities on the lymphographic radiographs.[4]

Partial replacement by *fat or fibrous tissue,* or a combination of both, is a well-known cause of false-positive lymphographic diagnoses in staging patients with pelvic tumors, because these changes are seen with increasing frequency in pelvic lymph nodes in older patients. However, many patients with malignant lymphoma (and particularly those with Hodgkin disease) are in a younger age group, and the lymph nodes at greatest risk are in the retroperitoneum rather than in the pelvis. Therefore, although fat and/or fibrous replacement can be the cause of a false-positive diagnosis, this is a lesser problem in patients with malignant lymphomas than in those with pelvic carcinomas.

Sinus histiocytosis (hyperplasia) is a nonspecific reactive process within lymph nodes in which there is a proliferation of histiocytes within the sinusoidal system. This entity can produce lymphographic abnormalities because the contrast media cannot enter portions of the sinusoidal system due to blockage by the proliferating histiocytes. Other processes, such as *infectious and inflammatory diseases* (e.g., microabscesses from granulomatous disease and noninfectious granulomata from sarcoidosis), can also produce architectural alterations that mimic involvement by lymphoma and other tumors. In general, these entities are unusual, and their preexisting presence is often known.

A particularly difficult differential diagnostic problem occurs when lymph nodes demonstrate a nonspe-

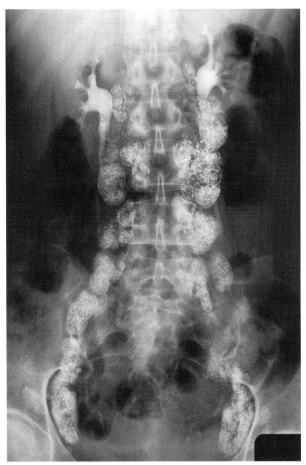

Figure 80-3. A 48-year-old woman with follicular mixed lymphoma. The staging lymphogram demonstrates all lymph nodes to be enlarged with a foamy internal architecture, interpreted as positive for lymphoma (confirmed by biopsy). This appearance is "typical" for follicular non-Hodgkin lymphomas, which frequently involve all visualized lymph node groups to a similar extent. (From Castellino RA, Goffinet DR, Blank N, Parker BR, Kaplan HS. The role of radiography in the staging of non-Hodgkin's lymphoma with laparotomy correlation. Radiology 1974;110:329–338. Used with permission.)

cific change known as *reactive follicular (lymphoid) hyperplasia.* In this condition, the follicles of the lymph node become enlarged and compress the adjacent sinusoidal system, so that at lymphography the lymph node demonstrates enlargement with a pronounced granular to frankly foamy pattern. This appearance exactly mimics the lymphographic appearance—as well as the low-power microscopy—of the follicular

lymphomas. It is only at high-power microscopy that the pathologist can distinguish the proliferating benign lymphocytes in the reactive follicle from the malignant lymphocyte in the malignant lymphoma follicle. Reactive follicular hyperplasia generally involves all nodal groups to the same extent, again much like many of the follicular non-Hodgkin lymphomas (Figs. 80-5 and 80-6). When confronted with this appearance (i.e., enlarged, plump nodes with a uniform, coarsely granular to minimally foamy architecture) in a patient with follicular non-Hodgkin lymphoma, one cannot make a confident interpretation. If the patient has Hodgkin disease or a diffuse non-Hodgkin lymphoma, then strong consideration should be given to this appearance representing reactive follicular hyperplasia. However, not surprisingly, at times this pattern can be caused by Hodgkin disease (particularly in the lymphocyte depletion subtype) or by diffuse non-Hodgkin lymphoma.

Reactive follicular hyperplasia, as a nonspecific finding, can be seen in the normal population (and therefore can occur coincidently in patients who have a concomitant malignancy); in this setting it is seen more frequently in young adults. It also can be seen in a variety of nonspecific inflammatory and immunologic processes, such as collagen vascular diseases and rheumatoid arthritis, immune deficiency diseases such as hypogammaglobulinemia and Wiskott-Aldrich syndrome, as a nonspecific response to systemic viral infections, and so forth (Figs. 80-7 and 80-8).[5]

Miscellaneous

Surveillance Abdominal Films

Following lymphography, the opacified retroperitoneal and pelvic lymph nodes retain sufficient contrast media so that accurate determination of size can be made on surveillance abdominal radiographs for periods of up to a year, and at times longer (Figs. 80-9 and 80-10). Because the nodes gradually lose the contrast media droplets, evaluation of internal architecture on surveillance studies is not possible (and will be misleading, because normal nodes will eventually develop an irregular to frankly "foamy" pattern of opacification). Instead, *the surveillance abdominal film only permits serial evaluation of lymph node size,* which

Figure 80-5. A 38-year-old woman with fever of unknown origin, splenomegaly, and abnormal liver function. The lymphogram shows bulky, enlarged, opacified nodes with a coarse, granular architecture, characteristic of nonspecific hyperplasia. At exploratory laparotomy, reactive follicular hyperplasia was found in excised paraaortic and splenic hilar lymph nodes, as well as in the spleen. (From Dunnick NR, Castellino RA. Lymphography in patients with suspected malignancy or fever of unexplained origin. Radiology 1977; 125:107–111. Used with permission.) ▶

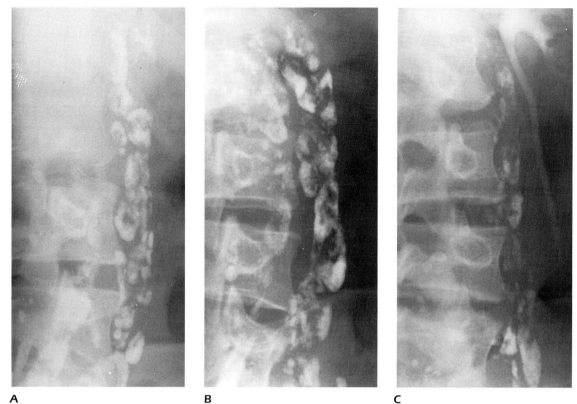

A B C

Figure 80-4. Left posterior projections of paraaortic lymph nodes in three different young adult men with nodular sclerosing Hodgkin disease. The visualized lymph nodes in each case are similar in appearance. The distinct filling defects in the somewhat globular but normal-size lymph nodes are commonly seen when a lymph node is involved with Hodgkin disease. The nodes in (A) indeed contained tumor; in (B), sinus hyperplasia; and, in (C), vascular transformation and fibrosis, each causing obliteration of portions of the sinusoidal system. (From Castellino RA, Billingham ME, Dorfman RF. Lymphographic accuracy in Hodgkin's disease and malignant lymphoma with a note on the "reactive" lymph node as a cause of most false-positive lymphograms. Invest Radiol 1974;9:155–165. Used with permission.)

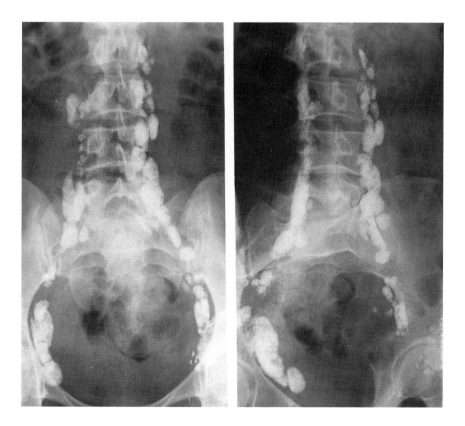

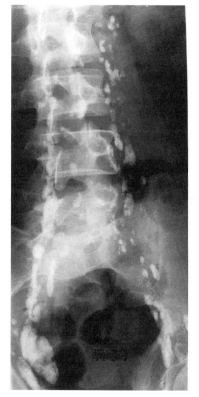

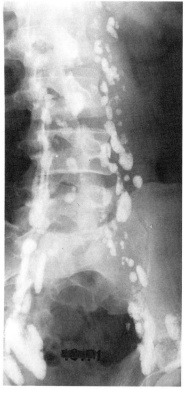

A   **B**

Figure 80-6. A 32-year-old man with stage IIA follicular lymphoma, treated by mantle radiotherapy. The initial lymphogram (A) is normal. A repeat lymphogram 2.3 years later (B), performed for routine reopacification, shows all lymph nodes to be larger and more granular than before, consistent with nonspecific reactive follicular hyperplasia. (From Castellino RA. Observations on "reactive (follicular) hyperplasia" as encountered in repeat lymphography in the lymphomas. Cancer 1974;34:2042–2050. Used with permission.)

is useful for monitoring the response to treatment of the originally involved lymph nodes or subsequent enlargement of normal-sized nodes due to disease relapse. The simple abdominal radiograph is thus a convenient monitor of the status of the residually opacified lymph nodes until the contrast medium retained in the nodes diminishes enough to prevent evaluation of size with confidence.[6]

Repeat Lymphography

A repeat lymphographic study can be performed when an insufficient amount of residual lymphographic con-

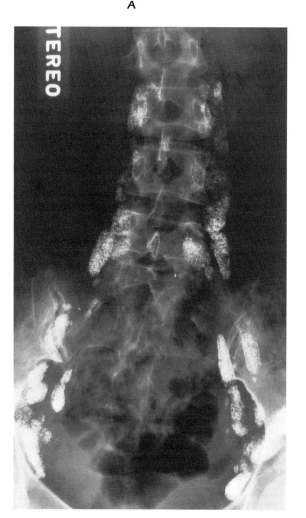

Figure 80-7. A 54-year-old woman with newly diagnosed non-Hodgkin lymphoma. The staging lymphogram demonstrates generalized minimal enlargement with a prominent granular to minimally foamy internal architecture, compatible with follicular non-Hodgkin lymphoma or nonspecific reactive follicular hyperplasia. This patient also had a long history of rheumatoid arthritis, and biopsy revealed reactive follicular hyperplasia.

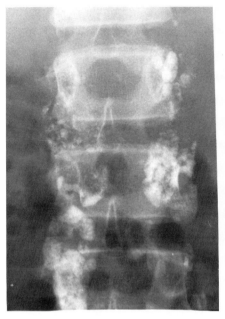
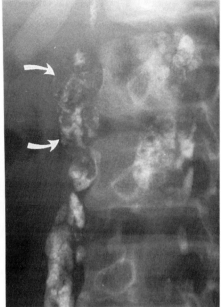

A **B**

Figure 80-8. A 12-year-old boy with nodular sclerosing Hodgkin disease. The staging lymphogram, anteroposterior (A) and right posterior oblique (B) projections, shows abnormal internal architecture of enlarged upper paracaval lymph nodes (*arrows,* B), suggesting Hodgkin disease. At laparotomy, these nodes contained eosinophils, presumably the result of prior parasitic infection, without evidence of Hodgkin disease. (From Parker BR, Blank N, Castellino RA. Lymphographic appearance of benign conditions simulating lymphoma. Radiology 1974;111:267–274. Used with permission.)

trast medium is retained in the nodes for confident evaluation of size.[7,8] In experienced hands, repeat lymphatic cannulation can be accomplished with equivalent success rates as for the initial study. The repeat lymphogram is interpreted using the same criteria as were used for the initial study, that is, the evaluation of lymph node architecture; however, it has the added advantage of having the prior lymphogram as a base-

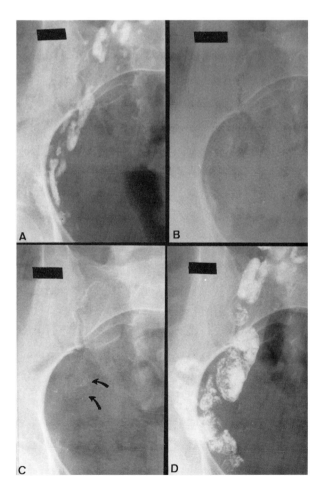

Figure 80-9. Patient with stage IIA Hodgkin disease. (A) The initial lymphogram is normal. (B) Surveillance films 11 months later show progressive loss of contrast from lymph nodes, which remain stable in size. (C) Six months later the minimal residual contrast media occupies a larger area than in (B, *arrow*), indicating interval lymph node enlargement. (D) This was confirmed by repeat lymphography 3 months later, which shows abnormal architecture compatible with Hodgkin disease (surgical proof). At this time, the patient was still clinically free of disease. (From Castellino RA, Cassady JR, Blank N, Kaplan HS. Roentgenologic aspects of Hodgkin's disease: II. Role of routine radiographs in detecting initial relapse. Cancer 1973;31:316–323. Used with permission.)

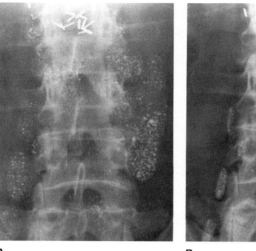
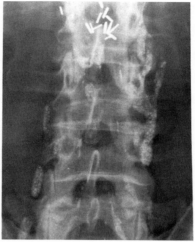
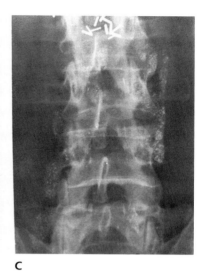

A   B   C

Figure 80-10. A 64-year-old man with previously treated non-Hodgkin lymphoma. (A) A routine surveillance abdominal film shows an interval increase in lymph node size from a prior study (not shown), indicating active disease. (B) Following therapy, a repeat abdominal film 3 months later shows a marked decrease in the size of the residually opacified lymph nodes, indicating a good therapeutic response.

(C) However, 2 months later another abdominal film shows a slight interval increase in the size of several nodes to the right of L4 and L5, indicating progression of disease. (From Castellino RA. Lymphography. In: Mass AA, Goldberg HI. Computed tomography, ultrasound, and x-ray. Univ. of California, 1979:105–123.)

line for comparison (Fig. 80-11). Some unique aspects related to repeat lymphography, based on the initial status of the opacified nodes and the influence of interval treatment since the initial lymphogram, are described below.

1. *Posttreatment effects.* Lymph nodes abnormal on the first lymphogram may demonstrate normal internal architecture at the time of repeat lymphography following therapy. However, not infrequently, previously abnormal nodes demonstrate persistent, although markedly improved, internal architectural abnormalities on repeat lymphography, caused by the residua of successfully treated disease.[9,10] This is not surprising, because foci of prior tumor that have completely responded to therapy may result in an area of scarring, with subsequent internal architectural distortion. Therefore, on repeat lymphography, persistent, although improved, internal architectural abnormalities in previously abnormal nodes are viewed with less concern than if the identical appearance were noted on a staging, pretreatment study. At times, the follow-up lymphogram serves as a baseline for subsequent surveillance with abdominal radiographs.

   In particular, normal nodes that have been previously irradiated, but also normal nodes in patients who have received chemotherapy, will at times demonstrate relatively poor and somewhat irregular opacification on repeat lymphography because

of the histologic changes induced by cytotoxic therapy. Thus nodes that appear normal on the pretreatment lymphogram may appear less well opacified ("washed out"), with an irregular pattern of opacification due to the effects of intervening therapy.

2. *Reactive (follicular) hyperplasia.* In patients who have received subtotal nodal radiotherapy, the lymph nodes that have not received irradiation may at times demonstrate a uniform increase in size and assume a globular shape and a markedly granular to minimally foamy internal architecture.[11] This process affects all nonirradiated nodes equally, presenting an image as if a "magnification radiograph" had been obtained of these same nodes before radiotherapy. This is seen particularly in adolescents and young adults, although it can occur in any age group. Histologically, these nodes demonstrate reactive follicular hyperplasia, a nonspecific finding. In clinical practice, because the unirradiated lymph nodes are at greatest risk for relapse, interval enlargement of these nodes on a repeat lymphogram (a similar phenomenon is at times seen on surveillance CT scans as well) is worrisome for disease relapse. The symmetry of the changes (increase in size and a pronounced granular architecture) should suggest benign reactive hyperplasia (Fig. 80-12). Relapse of disease more typically would be asymmetrical (or, if all nodes were involved, typically some would be involved to a greater extent than others) (Fig. 80-13).

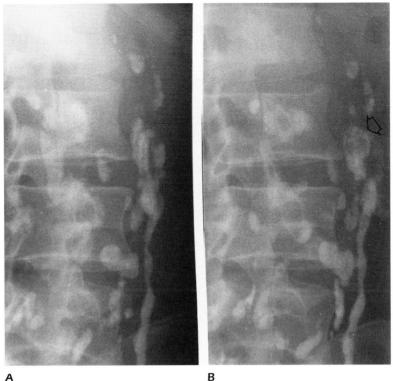

A

B

Figure 80-11. A 32-year-old man with stage IA nodular sclerosing Hodgkin disease, treated with local nodal radiotherapy to the left axilla. (A) The initial lymphogram is normal. (B) Repeat lymphogram 2.5 years later, performed for routine surveillance, shows one partially replaced ("rim sign") lymph node (*arrow*), interpreted as being tumor (biopsy-confirmed). (From Castellino RA, Fuks Z, Blank N, Kaplan HS. Roentgenologic aspects of Hodgkin's disease: repeat lymphangiography. Radiology 1973;109:53–58. Used with permission.)

Figure 80-12. An 11-year-old girl with Hodgkin disease. Following a normal (biopsy-proved) pretreatment lymphogram (A), she received radiation to the supradiaphragmatic, paralumbar, and upper common iliac lymph nodes. (B) A repeat lymphogram 2 years, 11 months later demonstrates posttreatment changes, that is, a decrease in the size and degree of opacification of the previously treated lymph nodes. The untreated lower iliac nodes have increased in size and in degree of granularity, a symmetric change interpreted as reactive hyperplasia. (C and D) Magnified detailed views of these lymph nodes (C is magnified view of A; D is magnified view of B). (From Castellino RA, Musumeci R, Markovits P. Lymphography. In: Parker BR, Castellino RA, eds. Pediatric oncologic radiology. St. Louis: Mosby, 1977. Used with permission.)

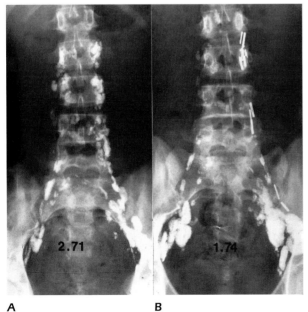

A   **B**

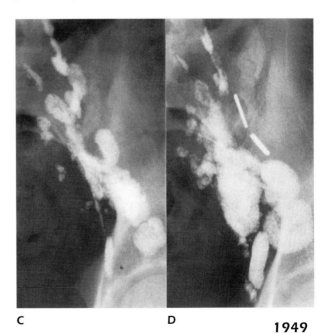

C   **D**

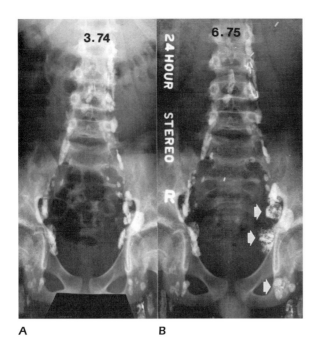

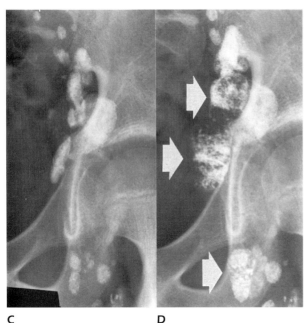

Figure 80-13. An 11-year-old boy with nodular sclerosing Hodgkin disease. Following a normal-appearing (biopsy-proved) pretreatment lymphogram (A), he received total nodal radiation therapy. A repeat study 1 year, 3 months later (B), performed for routine surveillance, showed interval increase in size and development of foci of abdominal internal architecture in the left external iliac and inguinal nodes (*arrows*), interpreted as representing disease relapse (biopsy-proved). (C and D) Magnified detailed views of these lymph nodes (C is magnified view of A; D is magnified view of B). (From Castellino RA, Musumeci R, Markovits P. Lymphography. In: Parker BR, Castellino RA, eds. Pediatric oncologic radiology. St. Louis: Mosby, 1977. Used with permission.)

Mycosis Fungoides

This cutaneous T-cell lymphoma, classified under the miscellaneous category of the NIH Working Formulation of non-Hodgkin lymphoma, is a malignant lymphoma of the skin that can eventually disseminate to lymph nodes and visceral organs. Lymphography has been used to stage these patients but has met with only limited success because the nodes draining the sites of skin involvement are frequently enlarged and show a markedly granular to foamy internal architecture on lymphography. At histology, dermatopathic lymphadenitis is present, which is a marked hyperplastic response within lymph nodes with deposition of melanin pigment, presumably as a nonspecific response to the primary skin disease. Although there does appear to be a clinical correlation between palpable lymphadenopathy (which can also be evaluated on lymphography) and clinical stage and prognosis, the performance of a lymphogram does not appear to contribute significantly to the management of these patients.[12,13]

Diagnostic Accuracy

During a 10- to 15-year period encompassing the 1970s, a number of institutions performed staging laparotomies in patients with newly diagnosed malignant lymphoma as part of comprehensive clinical trials. A splenectomy and biopsies of the liver and bone marrow were done, and multiple lymph nodes were excised during the laparotomy, and all material was subjected to histologic review. This information provided the opportunity to closely correlate the gross and microscopic appearances of the excised lymph nodes with the corresponding lymphographic images, providing not only detailed data on sensitivity, specificity, and accuracy rates but also insights about interpretive criteria.[14–18] Because the use of routine staging laparotomy

Table 80-3. Histopathologic Correlations of Lymphography in Newly Diagnosed, Previously Untreated Patients

	Hodgkin (n = 416)		Non-Hodgkin (n = 216)	
Sensitivity	100/117	(93%)	101/114	(89%)
Specificity	284/309	(92%)	88/102	(86%)
Accuracy				
Overall	384/426	(92%)	189/216	(88%)
Positive report	100/125	(80%)	101/115	(88%)
Negative report	284/291	(98%)	88/101	(87%)

Modified from Marglin S, Castellino RA. Lymphographic accuracy in 632 consecutive, previously untreated cases of Hodgkin disease and non-Hodgkin lymphoma. Radiology 1981;140:351–353. Used with permission.

Table 80-4. Histopathologic Correlations of CT and LAG in 121 Newly Diagnosed, Previously Untreated Patients with Hodgkin Disease

| | Paraaortic Nodes* | | | | Mesenteric Nodes | | Spleen | | Liver | |
	LAG		CT		CT		CT		CT	
Sensitivity	17/20	(85)	13/20	(65)	0/1	(0)	17/51	(33)	1/4	(25)
Specificity	85/87	(98)	80/87	(92)	90/91	(99)	53/70	(76)	117/117	(100)
Accuracy										
Overall	102/107	(95)	93/107	(87)	90/92	(98)	70/121	(58)	118/121	(98)
Positive report	17/19	(89)	13/20	(65)	0/1	(0)	17/34	(50)	1/1	(100)
Negative report	85/88	(97)	80/87	(92)	90/91	(99)	53/87	(61)	117/120	(98)

*LAG = lymphography. Numbers in parentheses are percentages. In seven patients, no retroperitoneal nodes were biopsied, and in an additional seven patients, the lymphographically positive nodes were not biopsied, leaving 107 cases for analysis.
From Castellino RA, et al. Computed tomography, lymphography, and staging laparotomy: correlations in initial staging of Hodgkin disease. AJR 1984;143:37–41. Used with permission.

Table 80-5. Histopathologic Correlations of CT and LAG in 24 Newly Diagnosed, Previously Untreated Patients with non-Hodgkin Lymphoma

| | Paraaortic Nodes* | | | | Mesenteric Nodes | | Spleen | | Liver | |
	LAG		CT		CT		CT		CT	
Sensitivity	14/14	(100)	12/14	(86)	10/15	(67)	5/11	(45)	2/3	(67)
Specificity	6/8	(75)	6/8	(75)	6/8	(75)	10/12	(83)	21/21	(100)
Accuracy	20/22	(91)	18/22	(82)	16/23	(70)	15/23	(65)	23/24	(96)

*LAG = lymphography. Numbers in parentheses are percentages.
From Castellino RA. Imaging techniques for extent determination of Hodgkin's disease and non-Hodgkin's lymphoma. In: Mirand EA, Hutchinson WB, Milich E, eds. 13th International Cancer Congress, part D. Research and treatment. New York: Alan R Liss, 1983:365–372. Used with permission.

markedly decreased in the early 1980s, less extensive information is available on the accuracy of CT scanning in staging these patients. There is no comparable histopathologic radiologic correlative database for MRI studies, which were brought into the clinical assessment process during the last half of the 1980s.

Table 80-3 summarizes the results of a long-term, prospective study of consecutive, previously untreated patients with Hodgkin disease and non-Hodgkin lymphoma who underwent lymphography followed by staging laparotomy.[14] The sensitivity, specificity, and overall accuracy, as well as predictive values, of lymphography in Hodgkin disease and in the non-Hodgkin lymphomas are high for radiologic tests evaluating the absence or presence of tumor at the time of presentation. Note that in Hodgkin disease most diagnostic errors consisted of false-positive studies, in which benign processes produced structural alterations within the lymph node that caused lymphographic appearances worrisome for involvement by tumor.[4] This is in contrast to the experience with solid tumors studied by lymphography, in which there are more interpretive errors due to false-negative diagnosis; that is, the

nodes are involved by "micrometastasis" too small to be detected with confidence on the lymphogram.

Table 80-4 provides a side-by-side comparison of the results of lymphography and CT scanning in 121 patients with Hodgkin disease (of which 107 had appropriate lymph nodes biopsied for radiologic histologic correlation) who underwent staging laparotomy.[19] These data indicate a statistically significant advantage of lymphography as compared to CT scanning. It should be noted, however, that experience with lymphographic interpretation was greatly enhanced by lymphographic-staging-laparotomy correlative experience obtained at Stanford over a number of years. Presumably these accuracy data would not be similar for many radiology groups with less lymphographic experience, whereas most radiology groups have comparable expertise in CT interpretation. It is clear that lymphography for staging malignant lymphomas continues to be performed less often, except in centers with large cancer populations where lymphographic expertise continues.[20]

Table 80-5 provides similar data for non-Hodgkin lymphoma.[21] Because routine staging laparotomies were stopped at an earlier date in non-Hodgkin lymphoma than in Hodgkin disease, the number of patients (24) is small, so that meaningful data are not available. However, the influence of LAG (and CT) results on staging and management was studied on 168 consecutive patients with newly diagnosed non-Hodgkin lymphoma.[22] In this analysis, all patients had bone marrow biopsy, and most had LAG (157, or 93 percent), abdominal pelvic CT (139, or 83 percent), or both (132, or 79 percent). The results of LAG and CT strongly influenced both the clinical (23 percent) and pathologic (14 percent) stages; importantly, these results influenced initial case management in 12 percent of all cases.

Lymphography has also been used in the management of children with malignant lymphomas. If the operators are experienced, the success rate in obtaining a diagnostic study is similar to that in adults. Accuracy data based on staging laparotomy results are also similar, although the need for precise information on disease distribution for radiotherapy planning often requires a formal staging laparotomy.[23–25]

References

1. Castellino RA. Hodgkin disease: practical concepts for the diagnostic radiologist. Radiology 1986;159:305–310.
2. Castellino RA. The non-Hodgkin lymphomas: practical concepts for the diagnostic radiologist. Radiology 1991;178:315–321.
3. National Cancer Institute sponsored study of classification of non-Hodgkin's lymphoma: summary and description of a working formulation for clinical usage. Cancer 1992;49:2112–2135.
4. Castellino RA, Billingham ME, Dorfman RF. Lymphographic accuracy in Hodgkin's disease and malignant lymphoma with a note on the "reactive" lymph node as a cause of most false-positive lymphograms. Invest Radiol 1974;9:155–165.
5. Parker BR, Blank N, Castellino RA. Lymphographic appearance of benign conditions simulating lymphoma. Radiology 1974;111:267–274.
6. Castellino RA, Cassady JR, Blank N, Kaplan HS. Roentgenologic aspects of Hodgkin's disease: II. Role of routine radiographs in detecting initial relapse. Cancer 1973;31:316–323.
7. Castellino RA, Fuks Z, Blank N, Kaplan HS. Roentgenologic aspects of Hodgkin's disease: repeat lymphangiography. Radiology 1973;109:53–58.
8. Dunnick NR, Fuks ZY, Castellino RA. Repeat lymphography in non-Hodgkin's lymphoma. Radiology 1975;115:349–354.
9. Markovits P, Blache R, Gasquet C, et al. Les images radiologiques des lymphographies faites après irradiation. Ann Radiol (Paris) 1969;12:835–847.
10. Markovits P, Blache R, Charbit A. A propos de l'aspect radiologique des lymphographies apres chimiotherapie dans les hematasarcomes: confrontation anatomo-radiologique. Ann Radiol 1970;13:539–558.
11. Castellino RA. Observations on "reactive (follicular) hyperplasia" as encountered in repeat lymphography in the lymphomas. Cancer 1974;34:2042–2050.
12. Castellino RA, Hoppe RT, Blank N, Young SW, Fuks Z. Experience with lymphography in patients with mycosis fungoides. Cancer Treat Rep 1979;63:581–586.
13. Hamminga L, Mulder JD, Evans C, Scheffer E, Meyer CJ, Van Vloten WA. Staging lymphography with respect to lymph node histology, treatment, and follow-up in patients with mycosis fungoides. Cancer 1981;47:692–697.
14. Marglin S, Castellino RA. Lymphographic accuracy in 632 consecutive, previously untreated cases of Hodgkin disease and non-Hodgkin lymphoma. Radiology 1981;140:351–353.
15. Kadin MR, Thompson RW. Lymphangiography—its practical value in surgically staged patients with Hodgkin's disease. West J Med 1974;120:193–199.
16. Kademian MT, Wirtanen GW. Accuracy of bipedal lymphography in Hodgkin's disease. AJR 1977;129:1041–1042.
17. Zaunbauer W, Haertel M, Fuchs WA. The diagnostic accuracy of lymphography in Hodgkin's disease. Fortschr Roentgenstr 1977;126:1–5.
18. Mansfield CM, Fabian C, Jones S, et al. Comparison of lymphangiography and computed tomography scanning evaluating abdominal disease in Stages III and IV Hodgkin's disease. Cancer 1990;66:2295–2299.
19. Castellino RA, Hoppe RT, Blank N, Young SW, Neumann C, Rosenberg SA, Kaplan HS. Computed tomography, lymphography, and staging laparotomy: correlations in initial staging of Hodgkin disease. AJR 1984;143:37–41.
20. North LB, Wallace S, Lindell MM, Jing BS, Fuller LM, Allen PK. Lymphography for staging lymphomas: is it still a useful procedure? AJR 1993;161:867–869.
21. Castellino RA. Imaging techniques for extent determination of Hodgkin's disease and non-Hodgkin's lymphoma. In: Mirand EA, Hutchinson WB, Milich E, eds. 13th International Cancer Congress: part D. Research and treatment. New York: Alan R Liss, 1983:365–372.
22. Pond GD, Castellino RA, Horning S, Hoppe RT. Non-Hodgkin lymphoma: influence of lymphography, CT, and bone marrow biopsy on staging and management. Radiology 1989;170:159–164.
23. Dunnick NR, Parker BR, Castellino RA. Pediatric lymphography: performance, interpretation, and accuracy in 193 consecutive children. Am J Roentgenol 1977;129:639–645.
24. Baker LL, Parker BR, Donaldson SS, Castellino RA. Staging of Hodgkin disease in children: comparison of CT and lymphography with laparotomy. AJR 1990;154:1251–1255.
25. Dudgeon DL, Kelly R, Ghory MJ, Halden WJ, Kaufman SL, Wharam M. The efficacy of lymphangiography in the staging of pediatric Hodgkin's disease. J Pediatr Surg 1986;21:233–235.

Index

Index